Oski's Essential Pediatrics

Oski's Essential Pediatrics

Second Edition

Editors

Michael Crocetti, M.D.

ASSISTANT PROFESSOR
DEPARTMENT OF PEDIATRICS
JOHNS HOPKINS BAYVIEW MEDICAL CENTER
BALTIMORE, MARYLAND

Michael A. Barone, M.D., M.P.H.

ASSISTANT PROFESSOR
DIRECTOR OF MEDICAL STUDENT EDUCATION
DEPARTMENT OF PEDIATRICS
JOHNS HOPKINS UNIVERSITY SCHOOL OF MEDICINE
DIRECTOR, PEDIATRIC MEDICAL EDUCATION
ST. AGNES HOSPITAL
BALTIMORE, MARYLAND

LIPPINCOTT WILLIAMS & WILKINS
A **Wolters Kluwer** Company
Philadelphia • Baltimore • New York • London
Buenos Aires • Hong Kong • Sydney • Tokyo

Acquisitions Editor: Anne M. Sydor
Developmental Editor: Jenny Kim
Supervising Editor: Mary Ann McLaughlin
Production Editor: Barbara Stabb
Manufacturing Manager: Ben Rivera
Cover Designer: Christine Jenny
Compositor: TechBooks
Printer: Quebecor World Taunton

530 Walnut Street
Philadelphia, PA 19106 USA
LWW.com

Printed in the USA

Library of Congress Cataloging-in-Publication Data

Oski's essential pediatrics / editors, Michael Crocetti, Michael A. Barone.—2nd ed.
p. ; cm.
Consolidated version of: Oski's pediatrics: principles and practice / editor-in-chief, Julia A. McMillan. 3rd ed. c1999.
Includes index.
ISBN 0-7817-3770-2
1. Pediatrics. I. Title: Essential pediatrics. II. Crocetti, Michael. III. Barone, Michael A. IV. Oski, Frank A. V. Oski's pediatrics.
[DNLM: 1. Pediatrics. WS 200 O82 2004]
RJ45.O85 2004
618.92—dc22

2004044104

Care has been taken to confirm the accuracy of the information presented and to describe generally accepted practices. However, the authors, editors, and publisher are not responsible for errors or omissions or for any consequences from application of the information in this book and make no warranty, expressed or implied, with respect to the currency, completeness, or accuracy of the contents of the publication. Application of this information in a particular situation remains the professional responsibility of the practitioner.

The authors, editors, and publisher have exerted every effort to ensure that drug selection and dosage set forth in this text are in accordance with current recommendations and practice at the time of publication. However, in view of ongoing research, changes in government regulations, and the constant flow of information relating to drug therapy and drug reactions, the reader is urged to check the package insert for each drug for any change in indications and dosage and for added warnings and precautions. This is particularly important when the recommended agent is a new or infrequently employed drug.

Some drugs and medical devices presented in this publication have Food and Drug Administration (FDA) clearance for limited use in restricted research settings. It is the responsibility of the health care provider to ascertain the FDA status of each drug or device planned for use in their clinical practice.

10 9 8 7 6 5 4 3 2 1

Contents

PART III
General Pediatrics

PART IV
Pediatrician's Companion: Things You Forget to Remember

Preface

As more and more information becomes available in Pediatrics, it is necessary to organize the fundamentals for those embarking in the field. With this in mind, we created this second edition of *Oski's Essentials of Pediatrics* by summarizing, reorganizing, and reformatting *Oski's Pediatrics: Principles and Practice.*

During the preparation of the manuscript, we commonly referred to the texts as the *Little Oski* and the *Big Oski*. Whatever the proper moniker of this book should be, it was created with the following in mind. Give the student and resident in Pediatrics a reference that is more comprehensive than the myriad summary "study-guides," but less intimidating than the ever-enlarging compendium pediatric texts. Stated another way, our goal was to produce a companion text with relevant, up to date, inpatient and outpatient topics likely to be encountered during a month on the wards or in the clinic. We hope that those who choose to use this book will feel that they have covered a topic in extensive (but not exhaustive) detail with an emphasis on the diagnosis and management of their patients. At those times when further detail is needed, particularly for epidemiology, etiology, or pathogenesis, the parallels with *Oski's Pediatrics: Principles and Practice* will help the reader use that text more efficiently.

In addition to our families, we would like to thank Ms. Jenny Kim of Lippincott Williams and Wilkins for her help during the preparation of this manuscript. Through personal hardship, Jenny was able to keep the project moving forward. Finally, thanks to Dr. Kevin Johnson and the late Dr. Frank Oski (a mentor with a capital "M" as some would say). Their preparation of the first edition of *Oski's Essentials of Pediatrics* led to the motivation to create this second edition.

Michael Crocetti, M.D.
Michael A. Barone, M.D., M.P.H.

Contributing Authors

Pasquale J. Accardo
Hoover Adger
Stuart P. Adler
Donald C. Anderson
Beth M. Ansel
Billy S. Arant, Jr.
Edwin J. Asturias
Robert L. Atmar
Carol J. Baker
Lewis A. Barness
Michael A. Barone
Phillip L. Berry
Marc L. Boom
Daniel C. Bowers
Kenneth M. Boyer
Mary L. Brandt
Warren K. Brasher
Eileen D. Brewer
J.Timothy Bricker
Marilyn R. Brown
Rebecca L. Byers
Arnold J. Capute
Richard O. Carpenter
Thomas O. Carpenter
John L. Carroll
James F. Casella
William J. Cashore
James T. Cassidy
Elizabeth A. Catlin
Frank Cecchin
Enrique Chacon-Cruz
John P. Cheatham
James D. Cherry
Myra L. Chiang
Murali M. Chintagumpala
J. Julian Chisolm, Jr.
Thomas G. Cleary
William D. Cochran
Gail J. Demmler
Martha B. Denckla
Elliot C. Dick
Harry C. Dietz III
William H. Dietz
Salvatore DiMauro
Patricia A. Donohoue
ZoAnn E. Dreyer
David J. Driscoll
Morven S. Edwards
Peyton A. Eggleston
Richard A. Ehrenkranz
Galal M. El-Said
B. Keith English
Jose A. Ettedgui
Ralph D. Feigin
Laurence Finberg
Marvin A. Fishman
Craig E. Fleishman
James D. Fortenberry
Richard A. Friedman
Arthur Garson, Jr.
Karen M. Gaudio
Daniel G. Glaze
W. Paul Glezen
Julius G. K. Goepp
Stuart L. Goldstein
Henry F. Gomez
Edmond T. Gonzales, Jr.
Richard J. Grand
Charles F. Grose
Ian Gross
Nicholas G. Guerina
Carl H. Gumbiner
Bryan E. Hainline
Neal A. Halsey
Margaret R. Hammerschlag
Paul E. Hammerschlag
Brian D. Hanna
I. Celine Hanson
James C. Harris
William R. Hayden
Robert A. Herzlinger
Leslie M. Higuchi
L. Leighton Hill
Lewis B. Holmes
Richard Hong
Walter T. Hughes
Ethylin Wang Jabs
W. Daniel Jackson
Joseph Jankovic
Victoria E. Judd
Arundhati S. Kale
Sheldon L. Kaplan
Kathleen A. Kennedy
Bradley Howard Kessler
John L. Kirkland
Rebecca T. Kirkland

Mark W. Kline
William J. Klish
Edward C. Kohaut
Daniel P. Krowchuk
Katherine S. Kula
Rebecca M. Landa
Marc H. Lebel
Howard M. Lederman
Mary M. Lee
Amy Feldman Lewanda
Carlos H. Lifschitz
Sarah S. Long
Martin I. Lorin
Gerald M. Loughlin
Penelope Terhune Louis
Lynn E. Luethke
Ruth Lynfield
Donald H. Mahoney, Jr.
Carole L. Marcus
M. Michele Mariscalco
Paul L. Martin
Edward O. Mason, Jr.
David O. Matson
Irene H. Maumenee
Kenneth L. McClain
Jonathan A. McCullars
Colston F. McEvoy
Julia A. McMillan
Dan G. McNamara
Laura R. Ment
Cynthia S. Minkovitz
Douglas K. Mitchell
John F. Modlin
Mary J. H. Morriss
W. Robert Morrow
Stewart H. Mostofsky
Kathleen J. Motil
Charles E. Mullins
James P. Nataro
William H. Neches
Edward J. Novotny, Jr.
Katherine L. O'Brien
Frank A. Oski
Frederick B. Palmer
Marc Paquet
Sang C. Park
Julie Thorne Parke
Wade P. Parks
Christian C. Patrick
Lori E. R. Patterson
Howard A. Pearson
Walter Pegoli, Jr.
Maria A. Pelidis
Alan K. Percy
Steven M. Peterec
Larry K. Pickering
Sharon E. Plon
Leslie Plotnick
David R. Powell
Arthur L. Prensky
Michael Recht
Vincent M. Riccardi
Lynne J. Roberts
Beryl J. Rosenstein
N. Paul Rosman
David R. Roth
Guillermo M. Ruiz-Palacios
Hugh A. Sampson
Pablo J. Sanchez
Mathuram Santosham
Joseph H. Schneider
Herbert Schneiderman
Paula J. Schweich
David T. Scott
Gwendolyn B. Scott
Bruce K. Shapiro
William T. Shearer
Jane D. Siegel
Norman J. Siegel
F. Estelle R. Simons
C. Wayne Smith
Nitsana A. Spigland
Paul D. Sponseller
Jeffrey R. Starke
Barbara W. Stechenberg
C. Philip Steuber
Janette F. Strasburger
Douglas R. Strother
John L. Sullivan
Larry H. Taber
Norman S. Talner
Jack L. Titus
Elias I. Traboulsi
Walter W. Tunnessen, Jr.
Jon E. Tyson
G. Wesley Vick III
Darryl C. De Vivo
Ellen R. Wald
W. Allan Walker
David S. Walton
Rebecca S. Wappner
Kent E. Ward
Joseph B. Warshaw
Steven L. Werlin
David E. Wesson
Bernhard L. Wiedermann
Robert Lee Williams
Michele Diane Wilson
Modena Hoover Wilson
Jerry A. Winkelstein
Lawrence S. Wissow
J. Timothy Wright
Michael J. Wright
Richard S. K. Young
Joseph H. Zelson
William T. Zempsky

PART

I

Pediatric Skills

CHAPTER 1

Pediatric History and Physical Examination

Adapted from Lewis A. Barness

HISTORY

Obtaining a complete history on a pediatric patient is not only necessary, but also leads to the correct diagnosis in the vast majority of children. The history is usually learned from the parent, the older child, or the caretaker of a sick child. After learning the fundamentals of obtaining and recording case history data, the nuances associated with interpreting information must be learned.

For the acutely ill child, a short, rapidly obtained report of the events of the immediate past may suffice temporarily, but as soon as the crisis is stabilized, a more complete history is necessary. A convenient method of obtaining a meaningful history is to ask systematically and directly all of the questions outlined in this chapter. After confidence is gained with experience, questions can be directed at specific problems and asked in an order designed to elicit more specific information about a suspected disease state or diagnosis. Some psychosocial implications will be obvious. More subtle details are often obtained by asking open-ended questions. Those patients with organic illness usually have short histories; those with psychosomatic illness generally have a longer list of symptoms and complaints.

During the interview, it is important to convey interest in the child, as well as the illness, to the parent. The parent should be allowed to talk freely at first and to express concerns in his or her own words. The interviewer should look directly either at the parent or the child intermittently and not only at the writing instruments or the record generated on the computer. A sympathetic listener who addresses the parent and child by name frequently obtains more accurate information than does a harried, distracted interviewer. Careful observation during the interview may uncover stresses and concerns that are not otherwise apparent.

GENERAL INFORMATION

Identifying data include the examination date; the patient's name, age and birth date, gender, and race; the referral source, if pertinent; the relationship of the child and informant; and some indication of the mental state or reliability of the informant. It is frequently helpful to include the ethnic or racial background, address, and telephone numbers of the informants.

CHIEF COMPLAINT

After the identifying data, the chief complaint should be recorded. Given in the informant's or patient's own words, the chief complaint is a brief statement of the reason why the patient is being seen. The stated complaint is often not the true reason the child was brought for attention. Expanding the question, "Why did you bring the child in?" to "What concerns you?" allows the informant to focus on the complaint more accurately. Carefully phrased questions can elicit information without prying.

HISTORY OF PRESENT ILLNESS

Next, the details of the present illness are recorded in chronologic order. For the sick child, it is helpful to begin, "The child was well until ___ days before this visit." This is followed by a daily documentation of events leading up to the present time including signs, symptoms, and treatment, if any. Statements should be recorded in number of days before the visit or specific dates, but not by days of the week, because chronology will be difficult to retrieve even a short time later. If the child is taking medicine, the record should indicate type and brand, the amount being taken, the frequency of administration, how well it has worked, and how long it has been taken.

For the well child, a simple statement such as "No complaints" or "No illness" suffices. A question about school attendance may be pertinent. If the past medical history is significant to the current illness, a brief summary is included. If information is obtained from old records, it should be noted.

PAST MEDICAL HISTORY

Depending on the age of the patient, some aspects of the past history that follow may not be pertinent. Obtaining the past medical history serves not only to provide a record of data that may be significant either now or later to the well-being of the child, but also to provide evidence of children who are at risk for health or psychosocial problems.

PRENATAL HISTORY

If a prenatal interview has been held (see following discussion), this information may already be available. Questions to be answered include those regarding the health of the mother during the pregnancy, especially in regard to any infections, other illnesses, vaginal bleeding, toxemia, or exposure to animals, any of which can have permanent effects on the embryo and child. The time and type of fetal movements should be determined. The record should include the number of previous pregnancies and their results; whether radiography was performed, what medications were taken, and whether the mother smoked or abused drugs or alcohol during the pregnancy; results of serology and blood typing of the mother and baby; and results of other tests such as amniocentesis. If the mother's weight gain was excessive or insufficient, this should also be noted.

BIRTH HISTORY

The duration of pregnancy, the ease or difficulty of labor, and the duration of labor may be important, especially if there is a question of developmental delay. The type of delivery (spontaneous, forceps-assisted, or cesarean section), type of anesthesia or analgesia used during delivery, attendance by other family members at delivery, and presenting part (if known) are recorded. Note the child's birth order (if there have been multiple births) and birth weight.

NEONATAL HISTORY

Many informants are aware of Apgar scores at birth and at 5 minutes, any unusual appearance of the child such as cyanosis or respiratory distress, and any resuscitative efforts that took place and their duration. If the mother was delayed in seeing the infant after birth, reasons should be sought. Jaundice, anemia, convulsions, dysmorphic states, and congenital anomalies or infections in the mother or infant are some of the reasons that viewing or handling of the newborn by the mother may be delayed. The time of onset of any of these abnormal states may be significant.

FEEDING HISTORY

Note whether the baby was breast- or bottle-fed and how well the baby took the first feeding. Poor sucking at the first feeding may be the result of sleepiness, but is also a warning sign of neurologic abnormality, which may not become manifest until much later in life. By the second or third feeding, even brain-damaged children usually nurse well.

If the infant has been bottle-fed, inquire about the type of formula used and the amount taken during a 24-hour period. At the same time, ask about the mother's initial reaction to her baby; the nature of bonding and eye-to-eye contact; and the baby's patterns of crying, sleeping, urinating, and defecating. Requirements for supplemental feeding, vomiting, regurgitation, colic, diarrhea, or other gastrointestinal or feeding problems should be noted.

Determine the ages at which solid foods were introduced and supplementation with vitamins or fluoride took place, as well as the age at which weaning occurred and the method used to wean. In addition, note the age at which baby foods, toddlers' foods, and table food were introduced, the response to these, and any evidence of food intolerance or vomiting. If feeding difficulties are present, determine the onset of the problem, methods of feeding, reasons for changes, interval between feedings, amount taken at each feeding, vomiting, crying, and weight changes. For an older child, ask the informant to supply some breakfast, lunch, and dinner (supper) menus; likes and dislikes; and response of the family to eating problems.

DEVELOPMENTAL HISTORY

Estimation of physical growth rate is important. Attempt to ascertain the birth weight and the weights at 6 months, 1 year, 2 years, 5 years, and 10 years. Lengths at similar ages are desirable. These data are plotted on physical growth charts. Any sudden gain or loss in physical growth should be noted particularly, because its onset may correspond to the onset of organic or psychosocial illness. It may be helpful to compare the child's growth with the rate of growth of siblings or parents.

Ages at which major developmental milestones were met aid in indicating deviations from normal. Such milestones include following a person with the eyes, holding the head erect, smiling responsively, reaching for objects, transferring objects, sitting alone, walking with support and alone, speaking the first words and sentences, and experiencing tooth eruption. Ages of dressing self, tying own shoes, hopping, skipping, and riding a tricycle and bicycle should be noted, as well as grade in school and school performance.

In addition, take note of the age at which bowel and bladder control was achieved. If problems exist, the ages at which toilet teaching began may also indicate reasons for problems.

BEHAVIOR HISTORY

Dependent on age, the amount of sleep and sleep problems and habits such as pica, smoking, and use of alcohol or drugs should be questioned. For a younger child, the informant should state whether the child is happy or difficult to manage and should indicate the child's response to new situations, strangers, and school. Temper tantrums, excessive or unprovoked crying, nail biting, and nightmares and night terrors should be recorded. For older children and adolescents, question the child regarding dating, dealing with the opposite sex, and parents' responses to menstruation and sexual development. Questions should be free of heterosexual assumption, direction of romantic interests, and gender of partners.

IMMUNIZATION HISTORY

The types of immunizations received with the number, dates, sites given, and reactions should be recorded as part of the history. In addition, it is helpful to record these immunizations with lot numbers on the front of the chart or in a convenient and obvious place.

HISTORY OF PAST ILLNESSES

Include a statement about the child's general health before the present encounter such as weight change, fever, weakness, or mood alterations. Specific inquiry is helpful regarding the results of any screening tests and any history of infectious or contagious diseases, or any other illness, as well as specific treatment, results, and residua. The history of each past illness should include dates of onset, course, and termination. If hospitalization or surgery was necessary, the diagnoses, dates, and name of the hospital should be included. Questions concerning allergies include the occurrence and type of any drug reactions, food allergies, hay fever, and asthma. Accidents, injuries, and poisonings should be noted.

REVIEW OF SYSTEMS

The review of systems serves as a checklist for pertinent information that might have been omitted. If information has been obtained previously, simply state, "See history of present illness" or "See history of past illnesses." Questions concerning each system may be introduced with a question such as, "Are there any symptoms related to . . . ?" Try to direct questions toward systems that relate to the chief complaint and history of present illness.

- Head (e.g., injuries, headache)
- Eyes (e.g., visual changes, crossed or tendency to cross, discharge, redness, puffiness, injuries, glasses)
- Ears (e.g., difficulty with hearing, pain, discharge, ear infections, myringotomy, ventilation tubes)
- Nose (e.g., watery or purulent discharge, difficulty in breathing through nose, epistaxis)
- Mouth and throat (e.g., sore throat or tongue, difficulty in swallowing, dental defects)
- Neck (e.g., swollen glands, masses, stiffness, symmetry)
- Breasts (e.g., lumps, pain, symmetry, nipple discharge, embarrassment)
- Lungs (e.g., shortness of breath, ability to keep up with peers, timing and character of cough, hoarseness, wheezing, hemoptysis, pain in chest)
- Heart (e.g., cyanosis, edema, heart murmurs or "heart trouble," pain over heart)
- Gastrointestinal (e.g., appetite; nausea; vomiting with relation to feeding, amount, color, blood- or bile-stained, or projectile;

number and character of bowel movements; abdominal pain or distention; jaundice)
- Genitourinary (e.g., dysuria, hematuria, frequency, oliguria, character of urinary stream, enuresis, urethral or vaginal discharge, menstrual history, attitude toward menses and opposite sex, sores, pain, sexual activity, birth control, sexually transmitted disease and protection, abortions)
- Extremities (e.g., weakness, deformities, difficulty in moving extremities or in walking, joint pain and swelling, muscle pain or cramps)
- Neurologic (e.g., headaches, fainting, dizziness, incoordination, seizures, numbness, tremors)
- Skin (e.g., rashes, hives, itching, color change, hair and nail growth, color and distribution, bruises or bleeds easily)
- Psychiatric (e.g., usual mood, nervousness, tension, drug use or abuse)

FAMILY HISTORY

The family history provides evidence for considering familial diseases as well as infections or contagious illnesses. A genetic type chart is easy to read and very helpful. It should include parents, siblings, and grandparents, with their ages, health, or cause of death. If problems with genetic implications exist, inquire about all known relatives. If a genetic type chart is used, pregnancies should be listed in a series and should include the health of the siblings (Fig. 1-1).

Family diseases such as allergy; blood, heart, lung, venereal, or kidney disease; tuberculosis; diabetes; rheumatic fever; convulsions; skin, gastrointestinal, behavioral, or mental disorders; cancer; or other diseases the informant mentions should be included. These diseases may have a heritable or contagious effect. Pertinent negative answers should also be included.

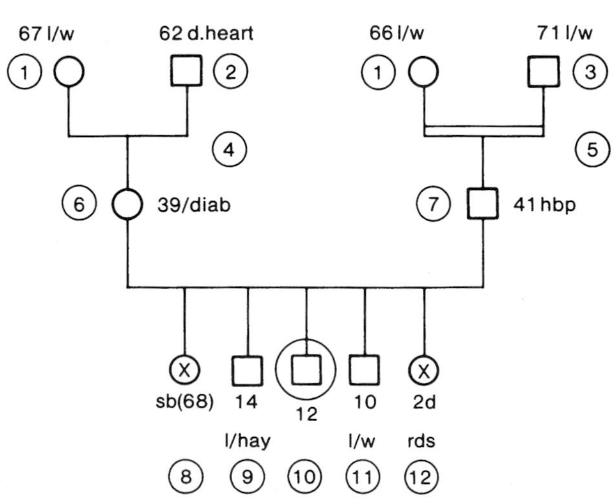

Figure 1-1. Genetic type chart. (*Circle*, female; square, male.) 1, maternal grandmother, 67 years old, living and well; paternal grandmother, 66, living and well. 2, Maternal grandfather, died at 62 of heart disease. 3, Paternal grandfather, 71, living and well. 4, Single horizontal line, married. 5, Double horizontal line, consanguineous marriage. 6, Mother, 39 years old, living, diabetic. 7, Father, 41 years old, living, hypertensive. 8, Stillbirth, died in 1968. 9, Male sibling, 14 years old, living, hay fever. 10, Patient, 12 years old (note light circle). 11, Brother, 10 years old, living and well. 12, Female, died at 2 days old of respiratory distress (year can be included).

SOCIAL HISTORY

Details of the family unit include the number of people in the habitat and its size, the presence of grandparents, the marital status of the parents, the significant caretaker, the total family income and its source, and whether the mother and father work outside the home. If it is pertinent to the current problems of the child, inquire about the family's attitude toward the child and toward each other, the type of discipline used, and the major disciplinarian. If the problem is psychosocial and only one parent is the informant, it may be necessary to interview the other parent and to outline a typical day in the life of the child.

HISTORY FROM THE CHILD

Even young children should be asked about their symptoms and their understanding of their problem. This also provides an opportunity to observe how the child interacts with the parent. For most adolescents, it is important to take part of the history from the adolescent alone after asking for his or her approval. Regardless of your own opinion, obtain the history objectively, without any moral implications, starting with open-ended questions related to the initial complaint and then directing the questions.

PHYSICAL EXAMINATION

Examination of the infant and young child begins with observing him or her and establishing rapport. The order of the examination should fit the child and the circumstances. Do not make sudden movements and first complete parts of the examination that require the child's cooperation. Painful or disagreeable procedures should be deferred to the end of the examination, and these should be explained to the child before proceeding. For the older child and adolescent, examination can begin with the head and conclude with the extremities. The approach is gentle but expeditious and complete. For the young, apprehensive child, chatter, reassurance, or other communication frequently permits an orderly examination. Some children are best held by the parent during the examination. For others, part of the examination may require restraint by the parent or assistant.

Because the entire child is to be examined, at some time all of the clothing must be removed. This does not necessarily mean that it must be removed at the same time. Only the part that is being examined needs to be uncovered, and then reclothed after examination of that part is complete. Except during infancy, modesty should be respected, and the child should be kept as comfortable as possible.

With practice, the examination can be completed quickly even in most critical emergency states. Only in those patients with apnea, shock, absence of pulse, or, occasionally, seizures is the complete examination delayed. Completion of the history can be accomplished during the physical examination. Talking to the parent frequently reassures the child. Praising the young child, explaining the parts of the examination to the older child, and reassuring the adolescent of normal findings facilitates the examination. Usually, if the examiner enjoys the spontaneity and responsiveness of children, the examination will be easier and more thorough.

MEASUREMENTS (VITAL SIGNS)

Temperature is taken in the axilla or rectum in the young child and by mouth after 5 or 6 years of age, when the child can understand how to hold the thermometer. Electronic thermometer probes inserted as usual or in the ear canal give rapid, accurate determinations. Elevated temperature occurs with infection, excitement, anxiety, exercise, hyperthyroidism, collagen-vascular disease, or tumor. Decreased temperature occurs with chilling, shock, hypothyroidism, or inactivity. Temperature may be decreased after taking certain drugs, with hypocortisolism, or with overwhelming infection.

The pulse rate can be obtained at any peripheral pulse (femoral, radial, or carotid) or by palpation over the heart. The normal rate varies from 70 to 170 beats per minute (bpm) at birth to 120 to 140 shortly after birth, and ranges from 80 to 140 at 1 to 2 years, from 80 to 120 at 3 years, and from 70 to 115 after 3 years. The sleeping pulse after the age of 2 years is normally about 20 bpm less than the awake pulse, but does not decrease with rheumatic fever or thyrotoxicosis. For each centigrade degree of temperature increase, the pulse rate increases approximately 10 bpm. The pulse rate is elevated with excitement, exercise, or hypermetabolic states and is decreased with hypometabolic states, hypertension, or increased intracranial pressure. Irregularity may be caused by sinus arrhythmia but can indicate underlying heart disease. Absence of the femoral pulse is a cardinal sign of postductal coarctation of the aorta.

RESPIRATORY RATE

The respiratory rate should be determined by observing the movement of the chest or abdomen or by auscultation of the chest. The normal newborn rate is 30 to 80 bpm; the rate decreases to 20 to 40 in early infancy and childhood and then to 15 to 25 in late childhood and adolescence. Exercise, anxiety, infection, and hypermetabolic states increase the rate; central nervous system lesions, metabolic abnormalities, alkalosis, depressants, and other poisons decrease the rate.

BLOOD PRESSURE

The blood pressure should be measured with a cuff, with the bladder completely encircling the extremity and the width covering one-half to two-thirds of the length of the upper arm or upper leg. The pressure should be recorded and compared with normal readings based on height. High systolic pressure occurs with excitement, anxiety, and hypermetabolic states. High systolic and diastolic pressures occur with renal diseases, pheochromocytoma, adrenal disease, arteritis, or coarctation of the aorta. Press and release the child's nail. Normally, color returns in less than 1 second, the capillary refill time. Color returns in 2 to 3 seconds with 50 to 90 mL/kg fluid depletion, and in more than 3 seconds with greater than 90 mL/kg fluid depletion. At more than 90 mL/kg fluid depletion, medical shock ensues.

HEIGHT, WEIGHT, AND HEAD CIRCUMFERENCE

To obtain height and weight recordings, the infant should be measured supine up to the age of 2 years and standing thereafter. Head circumference should be measured in all infants younger than 2 years and in those with misshapen heads, and measurements should be recorded with percentiles on a chart (Figs. 1-2 through 1-9).

Shortness may be caused by malnutrition, chronic illness, psychosocial deprivation, hormonal disorders, familial patterns, or syndromes with dwarfism. Gigantism may be the result of pituitary abnormalities. Compare sitting height and total height in dwarfs with standard measurements to determine the type of syndrome present.

Decreased weight can be caused by conditions similar to those that cause decreased height. In states of malnutrition, weight percentile is less than height percentile; head circumference remains normal unless the condition is severe and persists. Being overweight is usually exogenous and associated with increased height until epiphyseal closure. Being overweight as a result of endocrine disorders is associated with decreased linear growth.

GENERAL APPEARANCE

A statement should be recorded about the alertness, distress, general development, and nutrition of the child. Mental status, activity, unusual positions, or apprehension or cooperativeness may direct one to consider an acute or chronic illness or no illness at all. The child who lies quietly staring into space may be gravely ill. The child who lies quietly, but becomes irritable when held by the mother (paradoxic irritability), may have meningitis or pain in motion. Note any unusual odor, which may suggest the presence of a foreign body in one of the orifices, certain diseases, or toxins.

Skin

In examining the skin, record its color and turgor, the type of any lesions, and the condition of body and scalp hair and nails. Normal color of the skin is the result of the presence of melanin; depigmented areas are vitiligo; absence of pigment occurs in albinism. Cyanosis is caused by desaturation or abnormal forms of hemoglobin; jaundice is caused by excessive bilirubin deposited in the adipose tissue. Note the size and borders of nevi, which are usually darkly pigmented areas, and café au lait spots, which are brownish areas that may signal neurofibromatosis. White leaf-shaped spots suggest tuberous sclerosis. Ecchymoses or petechiae and scars may indicate abuse.

Swelling may be caused by edema. Lack of turgor occurs with dehydration or recent weight loss. Describe any rashes, many of which are characteristic of viral or bacterial infection.

Head and Face

Record the shape, symmetry, and any defects of the head; the distribution of hair; and the size and tension of the fontanelles. A large head may be an early sign of hydrocephalus or an intracranial mass. A small head may be the result of early closure of sutures or lack of brain development. For any deviation from normal head size, frequent measurements are necessary. The fontanelles are normally flat. The posterior fontanelle closes by 2 months of age, and the anterior fontanelle closes by 12 to 18 months of age. Unusual hair whorls are associated with severe intracranial abnormalities.

The face may appear distinctive for a number of syndromes. For example, unilateral facial paralysis may be associated with congenital heart disease. Coarse facies occur with storage diseases. Epicanthal folds occur in a number of syndromes including trisomy 21.

Eyes

Test vision grossly in the young child with brightly colored objects. In the older child, test with Snellen's E chart. Evaluate for strabismus by noting the position of the reflection of light on the

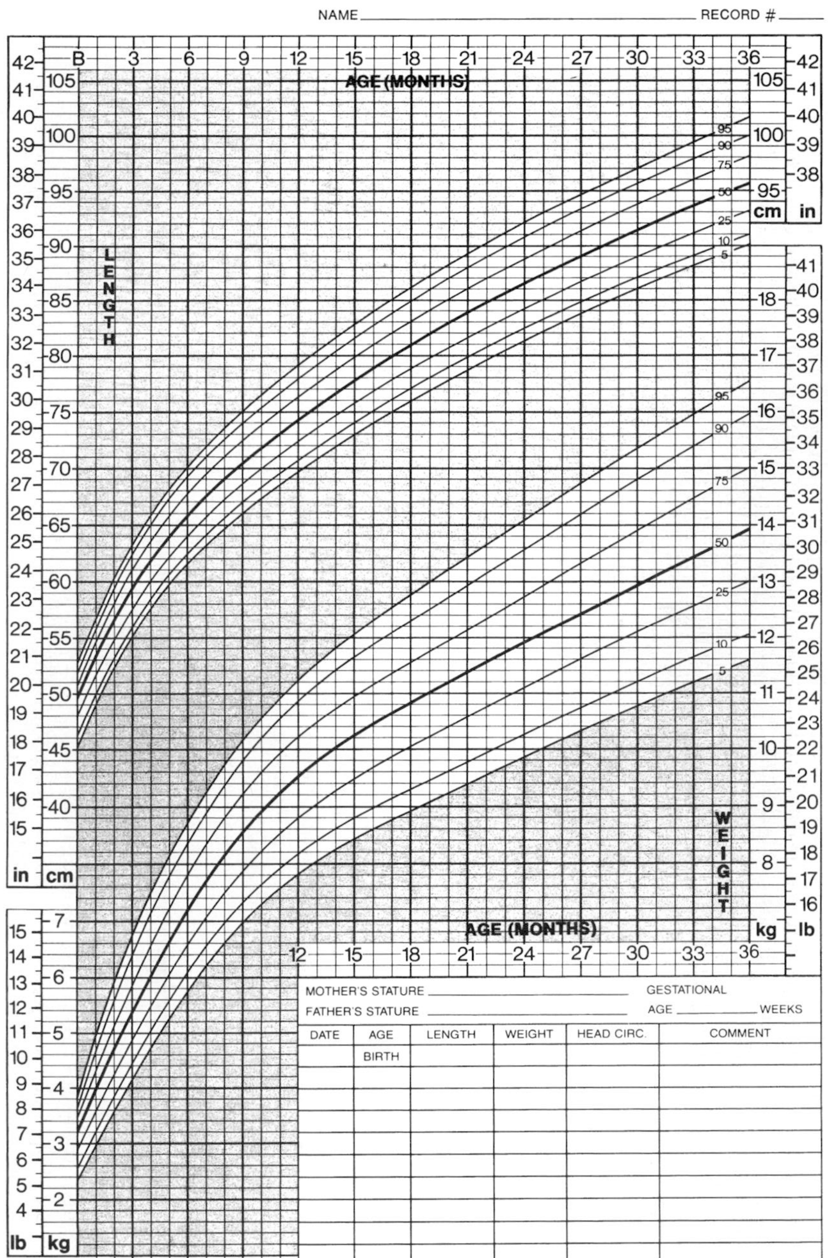

Figure 1-2. National Center for Health Statistics percentiles of physical growth in girls from birth to 36 months of age. (Copyright 1982 Ross Laboratories, Columbus, OH 43216. Adapted from Hamill PVV, Drizd TA, Johnson CL, et al. Physical growth: National Center for Health Statistics percentiles. Am J Clin Nutr 1979;32:607. Data from the Fels Research Institute, Wright State University School of Medicine, Yellow Springs, OH.)

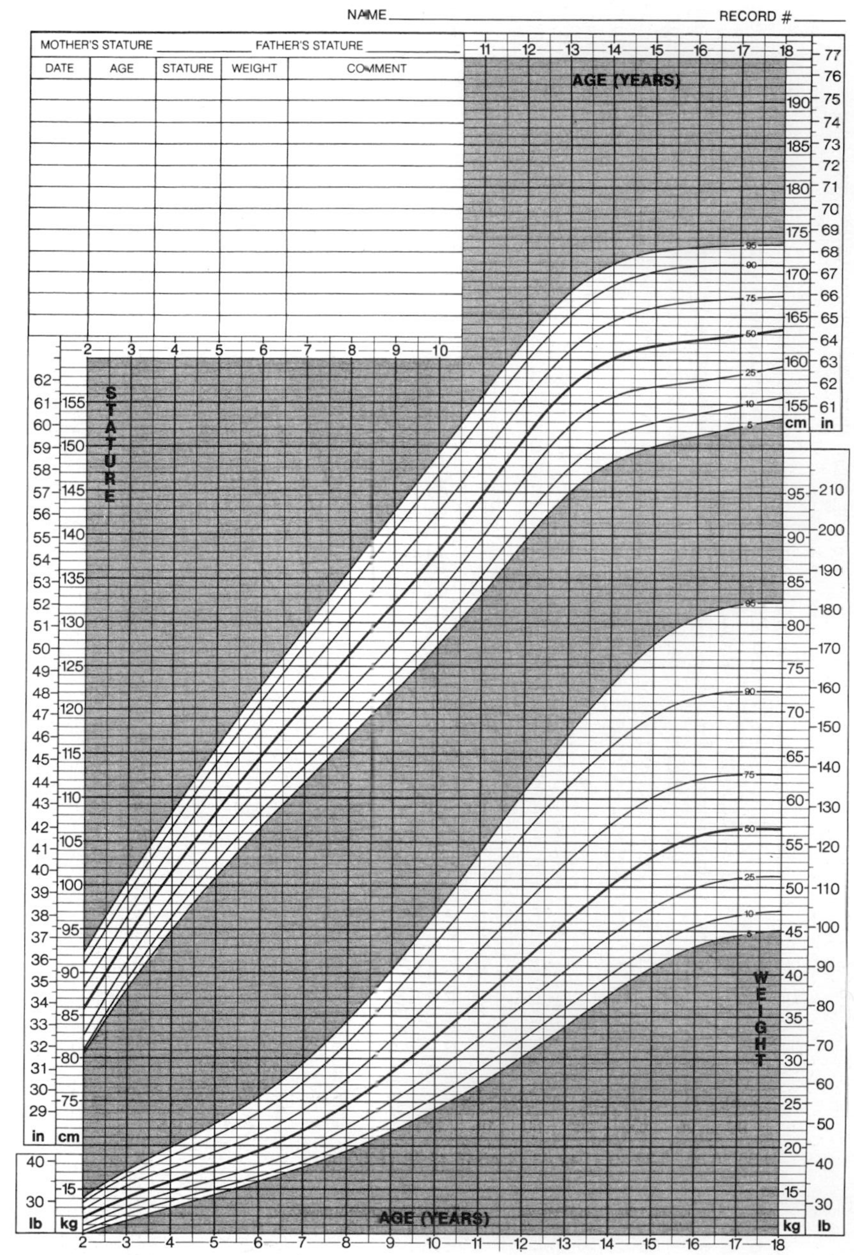

Figure 1-3. National Center for Health Statistics percentiles of physical growth in girls 2 to 18 years of age. (Copyright 1982 Ross Laboratories, Columbus, OH 43216. Adapted from Hamill PVV, Drizd TA, Johnson CL, et al. Physical growth: National Center for Health Statistics percentiles. Am J Clin Nutr 1979;32:607. Data from the National Center for Health Statistics, Hyattsville, MD.)

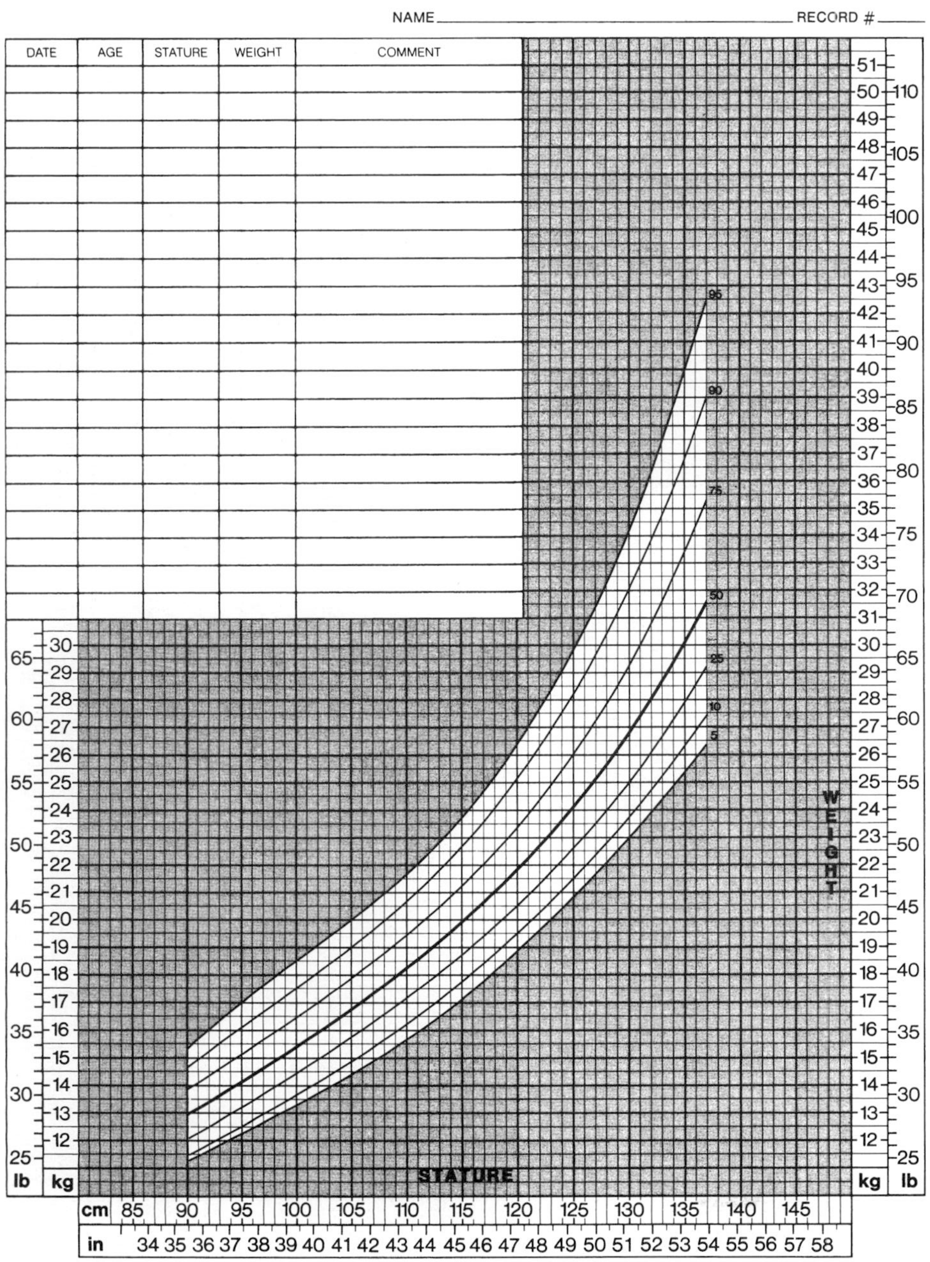

Figure 1-4. National Center for Health Statistics percentiles of prepubescent physical growth in girls. (Copyright 1982 Ross Laboratories, Columbus, OH 43216. Adapted from Hamill PVV, Drizd TA, Johnson CL, et al. Physical growth: National Center for Health Statistics percentiles. Am J Clin Nutr 1979;32:607. Data from the National Center for Health Statistics, Hyattsville, MD.)

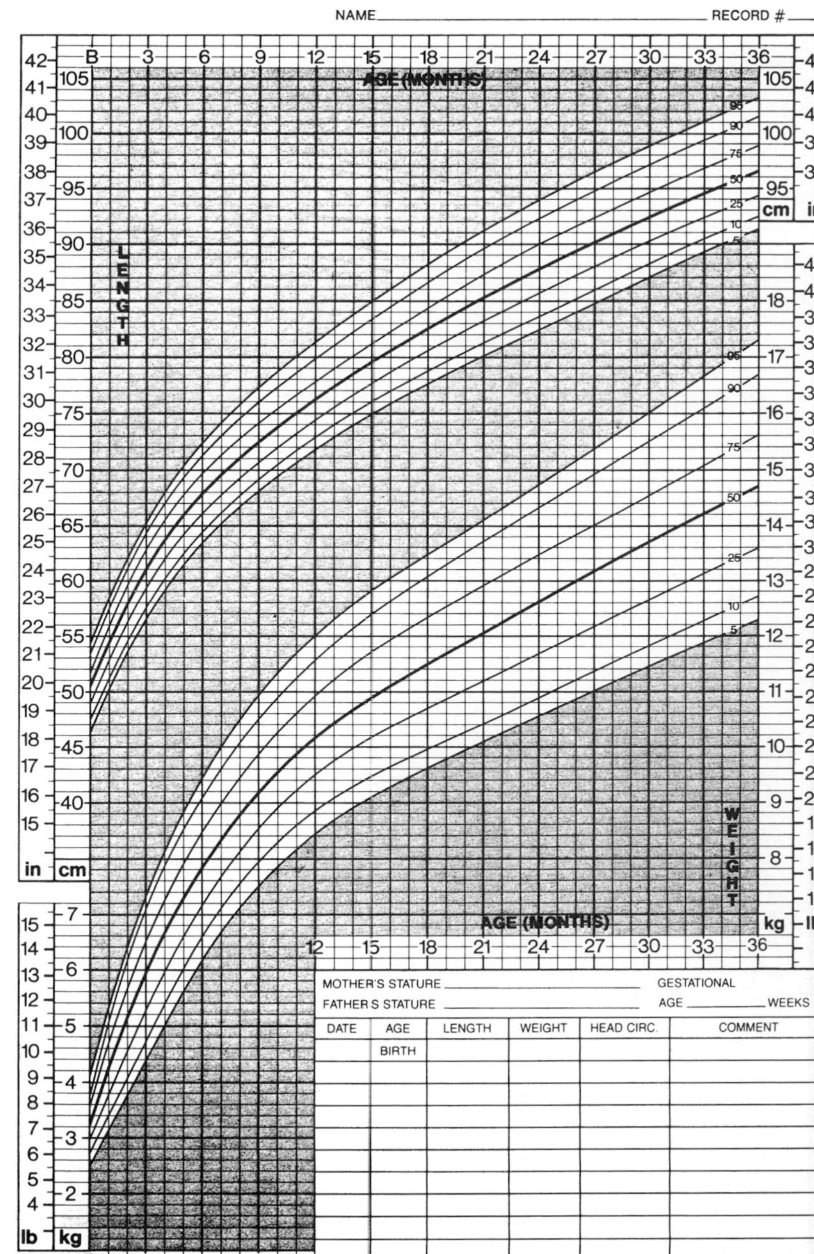

Figure 1-5. National Center for Health Statistics percentiles of physical growth in boys from birth to 36 months of age. (Copyright 1982 Ross Laboratories, Columbus, OH 43216. Adapted from Hamill PVV, Drizd TA, Johnson CL, et al. Physical growth: National Center for Health Statistics percentiles. Am J Clin Nutr 1979;32:607. Data from the Fels Research Institute, Wright State University School of Medicine, Yellow Springs, OH.)

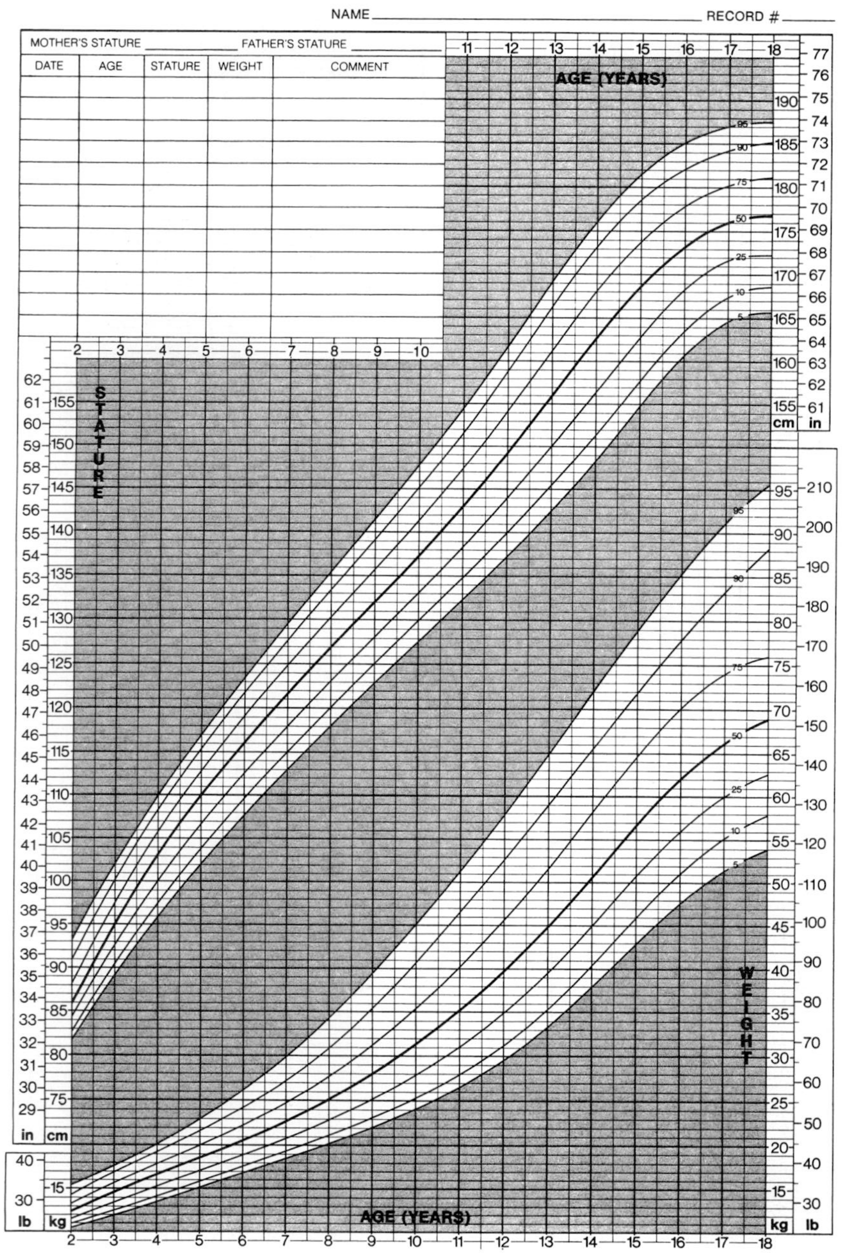

Figure 1-6. National Center for Health Statistics percentiles of physical growth in boys 2 to 18 years of age. (Copyright 1982 Ross Laboratories, Columbus, OH 43216. Adapted from Hamill PVV, Drizd TA, Johnson CL, et al. Physical growth: National Center for Health Statistics percentiles. Am J Clin Nutr 1979;32:607. Data from the National Center for Health Statistics, Hyattsville, MD.)

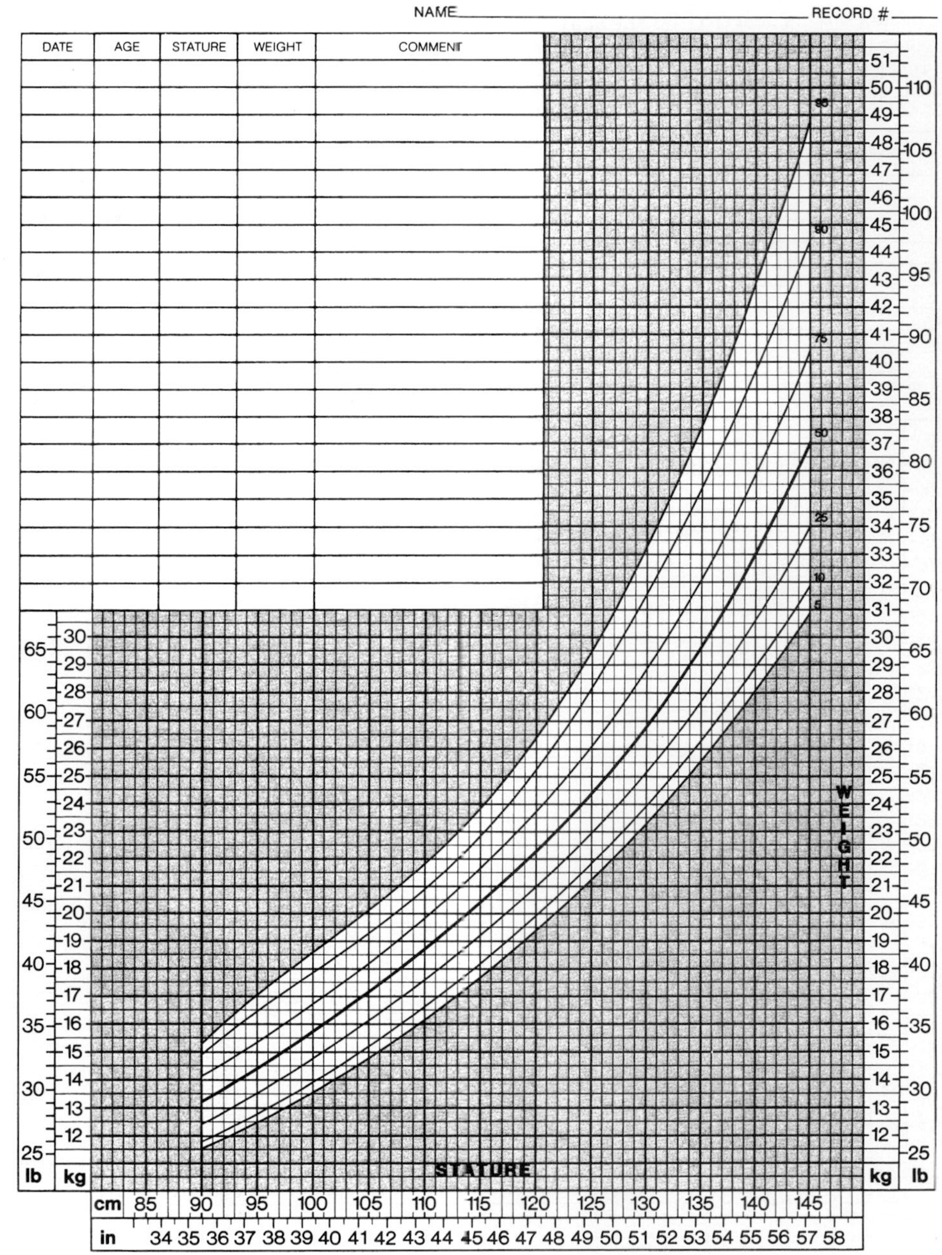

Figure 1-7. National Center for Health Statistics percentiles of prepubescent physical growth in boys. (Copyright 1982 Ross Laboratories, Columbus, OH 43216. Adapted from Hamill PVV, Drizd TA, Johnson CL, et al. Physical growth: National Center for Health Statistics percentiles. Am J Clin Nutr 1979;32:607. Data from the National Center for Health Statistics, Hyattsville, MD.)

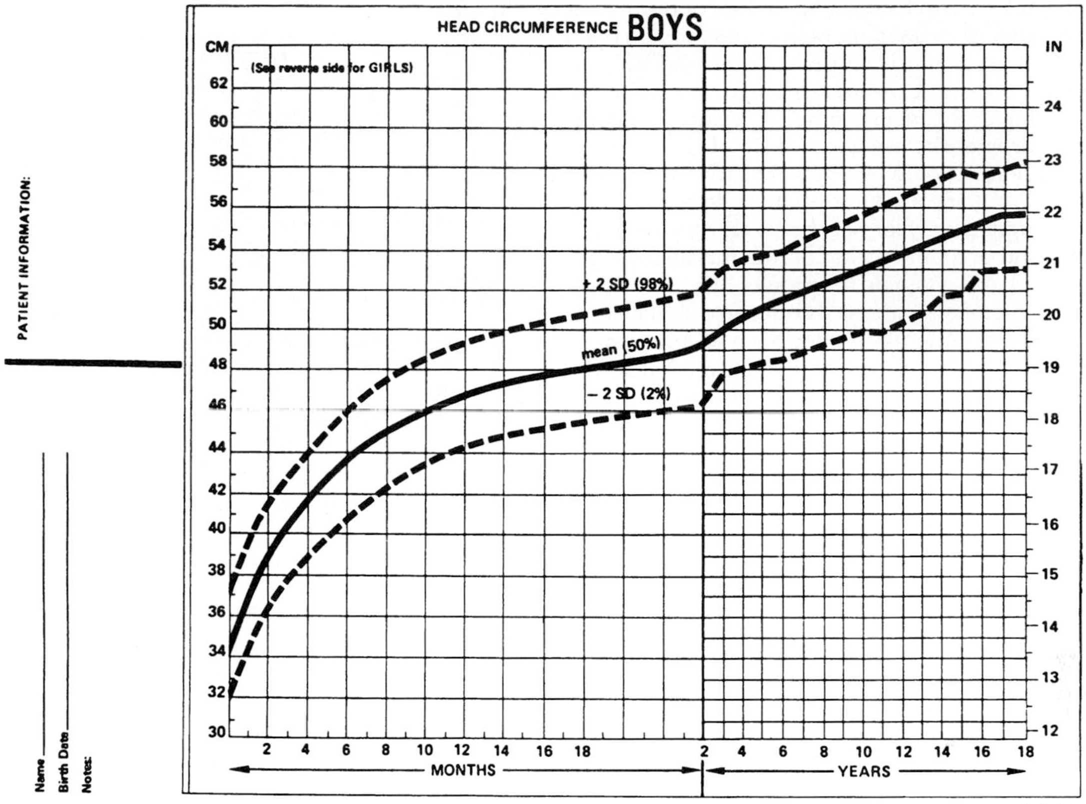

Figure 1-8. Head circumference in boys. (Reprinted with permission from Nellhaus G. Composite international and interracial graphs. Pediatrics 1968;41:106.)

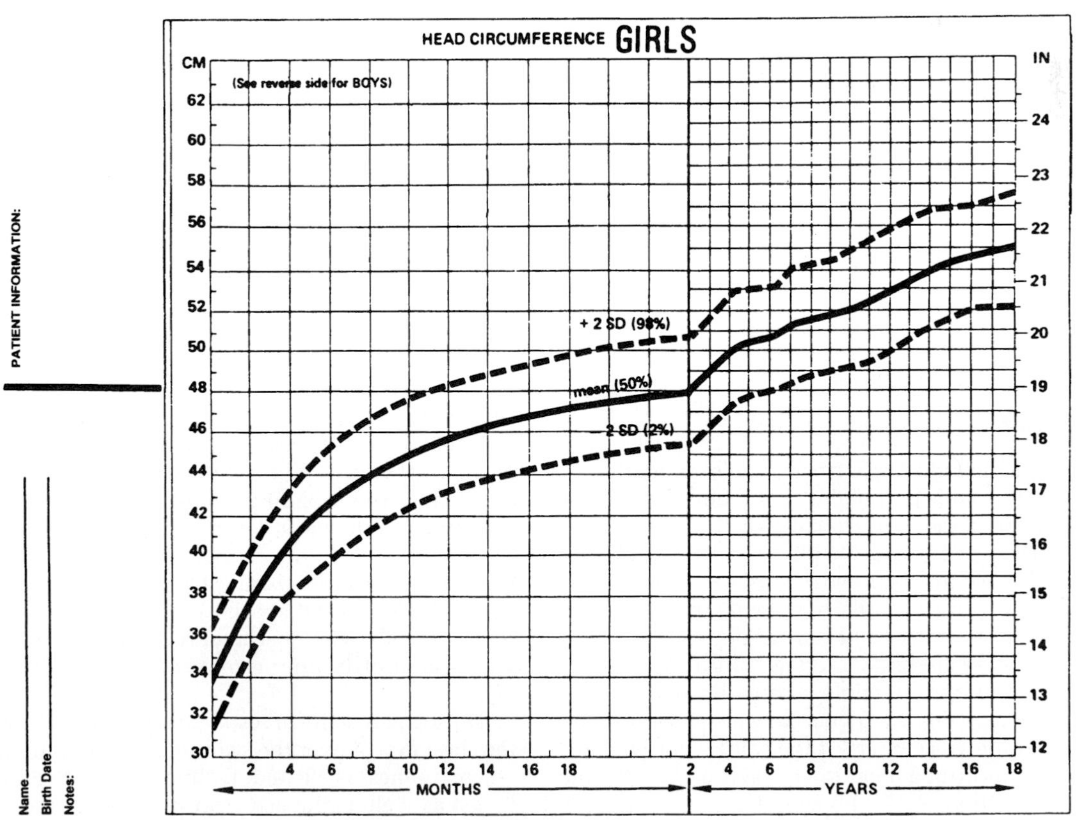

Figure 1-9. Head circumference in girls. (Reprinted with permission from Nellhaus G. Composite international and interracial graphs. Pediatrics 1968;41:106.)

cornea from a distant source. Evaluate the range of eye movements and the presence of nystagmus. Both eyelids should open equally. Failure to open is ptosis and may be caused by neurologic or systemic diseases. Upward slanting of the palpebral fissures with covering of the inner canthus (epicanthal folds) is a sign of Down syndrome. The conjunctivae should be pink, but not inflamed; the sclerae should be white. Examine the cornea for haziness (a sign of glaucoma) or opacities. Record the size and shape of the pupils, the color of the iris, and the response of the iris to light and accommodation. In the funduscopic examination, use a zero lens and note the presence of a red reflex, or hemorrhages or pigmented areas, and the size of the veins compared to the arteries. Any obstruction such as a corneal or lenticular cataract, will obliterate part or all of the red reflex. The disc borders should be sharp. They are blurred with increased intracranial pressure. The macula may not be clear, which is a sign of degenerative diseases. Obtain the corneal reflex by lightly touching the cornea with a piece of cotton. Failure to blink indicates trigeminal or facial nerve injury.

Ears

Note the position of the ears and abnormalities of the external ear, the pinna. Low-set ears may suggest the presence of renal agenesis. Tags and deformities are frequently associated with other minor or major anomalies. Grossly evaluate hearing, then proceed with examination of the inner ear. Pull the earlobe up and anteriorly. Grasp an otoscope equipped with a bright light so the hand rests on the child's head and moves with any movement of the head, and use the largest speculum that will fit into the canal. The canal should be clear, and the drum should be pearly gray in color and concave. A cone of light, the malleus, and sometimes the incus can be identified. If the bones are not visualized, the drum is not gray in color or is infected, or the drum is not concave, fluid may be in the ear. Fill the canal firmly with the speculum and give a short burst of air. The tympanic membrane should move. Lack of motion suggests serous or purulent otitis media.

Nose

Raise the tip of the nose and look up the nose with a bright light. Record discharges, bleeding, or deformities of the septum. The normal nasal mucosa is light pink. Tap on the maxillary and frontal sinuses for tenderness. Feel for air egress from both nares.

Mouth and Throat

The young child is usually most resistant during examination of the mouth and throat, so this part of the examination should be performed near the end of the visit. The child should be sitting so the tongue is less likely to obstruct the pharynx. Deformities or infections around the lips are recorded. Count the number and note the condition of the teeth. Similarly, note the condition and color of the tongue, buccal mucosa, palate, tonsils, and posterior pharynx. Normally, these are pink. Exudate indicates infection by bacteria, viruses, or fungi, but etiology cannot usually be determined by physical examination alone. Note also the presence of the gag reflex and the voice or cry. If the child seems hoarse, question the parent concerning the normal voice. Laryngitis can lead to airway obstruction. After the age of 2 years, children should not drool. Chronic drooling may suggest mental deficiency, but acute onset of drooling is a grave sign of epiglottitis or poison ingestion.

Neck

Feel in the neck for lymph nodes, which are normally nontender and up to 1 cm in diameter in both the anterior and posterior cervical triangles. Larger or tender nodes occur with local or systemic infection or malignancies. Feel the trachea in the midline. Feel for the thyroid. Other masses may be present and are always abnormal. Flex the neck. Resistance to flexion is a cardinal sign of meningitis, but this also occurs with severe infections around the neck or dislocation of the cervical vertebrae.

Lymph Nodes

In addition to the lymph nodes in the neck, palpate inguinal, epitrochlear, supraclavicular, axillary, and posterior occipital nodes. Normally, inguinal nodes may be up to 1 cm in diameter; the others are nonpalpable or less than 5 mm. Larger or tender nodes hold significance similar to that described for abnormal cervical glands.

Chest

Observe the chest for shape and symmetry. The chest wall is almost round in infancy and in children with obstructive lung disease. Respirations are predominantly abdominal until about 6 years of age when they become thoracic. Note suprasternal, intercostal, and subcostal retractions, which are signs of increased respiratory work. Swelling at the costochondral junctions is an indication of rickets. Edema of the chest wall occurs in children with superior vena cava obstruction. Asymmetry of expansion occurs with diaphragmatic paralysis, pneumothorax, or other intrathoracic abnormalities.

Breasts

Breasts are normally hypertrophied at birth; they regress within 6 months and develop with the onset of puberty. Development during adolescence is staged. Breast development in both boys and girls usually begins asymmetrically. Palpate for nodules, which may be cysts or tumors. Redness, heat, and tenderness usually indicate infection.

Lungs

Note the type and rate of the child's breathing. The rate of respiration varies, as described previously. Rapid rates, known as tachypnea, are associated with infection, fever, excitement, exercise, heart failure, or intoxicants. Slower rates are characteristic of intracranial lesions, depression caused by sedative drugs, heart block, or alkalosis. Cheyne-Stokes breathing, which is characterized by periods of deep, rapid respirations followed by slow, shallow respirations, is common in premature and newborn infants, and in those with intracranial or metabolic abnormalities. Dyspnea, or distress during breathing, is associated with flaring of the intercostal spaces and nares. Inspiratory dyspnea is more common with obstruction high in the respiratory system, and expiratory dyspnea is more common with lower respiratory diseases.

During percussion a resonant sound is obtained over most of the chest except over the scapulae, diaphragm, liver, and heart, where dullness is elicited. Dullness detects consolidation in the lungs, as well as the size and position of the liver and heart. Scratch percussion, which involves tapping the chest wall with a finger while listening with a bell stethoscope over the heart and liver, is especially useful in determining heart and liver size.

Increased resonance is found with increased trapped air, emphysema, or air in the pleural space (pneumothorax).

To auscultate the lungs, listen with a small bell in small children and with the diaphragm in older children. Normal breath sounds are bronchovesicular and inspiration is twice as long as expiration in young children; breath sounds are vesicular and inspiration is three times as long as expiration in older children. Breath sounds are decreased with consolidation or pleural fluid in the young child and increased with pneumonia in the older child. Fine crackles either in inspiration or expiration (rales) indicate foreign substances, usually fluid, in the alveoli or smaller bronchi, as occurs in bronchitis, pneumonia, or heart failure. Coarse extraneous sounds (rhonchi) are the result of foreign substances in the larger airways, as in crying or upper respiratory infection. Musical extraneous sounds (wheezes) are caused by air flow through compromised larger airways, as in asthma.

Heart

In addition to the heart's rate (pulse) and rhythm, and the blood pressure, note the size, shape, sound quality, and presence of murmurs when examining the heart. Precordial bulging is a sign of right-sided enlargement. A cardiac impulse may not be noted in a young child, but in a thin, active child, it may suggest the size and position of the heart. An apex beat outside the midclavicular line in the fifth interspace indicates cardiomegaly, which is a significant sign of heart disease or heart failure. Palpation and percussion were described previously. Auscultate both in the sitting and the supine positions. Determine the heart rate and rhythm if this was not done previously. Auscultate initially over the apex (mitral area), then over the lower right sternal border (tricuspid area), second left intercostal space at the sternal edge (pulmonary area), and second right intercostal space at the sternal edge (aortic area). Next, proceed to the remainder of the precordium, axillae, back, and neck. Note heart sounds and any arrhythmia. A loud first sound at the apex occurs with mitral stenosis, a loud second sound at the pulmonary area occurs with pulmonary hypertension, and a fixed split-second sound in the pulmonary area occurs with an atrial septal defect. Innocent murmurs are systolic, musical, or vibratory and of low intensity, and are usually heard at the third left interspace, just inside the apex, or beneath either clavicle. The latter is a venous hum that may be continuous and that disappears when the patient is supine. Diastolic murmurs are almost always significant. Significant systolic murmurs may be stenotic and are loudest in midsystole over the aortic or pulmonary areas. Regurgitant murmurs begin immediately after the first sound. Over the mitral or tricuspid area, they indicate valvular insufficiency. A continuous or uneven systolic murmur along the upper left sternal border indicates patent ductus arteriosus.

Abdomen

Observe the shape and tone of the abdomen. A flat abdomen may indicate diaphragmatic hernia; a distended abdomen may indicate intestinal obstruction or ascites; a board-like abdominal wall may indicate intraabdominal disease. Auscultate before percussing or palpating. Normally, peristaltic sounds are heard every 10 to 30 seconds. High-pitched frequent sounds occur with obstruction or peritonitis; absent sounds indicate ileus. Next, palpate gently, beginning in the left lower quadrant and proceeding to the left upper, right upper, right lower, and midline areas. Then palpate more deeply in the same areas and follow with palpation in the same areas with the unused hand pushing toward the front hand from the child's back. Feel especially for the liver in the right upper quadrant and the spleen in the left upper quadrant, and estimate their size. Any other masses are abnormal.

Transilluminate other masses to distinguish cystic from solid masses. Determine tenderness and attempt to locate the maximum point of any tenderness, which may indicate intraabdominal infection such as peritonitis, cystitis, or appendicitis; or rapid enlargement of organs, as occurs with enlargement of the liver in heart failure. Percuss to verify findings. Feel in the costovertebral angles to determine kidney size. Tenderness here usually indicates pyelonephritis. Percuss or palpate the bladder for size and tenderness.

Genitalia

A child's stage of pubertal development is estimated from the presence of pubic hair. Average adolescent development in girls proceeds as follows: breast development after 8 years of age, pubic hair after 12 years of age, increase in height velocity after 12 years of age, and menarche and axillary hair after 13 years of age. Average development in boys proceeds as follows: testicular enlargement at 11.5 years of age, pubic hair at 12.5 years of age, increase in height velocity at 14 years of age, and facial and axillary hair at 14.5 years of age. Variations in order of development suggest hormonal abnormalities. Modesty of the child should be respected during the examination, especially concerning examination of the breasts and genitalia.

Inspect the genitalia for urethral discharges, which are always pathologic and indicate infection anywhere in the genitourinary system.

In a girl, vaginal bleeding after the newborn period and before puberty may be the result of injury or a foreign body. Fused labia minora usually part with hygiene. Imperforate hymen causes hydrocolpos before puberty and hematocolpos after menarche. Vaginal discharge may be the result of injury or a foreign body in a young girl, is usually normal at the start of puberty, and suggests infection in an older girl. Adolescents with vaginal discharge, dysuria, lower abdominal pain, irregular bleeding, or sexual activity require a complete vaginal examination. The uterus in a younger child is palpated for size, shape, and tenderness with one hand over the lower abdomen and a finger of the other hand in the rectum. For an older child, the cervix is visualized with a vaginoscope or small speculum, and cultures are obtained.

In boys, testes should be in the scrotum after birth, although active cremasteric reflexes may empty the scrotum temporarily. The meatal opening should be slit-like and the urinary stream should be strong. Hydroceles, which do not reduce and do transilluminate, and hernias, which reduce but do not transilluminate, enlarge the scrotum. Testicular tenderness suggests torsion of the testis or epididymitis.

Rectum

Inspect the anus for fissures, inflammation, or lack of tone. The latter may indicate child abuse. The rectum is not examined routinely but is examined in all children with abdominal or gastrointestinal complaints including diarrhea, constipation, or bleeding from the rectum.

Extremities and Back

Asymmetry, anomalies, unusual size, pain, tenderness, heat, and swelling deformities of the extremities and back must be distinguished from congenital malformations, osteomyelitis, cellulitis, myositis or, rarely, rickets and scurvy. Joint heat, tenderness, swelling, effusion, redness, and limitation or pain on motion may indicate arthritis, arthralgia, synovitis or injury, or septic arthritis (which is a medical emergency). Observe the child walking and look for the presence of a limp. Clubbing of the fingers is a sign of chronic hypoxemia, as in congenital heart or chronic pulmonary diseases.

The spine should be straight with mild lumbar lordosis. Kyphosis, scoliosis, masses, tenderness, limitation of motion, spina bifida, pilonidal dimples, tufts of hair, or cysts may be caused by injury, malformation, infections, or tumors.

Weakness, tenderness, or paresis of the muscles suggests inflammatory muscle disease, congenital or metabolic neuromuscular diseases, or central nervous system abnormalities.

Neurologic Examination

Mental status and orientation help determine the acuteness of a child's illness depending on the environmental conditions. Position at rest and abnormal movements such as tremors, twitching, choreiform movements, and athetosis are characteristic of hyperirritability of the central nervous system. Incoordination of gait usually indicates cerebellar dysfunction. Kernig sign (inability to extend the leg with the hip flexed) and Brudzinski sign (flexing the neck with resultant flexion of the hip or knee) are indications of meningeal irritation.

Cranial nerves can be tested. Dysfunction of olfactory nerve I results in anosmia. Dysfunction of the trigeminal nerve V results in lack of sensation of the face and tongue. With peripheral facial nerve VII paralysis, neither the forehead nor the face moves. With nuclear VII paralysis, the forehead moves. Difficulty in swallowing and loss of pharyngeal reflexes are caused by dysfunction of the glossopharyngeal nerve IX or the vagus nerve X. Patients cannot contract the sternocleidomastoid or trapezius muscles with involvement of the spinal accessory nerve XI. The tongue protrudes to the involved side with hypoglossal nerve XII lesions.

Examination of tendon reflexes (biceps, triceps, patellar, and Achilles) is less important than is observation of general activity. Hyperactive reflexes indicate an upper motor neuron lesion or hypocalcemia. Decreased reflexes are seen in lower motor neuron lesions or the muscular dystrophies.

NEWBORN EXAMINATION

In the delivery room, a minimal examination is needed. The general appearance is noted and, at 1 and 5 minutes of age, an Apgar score is assigned (Table 1-1). A score of 7 or less indicates that an infant is at risk.

The infant is placed in a warmer. A small catheter is passed through both nares. Secretions are aspirated, and the tube is continued into the stomach and the stomach contents are aspirated. Easy passage of the catheter indicates patency of both nares. Passage into the stomach obviates blind pouch types of tracheoesophageal fistulas. The infant may urinate or defecate, indicating patency of these orifices. The mouth is inspected for cleft palate. Gestational age is assessed based on neurodevelopmental signs. Newborn care is then given and further examination is deferred to the nursery.

Preferably within the first few hours of birth, an admission newborn examination is performed in the presence of the parents. Develop a routine for the newborn examination so that critical areas are never omitted. In the first few hours of life, newborns are usually awake, but after 4 hours, they may be sleepy. The pressing question to be answered in the first examination is, "Is my child normal?" Although the order of the examination may vary, as with the history, initiate an order of recording for easy retrieval of information if it is needed later. See chapter 6 for a complete discussion of the newborn exam.

TABLE 1-1. Apgar Score

Rating	0	1	2
Appearance	Pale or blue	Body pink, extremities blue	Pink all over
Pulse	Absent	100	100
Grimace	None	Weak	Strong
Activity (tone)	Limp	Some flexion	Spontaneous movement
Respiratory effort	Absent	Hypoventilation gasping	Coordinated vigorous cry

CHAPTER 2

The Problem-Oriented Medical Record

Adapted from Herbert Schneiderman

The problem-oriented medical record (POMR) system was introduced in 1965 by Dr. Lawrence Weed as a means of correcting certain deficiencies in the traditional approach to medical record keeping. Enthusiastically endorsed by many clinicians, it has been used for patient care, student and house officer teaching, and medical audit. More recently, the POMR system has also been implemented by members of the allied health professions.

TRADITIONAL APPROACH

Courses in introduction to clinical medicine have used variants of the traditional scheme shown in Fig. 2-1. One takes a history from the patient or a parent and then performs a physical examination. This information provides the basis for producing a differential diagnosis. A differential diagnosis is a mutually exclusive list of diagnoses used to develop a diagnostic plan. The diagnostic plan generates clinical data. Analysis of the data leads to modification of the differential diagnosis, and this process continues until a definitive diagnosis is achieved. At that point, treatment begins.

Difficulties with the Traditional Approach

The traditional model is a rough guide to medical decision making that every clinician has learned to modify for practical purposes. As a model, it is heavily oriented toward making a diagnosis. Sometimes, however, a decision must be made in a situation in which the diagnosis is not the primary concern (e.g., a routine history of an infant hospitalized with bronchiolitis reveals that he or she has had no immunizations; a child with rheumatoid arthritis is not responding to aspirin therapy). Much of modern inpatient management is directed at patients with complex treatment problems; in the traditional model, these complexities do not receive sufficient recognition or emphasis.

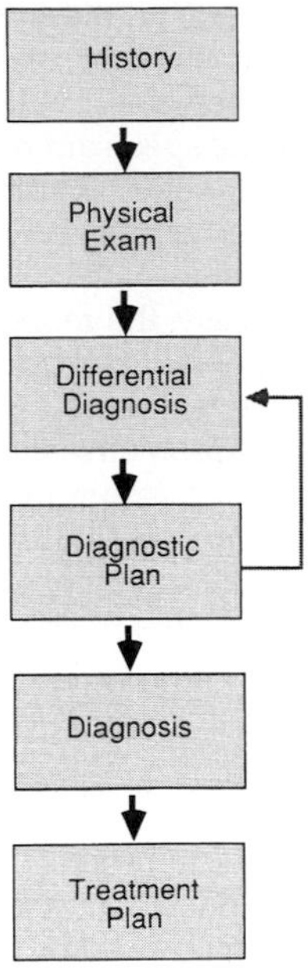

Figure 2-1. The traditional model of medical recording.

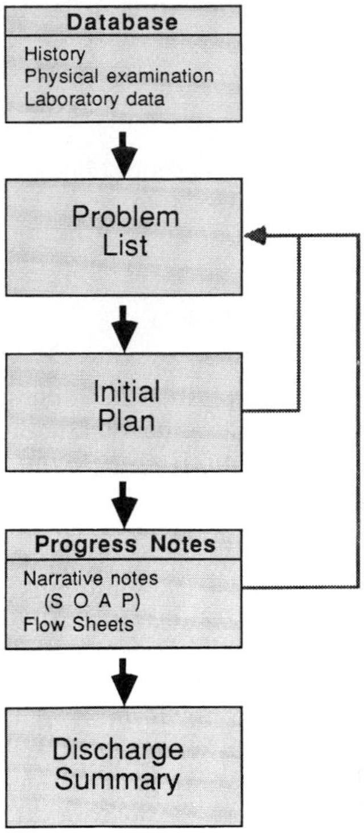

Figure 2-2. The problem-oriented medical record system. SOAP, *s*ubjective, *o*bjective, *a*ssessment, *p*lan.

Even when diagnosis is a central concern, the traditional model may present difficulties. It suggests that each patient has a single diagnosis when, in fact, a child may have concurrent diseases (e.g., a child with malabsorption also has pediculosis). Or, while one diagnostic problem is investigated, another is discovered (e.g., a child is undergoing evaluation for a pneumonia, and a complete blood count reveals a microcytic, hypochromic anemia).

The traditional model is even less helpful when a single disease or diagnosis has multiple components, each of which may present diagnostic problems (e.g., a patient with meningomyelocele has hydrocephalus and orthopedic deformities and is not urinating spontaneously).

Because the traditional model emphasizes diagnosis, the physician may formulate a diagnosis prematurely or ignore abnormal data that do not seem to relate to a current diagnostic formulation. In addition, some conventional diagnostic labels are insufficiently descriptive. The broad term *asthma* is equally likely to refer to the illness of a child who takes medication occasionally for symptoms or to another child who has had numerous hospitalizations and requires long-term maintenance on several drugs.

PROBLEM-ORIENTED MEDICAL RECORD SYSTEM

The POMR system, although not perfect, remedies some of the deficiencies of the traditional model. It facilitates identification and tracking of multiple diagnoses, diagnostic investigations, and therapeutic problems.

The POMR system consists of the following components: a database, problem list, initial plan, progress notes (which include narrative notes and flow sheets), and discharge notes (Fig. 2-2). First, a database is established, based partly on a patient's chief complaint. This database leads to the formulation of a complete problem list. Using this list, an initial plan of action is constructed. Progress notes are also structured by the problem list. Information gathered during investigation leads to modification of the problem list, or the patient may develop new problems as a consequence of treatment or from the natural course of the disease; these problems are added to the list. If the patient is hospitalized, the discharge summary is also organized according to the problem list.

Database

The database includes the history, physical examination, background information, and laboratory data. Data can be gathered into three groups: inquiry into the problem, routine screening, and general background information. Inquiry into the problem includes the traditional consideration of the present illness and pertinent parts of the physical examination. Routine screening consists of questions and items of the physical examination regarding problems unsuspected by the patient or parents (e.g., a child brought in with a running nose is found, after a routine developmental check, to have delayed speech). General background information includes family and social history, hobbies, and so forth.

The difference between inquiry and screening should be distinguished. In routine screening, tapping the knees of a healthy 2-year-old child to elicit deep tendon reflexes is of limited use; investigation of gross motor development is much more helpful. Testing for deep tendon reflexes in a comatose 2-year-old child, however, is an essential part of an inquiry into the problem.

The content of a structured inquiry into a problem varies with the problem. Similarly, routine screening and background information vary with the age, gender, race, and socioeconomic status and background of the patient. For example, a birth history or information on formula feeding is more useful in evaluating an infant than a husky 14-year-old child admitted for a sports injury. Likewise, abduction of the hips with the knees flexed is an important technique used to evaluate infants for hip dysplasia, but it is not particularly helpful in the routine evaluation of a normal 4-year-old child, for whom gait observation is more useful.

Problem List

Each of the patient's problems should be numbered and listed in the problem list, as in the following:

1. Pneumonia
2. Hypochromic microcytic anemia
3. Developmental delay by history
4. Behind in immunizations

A problem should be listed in its most definitive form, but it should not be a guess, no matter how inspired, based on incomplete data. If the first problem is a suspected meningitis manifesting as a bulging fontanelle, the problem should be listed as "1. Bulging fontanelle." If a lumbar puncture has already been done before the write-up and corroborates your suspicions, the problem should be recorded as "1. Meningitis". If the culture result is positive for *Streptococcus pneumoniae,* the problem should then be changed to "1. Pneumococcal meningitis," but the number (in this case, 1) should not be changed, for ease in reviewing the chart.

A diagnostic problem may have several manifestations. If the manifestations are minor, they can be listed as part of the same problem. If the manifestations are major and require careful, individual management, they should be treated as separate problems. For example, a single problem could be listed like this:

1. Meningitis with syndrome of inappropriate antidiuretic hormone (SIADH)

If the SIADH is severe, however, the list should specify two separate problems, as follows:

1. Meningitis
2. SIADH secondary to problem 1

The utility of a problem list is apparent when a disease process is complex and several different components each requires a decision. The following is an example of a problem list for a patient with meningomyelocele and concomitant illnesses:

1. Meningomyelocele
2. Hydrocephalus secondary to Arnold-Chiari malformation
3. Blocked ventriculoperitoneal shunt
4. Scoliosis with vertebral and rib abnormalities
5. Restrictive airway disease secondary to 4
6. Feeding difficulty secondary to 5
7. Bilateral equinovarus deformities secondary to 1
8. Neurogenic bladder secondary to 1
9. Family education regarding home care

This breakdown is not the only way to construct this problem list. For example, the Arnold-Chiari malformation could be designated as a separate problem, or problems 2 and 4 could be listed as secondary to 1. Minor variations in constructing a list are unimportant. What is important is to have a coherent, complete set of problems that help the clinician think and plan for the patient.

Initial Plan

In the traditional scheme, a differential diagnosis leads to a diagnostic plan, which results in a diagnosis. Then, a treatment plan is constructed. In real life, diagnostic and treatment decisions are made as soon as initial impressions (including differential diagnosis) are formed, and both types of planning usually continue concurrently. For example, if a lumbar puncture reveals 1,000 polymorphonuclear cells, a diagnosis of bacterial meningitis is made. The patient is taken off oral feeding, put on intravenous fluids, confined to bed, and treated with an antibacterial drug or drugs that cover the spectrum of possible organisms. If *S. pneumoniae* grows from blood and spinal fluid when cultures are taken, an antibiotic regimen is chosen that is best for that specific organism.

The more complex the case, the more likely it is that the traditional unstructured diagnostic and treatment plans will be incomplete and will omit needed items.

In the POMR system, the problem list serves to organize initial planning efforts, and the plan is numbered to correspond with the problems on the problem list, as shown in this example:

Problem List

1. Left lower lobe pneumonia with cough
2. Microcytic, hypochromic anemia
3. Developmental delay revealed by history
4. Behind on immunizations

Initial Plan

1. Chest radiography, blood culture, purified protein derivative (tuberculin)
2. Free erythrocyte protoporphyrin, stool guaiac, detailed nutritional history
3. Do developmental assessment before discharge

4a. Discuss routine health care with parents
4b. Give second diphtheria, tetanus, and pertussis and oral poliovirus vaccine immunizations on discharge

Specific plans are of three types: diagnostic, therapeutic, and patient and family education. In this system, "rule out iron deficiency anemia" is not a diagnosis or a problem but a plan to establish a diagnosis. The patient and family education component is extremely important and has been insufficiently stressed in medical education. If a problem has several components, it may be useful to categorize planning efforts by type. For example, if the problem is "failure to thrive," the planning efforts for that problem could be listed as follows:

- Diagnostic: complete blood count, blood urea nitrogen, liver function tests, intake and output, and nutritional analysis of daily feeding
- Therapeutic: regular infant diet
- Educational: teach parents parenting and feeding techniques and have social agency follow family

Progress Notes

NARRATIVE NOTES

Narrative notes are organized by the subjective, objective, assessment, plan (SOAP) method. Subjective information, including symptoms, comes from the patient. Objective information, including physical findings and laboratory data, is obtained from and by health professionals. Assessment is the interpretation of subjective and objective data. Plan is the action to be taken including diagnostic, therapeutic, and educational components, arrangements for services, and other steps.

An example of narrative notes for the problem "1. Sore throat" using the SOAP breakdown follows:

- Subjective: patient says throat feels better and she is hungry
- Objective: temperature is down to 99°F; throat culture grew beta-hemolytic streptococci
- Assessment: streptococcal pharyngitis
- Plan: continue penicillin for 8 more days

	January	February	March	April	May
BUN	10			8	
renal scan		normal			
VCU			normal		
urine culture	E. coli	E.coli	Klebsiella	negative	negative
prophylactic antibiotics				trimethoprim/ sulfa	→

Figure 2-3. Sample flow sheet for a child with a neurogenic bladder. BUN, blood urea nitrogen; VCU, voiding cystourethrogram.

In this case, the problem would now be redefined as "1. Streptococcal pharyngitis."

Entries do not need to be made every day for each SOAP category or each problem, as the following list shows:

1. Left lower lobe pneumonia
   Objective: day 3 on penicillin; patient is coughing less; temperature down to 100°F
4. Behind on immunizations
   Plan: discuss rationale for immunizations with parents; consider ordering a visiting nurse for a home visit after discharge

FLOW SHEETS

When variables such as blood urea nitrogen or bilirubin are repeated serially, it may be difficult to compare and analyze them from narrative notes, particularly if several types of measurements are being compared.

The flow sheet is an excellent way to record and assess serial observations. (In pediatrics, we have traditionally used variations of flow sheets—head circumference and growth charts—to display and compare data.) This type of record is particularly valuable when several variables such as laboratory tests, symptoms, and treatment, are monitored simultaneously. Fig. 2-3 is an example of a flow sheet for a child with a neurogenic bladder.

Discharge Summary

Discharge summaries are potentially excellent self-teaching tools providing physicians the opportunity to review and analyze a patient's hospitalization, the decisions made, and the outcomes. They are also important sources of information for the community health professionals who will care for the recently hospitalized child.

Unfortunately, discharge summaries are often dictated in a perfunctory manner to meet hospital regulations. Little thought is given to their use and, consequently, they are too long; contain irrelevant, unstructured, and unassessed material; and lack important information for future health care providers.

The discharge summary should be problem oriented. This requirement is perhaps less important for a child admitted for a single problem, which was successfully treated and is resolving, than it is for a child with multiple problems, some of which are still active at the time of discharge. All problems, active and inactive, should be listed. Information related to each problem can be organized into the categories of subjective, objective, and therapeutic. Sometimes a problem may be described best by combining elements of the subjective and objective in a concise narrative, as in the following example of a patient with pneumococcal pneumonia:

> The patient was admitted with a 3-day history of coughing and fever. On admission, dullness and rales were apparent posteriorly in the left lower lung field. Other physical findings were normal. The chest film showed left lower lobe pneumonia, and sputum culture grew *S. pneumoniae*.

Only those items from the medical history, physical examination, or laboratory data necessary for future analysis or management of the patient should be included. The degree of detail should vary with the types and complications of the problems. An episode of asthma successfully treated with a short course of inhalant bronchodilators and corticosteroids may be described briefly. It is pointless to include a series of all the blood gases taken during the child's hospitalization. These data, useful at the time they are drawn, are of little significance for the future management of the patient. On the other hand, if a child is admitted with a fever of unknown origin and is discharged without a diagnosis, the various radiographic films and laboratory test results that were obtained should be listed, even if the results were normal. What studies were done and what they showed at a particular time are important for the physician to know.

Again, as in the initial plan, a problem-oriented discharge summary makes it easier to record and review complicated management plans. Flow sheets may be useful as part of the discharge summary. Although they cannot be dictated, they can be copied and added to the summary.

SOME PROBLEMS IN USING THE PROBLEM-ORIENTED MEDICAL RECORD SYSTEM

Students working with the POMR system occasionally ask about the correct way to chart a situation in which there is interaction between problems, so that treatment for one problem may influence the treatment, or be the same as that, for a second problem. No hard and fast solutions exist. One should be clear about what one is planning and not worry excessively about the form. For example, restrictive airway disease in a small infant may affect the ability to feed. Proper treatment of the airway disease may also alleviate the feeding problem. The following are two ways of charting the plan:

Problem List

4. Restrictive airway disease
5. Feeding difficulty secondary to 4

Initial Plan

4. Request ear, nose, and throat consult for tracheotomy and assisted ventilation; this may also alleviate feeding problem
5. See plan for 4

or

4 and 5. Request ear, nose, and throat consult for tracheotomy and assisted ventilation; this may also alleviate feeding problem

Another difficulty exists for the isolated user. The POMR system is intended to be used by the entire health team. The intern writes the problem list, and the list is modified by the resident and attending physician. The resident and attending physician check for completeness and accuracy in formulation of problems, and the intern makes corrections. The same numbering system is used by all the physicians. Consultants, nurses, therapists, and social workers are also expected to stay within the framework for the sake of convenience and coherence.

This scenario may not occur in real life. Some physicians on a ward do not use the system at all; others use their own organization schemes or numbering sequence. The individual student or house officer may find it worthwhile to use the POMR system to organize his or her thinking and to impose an intelligent order on observations, problems, and plans.

FUTURE TRENDS

Dr. Weed devised the POMR with the view from the beginning that it could be used with computer technology. The increasing use of computer systems that implement the POMR has demonstrated limitations of the original method, and a number of researchers have designed or are designing new computer-based record systems that incorporate, modify, and expand the original ideas for use in primary-care and hospital-based settings. Among other possibilities, computerization should make it feasible to provide a link between problems and subproblems and interaction between problems. Computerization should also provide ways to display problems and supporting data in varying levels of detail and in different contexts. Such structured electronic problem-oriented records are promising tools for the improvement of medical care.

CHAPTER 3
Diagnostic Process

Adapted from Frank A. Oski

Diagnosis is one of the most important tasks of the clinician. Problem solving in medicine has been described, somewhat cynically, as "the process of making adequate decisions with inadequate information." If the diagnosis is correct and treatment is available, proper care usually follows. If no specific treatment is available, correct diagnosis is still important, because it provides a basis for prognosis and advice to patients or parents.

The need for a logical approach to medical diagnosis is vitally important to the economy of the United States, where health costs account for at least 10% of the gross national product. Former U.S. Secretary of Health, Education, and Welfare Joseph A. Califano observed that "the physician is the central decision maker for more than 70% of health care services." These decisions include that for hospitalization, duration of hospitalization, medications administered, and diagnostic tests used.

The cognitive processes used in making a diagnosis are not fully understood. Perhaps nowhere else in medicine do the art and science of medicine blend as imperceptibly as they do in the process of making a diagnosis.

Physicians use four basic approaches to reach a diagnosis: pattern recognition, sampling the universe, clinical algorithms, and hypothesis generation. Pattern recognition is the process by which a diagnosis is made based on physical clues or linkage identification. For example, a diagnosis of Down syndrome can be made by recognizing the physical findings that make up this genetic abnormality. Similarly, the diagnosis of Henoch-Schönlein purpura is immediately apparent if the rash has a characteristic pattern and distribution. Diagnosis by pattern identification requires familiarity with diseases through experience or study. The expression "the more you see, the more you know, and the more you know, the more you see" describes how pattern recognition develops. Linkage identification is a form of pattern recognition. A diagnosis is based on history and physical or laboratory findings. For example, the finding of a micropenis and hypoglycemia in a neonate would result in a prompt diagnosis of congenital hypopituitarism. A history of bloody diarrhea in association with a white blood cell count demonstrating more band forms than mature polymorphonuclear leukocytes would result in an immediate diagnosis of *Shigella* gastroenteritis. Skill in linkage identification, like pattern recognition, is gained by observation and study. The seemingly intuitive diagnosis, often the hallmark of the older physician, is usually a result of linkage identification.

Sampling the universe refers to the mindless ordering of laboratory studies in hopes that an abnormality will appear that can result in a diagnosis. This is a diagnostic process to be decried. In the United States, approximately $27 billion per year is spent on laboratory tests, and another $2 billion per year is spent on chest roentgenography. An estimated 20% to 60% of these tests are unnecessary. If the estimates are accurate, $6 to $12 billion per year is spent on procedures that do not aid in the diagnosis or treatment of illness. The amount spent specifically on pediatric patients is unknown.

Laboratory tests should be obtained only to support a hypothesis. If the history and physical diagnosis do not suggest an underlying organic disorder, no rationale exists for ordering a battery of laboratory tests in an attempt to uncover an occult disease. The evaluation of infants and children with failure to thrive is an example of this form of behavior. In a 1978 review of 2,607 laboratory studies performed on 185 patients with failure to thrive, Sills found that only 1.4% of the tests were of any positive diagnostic assistance, and all of them were specifically indicated by the history or physical examination.

A clinical algorithm is a protocol, presented as a flow chart, that contains branch points requiring decisions. The clinical algorithm enables the user to reach a diagnosis. The clinical algorithm is a byproduct of computer science and is based on the belief that the medical diagnostic process can be automated. A number of clinical situations have been adapted successfully to algorithms, but the majority has not. An example of a clinical algorithm is depicted in Fig. 3-1.

Early algorithms were comprehensive and required many laboratory tests and physical findings. Many of these procedures were found to be unnecessary, and algorithms were simplified. An algorithm is not merely a list of symptoms or diagnostic procedures, but a logical flow chart or decision table that helps clinicians make decisions. They often require a precise yes or no answer; not all clinical questions can be answered so crisply. "Maybe" or any other vague answer blocks the progression in the typical algorithm. Algorithms have not been developed for every clinical situation or patient complaint. Algorithms are not yet a substitute for decision analysis or hypothesis generation in the establishment of a diagnosis.

Hypothesis generation, the development of explanations for the patient's problem, is the most common and intellectually satisfying technique for arriving at a diagnosis. The development of hypotheses distinguishes the problem-solving process from mere data collection. The stockpiling of facts without a

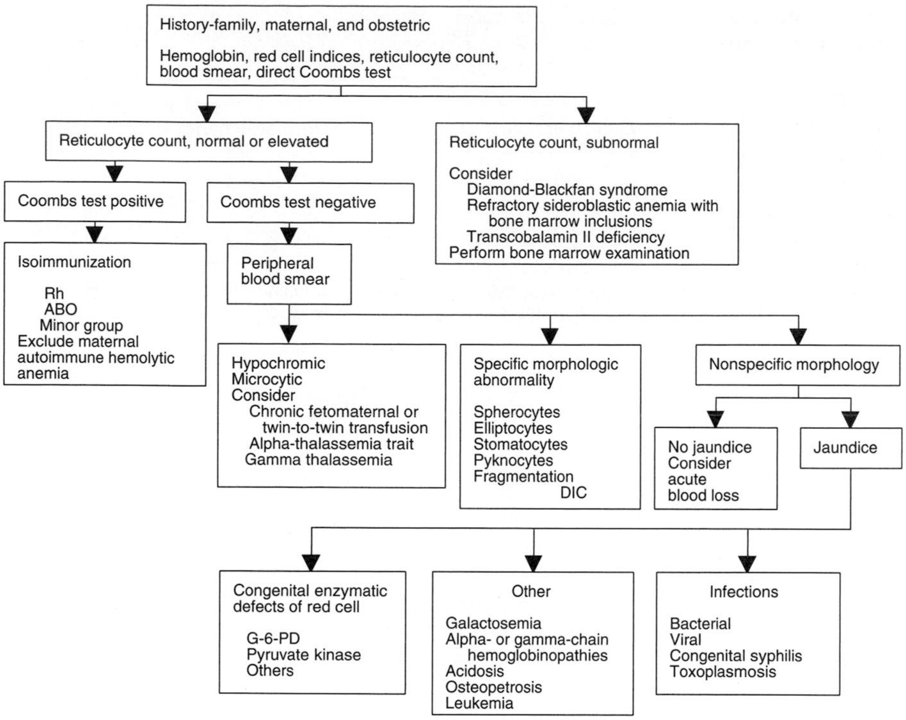

Figure 3-1. An approach to the differential diagnosis of anemia in the newborn. DIC, disseminated intravascular coagulation; G6PD, glucose 6-phosphate dehydrogenase. (Reprinted with permission from Oski FA, Naiman JL. *Hematologic problems of the newborn.* Philadelphia: Saunders, 1982:72.)

hypothesis has been likened to baseball statisticians with a great number of facts at hand but no way of determining what the facts really mean.

Hypotheses, or potential diagnoses, are generated early in patient encounters. Studies demonstrate that the competent physician begins to generate hypotheses the moment the chief complaint is heard. The generation of hypotheses continues as the remainder of the history unfolds. These hypotheses guide further inquiry. This immediate hypothesis generation directly contradicts the conventional strategy taught to medical students, which is to defer all hypotheses until history taking and physical examination are completed.

Many physicians use a common strategy to analyze presenting complaints. Initially, they interpret complaints anatomically; next, they interpret complaints physiologically; and finally, they interpret major symptoms pathophysiologically.

Fulginiti lists seven principles used to establish a clinical hypothesis:

- Common diseases and conditions occur commonly.
- A single process should be invoked to explain most of the data, if not all of it.
- Simple problems usually have simple explanations.
- Hypotheses should derive from the data and not be imposed on them.
- The hypothesis should be consistent with known pathophysiologic mechanisms.
- Serious consideration of an individual hypothesis should be based on its probability.
- Hypotheses may be formulated, accepted, rejected, or modified at any point in the course of problem solving.

As mentioned, research reveals that competent physicians tend to generate hypotheses the moment the chief complaint is heard. The same research demonstrates that a limited number of hypotheses are entertained simultaneously. More than five hypotheses usually are not actively retained, and never are more than seven considered. Investigation is often limited to the hypotheses that survive revisions that occur while the history and physical examination are performed. Several things can go wrong: The physician may retain hypotheses that are too general and often not easily tested; facts and findings may be ignored because they are inconsistent with a hypothesis; and physicians may be loath to generate new hypotheses after the initial list is formulated and equally loath to discard an existing one.

The human mind needs to perceive problems as having limited degrees of complexity. We oversimplify by assigning new information to existing hypotheses rather than forming new hypotheses, even when the information does not fit. The labeling of a condition as atypical or as a *form fruste* is an example of the parsimony of the human mind and is responsible for the slow recognition of new diseases.

SUGGESTED GUIDELINES FOR ESTABLISHING A DIAGNOSIS

- Always think of a number of diagnostic possibilities that are compatible with the chief complaint or the initial physical findings. Always consider the most common diagnosis first, but always include among your diagnoses those conditions, no matter how rare, for which treatment is available and which, if missed and untreated, would produce irreparable harm or even death to your patient.
- Form a reasoned plan for testing your hypothesis. Sequence laboratory tests to establish, or rule out, the most common diseases first, as well as the diseases requiring urgent treatment.
- Do not rush to make a diagnosis for which no treatment is available.
- Never perform a diagnostic procedure that is not related to any of your diagnostic possibilities (e.g., a urinalysis in a patient being evaluated for inspiratory stridor).
- Do not pursue a differential among diagnoses that will not alter your course of action.
- Always consider the harm that tests might do, as well as their costs. Balance the harm and the costs against the information that may be gained.

- Be constantly aware of the natural tendency to discount, or even disregard, evidence likely to eliminate your favored diagnosis.
- Never dismiss the possibility that a patient with multiple complaints or problems may have more than one disease. The chances of having two common diseases simultaneously are greater than the chance of having one rare disease.
- If you cannot rule out the possibility of the presence of a disease that would result in serious harm to the patient if left untreated, then treat the patient as if the disease was present.

Probability and utility should always guide your actions.

TABLE 4-1. Estimate of Caloric Expenditure or Volume of Maintenance Fluids*

Body weight (kg)	Caloric expenditure (kcal/kg/d) or maintenance fluids (mL/kg/d)
1–10	100/kg
11–20	1,000 plus 50/kg more than 10 kg
21–80	1,500 plus 20/kg more than 20 kg

* Example: Assume that a child is afebrile and minimally active. A 13-kg child needs 1,000 + 50 (13 − 10) = 1,150 kcal or mL/d.

CHAPTER 4
Fluid and Electrolyte Management

Adapted from Norman J. Siegel, Thomas O. Carpenter, and Karen M. Gaudio

PARENTERAL FLUID THERAPY

Most approaches to parenteral fluid therapy are empiric and based on clinical experience. When considering parenteral fluids for a patient, some general principles apply:

- Therapy must be individualized for every patient, a "cookbook" approach is discouraged.
- Calculations of the requirements for fluids and electrolytes are always estimates and cannot be assumed to be definitive.
- The patient's response to therapy is the best determinant of the success of any fluid therapy.

Parenteral fluid therapy is divided into three major components: maintenance therapy designed to maintain a state of hydration; deficit therapy designed to replace losses of electrolytes and water that occurred before a physician encountered the patient; and replacement therapy designed to replace ongoing losses after the patient has entered a therapeutic program.

Maintenance Fluids

Maintenance therapy is designed to replace the water and electrolytes that are lost under ordinary homeostatic conditions. Fluid requirements for maintenance therapy are best related to the metabolic rate and energy expenditures of the patient. Holliday and Segar demonstrated that the rate of caloric expenditure was relatively fixed for infants and children in three weight categories. In children weighing between 1 and 10 kg, the rate was 100 cal/kg; in those weighing between 11 and 20 kg, it was 50 cal/kg; and in those weighing between 21 and 80 kg, it was 20 cal/kg. Many of the initial programs for fluid therapy suggested that water would be expended at a rate of 120 mL/kcal of energy expenditure. Endogenous sources of water from oxidation, however, contribute 17 mL/100 kcal; and preformed water contributes 3 mL/100 kcal. Thus, 100 mL of exogenous water is needed for every 100 kcal of energy expended. Therefore, a child who weighs 13 kg would have an estimated maintenance fluid requirement of 1,150 mL/day: 1,000 mL would be for the first 10 kg, then 50 mL/kg for the next 3 kg equals 1,000 mL plus 150 mL, or a total of 1,150 mL/day. Similarly, this same patient would be expected to have a caloric expenditure of approximately 1,150 kcal/day (Table 4-1).

Beyond 80 kg, the proportion of body weight and water distribution diverges significantly, so that calculations extended beyond 80 kg are likely to be a significant overestimate of fluid requirements. From a practical perspective, the sliding scale in Table 4-1 can be converted to milliliters per kilogram per hour as follows by dividing the total daily volume to be administered by 24 or by the following convention: 1 to 10 kg, 4 mL/kg/hour; 11 to 20 kg, 40 mL/hour (for first 10 kg) + 2 mL/kg/hour (for each kilogram more than 10); and 21 to 80 kg, 60 mL/hour (for first 20 kg) + 1 mL/kg/hour (for each kilogram more than 20).

Maintenance fluids provide for losses from two major sources: evaporative (or insensible losses) and urinary losses. Insensible or evaporative losses amount to approximately one-third of the calculated maintenance fluids. Clearly, ambient temperature and humidity have a profound effect on the volume of fluid lost. An increase in insensible losses might be anticipated when children are hyperthermic or tachypneic. In the normal patient, evaporative fluid losses do not contain solutes and, therefore, the fluid required to replace this volume should be free of electrolytes.

Urinary losses will account for approximately two-thirds of the calculated maintenance requirement. In most clinical situations in which the patient might be expected to make a more dilute urine (diabetes insipidus, prematurity of birth, sickle cell disease), an appropriate increase in maintenance fluids must be provided. On the other hand, in those clinical situations in which it is not possible to dilute the urine to a specific gravity of 1.010 or an osmolarity of 300 mOsm/L [excessive or inappropriate antidiuretic hormone (ADH) release, congestive heart failure], the volume of maintenance fluids must be decreased appropriately.

Early empiric studies determined that approximately 2 to 3 mEq of sodium and chloride and 2 to 2.5 mEq of potassium for each 100 kcal expended or for each 100 mL of maintenance fluid were required to maintain normal electrolyte homeostasis and allow for growth. The addition of 5 g of dextrose in each 100 mL of fluid allows for the provision of approximately 20% of the caloric need when full maintenance fluid volume could be administered. Therefore, the parenteral fluid solution recommended for maintenance fluid therapy contains 25 to 30 mEq/L of sodium and chloride, 20 mEq/L of potassium, and 50 g/L of dextrose. A number of commercially available solutions meet the requirements for maintenance therapy (Table 4-2). For the purpose of maintenance therapy, a solution of D5 0.2 normal saline plus 20 mEq/L of potassium is recommended.

To monitor a patient's response to fluids, parameters such as change in body weight and change in serum sodium concentration should be used. For example, weight gain combined with a

TABLE 4-2. Electrolyte Composition of Common Parenteral Solutions

Electrolyte	NS	D5 0.5 NS	D5 0.2 NS	Ringer lactate	Plasma-lyte A
Na (mEq/L)	154	77	38	130	140
Cl (mEq/L)	154	77	38	109	98
K (mEq/L)	—	—	—	4	5
Glucose (g/L)	—	50	50	—	—
Lactate (mEq/L)	—	—	—	28	—
Acetate (mEq/L)	—	—	—	—	27

NS, normal saline.

decrease in serum sodium level or the development of peripheral edema suggests overhydration. Weight loss with a continuing increase in the serum sodium level or a persistent tachycardia would suggest inadequate fluid administration.

Because maintenance therapy provides for only 20% of the caloric expenditure, we should anticipate that our patient would lose weight at approximately 0.5% to 1.0% per day because of deficient caloric intake.

Disorders of Volume Depletion/Deficit Therapy

Illnesses such as diarrhea and vomiting frequently cause deficit states in children. A limited ability of the kidney in the premature infant and young child to concentrate the urine maximally makes them particularly susceptible to dehydration.

In evaluating a child who is dehydrated, three essential steps must be completed:

- The degree or severity of the dehydration must be estimated.
- The type of deficit must be determined.
- A plan for repair of the deficit must be developed and initiated.

Laboratory studies cannot accurately determine the severity or degree of dehydration. The only truly objective means of making such a determination is to know precisely the change in body weight that has occurred over a limited period. If weight change is available, it should be used. If weights are not available, the estimate of the degree of dehydration is made most often on the basis of clinical observation and experience. Table 4-3 lists a number of clinical features used in assessing the degree of dehydration. Note that similar findings represent different degrees of dehydration in older children as compared with infants. With mild degrees of volume depletion, the clinical signs are not very remarkable, and one relies largely on a history of excessive fluid losses. When the patient approaches a more moderate state of dehydration, the clinical findings become more apparent. For patients with severe dehydration, a nearly shock-like state occurs, which requires the initiation of resuscitative fluids expeditiously to prevent the development of irreversible metabolic changes.

TABLE 4-3. Evaluation of Severity of Dehydration

Examination	Older child 3%, infant 5%	Older child 6%, infant 10%	Older child 9%, infant 15%
Skin turgor	Normal	Tenting	None
Skin, touch	Normal	Dry	Clammy
Buccal mucosa/lips	Moist	Dry	Parched/cracked
Eyes	Normal	Deep set	Sunken
Crying, tears	Present	Reduced	None
Fontanelle	Flat	Soft	Sunken
Central nervous system	Consolable	Irritable	Lethargic
Pulse	Regular	Slightly increased	Tachycardia
Urine output	Normal	Decreased	Anuria

For practical purposes, three types of dehydration exist based on the serum sodium concentration: isotonic (serum sodium 130–150 mEq/L), hypotonic (serum sodium less than 130 mEq/L), and hypertonic (serum sodium greater than 155 mEq/L). The patient's measured serum electrolytes reflect the types of losses that have occurred. For example, in a patient who has hypotonic dehydration, losses have consisted of more sodium than water or that replacement fluid has contained an excess of free water. Similarly, for the patient with hypertonic dehydration, fluid losses have consisted of more water than electrolytes. This is particularly evident in certain types of diarrhea in which the electrolyte losses may be very low but the water losses are quite high. Differences can exist for corrective therapy for each type of dehydration.

An approach for rehydration is needed next and many interchangeable paradigms exist. The first phase of therapy (the *bolus*) should consist of the rapid infusion of an isotonic fluid (normal saline or Ringer's lactate). The rate of infusion is typically 1% to 2% of body weight (10–20 mL/kg) over 1 hour. If the patient is severely dehydrated, 3% to 5% of body weight (30–50 mL/kg) should be given over 1 to 2 hours and continued until cardiovascular signs are stable.

The second phase of therapy replaces the deficit of fluids and electrolytes that has occurred. This may be accomplished in several different ways, but certain principles must be observed.

- Total body repair requires a relatively prolonged period in all types of dehydration.
- Total body potassium losses cannot be replaced rapidly because potassium is predominantly an intracellular ion. Therefore, potassium should be added to the rehydration solution only after the patient has voided and then in concentrations that generally do not exceed 40 mEq/L or a rate of infusion of 0.5 mEq/kg/hour.
- A solution of "half" normal saline (technically 0.45%, often written as 0.5 NS or $^1/_2$ NS) is generally recommended during the period of rehydration to replace the accrued sodium deficit (even if the measured serum sodium is normal).
- The patient must be monitored carefully during the period of rehydration. Remember that the initial estimate of the degree of dehydration was perhaps based on subjective criteria.

Several approaches exist to this second phase of deficit therapy, but most prefer a system in which the patient is rehydrated in 24 hours. Such a system is not appropriate for infants and children with severe and/or hypertonic dehydration and a longer period of rehydration therapy is recommended. In 24-hour replacement, one-third of the maintenance volume plus one-half of the deficit is given over the first 8 hours of rehydration and two-thirds of the maintenance volume and one-half of the deficit is given in the subsequent 16 hours.

As stated above, hypertonic dehydration necessitates a change in the timing of deficit repair. Because the sodium deficit is less than in other forms of dehydration, it seems reasonable to give a smaller amount of sodium in the repair fluid. However, a very dilute solution given rapidly causes water shifts into the dehydrated hypertonic cell, is detrimental to cell function, and can cause cerebral edema. Therefore, the rate of fluid administration should be the primary concern and either D5 0.2 NS or D5 0.5 NS may be used. The volume of fluid to be given should be calculated as deficit (based on body weight multiplied by percent dehydration) plus maintenance requirements. This volume should be given over 24 to 48 hours (adjust maintenance volume accordingly). Also, in hypertonic dehydration, hypocalcemia, which occurs infrequently, should be watched for. If the patient is symptomatic, calcium gluconate can be given intravenously, slowly with the aid of a cardiac monitor.

Hyperglycemia can also occur in hypertonic dehydration due to reduced insulin secretion and decreased cell sensitivity to insulin. This complication is significant in evaluating the rate of decrease in serum sodium. A decrease in serum sodium of 0.5 mEq/L/hour or approximately 12 mEq/L/day is desirable. In evaluating the decline in serum sodium, care must be taken to account for the effect of hyperglycemia. When serum glucose is elevated, the measured serum sodium is suppressed by 1.6 mEq/L for each 100 mg/dL the serum glucose is more than 100 mg/dL. For example, serum sodium of 170 mEq/L with serum glucose of 600 mg/dL is an effective serum sodium of 178 mEq/L ($600 - 100 = 500$; $500 \times 1.6/100 = 8$).

In all types of dehydration, monitoring the patient and his or her response to therapy is essential. Fluids frequently need to be readjusted.

Phase 3 of deficit therapy is a transition toward maintenance fluid therapy. In addition to the usual maintenance therapy, one must provide for ongoing fluid losses from sources other than evaporative or urinary losses.

Replacement Therapy/Ongoing Losses

Fluids designed to replenish ongoing losses are usually termed *replacement therapy*. As the composition of the electrolytes in various body fluids can vary considerably from patient to patient, the electrolyte content of fluids should be specifically measured and replaced milliequivalent for milliequivalent and milliliter for milliliter. Practically, this is often done by replacing the previous 4-hour volume loss with the appropriate solution over the subsequent 4-hour period. In general, a consideration of replacing ongoing losses should occur when the total volume of the losses approaches 1% to 2% of body weight (10–20 ml/kg).

A full discussion of oral rehydration therapy is given in Chapter 193.

ELECTROLYTE DISORDERS

Sodium Disorders

HYPONATREMIA

The first step in evaluating children with hyponatremia (defined as a serum sodium concentration of less than 130 mEq/L) is to determine whether the low serum sodium level is an artifact. A low serum sodium level can be found if the blood sample has been drawn through an indwelling catheter that has not been cleared adequately, or if the sample is obtained upstream from a rapidly infusing intravenous fluid that is hypotonic. Hyperlipidemia causes an increase in serum solids and, concomitantly, a falsely low serum sodium value can be reported. In hyperglycemia, due to fluid shifts into the intravascular space, the serum sodium value may not reflect the effective sodium concentration. In this case, the true serum sodium level can be estimated by adding 1.6 mEq/L to the measured serum sodium value for each 100 mg/dL that the serum glucose is above normal values (usually assumed to be 100 mg/dL). An example is given previously (see discussion of hypertonic dehydration). Once it is certain that the serum sodium value obtained is not an artifact, careful systematic evaluation of the patient usually leads to a specific diagnosis.

In patients whose weight has decreased, a primary source of salt loss from sources such as urine, sweat, tears, or the gastrointestinal tract should be sought. If the salt loss is the result of any condition other than one affecting the kidney, the urinary sodium concentration should be reduced (usually less than 20 mEq/L). Gastrointestinal losses of sodium are frequently obvious (i.e., vomiting or diarrhea). In young children with cystic fibrosis, the loss of sodium in sweat can be substantial, and this site of sodium loss may not be evident until the diagnosis of cystic fibrosis is established. Because of concomitant losses of chloride, these infants frequently have a hypochloremic metabolic alkalosis.

When urinary sodium concentration is elevated, either an intrinsic or an extrinsic renal defect should be suspected. The differential diagnosis includes autosomal dominant polycystic kidney disease, acute interstitial nephritis, adrenal insufficiency (particularly if hyperkalemia is also present), and chronic diuretic therapy.

Patients with hyponatremia who have stable weight or manifestations of volume excess such as edema often have a primary defect in water excretion. Hyponatremia is difficult to develop by the intake of free water in older children and adults, but this can occur in younger infants due to their intrinsically lower glomerular filtration rate, which decreases the amount of hypotonic fluid presented to the renal tubules.

Other situations in which there is diminished free water excretion are those with augmented proximal reabsorption such as intravascular volume depletion, in which effective renal blood flow is decreased or disorders such as congestive heart failure, cirrhosis, or nephrosis.

Another cause of hyponatremia to be considered is the syndrome of inappropriate ADH secretion (SIADH). ADH increases the permeability of the renal collecting ducts to water; therefore, any condition that causes secretion of this hormone diminishes free water excretion and leads to the development of hyponatremia. In states of hyponatremia, ADH secretion should be reduced because of hypoosmolar extracellular fluid. If extracellular hypotonicity is combined with volume depletion, however, ADH may be released in response to baroreceptors. In patients whose weight is stable or increased, this response could not be invoked and release of ADH might be occurring in a nonphysiologic or inappropriate manner. Patients with SIADH do not manifest edema, although their total body weight may have increased, which appears to be related to the fact that SIADH is associated with overhydration of both the extracellular and intracellular spaces, along with a shift of sodium ion distribution.

Determining the specific cause for hyponatremia is essential for designing effective therapy. For those patients who are intravascularly volume depleted and hyponatremic, the primary therapy should be to replace salt and water losses by the administration of fluids. In patients who have a primary defect in free water excretion, the major aspect of therapy is to restrict fluid intake to provide an adequate amount of time for free water to be excreted.

Some patients with hyponatremia have central nervous system signs such as a clouded sensorium or seizures. In this situation, raising the serum sodium level to at least 125 mEq/L by the infusion of hypertonic sodium chloride may be appropriate. The infusion of approximately 12 mL/kg of a 3% saline solution can be estimated to raise the serum sodium level approximately 10 mEq/L.

HYPERNATREMIA

Hypernatremia, defined as a serum sodium level of more than 150 mEq/L, is an important and potentially serious problem that requires careful evaluation and management. Excessive water losses or the intake of salt can result in hypernatremia. Assessing the potential causes for hypernatremia relative to the patient's state of hydration is helpful. In a patient whose body weight is unchanged or increased slightly, it could be assumed that the hypernatremia is the result of a net increase in total body sodium that has not been accompanied by an appropriate amount of water. Typically, an increase in sodium intake would result in hypertonicity of plasma and stimulation of our thirst mechanism and ADH release. Concomitantly, these two factors would act to restore the plasma sodium to relatively normal values. Therefore, in the face of a normally functioning posterior pituitary and hypothalamus, it is unusual for sodium intake to be the primary cause of hypernatremia. Some patients who receive excessive sodium such as large volumes of sodium bicarbonate (which contains 1 mEq/mL), can develop a state of euvolemic hypernatremia. Such a condition would be maintained only to the extent that the offending agent was not recognized or that the patient was unable to respond and request additional free water. Unless the period of salt poisoning has been extensive, appropriate therapy for these patients involves eliminating the sodium intake and providing adequate free water to restore plasma tonicity. In a few patients, hypernatremia is termed *essential* or is related to central hypodipsia because of resetting of the osmolar receptors. These patients who may have extreme hypernatremia without significant clinical signs are rare. Most often, this disorder is seen in children who have had significant central nervous system insults.

Hypernatremia is often due to hypotonic fluid losses such as those occuring in patients with severe gastroenteritis, excessive sweating, or after the administration of diuretic agents. In each of these clinical settings, hypernatremia occurs only when inadequate free water has been provided.

Excessive free water losses can occur either because of an enhancement of insensible fluid losses or because of the inability of the kidney to retain water. For example, premature infants placed under a radiant warmer are particularly susceptible to the development of hypernatremia. Also, free water can be lost from the kidney either because of a lack of ADH secretion by the posterior pituitary (central diabetes insipidus) or because of the resistance of the collecting duct to respond to ADH (nephrogenic diabetes insipidus). Patients with diabetes insipidus frequently have polyuria despite significant dehydration.

The greatest risk in the treatment of patients with hypernatremia (correction of serum sodium) is the development of cerebral edema. As the extracellular sodium level decreases during therapy, water moves into brain cells and causes intracellular overhydration. This paradoxic rebound effect has been attributed to "idiogenic osmoles," such as trimethylamines, which are produced in response to chronic volume depletion. These intracellular osmolytes are neither generated nor dissipated rapidly. The accumulation of these intracellular osmolytes may be responsible for the paradoxic cerebral edema that is associated with rapid correction of hypernatremia. A slow, cautious rehydration program extended over 48 to 72 hours allows for progressive decrease in these compounds as extracellular tonicity is returned to normal.

Potassium Disorders

In evaluating patients with disorders of potassium, it must be remembered that, since most potassium is intracellular, the serum potassium concentration represents an extremely small portion of total body potassium and that alterations in the serum potassium level may not be a reflection of overall total body potassium balance. Consequently, those factors should be sought that can result in a change in serum potassium without having any effect on total body potassium.

HYPOKALEMIA

Hypokalemia, generally defined as a serum potassium level of less than 3.5 mEq/L, requires a systematic approach, which includes the following:

- An assessment of acid–base status and the possibility that hypokalemia is simply secondary to shifts of potassium from the extracellular to the intracellular space.
- An evaluation of potential lack of potassium intake, although it would have to be prolonged and fairly severe to produce total body potassium deficiency.
- An assessment of potential sources of potassium loss through either the gastrointestinal tract or sweating, in which case, the urinary potassium level should be quite low.
- Excessive losses of potassium through the kidney, in which case, the urinary potassium concentration should be elevated.

There is no practical and effective method for determining total body potassium status. The appearance of U waves on electrocardiography is a relatively crude and late-developing index of potassium balance.

In patients with alkalosis, hypokalemia occurs because of movement of potassium into cells as hydrogen ions move out of cells to buffer the extracellular alkalinity. Hypokalemic alkalosis can be seen in children with vomiting, and the concomitant volume depletion and stimulation of aldosterone secretion affect potassium loss further. Patients with diabetes mellitus may develop hypokalemia, due, in part, to the loss of potassium during the period of osmotic diuresis from their hyperglycemia and, in part, by the effect of insulin (which insulin drives potassium into cells) and correction of metabolic acidosis. Catecholamines can result in increased potassium removal into skeletal muscle producing a state of hypokalemia. Of note, beta-adrenergic agonists, which are used to treat bronchospasm and reactive airway disease, can produce transient hypokalemia because of their stimulation of potassium movement into cells. Hypokalemia has also been associated with periodic paralysis.

Hypokalemia in the face of total body potassium depletion occurs because of either inadequate potassium intake or excessive potassium losses. The kidney can reduce potassium excretion dramatically. Therefore, patients must either reduce their intake of potassium drastically or they must be kept on potassium-free parenteral fluids for a prolonged period to induce total body potassium deficiency.

Excessive loss of potassium through the gastrointestinal tract, sweat, or the kidney can cause hypokalemia. The intestines preferentially secrete potassium bicarbonate into the lumen and reabsorb sodium chloride. Therefore, in the setting of chronic or long-term diarrhea, potassium depletion can become a significant problem. Although sweat contains only approximately 10 mEq/L of potassium, losses through this route can be substantial when they are associated with heavy exercise. This can be exacerbated by volume depletion and activation of aldosterone secretion, as well as by release of catecholamines.

Potassium losses in the kidney increase when the peritubular potassium concentration increases or when the luminal potassium concentration decreases. In most clinical situations, it can be anticipated that the major defect in potassium homeostasis occurs in the distal nephron because this is the final regulatory site for potassium homeostasis. For example, an increase in flow through the distal nephron, which can be associated with volume expansion, increases potassium secretion. Potassium

TABLE 4-4. Assessment of Hyperkalemia

Spurious
Mechanical trauma to red blood cells during venipuncture
Marked leukocytosis (white blood cells $>10^5$ per microliter)
Thrombocytosis (platelets >500,000 per microliter)
Acidosis
Increased intake or tissue breakdown
Oral or parenteral fluid intake
Tissue catabolism
Succinylcholine
Diminished excretion/deposition
Renal insufficiency/diminished distal nephron function
Decreased aldosterone effect
Volume depletion
Drugs

secretion in this segment is also sensitive to sodium and chloride content. If the luminal chloride concentration is decreased or the luminal sodium concentration is increased, potassium entry into the tubular fluid will be enhanced. Diuretic agents, which increase the flow in the distal nephron, stimulate potassium secretion by several mechanisms including increased distal flow rate, increased luminal sodium and chloride concentration, and stimulation of aldosterone secretion.

Either primary or secondary hypermineralocorticoidism can stimulate sodium reabsorption in exchange for potassium and hydrogen. Primary hyperaldosteronism is relatively rare in children. Aldosterone secretion associated with hyperreninemia, secondary to renal artery stenosis, can result in hypokalemia and hypertension.

HYPERKALEMIA

Hyperkalemia, generally defined as a serum potassium concentration of more than 6.5 mEq/L, is a potentially life-threatening abnormality. Causes of hyperkalemia are shown in Table 4-4.

Various causes of hyperkalemia involve situations in which potassium is released from the intracellular site. The release of potassium from red blood cells that are injured during venipuncture can increase the serum potassium concentration significantly, often referred to as a hemolyzed sample. Lysis or breakdown of cells during the clotting process can also increase the serum potassium concentration. This may be the case in patients with marked leukocytosis or very high platelet counts. Cellular shifts of hydrogen and potassium ions in response to acid–base balance can be significant. Patients who are significantly acidemic may appear to have hyperkalemia even when their total body potassium is normal or depleted. This is particularly important in patients with diabetic ketoacidosis. Significant hyperkalemia can be expected to be associated with a decrease in muscle strength and the development of peaked T-waves on electrocardiography.

Hyperkalemia can be attributed to an increase in potassium intake or endogenous potassium from tissue catabolism. When the rate of tissue breakdown is extremely rapid or is combined with a mild degree of renal dysfunction, hyperkalemia may occur. Examples of this include the rapid hemolysis of red blood cells that is associated with autoimmune hemolytic anemia or an incompatible blood transfusion, the administration of cytotoxic agents to patients with malignant lymphomas, and severe tissue damage from trauma or rhabdomyolysis. If renal function, urine output, and the other adaptive mechanisms are intact, it is generally difficult to explain hyperkalemia on the basis of an acute potassium load. For example, mild hyperkalemia is a potent stimulus for aldosterone secretion and results in increased urinary flow rate. Thus, an acute potassium load can be excreted relatively efficiently and should not induce a significant sustained increase in serum potassium. Because of these adaptive mechanisms, the practice of giving "runs of K" intravenously to patients with hypokalemia is often ineffective and should rarely be done. In fact, the vast majority of the bolus of potassium can be found in the urine within 2 hours of administration.

Generally, the development of significant hyperkalemia should suggest a primary defect in potassium excretion. Patients with renal insufficiency are particularly susceptible to hyperkalemia. The plasma level of serum potassium in patients with renal failure is also related to the degree of metabolic acidosis, which is a common feature of chronic renal failure.

Reduction in aldosterone production or end-organ unresponsiveness to aldosterone leads to the development of hyperkalemia as seen in adrenal insufficiency or congenital adrenal hyperplasia. The administration of competitive inhibitors of aldosterone such as spironolactone in an attempt to spare potassium losses in association with diuretic administration may make patients more susceptible to hyperkalemia, particularly if they encounter an acute potassium load.

In situations in which renal perfusion has been diminished markedly such as severe volume depletion from diarrhea, delivery of sodium to the distal site is decreased. The diminished delivery of sodium to this nephron site decreases the rate of potassium secretion and makes the patient susceptible to hyperkalemia. In these states of profound volume depletion and decreases in renal perfusion, an associated metabolic acidosis is seen as well.

Last, drugs known to cause an impairment in the renin–aldosterone axis (such as Angiotensin-converting enzyme inhibitors) have been associated with the development of hyperkalemia. This effect probably occurs because of the diminished production of angiotensin II and the lack of stimulation of aldosterone secretion.

CHAPTER 5
Evaluating and Using Laboratory Tests

Adapted from Cynthia S. Minkovitz and Lawrence S. Wissow

Laboratory tests can be powerful aids in diagnosis and patient management, but many physicians know little about the tests they commonly order. The result is often extra expense and, at times, avoidable morbidity.

In this chapter, the term *test* means a laboratory or clinical procedure such as a urinalysis. The concepts discussed here can apply to most other procedures used to gather clinical information. For example, questions in a medical history can be considered tests for which performance characteristics can be defined and measured.

CHARACTERISTICS OF TESTS

Practical Considerations

Most of the time a variety of tests is possible. The ordering clinician must consider variations in their practicality such as cost, availability, risk to the patient, and speed of obtaining results.

The skill or equipment required to perform the tests may vary, requiring the clinician to choose carefully which laboratory or machine to entrust with the analysis. All laboratories, whether office based or reference labs, should have the highest standards of quality control.

Performance Characteristics of Tests

A test's precision reflects how much difference to expect if the same specimen was tested repeatedly. A test's precision is not always related to its accuracy (i.e., the relationship of test result to true value of the measured parameter). A machine can measure serum potassium with great precision, but values are meaningless if one does not recognize that hemolysis may render them inaccurate.

Two-by-Two Table

The following paragraphs refer to Fig. 5-1, the standard two-by-two cross-tabulation. Suppose test 1 is designed to detect disease X. The columns in Fig. 5-1 represent two groups of individuals: Those on the left (+) are known to have disease X; those on the right (−) are known to be free of the condition. The rows classify individuals based on results of test 1: The top row (+) counts all those whose test results were positive; the bottom row (−) counts all those whose test results were negative. Each cell (A, B, C, D) divides the group of tested individuals into four categories:

Cell	Have disease X?	Test result	Label
A	Yes	Positive	True-positive
B	No	Positive	False-positive
C	Yes	Negative	False-negative
D	No	Negative	True-negative

If the test worked perfectly, there would be 100% agreement between test results and true presence of disease (cells A and D only). This almost never occurs, which is a reminder when interpreting test results: A positive (or negative) test result does not guarantee that a disease is (or is not) present. The test only tells how great a chance exists that the disease is present.

Sensitivity and Specificity

Sensitivity is the likelihood that a test will be positive in the presence of a targeted disease. Sensitivity is A/(A + C) (Fig. 5-1). Test sensitivity is critical in screening for asymptomatic disease and ruling out specific diagnoses. When A is large compared to C [i.e., when A/(A + C) is greater than 0.99], relative confidence exists that if the result of test 1 is negative, an individual does

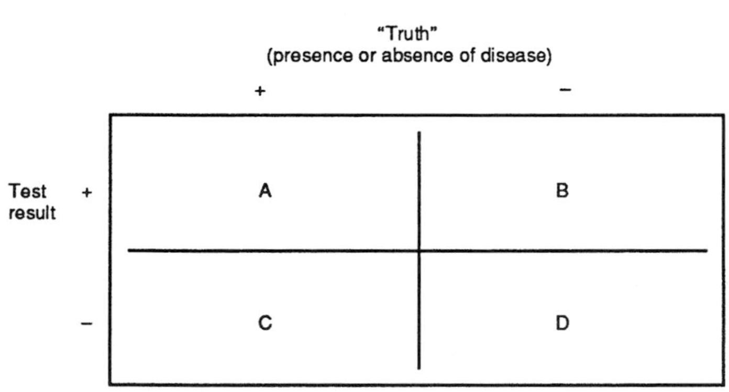

Figure 5-1. The two-by-two cross-tabulation used to describe basic test characteristics.

not have disease X. This does not make any claims for what a positive test result means.

Specificity is the likelihood of a test to be negative in individuals who do not have the disease. Specificity is defined as D/(B + D) (Fig. 5-1). Very specific tests are often used to confirm or rule in a suspected diagnosis. When D is very large compared to B [i.e., D/(B + D) is close to 1], a positive result is unlikely to occur in an individual who truly does not have disease X. Specificity alone does not make any claims for what a negative test result means.

Two important points about sensitivity and specificity are worth noting. First, for most tests, some range of results exists that is shared by individuals who have the disease and those who do not. Thus, if the definition of a positive and negative test result changes, so do the relative sizes of A, B, C, and D and, consequently, the test's sensitivity and specificity. For most tests, a change in definition that benefits sensitivity does so at the expense of specificity and vice versa. Only changing the test, not the definition, is likely to improve both simultaneously. Second, how a test is used is determined by where the *cut points* are placed. For example, screening tests are typically designed to have high sensitivity in order to identify all individuals with a condition (or at risk for a condition). In such cases, tests often use a low cut point so individuals are not missed; this is done at the expense of obtaining positive results in those without disease (false-positives, see below).

Predictive Value

Which patients have disease and which do not is rarely known, hence the need for diagnostic tests. What the clinician really wants to know is how likely a positive test means that disease is present or that a negative result means disease is absent. The way to express this is with two quantities, the test's positive and negative predictive values. Positive predictive value is the proportion of persons who test positive on test 1 and who actually have disease X, or A/(A + B) (Fig. 5-1), or the probability that disease X will be present given a positive test result. The negative predictive value is D/(C + D) (Fig. 5-1), or the probability that disease is not present given a negative test result.

A test's positive and negative predictive values vary with the prevalence of the disease in the population, for example, the use of enzyme-linked immunosorbent assays (ELISA) for human immunodeficiency virus (HIV). This test typically has a sensitivity that approaches 100% and a specificity of more than 99%. With a prevalence of HIV antibodies approaching 50% (Fig. 5-2), the positive and negative predictive values of the test are both nearly 100%. Fig. 5-3 shows how the same test performs in a population of male army recruits in whom the prevalence of HIV positivity is reported to be 0.16%. The positive predictive value of the test is 24%. In other words, for every true-positive result, approximately three are false-positive. Thus, HIV testing of low-prevalence populations requires sequential use of other tests, usually a repeat ELISA followed by a Western blot, to separate the true-positive from the false-positive results.

Likelihood Ratio

The likelihood ratio can help to assess the diagnostic benefit of a positive or negative test result. Unlike the predictive value, however, the likelihood ratio is independent of the prevalence of disease.

The likelihood ratio is a ratio of probabilities: the probability that the test result is positive in a person who really has the disease compared to the probability that the test result is positive in a person who does not have the disease. For example, a person

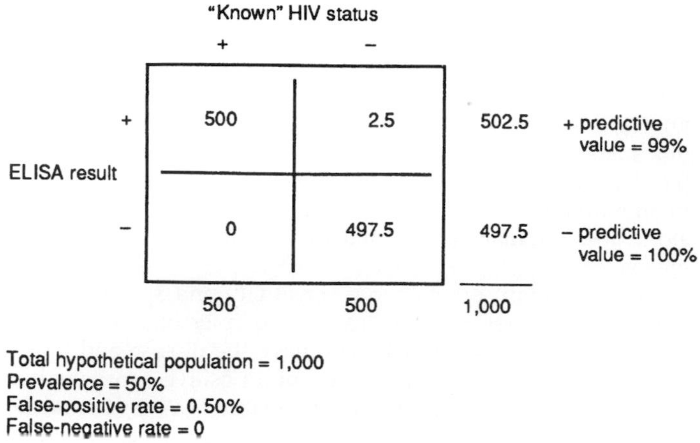

Figure 5-2. Hypothetical data for use of a single enzyme-linked immunosorbent assay (ELISA) test to detect antibodies to human immunodeficiency virus (HIV) in a high-prevalence population.

with disease X is so many times more likely to have a positive result on test 1 than is a person who does not have disease X. The chance that a person with disease X will have a positive test result is the same as A/(A + C) (Fig. 5-1), or the test's sensitivity. The chance that a person without disease X will have a positive test result is B/(B + D) (Fig. 5-1), or 1 minus the test's specificity.

Using a formula known as *Bayes' theorem,* the likelihood ratio can be used to calculate, for any level of disease prevalence or pretest chance that a patient has disease, the revised or posttest chance, given the test results that disease is present or absent.

Table 5-1 shows results of HIV antibody tests as a function of population prevalence of disease. For example, among female donors and male army recruits, it can be argued that the posttest chance of HIV infection is not increased to a point where the clinician knows more about whether the patient is infected or not. Among transfusion recipients, however, a substantial amount of information is gained. A relatively low 5% chance of HIV positivity jumps to a practically certain 91% chance.

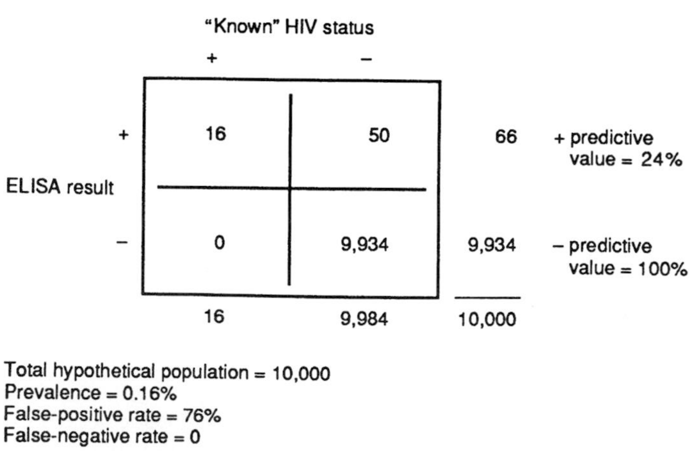

Figure 5-3. Hypothetical data for use of a single enzyme-linked immunosorbent assay (ELISA) test to detect antibodies to human immunodeficiency virus (HIV) in a low-prevalence population.

TABLE 5-1. Posttest Probabilities of Human Immunodeficiency Virus Seropositivity after a Single Enzyme-Linked Immunosorbent Asssay Test*

Population group	Pretest probability	Pretest odds	Posttest odds	Posttest probability
Hemophiliacs	0.50	1:1	200:1	0.99
Transfusion recipients	0.05	0.05:1	10:1	0.91
Male Army recruits	0.0016	0.0016:1	0.32:1	0.24
Female blood donors	0.0001	0.0001:1	0.02:1	0.02

* Based on a sensitivity of 100, a specificity of 99.5, and a likelihood ration of 200. *Pretest probabilities reprinted with permission from Meyer KB, Pauker SG. Screening for HIV: can we afford the false-positive rates?* N Engl J Med *1987;317:238.*

Using likelihood ratios illustrates the following point: When one is relatively certain that a patient does or does not have a disease, performing a diagnostic test adds little extra certainty to the diagnosis and, in fact, may confuse the issue rather than help.

CHOOSING TESTS FOR SCREENING

Screening is defined as testing for disease in an apparently healthy population or individual. The goal of screening is not to necessarily detect disease in individuals but to identify persons who are at risk and who warrant further testing. Commonly used pediatric screening tests include measurement of hematocrit to detect anemia and perinatal tests to detect inborn errors of metabolism.

The following questions will help the clinician decide whether the target disease is a suitable candidate for detection by screening.

- Is the disease serious enough to warrant the effort?
- Is the disease common enough, relative to its seriousness, to warrant mass testing of persons?
- Does the disease have a preclinical phase that allows it to be detected by a screening test?
- Is there any benefit such as improved prognosis, to detecting the disease in its preclinical phase?
- Are follow-up mechanisms such as counseling, available for persons who have positive screening results?

If a disease is suitable for screening, a test must be identified based on the following:

- The test must be easy to perform and interpret with good reproducibility and accuracy.
- The test should measure something definitely related to the condition, not non-specific finding.
- The test must have acceptably low risk, morbidity, and cost.

Most screening tests are designed to be highly sensitive. That is, a negative result indicates a low chance that the tested individual is at risk of having the target disease. A positive result, however, may mean only that the individual is somewhat more likely to have the disease. Further testing is usually required because simple, highly sensitive tests are not often very specific and will generate false-positive results. The best screening tests are both highly sensitive and highly specific.

PART

II

The Newborn

SECTION

A

The Normal Newborn

CHAPTER 6

Management of the Normal Newborn

Adapted from William D. Cochran
and Joseph H. Zelson

BIRTH AND NEWBORN ENVIRONMENT

Efforts are now made to create a natural and comfortable environment for childbirth in hospitals. A combination labor, delivery, and recovery room (occasionally even a postpartum room as well) has been incorporated into the construction of almost all new hospitals, and fathers and others close to the mother can now be present during the birthing process. Attempts to involve siblings in the birth have mostly failed, but no inherent reason exists why they should not participate if the family so desires. The labor bed should be comfortable, chairs should be available, and typical delivery room equipment (for possible maternal anesthesia and newborn resuscitation) should be as unobtrusive as possible. Mothers should be encouraged to hold and even nurse their infants as soon after delivery as possible. This provides assurance of normalcy, and maternal attachment may also be enhanced during the hyperalert state that characterizes the newborn in the early minutes after delivery.

Because newborns are warmer than their mothers by approximately 0.5°C, they are born vasodilated and tend to lose heat rapidly. Also contributing to their heat loss is evaporative heat loss in the often too cold delivery room environment. The newborn should be dried and wrapped and allowed skin-to-skin contact with the mother to decrease heat loss and encourage early bonding. A stocking cap placed immediately over the head while the rest of the infant is being dried helps to blunt this initial heat loss. Marked heat loss and consequent lowering of the infant's core temperature can cause an otherwise well infant to exhibit grunting respiration and cyanosis and to develop a measurable metabolic acidosis.

Apgar scores should be assigned, and a brief, but essential, examination of the baby should be done in the delivery room. This determines whether the infant can go to the regular nursery or needs a more acute care nursery. Major anomalies, labor or drug-induced asphyxia or depression, and expected or unexpected prematurity should be recognized in the delivery room. Babies with malformations need to be seen by the mother and father, with appropriate support and explanation.

INITIAL PHYSICAL EXAMINATION

A thorough examination by a physician or nurse practitioner should be done within 24 hours of birth. Use of warming lights during this examination keeps the infant warm and, hence, less fussy. Many perform the examination in front of the parents so they can ask appropriate questions. A full prenatal and delivery history should be available, as well as information provided by nurses concerning infant behavior and early feeding patterns. Evaluations by nursery nurses are done at least every 8 hours and usually much more frequently after admission or when deviations from normal such as persistent hypothermia, grunting and retracting, questionable cyanosis, hypotonia, or jitters are noted. Febrile infants with rectal temperatures of 100°F or higher need especially careful observation and evaluation.

Before fetal ultrasound in early and even later pregnancy became standard, 3% of all newborns were said to have a major malformation at birth. Unexpected anomalies such as those of the central nervous system, heart, skeleton, or gastrointestinal tract, may still be found. One should be alert for evidence of physical or hypoxic stress caused by the labor or the delivery process. The examiner should also be aware of risk factors such as infection (especially group B streptococcus) or hemolytic disease. The experienced examiner is alert for subtle signs related to newborn tone or level of arousal. An infant who becomes alert and stops moving or fretting in the presence of conversation can probably hear. Sudden bright lights will almost always cause a blink, initially providing assurance of at least some vision.

Experienced examiners evaluate the neurologic system throughout the examination using the infant's response to the general examination as an indicator of neurologic status. Painful components of the examination usually elicit an aversion response, the absence of which might indicate central nervous system pathology. Redressing or briefly holding and cuddling an infant usually quiets a crying infant, although using a pacifier is often the most effective method. The infant's general patterns of response may provide clues to underlying pathology. Sometime during the examination, the infant should be totally naked so his or her skin, posture, movements, proportions, and general behavior can best be evaluated.

Heart and Lungs

The heart and lungs are commonly examined first while, it is hoped, the infant is still quiet and unchilled. This part of the examination can be done with just the shirt pulled up and the diaper on, thus causing the least disturbance to, and chilling of, the baby. The infant should be examined for the presence of central cyanosis. Acrocyanosis of the hands, feet, and, occasionally, even lips (but a pink tongue) is normal, especially if the baby is cold.

All the rest of the skin should be pink. Heart sounds loudest on the right suggest dextrocardia or possibly a left pneumothorax. Rate and rhythm should be noted; a variable rate between 90 and 160 beats per minute is in the normal range. Some brief irregularities of rhythm, usually from premature ventricular contractions, are common, and if an isolated finding they are usually benign and transient. Systolic murmurs are common on the first day and usually reflect the closing ductus arteriosus or are simple flow murmurs. Persistent murmurs or murmurs accompanied by an overactive heart, or in the presence of a fixed rate with no vagal slowing with quieting, or accompanied by tachycardia need careful evaluation. Femoral pulses may be difficult to palpate but should be sought, especially in the presence of systolic murmurs, to rule out coarctation of the aorta. If they are not palpated, four extremity blood pressures should be done.

A pink, apparently well-oxygenated infant who is breathing quietly without retractions and grunting is immediately reassuring to the examiner. However, breath sounds on both sides of the chest should be listened for, if only briefly. Most infants breathe rather irregularly in the first day or two of life, and the depth of each breath varies as well. Their abdomens often rise and fall because they use their diaphragms more than intercostal muscles. Asymmetry, intercostal retractions, and tachypnea (a respiratory rate of more than 60) are worrisome if they are more than transient findings. Decreased heart sounds may suggest a pneumothorax.

Abdomen

Examination of the abdomen is best carried out with the infant naked. Again, observation is important. On the first day, the newborn abdomen is full and rounded, not asymmetric or scaphoid. Diastasis recti, nonunion of the two rectus muscles from the umbilicus to the xiphoid, often causes a mild herniation in the midline. The parents should be advised that this will resolve. Asymmetry, unless it is caused by a big stomach bubble (often just after eating or crying), may be a clue to an abnormal abdominal mass. A scaphoid abdomen, usually with accompanying increased respiratory effort, might indicate a diaphragmatic hernia with some of the abdominal contents up in the chest (most commonly the left). The veins in the skin over the upper abdomen often appear dilated. The cord and its three vessels will have been evaluated at delivery, but can be rechecked quickly. A two-vessel cord is accompanied by another major anomaly at least 10% of the time, so this should alert the examiner. The spleen is not usually palpable.

In the newborn, the liver edge can be evaluated best by approaching it from below with the thumb held flattened on the abdomen and placed between the midline and axillary line, beginning the palpation at the level of the umbilicus and progressing upward. The pad of the thumb, with its greater sensitivity, should pick up the liver edge as the infant inhales. Generally, the liver edge is felt 1 to 2 cm below the right costal margin. In infants with intrauterine growth retardation, the liver may not be palpable. Conversely, in infants of diabetic mothers, the edge may be as much as 4 cm below the costal margin.

Deep (and sometimes briefly painful) palpation is done to examine the kidneys. With careful bimanual palpation, the left kidney can almost always be palpated, the examiner placing the third finger of one hand posteriorly in the lowest left costovertebral angle and then trapping the left kidney against that finger with the index and third fingers of the other hand (Fig. 6-1). The lower pole of the normal right kidney is palpated only occasionally, but if the right kidney is enlarged, it will be noted. Finally, one should feel infraumbilically for the bladder, which most commonly is not felt. If the bladder is felt, it should be rechecked soon. If it is always palpable, it most probably means posterior urethral valves are obstructing urinary outflow (male infants) or, in rare cases, the infant has an atonic bladder. The examination should make note of the absence of masses.

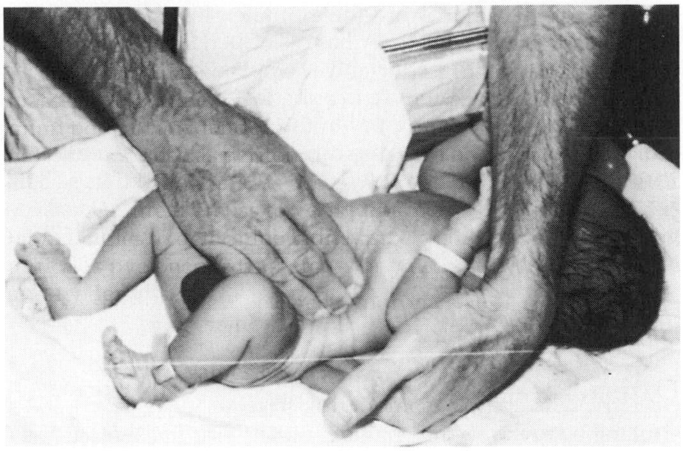

Figure 6-1. Palpation of the left kidney.

Genitalia and Anus

The labia majora in the term female infant are enlarged and, generally, almost completely cover the labia minora except in the clitoral region. The clitoris should be examined for size and palpated for diameter. Both labia should be spread, and the pale pink, glistening vaginal orifice should be examined for patency and discharge (usually creamy and white). An apparent imperforate hymen should be checked with a small soft catheter to see if it will slip by, because an enlarged Bartholin gland often mimics imperforation. The fourchette should be checked for any fistula. The labia majora should be palpated briefly for masses (which, when present, are most commonly an ovary). Vaginal discharge is normal and after the third day is occasionally hemorrhagic. In infants who were frank breech, the labia might be edematous and ecchymotic appearing.

In the male infant, the penis and foreskin should be examined for hypospadias, with consideration given to the size of the penis. A hooded foreskin may be present in a first-degree hypospadias. The scrotum's rugation and size should be noted. Testes should be palpated bilaterally and noted if present but not in the scrotum. Finding nonpalpable testes in any phenotypic male infant should raise a question of virilizing adrenal hyperplasia. Undescended testes are commonly found in male infants of less than 34 weeks' gestation. Commonly, hydroceles are present and should transilluminate. The testes should be located in those instances as well.

The anus should be checked for patency and position. Occasionally, large fistulae are mistaken for a normal anus.

Hips

Dislocated hips, although rare, are the most common hidden and quiescent anomaly and, unfortunately, if not diagnosed until the infant (or even child) starts to walk, can result in permanent disability. The hips are examined by placing the legs in a frog-leg position, with the third fingertip on the greater trochanter and the thumb pressing laterally and down on the inside of the knee until the knee is pressed against the mattress; meanwhile, the third finger is pushing up toward the examiner. In other words, the femoral head most commonly has dislocated following a vector that has a posterior, superior, and a lateral component, so to relocate it, the examiner is trying to bring the femoral head back up that vector. The knee abducted in the frog-leg position tightens the anterior segment of the hip capsule, thus creating a fulcrum that permits the head of the femur to move back into its socket. One sign of a dislocated hip is an asymmetric crease of skin folds under the buttock (Galeazzi sign). This sign is not helpful if bilateral dislocation exists. The possibility of undiagnosed dislocated hips should obviously be rechecked at follow-up physical examinations.

Extremities and Joints

All long bones should be palpated briefly for unexpected fractures. Joints should be assessed for range of motion and evidence of uterine deformation. The most common deformation is tibial bowing and the next most common is forefoot adduction, with a clubfoot being the most extreme. Any foot that can be corrected passively to a neutral position usually corrects spontaneously over time. Counting the fingers and toes avoids the embarrassment of being asked later, "Why does my baby have six toes?" The clavicles should be palpated for fracture, which, if present, heals spontaneously. Thought should be given to the length of the limbs; the fingers should extend as far as the lower buttocks when straightened. Infants presenting by breech often hold their legs in bizarre positions, but in a matter of days, the leg positions return to normal.

Head, Eyes, and Ears

Normal head circumference at term is between 33 and 38 cm. The head should be observed and palpated for the degree of molding and caput succedaneum (edema of the leading portion of the scalp in a vertex delivery). Occasionally, the degree of molding is marked but still benign (Fig. 6-2). A caput occasionally obscures a developing cephalohematoma (the latter caused by bleeding under the periosteum of a parietal bone). Cephalohematomas usually do not mature until day 2 or 3 of life and, being subperiosteal, never extend beyond the suture line as do caputs. The use of vacuum extraction sometimes makes it difficult to distinguish a caput from a cephalohematoma, but by day 3 of life, caputs usually disappear. Subgaleal hemorrhages are more common because of the increased use of vacuum extractions. They are fluctuant but cross suture lines. The parietal and coronal sutures should be examined for patency and mobility. If the head circumference is within normal limits, the diameter of the anterior fontanelle can vary from 1 to 5 or 6 cm. Very large anterior fontanelles may be associated with hypothyroidism. Craniotabes, a ping-pong ball feel over the parietal bones with pressure, is a rare but normal variant.

The eyes may be difficult to visualize because the caput edema has migrated to the lids. In subdued light, while sucking on a pacifier or being held vertically, most infants will open their eyes. The eye examination is done more easily on the day of discharge when the integrity of the iris, presence of a red reflex, and absence of cataracts can be evaluated. Disconjugate eye gaze is common in the neonatal period. Hemorrhages in the conjunctivae are common, especially after strong labor. The ears should be examined for shape, the presence of an outer canal, and for preauricular pits or tags.

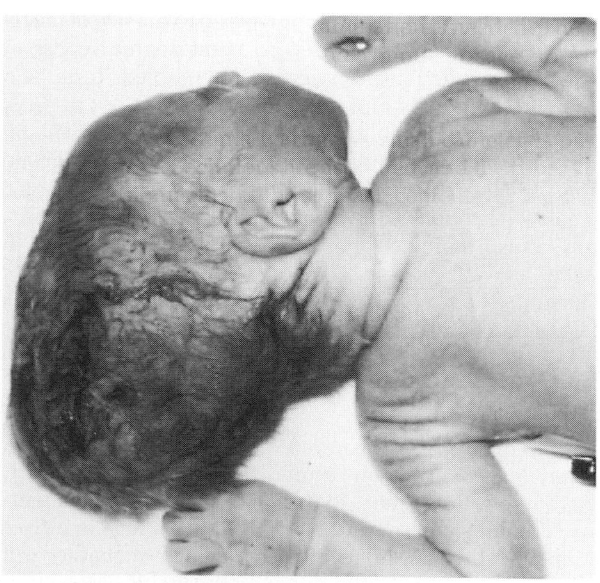

Figure 6-2. Molding of the head.

Neck and Mouth

Newborn infants may look like little football players because they have such short necks, so care must be exercised, tipping the chin up to rule out thyroid abnormalities, or sinus tracts of the thyroid or of the second or third branchial arch. The tongue and gums should be checked carefully. The mouth should be examined with a tongue blade and light, especially for palatal defects, which include bony clefts with an intact soft palate, a partial cleft, or a complete cleft of both the hard and soft palates. Visualization and palpation are usually necessary. Ebstein pearls are small, white cysts often seen close to the midline at the junction of the hard and soft palates. They soon disappear with sucking. Abnormalities of the gums are less common, and sublingual cysts are unusual. If cysts are present, temporizing is worthwhile to see if vigorous sucking causes them to break spontaneously. Asynclitism, in which the maxillary gum line is not parallel to the mandibular gum line, is common, and extreme cases are associated with temporary feeding problems. Asynclitism is often associated with arrest of descent during labor. Rarely, natal teeth are found. A short frenulum is not uncommon, and parents need to be reassured that such babies generally suck, feed, and speak normally.

Skin

Normal findings and variations on the first day include tiny milia (unbroken sweat glands), most commonly found on the nose, and petechiae, usually noted above the nipple line or on the head secondary to the pressure of labor or on the back from the traction of delivery. Occasionally, 0.5- to 1.0-cm vesicles or pustules, often broken, with no erythematous base are seen, usually clustered around the genitalia. Petechiae scattered more generally should prompt a more complete evaluation. Jaundice on the first day should always be considered abnormal. Mongoloid or blue spots up to 10 to 15 cm are often noted on the trunk or thighs of nonwhite infants. A nevus flammeus of the upper eyelids, at the nape of the neck, or, occasionally, extending down to the nose and upper lip is frequently seen but fades within a few weeks.

As part of gestational age dating, there are helpful variations to be recognized in the general appearance of a newborn's skin. The skin during late prematurity is still quite thin and, thus the infant's color is pinker (almost red) compared with that of a postterm infant whose epidermis is thicker and, at least in repose, appears pale with a faint pink tinge. Although some

TABLE 6-1. Common Reflexes of Newborns and Infants

Reflex	Newborn	2 months	4 months	6 months	8 months
Moro	Present/complete	Fading/partial			Absent
Stepping	Present	Fading		Absent	
Placing	Present	Fading		Absent	
Tonic neck	Present	Fading			
Rooting	Excellent	Fading		Absent	
Sucking	Present	Fading (replaced by purposeful activity)			
Head control	Poor but present	Improving		Good	
Palmar grasp	Excellent	Fading		Absent	
Plantar grasp	Excellent	Fading		Absent	
Triceps	Present				
Patellar	Present				

racial variation exists, lanugo (fine hair found especially on shoulders) is more common as prematurity increases. Vernix caseosa, the greasy, white, often quite copious material produced *in utero* by the exocrine glands, is most common after 35 weeks of gestation and is usually completely shed into the amniotic fluid after 40 to 41 weeks. Postterm infants either have none left on their skin or have it only in creases in the skin.

Neurologic Examination

The neurologic examination can be time consuming, so the examiner should decide what is necessary and in what depth it should be carried out depending on the individual circumstance. Neurologic assessment of the newborn usually includes at least a brief evaluation of most of the cranial nerves, peripheral motor activity and symmetry, general body tone, quality of the cry, level of alertness, and Moro response. Table 6-1 lists the more common reflexes tested. The neurologic examination is often done concurrently with the rest of the physical examination, noting how the infant responds throughout. Movement and symmetry of the facial muscles and movement symmetry and tone of the arms, legs, and trunk should be noted while handling the infant, with special attention to lack of movement of one arm or hand as a possible indicator of an Erb palsy. In rare cases, no hand movement indicates a Klumpke palsy. When the mouth and palate are checked, the infant's gag reflex should be noted. Body tone is most easily evaluated with the infant held up off the mattress face down, balanced over a hand on the chest. Held thus, the normal term infant generally holds the arms and legs flexed, and the head, although hanging down somewhat, has some degree of extension. With the infant in this position, the spine can be examined for anomalies such as pilonidal sinus tracts and neural tube defects. Variations of the infant's cry can be assessed for strength and quality.

Most so-called newborn reflexes such as the Moro reflex, decrease with repetition. The sucking and rooting reflexes can be assessed with a pacifier or a well-scrubbed or gloved finger. Lightly touching the upper lip laterally elicits the rooting response, with the mouth opening and the head turning toward the touch. The Moro response to being startled is characterized by extension of the arms with fingers extended, flexion of the thighs, grasping of the toes, and a strong cry, followed by folding of the arms and relaxation of the hands (Fig. 6-3). The Moro reflex can be elicited by dropping the end of the crib 10 to 20 degrees or by pulling the infant by the arms slightly off the bed, followed by a sudden release. The Moro reflex should be symmetric. The stepping and placing responses may be difficult to elicit until 2 or 3 days of age. The stepping reflex is elicited by placing and pushing the

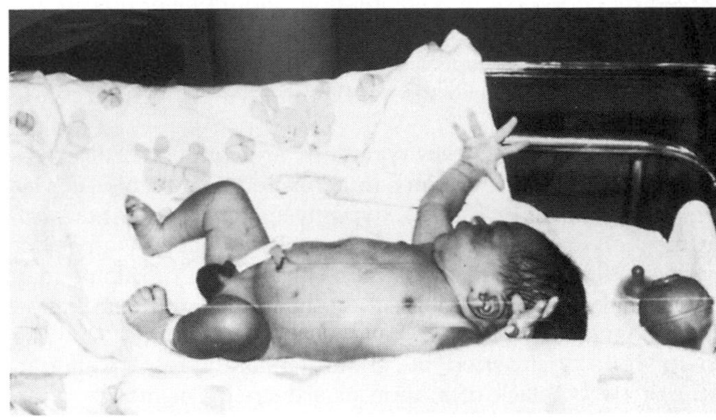

Figure 6-3. The Moro reflex.

infant's feet against the mattress and then leaning the infant far forward to flex the feet up toward the tibiae. With gentle rocking from side to side, the infant may take a few clumsy steps forward. (This is possibly a fetal reflex that may assist the fetus to the vertex position before delivery and may still be functioning in the early newborn period.) The placing response is brought out by holding the top of the infant's feet against the edge of the crib or a similar object. The infant will then lift that leg and place the foot on the object. A strong grasp reflex is generally present in both upper and lower extremities.

Normal reflexes are indicators more of peripheral than central neurologic integrity at birth and so cannot exclude occasional severe central nervous system pathology.

Measurements and Gestational Dating

All infants should be weighed carefully on standardized scales. Length and head circumference should be measured accurately. Body length is best measured on a measuring trough or board and should be reproducible to within 1 cm. Measurement done with a tape while the infant lies in the crib is less precise. Accurate measurements are important for gestational age assessment using standard grids.

Normal Variations

The examiner must decide whether particular variations of physical findings are within the normal range. For instance, most infants void within 24 hours and pass their first meconium stool by 48 hours, yet the great majority of term infants have both urinated and passed meconium by 12 hours or earlier. Concern about cardiac findings, especially murmurs, is common. A first-day grade 1 or 2 murmur associated with a heart rate of less than 160 at rest and no hyperdynamic activity, respiratory symptoms, or cyanosis may not require further workup. Murmurs lasting more than a day, however, especially when accompanied by other clinical symptoms, need further evaluation such as four-way blood pressure oximetry, a hyperoxia challenge, and possibly chest roentgenography, electrocardiography, and echocardiography. Acrocyanosis must be differentiated from general cyanosis. If the infant's tongue is pink, then general cyanosis is not present.

Respiratory variations include transient tachypnea (a rate greater than 60) or periodic breathing. If the tachypnea changes minute by minute and there are intervals when the rate is less than 60, that is a good prognostic sign. Periodic breathing, accompanied by periods of hypoventilation, should be of no concern as long as no color change accompanies the finding. Persistent expiratory grunting, especially if the infant is not cold, requires additional evaluation. Cyanosis accompanying only hard crying is not uncommon.

Central nervous system variations are common. For excessive irritability, the examiner must exclude problems such as previous hypoxia or trauma, hypoglycemia, drug withdrawal, or infection. If an irritable infant is easily soothed by a pacifier or by holding, the process is more likely benign. Infants may appear to be somnolent or stuporous after a long, hard labor. This behavior may wax and wane, with the infant "shutting down" for a brief period, but should generally resolve after an hour or two. A lack of motion or a decrease in motion of an arm or leg suggests nerve injury. Seizures are often difficult to diagnose and may be confused with the posturing and brief apnea some infants exhibit secondary to mucus or formula in the airway, but seizure activity usually involves the eyelids or hands and is usually clonic in nature. Also, when picked up, the infant with a seizure usually continues such behavior. An infant's cry can be high and piercing, as might be seen with central nervous system involvement, or hoarse, as might be seen with vocal cord paralysis or hypothyroidism, and yet it could be perfectly normal. Although the full-term newborn might be cold shortly after birth, the infant should be able to stabilize and maintain a normal temperature greater than 36°C after several hours of age, and an infant who cannot maintain temperature may need to be further evaluated.

BREAST-FEEDING AND FORMULAS

Breast-feeding of newborns has had a resurgence in the United States, and in many hospitals at least 75% of mothers breast-feed, at least initially. Initial feeding schedules ideally should be adjusted to the infant's demand. This is more easily accomplished when infants room-in with the mother, so this should be encouraged whenever feasible. Breast-feeding should begin within the first hour after birth—even in the delivery or birthing room. During the first hour, the baby is often alert, awake, and anxious to suck. Infants less than 2 to 3 days old should be fed at least every 2 to 3 hours during the day and evening and more frequently if awake and hungry.

Newborns often awake frequently for a number of sequential feedings before spacing out their next feeding to 2 to 3 hours. Within several days, they can often be so satiated by frequent day and evening feedings that they begin to space their feedings as long as 5 to 6 hours apart at night. As the mother's milk supply builds up naturally by day 3 or 4, more milk is taken per feeding, which lengthens the time between feedings. Infants should nurse for up to 15 minutes over the first 3 to 4 days, and mothers should try to offer both breasts at each feeding. By 1 week of age, many breast-fed infants are on a fairly definite schedule of approximately eight feedings per day.

Breast-feeding women need support and instruction by trained personnel (Table 6-2). Women who have had cesarean deliveries may take an extra day or two to establish their milk supply.

TABLE 6-2. Breast-Feeding for the First-Time Mother

What a breast-feeding mother needs to know before the delivery of her first baby:

1. Every full-term healthy newborn has a built-in 2 to 3-day food supply. Colostrum, the first milk, is lemony yellow and contains the mother's immunity, thus protecting the baby from many infections during the first 6 weeks of life. Colostrum could be considered the baby's first immunization that only a mother can provide.

   The larger volume of breast milk will usually "come in" on postpartum day 3 or 4. Its production depends on the frequent suckling of the baby and the mother's hormonal responses.

   Every baby is different! Some come out as "barracudas" and eat like a veteran from the first feed. Others we call "connoisseurs" take two to three sucks and stop a while and continually repeat this process. Anything in between is possible.
2. Every time you feed your baby you will be very thirsty. Drink 8 oz of clear liquid every time you feed your baby. As a bonus, you will not be constipated. Water is sufficient!
3. Your baby should not suck on only your nipple! The baby should suck in and nurse on the dark portion behind the nipple (the are- ola) as well. The nurse in the hospital can show you how to do this and the correct positions used in feeding the baby.
4. Your baby empties the breast in 6 to 8 minutes. The highest fat content is in the last portion of the feeding. We suggest that you feed the baby 10 minutes on one side, burp the baby, and then go 10 to 15 minutes on the second side. Burp after each breast, and alternate sides. A comfortable chair with arms and a pillow on which the baby can lie is most comfortable.
5. Until your milk comes in at day 3 or 4, feed every 3 hours or even more frequently if the child is fussy. Once the milk is in, you can feed every 2 to 4 hours. You require about 2 hours to replenish an adequate milk supply in each breast. After 3 hours, gently try to wake the baby during the day and feed. This may prevent the baby from turning day into night. Between midnight and six o'clock, let the baby "be the alarm clock."
6. When your milk comes in, you may for a period of time have more milk than the child needs. This is a good time to pump your breasts and store some breast milk in the freezer. Discuss this with your doctor or nurse. During a period at 2 to 4 weeks of age, the baby will feed more frequently for a few days. This may also occur at 6 to 8 weeks and 6 months.
7. One of the most frequent questions asked is, "How do I know I've given enough breast milk?" The baby should have six to eight wet diapers a day by day 5 or 6 and more than eight by 8 to 10 days. If a disposable diaper is used, put a fresh diaper in one hand and the used diaper in the other and compare the weights. With postpartum home visits, a probability weight checking will be available to you.
8. Until your nipples "toughen up" (at 10 days to 2 weeks), it is wise to try at least three different nursing positions (e.g., the common cradle position, lying flat beside the baby, and holding the baby in the "football" position) to prevent cracked nipples.

COMMON NEWBORN PROBLEMS

Many women have delayed having children until their late 20s or longer and so have prolonged their anticipation, as well as possibly heightened their expectations for a perfect child. Conversely, midteenage pregnancies now make up 5% to 10% of all births, and these young mothers need to finish school, as well as make the transition to adulthood and motherhood. Developing appropriate groupings of new mothers is an excellent educational technique. These groups can meet in the doctor's office at appropriate off-hour times or even in the home of one of the participants. Having the physician or nurse participating some or all of the time is helpful.

Temperament and Sleep

Excessive crying is one of the most common and exceedingly frustrating problems in the first 3 months of life and can become the bane of the parents and often of their doctor. Hunger or illness must be eliminated as the cause of excessive crying, so appropriate signs and symptoms of illness or partial starvation must be elicited by history and examination. Some babies need additional nonnutritive sucking, and it is probably preferable that they use a pacifier or their thumb rather than be very fussy or overfed. The choice between thumb and pacifier is for parents to decide; each has its benefits and disadvantages. Pacifiers, formerly not recommended for fear they would never be discarded and also might misalign permanent teeth, are now widely accepted and may offer relief. Thumb sucking generates the same value judgments; the thumb is always available but has the disadvantage of not being discardable. Generally, if the parents have no strong objection to either and feel that they will not be upset if the habit persists up to age 3 or 5 years, it is probably a worthwhile approach. For persistent crying, mothers can also be told that picking up their babies and holding and rocking them usually quiets them. However, most infants enjoy this bodily contact and motion, and it soon becomes a fixed habit. Holding a baby is important. No one can tell a set of parents how much holding is too much or not enough. A good guideline is to hold the baby as much as the parents want to, but not out of desperation or when the parents do not want to. The primary caregiver (usually the mother) should decide how much to let the baby cry, and those helping her should abide by her rules, thus helping to maintain consistency of care. Although crying is frustrating and worrisome, no evidence exists that it is physically or even psychologically harmful (at least to the baby). Some professionals recommend that the baby learn to soothe and quiet himself or herself at times. Crying can have many causes and does not necessarily mean a baby is hungry or in pain.

Demand and scheduled feedings both have proponents. Certainly, for the mother planning on breast-feeding her infant, a demand schedule for at least the first 3 to 5 days is accepted almost universally and is much more successful. In feeding on demand, the infant is put to the breast at the most appropriate time—when he or she is hungry and willing to suck the hardest—but not exhausted from crying. After the first few days, many recommend a schedule of sorts, but this is almost always more easily carried out when bottle-feeding.

Few people would dispute that a baby's parents are happier when the infant sleeps longer at night (and the longer the better, up to a point). Instructing a parent to wake the infant during days and evenings as frequently as the infant woke the parent the previous night soon moves the infant's longest sleep to the night hours. Unfortunately, although it is possible to make the longest sleep occur during the night, that sleep will not necessarily last for 6 to 8 hours. One alternative is a semidemand schedule (i.e., feeding the baby when he or she is hungry, but with certain limits—2 hours at the earliest and 3.5 hours at the latest for the first 2 weeks of life; thereafter allowing the infant to go up to 4.5 hours in the day between feedings until the baby sleeps through the night). Most infants can sleep through the night by 3 to 8 weeks of age.

Jaundice

Jaundice (Chapter 36, Neonatal Hyperbilirubinemia), with its potential marked hyperbilirubinemia, is more of a concern at present because mothers are being discharged from the hospital so soon after birth that the peak bilirubin level often occurs subsequent to discharge. Mothers should be alerted to this possibility, especially if they are breast-feeding, and inadequate intake with its consequent dehydration can accentuate jaundice.

Circumcision

Circumcision of newborn male infants continues, although there has been a slight decrease in the use of the procedure. In most instances, it is done for religious or cultural reasons. Although one or two reports have argued that less "urinary infection" is found in circumcised male infants, variation in the method of documentation (clean catch versus bladder taps) makes the evidence less conclusive. After circumcision, slathering the exposed raw glans with petroleum jelly at each diaper change for the next 3 days is all that is necessary. Superficial bleeding and minimal surface infection are normal. Babies do feel pain, and the need for and use of local anesthesia for circumcision is controversial and has both its proponents and opponents.

Umbilicus

Umbilical cord care ranges from careful application of an antibiotic ointment 2 or 3 times per day, through alcohol wipes once a day, to no care at all other than observation until the cord falls off. All evidence seems to indicate that the more aseptic the care, the longer the cord hangs on, so some superficial colonization may speed the process. Certainly, quick bathing of that abdominal area, even daily, seems a benign process. The concern for doctor and parents is the development of an omphalitis, which appears as reddened, thickened periumbilical skin, sometimes (ominously) accompanied by a palpable thickened falciform ligament.

Elimination

Frequency of stooling can vary from every feeding initially to every several days. Stools start as meconium, a dark tarry material shortly after birth, and soon make the transition to liquid or seedy yellow puddles. As long as a baby can pass stools without crying or blood, the process is probably normal. There will be an urge to pass stool or gas with each feeding because of the gastrocolic reflex, and passing large amounts of gas is normal. Many babies stop in the middle of a feeding and work and grunt to pass gas or a stool.

Siblings

Sibling rivalry, particularly on the part of the next youngest sibling, is probably a universal phenomenon, whether overt or covert. Its clinical presentation can vary from overt hostility to compensated expressions of love and affection, or even to internalized changes such as a return of bedwetting, thumb sucking, or increased dependency. Frequently, it manifests as attention-getting behavior directed at parents and not at the new infant. Parents should be informed of its myriad manifestations and counseled to be as consistent as possible in their planned response. Letting the older sibling participate, as much as is reasonable, in the care of the new infant seems to lessen his or her feelings of abandonment and neglect. Generally, the more scolding a parent does, the worse the behavior gets. Giving the child positive, not negative, attention is preferable and ignoring as much of the negative behavior as possible is generally a more rewarding strategy. Many books are available to help siblings accept the new baby and their own jealousy.

Environment and Work

Exposing a newborn to other adults and especially to siblings with possible contagious diseases is a common concern. Although most newborns seem less prone to viral illnesses (probably because of passive immunity from their mother) than do older infants or young children, it is wise to minimize such exposure. If a mother is sure that she has had chickenpox, her infant is probably as protected as she is. Whether a newborn with that background should be allowed to stay at home with an infected sibling is controversial but not prohibited by all. With no such maternal history, exposure should not be allowed until the older sibling has had the illness for at least 1 week. Probably avoiding contact with crowds and other unrelated toddlers for several weeks is judicious as a way to reduce risk of illness.

The conflict and guilt that many mothers feel when they work outside the home have always been present, but now they are becoming problems for most mothers because more and more women work. Many women have no apparent guilt at all, and they seem to handle the double role best. When it is a matter of absolute economic necessity, mothers seem less ambivalent about their absence from home. Whatever the circumstances, the possible ambivalence should be addressed openly, at least as a question.

SECTION

B

The Premature Newborn

CHAPTER 7

The Premature Newborn

Adapted from Steven M. Peterec
and Joseph B. Warshaw

DEFINITIONS AND TERMINOLOGY

Term infants are born between 38 and 42 weeks after the onset of the mother's last menstrual period. A *preterm* newborn is defined as an infant born before the start of the 38th week of gestation.

Low birth weight (LBW) describes infants with a birth weight of less than 2,500 g; very low birth weight (VLBW) describes infants with a birth weight of less than 1,500 g; and extremely low birth weight (ELBW) describes infants with a birth weight of less than 1,000 g.

The degree of maturation does not always parallel gestational age; birth weight may be small for gestational age or large for gestational age. Most, but not all, preterm infants are LBW, and most, but not all, LBW infants are preterm.

INCIDENCE AND CAUSES OF PRETERM DELIVERY

Preterm delivery affects approximately 400,000 births each year. The percentages of LBW and VLBW infants were 7.4% and 1.4% of births, respectively, in 1996.

TABLE 7-1. Factors Predisposing to Preterm Labor and Delivery

Spontaneous rupture of membranes
Chorioamnionic membrane infection
Fetal malformations
Fetal demise
Uterine overdistention
Polyhydramnios
Multiple gestation
Uterine anomalies and myomata
Retained intrauterine device
Faulty placentation
Placenta previa
Placental abruption
Cervical incompetence
Serious maternal disease
Maternal smoking and cocaine use
Elective induction
Unknown causes

Adapted from Cunningham FG, MacDonald PC, Gant NF, Leveno KJ, Gilstrap LC. *Williams' obstetrics,* 19th ed. Norwalk, CT: Appleton & Lange, 1993.

Risk factors for preterm delivery include poor prenatal care, low socioeconomic status, nonwhite race, maternal age less than 18 years or more than 40 years, low prepregnancy weight, and a history of previous preterm delivery or late abortion. Factors possibly responsible for preterm labor and delivery appear in Table 7-1.

SURVIVAL

The survival of preterm infants has improved steadily since the 1970s with greatest advances for infants with birth weights between 500 and 750 g. Survival of preterm infants is related to birth weight and gestational age. Most neonatal intensive care units (NICUs) consider 23 weeks' gestation to be the lower limit of viability. The decision whether to initiate resuscitative efforts for infants born near this gestational age, or for infants with birth weights of less than 500 to 600 g, is difficult.

PROBLEMS OF PREMATURITY

The multitude of problems experienced by preterm infants are primarily caused by functional immaturity of various organ systems. The degree of functional immaturity (and thus the frequency and severity of neonatal morbidities) is inversely related to gestational age and birth weight. Table 7-2 demonstrates this relationship for selected neonatal morbidities. Many of the problems of preterm newborns are partly or largely iatrogenic. Perhaps the most obvious example of this is ventilator-induced lung trauma and the development of chronic lung disease. Other examples are presented in Table 7-3. Many of the problems of prematurity resolve with growth and maturation with exceptions being possible long-term growth restriction and neurodevelopmental and pulmonary sequelae.

Gestational Age Assessment

An accurate determination of gestational age is an important component of care of the preterm neonate for, among other reasons, decisions regarding interventions at the limits of viability and anticipation as to the pharmacokinetics of certain drugs.

After delivery, examination of the newborn is used to confirm obstetric dates or to establish gestational age. A modified version of the Ballard score is shown in Fig. 7-1. Scores are given for physical and neuromuscular maturity, then added to estimate a gestational age to within 2 weeks.

TABLE 7-2. Neonatal Morbidity According to Birth Weight of 4,279 Infants Born at Centers Participating in the National Institute of Child Health and Human Development Neonatal Research Network*

	Birth weight (g)			
	501–750	751–1,000	1,001–1,250	1,251–1,500
Respiratory distress syndrome	89	83	58	39
Chronic lung disease	23	26	16	8
Indomethacin for patent ductus arteriosus	45	48	30	17
Late septicemia	31	31	22	9
Grade III or IV intraventricular hemorrhage	25	16	8	3
Periventricular leukomalacia	10	10	8	5
Necrotizing enterocolitis stage II or higher	6	6	5	4

*Data expressed as percentages.
Adapted from Fanaroff AA, Wright LL, Stevenson DK, et al. Very-low-birth-weight outcomes of the National Institute of Child Health and Human Development Neonatal Research Network, May 1991 through December 1992. *Am J Obstet Gynecol* 1995;173:1423.

Specific Problems of Prematurity by Organ System

RESPIRATORY FUNCTION

Impaired respiratory function is usually the most urgent concern shortly after the delivery of a preterm newborn. The incidence and severity of lung immaturity are inversely related to gestational age. Preterm infants may also have decreased central respiratory drive leading to central apnea. The preterm neonate's airway is also less stable. Finally, with decreasing gestational age, ventilatory muscle mass decreases and chest wall compliance increases. VLBW infants may not be able to perform the work necessary for effective ventilation.

CARDIOVASCULAR FUNCTION

Cardiac insufficiency is usually caused by the persistence of a patent ductus arteriousus (PDA), or myocardial dysfunction due sepsis, asphyxia, or congenital heart disease.

In utero, the ductus arteriosus is patent and allows the majority of the right ventricular output to bypass the pulmonary circulation by shunting blood from the pulmonary artery to the descending aorta. After birth, the plasma oxygen tension increases sharply, effecting a reactive vasoconstriction of the ductus arteriosus, which is functionally closed within 10 to 15 hours of birth in most term neonates. Closure of the ductus arteriosus is delayed in preterm neonates. As pulmonary vascular resistance decreases, a PDA may cause shunting of blood from the aorta to the pulmonary artery (left to right) with subsequent myocardial stress, pulmonary congestion, and systemic underperfusion. A PDA may worsen the course of respiratory distress syndrome, increase the incidence of bronchopulmonary dysplasia, cause congestive heart failure, and through "steal" of systemic blood flow, increase the risk of necrotizing enterocolitis, cerebral ischemia, and intraventricular hemorrhage. Neonates with a PDA typically have a systolic or continuous murmur, hyperactive precordium, increased pulse pressure, and bounding pulses.

Pharmacologic closure of PDA with indomethacin, an inhibitor of prostaglandin synthesis, may be attempted. Surgical closure is the final and definitive treatment option but has the associated risks of surgery.

TABLE 7-3. Examples of Secondary Disorders of Preterm Infants That Result from the Treatment of Primary Disorders

Primary disorder	Intervention	Secondary disorder
Respiratory distress syndrome	Mechanical ventilation	Chronic lung disease Air leak syndromes
Chronic lung disease	Corticosteroid therapy	Growth impairment Hyperglycemia Hypertension
	Diuretic therapy	Electrolyte imbalance Nephrocalcinosis Osteopenia
Patent ductus arteriosus	Indomethacin	Renal dysfunction
Gastrointestinal immaturity	Parenteral hyper-alimentation	Cholestasis
	Central venous catheter	Bacteremia, sepsis
Multiple organ dysfunction	Laboratory tests	Anemia

FLUIDS, ELECTROLYTES, AND NUTRITION

Premature infants have low body fat, high total body water, and a large surface area-to-body mass ratio. After birth, neonates lose body weight due to a loss of body water. This weight loss is associated with a diuretic phase and is part of the normal adaptation to extrauterine life. Neonates with lower birth weights lose a greater proportion of their body weight. Some of this weight loss is related to transepidermal water loss and depends on body size, gestational age, and skin thickness, as well as a number of environmental factors. Smaller, less mature infants have substantially higher transepidermal water loss because of their thin, poorly developed skin, low subcutaneous body fat deposits, and high surface area-to-body mass ratios. With increasing postnatal age, the stratum corneum of the skin keratinizes and becomes less permeable. Transepidermal fluid losses can be limited by increasing ambient humidity or through the use of heat shields, membranes, dressings, or topical agents.

The provision of maintenance fluids to the preterm neonate must be individually tailored. After selecting a particular fluid infusion rate, adjustments must be made based on serial weights, electrolytes, and urine output. Weight loss greater or less than that expected from normal contraction diureses mandates compensatory decreases or increases in fluid infusion.

Maintenance electrolyte requirements are generally 2 to 3 mEq/kg/day of sodium and 1 to 3 mEq/kg/day of potassium

Neuromuscular maturity

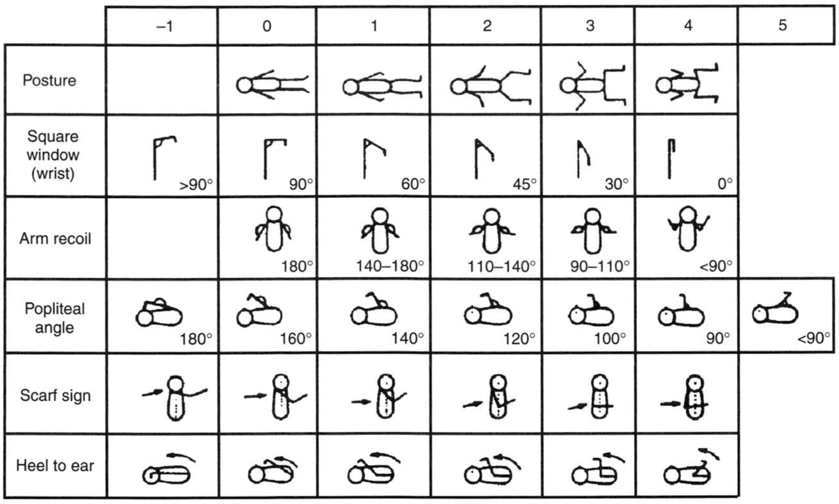

-1
0
1
2
3
4
5
Posture
Square window (wrist)
>90°
90°
60°
45°
30°
0°
Arm recoil
180°
140–180°
110–140°
90–110°
<90°
Popliteal angle
180°
160°
140°
120°
100°
90°
<90°
Scarf sign
Heel to ear

Physical maturity

	-1	0	1	2	3	4	5
Skin	Sticky, friable, transparent	Gelatinous, red, translucent	Smooth, pink; visible veins	Superficial peeling and/or rash, few veins	Cracking pale areas, rare veins	Parchment, deep cracking, no vessels	Leathery, cracked, wrinkled
Lanugo	None	Sparse	Abundant	Thinning	Bald areas	Mostly bald	
Plantar surface	Heel–toe 40–50 mm: –1 <40 mm: –2	>50 mm No crease	Faint red marks	Anterior transverse crease only	Creases anterior 2/3	Creases over entire sole	
Breast	Imperceptible	Barely perceptible	Flat areola, no bud	Stippled areola 1–2 mm bud	Raised areola 3–4 mm bud	Full areola 5–10 mm bud	
Eye/ear	Lids fused loosely: –1 tightly: –2	Lids open; pinna flat, stays folded	Slightly curved pinna; soft; slow recoil	Well-curved pinna; soft but ready recoil	Formed and firm, instant recoil	Thick cartilage, ear stiff	
Genitals: male	Scrotum flat, smooth	Scrotum empty, faint rugae	Testes in upper canal, rare rugae	Testes descending, few rugae	Testes down, good rugae	Testes pendulous, deep rugae	
Genitals: female	Clitoris prominent, labia flat	Prominent clitoris, small labia minora	Prominent clitoris, enlarging minora	Majora and minora equally prominent	Majora large, minora small	Majora cover clitoris and minora	

Maturity rating

Score	Weeks
–10	20
–5	22
0	24
5	26
10	28
15	30
20	32
25	34
30	36
35	38
40	40
45	42
50	44

Figure 7-1. Expanded New Ballard Score for determining gestational age by assessments of physical and neuromuscular maturity. (Reprinted with permission from Ballard JL, Khoury JC, Wedig K, Wang L, Eilers-Walsman BL, Lipp R. New Ballard Score, expanded to include extremely premature infants. *J Pediatr* 1991;119:417.)

starting at a few days of life after isotonic fluid contraction has occurred.

The rate of fetal weight gain increases during the second half of pregnancy: Weight gain is approximately 10 g/day from 20 to 22 weeks' gestation, 20 g/day from 28 to 30 weeks' gestation, and 30 g/day from 34 to 36 weeks' gestation.

Energy requirements in the neonatal period are partitioned into several components. Energy expended on basal metabolism (or *resting caloric expenditure*) is used to maintain fundamental cellular and tissue processes in the resting, unfed state in a thermoneutral environment. The basal metabolic rate is approximately 50 kcal/kg/day. The thermic effects of feeding (or *specific dynamic action*) is the energy expended above the basal metabolic rate in response to feeding and includes the transport and conversion of absorbed nutrients into their storage forms. Growth of 10 to 15 g/kg/day requires approximately 40 to 75 kcal/kg/day more than the 50 kcal/kg/day maintenance expenditure. Although total requirements vary, adequate weight gain can usually be achieved by providing 100 to 120 kcal/ kg/day to growing preterm infants. Some infants, especially those with chronic lung disease, need a greater number of calories. Infants who are unable to tolerate enteral feeds should be started on parenteral nutrition to maintain positive nutritional balance.

The rate of neonatal weight gain is usually plotted against postnatal growth curves such as those shown in Fig. 7-2. These curves do not necessarily reflect optimal growth as they were generated in sick infants before modern advances in neonatal care. The growth in neonatal head circumference and length is important to follow. Growth in head circumference reflects brain growth, which unfortunately does not always parallel somatic growth. Growth in length reflects skeletal growth.

ENDOCRINE AND METABOLIC FUNCTION

In utero, glucose is transported across the placenta at a rate of approximately 4 to 6 mg/kg/minute. At delivery, preterm neonates have limited glycogen stores, impaired gluconeogenesis, and limited alternative fuels. Common problems such as respiratory distress, sepsis can quickly deplete energy stores. Preterm infants are often started on intravenous glucose infusions shortly after delivery to avoid hypoglycemia. An infusion of 10% dextrose at 80 mL/kg/day provides 5.6 mg/kg/minute of glucose, which usually maintains euglycemia.

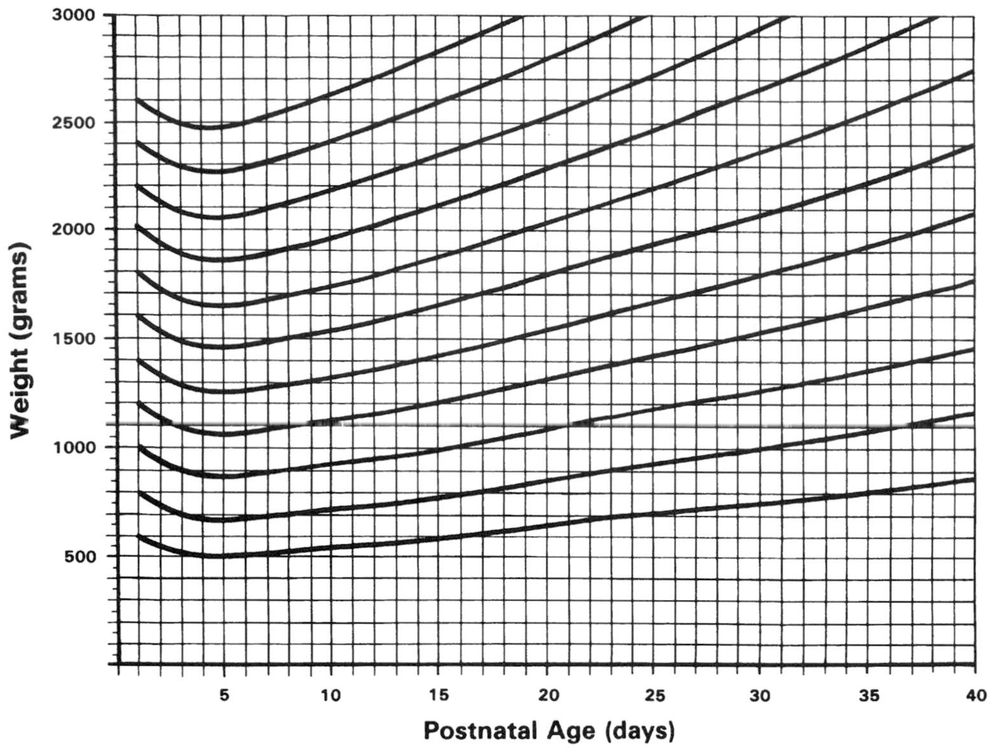

Figure 7-2. Postnatal growth grid including growth curves for 100-g birth-weight groups. Derived from postnatal body weight changes in 385 surviving infants with birth weights less than 2,500 g. (Reprinted with permission from Shaffer SG, Quimiro CL, Anderson JV, Hall RT. Postnatal weight changes in low-birth-weight infants. *Pediatrics* 1987;79:702.)

Hyperglycemia is less frequent in preterm infants, but can occur with stress or as carbohydrate intake is increased for nutritional support. Insulin therapy may be required.

Hypocalcemia is also a common problem in preterm infants, particularly those who are septic, asphyxiated, or growth retarded. Calcium can be provided empirically in the initial maintenance fluids of VLBW infants, or serum levels (preferably of ionized calcium) can be followed until routine intravenous hyperalimentation or feedings are begun.

HEMATOLOGIC FUNCTION

Anemia is a frequent problem in the preterm neonate and occurs due to phlebotomy losses, a shortened red blood cell lifespan in preterm infants (approximately 35–50 days, in contrast to 60–70 days in the term infant), and a relatively diminished erythropoietin output in response to anemia. Anemia of prematurity appears to be most likely caused by inadequate production of erythropoietin. Preterm neonates experience an earlier and deeper nadir in hemoglobin and hematocrit than do term neonates experiencing physiologic anemia at 10 to 12 weeks of age. A VLBW infant may commonly receive transfusions of packed red blood cells during hospitalization in the NICU. Indications for transfusion include not only the level of hemoglobin or hematocrit, but also other factors such as the amount of respiratory support required or the presence of other clinical problems such as sepsis. In addition to trying to limit phlebotomy, exogenous erythropoietin therapy has been shown to stimulate erythropoiesis and decrease transfusion requirements.

Indirect hyperbilirubinemia is an extremely common problem in the preterm neonate and is discussed at length in Chapter 36.

INFECTIOUS DISEASE

Infection of the preterm neonate is much more common than infection of the term neonate. Late onset nosocomial sepsis by coagulase-negative staphylococci and fungi is a significant problem in preterm infants with percutaneous central venous catheters. Specific neonatal infections are discussed in Part II, Section G.

NEUROLOGIC FUNCTION

The preterm newborn is at higher risk of a number of neurologic problems including intraventricular-periventricular hemorrhage, periventricular leukomalacia, retinopathy of prematurity, and hearing loss. Even preterm infants without identifiable neuroimaging abnormalities may have subsequent neurodevelopmental problems. The incidence of intraventricular hemorrhage among VLBW infants is approximately 30% to 35% and is thus a major cause of morbidity and mortality.

GASTROINTESTINAL FUNCTION

Because of functional immaturity, as well as other concurrent illnesses, feeding the very preterm infant is often quite difficult. Dilute feeds are initially given in small volumes, and tolerance is assessed by monitoring gastric residuals, the abdominal examination, and the stooling pattern. Necrotizing enterocolitis usually occurs only after a preterm infant has been fed. Infants who do not tolerate enteral feeds and receive prolonged parenteral nutritional support are at risk of developing cholestasis. The time of first stool passage is delayed in preterm infants.

Criteria for Discharge of Preterm Neonates

The myriad problems above may lead to neonatal mortality or long-term morbidity. With the exception neurologic sequelae, however, most problems, even many pulmonary problems, steadily improve and disappear with time and growth. Many NICUs transfer "feeding and growing" infants from an intensive care room to a step-down room or unit. A number of milestones must then be reached before a preterm neonate is considered ready for discharge home (Table 7-4).

TABLE 7-4. Guidelines for Discharge of Preterm Neonates from the Newborn Special Care Unit, The Children's Hospital at Yale–New Haven

Weight greater than approximately 1,850 g
Postconceptional age >35 weeks completed
Maturational milestones met
No apnea of prematurity requiring intervention for >7 days (off respiratory stimulants for >7 days)
Maintaining temperature in crib
Feeding by mouth
Gained weight at least 2–3 days while in crib conditions and fed by mouth
No acute illness requiring ongoing hospital care
Chronic lung disease is capable of outpatient management
Retinopathy of prematurity is of a severity that can be followed as an outpatient
Home social situation acceptable
Parental teaching accomplished
Parents roomed-in overnight in complicated cases
Cardiopulmonary resuscitation training in selected cases
Predischarge tests and procedures completed
Hearing test
Eye examination
Immunizations up to date
Respiratory syncytial virus immunoprophylaxis up to date if in respiratory syncytial virus season
Central lines removed
Inguinal hernias, if they were present, have been repaired
Ileostomy, if present after necrotizing enterocolitis, has been taken down
Circumcision of boy performed, if desired by parents
Outpatient follow-up arranged, and pediatrician up to date on infant's status

Most neonates are observed until a postconceptional age of at least 35 weeks. Many ELBW infants require hospitalization until their estimated date of confinement or beyond.

SPECIAL ISSUES

Environment

Exposure to noise in the NICU may result in cochlear damage and disrupt normal growth and development of preterm infants. Babies should not be exposed to noise levels of more than 45 dB. Excessive ambient light may also be detrimental to the preterm infant. Mounting evidence suggests that increased physical contact between the preterm infant and his or her parents is beneficial. "Kangaroo care" of preterm infants, in which they are held directly against their parent's naked chest for periods of time, may decrease the frequency of apnea, enhance breast-feeding, and lead to improvement in other physiologic parameters. Appropriate analgesia for painful procedures is indicated, as it would be for term neonates and older children.

Parental Support

Psychosocial issues and parental support are important in the care of any child. Preterm delivery with or without intensive care nursing heightens the anxiety associated with childbirth. Even the delivery of a relatively stable and uncomplicated preterm infant may be the most unsettling, anxiety-provoking event that the parents have ever faced. Moreover, the consequences of preterm delivery may permanently affect the family's quality of life.

No situation is more stressful for parents than the need to make end-of-life decisions. Preterm neonates, especially those born near the limits of viability, may become so ill that continued medical care becomes futile. In these cases, most neonatologists recommend withdrawal of medical support. Effective and compassionate communication with the family is essential in such situations. The provision or withholding of resuscitative efforts for neonates born near the limits of viability is another difficult, ethical issue often dealt with in the care of preterm infants.

Economics

Neonatal intensive care is one of the most expensive types of hospital care. Cost is clearly related to birth weight and survival rate. The allocation of extensive resources to preterm neonates, especially those born near the limits of viability, remains controversial. Prenatal care, which improves neonatal outcome, demonstrates greater cost effectiveness. In 1985, it was estimated that for every dollar spent on prenatal care, $3 was saved in the first year after delivery and an additional $10 was saved over a lifetime.

OUTCOME

The outcome of LBW infants with birth weights of more than 1,000 g is generally good in terms of both morbidity and mortality. The long-term outcome of infants with lower birth weights, however, particularly of those with birth weights of less than 750 g, remains concerning.

Predicting which LBW neonates are at risk for long-term neurodevelopmental impairment is difficult. Earlier gestational age, lower birth weight, perinatal asphyxia, microcephaly, early abnormal neurologic signs (especially seizures), intracranial hemorrhage, and ischemic brain lesions such as periventricular leukomalacia clearly convey a poorer prognosis.

Unfortunately, early intervention in the first 3 years after neonatal discharge (including frequent home visits and parental education) has resulted in little long-term improvement in full-scale IQ, behavior, or health at 5 years of life, particularly for infants with birth weights of less than 2,000 g. By school age, VLBW infants have had a greater number of medical problems (including respiratory conditions), poorer growth, more surgical procedures, and more hospitalizations than matched children born at term.

CHAPTER 8
Neonatal Intensive Care

Adapted from Richard A. Ehrenkranz

DELIVERY ROOM RESUSCITATION

Adaptation from the intrauterine to the extrauterine environment demands major physiologic changes. For example, *in utero* the human fetus is totally dependent on the mother for respiratory gas exchange, nutrient supply, waste product removal, and thermoregulation. After delivery, the neonate's lungs must replace the placenta as the site of respiratory gas exchange; stored glycogen and absorption of nutrients by the gastrointestinal tract provide for metabolic homeostasis and growth; the task of waste elimination is taken over by the gastrointestinal tract and kidneys with the latter also responsible for the maintenance of water and electrolyte balance; and the neonate must be prepared to supply energy to maintain body temperature. In most newborn infants (approximately 85%–90%), these changes proceed smoothly, and the infants require little or no assistance after delivery. However, a few require help and close observation until they complete the transition successfully, and the occasional infant fails completely to adapt. The main goals of delivery room resuscitation are the establishment of respiratory activity with gas exchange and the conversion from the fetal to the neonatal circulation.

Apgar Score

In 1953, Dr. Virginia Apgar proposed a method of evaluating the newborn infant in the delivery room based on five easily determined signs. This evaluation, known as the *Apgar score* (Table 8-1), gives a rating of 0, 1, or 2 to each sign. A score of 10 indicates that the infant is in the best possible condition, whereas a score of less than 3 implies moderate to severe asphyxia. Currently, a score is assigned at 1 and 5 minutes. The 1-minute score is a guide to the infant's well-being. It indicates the degree of asphyxia and had been previously used to suggest appropriate resuscitative measures. In practice, the infant's respiratory activity, heart rate, and color are the best indicators of the need for resuscitation, not the 1-minute Apgar score. Although the 5-minute score had been thought to correlate with neonatal morbidity, it more accurately indicates the response to resuscitative efforts. If the Apgar score at 5 minutes is still less than 7, additional scores every 5 minutes for a total of 20 minutes have been recommended to assess response and the appropriateness of continued resuscitative measures.

Resuscitation in the Delivery Room

Figure 8-1 is an algorithm of the delivery room assessment and management recommended by International Liason Committee on Resuscitation. As soon as the infant's head is delivered, the mouth, nose, and pharynx should be gently suctioned. After the rest of the infant is delivered and the umbilical cord is clamped and cut, the infant is transferred in a head-down position and placed under a radiant heater on a resuscitation table in the supine or side-lying position. Most infants begin to cry between the time the body is delivered and the cord is cut.

On the radiant warmer, the neonate is quickly and thoroughly dried. This should minimize evaporative heat loss, while placement under a preheated radiant warmer should minimize radiant and convective heat loss. The mouth and nose are then gently suctioned with a bulb syringe or a suction catheter. The mouth is suctioned first to prevent aspiration. Blind deep or vigorous nasopharyngeal suctioning with a suction catheter can result in laryngeal spasm and increased vagal tone with apnea and bradycardia. For this reason, unless meconium staining of the amniotic fluid exists, deep suctioning of the oropharynx should be delayed for several minutes until normal ventilation has been established.

If respiratory activity is inadequate, however, additional tactile stimulation should be provided by flicking the heel or slapping the sole of the infant's foot or by rubbing the infant's back. The activities performed up to this point—drying the infant, suctioning the airway, and providing tactile stimulation—should be completed within 30 seconds.

If the infant has adequate spontaneous respiratory activity, then the heart rate is evaluated. Heart rate can be determined by auscultation or palpation of the umbilical cord or of the brachial artery. If the infant's heart rate is adequate, more than 100 *beats per minute* (bpm), then color is evaluated. Free-flow oxygen should be given to the infant with central cyanosis who is breathing spontaneously and has a heart rate of more than 100 bpm. Free-flow oxygen is unnecessary for infants with only peripheral cyanosis (acrocyanosis).

If the infant is apneic or if the infant's respiratory effort is insufficient to maintain a heart rate of more than 100 bpm, positive-pressure bag and mask ventilation with oxygen should be initiated promptly. After a 20- to 30-second period of ventilation at a rate of 40 to 60 breaths per minute, the infant's heart rate should be evaluated. If the heart rate is more than 100 bpm and if the infant displays spontaneous breathing activity, positive-pressure ventilation can be discontinued; free-flow oxygen should be provided until the infant remains pink. If the heart rate is between 60 and 100 bpm, positive-pressure bag and mask ventilation should be continued, and the infant's heart rate should be reevaluated after another 30 seconds. If the heart rate is less than 60 and not increasing after the initial period of ventilation, positive-pressure ventilation should be continued, and chest compressions should be initiated. Alternatively, if an individual skilled at endotracheal intubation is present in the delivery room, the infant can be intubated and the heart rate response to positive-pressure ventilation by bag and endotracheal tube can be used to determine the need for chest compressions.

Chest compressions should be performed on the lower third of the sternum and the depth should be approximately one-third the antero-posterior diameter of the chest. There are two methods. In one method, both thumbs are placed over the middle third of the sternum, and the other fingers encircle and support the back. The thumbs are positioned on the sternum just below the imaginary line drawn between the nipples; thumbs may have to be superimposed with very low-birth-weight (*VLBW*) infants. Alternatively, compressions could be administered with the ring and middle fingers of one hand placed on the sternum approximately one finger breadth below the nipple line; the other hand could be used to support the infant's back. The lowest portion of the sternum should not be compressed, because abdominal organs might be injured.

TABLE 8-1. Apgar Score

Sign	0	1	2
Heart rate	Absent	Slow (<100 beats per minute)	>100 beats per minute
Respiratory effort	Absent	Irregular weak cry	Regular, strong cry
Muscle tone	Flaccid	Some flexion of upper extremities	Well-flexed active motion
Reflex irritability	No response	Grimace	Cough or sneeze
Color	Central cyanosis	Peripheral cyanosis	Completely pink

Adapted from Apgar V. A proposal for a new method of evaluation of the newborn infant. *Curr Res Anesth Analg* 1953;32:260.

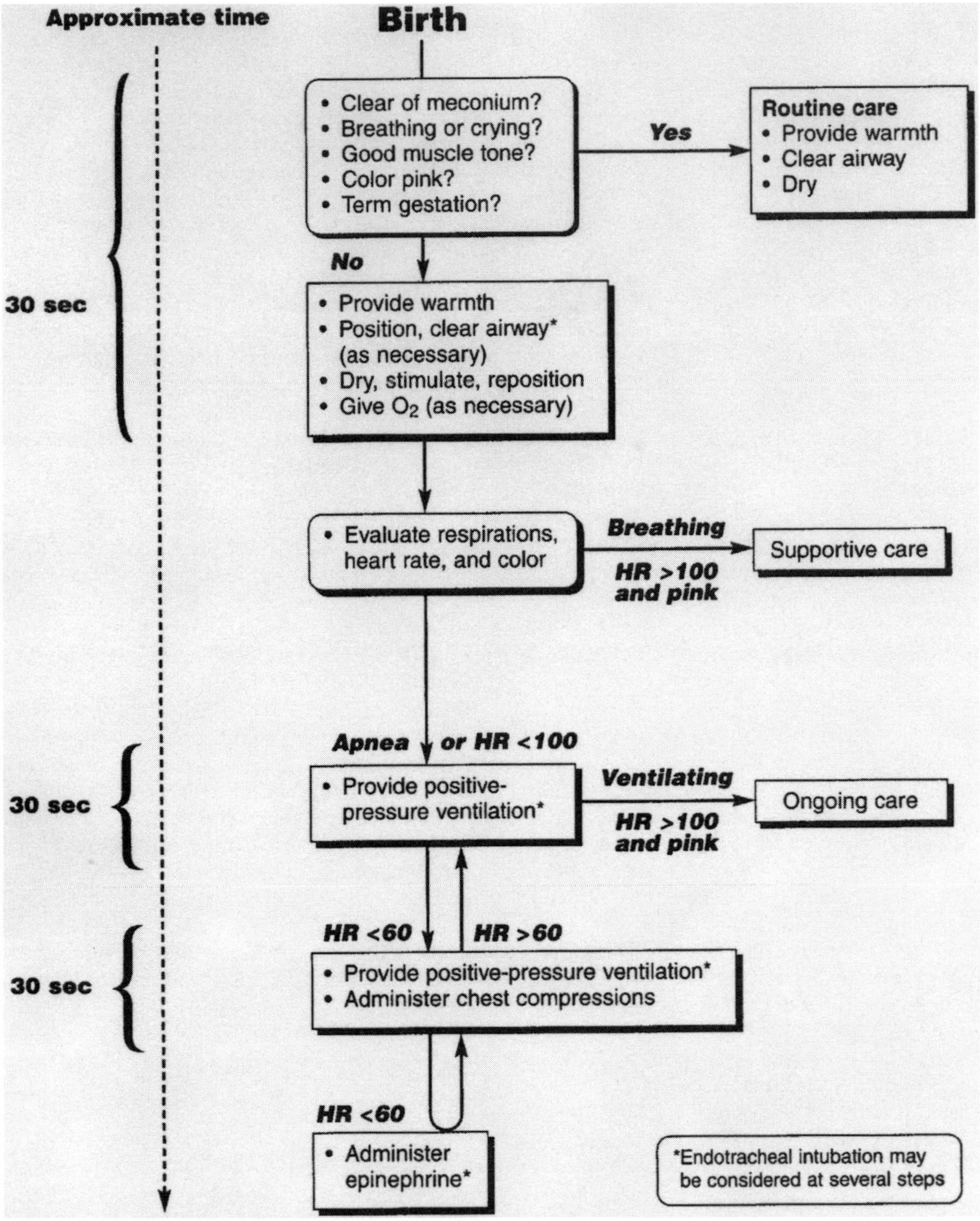

Figure 8-1. Algorithm for resuscitation of the newly born infant (Reprinted with permission from Niermeyer S, Kattwinkel J, Van Reempts P, et al. International Guidelines for Neonatal Resuscitation: An Excerpt From the Guidelines 2000 for Cardiopulmonary Resuscitation and Emergency Cardiovascular Care: International Consensus on Science. Pediatrics. 2000;106(3). http://www.pediatrics.org/cgi/content/full/106/ 3/e29).

If the heart rate improves and climbs to more than 80 bpm after approximately 30 seconds of chest compressions and ventilation, chest compressions can be discontinued. In most cases, positive-pressure ventilatory assistance should be continued until the infant has been transferred to the NICU, where blood pressure, perfusion, arterial blood gases, and acid–base status can be evaluated. If the infant's heart rate does not improve and remains less than 60 bpm after a 30- to 60-second period of adequate positive-pressure ventilation with oxygen and chest compressions, epinephrine should be given. Although epinephrine can be given intravenously, administration via the endotracheal tube is easier (0.1 to 0.3 mL/kg of a 1:10,000 solution, intravenously or endotracheally). Doses of epinephrine may be repeated every 5 minutes if required.

Naloxone hydrochloride (Narcan) may be indicated to reverse respiratory depression associated with a history of maternal narcotic administration within the 4 hours immediately preceding delivery. Naloxone, a competitive narcotic antagonist with a duration of action of 1 to 4 hours, can be administered (0.1 mg/kg per dose) intravenously, endotracheally, intramuscularly, or subcutaneously. Therefore, infants who are treated must be monitored closely for recurrent respiratory depression; repeated doses may be given. Administering naloxone to the infant of a narcotic-addicted mother may precipitate seizures.

Sodium bicarbonate should be given when a significant metabolic acidosis has been documented or is assumed to be present. Sodium bicarbonate should not be given unless the infant is being adequately ventilated, because it causes the arterial PCO_2 to increase. The increased PCO_2 results from the spontaneous conversion of bicarbonate to water and carbon dioxide following its addition to a closed acidotic system, which is analogous to a poorly ventilated patient.

A volume expander should be considered when evidence exists of acute bleeding with signs of hypovolemia in an infant requiring resuscitation. A volume of 10 mL/kg of 5% albumin, normal saline, or Ringer's lactate can be infused over approximately 10 minutes; O-negative whole blood or packed red blood cells may also be given, but these may not be as readily available as the other fluids.

During a neonatal resuscitation in the delivery room, vascular access is most readily achieved by inserting a fluid-filled umbilical catheter (or feeding tube) into the umbilical vein. The tip of the catheter should lie just below the surface of the abdominal wall at a location at which free flow of blood is present. Inserting the catheter farther into the umbilical vein might position the catheter tip within a branch of the portal vein, and infusing resuscitative solutions into that vessel might result in liver damage.

In summary, delivery room resuscitation involves the same sequence used during any cardiopulmonary resuscitation: The airway is established, breathing is initiated, circulation is supported, and then, if necessary, drugs are given.

Ventilatory Equipment for Resuscitation

Two standard types of ventilation bags exist, a self-inflating bag and an anesthesia bag. The self-inflating bag refills itself because of its elasticity, *independently* of gas flow. An intake valve or a series of valves at one end of the bag allows it to be rapidly reinflated. However, unless this type of bag is fitted with an oxygen reservoir that surrounds the intake valve(s), oxygen flowing into the bag is diluted by the air that is reinflating the bag, and high concentrations of oxygen cannot be delivered. Although the self-inflating feature makes this bag easier to use, some self-inflating bags deliver oxygen only when they are compressed. Self-inflating bags that permit free-flow oxygen are preferable.

The anesthesia bag is reinflated by a continuous flow of air or oxygen from a compressed gas source. Delivery of an adequate ventilatory volume requires that the bag be refilled sufficiently between breaths. This is a function of the rate of air/oxygen gas flow into the intake port, adjustment of a flow control or exit valve, and the soundness of the seal between the infant and the facemask or endotracheal tube. If ventilation is interrupted and the mask is removed from the infant's face or the bag is disconnected from the endotracheal tube, the bag promptly deflates; it must be allowed to reinflate before positive-pressure ventilation can be restarted. However, this is a flow-through system, and facial oxygen can be provided by directing the ventilation port (with or without a mask) toward the infant's face. The anesthesia bag can deliver very high inspiratory pressures, so a pressure gauge must be included within the respiratory circuit so that peak inspiratory pressures can be monitored.

Facemasks and endotracheal tubes should be available in sizes appropriate for preterm and term neonates. Facemasks should conform to the infant's facial features and should form a tight seal while covering the nose and mouth. The largest endotracheal tube that fits easily into the trachea should be used during intubation: the smaller the tube, the greater the airway resistance and the more difficulty in suctioning during pulmonary toilet. The tube should be noncuffed; cuffed tubes have been associated with subglottic and tracheal necrosis in neonates. Appropriate endotracheal tube size (internal diameter) is a function of body weight: body weight less than 1,000 g, 2.5 mm; 1,000 to 2,000 g, 3.0 mm; 2,000 to 3,500 g, 3.5 mm; and more than 3,500 g, 4.0 mm. In addition, many endotracheal tubes have a black line above the tip of the tube ranging from approximately 2 cm with 2.5-mm tubes to approximately 3.5 cm with 4.0-mm tubes. If this line is placed at the level of the vocal cords, the tip of the tube should be above the carina and in the midtrachea.

Laryngoscopy and Endotracheal Intubation

To facilitate endotracheal intubation, the infant should be lying supine under the radiant warmer of the resuscitation table with a rolled or folded towel under the shoulders to produce slight neck extension (Fig. 8-2). In this position, the infant's chin is slightly extended as if sniffing the air. Hyperextending the infant's neck usually obstructs visualization of the glottic opening and the vocal cords. The infant's head is steadied by the operator's right hand or by an assistant. The laryngoscope is held between the thumb and first finger of the operator's left hand and the infant's chin is grasped firmly with the second and third fingers of that hand. During intubation, the infant's heart rate is monitored by auscultation or with a cardiac monitor. The appropriate-sized blade of a lighted laryngoscope is inserted near the right corner of the infant's mouth and advanced between the tongue and palate for approximately 2 cm. As the blade advances, it should be moved to the left side of the mouth. This maneuver moves the tongue to the left of the blade and permits visualization of the base of the tongue and epiglottis.

The blade is advanced into the vallecula, the space between the base of the tongue and the anterior surface of the epiglottis. Gentle elevation of the tip of the blade lifts the epiglottis anteriorly revealing the glottic opening. In addition, the fourth or small finger of the left hand can press on the hyoid bone to move the larynx posteriorly and expose the glottis. Then, under direct visualization, the endotracheal tube is inserted along the right side of the blade into the trachea, approximately 2 to 3 cm below the level of the vocal cords (when applicable, the black line on the tube should be at the level of the vocal cords). The laryngoscope blade is then removed while the position of the tube is maintained by the right hand on the infant's face.

When intubation is complete, the lungs should be expanded with a ventilation bag or by mouth. Tube placement should be confirmed by auscultatory evidence of equal, bilateral breath sounds over the axillary regions and symmetric chest movement. Unequal breath sounds and chest excursions suggest that the tube is probably in the mainstem bronchus of the lung producing the louder breath sounds. In that case, the tube should be withdrawn until breath sounds improve and become equal. Once the tube is secured, a chest roentgenograph should be obtained to confirm tube position.

Meconium Staining of the Amniotic Fluid

Meconium staining of the amniotic fluid occurs 10% to 12% of all deliveries. The presence of meconium in the amniotic fluid may indicate fetal distress. Aspirated meconium in the mouth and pharynx can lead to *meconium aspiration pneumonia*. Because of this, in a delivery in which the amniotic fluid is stained with meconium, the upper airway (nose, mouth and pharynx) should be cleared in the intrapartum period when the head is delivered. The infant is then brought immediately to the resuscitation table, and additional suctioning of the airway may be performed.

If the infant is breathing and active, vigorous drying should be avoided, and suctioning the trachea is not indicated as it may cause more harm than good.

If the infant has inadequate respiratory effort of a heart rate less than 100, immediate tracheal suctioning is performed via a meconium aspirator or an endotracheal tube affixed with a suction adapter connected to mechanical suction (maximum pressure of 100 mm Hg). The duration of suction can be regulated via the thumb control port on the meconium aspirator. The meconium aspirator or endotracheal tube is slowly withdrawn as suction is applied. Suction catheters inserted through the endotracheal tube may be inadequate to remove thick, tenacious meconium and, therefore, are not recommended. When possible, ventilatory stimulation or positive-pressure ventilation is not begun until meconium is no longer removed by tracheal suction.

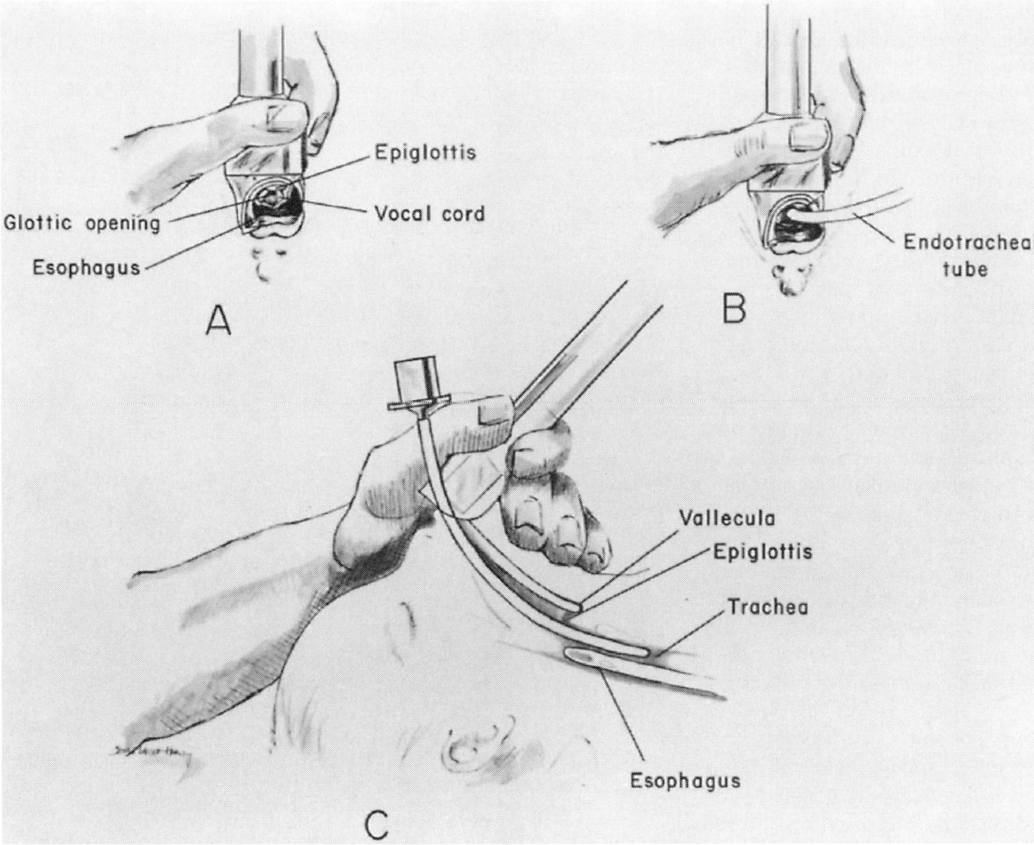

Figure 8-2. Technique of endotracheal intubation. **A:** Direct laryngoscopy. Note the glottic opening below the epiglottis and between the vocal cords. The esophagus is posterior to the glottis. **B:** Insertion of the endotracheal tube through the glottic opening from the right corner of the mouth. **C:** The endotracheal tube is within the trachea. Note that the tip of the laryngoscopy blade is in the vallecula above the anterior surface of the epiglottis, and that the esophagus is below the trachea. (Reprinted with permission from Ehrenkranz RA. Delivery room emergencies and resuscitation. In: Warshaw JB, Hobbins JC, eds. *Principles and practice of perinatal medicine: maternal-fetal and newborn care.* Menlo Park, CA: Addison-Wesley, 1983:209.)

Special Problems Interfering with Delivery Room Resuscitation

VLBW preterm infants may lack the strength to maintain adequate respiratory effort and may require respiratory assistance in the delivery room to sustain gas exchange. Some of these infants may be further depressed by sepsis or pneumonia caused by clinical amnionitis or by maternal therapies such as magnesium sulfate used to treat preterm labor or preeclampsia or eclampsia. Because the incidence of respiratory distress syndrome is substantial in infants at 30 weeks of gestation or less, some clinicians prophylactically begin surfactant replacement therapy in the delivery room if the infants have been intubated.

As many as 3% of full-term infants develop a spontaneous pneumothorax or pneumomediastinum after a normal spontaneous vaginal delivery. This air leak develops as a complication of the intrathoracic pressure generated by the infant during the initial respiratory efforts. Although a pneumomediastinum may produce tachypnea, it rarely results in significant respiratory difficulty. A pneumothorax interferes with the establishment of respiratory activity only if it is large and under tension producing mediastinal shift and compromising circulation and the contralateral lung.

The presence of a scaphoid abdomen, immediate cyanosis, and respiratory distress suggests the presence of a diaphragmatic hernia. Diaphragmatic hernias usually occur on the left side of the thorax inhibiting the normal growth and development of the left lung and often inhibiting the growth and development of the right lung because of displacement of the mediastinum and the heart to the right. Breath sounds are diminished or absent on the left, and the heart sounds are heard in the right chest. Endotracheal intubation should be performed quickly, because respiratory activity and cardiac function will be further compromised as the bowel fills with gas.

Congenital anomalies such as bilateral choanal atresia, laryngeal webs, and other obstructive malformations of the epiglottis, larynx, or trachea prevent air exchange. If respiratory movements are observed but no air movement occurs when the infant's mouth is closed, the mouth and posterior pharynx should be cleared of secretions, an oral airway should be established, and the patency of each choana should be determined by attempting to pass a suction catheter through each nostril into the posterior oropharynx. If effective air exchange is not achieved, laryngoscopy and endotracheal intubation should be performed.

Nonimmune hydrops fetalis, a condition implying an excess of total body water that is not associated with a circulating antibody against a red blood cell, may hinder the establishment of effective respiratory activity. The excessive accumulation of extracellular fluid includes subcutaneous edema, pleural and pericardial effusions, ascites, polyhydramnios, and placental thickening.

NEWBORN INTENSIVE CARE UNIT ADMISSION ROUTINES, MONITORING, AND PROCEDURES

On admission to the NICU, every infant should be weighed; vital signs, including an apical pulse, respiratory rate, blood pressure, and axillary temperature, should be obtained; and a capillary hematocrit (or hemoglobin) and blood sugar (e.g., with glucose oxidase-impregnated reagent strips) should be measured. Vitamin K_1 (0.5–1.0 mg) should be given intramuscularly and ophthalmic prophylaxis should be given (0.5%

erythromycin ophthalmic ointment, 1% tetracycline ophthalmic ointment, or 1% silver nitrate). Surface electrodes should be placed, and monitoring of cardiac function should be initiated. After axillary temperature is determined on admission, body temperature can be monitored continuously with a skin temperature probe (or thermistor) or with serial axillary temperature measurements. Environmental temperature should be adjusted to maintain the skin or axillary temperature between 36.0°C and 36.5°C. Oxygen consumption has been shown to be minimized with such an environmental temperature (neutral thermal environment).

Any infant who has respiratory distress or who requires supplemental inspiratory oxygen after delivery should be monitored expectantly with a pulse oximeter or transcutaneous oxygen and carbon dioxide electrodes. Depending on the severity of the respiratory distress, an arterial blood gas measurement should be considered, and the need for mechanical ventilatory assistance and placement of an umbilical (or peripheral) arterial catheter for serial arterial blood gas measurements evaluated.

Serial blood pressure monitoring should be done on infants who are unstable. Noninvasive blood pressure measurements can be performed by monitors that inflate a blood pressure cuff at preset intervals and then display systolic, diastolic, and mean blood pressure and heart rate. Continuous blood pressure monitoring can be performed from an arterial catheter with a pressure transducer.

The age at which enteral feedings are initiated depends on factors such as the infant's birth weight and gestational age, a history of fetal distress, and the presence and severity of respiratory distress. Intravenous fluids and parenteral nutrition solutions should be provided until enteral feedings are well established to maintain normal fluid and electrolyte status and to approach nitrogen and caloric needs. Enteral feedings in VLBW infants are often delayed for at least 24 hours; then small volumes are offered by nasogastric tube if the infant's condition is stable. Enteral feedings are slowly increased in caloric density and then volume as tolerated; parenteral nutrition is maintained and slowly decreased as enteral feedings advance.

CHAPTER 9

Follow-up of Infants Discharged from the Newborn Intensive Care Unit (NICU)

Adapted from David T. Scott and Jon E. Tyson

The need for follow-up programs for high-risk newborns has now been widely accepted. Most follow-up programs offer some synthesis clinical service to the patient while performing clinical research on developmental outcome measures. Whenever feasible, follow-up should be provided for infants with any of the neonatal problems listed in Table 9-1.

For infants who have primary pediatricians skilled in managing disorders such as bronchopulmonary dysplasia, short gut syndrome, and the sequelae of intracranial hemorrhage and hypoxic-ischemic encephalopathy, follow-up clinics may need to provide no more than standardized neurodevelopmental assessments. However, indigent populations have the most limited access to health care and the highest prevalence of neurodevelopmental morbidity. For indigent populations, the provision of comprehensive medical care in the follow-up clinic may be important, both to manage health problems and to reduce loss to follow-up.

TABLE 9-1. Some Indications for Newborn Follow-up Referral

Birth weight of 1,250 g or less
Treatment with mechanical ventilation for 12 hours or longer
Bronchopulmonary dysplasia
Recurrent apneic episodes at or beyond 38 weeks' postconceptional age
Grades 2 to 4 intraventricular hemorrhage, intracerebral lesions, or ventriculomegaly by sonogram or computed tomography
Seizures or persistent neurologic abnormality
Meningitis
Cystic white-matter disease
One or more major congenital anomalies
Any problem requiring major surgery in the neonatal period

MEDICAL EVALUATION AND CARE

Routine medical care for high-risk infants includes administration of immunizations and evaluation of growth, vision, and hearing. Immunizations for preterm infants should be given at the same postnatal age as for term infants. Growth is assessed in much the same manner as for full-term infants, except that more stable growth trajectories and better predictions of later growth status are generally obtained by plotting growth measures on a postterm (corrected) age scale. The American Academy of Pediatrics (AAP) recommends that vision examinations be provided to all premature infants who receive oxygen therapy. If no retinopathy has been identified, periodic eye examinations should be performed until the retina is mature (usually by 2–3 months after term); if retinopathy has been identified, eye examinations should continue until the disease process is stable or resolving. Universal hearing screening generally occurs in all infants but is particularly important in infants who meet some of the characteristics in Table 9-2.

NEUROLOGIC ASSESSMENTS

Several methods of neurologic assessment have been described, both for the neonatal period and for the ensuing months. The method most familiar to practicing physicians focuses on infant reflexes and posture. However, this method may not be adequate for early identification of subtle findings. Many infants

TABLE 9-2. Some Indications for Audiologic Evaluation

Birth weight of less than 1,500 g
Potentially toxic levels of bilirubin
Congenital malformations involving the external ear, palate, face, or skull
Congenital nonbacterial infections
Meningitis
Prolonged administration of aminoglycosides or other ototoxic drugs
Family history of hearing loss

with suspect or mild neurologic findings (e.g., mild hypotonia, mild hypertonia of the legs) subsequently become normal. This fact has led some follow-up investigators to describe a transient dystonia that appears and then resolves spontaneously during the first year. In the National Collaborative Perinatal Project sample, however, 84% of infants with moderate or severe quadriplegia at 1 year and 87% of those with moderate or severe hemiparesis at 1 year were classified as having cerebral palsy at 7 years.

DEVELOPMENTAL ASSESSMENTS

Most newborn follow-up programs at tertiary medical centers have used the Bayley Scales of Infant Development and the Bayley Scales of Infant Development, Second Edition (BSID-II). These tests are the products of decades of refinement and restandardization. Both editions of the Bayley Scales were standardized on large national samples constructed to be representative of the U.S. population.

Both editions of the Bayley Scales generate age equivalents and developmental indexes in both the cognitive and motor domains. The age equivalents are the age for which a given level of performance would be typical. The mental and motor indexes are standardized scores that are distributed in the same manner as IQ scores with a population mean of 100 and standard deviations of either 16 (1969 edition) or 15 (1993 edition). These indexes permit comparison of a given infant with other infants of the same age. When evaluating premature infants, most developmental clinicians now use the infant's postterm or corrected age (i.e., the age computed from the child's due date), so that the comparison will be with other infants of the same biological (postconceptional) age.

CHOICE OF AN AGE SCALE

Early follow-up studies often calculated the age of premature children from the date of their premature birth. Thus, premature children were compared with full-term children who were the same postnatal age but a more advanced postconceptional age. Not surprisingly, the full-term children were almost always taller, heavier, and more advanced developmentally. Other studies have attempted to put premature children on the same biological footing as the full-term controls by using the child's postterm or *corrected age*.

Although the use of the postterm age for premature children has gained ever-wider acceptance, the age range over which it should be used is controversial. In some early studies in which the degree of prematurity was modest and the samples were small, the use of the postterm age did not seem to make a significant difference after 1 or 2 years, and the investigators, thus changed from the corrected age scale to the chronologic age scale after that point. However, as more survivors with greater and greater degrees of prematurity were studied, the effects of using the corrected versus the chronologic age could be seen at progressively later ages. For this reason, some investigators and clinicians now use the postterm age indefinitely.

NEUROLOGIC AND DEVELOPMENTAL INTERVENTIONS

Since the early 1960s, several early intervention programs have been developed in an effort to promote normal development, particularly for socioeconomically disadvantaged children. The efficacy of these programs, which typically include physical therapy, occupational therapy, as well as speech and language therapy, remains questionable.

One well-controlled, multisite, randomized clinical trial is the Infant Health and Development Program (IHDP). At each of eight clinical sites, premature, low-birth-weight (LBW) children were randomly assigned either to a follow-up group or to an intervention group. Children in the follow-up group received medical follow-up care and blinded developmental evaluations; children in the intervention group received the same follow-up services and a broad-spectrum early intervention program for the infants and their families.

At 3 years postterm age, differences were found in each of the three IHDP outcome domains. In the cognitive domain, large IQ effects were noted: Among children with birth weights between 2,001 and 2,500 g, intervention children exhibited a cognitive advantage of 13.2 IQ points; among children with birth weights of 2,000 g or less, the IQ advantage was 6.6 points. Secondary analyses suggested that the IQ effects were largest for children from disadvantaged families. In the behavior domain, there was a small but significant tendency for the mothers of intervention children to report fewer behavior problems than the mothers of follow-up children. In the health domain, mothers of children with birth weights of 2,000 g or less reported more illnesses and health conditions for intervention children than for follow-up children; no differences were found on a measure of serious health conditions, however.

The IHDP sample was reassessed in two follow-up studies beyond age 3 years (the age at which the intervention ended). At age 5 (2 years after the intervention ended), no significant differences were found in the behavior or health domains. In the cognitive domain, no significant differences remained in the lighter birth-weight stratum (less than or equal to 2,000 g), although modest but significant residual differences were found in the heavier birth-weight stratum. At age 8 (5 years after the end of the intervention program), there were, again, no significant differences in the behavior or health domains. But in the cognitive domain, the heavier birth-weight stratum showed a significant 4.4-point IQ advantage in the intervention groups; a somewhat larger treatment effect was found on a standardized vocabulary test. Thus, early intervention programs appear to enhance the developmental progress of LBW premature infants, but the treatment effects may diminish over time once the intervention is withdrawn.

SECTION

C

Respiratory System

CHAPTER 10

Causes of Respiratory Distress in the Newborn

Adapted from Ian Gross

Respiratory distress is a common presentation of disease in the newborn infant. The term is used to describe a constellation of easily observable physical signs including rapid breathing (more than 60 breaths per minute), cyanosis, retractions (sucking in of the skin between the ribs, under the ribs, or above the sternum with each breath), flaring of the nostrils, and a grunting sound on expiration. Many causes are responsible for these signs, and their presence is an indication that further observation or investigation is necessary. The causes of respiratory distress in the newborn include the following:

A. Airway obstruction
   1. Choanal atresia
   2. Congenital stridor (may be caused by congenital defects such as laryngomalacia, tracheomalacia, laryngeal webs, or aberrant vessels compressing the airways)
B. Pulmonary disorders
   1. Respiratory distress syndrome (hyaline membrane disease)
   2. Transient tachypnea
   3. Pneumonia
   4. Aspiration syndromes
   5. Persistent pulmonary hypertension
   6. Air leak: interstitial emphysema, pneumothorax, or pneumomediastinum
   7. Congenital malformations (e.g., diaphragmatic hernia, pulmonary hypoplasia, congenital lobar emphysema, tracheoesophageal fistula)
   8. Atelectasis
   9. Pulmonary hemorrhage
   10. Chronic lung disease (bronchopulmonary dysplasia, Wilson-Mikity syndrome)
C. Nonpulmonary causes
   1. Cardiac disease
   2. Metabolic acidosis
   3. Central nervous system disorders
   4. Hypothermia or hyperthermia

Babies may breathe rapidly during the first few hours after birth. This phenomenon is related to the clearing of lung fluid from the airways and the cardiopulmonary adjustment to extrauterine life. Tachypnea may also be associated with transient conditions such as hypothermia. Isolated tachypnea, which is not associated with cyanosis, may be managed by observation only during the first few hours of life. If the tachypnea persists or is associated with other evidence of respiratory distress, further investigation is indicated. This analysis usually includes a radiograph of the chest and determination of arterial blood gas levels or of blood oxygen saturation.

Because respiratory distress is caused by many factors that cannot be differentiated by clinical examination alone, a chest radiograph is indicated in any infant who has significant respiratory distress. A sudden deterioration in respiratory status is also an indication for obtaining a chest radiograph to rule out conditions that require urgent treatment, such as pneumothorax. Very early chest films (in the first 2–4 hours after birth) are often not helpful in differentiating the various forms of parenchymal lung disease, because the presence of lung fluid tends to produce a hazy appearance or diffuse fine infiltrates. Early radiographs are useful, however, for excluding conditions that require surgical intervention such as diaphragmatic hernia and air leaks.

If there is no clear-cut pulmonary cause for the respiratory distress, it will also be necessary to exclude the presence of cardiac disease. This can usually be done by chest radiograph, electrocardiogram, and echocardiogram. In some respiratory conditions (e.g., persistent pulmonary hypertension), the echocardiogram is not only useful for excluding heart disease, but also plays a role in the diagnosis and management of the pulmonary disorder. Occasionally, it is useful to determine the response to inhalation of 100% oxygen. In the presence of lung disease, the arterial Po_2 should increase after the inhalation of high concentrations of inspired oxygen, whereas with a fixed cardiac right-to-left shunt, there will be little increase in Po_2. This procedure carries the risk of causing closure of a patent ductus arteriosus in a ductal-dependent cardiac lesion.

CHAPTER 11
Transient Tachypnea of the Newborn

Adapted from Ian Gross

Transient tachypnea of the newborn (also called retained fetal lung fluid, wet lung, or respiratory distress syndrome type II) is a benign, self-limited condition seen primarily in full-term infants. It is believed to result from delay in the reabsorption of fetal pulmonary fluid. An association is seen between delivery by cesarean section and the development of this condition, possibly because of the compression of the chest during vaginal delivery and the mechanical "wringing out" of fetal lung fluid. These infants have respiratory distress shortly after birth. The features are tachypnea, mild retractions, and (sometimes) cyanosis. The clinical course is usually transient and mild with resolution of the problem in 24 to 48 hours. In some infants, the condition is more severe and may persist for 72 hours or longer.

The diagnosis is made by radiography. The classic appearance is that of a well-aerated lung with streaky markings radiating out from the hila (starburst appearance) and small amounts of fluid in the fissures, particularly the right middle fissure. The major condition from which transient tachypnea must be differentiated is pneumonia. Differentiation can sometimes be difficult in prolonged cases of transient tachypnea, although resolution is usually more rapid than with pneumonia.

Treatment is essentially symptomatic. Blood gas levels or oxygen saturation are monitored, and oxygen is administered to maintain a P_ao_2 of 60 to 80 mm Hg. Occasionally, a brief period of mechanical ventilation may be necessary. If the diagnosis of pneumonia cannot be excluded, antibiotics are given, although transient tachypnea itself does not require antibacterial treatment. This condition is not associated with long-term sequelae such as bronchopulmonary dysplasia, and the prognosis is excellent.

CHAPTER 12
Apnea

Adapted from Robert A. Herzlinger

Apnea is defined as a respiratory pause of 20 seconds or longer, or a shorter pause associated with cyanosis, abrupt pallor or hypotonia, or bradycardia. Apnea is an extremely common finding in premature infants. Approximately 25% of infants weighing less than 2,500 g at birth, 50% weighing less than 1,500 g, and 84% of those weighing less than 1,000 g have significant apnea. Apnea decreases with increasing postconceptual age and usually resolves by 35 to 36 weeks' postconceptual age.

Apnea can be classified into three types: Central apnea (10%–25%) is characterized by absence of both chest wall movement and nasal air flow; obstructive apnea (10%–20%) is associated with chest wall movement without nasal air flow; and mixed apnea (50%–70%) has both obstructive and central components. The location of the obstruction is usually at the level of the pharynx. Periodic breathing is another manifestation of immature ventilatory control defined as regular cycles of breathing interrupted by regular pauses of 5 to 10 seconds in duration. This breathing pattern also decreases in frequency with increasing postnatal age. Periodic breathing is considered normal in preterm and term infants.

ETIOLOGY

The most common cause of apnea is apnea of prematurity (Table 12-1), which is attributed to immaturity of the ventilatory control mechanism. Delayed brainstem auditory evoked responses have been noted in premature infants with apnea compared with controls. Functional obstruction of the upper airway has been attributed to dyscoordination of brainstem control of pharyngeal patency and diaphragmatic contractions. Inhibitory respiratory reflexes may predispose to apnea. The physiologic consequences of severe apnea include hypoxemia, hypercarbia, reflex-induced bradycardia, hypotension, and a decrease in cerebral blood flow. Although apnea of prematurity is not thought to have long-term consequences, severe prolonged spells may induce hypoxic ischemic central nervous system injury. In the face of an immature and unstable ventilatory control mechanism, a wide variety of conditions can induce apnea in premature infants. A full-term infant may develop apnea as a consequence of these underlying disorders as well. In contrast to premature infants, a specific

TABLE 12-1. Causes of Apnea

Apnea of prematurity
Central nervous system disorders
Intraventricular/periventricular hemorrhage
Subarachnoid hemorrhage
Infarction
Seizures
Structural anomalies
Central hypoventilation syndrome
Cardiorespiratory disorders
Respiratory distress syndrome
Bronchopulmonary dysplasia
Patent ductus arteriosus
Metabolic disorders
Hypoglycemia
Electrolytic imbalance
Inborn errors of metabolism
Hematologic disorders
Anemia
Infection
Sepsis/meningitis
Respiratory syncytial virus
Gastrointestinal disorders
Necrotizing enterocolitis
Gastroesophageal reflux
Medications
Phenobarbital
General anesthesia
Prostaglandin E_1
Airway obstruction
Craniofacial anomalies
Choanal atresia
Pierre Robin syndrome
Achondroplasia
Secretions
Neck flexion
Stimulation of inhibitory reflexes
Feeding-associated apnea
Thermoregulatory
Rapid warming

etiology is more likely to be found in the term or near-term infant with apnea.

EVALUATION AND MANAGEMENT

All infants at risk for apnea of prematurity (i.e., those of less than 34 weeks' gestation) require cardiac and thoracic impedance monitoring when admitted to the nursery. Because this technology may fail to detect significant hypoxemic episodes in premature infants, pulse oximetry is indicated for these infants. Apnea of prematurity is a diagnosis of exclusion. A careful history and physical examination directs further evaluation. An investigation for sepsis or meningitis should be performed in infants with other signs and symptoms of sepsis, in infants with apnea beyond 34 weeks' gestation, in infants with sudden onset of apnea, and infants with severe episodes. Apnea associated with gastroesophageal reflux frequently occurs after feedings while the infant is awake and may be associated with regurgitation. When apnea is a manifestation of seizures, other seizure signs are frequently noted such as staring gaze and increased tone. Dyscoordination of suck, swallow, and breathing present with apnea episodes during feedings. They usually resolve with increasing postconceptual age.

Management of apnea of prematurity is determined by the frequency and severity of the episodes. If these are mild and not associated with cyanosis and bradycardia, they may be treated with gentle stimulation, clearance of secretions from the airway, and avoidance of neck flexion. The prone position has been associated with decreased frequency of apneic episodes. If significant apnea persists, methylxanthines are indicated. These medications are effective against mixed, central, and obstructive apnea. The proposed mechanisms of action of methylxanthines include (a) increased minute ventilation, (b) increased CO_2 responsiveness, (c) enhanced diaphragmatic contractility, (d) improved pulmonary mechanics, and (e) decreased hypoxic ventilatory depression. Theophylline is the most commonly used agent. Theophylline is given in a loading dose of 4 to 6 mg/kg followed by a maintenance dosage of 1.5 to 3.0 mg/kg every 8 to 12 hours. Trough blood levels are monitored, and the dosage is adjusted accordingly. The therapeutic level is 7 to 12 μg/mL. Toxicity may occur when levels exceed 15 μg/mL and usually presents with tachycardia, irritability, and vomiting. Caffeine citrate, which is given orally, has a longer half-life and a wider therapeutic range and may be used as an alternative to theophylline. The loading dose of caffeine citrate is 20 to 40 mg/kg orally, followed by a maintenance dose of 5 to 8 mg/kg per dose orally given every 24 hours. The therapeutic trough serum concentration is 5 to 25 μg/mL. Concentrations greater than 40 to 50 μg/mL may be associated with toxicity. Persistent apnea, despite methylxanthine therapy, is an indication for nasal continuous positive airway pressure, which is effective for obstructive and mixed apnea spells. The proposed mechanism of action for continuous positive airway pressure involves stabilization of the upper airway and chest wall, as well as reducing inhibitory respiratory reflexes and increasing functional residual capacity. Intubation and mechanical ventilation are indicated if significant apnea persists despite the previously mentioned measure. Packed red blood cell transfusions (15 mL/kg) may reduce apnea when the hematocrit level is less than 30%.

Newer pharmacologic agents proposed for the treatment of apnea unresponsive to methylxanthines include doxapram, a peripheral chemoreceptor stimulant, and primidone, a deoxybarbiturate. Their safety and effectiveness in the treatment of apnea have not been established.

Infants with apnea of prematurity may be discharged home if they are more than 35 to 36 weeks' postconceptual age and have remained apnea-free for 7 to 10 days. The vulnerability of the respiratory control mechanism persists in premature infants who are at risk for recurrent apnea if exposed to stresses such as respiratory syncytial virus infection, sepsis, or general anesthesia. Although the incidence of sudden infant death syndrome (SIDS) increases with decreasing gestational age, parents should be reassured that apnea of prematurity is not an independent risk factor for SIDS.

Predischarge cardiorespiratory recordings have not been predictive of subsequent apneic episodes in very low-birth-weight infants, nor are these recordings predictive of SIDS. Home monitoring may be used to shorten the hospitalization of premature infants with persistent apnea beyond 36 weeks' postconceptual age. The home monitor may be discontinued if no significant episodes occur for 2 to 3 months. Apnea of prematurity, which resolves before 36 weeks' postconceptual age, is not, in itself, an indication for home monitoring. Premature infants should have pulse oximetry monitoring in car seats before discharge because apnea and desaturation spells have been reported with these devices. Although term infants should be placed on their sides or backs when sleeping to reduce SIDS, the appropriate sleeping position for preterm infants has not been established.

CHAPTER 13
Pneumonia

Adapted from Ian Gross

Pneumonia in the newborn period may arise during the first 2 to 3 days after birth (early-onset) or after the first week (late-onset). It may occur as an isolated infection or in association with septicemia. Pneumonia that develops shortly after birth is probably acquired *in utero,* or intrapartum by hematogenous spread from the mother, by ascending infection from the vagina and cervix, or by aspiration of contaminated secretions immediately after birth. Late-onset pneumonia, similar to other nosocomial infections in the newborn unit, can be transmitted by the infant's caretakers. The most common pathogens are group B streptococci and gram-negative organisms such as *Escherichia coli* and *Klebsiella,* but a wide variety of organisms may be involved.

CLINICAL CHARACTERISTICS

Infants with early-onset pneumonia usually have respiratory distress during the first few hours after birth. If they are premature, the symptoms may be indistinguishable from those of respiratory distress syndrome (RDS). Features that suggest pneumonia rather than RDS include maternal chorioamnionitis, prolonged rupture of the membranes, early onset of apnea, and poor perfusion and shock. The amniotic fluid lecithin-sphingomyelin ratio, if available, is also useful in differentiating pneumonia from RDS (a "mature" ratio rules out RDS).

The clinical course of neonatal pneumonia varies considerably. Some infants have fulminant disease with a rapid downhill course and early death. More commonly, moderate respiratory distress develops and assisted ventilation may be required for a few days, after which the baby recovers. The course may be different from that of RDS, which tends to become progressively

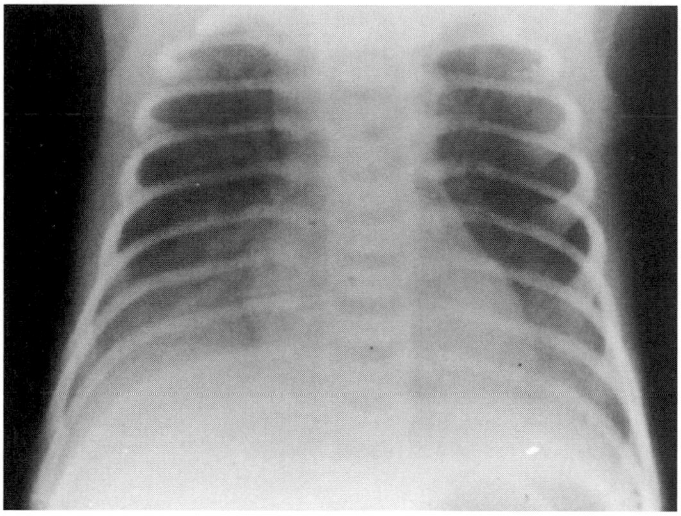

Figure 13-1. Bilateral lobar consolidation in an infant with pneumonia.

more severe and to peak at 48 to 72 hours; pneumonia usually follows a more level course. In addition to parenchymal lung disease, some infants also have severe pulmonary hypertension, presumably secondary to pulmonary vasospasm, with right-to-left shunting of blood. This complication is associated with significant morbidity and mortality.

RADIOGRAPHIC APPEARANCE

At least four different radiographic appearances have been described in newborn infants with pneumonia and include extensive coarse infiltrates scattered throughout both lungs and lobar consolidation (Fig. 13-1). Also possible is an RDS-like pattern (Fig. 13-2); the radiographic appearance of pneumonia in premature infants, particularly that caused by the group B streptococci, may be indistinguishable from that seen in RDS. It is possible that some of these infants have both RDS and pneumonia. Additionally, scattered small infiltrates may develop in one or both lungs (more commonly in mature than in premature infants).

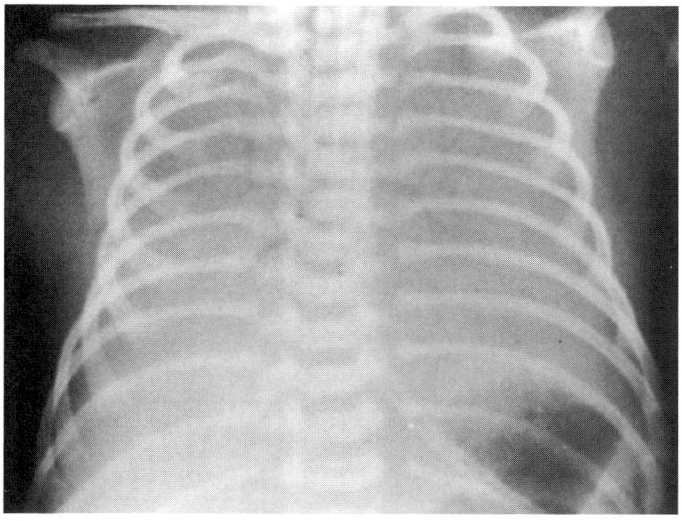

Figure 13-2. Respiratory distress syndrome-like pattern in a premature infant with pneumonia. The radiodensity of the lungs is increased greatly resulting in an opacified appearance.

DIFFERENTIAL DIAGNOSIS

In the full-term infant with a few scattered lung infiltrates on the chest radiograph, pneumonia must be differentiated from transient tachypnea of the newborn. The respiratory distress of pneumonia usually persists for a few days, whereas transient tachypnea is more likely to resolve within 48 hours. In the premature infant with a radiographic appearance consistent with RDS, it may not be possible to distinguish the two conditions, at least in the early stages. The use of cultures to identify the organism is not often helpful. Unless there is associated septicemia, blood cultures will be negative.

TREATMENT

Since the 1970s, the improved survival of infants with serious neonatal infections has been related to advances in supportive techniques, as well as antibiotic therapy. Because a precise bacterial diagnosis is usually not available, broad-spectrum coverage (e.g., with a penicillin and an aminoglycoside) is instituted for 7 to 10 days. If gentamicin is used, peak and trough levels of this antibiotic in the blood should be determined to ensure that the dose and frequency of administration are appropriate.

In those infants who demonstrate evidence of pulmonary hypertension and right-to-left shunting, nitric oxide inhalation can be very effective. (If nitric oxide is not available, infusion of tolazoline may be used by physicians who have experience with this vasodilator and its complications.) In a few infants, the pulmonary hypertension is so severe and intractable that institution of extracorporeal membrane oxygenation (ECMO) is indicated.

Most infants with pneumonia do well and survive without long-term sequelae. Patients who require prolonged ventilation with high peak inspiratory pressures and high oxygen concentrations may develop chronic lung disease.

CHAPTER 14

Meconium Aspiration Syndrome

Adapted from Ian Gross

Meconium is passed into the amniotic fluid in approximately 10% of all births. Although passage of meconium may be associated with intrauterine fetal hypoxia, it also occurs in normal deliveries in the absence of asphyxia. Meconium aspiration is not seen in premature infants of less than 34 weeks' gestation, as these infants rarely demonstrate meconium-stained amniotic fluid. It is more common in postmature babies.

It is important that infants who are born covered with thick meconium and have not yet cried vigorously should have adequate aspiration of the meconium from their pharynx and trachea immediately after birth.

Meconium that has not been cleared from the trachea migrates peripherally and obstructs the smaller airways. Partial occlusion may result in a one-way valve effect with distal hyperinflation. Alternatively, the small airways may be blocked completely leading to atelectasis. In some infants, persistent pulmonary hypertension develops, which considerably complicates therapy.

Clinical signs of meconium aspiration in infants include respiratory distress and an overdistended chest. Coarse rales may be heard. The chest radiograph reveals hyperinflation of the lungs with patchy infiltrates. Because of the air-trapping effect of meconium in the airways, pneumothorax is common, occurring in 20% to 50% of cases.

Management of these patients is symptomatic. They require oxygen supplementation and, frequently, ventilator therapy. The diffuse small airway obstruction often necessitates the use of high peak inspiratory pressures to maintain adequate ventilation. If conventional ventilator therapy is failing, or if very high airway pressure is required, a trial of high-frequency ventilation is indicated. Some reports have suggested that administration of surfactant to these infants is beneficial. It is possible that there is secondary surfactant deficiency due to hypoxia and acidosis, analogous to the surfactant deficiency in adult RDS, or shock lung. The use of antibiotics is controversial; some neonatologists do not use antibiotics in uncomplicated cases of meconium aspiration, whereas others do because of concern for secondary infection.

CHAPTER 15
Respiratory Distress Syndrome

Adapted from Ian Gross

INCIDENCE

The incidence of respiratory distress syndrome (RDS) varies from country to country throughout the world. It depends on the gestational age of the newborn infant and whether the infant's mother received antenatal glucocorticoid treatment. In general, the incidence of RDS in infants born before 30 weeks' gestation is approximately 60% in infants who have not been exposed to antenatal glucocorticoids and about 35% in infants who have received an adequate course of glucocorticoid therapy. Between 30 and 34 weeks' gestation, the incidence is approximately 25% in untreated or inadequately glucocorticoid-treated infants and approximately 10% in infants who have received a full course of treatment. In premature infants of more than 34 weeks' gestational age, the incidence is approximately 5%, and RDS is rare in full-term infants.

FACTORS MODIFYING THE RISK OF RESPIRATORY DISTRESS SYNDROME OF THE NEWBORN

The factors associated with an increased risk of RDS include prematurity, maternal diabetes (classes A–C), delivery by cesarean section without antecedent labor, perinatal asphyxia, second twin, and history of a previous infant with RDS. The increased incidence of RDS in infants of diabetic mothers may be related to the hyperglycemia, increased ketones, or hyperinsulinemia that occurs during fetal life. Because labor enhances surfactant production, infants born by cesarean section that is not preceded by labor have an increased incidence of RDS. Acute asphyxia with hypoxia and acidosis appears to inhibit surfactant production. The incidence of RDS is higher in a second-born twin, as are a variety of other problems; whether this finding is related to asphyxia is not clear. Finally, there appears to be a familial tendency toward RDS, and a history of a sibling with RDS places a subsequent premature infant at higher risk.

Also, certain conditions decrease the incidence of RDS such as long-term maternal stress (e.g., toxemia, hypertension), intrauterine growth retardation, maternal infection, maternal heroin exposure, and glucocorticoid treatment. Chronic low-grade maternal stress, as opposed to acute asphyxia, accelerates lung maturation by a mechanism that is not entirely clear. It is possible that hormones such as glucocorticoids are involved.

PATHOGENESIS

Current concepts of the pathogenesis of RDS are illustrated in Fig. 15-1. The basic deficit is immaturity of surfactant production and lung structure. This results in a lung that is stiff and prone to atelectasis. Blood continues to perfuse the poorly ventilated areas resulting in a right-to-left shunt and hypoxemia. The hypoxemia, in turn, causes a metabolic acidosis as a result of poor tissue oxygenation. In the presence of hypoxemia and acidosis, the pulmonary arterioles tend to constrict producing increased pressure in the pulmonary circulation. Furthermore, hypoxemia and acidosis inhibits the continued production of surfactant. Alveolar disruption and necrosis also occur resulting in leakage of fluid and fibrin from the pulmonary capillaries into the alveolar space. This fluid and fibrin exudate eventually coalesces to form intraalveolar eosinophilic hyaline membranes characteristic of this disease. If the ductus arteriosus is patent, as it usually is during the first day after birth in premature infants, blood may flow from right to left. If aortic pressure exceeds pulmonary artery pressure, however, flow will be from left to right,

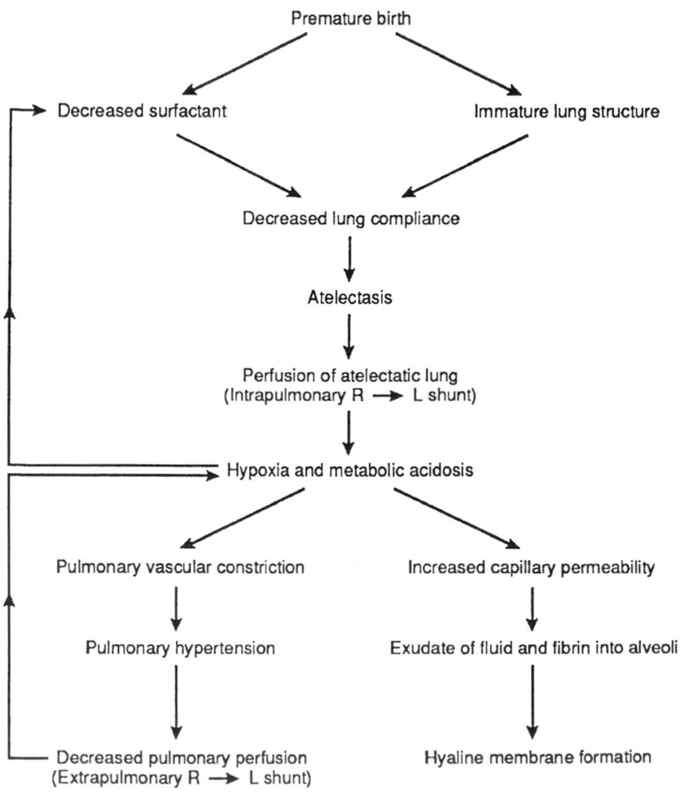

Figure 15-1. The pathogenesis of respiratory distress syndrome of the newborn.

and flooding of the lungs with pulmonary edema may ensue. This complication will further decrease lung compliance.

CLINICAL CHARACTERISTICS

The clinical course of uncomplicated RDS usually follows a fairly consistent pattern. The infant demonstrates signs of respiratory distress that become worse during the first few hours after birth. In some infants, especially those who are extremely immature, the respiratory distress may be severe from the start. The disease then progresses for 48 to 72 hours, reaches a peak, and starts to improve. The onset of recovery is often associated with diuresis. This classic course may not occur, however, in infants with very low birth weights (VLBWs) or those who are very sick. With the use of ventilators and high oxygen concentrations, oxidant or mechanical injury may induce secondary lung damage, and a prolonged respiratory illness may ensue.

Infants with RDS initially have the classic features of respiratory distress in the newborn (i.e., tachypnea, flaring of the nose, retractions of the chest, cyanosis, and grunting). Radiographs taken at approximately 6 hours after birth reveal evidence of diffuse atelectasis and loss of lung volume (Fig. 15-2). The lung fields, which are relatively opaque, have been described as resembling ground glass or being reticulogranular. Because the lung fields are radiodense, the heart border may be obscured. In addition, air within the bronchi stands out in contrast to the lung fields as "air bronchograms" that may extend down to the diaphragm. This radiographic picture, although characteristic of RDS, may also be seen in neonatal pneumonia in premature infants, and it may be impossible to distinguish RDS from pneumonia on radiographic grounds.

The differential diagnosis of RDS includes other causes of respiratory distress in the premature infant. The condition with which it is most likely to be confused is group B streptococcal pneumonia, which may mimic RDS in almost every respect. At times, it may be possible to differentiate these two disorders only retrospectively by reviewing the course and pattern of the illness.

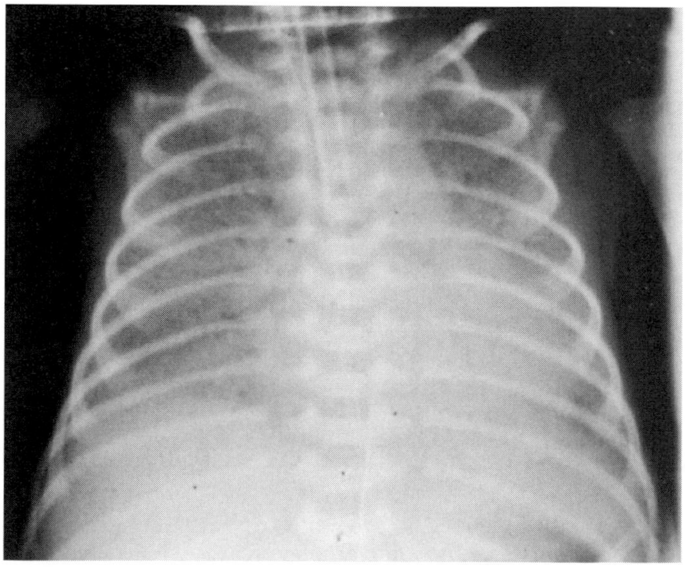

Figure 15-2. Roentgenogram of the chest of an infant with respiratory distress syndrome. Note the diffusely opaque lung fields and the indistinct cardiac outline. Radiolucent "air bronchograms" can also be seen.

MANAGEMENT OF RESPIRATORY DISTRESS SYNDROME OF THE NEWBORN

Respiratory Care

A major role of neonatal intensive care units is providing respiratory care to infants with RDS. The level of intervention required depends on the severity of the respiratory distress. This is determined primarily by the arterial blood gas levels and by the amount of supplemental oxygen that the infant needs to maintain an adequate arterial oxygen tension (P_aO_2). The goal of therapy is to keep the P_aO_2 in the range of 45 to 70 mm Hg, the P_aCO_2 between 35 and 55 mm Hg, and the pH at more than 7.25.

Although P_aO_2 values of 45 to 70 mm Hg are lower than those observed in healthy full-term infants, they are used primarily because premature infants are susceptible to oxygen injury to their eyes (retinopathy of prematurity), and this range is generally thought to be safe. In addition, lower P_aO_2 levels require the administration of lower concentrations of inspired oxygen. High concentrations of inspired oxygen play a role in the pathogenesis of pulmonary oxygen toxicity, which results in bronchopulmonary dysplasia. P_aO_2 levels lower than 35 mm Hg, however, can result in tissue hypoxia and metabolic acidosis. Thus, the P_aO_2 values used are a compromise designed to avoid hypoxia at the low end and oxygen injury to the eyes and lungs at the high end.

The specific indications for, and methods of, respiratory support vary from center to center, but the following guidelines reflect common practice. If the baby requires supplemental oxygen to maintain the P_aO_2 in the 45 to 70 mm Hg range, assisted ventilation is initiated. Depending on the severity of the respiratory distress, this may be by continuous positive airway pressure (CPAP) or intubation and ventilation. If the respiratory distress is judged to be mild (breathing not excessively labored, P_aCO_2 less than 55 mm Hg, inspired oxygen concentration [FIO_2] less than 0.35–0.40, no acidosis) the first step is to deliver CPAP via nasal prongs, which are small catheters inserted into the nostrils and connected to a source of air and O_2. CPAP is generated by partially occluding expiration so that there is a distending pressure within the airways. This promotes oxygenation by increasing the functional residual capacity and preventing alveolar collapse at the end of expiration. If nasal CPAP is inadequate (e.g., if the infant is laboring to breathe, the P_aCO_2 is greater than 60 mm Hg and rising, respiratory acidosis is developing), or if the FIO_2 required is greater than 0.4 to 0.5, the infant is intubated and ventilated via an endotracheal tube. At this stage, surfactant therapy should also be initiated (see later). If the respiratory distress is moderate or severe from the start, the infant is immediately intubated and ventilated, and surfactant is administered soon thereafter.

Because the premature lung is extremely fragile and may be injured by inspired oxygen or pressure from mechanical ventilation, the aim of therapy should be to provide adequate oxygenation by using as gentle a mode of ventilation as possible. Many newborn units, accordingly, will accept a P_aCO_2 in the range of 50 to 55 mm Hg or even higher, as long as the pH is not less than 7.20 to 7.25, rather than increase the peak inspiratory pressure to reduce the P_aCO_2. This approach is known as permissive hypercapnia. There is an increasing tendency to accept blood gas levels that might not be considered optimal in the full-term infant or older child to prevent pressure injury to the lungs.

As the lungs start to recover and compliance improves, usually after 2 to 4 days, respiratory support can be progressively reduced and the infant can be weaned from the ventilator. After extubation, application of CPAP by nasal prongs is often helpful in the transition to unsupported breathing.

The role of high-frequency ventilators (primarily oscillators) in the management of RDS is still being evaluated. These ventilators are believed to work by augmented diffusion and provide an extremely high respiratory rate (e.g., 900–1,200 breaths per minute) with very low tidal volumes. High PEEP settings are used to produce a mean airway pressure that is sufficient to inflate the lungs adequately. Randomized trials have demonstrated that high-frequency oscillation is an effective therapy for infants with pulmonary interstitial emphysema. In addition, many centers will try high-frequency ventilation if conventional therapy is failing. The role of high-frequency ventilation in the routine management of RDS is the subject of ongoing study.

Surfactant Therapy

The successful use of pulmonary surfactant preparations for the prevention or amelioration of RDS represents one of the major advances in neonatal care since the late 1980s. (The composition of surfactant is described in Chapter 38.) Surfactant preparations are generally administered as liquid suspensions that are instilled into the lungs via an endotracheal tube. For this reason, surfactant therapy is confined to infants who are intubated and ventilated. Two approaches to surfactant therapy have evolved. Prevention therapy refers to the administration of surfactant immediately after birth in the delivery area to premature infants at risk for RDS. Rescue or treatment therapy refers to the administration of surfactant to infants with diagnosed RDS; the first dose is usually given within a few hours after birth.

Large, multicenter trials have demonstrated the effectiveness of modified natural and artificial surfactants for the prevention or treatment of RDS. Studies in which up to four doses were administered during the first 48 hours after birth have consistently demonstrated a 30% to 40% reduction in mortality from all causes and an even greater decrease in the rate of death from RDS. This reduction in mortality was observed with both artificial and natural surfactants, whether they were given as prevention or as rescue therapy. Other benefits common to all therapies were a decrease in the amount of ventilator support needed and in the incidence of pulmonary air leaks (interstitial emphysema and pneumothorax). There was also a lower incidence of RDS in the prevention studies. (Rescue therapy is given only to infants with RDS.) A disappointing finding was the absence of a consistent decrease in bronchopulmonary dysplasia in surviving infants. This may be due to increased survival of sicker infants who would be at high risk for this complication.

Subsequent studies have compared the effectiveness of prevention versus rescue therapy. Potential advantages of prevention therapy include better distribution of surfactant in lung fluid that has not yet been absorbed and administration before lung injury from ventilation occurs. Potential disadvantages include the fact that many premature infants do not develop RDS and, therefore, would be treated unnecessarily with an expensive agent; the possibility of treating a baby who is not yet stabilized, which can complicate delivery room resuscitation; and the inability to check endotracheal tube position carefully before therapy is initiated. Studies comparing the two modes of treatment directly have shown that prevention tends to be more effective than rescue for babies of less than 26 weeks' gestation at birth. The benefits were decreased mortality and pneumothorax. Prevention therapy should only be administered to extremely premature infants at high risk of developing RDS by personnel capable of dealing with the complications of such therapy. More mature infants should be stabilized and surfactant therapy initiated as soon as clinical signs of RDS are apparent. In all cases, treatment should be initiated as soon as it is safe and feasible, and many centers now use early post-stabilization treatment for all infants.

Surfactant therapy has been associated with few complications. There has been no consistent impact on the incidence of infection, severe intraventricular hemorrhage, retinopathy of prematurity, patent ductus arteriosus, or necrotizing enterocolitis, although individual studies have reported increases or decreases in some of these conditions. In addition, no evidence suggests the development of antibodies to surfactant proteins in the serum of infants who have received natural surfactant therapy. Long-term follow-up studies have shown benefits in pulmonary function and neurologic status.

Other Aspects of Treatment

Other components of treatment are also important. Body temperature should be maintained by caring for the infant on a radiant warmer or in an incubator. Initially, fluids and calories will have to be provided intravenously, as infants who are breathing rapidly do not tolerate oral or nasogastric feedings. For the first day after birth, the infant may be given an intravenous glucose solution. After that, intravenous amino acid, glucose, and lipid solutions are usually administered. Very immature infants may require more prolonged total parenteral nutrition via a central vein. The fluid volume will depend on the gestational age of the infant and on the type of environment in which the infant is being nursed. Very immature infants, particularly those who are managed on radiant warmers, may require large fluid volumes.

Antibiotics are generally administered, not because RDS is an infectious condition or to prophylactically cover invasive procedures such as catheters, but because, in many cases, pneumonia cannot be excluded or signs of maternal infection are evident.

Sodium bicarbonate should be used sparingly. Overuse carries the risk of inducing hypernatremia and may precipitate an intraventricular hemorrhage, particularly if it is given in bolus form. Acidosis should be treated initially by optimizing ventilation. A persistent metabolic acidosis with a pH of less than 7.20 can be treated with a slow, dilute bicarbonate infusion of 1 to 2 mEq/kg. Persistent acidosis is also an indication to assess general perfusion and to determine if a significant patent ductus arteriosus is present. The latter should be treated by indomethacin therapy or by surgical ligation if indomethacin is not effective.

COMPLICATIONS

The major complications of RDS are related to therapy. Air leak is caused by increased airway pressure from ventilation or CPAP. Chronic lung disease (bronchopulmonary dysplasia) is believed to result from injury to the lungs by oxygen and ventilator pressure. The fragile lung of the extremely premature infant is particularly susceptible to injury, so the incidence of bronchopulmonary dysplasia is greatly increased in infants with birth weights of less than 1,250 g. Bronchopulmonary dysplasia is reviewed in Chapter 16. Catheter complications arise from the insertion of a catheter into the aorta, which can result in thromboembolic complications such as hypertension due to renal arterial thrombosis, necrotizing enterocolitis, and infarction of other organs. Additionally, an increased incidence of intraventricular hemorrhage is seen in infants with RDS. The mechanism may be related to intravascular pressure swings. Because RDS occurs in premature infants who are treated with oxygen, they are at particular risk for retinopathy of prematurity. Like bronchopulmonary dysplasia, this complication occurs mainly in infants with birth weights of less than 1,250 g.

PREVENTION OF RESPIRATORY DISTRESS SYNDROME OF THE NEWBORN

Three approaches are possible in the prevention of RDS in premature infants: antenatal prediction of fetal lung maturity, pharmacologic acceleration of fetal lung development, and prevention therapy with surfactant (see previous discussion). The best approach is prevention of prematurity itself.

Antenatal Prediction of Fetal Lung Maturity

The fetal lung secretes surfactant into the amniotic fluid. Examination of the amniotic fluid can reveal whether the lung is synthesizing surfactant-associated phospholipids in quantities sufficient to support respiration. This is done most commonly by measuring the lecithin-sphingomyelin (LS) ratio and by determining whether phosphatidylglycerol (PG), another surfactant-related phospholipid, is detectable. Lecithin (or phosphatidylcholine) is the most abundant component of surfactant, and the lecithin in amniotic fluid is derived from the fetal lung, whereas the sphingomyelin is derived from nonpulmonary sources. As the lung matures, the LS ratio increases. When this ratio is greater than 2, the fetal lungs are almost invariably mature; a ratio of 1.5 to 2.0 is indeterminate; and a value of less than 1.5 predicts immaturity. The test errs on the side of overpredicting immaturity. If there is no PG in the amniotic fluid and the LS ratio is less than 1.5, an obstetrician considering an elective delivery may decide to delay until such time as the lung is mature.

Measurement of surfactant-specific proteins (SP; particularly SP-A) in the amniotic fluid has been used experimentally to evaluate lung maturity and appears to be a good indicator. Rapid and relatively simple enzyme linked immunosorbent assays may increase the clinical use of this test in the future. Determination of gestational age by ultrasound measurements such as the biparietal diameter of the head, are also useful for preventing inadvertent early elective delivery with the associated risk of RDS.

Pharmacologic Acceleration of Fetal Lung Maturation

Fetal lung development is known to be controlled by multiple factors. Agents that have been demonstrated to enhance lung maturation include glucocorticoids, thyroid hormones, growth factors (such as epidermal growth factor), transcription factors (such as thyroid transcription factor), and cyclic adenosine monophosphate. Most of this information has come from animal studies, but a substantial body of evidence indicates that glucocorticoids accelerate lung maturation in humans, and these agents have been used clinically since the 1970s for this purpose. Because glucocorticoids act by enhancing RNA transcription and protein synthesis, which is a process that takes time, they are most effective if the infant is delivered more than 24 hours after the initial dose. The benefits of glucocorticoids decrease if the infant is not delivered within 7 days.

When they are administered appropriately, antenatal glucocorticoids reduce the incidence of RDS by approximately 50%. Other clinically important benefits of antenatal glucocorticoid therapy include decreased early neonatal deaths, intraventricular bleeds, necrotizing enterocolitis, and a tendency to better neurologic outcome at follow-up.

It is recommended that antenatal steroids should be used in all cases of threatened premature labor before 34 weeks' gestation, if immediate delivery is not anticipated and there is evidence of pulmonary immaturity, or pulmonary maturity is unknown. The usual regimen is to administer betamethasone or dexamethasone, glucocorticoids that cross the placenta readily, for a period of 48 hours. If the infant is not delivered within 7 days, another course of glucocorticoids may be necessary if threatened premature labor occurs again.

CHAPTER 16
Bronchopulmonary Dysplasia

Adapted from Kathleen A. Kennedy and Joseph B. Warshaw

Most neonates with acute lung disease recover completely within the first week of life. Some of these infants, however, develop chronic respiratory disease characterized by tachypnea, dyspnea, hypoxemia, and hypercarbia. In 1967, Northway and colleagues first described the clinical, radiologic, and pathologic manifestations of chronic lung disease in survivors of hyaline membrane disease (HMD) and introduced the term *bronchopulmonary dysplasia* (BPD). These authors postulated that the disease was caused by oxygen toxicity and ventilator-induced barotrauma superimposed on the healing infant lung. As neonatal intensive care has become more sophisticated, the survival of very low-birth-weight (VLBW) infants has increased dramatically, and chronic lung disease is now seen in very small infants who did not have HMD. Although the birth weight-specific incidence of BPD seems to have remained fairly stable with increasing survival rates, the result of this increased survival is an increase in the absolute numbers of survivors with BPD. The effect of BPD in the population is difficult to determine because the incidence varies according to the definition used and the population studied. In a population-based study from New Zealand, chronic lung disease (CLD), defined as an oxygen requirement at 28 days' postnatal age or 36 weeks' postmenstrual age, occurred in 39% and 23% of 500- to 1,499-g survivors, respectively. In a retrospective study of 1,625 infants with birth weights between 700 and 1,500 g treated in eight major medical centers in the United States, the incidence of CLD, defined as an oxygen requirement at 28 days of age, ranged from 6% to 33% in the different medical centers. Within the entire study population, lower birth weight, white race, and male gender were identified as risk factors for the development of CLD, but differences in patient populations did not account fully for the discrepancies in the incidence of CLD among the different medical centers. Although these observations suggest that certain aspects of patient management may alter the risk for CLD, no single cause or preventive measure is likely to be identified for this complex disease process.

DIAGNOSIS

The diagnosis of BPD is suspected when a neonate with acute lung disease fails to follow the anticipated course of resolution or has a gradual increase in oxygen and ventilator requirements during the first month of life. In 1979, Bancalari et al. characterized the disease as tachypnea, retractions, and supplemental oxygen requirement for more than 28 days in infants who had received positive-pressure ventilation for at least 3 days in the first week of life. Associated chest radiographic findings included strand-like densities in both lung fields alternating with areas of normal or increased lucency. The diagnosis of BPD must be made on the basis of both clinical and radiographic characteristics. No specific tests exist that can be used to confirm the diagnosis. The diagnosis of CLD has usually been defined on the basis of clinical criteria only. The distinction between unresolved acute lung disease and CLD persisting until 28 days of age is arbitrary, based, in part, on the likelihood that pulmonary dysfunction that persists for at least 4 weeks will be associated with increased long-term morbidity and mortality. The distinction can be problematic when considering therapeutic modalities begun at 1 to 3 weeks of age in infants with pulmonary dysfunction or when classifying deaths from respiratory failure at 1 to 4 weeks of age. A more stringent diagnostic criterion for CLD, oxygen therapy at 36 weeks' corrected postnatal gestational age, has been recommended because this definition has been shown to be a more specific predictor of long-term pulmonary morbidity in VLBW infants.

Cystic fibrosis and $alpha_1$-antitrypsin deficiency rarely cause pulmonary symptoms in the first weeks of life. Neonates with these genetic disorders, who also have acute lung injury shortly after birth, may subsequently experience slowly progressive CLD, however. Sweat chloride analysis, genetic screening, or determination of serum $alpha_1$-antitrypsin levels is required to distinguish these disorders from BPD. These evaluations should be considered for infants with progressively worsening CLD.

Patent ductus arteriosus commonly presents during the resolution of HMD in very premature infants. At this stage, increased pulmonary blood flow from a patent ductus can cause prolonged oxygen and ventilator requirements similar to the clinical course observed in infants with evolving BPD. The diagnosis and hemodynamic significance of a patent ductus arteriosus can usually be determined by physical examination and echocardiography.

Viral pneumonia acquired in the early neonatal period can cause progressive hypoxemia and respiratory failure. The diagnosis can be confirmed with nasopharyngeal viral cultures or urine culture for cytomegalovirus.

COMPLICATIONS

Pulmonary hypertension and cor pulmonale can result from many forms of chronic pulmonary disease including BPD. Mortality is high in infants with severe BPD and cor pulmonale, so therapeutic endeavors should be directed toward preventing the development of cor pulmonale. Pulmonary arterial pressure can be decreased by increasing oxygen administration in infants with BPD.

Infants with BPD have an increased susceptibility to severe bacterial and viral pneumonia. In the first year after hospital discharge, many infants with BPD are readmitted for pulmonary exacerbations. Respiratory syncytial virus and pertussis infections can be fatal in infants with BPD.

Congestive heart failure with pulmonary and systemic venous congestion frequently complicates the treatment of infants with BPD. The etiology of left-sided heart failure in infants with BPD is uncertain. Fluid tolerance varies greatly and must be determined on an individual basis.

MANAGEMENT

Although exposure to high concentrations of oxygen is thought to be a contributing factor in the pathogenesis of BPD, chronic administration of oxygen is one of the most important aspects in the management of CLD in infants. Maintaining a P_aO_2 greater than 60 mm Hg or an O_2 saturation greater than 90% should reduce the risk of cor pulmonale from chronic hypoxemia. Many infants have decreased oxygenation during sleep and feedings and may require additional oxygen therapy during these times.

Pulmonary and systemic edema develop in many infants with BPD when excessive parenteral fluid is administered, and chronic fluid restriction has become almost routine in the management of infants with BPD. Because respiratory infection or hypoxemia predisposes the infants to pulmonary edema, isolated episodes of pulmonary edema do not necessarily warrant chronic restriction of enteral fluid intake. Fluid given enterally is generally tolerated better than fluid given parenterally. This observation suggests that passive absorption of fluid from the gastrointestinal tract is controlled by osmotic forces. Modest fluid (140–160 mL/kg/day) and sodium (2–3 mEq/kg/day) restriction may decrease oxygen requirements and respiratory work in these infants. Severe fluid restriction at the expense of adequate nutrition is not indicated.

Although diuretic therapy is used commonly in infants with BPD, the diuretic and nondiuretic cardiopulmonary effects of chronic diuretic therapy in these infants have not been explored fully. Diuretic therapy may allow for increased fluid administration, and diuretic agents have been shown to improve pulmonary mechanics in infants with BPD. Long-term benefits of diuretic therapy in these infants are uncertain. The efficacy of furosemide versus thiazide diuretics in infants with BPD is unknown, and careful attention must be given to electrolyte balance when diuretics are used in these infants. Replacement of potassium and chloride may be necessary to prevent metabolic alkalosis and hypoventilation during diuretic therapy. Sodium supplementation enhances fluid retention and defeats the purpose of diuretic therapy. Calcium wasting may exacerbate osteopenia of prematurity in infants treated with diuretics.

Infants with BPD have increased airway resistance and increased work of breathing compared with age-matched control infants. Some of these infants have bronchial hyperreactivity that responds favorably to bronchodilator therapy with theophylline or beta-adrenergic agonists. Response to bronchodilator therapy has been demonstrated in infants as young as 2 weeks' postnatal age.

Adequate nutrition is necessary for lung growth and repair, but meeting nutritional needs is often a challenge in infants with BPD. Infants with BPD have tachypnea and increased respiratory effort, and they may require more calories for adequate growth than do infants without respiratory disease. The caloric needs of an individual infant should be determined by the intake required to achieve a sustained weight gain of at least 10 g/kg/day. Some infants may require as much as 150 kcal/kg/day. If oral or nasogastric feedings are not tolerated, prolonged peripheral parenteral nutrition rarely provides adequate calories and central parenteral nutrition should be considered. Supplemented formulas can be used to increase caloric intake in infants who cannot tolerate increased feeding volumes because of congestive heart failure or gastroesophageal reflux. Respiratory infections should be prevented, if possible, by avoiding exposure of the infant to other patients, hospital personnel, and family members with viral symptoms. When viral respiratory infections occur in infants with BPD, requirements for oxygen, bronchodilator therapy, and diuretics are often increased for at least 1 week. If respiratory failure develops, requiring the reinstitution of ventilator therapy, the mortality is high and recovery may be very prolonged.

SECTION

D

Cardiovascular System

CHAPTER 17

Critical Cardiac Disease in Infants

Adapted from Norman S. Talner and Craig E. Fleishman

Life-threatening cardiac disease in newborn infants occurs in some 3 in 1,000 live births. Ventricular septal defects, patent ductus arteriosus, transposition of the great arteries, tetralogy of Fallot, hypoplastic right-heart syndrome (tricuspid and pulmonary atresia), critical pulmonary stenosis with right-to-left atrial shunting, hypoplastic left-heart syndrome, and coarctation of the aorta account for a majority of the lesions. When these lesions are classified on the basis of their fundamental physiologic disturbance, they fall into three major categories. These include hypoxemia (transposition, tetralogy, hypoplastic right-heart syndrome, and critical pulmonic stenosis), impaired systemic perfusion (hypoplastic left-heart syndrome, coarctation), and the large-volume left-to-right shunt (ventricular septal defect, patent ductus arteriosus). Additional life-threatening situations of importance in the differential diagnosis of these conditions include common mixing lesions (single ventricle, common atrium, truncus arteriosus), anomalies of pulmonary venous return, and persistent pulmonary hypertension.

SPECIAL PROBLEMS IN MANAGEMENT

Congestive Heart Failure

Congestive heart failure in fetuses is manifest as hydrops fetalis. This condition can arise from regurgitant lesions of the right-sided AV or semilunar valves, large systemic arteriovenous fistulas, myocardial disease, severe anemia, and prolonged tachyarrhythmias. Systemic venous congestion from the elevated right-sided filling pressures and volumes results in hepatomegaly and the accumulation of fluid in serous cavities and may progress to generalized anasarca. Although the overall prognosis for survival is poor when hydrops develops, some infants have been salvaged by transplacental therapy for life-threatening cardiac arrhythmias with digoxin, propranolol, or procainamide. Intrauterine transfusions have also improved the hemodynamic status of fetuses with severe hemolytic disease. In preterm infants, particularly those with birth weights of less than 1,500 g, patency of the ductus arteriosus can produce the clinical picture of congestive heart failure and complicate treatment of the respiratory distress syndrome. The classic clinical findings (bounding arterial pulsations, continuous murmur) may be absent in such infants, and diagnosis may rest on Doppler-derived flow velocity determinations demonstrating left-to-right shunting via the ductus into the pulmonary artery. Management of the problem in such infants consists of the intravenous administration of indomethacin, which inhibits prostaglandin synthesis, if platelet counts are adequate and renal function is intact. In instances in which a course of indomethacin therapy does not produce ductal closure, surgical ligation is necessary.

When congestive heart failure accompanies an acute low-perfusion state (coarctation, hypoplastic left heart) in which systemic blood flow depends on continued patency of the ductus arteriosus, the administration of PGE1, which will dilate the ductus arteriosus, may restore tissue perfusion. Restoration of systemic perfusion is the key. In addition to PGE1, this clinical state requires a titratable inotropic agent such as dopamine or dobutamine, to support myocardial function.

Congestive heart failure is encountered most frequently in infants with large-volume left-to-right shunts (ventricular septal defects, AV canal defects, patent ductus arteriosus). Treatment of such infants requires interventions to lessen pulmonary and systemic venous congestion, while attempts are made to improve systemic blood flow to allow for body growth. Furosemide is the diuretic agent used most widely to promote salt and water loss, and it may be required two to three times a day in the management of severe pulmonary edema. Spironolactone is a valuable adjunct to diuretic therapy, as it tends to reduce potassium loss. Serum electrolyte levels must be monitored when the loop diuretics are used on a frequent basis.

The use of cardiac glycosides in the treatment of the high-output congestive heart failure that accompanies a large-volume left-to-right shunt is somewhat controversial. The need for an inotropic agent has been challenged because myocardial contractility is not impaired. Nevertheless, more than 50% of affected infants appear to improve clinically. This improvement may be explained on the basis of withdrawal of adrenergic support, thus decreasing oxygen demands. Supporting this hypothesis is the fall in oxygen consumption seen in some patients with a favorable clinical response to cardiac glycosides, along with a decrease in the levels of circulating catecholamines. Vasodilator therapy has also been introduced into the management schema for infants with large ventricular or AV septal defects and dilated congestive cardiomyopathies. With vasodilatation and a lessening of left ventricular afterload, the left-to-right shunt, if present, may diminish, whereas systemic blood flow increases. Vasodilators in clinical use include sodium nitroprusside for intravenous use and angiotensin-converting enzyme inhibitors that may be used orally. Supportive measures for these infants include oxygen administration, maintenance of a semiupright position, correction of relative anemia, intravenous hyperalimentation and, possibly, the use of a ventilator if respiratory failure is present. A poor clinical response, however, warrants early surgical repair of the defect.

Infants with a dilated cardiomyopathy should be evaluated for the presence of carnitine deficiency (serum, skeletal muscle), as replacement therapy with l-carnitine may be lifesaving by restoring myocardial oxidative function. In other situations, the ultimate management may be heart transplantation.

Persistent Pulmonary Hypertension

Elevation of pulmonary artery pressures and an increase in pulmonary vascular resistance can complicate the management of some of the clinical problems encountered during the newborn period. Persistent pulmonary hypertension may occur rarely as a primary abnormality of the pulmonary vascular bed or may be seen accompanying pulmonary disorders (infections, lung hypoplasia, respiratory distress syndrome), diaphragmatic hernias, and certain congenital and acquired cardiac diseases such as large-volume left-to-right shunts, anomalies of pulmonary venous return with pulmonary venous obstruction, and cardiomyopathies. What has become apparent is that chronic intrauterine asphyxia can produce structural alterations in the pulmonary vascular bed, which may result in significant postnatal problems in oxygenation caused by a restricted pulmonary circulation and persistent right-to-left shunting via fetal flow channels. Meconium aspiration at delivery may be the only terminal event in a more chronic intrauterine asphyxial state.

The treatment of affected infants rests on establishing the underlying diagnosis and using therapeutic strategies aimed at increasing oxygen transport, improving ventilatory function, preserving or augmenting cardiac output, and attempting interventions that may lower pulmonary vascular resistance (decreasing blood viscosity, diminishing ventricular filling pressure, surgically relieving pulmonary venous obstruction, and producing vasodilatation).

A rational approach to diagnosis and management in such patients includes determination of the arterial blood gas tensions and pH level to define the degree of hypoxemia and the ventilatory status. Next, clinicians should assess the presence or absence of respiratory distress (retractions, grunting, alar flaring, and use of the accessory muscles of respiration). Usually, ventilatory support is required if severe hypoxemia dominates the clinical picture; this condition can be assessed best with an indwelling arterial line (umbilical artery) and simultaneous sampling of arterial blood for P_aO_2 from this site and the right radial artery with as little disturbance of the infant as possible. Pulse oximetry offers a noninvasive alternative to this approach. When the descending aortic saturation is less than the right radial saturation, right-to-left ductal shunting is present, and pulmonary vascular resistance has to exceed systemic vascular resistance. The pH and PCO_2 values also aid in patient evaluation. Elevation of P_aCO_2 suggests significant compromise of ventilatory function. A metabolic acidemia can be associated with a low P_aO_2 (less than 35 mm Hg) or with decreased systemic perfusion and relatively normal P_aO_2 values. If the descending aortic and right arm saturation tensions are equal, the ductus could still be shunting, but this condition is masked by right-to-left shunts at more proximal sites such as the foramen ovale and lungs.

The state of perfusion must also be checked by palpation of the peripheral arterial pulses, capillary refill, and skin temperature. If perfusion is compromised, management must include provision of volume and inotropic support to restore perfusion of regional circulations. If perfusion and ventilation are not compromised, the clinician can proceed directly to determination of the site of right-to-left shunting.

The hyperoxia test (response to FiO_2, 1.0) has been touted as a way to separate a cardiac problem from one involving the lungs or pulmonary circulation. However, interpretation of an increase in PO_2 or oxygen saturation is subject to error. Impressive increments have been observed in the face of cardiac disease and little or no response in association with severe lung disease. Therefore, we recommend that part of the assessment, before vasodilator therapy is instituted, include echocardiography performed by a cardiologist experienced in the evaluation of critically ill newborns. A chest film focused on heart size, lung vascularity, and other malformations (e.g., diaphragmatic hernia) is useful as part of the clinical evaluation. An ECG examined for evidence of myocardial ischemia (ST-T wave changes) and myocardial enzyme levels can also aid in establishing a specific diagnosis.

Treatment of affected patients is based on approaches aimed at raising arterial oxygen content and tension. The latter are functions of the following variables: pulmonary capillary oxygen content, cardiac output, the right-to-left shunt, and oxygen extraction. Each of these is capable of being manipulated given that a change in one of these factors may influence one of the other variables. For example, increasing P_aO_2 by positive-pressure ventilation may impede venous return and diminish cardiac output. On the other hand, raising cardiac output (e.g., with inotropic agents) may increase metabolic demands and intrapulmonary right-to-left shunting.

Raising the inspired oxygen concentration may have a number of beneficial effects. An increase in dissolved oxygen permits nearly a 10% rise in oxygen saturation, even in the face of a fixed right-to-left shunt. Furthermore, oxygen is capable of dilating constricted pulmonary resistance vessels. The only situation in which oxygen administration may be deleterious is one exhibiting duct-dependent systemic blood flow (see Low-Perfusion States). This disorder will not take place in such conditions as pulmonary atresia, however, in which duct-dependent pulmonary perfusion occurs because pulmonary flow is limited, and oxygen saturation will rise only minimally; it's not enough to compromise the caliber of the ductus.

The hematocrit is another factor that can alter the response of the pulmonary vascular bed by its effect on blood viscosity. Hyperviscosity of more than 65% (a hematocrit of greater than 65%) will raise pulmonary vascular resistance and increase right-to-left shunting. A low hematocrit, on the other hand, limits its oxygen-carrying capacity. Therefore, keeping the hematocrit in the range of 40% to 50% is appropriate. The provision of ventilatory support can lower an elevated P_aCO_2 to normal or low levels, whereas areas of alveolar collapse may be inflated, thereby raising the level of P_aO_2. If the potential deleterious effects of positive-pressure breathing on cardiac output are taken into consideration and various ventilatory maneuvers are tried while P_aO_2 and P_aCO_2 are monitored, an increase in P_aO_2 can be achieved while circulatory function is maintained.

Provision of an adequate cardiac output is essential in the treatment of patients with severe hypoxemia. Usually, hypoxemia can be tolerated, at least for short periods of time, if cardiac output is maintained, as in the case of infants with congenital heart disease. The combination of low cardiac output and hypoxemia, however, cannot be tolerated.

Cardiac output can be increased by volume infusions of whole blood, if blood loss is a problem, or infusions of electrolyte or albumin solutions when hemoglobin does not have to be replaced. If contractility is decreased, as assessed through echocardiographic evaluation, an inotropic agent such as dopamine or dobutamine, should be administered. These have primarily $beta_1$

receptor function (increased contractility and vasodilation) and cause little change in heart rate.

Vasodilators have been used widely in the treatment of infants with persistent pulmonary hypertension with varying degrees of success. The major risk of such therapy relates to the possibility of producing systemic hypotension, thereby worsening the clinical picture. Furthermore, its injudicious use in patients whose hypoxemia is on a cardiac basis (duct-dependent pulmonary blood flow) can induce further right-to-left shunting and worsen the metabolic status.

Reduction in right-to-left shunt flow may be achieved by improving ventilation, particularly in those with impaired ventilation and stiff lungs. Oxygen extraction may be decreased by diminishing oxygen demands or by lessening the work of breathing and decreasing overall metabolic demands.

Conservative management consisting of some (but not a marked degree of) hyperventilation, provision of adequate volume, support of the myocardium, and increased inspired oxygen concentrations appears to result in reasonable survival data. Extracorporeal membrane oxygenation has also yielded encouraging results, but this approach is expensive, requires specialized personnel, and has raised concern relative to the long-term central nervous system effects of ligation of a carotid artery, which is required for the procedure. The introduction of inhaled nitric oxide (NO), a potent vasodilator, offers a novel approach to disorders of the pulmonary circulation. Experience has been gained on the acute effects of inhalational NO (endothelial relaxing factor) in term neonates with severe persistent pulmonary hypertension. Endothelial-derived NO modulates pulmonary vascular smooth-muscle tone in experimental animal models of pulmonary hypertension and appears to influence the postnatal decline in pulmonary vascular resistance. Inhaled NO diffuses from the alveolar space to pulmonary vascular smooth muscle, stimulates cyclic guanosine monophosphate production, and induces vasodilation. NO does bind to hemoglobin forming methemoglobin that is then excreted as urinary nitrite. Successful use of NO offers the possibility of avoiding or, at least limiting, the use of extracorporeal membrane oxygenation lessening the requirements for high oxygen concentrations and airway pressures and, thus, lowering the risk of acute and chronic lung injury.

SECTION

E

Gastrointestinal System

CHAPTER 18

Sucking and Swallowing Disorders and Gastroesophageal Reflux

Adapted from Colston F. McEvoy

SUCKING AND SWALLOWING

Pharyngeal swallowing is observed as early as 10 to 11 weeks' gestation and suckling is seen at 18 to 24 weeks. Late-term fetuses swallow amniotic fluid at a rate equal to that of fetal urination. Interruptions in fetal ingestion of amniotic fluid due to gastrointestinal tract obstruction or neurologic abnormalities can upset this balance and result in polyhydramnios. In premature infants, a mature sucking pattern sufficient to support total oral intake of calories is usually not achieved until 34 weeks' gestation. Coordination of sucking, swallowing, and breathing is a prerequisite to successful oral feeding.

The causes of dysfunctional sucking and swallowing are varied (Table 18-1) and often result in poor growth due to inadequate oral intake and respiratory complications from aspiration. Neuromuscular disease, usually characterized by hypotonia, may cause diminished suck or discoordinated swallow. Structural anomalies or lesions of the mouth, pharynx, or larynx often interfere with the mechanics of sucking and swallowing. At the level of the esophagus, congenital abnormalities, stricture, mucosal inflammation, or extrinsic compression may result in swallowing difficulty.

Achalasia is a motility disorder of the esophagus characterized by a functional obstruction of the gastroesophageal junction. The estimated incidence in the general population is 1 in 100,000 per year; however, only 5% of cases occur in children younger than 5 years. Achalasia can occur in families, although the mode of inheritance is unclear. Children often present with vomiting, regurgitation, or dysphagia. The vomiting frequently begins with solids and progresses to liquids as well. Children, thus affected, may also have recurrent pulmonary infections and failure to thrive. An upper gastrointestinal examination may suggest the diagnosis by showing a characteristic "beaking" or tapering of the distal esophagus with varying degrees of esophageal dilation. The diagnosis is made by manometry, which shows abnormal relaxation of the lower esophageal sphincter, absent peristalsis, and elevated intraesophageal pressure. Treatment of achalasia consists of either balloon dilation or a surgical myotomy of the lower esophageal sphincter muscles.

TABLE 18-1. Causes of Abnormal Sucking and Swallowing in the Newborn Period (Birth to 28 Days)

Structural anomalies
General
Micrognathia
Cleft palate
Macroglossia
Ranula
Lingual hygroma
Lingual hemangioma
Lingual thyroid
Dermoid cyst (lingual)
Choanal atresia or stenosis
Pharyngeal cyst
Laryngeal cleft
Esophageal anomalies
Syndromes
Pierre-Robin
Trisomy 21
Trisomies 13–15
Congenital hypothyroidism
Glycogen storage disease, type II
Neurologic
Congenital
Möbius syndrome
Werdnig-Hoffmann disease
Neonatal myasthenia gravis
Familial dysautonomia
Acquired
Birth asphyxia
Bulbar palsy
Palatal paralysis
Cricopharyngeal achalasia
Recurrent laryngeal nerve paralysis
Botulism
Kernicterus
Tetanus neonatorum
Sedation
Muscular
Congenital
Benign congenital hypotonia
Myotonic dystrophy
Muscular dystrophy
Amyotonia congenita
Acquired
Hypocalcemia
Hypomagnesemia
Hypokalemia
Hypophosphatemia

Modified from Gyboski J, Walker WA, eds. *Gastrointestinal problems in the infant*, 2nd ed. Philadelphia: Saunders, 1983.

GASTROESOPHAGEAL REFLUX

Gastroesophageal reflux (GER) is defined as the spontaneous regurgitation of gastric contents into the esophagus. This process occurs physiologically in young infants, the majority of whom have mild symptoms that resolve with age. GER is pathologic (GER disease) in infants who experience complications or in older children and adults. The proposed mechanisms for physiologic reflux include increased transient relaxations of the lower esophageal sphincter (LES), delayed gastric emptying, and an intraabdominal-LES pressure differential. In addition to these factors, lower basal LES tone and esophageal dysmotility may contribute to pathologic reflux.

The typical clinical presentation of the infant with uncomplicated GER is a "happy spitter" who effortlessly brings up small amounts of milk after feedings but grows well. This usually begins in the first few weeks of life and resolves by 9 to 24 months. GER is fairly common in premature infants, especially those with respiratory disease. In infants with more significant regurgitation or frank vomiting, other etiologies such as obstruction, infection, and metabolic or neurologic disease should be ruled out before the diagnosis of GER is made. Older children and adolescents with GER disease present less frequently with vomiting. Commonly, they complain of heartburn, regurgitation, and acid taste. Infants and children with neurologic impairment have a high incidence of chronic reflux, which often results in complications.

Esophagitis is a complication of GER that, when severe, can lead to bleeding and anemia, stricture formation, or metaplasia (Barrett's esophagus). Infants with esophagitis present with feeding refusal or irritability and arching with feedings. Older children report pain or feeling as though food gets stuck when swallowing. The inflammation of the esophageal mucosa is the result of injury from chronic gastric acid exposure and causes further esophageal dysmotility, thereby exacerbating the regurgitation or vomiting. Significant reflux can cause failure to thrive in infants who do not retain enough formula to meet their caloric needs or limit their intake secondary to discomfort. Perhaps one of the most worrisome complications of reflux is its association with respiratory disease. Clearly, some infants aspirate gastric contents during an episode of reflux. Usually, these children have underlying neurologic disease that compromises their ability to protect their airway. In addition, these neurologically impaired children may aspirate oral contents owing to an uncoordinated swallowing mechanism. Subclinical reflux may be the cause of refractory asthma or repeated episodes of pneumonia in some children. Conversely, the coughing associated with chronic respiratory disease such as asthma or cystic fibrosis, may induce reflux by increasing intraabdominal pressure above that of the LES. Apnea or apparent life-threatening events in infants have been associated with GER, although proving a cause-and-effect relationship is very difficult. Other conditions attributed to GER include recurrent otalgia, dental caries, and Sandifer syndrome, a posturing with the head tilted or twisted.

In most infants, the diagnosis of GER can be made on the basis of clinical history and findings. For significant vomiting, a barium study of the upper gastrointestinal tract can rule out obstruction, hiatal hernia, or esophageal stricture. This radiologic test is not an accurate assessment of reflux, which can be missed or iatrogenically provoked in an upset child. The gold-standard diagnostic test is continuous esophageal pH monitoring to detect the presence of gastric acid in the normally neutral distal esophageal lumen. It enables measurement of the frequency and duration of reflux episodes. This study is most helpful in diagnosing occult GER in patients who present with possible complications or to correlate reflux episodes with certain symptoms. To determine the relationship of reflux with apnea, a pH study is best performed as part of a multichannel pneumocardiography test. Reflux esophagitis is diagnosed by endoscopy with biopsy. The esophageal mucosa may appear endoscopically normal in mild to moderate esophagitis, but characteristic histologic findings are diagnostic.

Treatment of reflux is conservative in most uncomplicated cases and consists of postural management and modification of feedings. A head-elevated, prone position has been shown to decrease reflux in infants. Studies have shown that the traditional reflux therapy of placement in an infant seat is detrimental rather than beneficial. Thickening of the feedings and giving smaller volumes may reduce clinical symptoms of GER. Some infants, particularly those with a family history of atopy, may have exacerbated symptoms due to a cow's-milk or soy-protein intolerance and will benefit from a switch to a protein hydrolysate formula or from placing the breast-feeding mother on a restricted diet. A continuous infusion of formula through a nasogastric, gastrostomy, or jejunal tube may be beneficial in treating poor weight gain resulting from severe reflux. Pharmacologic therapy is aimed at acid reduction to treat or prevent peptic esophagitis and at enhancement of gastric emptying and LES tone with a prokinetic agent. Depending on the severity of GER disease, acid suppression can be achieved with antacids given an hour before and after feedings, an H_2 antagonist, or a proton pump inhibitor. Metaclopramide is a prokinetic agent used to treat GER in pediatric patients. It is associated with side effects of sedation and occasionally extrapyramidal reactions. Surgical therapy is reserved for severe reflux disease that is refractory to medical management or has life-threatening complications such as aspiration pneumonia. This procedure, the most common of which is the Nissen fundoplication, involves wrapping the gastric fundus around the distal esophagus to prevent reflux and has its complications (e.g., gas-bloat, retching, dumping syndrome, breakdown of the wrap, herniation into the thorax, or obstruction secondary to adhesions).

CHAPTER 19
Necrotizing Enterocolitis

Adapted from Kathleen J. Motil

Necrotizing enterocolitis (NEC) is a common gastrointestinal emergency in neonatal intensive care units. A classification scheme divides NEC into an idiopathic variety (both sporadic and epidemic), a variety that is associated with precipitating factors such as administration of hypertonic agents into the GI tract (for example, drugs and certain nutritional formulas), and a type associated with GI pathology such as intestinal obstruction.

The overall incidence of necrotizing enterocolitis is 2.4 in 1,000 live births or 2.1% of all admissions to neonatal intensive care units. The incidence of necrotizing enterocolitis averages 3% to 4% in infants whose birth weight is less than 2,000 g and decreases significantly to 1% in infants whose birth weight is greater than 2,000 g. Both genders are affected equally.

ETIOLOGY AND PATHOGENESIS

The etiology of idiopathic necrotizing enterocolitis is unknown but is probably mulitfactorial. The features most commonly implicated are ischemic insult to the gastrointestinal tract, the presence of bacterial or viral organisms in the tract, the availability of intraluminal substrate (usually formula or human milk) to promote bacterial proliferation or induce mucosal injury, and altered host defense. Other factors such as inflammatory mediators (cytokines), oxygen radicals, and bacterial fermentation products and toxins are thought to propagate the disease process.

Ischemia possibly contributes to the pathogenesis of necrotizing enterocolitis in the human infant. The regulation of mesenteric blood flow to the gastrointestinal tract in infants is thought to mimic the "diving reflex" in aquatic animals. During hypoxic conditions, the brain and heart are protected from ischemic damage by shunting blood away from the mesenteric, renal, and peripheral vascular beds causing possible ischemic damage in these compromised areas. With resuscitation, perfusion rebounds, leading to vascular congestion and mucosal hemorrhages secondary to ischemic injury to the blood vessels. Many perinatal events such as birth asphyxia, respiratory distress syndrome, apnea, and patent ductus arteriosus predispose the neonate to hypoxia. The theory of hypoxic/ischemic injury to the GI tract is not adequate to fully explain the pathogenesis of NEC because some infants with no evidence of these risk factors have the disorder.

The intestinal microflora provide an additional component in the development of ischemic necrosis of the intestinal tract. However, the role of gastrointestinal microorganisms in the pathogenesis of NEC remains unclear. Microorganism invasion of tissue may occur after ischemic damage to the mucosal barrier of the gastrointestinal tract. A number of bacterial, viral, and fungal organisms have been isolated in outbreaks of necrotizing enterocolitis. Bacterial organisms such as *Escherichia coli*, *Klebsiella pneumoniae*, *Pseudomonas*, and *Clostridium difficile*, have been recovered from the blood and peritoneal cavities of some one-third of all infants with necrotizing enterocolitis. Virus particles have been identified concurrently in the feces of infants with necrotizing enterocolitis and their mothers, the midwives, and the nursing staff involved in treatment of the infants. Fungi have also been isolated from infants born to immunocompromised mothers.

Inflammatory mediators may further aggravate the injury induced by infectious agents. Bacterial endotoxin can directly initiate the production of tumor necrosis factor. This cytokine, in turn, stimulates the production of the interleukins and platelet-activating factor. These inflammatory mediators act synergistically to produce intestinal injury similar to that found in necrotizing enterocolitis.

Milk feedings have also been implicated in the pathogenesis of neonatal necrotizing enterocolitis. Approximately 93% of all infants in whom necrotizing enterocolitis develops have been fed enterally. Human milk and commercial formulas serve as substrates for bacterial proliferation in the gastrointestinal tract. Because neonates partially malabsorb the carbohydrate and fat constituents in milk, reducing substances, organic acids, carbon dioxide, and hydrogen gas may be produced by the bacterial fermentation of these nutrients. Although milk feedings are often felt to be a contributory factor in the development of necrotizing enterocolitis, the disease may develop in some infants who have never been fed. Studies suggest that feedings do not adversely affect the incidence of necrotizing enterocolitis. Furthermore, withholding feedings does not reduce the incidence of necrotizing enterocolitis.

Necrotizing enterocolitis may result from direct mucosal injury induced by hyperosmolar formulas. Although such formulas are rarely used in neonatal nurseries, medications that are frequently administered orally may contain hypertonic additives that irritate the intestinal mucosa and precipitate disease. Other hyperosmolar agents instilled directly into the bowel for diagnostic studies such as Renografin-76 (66% meglumine diatrizoate, 10% sodium diatrizoate), may precipitate necrotizing enterocolitis.

Immunologic and gastrointestinal immaturity in the neonate may play a role in the development of necrotizing enterocolitis. At birth, the human intestinal mucosa has no secretory immunoglobulin A (IgA), the major gastrointestinal immunoprotective antibody. Human milk contains immunocompetent cells and secretory IgA. Some studies support a protective role of human milk in the prevention of necrotizing enterocolitis.

PATHOLOGY

Neonatal necrotizing enterocolitis may be characterized broadly as intestinal infarction. This disorder primarily affects the terminal ileum and colon, although (in severe cases) the entire gastrointestinal tract may be involved. On gross examination, the bowel is distended and hemorrhagic. Subserosal collections of gas may or may not be present along the mesenteric border. Gangrenous necrosis, with or without perforation, may be present on the antimesenteric border.

PREDISPOSING FACTORS

Risk factors for the development of NEC are shown in Table 19-1. Prenatal risk factors for infants less than 2000 grams include maternal age older than 35 years and premature rupture of membranes. Perinatal risk factors include maternal anesthesia at delivery and depressed Apgar scores at 5 minutes. Postnatal risk factors include patent ductus arteriosus, the use of

TABLE 19-1. Proposed Risk Factors Associated with Necrotizing Enterocolitis

Group I: preterm infants <2,000 g
Prenatal
Maternal age >35 years
Maternal infection treated with antibiotics
Premature rupture of membranes >24 hours before delivery
Perinatal
Maternal anesthesia at delivery
Normal Apgar score at 1 minute, low at 5 minutes
Postnatal
Patent ductus arteriosus
Administration of intravenous glucose or total parenteral nutrition before onset of disease
Gavage feeding
Absence of prophylactic oral antibiotics before the onset of disease
Transport to community hospital from regional neonatal intensive care unit
Cocaine exposure
Group II: older infants >2,000 g
Perinatal
Polycythemia
Respiratory distress
Hypoglycemia
Postoperative repair of abdominal wall defects and gastrointestinal tract lesions

total parenteral nutrition or gavage feedings, and the absence of prophylactic oral antibiotics before the onset of necrotizing enterocolitis. Additional risk factors have been identified for infants who average more than 2,000 g at birth. Polycythemia (peripheral venous hematocrit greater than 65%) is the most common predisposing factor. Respiratory distress and hypoglycemia (serum glucose level less than 30 mg/dL) also occur more frequently in this group of infants. Although NEC can occur in larger infants, prematurity is thought to be one of the most important factors that predisposes the neonate to this disorder.

CLINICAL FEATURES

Nearly three-fourths of all infants with necrotizing enterocolitis are born prematurely. The onset of symptoms occurs within the first 5 days of life in 44% of infants, although symptoms may occur as early as the first day and as late as the fourth week after birth.

Feedings with either human milk or commercial formulas have been instituted in nearly all infants in whom necrotizing enterocolitis develops. Gastric distention and feeding intolerance (characterized by signs and symptoms such as vomiting, diminished bowel sounds, diarrhea, hematochezia) are the earliest presenting symptoms of the disease. Systemic manifestations include temperature instability, lethargy, apnea, respiratory failure, and hypotension. Lethargy, severe acidosis, sepsis, disseminated intravascular coagulation, and shock may supervene rapidly.

Subclinical necrotizing enterocolitis is suspected (but not confirmed) in approximately 25% of cases, and the symptoms resolve gradually. Between 25% and 40% of cases exhibit fulminant progression of the disease with evidence of perforation and peritonitis.

LABORATORY AND RADIOGRAPHIC STUDIES

Laboratory studies may demonstrate a decreased platelet count, increased prothrombin and partial thromboplastin times, and other evidence of disseminated intravascular coagulation. An absolute neutrophil count of less than 1,500 per cubic millimeter is associated with a poor prognosis. Stool guaiac for blood may be positive. Hyponatremia and persistent metabolic acidosis are nonspecific but may suggest the presence of sepsis or necrotic bowel.

Blood cultures and cerebrospinal fluid cultures should be obtained if sepsis or meningitis is suspected. Stool cultures generally show the presence of normal enteric flora.

An abdominal film in the supine, decubitus, or upright position may show the presence of *pneumatosis intestinalis* (the hallmark of necrotizing enterocolitis) and edema of the bowel wall, dilatation of loops of bowel, ascites, portal vein gas, or free air in the peritoneum. Fixed loops of bowel on serial abdominal x-rays are an ominous feature suggesting intestinal perforation. Abdominal ultrasonography may prove useful for identifying gangrenous bowel and impending perforation.

The diagnosis of necrotizing enterocolitis is confirmed when the following triad of clinical features is present: abdominal distention, hematochezia, and pneumatosis intestinalis.

DIFFERENTIAL DIAGNOSIS

The differential diagnosis of necrotizing enterocolitis includes anal fissures, pneumatosis coli, infectious enterocolitis, neonatal appendicitis, intestinal obstruction, spontaneous perforation, and Hirschsprung disease.

Anal fissures have been reported in conjunction with necrotizing enterocolitis, but a cause-effect relationship is unclear. A high index of suspicion for NEC is required when premature infants have rectal bleeding or guaiac-positive stools, even in the presence of anal fissures.

Pneumatosis coli is a benign form of necrotizing enterocolitis seen primarily in premature infants. Clinical features include gastric residua and vomiting (in some patients), transient episodes of lethargy and apnea, mild abdominal distention, and frank blood in the stools. Radiographic studies demonstrate intramural intestinal gas limited to the colon and the absence of small bowel dilatation and pneumatosis. Recovery is complete within 3 days, and no sequelae are apparent. This entity can be differentiated from classic necrotizing enterocolitis by its clinical course.

Infectious enterocolitis may be attributed to a number of pathogenic organisms including *Salmonella, Shigella, Campylobacter,* and *C. difficile*, some of which have also been associated with necrotizing enterocolitis. Stool cultures should be obtained to identify the presence or absence of these organisms.

Neonatal appendicitis may masquerade as necrotizing enterocolitis. This entity is rare in newborn infants, however, presumably because of the persistence of the funnel-shaped configuration of the fetal appendix, which is less prone to obstruction. Findings at laparotomy, if necessary, will distinguish between neonatal appendicitis and necrotizing enterocolitis.

Gangrenous enterocolitis or perforation may be associated with intestinal obstruction resulting from intussusception, meconium ileus, ileal atresia, volvulus, or milk curds. Similarly, Hirschsprung disease may present as fulminant enterocolitis with colonic obstruction, diarrhea, and sepsis.

TREATMENT

The treatment of infants with necrotizing enterocolitis is based on a method of clinical staging at the time of diagnosis (Table 19-2). Infants classified as having stage I or stage II disease require appropriate diagnostic studies and vigorous medical therapy, whereas infants categorized as having stage III disease require surgical intervention.

The medical treatment of necrotizing enterocolitis is primarily supportive. When the diagnosis is suspected, oral feedings should be withheld and nasogastric suction and intravenous fluid should be instituted. Initial laboratory studies should be obtained as above, and the stools should be checked for occult blood. Total parenteral nutrition should be provided to maintain the nutritional status of the infant. Parenteral antibiotics that cover a broad spectrum of aerobic and anaerobic organisms should be administered. The choice of antibiotic therapy will often depend on the resistance patterns of individual institutions but should be directed at enteric organisms, as well as anaerobes. Combinations of ampicillin and an aminoglycoside (with or without clindamycin) are often used. Cephalosporins such as cefoxitin may also be used.

Serial abdominal films of infants in the supine and left lateral decubitus positions (the latter to allow free air to rise over the liver) are recommended every 6 to 8 hours, as needed, and serve as the best guide in following the course of the disease. If the illness progresses no further and the pneumatosis resolves, nasogastric suction may be discontinued. Oral feedings may be resumed gradually within 10 to 14 days after the acute illness.

Surgical intervention is necessary when the disease involves the full thickness of the bowel wall resulting in gangrene or frank

TABLE 19-2. Staging Criteria for the Treatment of Necrotizing Enterocolitis

Stage	Systemic	Intestinal	Radiologic	Treatment
I. Suspect	Lethargy, temperature instability, apnea, bradycardia	Gastric residual, emesis, abdominal distention, hematochezia	Ileus, intestinal dilation	Parenteral nutrition, nasogastric suction, antibiotics
II. Definite—same features as stage I plus				
A. Mildly ill	—	Absent bowel sounds	Pneumatosis intestinalis	—
B. Moderately ill	Metabolic acidosis, thrombocytopenia	Abdominal tenderness	Portal vein gas	$NaHCO_3$
III. Advanced—same features as stage II plus				
A. Shock	Respiratory arrest, hypotension, disseminated intravascular coagulation, combined respiratory metabolic acidosis	Peritonitis	Ascites	Intravenous fluids, isotropic agents, paracentesis
B. Bowel perforation	—	—	Pneumoperitoneum	Surgery

perforation. The surgical goal is to stabilize gross peritoneal infection without sacrificing bowel length. The indications for surgery include rapid clinical deterioration of the patient intestinal, a palpable abdominal mass; intestinal obstruction or peritonitis (often seen with progressive erythematous discoloration of the abdominal wall).

Operative procedures may range from a segmental resection to no resection with placement of a drain. A primary anastomosis may be possible if a limited resection is performed, although many infants will require a staged procedure involving resection and proximal enterostomy with distal mucous fistula formation, followed by closure 8 to 12 weeks later. When the disease process is extensive, only unquestionably necrotic or frankly perforated bowel should be excised.

COMPLICATIONS

Acute complications include sepsis (60%), peritonitis (20%–30%), abscess formation, thrombocytopenia, disseminated intravascular coagulation, and intestinal or extraintestinal bleeding. Antibiotic therapy, fresh-frozen plasma, platelet concentrates, and red cell or exchange transfusion may be necessary. Aggressive, advanced life support resuscitative measures such as mechanical ventilation may be needed in the very ill infant.

The late complications of necrotizing enterocolitis include stenosis, stricture formation, intestinal atresia, pericolic abscess, enterocele, enterocolic fistula, and short gut syndrome. Intestinal stenoses and strictures occur in 9% to 36% of infants treated medically and less frequently in those treated surgically. Approximately 80% of strictures occur in the colon, predominantly on the left side. Strictures are treated surgically. The procedures of choice are resection and primary anastomosis. Significant malabsorption may occur postoperatively in some 10% of patients with necrotizing enterocolitis because the amount of small bowel remaining after surgery is insufficient. This is often referred to as the *short-gut syndrome*. Prolonged parenteral or enteral nutrition may be required for survival.

PROGNOSIS

The prognosis for necrotizing enterocolitis has improved considerably since the late 1980s, as a result of advances in the care of critically ill infants, earlier diagnosis and treatment, and the institution of a standard aggressive approach in the treatment of this disorder. Currently, the overall survival rate is 70% to 80%. The prognosis is adversely affected by the degree of prematurity and the persistence of respiratory problems requiring ventilatory support. Late-onset necrotizing enterocolitis has a better prognosis than does the early-onset form.

SECTION

F

Neonatal Neurology

CHAPTER 20
Brachial Plexus Palsy

Adapted from Paul D. Sponseller

The brachial plexus is composed of contributions from nerve roots C5 to T1. Most severe injuries to the area involve lateral flexion of the neck or downward pressure on the shoulder, which may occur during a difficult delivery. Therefore, it is common for the upper portions of the plexus (C5-7) to be stretched. This stretching causes denervation of the shoulder abductors and elbow flexors, which results in gradual joint contractures if it is not treated. These brachial plexus injuries are known as *Erb-Duchenne palsies*. The lower plexus (C7–T1) can be affected by excessive abduction-traction and has a poorer prognosis; this is the rarest occurrence, and it is called *Klumpke palsy*. Such cases result in loss of function of the elbow extensors, wrist flexors, and finger muscles and possibly in a Horner syndrome. Occasionally, the entire plexus may be involved.

Factors associated with brachial plexus palsy include shoulder dystocia, breech position, high birth weight, and prolonged labor. The incidence is 1 to 3 in 1,000 births. The site of injury may be at any level from the origin of the nerve roots to the plexus itself, but even root lesions may resolve spontaneously. On physical examination, the early typical Erb palsy appears as an arm that is rotated internally at the shoulder, extended at the elbow, and flexed at the fingers. Initially, passive range of motion should be full.

Skeletal injuries such as clavicle fractures and proximal humerus separations should be ruled out radiographically, although they can often be differentiated by guarding on testing of passive motion and the presence of Moro response. Because of the trauma, palsy and skeletal injury may coexist.

Treatment involves maintenance of motion and transfers of tendon in those rare, severe cases in which function does not return. With current obstetric practice, 92% of palsies resolve completely by the time affected infants reach 3 months of age, and 95% of such infants eventually recover fully. Physical therapy should be used initially to maintain range of motion. Splinting, in most cases, results in contractures, although later functional splinting of the hand may have a role. For patients with persistent weakness at age 3 months, electromyography and possibly myelography may help to identify those rare cases in which nerve grafting is required. Cases detected later may benefit from osteotomy or contracture release and tendon transfer, especially to restore shoulder external rotation.

CHAPTER 21
Intraventricular Hemorrhage of the Preterm Infant

Adapted from Laura R. Ment

Intraventricular hemorrhage (IVH), or hemorrhage into the germinal matrix tissues, with possible rupture into the ventricular system and parenchyma of the developing brain, remains a major problem of preterm neonates and is believed to be the result of alterations in cerebral blood flow (CBF) to a damaged germinal matrix capillary bed. Figure 21-1 illustrates a model for the development of IVH. Because the germinal matrix begins to involute after 34 weeks of gestation, germinal matrix hemorrhages (GMH) and IVHs are lesions of preterm infants, and the incidence of GMH/IVH in infants of less than 1,500-g birth weight is now reported to range from 15% to 30%. Seizures, hydrocephalus, periventricular leukomalacia (PVL), and neonatal death are more frequent in infants with GMH/IVH than in those without hemorrhage when matched for birth weight or gestational age. In addition, although the long-term neurodevelopmental outcome for those infants with lower grades of hemorrhage remains unclear, most observers agree that infants with parenchymal involvement of hemorrhage are at higher risk for neurodevelopmental handicap.

Cranial ultrasonography is the method of choice for diagnosis of GMH/IVH in newborn special care units. A standard grading system, which was originally applied to the computed tomographic scan, has been adapted to cranial ultrasonography examinations (Table 21-1). The most common site for parenchymal involvement of hemorrhage is the frontal region; many hemorrhages occur bilaterally. Less commonly, the caudate nuclei and occipital periventricular white-matter regions are involved.

In most newborn intensive care units, echoencephalography is performed on postnatal days 2 to 3 and is then repeated during the second postnatal week to screen preterm neonates of 1,500 g or less or of 34 weeks' gestational age or less for GMH/IVH.

OUTCOME AND TREATMENT

Infants with GMH/IVH are at risk for the development of posthemorrhagic hydrocephalus (PHH) and are known to

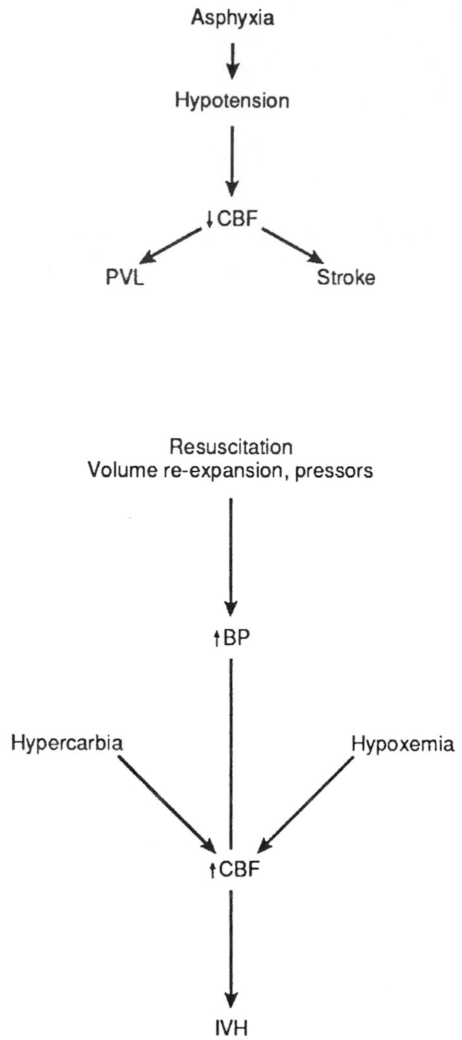

Figure 21-1. Model for the development of intraventricular hemorrhage in the preterm infant. BP, blood pressure; CBF, cerebral blood flow; IVH, intraventricular hemorrhage; PVL, periventricular leukomalacia.

TABLE 21-1. Grading System for Neonatal Intraventricular Hemorrhage

Grade	Description
I	Germinal matrix hemorrhage
II	Blood within but not distending the lateral ventricular system
III	Blood filling and distending the ventricular system
IV	Parenchymal involvement of hemorrhage with or without any of the above

Adapted from Papile LS, Burstein J, Burstein R, et al. Incidence and evolution of the subependymal intraventricular hemorrhage: a study of infants with weights less than 1500 grams. *J Pediatr* 1978;92:529.

have higher incidences of neonatal seizures and PVL (Fig. 21-1), as compared with preterm infants without hemorrhage matched for birth weight or gestational age. Finally, most investigators agree that those infants with parenchymal involvement of GMH/IVH are at high risk for neurodevelopmental handicap.

PHH (Fig. 21-2) is the combination of ventriculomegaly (diagnosed by serial echoencephalography studies) and increased intracranial pressure. PHH is generally a communicating hydrocephalus with a block at the level of the arachnoid villi or, less commonly, at the foramina of Luschka and Magendie in the posterior fossa. Hydrocephalus results when the blood and protein in the cerebrospinal fluid produce a chemical arachnoiditis that may be transient or, less commonly, permanent. A small percentage of infants with IVH will have a noncommunicating hydrocephalus with a block at the level of the aqueduct secondary to an ependymal reaction similar to that of the arachnoid or an acute clot. Infants with the latter type of hydrocephalus will require neurosurgical intervention, whereas the treatment for neonates with communicating PHH (at least initially) is medical.

All infants with intraventricular blood require close ultrasonographic monitoring of ventricular size (Fig. 21-3). These patients should undergo frequent head circumference

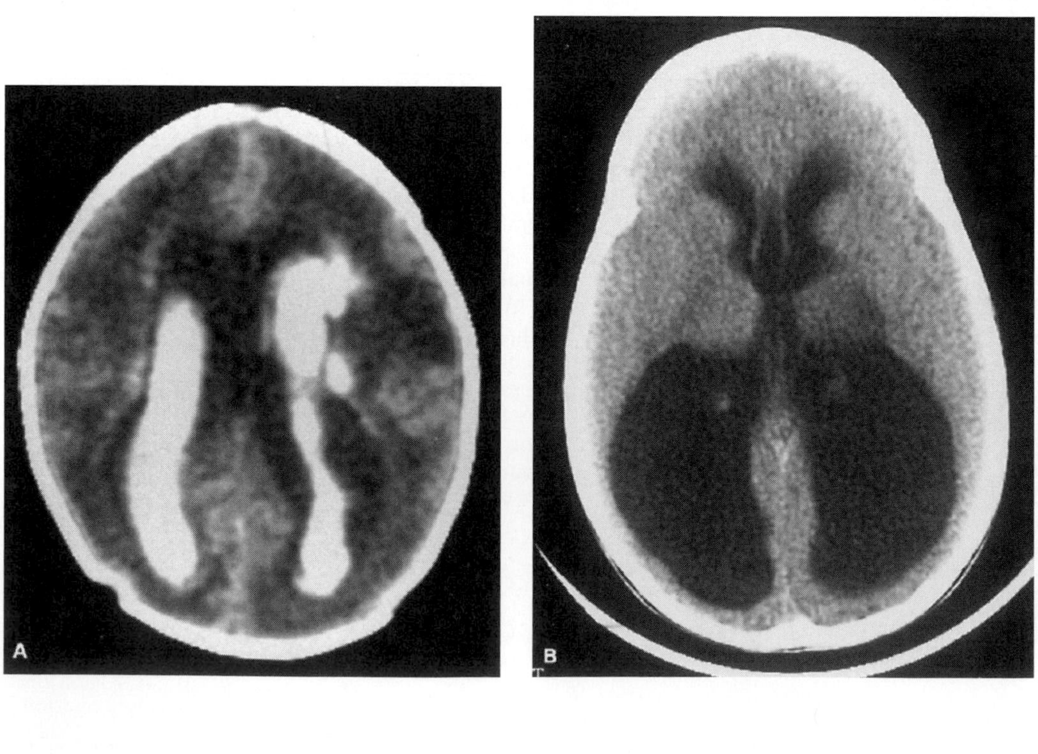

Figure 21-2. A: Computed tomographic scan of preterm infant of 28 weeks' gestational age with bilateral intraventricular hemorrhage. **B:** Repeat computed tomographic scan—performed because of rapidly increasing occipitofrontal head circumference, lethargy, and increasing apneic spells—demonstrated ventriculomegaly. Lumbar puncture revealed an opening pressure of greater than 200 mm of water consistent with the diagnosis of posthemorrhagic hydrocephalus.

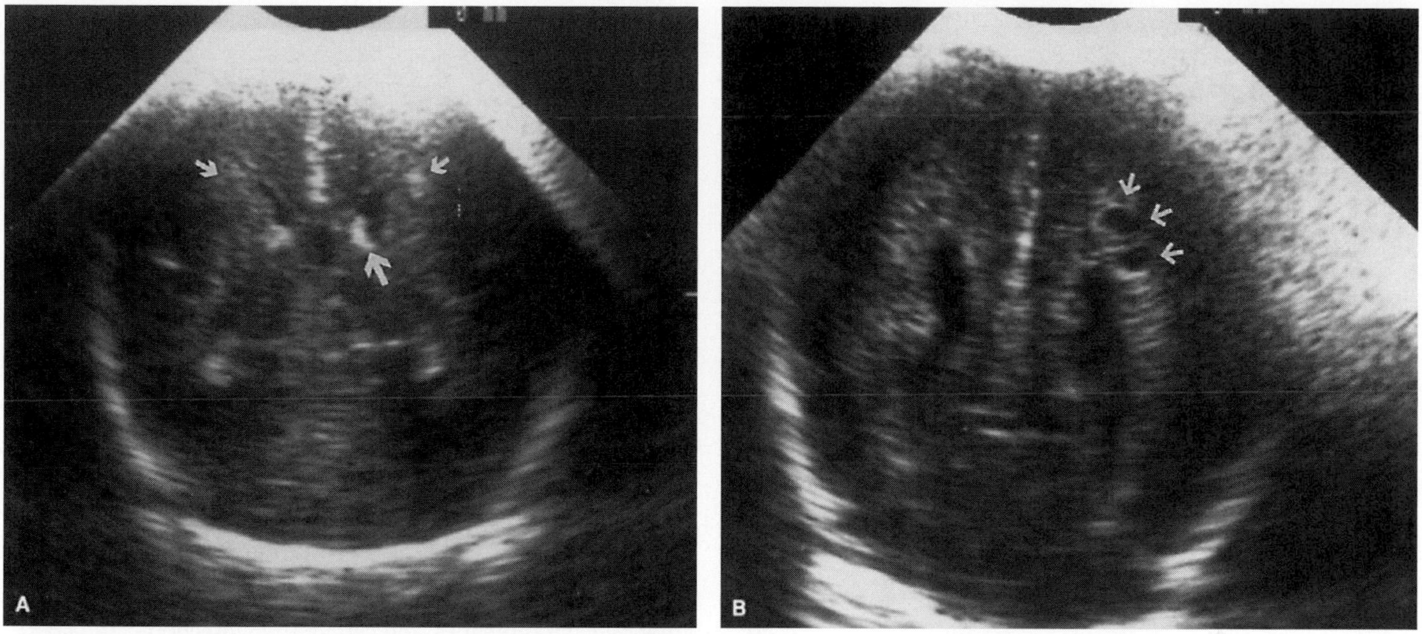

Figure 21-3. Coronal cranial ultrasonographic studies of a 1,000-g boy of 29 weeks' gestation with bloody spinal fluid. **A:** Ultrasonography on the second postnatal day demonstrated left-sided intraventricular hemorrhage (*large arrow*) and periventricular echodensities bilaterally (*small arrows*). **B:** Follow-up study 1 week later revealed periventricular cystic lesions consistent with the diagnosis of periventricular leukomalacia (*arrows*).

measurements and cranial ultrasonographic examinations for determination of ventricular size. Because prolonged increased intracranial pressure may result in apnea, vomiting, lethargy, and (ultimately) optic atrophy, the intracranial pressure of infants with head circumferences crossing the expected growth curves and those infants demonstrating evidence for increasing ventricular size should be checked and, when the diagnosis is confirmed, treatment should be provided. The standard treatment protocol for infants with communicating hydrocephalus includes lumbar punctures with removal of cerebrospinal fluid to normalize intracranial pressure and frequent ultrasound checks of ventricular size. Alternatively, for those infants with evidence of noncommunicating hydrocephalus or intraparenchymal involvement of hemorrhage and shift of the cerebral midline, ventricular taps or the insertion of ventricular catheters with reservoirs performed by neurosurgical personnel are indicated, and the placement of a ventriculoperitoneal shunt may ultimately be necessary.

In many large series of preterm neonates, the incidence of motor handicaps appears to be low. These abnormalities include spastic diplegia, hemiparesis, and (rarely) spastic quadriparesis. Many infants with spastic diplegia have neuroimaging evidence for PVL or low-pressure cerebral ventriculomegaly, but only 50% to 60% of infants with these cranial ultrasonographic findings at term will be found to suffer motor handicap at age 3 years.

Although many investigators doubt the existence of differences in the developmental outcome of infants with grade I, II, or III IVH (as compared with infants with no known evidence of hemorrhage in the neonatal period), data suggest that the rate of cognitive deficits may increase with the grade of IVH in this patient population. Infants with parenchymal involvement of hemorrhage, or grade IV IVH, experience a wide range of outcomes; review of the literature suggests that 50% to 85% of all neonates with grade IV IVH will have motor and cognitive handicaps.

INTERVENTION STUDIES

A variety of measures has been suggested to prevent GMH/IVH. Clearly, the most important way to prevent the disorder is to prevent preterm birth. When that is not possible, the preferable approach is transport of the mother and fetus to a regional perinatal center specializing in high-risk obstetric care; "outborn" infants have consistently higher rates of GMH/IVH than do those infants who are "inborn." In addition, antenatal corticosteroid exposure has a clear role in reducing the incidence of IVH in preterm infants.

Abrupt increases in blood pressure and, thus, changes in CBF should be avoided. Blood pressure and transcutaneous Po_2 should be monitored continuously to avoid hypotension and hypoxemia. Hypercapnia should be avoided similarly. The role of the patent ductus arteriosus and its abrupt closure in the genesis of IVH has long been debated, and it appears that pharmacologic closure promotes smoother changes in blood flow than do surgical procedures.

Finally, multiple pharmacologic intervention trials have sought to prevent GMH/IVH. The drugs used include phenobarbital, indomethacin, ethamsylate, vitamin E, and pancuronium bromide (Pavulon), among others. These agents lower CBF, alter the metabolic rate, scavenge free radicals, stabilize capillary membranes, and prevent fluctuations in CBF, respectively. Only low-dose indomethacin (0.1 mg/kg at 6–12 postnatal hours by slow intravenous infusion over 20–30 minutes and repeated 24 and 48 hours thereafter) has been demonstrated in multiple single-institution studies and a multicenter trial both to lower the incidence and to decrease the severity of IVH.

CHAPTER 22
Neonatal Seizures

Adapted from Edward J. Novotny, Jr.

Seizures are an important sign of neurologic disease in the newborn. Their incidence varies between 1% and 20%. Neonates with neurologic dysfunction are frequently critically ill and may exhibit abnormal motor phenomena, autonomic instability, and alteration in consciousness. Abnormal motor activities, including posturing, clonus, choreoathetosis, dystonia, and seizures, are frequently seen in these newborns. A classification of neonatal seizures is shown in Table 22-1. Differentiation between seizures and other abnormal behaviors [nonepileptic seizure-like events (NESLEs)] is traditionally made on clinical grounds.

Several clinical attributes are helpful in differentiating NESLEs from epileptic seizures. Infants with clonic seizures have slower, more rhythmic motor activity that cannot be stopped by restraint, whereas infants with tremors and clonus have rapid, irregular motor activity that ceases with restraint and change in posture of the limb. Various tactics such as touching the infant or making a sudden loud noise nearby, can typically induce tremor, clonus, and other nonepileptic motor automatisms. Another clinical characteristic that aids in distinguishing epileptic events from NESLEs is the fact that epileptic seizures are typically accompanied by changes in heart rate, respiratory pattern, pupil size, and blood pressure. An isolated episode of apnea is rarely an epileptic seizure, although apnea is seen frequently in epileptic seizures in association with other clinical signs. Many other causes of apnea in term and preterm infants should be excluded before an epileptic seizure is considered as the etiology.

ETIOLOGY AND DIAGNOSIS

Perinatal asphyxia, central nervous system (CNS) infections, intracranial hemorrhages, and cerebral infarcts account for approximately 90% of the disorders that are responsible for neonatal seizures. Developmental anomalies, acute metabolic disorders, and rare inborn errors of metabolism are less common etiologies. Identification of the latter two etiologic categories is crucial, because treatment is altered to management of the underlying disease.

Initial evaluation of the newborn with seizures should begin with a thorough history, with emphasis on prenatal and perinatal drug exposure, details of labor and delivery, presence of maternal infection, maternal metabolic status, and family history of seizures. Early assessment of cardiorespiratory status and stabilization are critical. A careful, general physical examination and a detailed neurologic examination are required. Funduscopic examination for retinal pathology indicating intracranial hemorrhage or CNS infection should be performed. Evaluation for hepatosplenomegaly and a thorough cardiovascular examination, including auscultation of the head for arteriovenous malformations, are necessary.

Initial investigations should include neuroimaging; cerebrospinal fluid examination; serum electrolyte determinations; calcium, magnesium, creatine, blood urea nitrogen, and glucose measurements; a complete blood count; and arterial blood gas determinations. Serum ammonia and hepatic enzyme concentrations, as well as other metabolic studies, should be obtained in selected cases. Neuroultrasound is an excellent initial technique with which to investigate the neuroanatomy, but computed tomography and magnetic resonance imaging are often required. Magnetic resonance imaging studies in premature and term infants have shown that exquisite, high-resolution images of the brain can be acquired easily. This neuroimaging method is clearly superior to computed tomography for the illustration of cerebral infarcts, CNS anomalies, and certain CNS infections.

In neurophysiologic investigations of neonates with seizures, the optimal time to obtain an EEG is while the clinical event in question is observed. This is obviously impractical, and an EEG should be obtained in the interictal period as soon as possible. EEGs obtained between seizures (interictally) provide important information about neurologic prognosis, especially if serial recordings are performed. Specific EEG patterns are observed in herpes simplex encephalitis and in certain metabolic diseases and congenital malformations. Persistent focal abnormalities seen on the EEG are correlated highly with structural CNS pathology. If intensive neurophysiologic monitoring is available, it can be used to identify whether an event is an epileptic seizure, although controversy exists about whether the lack of surface EEG epileptic activity excludes a particular event from being an epileptic seizure.

Certain types of seizures are seen in infants with specific disorders. For example, persistent partial motor seizures are typically noted in infants with strokes or congenital malformations. Clonic seizures are also commonly seen in infants with hypocalcemia, although the incidence of this disorder has decreased dramatically since the 1960s. Both subtle and tonic seizures are seen more often in infants with hypoxic-ischemic encephalopathy.

Several specific epileptic syndromes are noted primarily in the neonatal period. These include benign neonatal convulsions, which occur in full-term infants, usually beginning on the fifth day of life. These seizures are self-limited and resolve spontaneously in a few weeks. Benign neonatal familial convulsions is a rare disorder with an autosomal dominant pattern of inheritance in which seizures begin during the first week of life and usually resolve in the first few months. Early myoclonic encephalopathy begins in the first few weeks of life with generalized and multifocal myoclonic seizures and depression of consciousness. Several metabolic disorders, including nonketotic hyperglycinemia and D-glycericacidemia, have been identified in infants with this clinical syndrome. Finally, early infantile encephalopathy with burst suppression is observed in infants who primarily have tonic seizures and a progressive deterioration in neurologic function in the first month of life.

TABLE 22-1. Classification of Neonatal Seizures

Epileptic seizures
Focal clonic
Focal tonic
Myoclonic
Nonepileptic seizurelike events
Generalized tonic
Myoclonic
Fragmentary
Motor automatisms
Oral-buccal-lingual
Ocular
Complex movements
Apnea

TREATMENT

Treatment with antiepileptic agents should be withheld in infants who have generalized tonic and subtle seizures, especially in the case of subtle seizures occurring in a full-term infant. Initial management of the newborn with suspected seizures includes rapid assessment and stabilization of respiratory and cardiovascular status. This should be followed immediately by determination of glucose and electrolyte status including measurement of the serum calcium level. Initial bedside measurement of the glucose level should be performed and, if it is abnormal, 2 to 4 mL/kg of $D_{25}W$ glucose should be given parenterally. Giving 1 mL/kg of 10% calcium gluconate parenterally should treat hypocalcemia. Next, evaluation for a CNS infection is indicated by examination of the cerebrospinal fluid. Neuroimaging should be performed to exclude any structural neuropathology such as an intracranial hemorrhage, CNS anomaly, or cerebral infarct.

If the clinical seizures seen are definite epileptic seizures, treatment with either a benzodiazepine or phenobarbital is indicated. Phenobarbital should be given at a dose of 15 to 20 mg/kg intravenously. If the seizures persist, 15 to 20 mg/kg of phenytoin should be administered intravenously at a rate of 1 mg/kg/minute. Close monitoring of the blood pressure, electrocardiogram results, and respiratory status is required with administration of this drug. If a question exists as to whether the events are epileptic seizures, treatment with a benzodiazepine should be considered, because these agents have a rapid onset of action and short half-lives. Finally, primidone, valproic acid, lidocaine, and pentobarbital have all been used in the treatment of intractable seizures in the neonatal period. Use of these agents should not be considered unless the seizures are well documented both clinically and electrophysiologically. Infants with documented intractable epileptic seizures in the neonatal and infantile period should be given a trial of pyridoxine. This vitamin is an important cofactor for several enzyme systems including the enzymes responsible for metabolism for the putative amino acid neurotransmitters. Fifty to 100 mg of pyridoxine should be given parenterally while the infant's EEG is being monitored. Infants with pyridoxine-dependent seizures have a dramatic improvement in their EEG with the administration of pyridoxine.

The duration of therapy should be guided by the risk of recurrence of seizures and the possible toxicity induced by treatment. Infants with cerebral malformations and significant structural lesions are at high risk for continuing to have seizures, whereas those infants with hypoxic-ischemic encephalopathy or a metabolic cause have a much lower risk of recurrence. If the neurologic examination and the interictal EEG results are normal, the chance of the infant having later seizures is small. Concerns regarding the effects of drugs on the developing nervous system have also dictated that the duration of therapy be kept to a minimum. Antiepileptic therapy is discontinued in most infants before they are discharged from neonatal intensive care and is rarely continued for more than 8 weeks after discharge. EEGs obtained after the acute illness and in the first weeks of life aid in deciding whether to continue antiepileptic therapy, in assessing the risk of the development of epilepsy, and in determining the long-term neurologic outcome.

CHAPTER 23
The Floppy Infant and the Late Walker

Adapted from Richard S. K. Young

HISTORY

In the diagnosis of neurologic disease, the patient's history furnishes clues to the nature of the disorder, and the physical examination and laboratory tests provide confirmation. When the history of an infant with hypotonia is taken, information regarding any family history of neuromuscular disease, the quality of the fetal movements, and the presence of hydramnios should be obtained. The child's pattern of growth and his or her ability to feed should be elicited. Figure 23-1 presents algorithms for general diagnostic approaches to hypotonia.

PHYSICAL EXAMINATION

A general physical examination of any infant with suspected neurologic disease is essential to rule out motor delays caused by systemic disease. It should be determined whether congestive heart failure (dyspnea, edema, organomegaly) may be responsible for weakness or fatigue. The child should be examined for dysmorphic features (suggestive of a chromosomal abnormality) and for signs of endocrinopathy (umbilical hernia, dull cry, brittle hair).

Weakness typically begins in the proximal large muscles of the neck and in the pectoral and pelvic girdles producing poor head control in the infant and delay in walking in the older child. The muscles should be inspected for bulk, atrophy, fasciculations, and symmetry. The presence of fasciculations in the tongue muscle is evidence of denervation. The muscle stretch reflexes should be tested, and it should be determined whether sensation is intact.

NEUROLOGIC EVALUATION

Based on the results of the history and physical examination, the physician should first determine whether a problem exists or whether a child is simply at the lower limits of normal. If a neuromuscular disorder is suspected, it should be decided whether the lesion is central (spasticity correlates with upper motor neuron involvement) or peripheral (hyporeflexia correlates with lower motor neuron arc). The pediatrician should think anatomically about each element of the motor system and determine its degree of involvement beginning with the cerebral cortex and proceeding along the corticospinal tract to the muscle fiber.

CENTRAL NERVOUS SYSTEM

Cerebral injuries or malformations are the most common cause of weakness (central hypotonia). Cerebral conditions that may result in a floppy infant include hypoxic-ischemic encephalopathy, intracranial infection, cerebral hemorrhage, cerebral trauma, metabolic disorders, cerebral malformations, and chromosomal malformations. Children with these disorders may have seizures

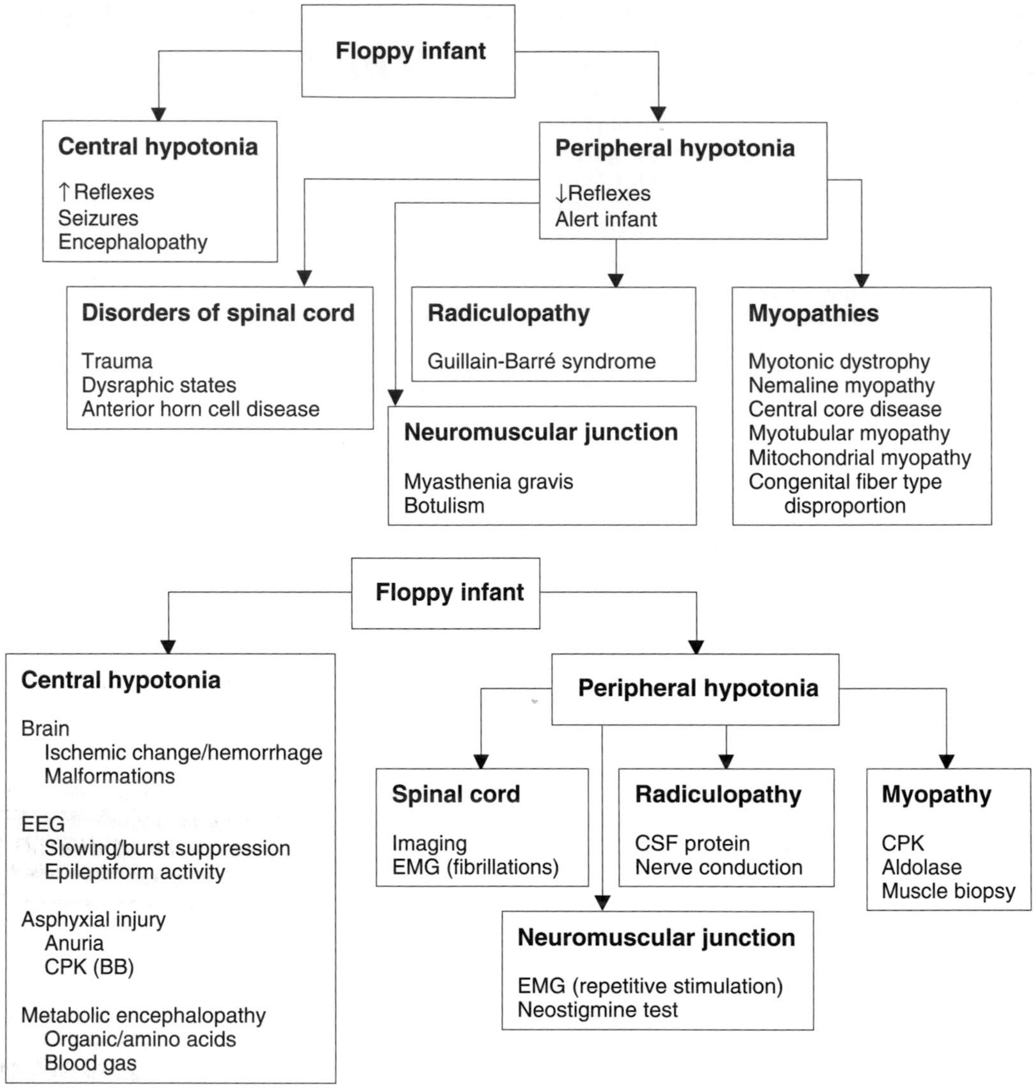

Figure 23-1. Algorithms illustrating general diagnostic approaches to hypotonia. CPK (BB), isoenzyme of creatine phospokinase containing two B subunits; CSF, cerebrospinal fluid; EEG, electroencephalogram; EMG, electromyelogram.

or other signs of cerebrocortical dysfunction. Central, as opposed to peripheral, causes of weakness result in spasticity with ankle clonus, crossed adductor reflex, Babinski sign, and fisting. Strabismus may also suggest central nervous system dysfunction causing floppiness in an infant.

SPINAL CORD

The most common causes of spinal cord disease producing a floppy infant are trauma, dysraphism (myelomeningocele), and degeneration of the anterior horn cells (Werdnig-Hoffmann Syndrome). Cervical spinal cord injury may result from tearing or shearing of the spinal cord during delivery of a large infant. Tumors or infections of the spinal cord are less common. Seesaw respirations are a sign of diaphragmatic breathing and indicate that the lesion is above the C4 level (emergence of the phrenic nerve). Widespread degeneration of anterior horn cells may also produce diaphragmatic breathing.

RADICULOPATHIES

Acute inflammatory polyneuropathy (Guillain-Barré syndrome) is an infrequent cause of weakness in the infant and young child. The disorder results from a postinfectious immune attack on the Schwann cells producing demyelination of peripheral nerves. Because of the interruption of the lower motor neuron arc, areflexia is present. The diagnosis is established by the presence of elevated protein levels in the cerebrospinal fluid and delay in nerve conduction. Intravenous immunoglobulin has been advocated as a therapy for Guillain-Barré syndrome.

Plasmapheresis has not gained wide acceptance because the prognosis of Guillain-Barré syndrome in children is generally benign.

DISORDERS OF THE PERIPHERAL NERVES

Peripheral nerve disease, other than Guillain-Barré syndrome, seldom causes weakness in the neonatal period. Disorders of the peripheral nerves occur sporadically (Leigh disease, Riley-Day syndrome or familial dysautonomia, and Möbius syndrome), although Dejériné-Sottas disease is inherited in an autosomal recessive manner.

DISORDERS INVOLVING THE NEUROMUSCULAR JUNCTION

Disorders of the neuromuscular junction may cause an infant to be floppy or an older child to be a late walker (Table 23-1).

TABLE 23-1. Neonatal Diseases of the Neuromuscular Junction

Myasthenia gravis
Transient, congenital
Metabolic disease
Hypermagnesemia
Toxins
Kanamycin, gentamicin, neomycin, streptomycin, polymyxin
Infantile botulism

DISORDERS OF MUSCLE

Muscle disorders include myotonic dystrophy, nemaline myopathy, central core disease, myotubular myopathy, mitochondrial disease, Duchenne's muscular dystrophy. See Chapter 225 for a complete discussion of myopathis disorders.

SECTION

G

Bacterial and Viral Infections

CHAPTER 24
Neonatal Sepsis

Adapted from Pablo J. Sánchez and Jane D. Siegel

The terms *neonatal sepsis* and *sepsis neonatorum* refer to invasive bacterial infections that involve primarily the bloodstream in infants during the first month of life. As a relatively compromised host, the neonate does not localize infection well, and invasion of the meninges occurs in approximately 10% to 25% of infants with bacteremia. Before the widespread implementation of the 1996 guidelines for intrapartum chemoprophylaxis for the prevention of infections caused by group B streptococcus (GBS), the incidence of neonatal sepsis in the United States varied from 1 to 10 per 1,000 live births with an average of 2 or 3 per 1,000. Although these infections are relatively uncommon, they may be associated with case-fatality rates of 15% to 30% and substantial morbidity in surviving infants. The pediatrician must be familiar with the etiologic agents, pathogenesis, and clinical manifestations of neonatal sepsis so that appropriate cultures can be obtained and effective antimicrobial therapy is initiated promptly.

TABLE 24-1. Pathogens Most Frequently Associated with Sepsis Neonatorum

Years	Most frequent	Other
1928–1932	beta-Streptococcus	*Staphylococcus aureus, Escherichia coli*
1933–1943	Group A streptococcus	*E. coli*
1944–1957	*E. coli*	*Pseudomonas aeruginosa*
1958–1965	*E. coli* (*S. aureus*)	*Pseudomonas* species, *Klebsiella-Enterobacter*
1966–1978	Group B streptococcus	*E. coli, Klebsiella-Enterobacter*
1979–1990	Group B streptococcus, *E. coli*	Coagulase-negative staphylococci, methicillin-resistant *S. aureus,** gram negatives, enterococcus, *Candida*

*Nosocomial outbreaks in some nurseries.
Adapted from Freedman RM, Ingram DI, Gross I, et al. A half century of neonatal sepsis at Yale, 1928–1978. *Am J Dis Child* 1981;135:140.

ETIOLOGY

Before 1996, the incidence of neonatal sepsis varied little over the years, but the predominant pathogens changed considerably from one decade to the next (Table 24-1). In the 1970s, GBS emerged and persisted through the 1990s as the predominant pathogen in most U.S. nurseries. A recent study of very low-birth-weight (VLBW) infants however, shows decling rates of GBS sepsis and increasing rates of gram negative (primarily *Escherichia coli*) sepsis. Although there has been a shift in serotype distribution, no change in virulence of GBS isolates has been documented.

Although GBS and *E. coli* account for at least 60% to 70% of all infections, several other pathogens are noteworthy. *Staphylococcus aureus, Klebsiella-Enterobacter, Serratia, Salmonella,* and *Pseudomonas* species are most frequently isolated from infants with late-onset infections, especially during nosocomial outbreaks. Methicillin-resistant *S. aureus,* vancomycin-resistant enterococcus, and gram-negative bacilli that are resistant to third-generation cephalosporins or aminoglycosides are particularly difficult to eradicate from nurseries for low-birth-weight (*LBW*) infants. The incidence of *Listeria monocytogenes* is highly variable with temporal clustering related to maternal infection associated with food-borne outbreaks.

Several other pathogens may play a role in neonatal sepsis. These include non–group D, alpha-hemolytic streptococcus, group D streptococci (both enterococcal and nonenterococcal), *Streptococcus pneumoniae, Neisseria meningitidis, Haemophilus influenzae* (mostly nontypable strains), and groups A, C, and G streptococci.

Coagulase-negative staphylococci and *Candida* species may be isolated from septic, premature infants who have prolonged stays in the intensive care unit. Coagulase-negative staphylococci account for more than 40% of late-onset infections in the neonatal intensive care unit. *Candida* species are associated with 5% to 10% of late-onset infections in most LBW nurseries.

Overall case-fatality rates for neonatal sepsis have decreased from 90% in the 1930s to 15% to 25% in the 1980s and further to 5% to 20% in the 1990s. This decrease is a result of earlier recognition of the nonspecific signs of sepsis and improved supportive care of the overwhelmed infant, as well as development of more active antimicrobial agents.

EPIDEMIOLOGY

Our knowledge of the epidemiology of perinatally acquired bacterial infections is based on extensive studies of the GBS and, to a lesser extent, *E. coli*. The gastrointestinal tract is the major site of asymptomatic colonization with both the GBS and *E. coli* for mother and infant. GBS may be isolated from the gastrointestinal or genitourinary tract in 5% to 30% of pregnant women. Younger, sexually experienced women from lower socioeconomic backgrounds have higher colonization rates. This organism is sexually transmitted, therefore, men can also be colonized in the urethra and pharynx. GBS are suppressed but not eradicated from mucosal surfaces by treatment with antibiotics.

In the absence of antibiotic treatment, between 40% and 70% of infants whose mothers are colonized at delivery become colonized themselves with GBS by one of three mechanisms:

- Transplacental transmission in the presence of maternal bacteremia
- Ascension from the vagina and cervix through microscopic leaks in the amniotic membranes or through frankly ruptured membranes
- Surface contamination during passage through the birth canal

The risk of transmission increases when the density (inoculum) and number of sites of maternal colonization are increased; the risk is not influenced by route of delivery. Invasive disease develops in only one of every 50 to 75 colonized infants. Community acquisition of GBS by the neonate after discharge from the nursery may occur, but it is rare. These rates of colonization and disease are comparable for the pathogenic strains of *E. coli* that are associated with 75% of neonatal meningitis cases caused by *E. coli* and 40% of sepsis cases caused by *E. coli*.

Listeria monocytogenes is a worldwide soil organism with a large animal reservoir. A mechanism of transfer from animal to human has not been proved. An outbreak of perinatal listeriosis associated with ingestion of contaminated coleslaw supports the hypothesis that vegetables contaminated by manure fertilizer obtained from infected animals are the source of human gastrointestinal tract colonization. Studies of pregnant women in epidemic areas have identified colonization rates of 5% to 8% with the gastrointestinal tract rather than the genital tract being the site of carriage of *L. monocytogenes*.

TABLE 24-2. Risk Factors for the Development of Sepsis Neonatorum

Obstetric
Prematurity
Prolonged rupture of membranes
Internal monitoring devices
Twin pregnancy
Maternal urinary tract infection
Maternal fever
Maternal bacteremia
Chorioamnionitis
Structural virulence factors
Capsular polysaccharide
Surface proteins
Cell wall components
Adhesins
Protease
Neuraminidase
Endotoxin (lipid A)
Extracellular toxin
Impaired host defenses
Specific humoral antibody
Complement
Fibronectin
Neutrophil supply
Opsonophagocytosis
Chemotaxis

PATHOGENESIS

Risk factors for the development of invasive bacterial infections may be categorized generally as obstetric, structural virulence factors of pathogenic strains of bacteria, and as impaired host defenses (Table 24-2). The presence of any of these risk factors is associated with a tenfold or greater increased risk of developing systemic infection.

Boyer and coworkers' 1983 epidemiologic studies of GBS revealed significantly increased attack rates (7.6 per 1,000 live births) associated with the following conditions: birth weight of less than 2,500 g, rupture of membranes for more than 18 hours, and maternal intrapartum fever higher than 37.5°C. A rate of 26.2 per 1,000 live births was observed in infants who weighed 1,000 g or less. Similar associations have been observed with other neonatal pathogens. Detection of GBS bacteriuria during pregnancy may be a means of identifying the heavily colonized woman whose infant is at increased risk of developing infection. Based on additional epidemiologic studies, the presence of at least one of the following risk factors is an indication for intrapartum GBS chemoprophylaxis: history of a previous infant with GBS disease, GBS bacteriuria during pregnancy, gestation less than 37 weeks, chorioamnionitis and maternal fever of 38.0°C or higher, membranes ruptured more than 18 hours, and maternal GBS colonization documented at 35 to 37 weeks' gestation.

The infant is occasionally able to eliminate GBS from the bloodstream without antibiotic therapy. Such transient bacteremias, however, are unpredictable. Delayed clearance from the bloodstream allows pathogens to multiply and cause either disseminated or focal disease.

CLINICAL MANIFESTATIONS

The clinical signs of bacterial infection in the neonate are presented in Table 24-3. These signs are distinctively nonspecific and may be associated with viral infections or with noninfectious

TABLE 24-3. Nonspecific Signs of Sepsis

Temperature instability
Respiratory distress
Feeding intolerance
Vomiting
Abdominal distention
Diarrhea
Jaundice
Pallor
Skin rash, petechiae
Hypotension
Tachycardia
Apnea and bradycardia
Irritability
High-pitched cry
Lethargy
Weak suck
Convulsions
Bulging of full fontanelle

disorders. Because the neonate is an impaired host, the clinical course is unpredictable and, can be, rapidly progressive. The presence of any of these signs alone or in combination may be an indication for complete evaluation to rule out sepsis and prompt initiation of empiric antimicrobial therapy.

Early-Onset Syndrome

Clinical manifestations of the GBS early-onset syndrome may be present at birth or appear at any time in the first week of life, but 95% of infants with early-onset infection present within the first 72 hours of life. Of the reported patients, 80% are term infants. Onset is usually sudden and follows a fulminant course with the primary focus of inflammation in the lungs. In 60% of infected patients, chest roentgenography shows a reticulogranular pattern with air bronchograms indistinguishable from that seen with hyaline membrane disease that is not complicated by infection. Gram-positive cocci may be seen within the hyaline membranes at postmortem examination. Persistent pulmonary hypertension may complicate the respiratory tract disease. In the most severe cases, apnea, hypotension, and disseminated intravascular coagulation cause rapid deterioration and result in death within 24 hours. Even prompt administration of antibiotics and aggressive supportive therapy may be unsuccessful in these overwhelmed infants. The case-fatality rate has been as high as 40% to 80%, but it is now 5% to 15% because of early recognition and the availability of advanced intensive care facilities. Serotypes Ia and III are associated with most cases of early-onset GBS disease when meningitis is not present. Groups D and G streptococci and nontypable *H. influenzae* are associated with a similar syndrome. Rarely, a transient GBS bacteremia may occur and produce mild, if any, clinical symptoms. If untreated, however, most bacteremia results in metastatic infection and fulminant disease. Meningitis may occur in 10% to 25% of bacteremic infants but is rarely present at birth.

The early-onset syndrome associated with *L. monocytogenes* has several distinguishing features. Often a flu-like illness occurs in the mother just before delivery, and the maternal blood culture results may be positive. In the infant, the lung is the primary focus of infection, but hepatosplenomegaly, purulent conjunctivitis, a skin rash consisting of irregular macules and papules or pustules in a truncal distribution, petechiae, and small granulomas on the posterior pharynx are characteristic of listeriosis. Chest roentgenography shows a distinct reticulonodular pattern of bronchopneumonia that is pathognomonic for this infection. The case-fatality rate is 40% to 80%.

Late-Onset Syndrome

The late-onset syndrome associated with GBS and *L. monocytogenes* usually occurs in infants 8 to 30 days of age, but it may be seen as late as 12 to 16 weeks, especially in premature infants. The onset is most often insidious, and the affected infants present with the nonspecific signs of sepsis. Meningitis is the most characteristic finding. GBS is known for its broad variety of foci, the most notable of which are osteomyelitis, septic arthritis, skin and soft tissue lesions, endocarditis, peritonitis, omphalitis, and pericarditis.

DIAGNOSIS

Whenever bacterial infection of the neonate is suspected, cultures of blood, cerebrospinal fluid, urine, and infected body fluids that are normally sterile or an aspirate from an infected soft tissue site or bone should be obtained before initiating antimicrobial therapy. Using more advanced blood culture technology, true pathogens are always recovered within 48 hours. Bacteria such as coagulase-negative staphylococcus or viridans streptococci, which are common contaminants, are more likely to be pathogens if isolated within 48 hours of incubation and if the same organism is isolated from blood cultures obtained from two separate sites.

Cultures of mucosal surfaces are not helpful in distinguishing the infected from the colonized infant. Similarly, gastric aspirate cultures reflect the maternal environment and do not distinguish the infected from the colonized infant. The polymorphonuclear leukocytes present in the gastric aspirate are of maternal origin and may reflect fetal stress of noninfectious origin. In contrast, culture of the tracheal aspirate obtained at the time of intubation has been useful in identifying the etiologic agent of early-onset neonatal pneumonia. Beyond the initial endotracheal tube placement, tracheal aspirates are less helpful because bacteria frequently colonize the tube without causing disease.

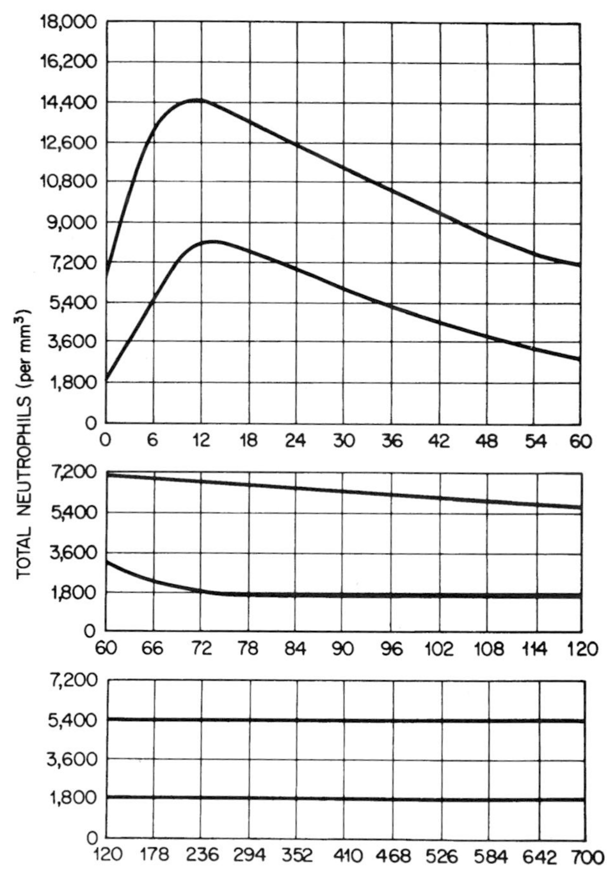

Figure 24-1. Normal total neutrophil counts after correction for nucleated red blood cells in neonates from birth to 700 hours of age. Formula for correction is as follows:

$$WBC = WBC_{CC} \times \frac{100}{NRBC + 100}$$

where WBC = corrected white blood cell count; WBC_{CC} = Coulter counter white blood cell count; NRBC = nucleated red blood cells. (Adapted from Manroe BL, Rosenfeld CR, Weinberg AG, Browne R. The neonatal blood count in health and disease. I. Reference values for neutrophilic cells. *J Pediatr* 1979;95:89; reprinted from House Staff Nursery Manual, Division of Neonatal-Perinatal Medicine, Southwestern Medical School, Dallas, TX, revised 1985.)

Because of poor sensitivity and specificity, latex particle agglutination tests are rarely helpful for clinical decision making and their use is discouraged in the child who has not yet received antibiotics.

Although many other tests have been studied such as C-reactive protein, ESR, and specific interleukin levels, the leukocyte count and differential continue to be used as a reliable indirect indicator of bacterial infection. After correction of the Coulter leukocyte count for the presence of nucleated red blood cells, the absolute total neutrophil count and the ratio of immature-to-total neutrophils are compared with normal standards for age (Figs. 24-1 and 24-2). Neutropenia is more likely than neutrophilia to be associated with neonatal sepsis. Pregnancy-induced hypertension or asphyxia in the absence of infection, however, may produce neutropenia in the absence of infection. The neutropenia of infection does not persist for more than 36 hours, whereas the neutropenia observed with noninfectious conditions may persist through the first 3 postnatal days and the ratio of immature-to-total neutrophils remains normal in the absence of infection. The most useful indicator of bacterial infection is an immature-to-total neutrophils ratio of 0.2 or more. An immature-to-total neutrophils ratio of 0.8 or more indicates depletion of bone marrow reserves and a poor prognosis for survival. The leukocyte count and immature-to-total neutrophils ratio determinations should be repeated after 12 hours, because studies in both animals and human infants demonstrate that the leukocyte count may be normal at the onset of GBS sepsis but becomes abnormal during the next 4 to 8 hours.

Chest roentgenography should always be obtained as part of the diagnostic evaluation of the infant with suspected sepsis and signs of respiratory tract disease. Other radiographic studies may be indicated by the specific clinical condition. Sonography, computed tomography, and magnetic resonance imaging are the most useful imaging techniques in this age group. Technetium bone scans have a high rate of false-negatives in very young infants, and gallium scans are discouraged because of the large amount of radiation.

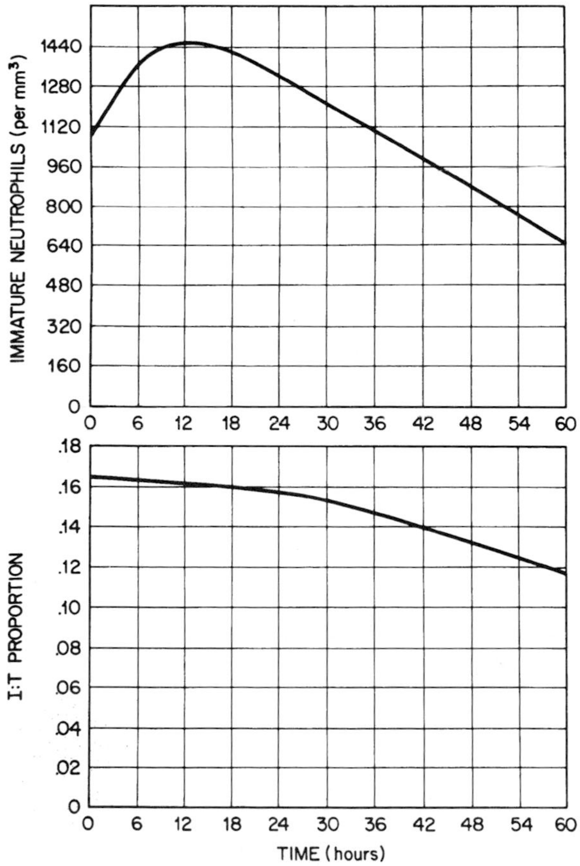

Figure 24-2. Normal total immature neutrophil counts and ratios of immature to total neutrophils (I:T) in neonates from birth to 60 hours of age. All bands and cell forms less mature than bands are classified together as immature neutrophils. (Adapted from Manroe BL, Rosenfeld CR, Weinberg AG, et al. The differential leukocyte count in the assessment and outcome of early onset group B streptococcal disease. *J Pediatr* 1977;91:632; reprinted from House Staff Nursery Manual, Division of Neonatal-Perinatal Medicine, Southwestern Medical School, Dallas, TX, revised 1997.)

THERAPY

The decision to initiate antimicrobial therapy in the neonate is based on the likelihood that an infant's clinical signs are a manifestation of infection, or that the normal-appearing infant is at high risk for developing infection within the first few hours of life. Because of the increased risk of infection and the subtlety of clinical manifestations of infection in premature infants, antimicrobial therapy should be strongly considered in the premature infant with only a single obstetric or clinical risk factor. In contrast, the asymptomatic term infant with only obstetric risk factors presents more of a dilemma. The approach recommended by the Centers for Disease Control and Prevention (CDC) (2002) for the management of a neonate whose mother received intrapartum antimicrobial GBS prophylaxis is shown in Fig. 24-3. The goal of this scheme is to identify and treat all infected infants but to avoid excessive investigation and treatment of uninfected infants. It must be emphasized that this algorithm is not an exclusive course of management. Variations that incorporate individual circumstances or institutional preferences may be appropriate.

Omission of a lumbar puncture in asymptomatic term infants with only a single risk factor who are evaluated in the first few hours after delivery is unlikely to jeopardize the diagnosis of meningitis, because term infants with *in utero* meningitis are almost always symptomatic at birth. If, however, the initial blood culture result becomes positive in an infant who did not have a lumbar puncture as part of the initial diagnostic evaluation, the lumbar puncture should be performed to be certain that meningitis has not developed. Lumbar puncture should also be considered in the evaluation of infants whose mothers received intrapartum antibiotics and have signs of infection but whose blood culture results are sterile. Furthermore, development or worsening of clinical signs of infection is an indication for immediate reevaluation and completion of the sepsis workup with lumbar puncture and initiation of antimicrobial therapy.

The choice of antimicrobial agents is determined by several factors: the likely etiologic agent, susceptibility patterns within a specific nursery, central nervous system penetration, toxicity, and the infant's hepatic and renal function. The regimen favored for empiric therapy of early-onset sepsis within the first 5 days of life is ampicillin and an aminoglycoside. Ampicillin is recommended rather than penicillin for its activity against *L. monocytogenes* and enterococci. Gentamicin remains the aminoglycoside of choice in most U.S. nurseries. Third-generation cephalosporins such as cefotaxime and ceftazidime should *not* be used routinely for empiric therapy of suspected sepsis because of the rapid emergence of resistance associated with heavy usage within a closed unit. Specific indications for usage of these newer drugs include gram-negative meningitis, prevalence of multidrug-resistant gram-negative rods, persistent

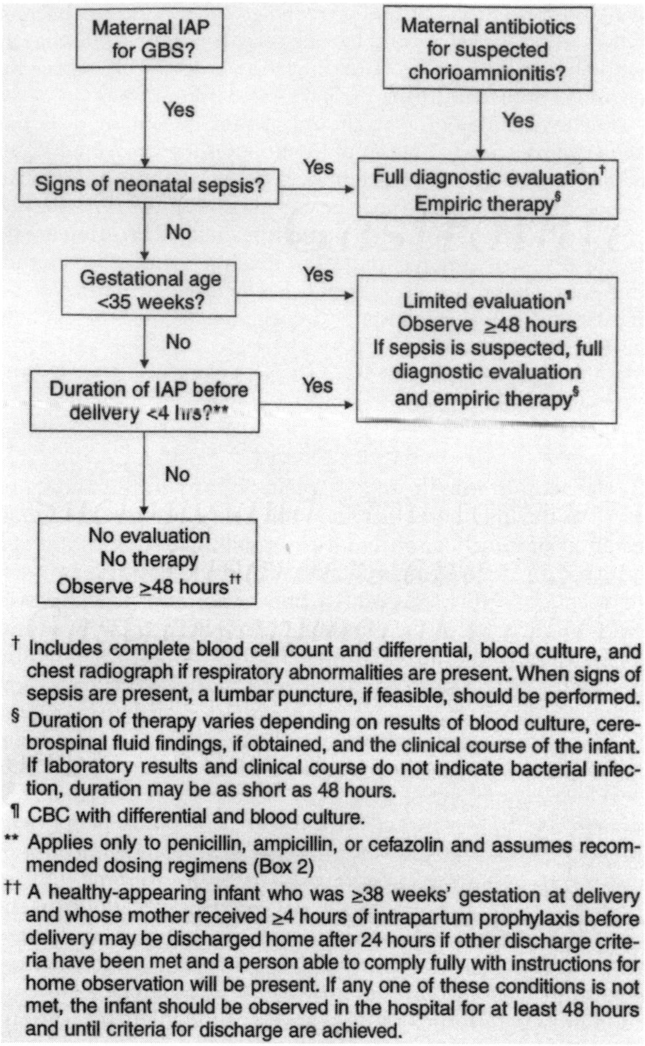

Figure 24-3. Sample algorithm for management of a newborn whose mother received intrapartum antimicrobial agents for prevention of early-onset group B streptococcal disease or suspected chorioamnionitis. This algorithm is not an exclusive course of management. Variations that incorporate individual circumstances or institutional preferences may be appropriate (Reprinted with permission from Centers for Disease Control and Prevention. Prevention of Perinatal Group B Streptococcal Disease. MMWR 2002;51(No. RR-11):13).

gram-negative bacteremia, poor clinical response to aminoglycosides, and extensive deep tissue infection or abscess. The decreased activity of aminoglycosides under acidic and anaerobic conditions characteristic of abscesses and deep tissue infections makes this class of drugs less effective for the treatment of such infections. When a third-generation cephalosporin is administered before identification of the infecting pathogen, ampicillin should be administered additionally because cephalosporins are inactive against *L. monocytogenes* and enterococci.

Beyond 5 days of age in the hospital environment, staphylococci become more likely pathogens requiring substitution of ampicillin with oxacillin, or with vancomycin if methicillin-resistant *S. aureus* is present within the nursery, or if foreign bodies (e.g., central venous catheters, shunts) are present, and the risk of coagulase staphylococci is increased. Virtually all coagulase-negative staphylococci are resistant to nafcillin, oxacillin, and clindamycin and require vancomycin treatment when they are true pathogens. Vancomycin use is a risk factor for the acquisition of vancomycin-resistant enterococcal infections. Thus, if no gram-positive organisms that are susceptible to vancomycin only (i.e., methicillin-resistant *S. aureus*, coagulase-negative staphylococci, ampicillin-resistant enterococci) are isolated by 48 hours, vancomycin should be discontinued. Obtaining two blood cultures from separate sites is helpful in distinguishing contaminants from true pathogens. Vancomycin treatment has been associated with delayed sterilization of cerebrospinal fluid in infants with GBS meningitis; therefore, ampicillin should be included if a vancomycin and aminoglycoside regimen is initiated, and GBS meningitis is likely.

The usual duration of treatment for most uncomplicated bacterial infections is 7 to 10 days. Longer courses (14 or 21 days or longer) are indicated for the treatment of meningitis and septic arthritis and osteomyelitis. The intravenous route of drug administration is preferred, but similar amounts of drugs (area under the curve) may be delivered after intramuscular injections in infants with adequate muscle mass and stable cardiovascular function. Bacterial disease is documented by culture in approximately 10% of infants with suspected sepsis. Therefore, a 7-day course of antimicrobial therapy is often completed in infants whose bacterial cultures are sterile at 48 hours when no other explanation for the infant's clinical condition exists, and an apparent response to therapy has occurred.

Provision of general supportive care to the septic infant is of utmost importance in optimizing the outcome. The need for ventilatory support, volume expansion with fresh-frozen plasma, replacement of blood or platelets, correction of electrolyte and other metabolic abnormalities, and early initiation of hyperalimentation must be determined. Increasing attention

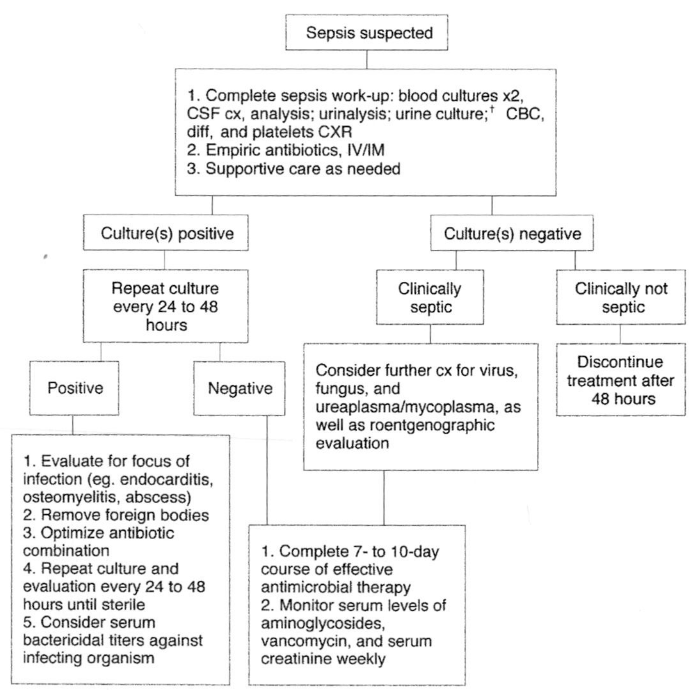

Figure 24-4. Recommended approach to the diagnostic evaluation and treatment of the neonate with suspected sepsis. †Urine cultures are rarely positive in the first 48 hours of life and may be omitted from the workup at that age. Subsequently, suprapubic bladder aspiration is the preferred method. CBC, complete blood count; CSF, cerebral spinal fluid; CXR, chest roentgenographic examination; diff, differential blood count; IM, intramuscularly; IV, intravenously.

has been directed toward enhancement of the neonate's deficient host responses. Intravenous immunoglobulin (IGIV) is a possible adjunctive therapy. Administration of IGIV preparations may improve neutrophil use and egression of neutrophils from the bone marrow and prevent bone marrow depletion, as well as provide specific deficient antibodies and improved opsonophagocytosis. A beneficial effect is observed only if immunoglobulin is given early in the course of disease in animal models. A meta-analysis of 110 evaluable cases of neonatal sepsis in three studies showed a significant decrease in acute mortality for neonates with sepsis who received a single dose of IGIV at the onset of clinical signs in addition to standard therapies.

An approach to the evaluation and treatment of neonates with suspected sepsis is shown in Fig. 24-4.

PREVENTION

Studies of prevention of neonatal infections have focused on GBS because of its greater prevalence and immunogenicity than the other common pathogen, *E. coli* K1. Both chemoprophylaxis and immunoprophylaxis measures have been under investigation. Intrapartum administration of ampicillin and gentamicin to women with chorioamnionitis has improved neonatal outcome. The reader is referred to the revised GBS Prevention Guidelines published by the CDC. These can be viewed at http://www.cdc.gov/mmwr/PDF/rr/rr5111.pdf Ultimately, a polyvalent GBS vaccine may prove to be the most effective prevention strategy.

CHAPTER 25
Meningitis

Adapted from Marc H. Lebel

EPIDEMIOLOGY

The incidence of neonatal bacterial meningitis is approximately 0.5 cases per 1,000 live births. The rates vary according to nursery and predisposing maternal and infant risk factors. The incidence of meningitis in low-birth-weight (LBW) infants is approximately three times that of infants with birth weight greater than 2,500 g. The other risk factors associated with an increased incidence of neonatal bacteremia and meningitis include premature or prolonged rupture of membranes, maternal fever or chorioamnionitis, and traumatic delivery. Group B streptococcus and *Listeria monocytogenes* can present with early-onset and late-onset diseases. Late-onset infections (after 7 days of life) are more often associated with meningitis.

MICROBIOLOGY

Group B streptococci and *Escherichia coli* are the two most frequent pathogens causing meningitis. *L. monocytogenes* is also an important but less frequently encountered pathogen. In some institutions, nonenterococcal group D streptococci cause a substantial proportion of meningitis cases. *Enterobacter* species, *Salmonellae* species, and other gram-negative bacilli are infrequently encountered. *Citrobacter diversus* can cause sporadic or epidemic meningitis in the neonate. *Staphylococcus* and *Candida* species occasionally cause meningitis in the sick premature infant who is subjected to invasive supportive management and monitoring devices. Common pathogenic organisms (*Haemophilus influenzae* type b, *Neisseria meningitidis*, and *Streptococcus pneumoniae*) of meningitis in older infants and children are infrequent causes of meningitis in the neonate.

PATHOGENESIS

Most cases of meningitis result from hematogenous dissemination. Factors that predispose to bacteremia also predispose to meningitis; up to one-third of infants with bacteremia develop meningitis. Rarely, meningitis is secondary to extension from infected skin through the soft tissues and skull (e.g., infected cephalhematoma). Infants with congenital malformations of the neural tube such as meningomyeloceles, can be infected by direct spread from skin surfaces.

Many organisms causing meningitis in the newborn possess specific surface antigens. The K1 polysaccharide of *E. coli* is present in 75% to 85% of strains isolated from neonates with meningitis. The BIII polysaccharide of group B streptococci is recovered from 30% of early-onset and 90% of late-onset strains causing neonatal meningitis. Type IVb strains of *L. monocytogenes* account for most meningitis cases.

The K1 antigen of *E. coli* confers resistance to phagocytosis and does not activate the alternate complement pathway. Immunochemical similarities exist between glycopeptides of the brain containing sialic acid and the capsular polysaccharide of *E. coli* K1 strains. Specific antibodies to the K1 antigen, however, appear to be highly protective against sepsis and meningitis. Delayed clearance of *E. coli* because of decreased phagocytosis may allow replication of the organism in the blood to a concentration of 1,000 or more organisms per milliliter, a concentration associated with an increased incidence of meningitis.

The capsular polysaccharide of serotype III of the group B streptococci seems to mediate resistance to phagocytosis; strains expressing this antigen adhere to buccal epithelial cells of neonates better than to those of adults. The presence of type-specific antibodies is necessary for opsonization of type Ia, II, and III strains, and high concentrations appear to confer resistance to the newborn infant. Phagocytosis of the organism is normal in the presence of type III polysaccharide, but chemiluminescence of neutrophils is decreased when exposed to this antigen; however, this decrease in chemiluminescence has also been found with other pathogens.

The pathogenesis of late-onset disease caused by group B streptococci is unclear. In most instances, serotype III is the infecting pathogen. Predisposing risk factors are usually absent. A history of preceding respiratory tract infection is present in many patients. This infection may alter the nasopharyngeal epithelium and facilitate invasion by the streptococci.

PATHOLOGY

The pathologic findings of meningitis in neonates are similar to those found in older children. A diffuse purulent leptomeningitis is almost always found and is more pronounced at the base of the brain. In the acute phase of the illness, brain edema is frequently present, but cerebral herniation is uncommon. Vasculitis is common with resultant thrombosis and possibly infarct of brain tissue. Brain abscesses can develop in these areas and can involve multiple lobes. Ventriculitis is present in three-fourths of infants, and hydrocephalus develops in approximately one-third. Subdural effusions rarely occur in the neonate. Leukomalacia with porencephaly can develop as a result of tissue anoxia.

CLINICAL MANIFESTATIONS

The clinical manifestations of meningitis in the newborn infant are often nonspecific and indistinguishable from those of sepsis. Meningitis should always be considered when the diagnosis of bacteremia is suspected. The cardinal signs of meningitis in older children such as stiff neck and Kernig and Brudzinski signs, are absent in most infants.

The most frequent signs are temperature instability, respiratory distress, irritability, lethargy, and poor feeding or vomiting. Seizures occur in 40% of newborn infants with meningitis. Other signs include a bulging fontanelle, hyperactivity or hypoactivity, alteration of the level of consciousness, tremor, twitching, apnea, stiff neck or opisthotonos, hemiparesis, and cranial nerve palsy.

DIAGNOSIS

The diagnosis of meningitis is based on examination and culture of the CSF. In most instances, when sepsis is suspected, a lumbar puncture should be performed at the time of the sepsis workup. In a critically ill child, however, the lumbar puncture can be postponed until the cardiorespiratory condition is stable. Although CSF cultures may be sterile in the infant who has received antibiotics before diagnosis, examination of the CSF for cellular and biochemistry values and for antigen detection is almost always indicative of meningitis.

A Gram-stained smear of CSF should be made for all infants, because grossly clear fluid with only a few cells can contain many bacteria. Gram stain or acridine orange smear of CSF reveals bacteria in at least 80% of infants with culture-proven meningitis. Because of the low concentrations of organisms (i.e., 10^3 colony-forming units per microliter of CSF), most Gram stain smears of CSF from infants with *L. monocytogenes* meningitis do not reveal the gram-positive bacillus.

The CSF laboratory findings in the neonate differ from those in older children (Table 25-1); this difference may be a result of an increase in the permeability of the blood–brain barrier (i.e., cerebral capillary endothelial cells). By 1 month of age, an infant's leukocyte count should be in the range of 0 to 5 cells per microliter. An overlap exists in the different cellular and biochemical characteristics between the infants with and without meningitis. Fewer than 1% of infants with proven meningitis, however, have an initial CSF examination that is completely normal. Simultaneous concentrations of blood and CSF glucose should be obtained, because low CSF glucose can reflect concurrent hypoglycemia, and a CSF-to-blood glucose ratio of less than 0.6 (60%) should be considered abnormal. The CSF leukocyte count is elevated in most newborns with meningitis, and polymorphonuclear leukocytes are preponderant except in some patients with listerial meningitis. The protein concentration may not be elevated at the time of diagnosis.

Blood culture specimens should be obtained from every patient; 85% of neonates with bacterial meningitis have positive blood culture results at the time of presentation.

TABLE 25-1. Normal Values for Cerebrospinal Fluid Examination in Neonates

	Term	Preterm[a]
Leukocyte count per microliter	7 (0–32)[b]	8 (0–29)
Percent of polymorphonuclear leukocytes	61	57
Protein (mg/dL)	90 (20–170)	115 (65–150)
Glucose (mg/dL)	52 (34–119)	50 (24–63)
Cerebrospinal fluid–to–blood glucose ratio	51% (44–248%)	75% (55–105%)

[a]Preterm is less than 38 weeks' gestation.
[b]Mean (range).
Adapted from Sarff LD, Platt LH, McCracken GH Jr. Cerebrospinal fluid evaluation in neonates: comparison of high risk infants with and without meningitis. *J Pediatr* 1976;88:273.

THERAPY

After CSF and blood cultures are obtained, antibiotic therapy should be initiated promptly with ampicillin and an aminoglycoside such as gentamicin or amikacin, or ampicillin and cefotaxime, in meningitis dosages. Therapy should be adjusted depending on results of cultures and susceptibility testing. For group B streptococcal or *L. monocytogenes* infection, 14 days of ampicillin or penicillin therapy is adequate in the patient without complications. However, some experts suggest a 21-day course of treatment. The addition of an aminoglycoside to ampicillin has been suggested by some authors because of synergistic activity against group B streptococci and *Listeria* species, especially if the strain demonstrates *in vitro* tolerance (i.e., a 32-fold difference between the minimal inhibitory concentration and minimal bactericidal concentration). No clinical studies have proven superiority of one regimen over another.

For gram-negative enteric meningitis, ampicillin and gentamicin have been used extensively since the 1970s. Delayed CSF sterilization for 3 or more days occurs in one-half of infants with meningitis caused by gram-negative pathogens. Because a poor prognosis is correlated directly with duration of positive CSF cultures for more than 3 days, many therapeutic regimens have been evaluated in an effort to improve the rate of bacteriologic response. Intrathecal and intraventricular antibiotic therapy is not recommended for neonatal meningitis.

The third-generation cephalosporins offer potential advantages for therapy of meningitis in the neonatal period. They possess extraordinary *in vitro* activity against gram-negative enteric bacilli (including most of the causative pathogens of neonatal meningitis), achieve high serum concentrations, and penetrate well into the CSF. They appear to be safe and well tolerated and lack the nephrotoxicity and ototoxicity associated with the use of aminoglycosides. Except for moxalactam, the third-generation cephalosporins are active against most streptococci but are inactive against *L. monocytogenes* and enterococci. Only ceftazidime provides adequate activity against *Pseudomonas aeruginosa*.

Cefotaxime is preferred for therapy of neonatal meningitis over other new-generation cephalosporins because of more extensive experience with this drug in the neonatal period, and because it does not substantially alter the bowel flora. Extensive or exclusive use of a cephalosporin in a closed newborn unit, however, may lead to rapid emergence of resistance. Outbreaks of cefotaxime-resistant *Enterobacter cloacae* infections have been described shortly after beginning routine therapy with cefotaxime for suspected sepsis in two neonatal intensive care units. These agents should be used selectively and as alternatives to the conventional regimen. Because of high biliary excretion and marked alteration of the normal intestinal flora and because of the potential concern for displacement of bilirubin, ceftriaxone should not be used in the newborn infant.

For gram-negative enteric meningitis, the duration of therapy should be 21 days or longer and should continue for at least 14 days after the first sterile CSF culture result. No published data exist on the efficacy of dexamethasone adjunctive therapy in neonatal meningitis. Corticosteroids cannot be recommended for infants with neonatal meningitis.

For premature infants hospitalized in the nursery for prolonged periods, staphylococci, enterococci, and gentamicin-resistant gram-negative organisms are potential pathogens. An alternative antimicrobial regimen should be considered. A combination of ampicillin and cefotaxime or ceftazidime could be used as initial empiric therapy. When an indwelling vascular catheter or a ventriculoperitoneal shunt is in place or when *S. epidermidis* and methicillin-resistant *S. aureus* are frequent causes of infection, vancomycin plus amikacin or vancomycin plus cefotaxime can be used initially. Metronidazole is indicated for treatment of central nervous system infection caused by *B. fragilis*.

Another CSF culture should be made after 48 to 72 hours of therapy to ensure sterility of the CSF. If culture results are positive after 48 hours for group B streptococci and 72 hours for coliform organisms, the susceptibilities of the pathogen should be reviewed. Cranial sonography, computed tomography (CT), or magnetic resonance imaging (MRI) should be considered. In all cases of meningitis caused by *C. diversus*, cranial CT or MRI scans should be obtained because of the frequent association with brain abscesses. In patients with an uncomplicated course of gram-negative meningitis, cranial CT or MRI scans should be obtained before discharge. The duration of antibiotic therapy for brain abscess should be at least 4 to 6 weeks depending on clinical evolution and resolution of the lesion based on repeated tomography. Neurosurgery should be considered early for needle aspiration of the abscess to identify the etiologic agent and to provide drainage or excision of the abscesses. Aminoglycosides are not very effective because of decreased activity in abscess cavities that have a low pH and anaerobic conditions.

Supportive care of the newborn is similar to that of the septic infant. Careful neurologic examination should be performed daily and the head circumference measured. Seizures should be controlled with intravenously administered phenobarbital or phenytoin. The serum electrolytes should be followed for detection of hyponatremia as a result of inappropriate secretion of antidiuretic hormone; fluid restriction is instituted if this condition develops. Some newborns with group B streptococcal meningitis develop diabetes insipidus during the course of the illness. Serum concentrations of aminoglycosides in the newborn period are unpredictable, especially for the LBW premature infant, and should be routinely determined to achieve therapeutic concentrations and avoid toxicity. Every infant should have a brainstem-evoked response audiogram at discharge or within 6 weeks after discharge from the hospital to detect hearing impairment.

PROGNOSIS

Despite improvement in intensive care facilities and excellent *in vitro* activity of the third-generation cephalosporins, meningitis in the neonatal period is still a devastating disease. The case-fatality rate remains approximately 15% to 30% depending on the causative pathogen, predisposing risk factors, and availability of intensive care facilities.

A poor outcome is associated with presence of coma at admission, persistent seizures, low birth weight, ventriculitis, duration of positive CSF culture results, very low or very high CSF leukocyte count, protein concentration higher than 500 mg/dL, and presence of brain abscess. For group B streptococcus, approximately 15% to 20% of survivors have major sequelae including spastic quadriplegia, profound mental retardation, hemiparesis, deafness, or blindness. Hydrocephalus develops in 11% of cases, and 13% have a seizure disorder. Survivors without major sequelae on physical examination, however, seem to function within normal limits and comparably with their siblings.

Sequelae are found in 35% to 50% of survivors of gram-negative meningitis. Ten percent have severe sequelae as defined by failure to develop beyond the age at which the disease occurred or required custodial care. Approximately 25% to 35% have mild to moderate sequelae, which many times do not interfere with adequate, albeit delayed, development. Hydrocephalus develops in one-third of patients. The prognosis of infants with brain abscesses is generally poor.

CHAPTER 26

Skin and Soft Tissue Infections

Adapted from Pablo J. Sánchez and Jane D. Siegel

The most common manifestations of skin and soft tissue bacterial infections are presented in Table 26-1. Most of these conditions occur beyond the first 3 days of life. The most frequently observed conditions are pustular lesions (impetigo neonatorum) caused by *Staphylococcus aureus* that cluster around the umbilicus and diaper area and are not usually associated with fever or systemic illness. Gram-positive cocci and polymorphonuclear leukocytes present on Gram-stained smear examination distinguish pustules from erythema toxicum, in which case only eosinophils are seen on smear. If only a few lesions are present, they are treated effectively by cleansing alone or cleansing followed by application of a topical antibiotic ointment. More extensive lesions may be treated with oral cephalexin for 5 days.

Staphylococcal scalded skin syndrome, or Ritter disease, is a much more extensive, exfoliative disease caused by phage group II staphylococci. These organisms elaborate an exotoxin that causes intraepidermal cleavage at the stratum granulosum. Infants first present with a tender, sunburn-like erythematous rash, then bullae develop with desquamation of large areas of skin. The presence of a Nikolsky sign (desquamation of the superficial layer of skin after light pressure over areas that appear to be uninvolved) is pathognomonic. The site of toxin production is distal from the area of involvement and is usually the conjunctiva, nasopharynx, umbilicus, or circumcision site.

TABLE 26-1. Infections of the Skin and Soft Tissues

Pustules
Impetigo
Scalded skin syndrome (Ritter disease)
Abscess of skin, scalp, breast
Omphalitis
Cellulitis
Adenitis
Necrotizing fasciitis
Echthyma gangrenosum

Staphylococcal bacteremia and superinfection are absent. These infants require intravenous antibiotic therapy to eliminate carriage of the toxin-producing staphylococci.

Toxic shock syndrome is associated with a unique toxin produced by certain strains of *S. aureus*. The focus of infection may not always be apparent. Clinical manifestations in neonates are similar to those seen in older children and adults: sunburn-like rash with mild desquamation occurring in the second week of illness and multiorgan system involvement with cardiovascular instability. Blood culture results are usually sterile, and the toxin-producing staphylococci may be recovered from mucosal surfaces or sites of tissue infection. Intravenous antibiotics and aggressive supportive care are required. Fluid requirements are greater than estimated because of severe capillary leak.

Scalp abscess is a complication of fetal monitoring with scalp electrodes. Any of the microorganisms present in the birth canal may be implicated. Superficial abscesses are treated locally with incision, drainage, and cleansing with an antibacterial solution. The presence of cellulitis requires systemic antibiotics. An infected cephalohematoma should be distinguished from a large superficial scalp abscess, because an infected cephalohematoma may be complicated by an underlying osteomyelitis.

Breast abscess is a well-localized lesion that is usually unilateral and presents more commonly in female infants with few if any systemic signs. The only clinical findings are swelling with erythema and warmth. Although group B streptococcus and *S. aureus* are the most common agents, gram-negative enteric bacilli have also been isolated. Rarely, bacteremia may be present. A diagnostic aspiration of the abscess should be performed and the infant should be treated with parenteral antibiotics. The choice of agent(s) can be made based on a Gram-stained smear of the drainage. If gram-positive cocci are seen, it is not necessary to provide gram-negative coverage. Incision and drainage, when required, should be carried out by a skilled pediatric surgeon to avoid damage to normal breast tissue in female infants.

In a term baby who is afebrile, minimal drainage from the umbilicus with mild erythema may be treated with local care and orally administered cephalexin or amoxicillin and clavulanate potassium. A wet, malodorous umbilical cord with minimal inflammation is usually associated with group A streptococcus and may be treated with a single intramuscular injection of benzathine penicillin G or a 5- to 7-day course of penicillin, or a semisynthetic penicillin (oxacillin or nafcillin), or cefazolin if concomitant *S. aureus* infection exists. More severe infection with bacteremia, cellulitis, necrotizing fasciitis, or peritonitis, however, may be associated with any of the neonatal pathogens and, therefore, requires treatment with broad-spectrum antibiotics for 10 to 14 days. Anaerobes, especially *Clostridium* species, may be important pathogens in severe necrotizing omphalitis; therefore, clindamycin or metronidazole should be included in the antibiotic regimen.

A characteristic syndrome of submandibular cellulitis or lymphadenitis has been described in infants with group B streptococcal bacteremia. These infants present at 2 to 10 weeks of age with the nonspecific signs of sepsis, fever, and a characteristic swelling with overlying erythema in the submandibular or submental area. Occasionally, the focal cellulitis appears during the first few hours after the patient is admitted to the hospital for treatment of suspected sepsis without a focus. Group B streptococcus is isolated from blood and tissue aspirate, and meningitis is not usually present. Response to parenteral antibiotic therapy is prompt.

Overwhelming sepsis and shock are associated with necrotizing fasciitis and ecthyma gangrenosum. An indurated area of skin with violaceous discoloration, overlying bullae, and rapid progression to necrosis is characteristic of necrotizing fasciitis. Group B streptococcus alone, or mixed bacteria, are associated with this process. Extensive debridement and broad-spectrum antimicrobials are required to control the systemic toxicity. This is the most serious infectious complication of circumcision. Ecthyma gangrenosum is a manifestation of vasculitis of the cutaneous blood vessels associated with *Pseudomonas aeruginosa* bacteremia or, less commonly, other gram-negative bacilli such as *Serratia* species. The lesion first appears as a vesicle on an erythematous base, then forms a well-demarcated area of induration with a necrotic center. The infecting organisms may be isolated from the skin lesion. Treatment of the septicemia with parenteral therapy is required.

Failure of *S. aureus* skin or soft tissue infections to respond to cephalosporins or semisynthetic penicillins may be caused by strains of methicillin-resistant *S. aureus* (MRSA). Therefore, it is helpful to know whether MRSA is considered endemic in the local hospital or community. Topical mupirocin ointment may be used for superficial MRSA infections. No oral antimicrobial agents that are effective against MRSA are appropriate for use in the neonate. Serious systemic MRSA infections require treatment with vancomycin.

S. aureus, and especially MRSA, infections in the first few weeks of life should be reported to the birth nursery to facilitate recognition of an outbreak in the nursery. Although infections this early in life are most often hospital-acquired, increasing numbers of community-acquired MRSA infections are reported in children without identifiable risk factors.

CHAPTER 27

Urinary Tract Infections

Adapted from Marc H. Lebel

EPIDEMIOLOGY

In infants less than 2 months of age presenting with fever, urinary tract infection is found in 8% to 10% of patients. Some studies indicate an increased susceptibility to urinary tract infections in uncircumcised male infants. Other reports suggest that breastfeeding is associated with a lower incidence of infection.

PATHOGENESIS

Urinary tract infections can be acquired by hematogenous infection of the kidney in association with neonatal bacteremia or by the ascending route via the genitourinary tract. The short female urethra is thought to allow for ascending infection and explains the higher frequency of infection in girls older than 3 months. In the uncircumcised male infant, accumulation of bacteria in preputial folds with meatal contamination is likely. Specific fimbrial receptors on the foreskin and along the urethra may allow for ascending infection. Malformations of the urinary tract may predispose to infection. Between 5% and 20% of infants presenting with urinary tract infection have an underlying malformation of the urinary tract.

In infants, 50% to 70% of *Escherichia coli* strains causing urinary infection belong to one of the eight common pyelonephritogenic O serotypes found in older patients. Furthermore, *E. coli* can attach to specific receptors on uroepithelial cells. *E. coli* strains isolated from infants with urinary tract infection show a higher percentage of P and X fimbriation and more type 1 pili than found in matched control patients. Other recognized *E. coli* virulence factors include hemolysin production, colicin production, resistance to serum bactericidal activity, and the ability to acquire iron.

MICROBIOLOGY

E. coli is the most frequent pathogen causing 75% to 85% of infections. Other gram-negative organisms such as *Klebsiella pneumoniae, Enterobacter* species, *Proteus vulgaris,* and *Pseudomonas aeruginosa* are encountered less often. Gram-positive bacteria (including enterococci, group B streptococci, and *Staphylococcus* species) are uncommon pathogens in neonates. Candidal infections are seen in debilitated newborns as part of disseminated candidiasis or in the presence of an indwelling urinary catheter. A few patients have been reported with mixed bacterial infections.

CLINICAL MANIFESTATIONS

Few specific symptoms or signs of urinary tract infection are recognizable in the newborn period. Conversely, clinical manifestations vary widely, and many infants are completely asymptomatic. When symptoms are present, they often consist of fever, irritability, decreased feeding, and lethargy. Some patients present with diarrhea, vomiting, or weight loss. Jaundice is seen in approximately 7% of cases and can be accompanied by hepatomegaly and splenomegaly. The genitalia should be carefully inspected and the abdomen palpated gently to detect malformations or enlargement of the kidneys and bladder. Occasionally, an alert caretaker notices crying on urination (i.e., dysuria).

DIAGNOSIS

The diagnosis of urinary tract infection is based on examination and culture of an appropriately collected urine specimen. A urine culture should be included in the sepsis workup of all infants older than 72 hours of age. Within the first 3 days of life, urinary tract infection occurs secondary to bacteremia; therefore, such infants are identified by blood culture. The most reliable test is when urine is obtained by suprapubic bladder puncture. This technique is safe and easy; bleeding or perforation of the bowel occurs rarely. Dehydration, abdominal distention, and a bleeding diathesis are contraindications for suprapubic aspiration. To optimize the yield of a successful tap, the aspiration should be done 30 to 60 minutes after the infant has voided. Any bacterial growth in cultures obtained by a suprapubic puncture is considered significant. In one study evaluating urine cultures obtained by suprapubic aspiration, 55% of children had fewer than the traditional 100,000 colonies per microliter and 9% had fewer than 10,000 colonies per microliter. Furthermore, mixed cultures and unusual organisms such as *Staphylococcus epidermidis* were occasionally seen. Catheterization of the bladder is a valuable and safe procedure when suprapubic aspiration is unsuccessful.

The simplest method of collecting a urine culture is by application of a sterile plastic bag after careful disinfection of the perineum; the bag is removed shortly after the child has voided. If more than 30 to 60 minutes elapses after the bag is applied or if stool is passed, the procedure must be repeated. Results of urine cultures obtained by bagged specimens are helpful when they are sterile, but a positive result is not necessarily indicative of infection because of frequent contamination during the collection process. Therefore, this method of obtaining a urine culture should be considered as a screening technique and the diagnosis must always be confirmed by a better method for urine culture. Preferably, a urine specimen should be obtained for culture by suprapubic aspiration or catheterization before initiation of antibiotics in infants evaluated for possible sepsis.

Pyuria (more than 10 leukocytes per high-power field) occurs in 75% of infants with proven urinary tract infection. Hematuria and proteinuria may be present. Gram-stained smear of urine sediment reveals bacteria in 80% of cases (including patients without pyuria). Some infants with proven infection, however, have a completely normal urinalysis result. An elevation of blood urea nitrogen and creatinine concentrations and electrolyte abnormalities can be secondary to dehydration or underlying renal abnormalities.

The peripheral leukocyte count is variable, and approximately one-third of patients have a preponderance of polymorphonuclear leukocytes and immature forms. Bacteremia is present in 20% to 30% of infants depending on postnatal age. Concurrent meningitis is rare but must be ruled out in the septic-appearing newborn. Sterile pleocytosis is seen occasionally.

THERAPY

The initial therapy should be given parenterally because of the frequent association with bacteremia in the newborn period. Ampicillin and an aminoglycoside are appropriate before culture and *in vitro* susceptibility results are available. If an infection with *S. aureus* such as a renal abscess, is suspected, a penicillinase-resistant penicillin (methicillin, oxacillin, nafcillin) should be started. When blood and cerebrospinal fluid (if obtained) culture results are sterile, the usual doses of antibiotics can be reduced. Repeat urine cultures should be done after 48 hours of therapy to document sterilization. Most patients respond promptly to antimicrobial therapy becoming afebrile in 1 to 2 days. If clinical response or urine sterilization is delayed, an immediate evaluation for urologic obstruction or abscess must be made and the pathogen's *in vitro* susceptibilities reviewed. Therapy should be continued for 14 days in the uncomplicated patient and a repeat urine culture is performed 1 week after discontinuation of antibiotic therapy.

Aminoglycoside drug concentrations should be determined if they are used for more than 2 days or if blood urea nitrogen and creatinine concentrations are elevated.

Radiologic evaluation of the urinary tract is essential for all infants with their first episode of infection to detect underlying anatomic lesions. Although some investigators feel its use is low yield (if the patient has had a normal prenatal ultrasound), renal ultrasound scan is used as an early screening procedure because the imaging does not depend on good renal function, and it is a safe and noninvasive procedure. A voiding cystourethrogram should be performed. This examination can be performed before the end of therapy when the patient is afebrile and the urine is sterile or, for the reliable family, it may be scheduled as an outpatient. Approximately 50% of infants with urinary tract infection have some abnormalities seen on radiologic evaluation, vesicoureteral reflux being the most common abnormality encountered. DMSA scintigraphy is more sensitive to detect renal involvement and renal cortical scarring and to assess quantitative differential renal function. It should be used if imaging evidence of pyelonephritis is desired.

PROGNOSIS

The goal of management is to prevent progressive renal damage and its consequences. Children should have regular follow-ups including repeated urine cultures. For infants with reflux, sonography and voiding cystourethrography or radionuclide scan should be repeated 6 to 12 months later regardless of whether infection occurs in the interim. Chemoprophylaxis with trimethoprim-sulfamethoxazole is provided to all infants with grade II or greater reflux and to those infants with frequent urinary tract infections regardless of the urologic status. In the first month of life, amoxicillin is used for prophylaxis because of the potential toxicity of sulfonamides in this age group. The incidence of recurrent infection is 20% to 30%, and almost all recurrences happen during the first year. Minimal or moderate (not involving calyceal system) reflux eventually disappears in most infants. Medical management, however, should be coordinated with a pediatric urologist for infants with more severe reflux. The role of circumcision in prevention of urinary tract infection in male children should be individualized.

CHAPTER 28

Group B Streptococcal Disease

Adapted from Carol J. Baker

Lancefield group B streptococcus emerged in the early 1970s as the most frequent cause of neonatal sepsis and meningitis. The reason for this shift in etiologic agents associated with neonatal sepsis remains unknown despite considerable advances in our understanding of bacteriologic and immunologic properties of this organism and the pathophysiology, treatment, and prevention of the infections it causes. Group B streptococci also cause pregnancy-related morbidity and invasive infections in nonpregnant adults with underlying medical conditions such as diabetes mellitus, malignancy, immunodeficiency, or neurologic, hepatic, or renal insufficiency. Nearly one-half of the group B streptococcal invasive infections occur in neonates and young infants.

BACTERIOLOGY AND EPIDEMIOLOGY

Streptococcus agalactiae, or group B streptococcus, is a facultative, encapsulated, gram-positive diplococcus that produces a narrow zone of beta-hemolysis on sheep blood agar surrounding flat, grayish white, mucoid colonies. Nonhemolytic and alpha-hemolytic strains have been isolated infrequently (1%) from humans with systemic infection.

All strains of group B streptococci share the group B-specific cell wall carbohydrate antigen originally defined by Lancefield. The strains may be classified into nine serotypes on the basis of capsular polysaccharides (type-specific antigens) and a surface protein, c. The polysaccharide antigens are designated Ia, Ib, II to VII. Strains possessing both the Ia polysaccharide antigen and the c protein antigen are now designated Ia/c (formerly, Ic). The c protein is found on all type Ib, up to 60% type II, and occasional III, IV, and V strains. Surface proteins identified as R and X antigens are found on some strains but do not seem to be associated with virulence. The capsular polysaccharides are the major virulence factor for group B streptococci. Antibodies to these structures are protective for homologous but not heterologous serotypes. The c protein is also a virulence factor, and antibodies to c protein are protective against experimental challenge with strains containing this antigen. Some *in vitro* evidence suggests that the extracellular enzyme hemolysin may also relate to virulence.

Group B streptococci may be recovered frequently from the lower genital and gastrointestinal tracts of pregnant women, but their presence is rarely associated with symptoms before rupture of membranes or labor. Reported carriage rates of group B streptococci in parturients vary from 5% to 40%. Variations are due not only to differences in age, ethnic origin, and geographic location, but also to the site and number of culture specimens taken and to differences in bacteriologic methods for growth and isolation. Colonization rates are higher in teenagers and African-American women as compared to white and Hispanic women, and rates are significantly lower in women who are Asian, Native American, or Alaskan.

Transmission of group B streptococci to the neonate can occur whenever a delivering mother harbors the organism. Exposure may occur by ascending infection through ruptured or (rarely) intact amniotic membranes or by surface contamination as the infant descends through the birth canal. Vertical transmission accounts for asymptomatic infection (or colonization) in approximately 55% of infants born to mothers carrying group B streptococci at delivery. Despite the high rate of transmission and colonization in newborns, overall, only 1% to 2% of infants born to mothers with colonization develop invasive infection. Initial colonization may persist for weeks to months at various mucous membrane sites, but acquisition of the organism by neonates after hospital discharge, although it may occur, is uncommon.

Clinically and epidemiologically, neonatal group B streptococcal infection can be divided into two distinct syndromes on the basis of onset age. Early-onset disease appears within the first 7 days of life and occurs in 1.3 to 3.7 of 1,000 live births, although the incidence has fallen in centers where maternal intrapartum chemoprophylaxis is given. Nearly 90% of early-onset cases and almost all fatal infections occur during the first day of life. Maternal factors increasing risk for early-onset disease are group B streptococcal bacteriuria during pregnancy, preterm delivery, intrapartum fever, prolonged rupture of membranes, and (perhaps) African-American origin and age younger than 20 years. Attack rates are related inversely to birth weight, but most neonates (80%) with early-onset disease are born at 37 or more weeks of gestation. Late-onset disease, which occurs after 7 days of age, is documented in several studies to affect 0.6 to 1.7 of 1,000 live births. Except for preterm delivery, the obstetric complications commonly accompanying early-onset disease are not factors associated with the later presentation of infant group B streptococcal infection. Late late-onset (greater than 3 months) disease was described in very low-birth-weight (VLBW) infants who remain hospitalized and susceptible, presumably through colonization at mucous membrane sites and by virtue of immature immune status. Another group of infants with late late-onset infection are those with human immunodeficiency virus infection. Late late-onset cases may account for up to 20% of group B streptococcal cases beyond the first week of life. Low levels of maternally derived serum IgG antibody directed against group B streptococcal capsular polysaccharide at delivery also increase the risk for invasive disease, no matter the age at onset.

CLINICAL PRESENTATIONS

Early-onset infection usually appears at or within hours of birth (Table 28-1). The highest attack rate is observed in preterm

TABLE 28-1. Comparison of Early- and Late-Onset Group B Streptococcal Infection in Neonates

	Early-onset	Late-onset	Late late-onset
Mean age at onset of symptoms	8 hr	27 d	>3 mo
Incidence	1.3–3.7 per 1,000 live births	0.6–1.7 per 1,000 live births	Unknown
Maternal obstetric risks for sepsis	Common	Uncommon	Common
Common clinical presentations	Pneumonia (40%); meningitis (10%); bacteremia without focus (45%)	Bacteremia without focus (55%); meningitis (35%); osteomyelitis arthritis (5%)	Same as late-onset
Common serotypes	I (Ia, Ib/c, Ia/c), III, V	III (80%)	Unknown
Case-fatality rate	5–10%	2–5%	Low

infants born to women with known obstetric factors posing risk for neonatal sepsis. Clinical syndromes include bacteremia without a focus, pneumonia, and meningitis. Pneumonia and meningitis are typically accompanied by bacteremia. It has been estimated that a single blood culture is sterile in 10% of cases. Respiratory signs such as tachypnea, grunting, retractions, and cyanosis, or an unexpected apneic episode in a previously healthy, term neonate, are the first clues of illness in most infants regardless of the primary focus of infection. Poor perfusion is a presenting finding in some one-fourth of cases and may be found at birth in infants with *in utero* onset of infection. Nonspecific signs such as lethargy, poor feeding, tachycardia, jaundice, and fever, occur most often in term infants without respiratory symptoms. Features predictive of fatal outcome are birth weight of less than 2,500 g, pleural effusion in initial chest radiograph, absolute neutrophil count less than 1,500 per cubic millimeter, apnea, hypotension in the first 12 hours, and initial blood pH of less than 7.25.

Forty percent of neonates with early-onset group B streptococcal infection have pulmonary findings. One-third of these infants demonstrate radiographic evidence of congenital pneumonia with distinct infiltrates, and approximately one-half have findings typical of hyaline membrane disease. Reports describe neonates with early-onset group B streptococcal sepsis manifested by respiratory distress, persistent fetal circulation (or persistent pulmonary hypertension), and a normal chest radiograph. After the development of sepsis, some infants develop hypoxemia and multiorgan system failure.

Group B streptococcal meningitis is clinically indistinguishable from bacteremia with or without pulmonary involvement. For this reason, lumbar puncture for cerebrospinal fluid (CSF) studies and culture is always required for accurate diagnosis and appropriate therapy. Reports indicate that this focus of infection has decreased frequency from some 25% to 5% of cases. Although seizure activity may develop in half of neonates with group B streptococcal meningitis, it is rarely the presenting symptom. Prolonged seizure activity, focal neurologic signs, or coma are associated with poor outcome, as is the occurrence of shock, neutropenia, or a CSF protein level greater than 300 mg/dL.

Late-onset group B streptococcal infection is observed in infants at 8 days to 12 weeks of age and has diverse clinical manifestations. The mean age at onset is approximately 24 days, unless the infant was born before 32 weeks' gestation when presentation may extend until 5 to 7 months. The obstetric and early neonatal course is usually uneventful. Although some infants exhibit only fever and mild irritability, others have a few hours of illness culminated by septic shock, neutropenia, and death. As with early-onset infection, infants may present with bacteremia without a focus or may have localization to the central nervous system, skeletal system, soft tissues, or a variety of other foci.

When first described, the most frequent clinical manifestation of late-onset group B streptococcal infection was meningitis. Now bacteremia without a focus is the most frequent presentation (55% of cases), perhaps reflecting earlier diagnosis and therapy. Infants with late-onset group B streptococcal syndrome have comparatively fewer respiratory symptoms than do their early-onset counterparts, but a preceding or concurrent upper respiratory infection is noted in 20% to 30%. In those infants with meningitis (35% of cases), the course may often be complicated by seizures, diminished perfusion, or apnea, but anticipatory care with timely and appropriate interventions prevents additional morbidity. Meningitis may result in serious intracranial complications such as focal cerebritis, vascular thrombosis, obstructive ventriculitis, and subdural empyema, but these complications are uncommon.

Group B streptococcal osteomyelitis (mean, 31 days) follows an indolent course with few systemic signs. Decreased use of the involved extremity and pain with passive movement are typical findings. Infants often have a relatively long history before diagnosis (mean, 9 days). Bacteremia is unusual. Unlike other pathogens causing neonatal osteomyelitis, group B streptococcus has a predilection for the proximal humerus; the femur is the second most common site involved. Rarely is more than a single bone involved. Up to 70% of infants have accompanying pyarthrosis of the adjacent joint. Group B streptococcal septic arthritis without osteomyelitis occurs almost exclusively in the lower extremities and usually involves the hip joint. Onset of illness is acute (mean duration of symptoms before diagnosis, 1.5 days), and concurrent bacteremia is usual.

A variety of foci of late-onset group B streptococcal infection has been reported, but these are uncommon in comparison to bacteremia without a focus, meningitis, and bone and joint infection. Infants with facial or submandibular cellulitis due to group B streptococci have been described, as have other soft tissue infections that include necrotizing fasciitis, omphalitis, and scalp and breast abscesses.

PATHOPHYSIOLOGY

Genital or gastrointestinal colonization in mothers at delivery provides infants exposure by the ascending route. This is the necessary prelude of early-onset group B streptococcal infection. The degree of risk correlates directly with the degree (inoculum) of maternal colonization (heavy or light). A direct relationship between length of membrane rupture before delivery and risk of invasive infant disease has also been documented and, because amniotic fluid readily supports the replication of group B streptococci, the longer the interval, the higher is the inoculum. Invasion of reparative epithelium, pulmonary interstitium, endothelium of the pulmonary vessels, and (finally) bacteremia presumably follow aspiration of infected amniotic fluid or birth canal contents. Several case series indicated that 36% to 65% of infants are symptomatic at birth indicating that infection often begins *in utero*. In late-onset infection, adherence of group B streptococci to epithelium in the upper respiratory or gastrointestinal tract and resulting in colonization is presumably the first step in pathogenesis. Surface proteins have been implicated as adhesins, but their role may be defined only by creation of specific mutants. The mechanisms by which organisms replicating at mucosal surfaces invade are not elucidated, but the presence of capsule is crucial.

Evasion of host defenses is critical to the survival and replication of group B streptococci *in vivo*. When compared to immune effector mechanisms in adults and older infants, neonates (especially preterm infants) are developmentally deficient. Group B streptococci elaborate surface molecules including capsule, which inhibit host defenses. Pulmonary alveolar macrophages and monocytes [but not polymorphonuclear leukocytes (PMNLs)] are recruited into the alveoli of infants with early-onset infection, but the capsular polysaccharide attenuates this response. This decreased ability to recruit host cells effectively correlates with decreased pulmonary clearance. Once bacteremia ensues, the capsule of the organism, which is necessary for virulence in animal models of lethal bacteremia, inhibits deposition of complement and phagocytosis by PMNLs. In the absence of a sufficient quantity of type-specific antibodies directed against the capsular polysaccharide or complement, phagocytosis of group B streptococci by PMNLs is minimal.

Inflammatory mediators play a major role in the pathogenesis of group B streptococcal sepsis. Once invasive infection is established, ongoing replication and digestion of organisms can instigate host inflammatory responses that may be deleterious. Neonates recovering from group B streptococcal disease have circulating immune complexes that may contribute to end-organ damage. These immune complexes also elicit inflammatory mediators such as leukotriene B_4 and interleukin-6 (IL-6). Group B streptococcal cell wall components, particularly peptidoglycan, elicit tumor necrosis factor-alpha (TNF-α), IL-1, IL-6, and granulocyte colony-stimulating factor. TNF-α is found in the acute serum of up to 50% of infants with group B streptococcal sepsis.

DIFFERENTIAL DIAGNOSIS

The clinical manifestations of early-onset group B streptococcal infection resemble those of neonatal sepsis resulting from other pathogens. In the preterm infant, the clinical and radiographic distinction between group B streptococcal pneumonia and hyaline membrane disease at onset of illness is impossible. Helpful features suggesting group B streptococcal pneumonia in this kind of patient are maternal risk factors for sepsis, apnea, and shock within the first 24 hours of life, an Apgar score of less than 5 at 1 minute, neutropenia, and cardiomegaly or pleural effusion by chest radiograph. None of these features, however, is specific for group B streptococci, and each may be observed with other etiologic agents causing early-onset neonatal pneumonia. Because clinical findings alone cannot identify the 5% of infants with meningeal involvement, each infant with clinical signs of sepsis requires a lumbar puncture.

The differential diagnosis for late-onset group B streptococcal infection depends somewhat on the focus of infection. Infants who have bacteremia without a focus may present with nonspecific signs and fever, and they may be thought to have a viral illness. Only a high index of suspicion and collection of blood and CSF culture specimens will lead to a specific diagnosis. The relative lack of systemic findings in an infant with a metaphyseal lytic bone lesion, especially of the humerus, strongly suggests group B streptococcal osteomyelitis. Until group B streptococci are isolated from a bone aspirate or biopsy sample of the affected area, however, other etiologic agents such as *Staphylococcus aureus* and gram-negative enteric agents must be considered. The diversity of clinical presentations of late-onset group B streptococcal infection requires that it be appreciated as a possible etiologic agent in unknown infection at any site in infants 1 to 12 weeks of age. Isolation of group B streptococci from a normally sterile body site (blood, CSF, bone, synovial fluid, urine) is the only way to prove invasive group B streptococcal infection. Isolation of the organism from skin or mucosal surfaces is not diagnostically significant.

COMPLICATIONS AND SEQUELAE

Complications of infant group B streptococcal infection range from negligible functional deficits in infants with septic arthritis to profound neurologic consequences of severe meningitis. The mortality rate for early-onset infection is estimated to be 10% to 15% and, for late-onset disease, from 2% to 6%. Three series reported sequelae in survivors of group B streptococcal meningitis up to 8 years after illness. Major neurologic sequelae including global mental retardation, spastic quadriplegia, uncontrolled seizures, cortical blindness, deafness, hydrocephalus, and hypothalamic dysfunction occurred in 17% to 21%. Less severe sequelae such as spastic or flaccid paresis of one limb, speech and language delay, controlled seizure disorders, unilateral deafness, and mild cortical atrophy seen by computed tomography of the head, were found in some 20%. Relapse or recurrence of infection of both the early- and late-onset type have been reported in 1% to 5% of cases. In a few cases, however, circumstances (maternal mastitis, undrained abscess, congenital heart disease in an infant with endocarditis and underlying immune deficiency) may predispose infants to recurrence. In the majority, the reason for recurrence is not apparent. The opportunity for recurrent infection with optimal therapy exists in most patients, because intravenous therapy with beta-lactam antibiotics does not eliminate mucous membrane infection with group B streptococci. Also, most infants do not develop protective immunity after recovery from sepsis or meningitis. Thus, the opportunity for recurrent bacteremia exists, sometimes with dissemination to focal sites, including the meninges. Molecular techniques have shown that the majority of these recurrent infections are due to the strain implicated in the first episode suggesting persistent mucosal colonization as the underlying source.

TREATMENT AND PREVENTION

Penicillin G is the drug of choice for group B streptococcal infections because isolates remain uniformly susceptible. They are also susceptible *in vitro* to first-, second-, and third-generation cephalosporins, semisynthetic penicillins, and vancomycin. Resistance of group B streptococci to the aminoglycosides, colistin, bacitracin, trimethoprim-sulfamethoxazole, and metronidazole is uniform. However, susceptibility of group B streptococci to penicillin G is related directly to the inoculum size. The high inoculum often found in the CSF of infants with meningitis suggests that these infants may require substantially higher antibiotic concentrations in the CSF to inhibit growth. The combination of an aminoglycoside (usually gentamicin) with penicillin G or ampicillin is synergistic in killing group B streptococci *in vitro*. Ampicillin and gentamicin produce rapid killing of group B streptococci and are recommended for initial treatment of group B streptococcal infection and for maternally acquired sepsis of unknown etiology in the infant younger than 1 month. Once group B streptococci are identified in cultures, therapy may be modified to penicillin G alone. Delay in sterilizing CSF (achieved in 95% of patients within 24 to 36 hours) may be related to inadequate antibiotic dose or an unexpected suppurative focus. Ampicillin and gentamicin should be continued until sterilization of the CSF has been documented by repeat lumbar puncture, at which time the regimen may be changed to penicillin G alone.

The optimal dose of penicillin G for treatment of group B streptococcal meningitis has not been investigated, but several facts argue for the use of high-dose therapy. Group B streptococci have relatively high minimal inhibitory concentrations to penicillin G, especially in considering levels achievable in the CSF. Infants with group B streptococcal meningitis often have a high group B streptococcal inoculum in the CSF, which would increase the minimal bactericidal concentration. Reported cases of relapse have been associated primarily with doses of penicillin G of less than 200,000 U/kg/day. Finally, penicillin G is safe in neonates in doses up to 600,000 U/kg/day. For these reasons, penicillin G at a dose of 400,000 to 500,000 U/kg/day or ampicillin, 300 mg/kg/day, is recommended for treatment of group B streptococcal meningitis. Doses of approximately one-half these amounts are suggested for treatment of noncentral nervous system infections. Therapy for 10 days is adequate for pneumonia, bacteremia without a focus, and most soft tissue infections. Two to 3 weeks of treatment are suggested for meningitis and septic arthritis, and 3 to 4 weeks for osteomyelitis, endocarditis, and ventriculitis. These recommendations, however, must be tailored to each case.

Efforts to prevent neonatal group B streptococcal infection have aimed either to decrease frequency of group B streptococcal exposure of infants at birth or to alter their immune status. Most widely investigated are attempts to eliminate infant exposure during birth. The first evaluated approach was to attempt to eliminate maternal colonization during pregnancy. Courses of oral ampicillin or penicillin (with or without concurrent treatment of sexual partners) during the third trimester of pregnancy were ineffective in decreasing colonization at delivery. Next, several control clinical trials using intravenous ampicillin or penicillin G during labor in women known to carry group B streptococci significantly reduced both vertical transmission of group B streptococci and early-onset disease in neonates.

In 1996, the Centers for Disease Control and Prevention (CDC), in conjunction with other agencies, published a document on the prevention of perinatal Group B strep disease. This document was updated in 2002 and can be viewed at http://www.cdc.gov/mmwr/PDF/rr/rr5111.pdf Prior to the 2002 update, selection of women for intrapartum antibiotic prophylaxis was based on one of two strategies: culture-based screening for group B streptococcal colonization or detection (at admission for delivery) of one or more risk factors known to enhance risk for neonatal disease. The culture-based method is now recommended as it is at least 50% more effective than the risk-based approach. This culture-based method requires processing of lower vaginal and rectal swab specimens in selective broth medium after collection at 35 to 37 weeks' gestation. All colonized women would be offered intrapartum penicillin G. If the screening results are unknown, only women who are delivering at 37 weeks' gestation or less, have rupture of membranes for more than 18 hours, or have intrapartum fever of at least 38°C would be given chemoprophylaxis. Because most women who are offered prophylaxis will likely choose it, this method could reduce disease in term infants whose mothers have no recognizable risk factor other than colonization (up to 30% of cases). The CDC now recommends that all women be screened at 35–37 weeks' gestation. Under the older risk factor-based strategy (in which no screening cultures were performed), women with one or more of the following were candidates for prophylaxis: previous infant with invasive disease, bacteriuria with group B streptococcus during the pregnancy, labor at less than 37 weeks' gestation, membrane rupture 18 or more hours before delivery, or intrapartum fever. Although some centers still use the risk factor approach, it likely prevents fewer cases of neonatal GBS. Some series have shown that as many as 25–60% of neonatal GBS cases can be term infants without recognizable maternal risk factors.

CHAPTER 29
Cytomegalovirus

Adapted from Pablo J. Sánchez and Jane D. Siegel

Cytomegalovirus (CMV) has worldwide distribution and is the most common cause of congenital infections. CMV occurs in 0.4% to 2.4% of all live births. Acquisition of CMV is nearly always asymptomatic in the immunocompetent host. Seroprevalence studies indicate that an inverse relationship exists between socioeconomic status and development of infection. CMV seropositivity in women of childbearing age varies in the United States from 45% in higher socioeconomic groups to 70% in crowded areas with substandard living conditions; this figure increases to nearly 100% in developing countries. Two likely sources of primary CMV infection for pregnant women are infected sexual partners and young children in day-care centers.

TRANSMISSION

Perinatal transmission of CMV can occur *in utero*, during delivery, or postnatally. *In utero* infection occurs transplacentally during maternal viremia. Primary CMV infection acquired during pregnancy is associated with a 30% to 40% risk of congenital infection with more severe fetal effects when maternal infection occurs in the first half of pregnancy. However, symptomatic disease is present in only 10% to 15% of these infants. CMV can also be transmitted to the fetus after reactivation of latent infection in the mother. Approximately 0.2% to 2.0% of infants born to women who are seropositive before becoming pregnant are infected *in utero*, but they do not have clinically apparent disease at birth. Transmission of CMV to the newborn infant may also occur intrapartum from contact with infected cervical secretions. In the postpartum period, maternal-infant transmission of CMV occurs during breast-feeding, because 20% to 40% of seropositive women shed CMV into their breast milk. Asymptomatic infection occurs in 60% of infants fed infected breast milk and is usually the result of reactivation of CMV infection in a seropositive mother.

An important iatrogenic source of CMV infection is transfusion of blood that has not been treated to remove viable CMV from a seropositive donor to a seronegative infant. Under such conditions, the incidence is 10% to 30% and usually occurs in infants who weigh less than 1,300 g. The risk of infection is related to the volume of transfused blood, number of donors, and elevated complement fixation titers to CMV in donor blood. Horizontal transmission of CMV in a neonatal intensive care unit has been documented but is rare.

CLINICAL MANIFESTATIONS

Cytomegalic inclusion disease is the most serious but least common manifestation of congenital CMV infection. This syndrome is characterized by multiorgan involvement with the reticuloendothelial and central nervous systems most frequently affected. Typical clinical features of cytomegalic inclusion disease include intrauterine growth retardation, hepatosplenomegaly, jaundice, petechiae or purpura, microcephaly, chorioretinitis, and cerebral calcifications (Table 29-1). These features may occur singly or in combination.

Hepatomegaly with direct hyperbilirubinemia and mild elevation of serum transaminase levels are the most common abnormalities noted in the newborn period. Hepatitis usually resolves in the first year of life, and development of cirrhosis is rare. Splenomegaly is common and may be the only abnormality present at birth. Thrombocytopenia with petechiae is usually transient but may persist through the first year of life. "Blueberry muffin" spots are palpable, discrete, well-circumscribed, bluish purple lesions on yellow jaundiced skin. These are often mistaken for purpura; they represent dermal erythropoiesis in the more severely affected infants.

Central nervous system infection with CMV can result in encephalitis and abnormal brain development with seizures and an elevated protein content in the cerebrospinal fluid (CSF). Cerebral calcifications occur in as many as 50% of newborns with physical examination findings of CMV; their occurrence dates the maternal infection to the first trimester of pregnancy. The calcifications typically occur in the periventricular areas (Fig. 29-1) but may also occur within the brain parenchyma and particularly in the basal ganglia. Arrested brain growth results in microcephaly, and obstruction of the fourth ventricle may result in hydrocephalus. Ocular defects include chorioretinitis, strabismus, optic atrophy, microphthalmia, and cataracts.

The most common manifestation of congenital CMV infection is sensorineural hearing loss resulting from direct viral invasion of the inner ear. It occurs in 60% of infants with symptomatic congenital infection and in approximately 5% of infants with otherwise asymptomatic infection at birth. The hearing

TABLE 29-1. Frequency of Clinical Findings in Infants with Congenital Infections

Clinical findings	Congenital infection				
	Rubella	*Toxoplasma*	*CMV*	*Syphilis*	*HSV*
Intrauterine growth retardation	**+++**	±	++	++	±
Reticuloendothelial system					
Jaundice	+	++	**+++**	+++	+
Hepatitis	±	+	+++	+++	+
Hepatosplenomegaly	+++	++	**+++**	**+++**	+
Anemia	+	+++	++	+++	−
Thrombocytopenia	++	±	**+++**	++	+
Disseminated intravascular coagulation	−	−	±	−	++
Adenopathy	++	++	−	++	−
Dermal erythropoiesis	+	−	+	−	−
Skin rash	−	+	−	**++**	**+++**
Bone abnormalities	++	−	±	**++**	−
Eye					
Cataracts	**++**	±	±	±	−
Retinopathy	++	**+++**	**+**	±	**+++**
Microphthalmia	+	±	±	−	±
Central nervous system					
Microcephaly	+	+	**++**	−	±
Meningoencephalitis	++	+++	+++	++	**+++**
Brain calcification	±	**++**	++	−	+
Hydrocephalus	−	**++**	±	±	++
Hearing defect	+++	+	+++	+	−
Pneumonitis	++	+	±	+	±
Cardiovascular					
Myocarditis	+	±	±	±	−
Congenital defect	**+++**	−	−	−	−

±, rare; +, 5% to 20%; ++, 20% to 50%; +++, more than 50%; □, prominent feature of particular infection; CMV, cytomegalovirus; HSV, herpes simplex virus.

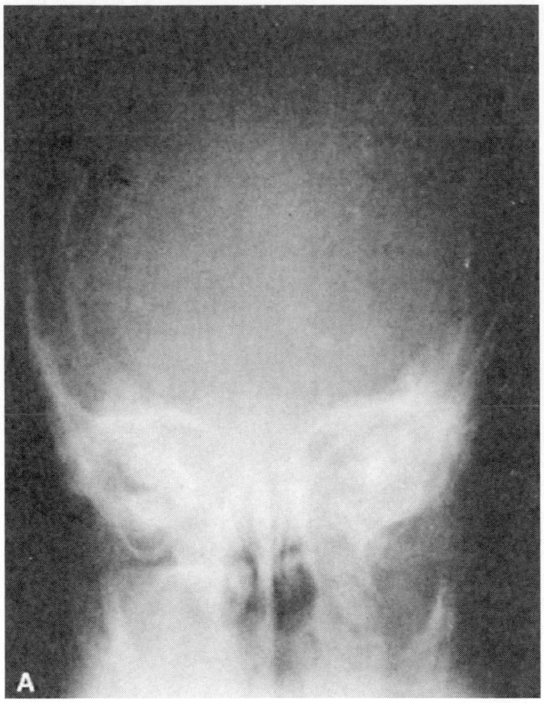

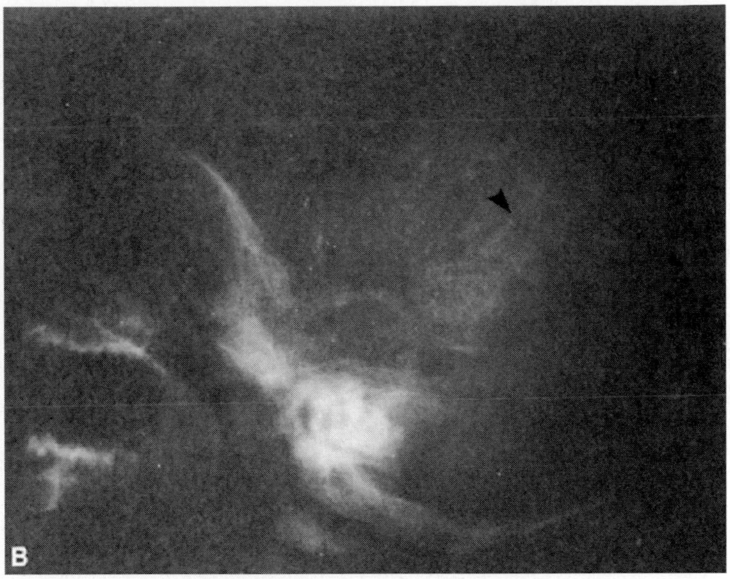

Figure 29-1. Anteroposterior (A) and lateral (B) skull roentgenograms demonstrating cerebral calcifications (arrow) lining the ventricles in a neonate with congenital cytomegalovirus infection (Reprinted with permission from Sanchez PJ and Siegel JD. Cytomegalovirus. In: McMillan JA, DeAngelis CD, Feigin RD, et al, eds. Oski's Pediatrics, Principles and Practice. Philadelphia: Lipponcott, Williams and Wilkins, 1999.)

loss may be unilateral and unsuspected until the third year of life.

A diffuse interstitial pneumonitis occurs in less than 1% of newborns with cytomegalic inclusion disease. Bone abnormalities in CMV infection consist of longitudinal radiolucent streaks in the metaphysis of long bones ("celery stalk" appearance), particularly the distal femur and proximal tibia. Generalized osteopenia with irregular metaphyseal fragmentation has also been described. Defective enamelization of the deciduous teeth occurs in 40% of symptomatic newborns and in 5% of infants with asymptomatic infection at birth.

Attempts have been made to implicate CMV in congenital cardiovascular, genitourinary, gastrointestinal, and musculoskeletal anomalies. Overall, the teratogenicity of CMV remains in doubt, although CMV has been associated with inguinal hernias in boys.

The type of maternal infection during pregnancy (i.e., primary or recurrent infection) and whether the newborn has clinical manifestations of CMV infection are the two most important factors with respect to prognosis. It was found that 25% of infants born to mothers who had a primary CMV infection during pregnancy manifest some neurodevelopmental sequelae, whereas only 8% of infants born after a maternal recurrent infection have sequelae.

CMV infection acquired at delivery is manifested by an afebrile pneumonia in 50% of exposed infants or, rarely, hepatitis or encephalitis after an incubation period of 4 to 12 weeks (mean, 8 weeks). In full-term infants, the disease tends to be mild and does not result in late neurologic sequelae. On the other hand, in premature infants with birth weights less than 1,500 g, perinatally acquired CMV infection may be more severe. CMV pneumonitis in these infants has been associated with development of chronic lung disease. Moreover, administration of dexamethasone for chronic lung disease in CMV-infected preterm infants has been associated with progression of their CMV disease.

DIAGNOSIS

The diagnosis of congenital and perinatal CMV infection is best confirmed by isolation of the virus from the urine (Table 29-2). Culture of saliva has been reported to be as sensitive as urine for detection of congenital CMV infection and represents a convenient and suitable alternative. Isolation of CMV from amniotic fluid has also been used to document *in utero* infection. All infants with congenital CMV infection have high titers of virus in their urine and pharynx at birth. Viral excretion in the urine persists for years, but the titer decreases markedly after 3 months. Pharyngeal shedding is not as prolonged. In infants infected with CMV perinatally, viruria and pharyngeal shedding appear after an incubation period of 4 to 12 weeks.

To diagnose congenital CMV infection accurately, cultures should be obtained within the first 2 weeks of life. After 3 weeks, viral shedding can occur from congenital, perinatal, or postnatally acquired infection. Polymerase chain reaction performed on such clinical specimens as blood, CSF, and urine has been found to be highly sensitive and specific for the detection of CMV DNA. Polymerase chain reaction is probably the preferred method for detection of CMV in CSF. Its detection in CSF has been associated with a more severe neurologic outcome.

Serologic studies have a limited role in the diagnosis of congenital CMV infection and are not recommended. The presence of CMV-specific IgG antibody denotes passively transferred maternal antibodies. On serial determinations, antibody titers to CMV in most congenitally infected infants show either a rapid or gradual decline to low levels between 4 months and 2 years of age. A minimum of infected infants demonstrates persistence of the high initial titer. An increase in titer has not been demonstrated in these infants, despite continued shedding of the virus. False-negative antibody levels determined by the complement fixation method have been seen in infected infants. Although the CMV-IgM immunofluorescent test detects 76% of congenitally infected infants, a false-positive rate of as high as

TABLE 29-2. Methods of Diagnosis of Congenital and Perinatal Infection

	Isolation of organism	Antigen detection	Measurement of antibody	Polymerase chain reaction
Cytomegalovirus	++	+	NR	±
Herpes simplex virus	++	+	NR	++
Varicella-zoster	±	±	++	±
Epstein-Barr virus	±	–	++	±
Rubella	±	±	++	–
Toxoplasmosis	±	–	++	++
Syphilis	±[a]	±	++	±
Human immuno-deficiency virus	±	+	NR	++
Hepatitis				
A	–	–	++	–
B	–	++	++	±
Delta	–	++	++	–
C	–	–	++	±
Neisseria gonorrhoeae	++	–	–	–
Chlamydia trachomatis	±	++[b]	+[c]	±
Mycoplasmas	++	–	±	±

–, not available; +, alternative method but usually less helpful; ++, preferred method; ±, possible, but may not be performed routinely by clinical laboratories; NR, not recommended.
[a]Spirochetes visualized by dark-field examination of suspected lesions.
[b]Preferred for conjunctivitis.
[c]Pneumonia only.

21% has been documented. Commercially available enzyme-linked immunosorbent assays that measure CMV-IgG have excellent reliability, but false-positive test results remain a problem with the CMV-IgM enzyme-linked immunosorbent assays. To interpret test results, the accuracy of the specific kit used must be known.

TREATMENT

At present, no antiviral agent is approved for treatment or prevention of congenital CMV infection. A clinical trial is ongoing to determine the safety and efficacy of intravenous ganciclovir (6 mg/kg every 12 hours) for treatment of infants with gestational age greater than or equal to 32 weeks (birth weight greater than or equal to 1,200 g) who have congenital CMV infection of the central nervous system. Toxicity of ganciclovir includes neutropenia and thrombocytopenia, and it has the potential to impair spermatogenesis. Moreover, treatment at birth of CMV-infected infants who are already symptomatic may be too late to prevent the long-term neurologic sequelae.

PREVENTION

Routine serologic screening is not recommended for women of childbearing age because no prophylactic or therapeutic interventions are available during pregnancy. Meticulous adherence to standard precautions, especially hand washing after exposure to urine or saliva from young infants and toddlers and immunocompromised patients, is the most effective means of preventing primary CMV infection in pregnant women. Pregnant women are not excluded from caring for patients who are known to have CMV infection because of the ubiquity of CMV and the demonstration that health care workers do not have higher rates of seroconversion than control subjects.

Transfusion-acquired CMV infection is eliminated by administration of CMV antibody-negative blood products to infants less than 1,500 g in birth weight. In many neonatal intensive care units, leukofiltration of blood to remove the white blood cell fraction has been used successfully to minimize the risk of CMV acquisition. Frozen deglycerolized red blood cells are also a suitable alternative, because they lack viable leukocytes. Similarly, freezing expressed breast milk at −20°C for 3 to 7 days effectively kills CMV.

CMV vaccine may ultimately be the best preventive strategy, but vaccine development remains investigational.

CHAPTER 30
Herpes Simplex Virus

Adapted from Pablo J. Sánchez and Jane D. Siegel

The estimated rate of occurrence of neonatal herpes simplex virus (HSV) infection in the United States is approximately 1 per 3,000 to 20,000 deliveries per year. Most neonatal infections are caused by HSV-2 with some 25% to 30% caused by HSV-1. The seroprevalence of HSV-2 antibodies among American women of childbearing age is 20% to 30%. However, only 5% of these seropositive women have a history of genital HSV infection. It is, therefore, not surprising that 70% of infants who develop HSV infection are born to women with asymptomatic HSV genital infection at the time of delivery and have neither a history of genital herpes nor a sexual partner with genital HSV infection. The frequency of asymptomatic shedding of HSV at the time of delivery varies from 0.01% to 0.39%. Among women with a past history of genital HSV infection, asymptomatic excretion at delivery is approximately 1% to 2%. Among those who had a primary infection during pregnancy, viral shedding at delivery is 36%. If HSV is diagnosed before the pregnancy and clinical recurrences have been fewer than six per year, the risk of reactivation at delivery is 10%. If there have been six or more episodes of HSV infection per year, then the risk of reactivation at delivery increases to 25%. Most importantly, however, one is unable to reliably predict viral shedding at delivery in any of these women.

TRANSMISSION

Acquisition of HSV by the infant can occur *in utero,* during delivery, or after birth. *In utero* infection with HSV accounts for approximately 5% of cases. Transmission occurs either transplacentally during a maternal viremia or by an ascending route from an infected maternal genital tract. The virus may pass through microscopic tears in the amniotic membranes to produce infection in infants delivered by cesarean section with intact membranes. HSV has been isolated from the blood of a pregnant woman with primary HSV infection, as well as from amniotic fluid, placenta, umbilical cord blood, and fetal tissue obtained at the time of spontaneous abortion. *In utero* acquisition of HSV, presumably from a transplacental route, is also suggested by reports of congenital malformations in infants born to women with genital herpes infection during pregnancy.

Transmission of HSV to the newborn infant usually occurs at delivery (85% of cases). Risk of neonatal infection is higher with primary maternal HSV infection than with recurrent infection (30%–50% versus 3%) because of the infant's prolonged exposure to large quantities of virus in the absence of protective neutralizing and antibody-dependent cellular cytotoxicity antibodies (Table 30-1). Prematurity, duration of rupture of amniotic membranes greater than 4 to 6 hours, and use of a scalp electrode for fetal heart rate monitoring also increase the risk of HSV infection.

Postnatal transmission of HSV (10% of cases) to the newborn infant may occur after contact with a maternal breast lesion during breast-feeding or from direct contact with other family members or, rarely, with health care workers who have active herpes labialis lesions. Nosocomial transmission of HSV in newborn nurseries has been documented by restriction endonuclease analysis of viral isolates, but it is rare.

CLINICAL MANIFESTATIONS

Clinical manifestations of intrauterine HSV infection are present at birth or within the first 48 hours of delivery. Skin vesicles with scars are common. Seizures, microcephaly, hydranencephaly, porencephaly, intracranial calcifications, microphthalmia, hepatomegaly with or without splenomegaly, and abnormalities on bone roentgenography may be seen. The adrenal gland is frequently involved, and chorioretinitis is either present at birth or develops in the first week of life.

Neonatal HSV infection acquired at birth is categorized by extent of disease: disseminated disease with or without evidence of central nervous system, skin, eye, and mouth involvement; central nervous system disease (encephalitis) with or without skin, eye, and mouth involvement; and localized infection of the skin, eye, mouth, or a combination of the three without visceral organ or central nervous system involvement. Subclinical infection may occur but is uncommon.

TABLE 30-1. Maternal Genital Herpes Infection and Risk of Perinatal Transmission

	Genital herpes simplex virus infection	
	Primary	***Recurrent***
Risk of perinatal transmission	30–50%	3%
Site of viral shedding	Cervix	Labia
Duration of viral shedding	3 wk	2–5 d
Quantity of virus shed	Large	Small
Neutralizing antibody	Absent	Present

Disseminated disease currently accounts for 25% of neonatal HSV infection. The average onset of illness is between 9 and 11 days of life, and the principal organs involved are the liver and adrenal glands. Approximately 50% of infants manifest central nervous system involvement from hematogenous spread of the virus, and 80% manifest skin, mouth, or eye lesions. The presenting signs and symptoms are nonspecific and include fever, lethargy, respiratory distress, apnea, jaundice, seizures and, in the most severe cases, shock with disseminated intravascular coagulation. Splenomegaly is often present. Pneumonitis, pleural effusion, and roentgenographic lesions in long bones may also occur. Without therapy, the case-fatality rate exceeds 80%. Most survivors develop psychomotor retardation and ocular defects.

Central nervous system disease from axonal transmission of virus accounts for approximately 30% of neonatal HSV infections. Clinical manifestations typically occur at 11 to 17 days of life and include lethargy, irritability, bulging fontanelle, focal or generalized seizures, and coma. Forty percent of infants have no skin vesicles. Examination of the cerebrospinal fluid (CSF) reveals an elevated leukocyte count with a predominance of lymphocytes and an elevated protein content. Red blood cells are occasionally present indicating hemorrhagic brain involvement. A normal cell count and protein concentration, however, may be found on the initial lumbar puncture. Mortality in untreated infants with localized central nervous system disease is 40% to 50%. Most survivors have neurologic sequelae consisting of seizures, spastic quadriplegia, hydrocephaly, porencephalic cyst, and psychomotor retardation.

Localized diseases of skin, eye, mouth, or all three occur in 45% of infants with HSV infection. The hallmark of neonatal HSV infection is the discrete vesicular lesions that occur in 90% of infants with localized infection. The vesicles usually appear first on the presenting part of the body that was in direct contact with the virus during delivery. Approximately 70% of untreated infants who present with skin vesicles develop disseminated infection or have progression of disease to involve the eyes or central nervous system. The majority of infants with skin lesions usually suffer recurrences during the first 6 to 12 months of life. Ocular involvement with HSV is manifested by keratoconjunctivitis, uveitis, chorioretinitis, cataracts, and retinal dysplasia. Sequelae of ocular HSV infection include corneal ulceration, microphthalmia, optic atrophy, and blindness. Three or more skin recurrences with HSV-2 in the first 6 months of life have been associated with an increased risk of abnormal development.

DIAGNOSIS

The preferred diagnostic method is isolation of HSV from skin vesicles, buffy coat, brain tissue, CSF, stool, urine, throat, nares, or conjunctivae. HSV has been isolated from the CSF in as many as 25% to 40% of cases of encephalitis. When mucocutaneous lesions are present, scraping from the base of a vesicle may reveal intranuclear inclusions and multinucleated giant cells by Tzanck test or Wright stain in 60% to 70% of cases; specific HSV antigen may be detected by immunofluorescence in 70% to 80% of cases.

The diagnosis of HSV encephalitis has been greatly improved by the development of the polymerase chain reaction (PCR) for detection of HSV DNA in CSF. HSV DNA can be detected by PCR in the majority of culture-positive CSF samples even after

1 week of acyclovir therapy. Other tests that aid in the detection of central nervous system abnormalities include electroencephalography, computed tomography, and magnetic resonance imaging (MRI). The characteristic electroencephalographic abnormality is a periodic slow and sharp wave discharge; more commonly, multiple independent foci of periodic activity are present. Computed tomographic scan may be normal early in the course of the disease with characteristic abnormalities appearing 3 to 5 days later. The most frequently observed findings in the acute phase are patchy areas of low attenuation in both cerebral hemispheres, or hemorrhage or calcification in the thalamus, insular cortex, periventricular white matter, and along the corticomedullary junction. Late findings include multicystic encephalomalacia and ventriculomegaly as a result of brain atrophy and destruction. MRI is more sensitive in detecting early abnormalities in the periventricular white matter and in defining the extent of parenchymal lesions.

TREATMENT

Two antiviral agents, acyclovir and vidarabine, have decreased the mortality and improved the outcome of neonatal HSV infection. Antiviral therapy is initiated when the clinical features heighten the index of suspicion, or when a neonate with negative bacterial culture results is not responding to broad-spectrum antibiotics. HSV may be recovered from brain biopsy specimens even after 24 to 48 hours of antiviral therapy. Acyclovir is the preferred therapy. A range of doses may be used depending on the severity of the infection. Acyclovir is administered intravenously for a minimum of 14 to 21 days. The latter is preferred for treatment of encephalitis, because increasing evidence shows early relapse or recurrence after shorter durations of therapy. Approximately 2% of infants treated with antiviral therapy for 10 to 14 days have recurrence of infection leading to central nervous system disease. No data or experience exists on the use of famciclovir or valacyclovir in neonates. Ocular HSV infection requires topical antiviral medication.

The mortality with disseminated disease has been reduced from 85% in untreated infants to 57% in infants treated with either acyclovir or vidarabine; 60% of these infants are normal at 1 year of age. Among infants with central nervous system disease, mortality without therapy is 50%, but among treated infants, it has decreased to 15%, although only 30% are normal on follow-up examination at 1 year of age. No deaths have occurred among treated infants with localized infection of the skin, eye, or oral cavity, and 94% of infants are normal at 1-year follow-up examination.

PREVENTION

Delivery of the infants of pregnant women with active genital herpes by cesarean section within 4 to 6 hours of rupture of amniotic membranes is the only intervention shown to prevent neonatal HSV infection. Nonetheless, 33% of neonates diagnosed with HSV infection are delivered by cesarean section. The use of fetal scalp electrodes, forceps, and maneuvers that might cause a break in the infant's skin during delivery should be avoided.

Results of antepartum genital HSV cultures from pregnant women with a history of genital herpes do not predict the infant's risk of exposure to HSV at delivery. Even if asymptomatic, infants born by vaginal delivery or cesarean section after prolonged rupture of membranes in the presence of active genital herpes lesions should have appropriate cultures for HSV taken 24 to 36 hours after delivery. Virus present at this time represents active replication and invasive infection, whereas virus isolated from mucous membrane cultures obtained at birth may only reflect surface contamination. If the mother has primary genital herpes and the infant is premature or has had invasive instrumentation or skin laceration during delivery, prophylactic or anticipatory antiviral therapy is recommended. If the mother has recurrent genital herpes and no other risk factors are present, antiviral therapy is withheld until culture results are known or clinical signs of disease develop. Antiviral therapy is initiated if HSV is isolated from any infant culture. This approach is widely recommended, but its efficacy is not known.

CHAPTER 31
Neonatal Syphilis

Adapted from Pablo J. Sánchez and Jane D. Siegel

Congenital syphilis, a result of fetal infection with *Treponema pallidum,* remains a major public health problem in the United States. From 1977 through 1990, a steady increase was seen in the incidence of primary and secondary syphilis among women in the United States. This increase was greatest among African-Americans and Hispanics of lower socioeconomic status who resided in large urban areas such as Detroit, Houston, Baltimore, Miami, and New York City. A major contributor to the increase of syphilis in these populations was the exchange of illegal drugs (notably crack cocaine) for sex with multiple partners whose identities were not known. Partner notification, a traditional syphilis-control strategy, was impossible to implement. Moreover, these women rarely sought prenatal care.

Subsequently, the number of cases of early congenital syphilis reported to the Centers for Disease Control and Prevention (CDC) increased from 108 in 1978 to more than 4,000 cases in 1991. This dramatic increase was caused by both an increase in actual cases and the use of revised reporting guidelines. Beginning in 1989, the surveillance definition for congenital syphilis was broadened. The new definition includes not only all infants with clinical evidence of active syphilis, but also asymptomatic infants and stillbirths born to women with untreated or inadequately treated syphilis. Use of the new surveillance case definition increases the number of confirmed or presumptive cases of congenital syphilis by almost four times.

During the 1990s, a decrease in early syphilis was noted; this finding has heightened expectations for the eventual control and even elimination of the disease in the United States.

TRANSMISSION

Pregnant women with primary or secondary syphilis are at highest risk of delivering infected infants. Transmission of infection to the fetus usually occurs transplacentally from maternal spirochetemia, but the neonate can also be infected through contact with a genital lesion at the time of delivery. Although congenital infection can occur anytime during gestation, the risk of fetal infection increases as the stage of pregnancy advances.

CLINICAL MANIFESTATIONS

Syphilis during pregnancy is associated with premature delivery, spontaneous abortion, stillbirth, nonimmune hydrops, perinatal death, and two characteristic syndromes of clinical disease, early and late congenital syphilis. *Early congenital syphilis* refers to those clinical manifestations that appear within the first 2 years of life. Those features that occur after 2 years are designated as *late congenital syphilis*. The clinical manifestations and laboratory findings of early congenital syphilis may be present at birth or may be delayed for several months if the infant remains untreated (Table 29-1 and Table 29-2). The physical signs are a direct result of active infection and inflammation.

Infants with congenital syphilis may be growth restricted at delivery. Hepatitis with hepatosplenomegaly occurs in 50% to 90% of affected infants. Liver abnormalities may require more than 1 year to resolve; cirrhosis is rare. Generalized nontender lymphadenopathy occurs in 20% to 50% of cases with characteristic involvement of the epitrochlear nodes. Hemolytic anemia with a negative Coombs test result is common. The peripheral leukocyte count can show either leukopenia or leukemoid reaction. Thrombocytopenia with petechiae and purpura occurs in approximately 30% of infants and may be the sole manifestation of congenital infection.

Mucocutaneous lesions are specific for congenital syphilis and occur in 40% to 60% of affected infants. The rash of congenital syphilis is usually maculopapular and located on the extremities. The lesions are initially oval and pink but then turn coppery brown and desquamate. Desquamation occurs mainly on the palms and soles. A characteristic vesicular bullous eruption known as *pemphigus syphiliticus* may develop with erythema, blister formation, and eventual crusting as healing occurs. Nasal discharge associated with rhinitis or "snuffles" is initially watery, but it may become thick, purulent, and even tinged with blood (Fig. 31-1). Nasal discharge and vesicular fluid contain large concentrations of spirochetes and are highly infectious.

Bone roentgenography shows skeletal abnormalities consisting of osteochondritis, periostitis, and osteitis in 80% to 90% of infants (Fig. 31-2). These abnormalities tend to be multiple

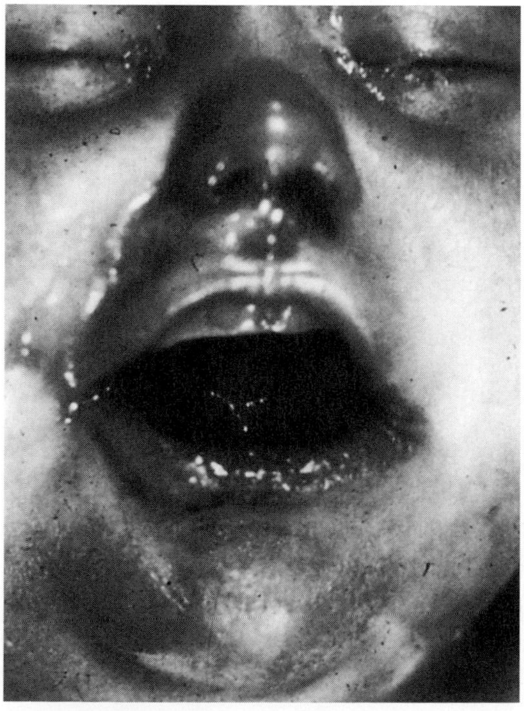

Figure 31-1. Sniffles or rhinitis in an infant with early congenital syphilis. This mucous discharge develops after the first week of life. (Courtesy of Dr. George H. McCracken, Jr., Dallas, TX.)

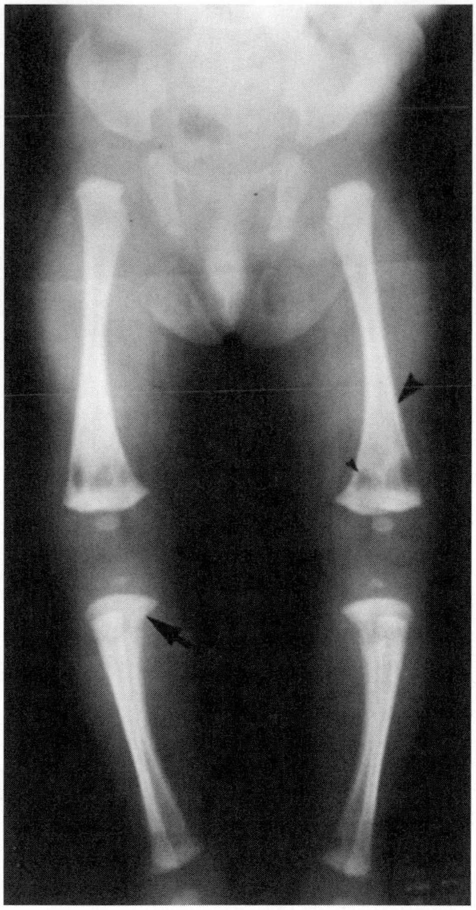

Figure 31-2. Bony lesions of early congenital syphilis: symmetric periostitis (*large arrow*); radiolucent metaphyseal area of osteochondritis (*small arrowhead*); bilateral metaphyseal defects on the upper medial aspect of the tibia; and Wimberger sign (*large arrowhead*). Similar changes may occur at the upper ends of the humeri. (Courtesy of Dr. Guido Currarino, Dallas, TX.)

and symmetric with the lower extremities involved more often than the upper extremities. The long bones (tibia, humerus, femur), ribs, and cranium are principally affected. Bilateral demineralization and osseous destruction of the proximal medial tibial metaphysis are referred to as *Wimberger sign* (Fig. 31-2). Periostitis requires 16 weeks for roentgenographic demonstration and consists of multiple layers of periosteal new bone formation in response to diaphyseal inflammation. Osteitis is the celery stalk appearance of long bones resulting from involvement of the medullary canal with resultant diaphysitis. After several months, complete healing of the affected bones occurs, even without antibiotic therapy.

Neurosyphilis occurs in 40% to 60% of infants with congenital syphilis. Two types of central nervous system involvement are described. Acute syphilitic leptomeningitis occurs in early infancy. Chronic meningovascular syphilis with progressive hydrocephalus, cranial nerve palsies, and cerebral infarction secondary to endarteritis usually presents toward the end of the first year of life. Cerebrospinal fluid (CSF) examination reveals pleocytosis with an elevated protein content and a reactive VDRL test result.

Ocular findings include chorioretinitis, cataract, glaucoma, and uveitis. Nephrosis with generalized edema, ascites, and proteinuria usually occurs at 2 to 3 months of age as a result of immune complex deposition in the renal glomeruli. Other less common manifestations include pneumonitis, pneumonia alba,

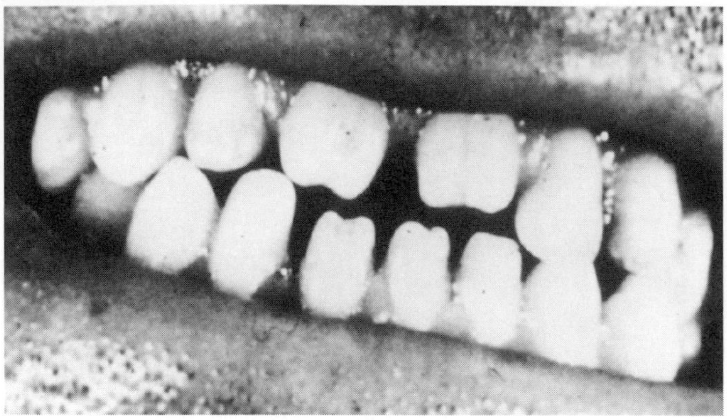

Figure 31-3. Hutchinson teeth in a child with late congenital syphilis. (Courtesy of Dr. George H. McCracken, Jr., Dallas, TX.)

myocarditis, pancreatitis, and inflammation and fibrosis of the gastrointestinal tract leading to malabsorption and diarrhea.

The clinical manifestations of late congenital syphilis result from ongoing inflammation or from scars caused by infection of early congenital syphilis. Development of the characteristic lesions is prevented by treatment during pregnancy or within the first 3 months of life. Infants with late congenital syphilis are not infective.

Dental stigmata result from the inflammatory response to *T. pallidum* infection in the developing permanent teeth during late gestation. The affected permanent upper central incisors (Hutchinson teeth) are small, widely spaced, barrel shaped, and notched with thinning and discoloration of the enamel (Fig. 31-3). The first 6-year lower molars (mulberry or Moon molars) may also be affected. The top surface has many small cusps instead of the usual four. Enamelization is defective. Infection before the 18th week of gestation may result in involvement of deciduous teeth, which are then misshapen, hypoplastic, and prone to dental caries.

The sequela of periostitis of the skull is frontal bossing, of the tibia is saber shins, and of the clavicle is Higouménakis sign with sternoclavicular thickening. Clutton joints, or painless synovitis and hydrarthrosis without involvement of the adjacent bones, are rare. Osteochondritis affecting the otic capsule may lead to cochlear degeneration and fibrous adhesions resulting in eighth nerve deafness, for which corticosteroid treatment may be beneficial.

The sequelae of syphilitic rhinitis include rhagades and short maxilla with a high palatal arch. If the inflammation of the nasal mucosa extends to the underlying cartilage and bone, perforation of the palate and nasal septum occurs resulting in a "saddle nose" deformity.

Late ocular manifestations include uveitis and interstitial keratitis. Interstitial keratitis usually appears at puberty and is not affected by penicillin therapy. Although corticosteroid treatment may be beneficial, keratitis often has a relapsing course and may lead to corneal clouding and blindness. Possible sequelae of central nervous system infection include mental retardation, hydrocephalus, seizure disorder, cranial nerve palsies, paralysis, and optic nerve atrophy.

DIAGNOSIS

The diagnosis of congenital syphilis is established by the observation of spirochetes in body fluids or tissue and suggested by serologic testing results. *T. pallidum* may be identified by dark field microscopy, fluorescent antibody, or silver stain of mucocutaneous lesions, nasal discharge, vesicular fluid, amniotic fluid, placenta, umbilical cord, or tissue obtained at autopsy. Involvement of the umbilical cord may result in a severe inflammatory reaction within its matrix, which is termed *necrotizing funisitis*.

Serologic tests for syphilis are classified into nontreponemal and treponemal tests. Nontreponemal tests include the VDRL test and the rapid plasma reagin (RPR) test. The same nontreponemal test should be performed on the mother and infant so that accurate comparisons can be made. A diagnosis of congenital syphilis is supported by an infant's nontreponemal antibody level that is four or more times that of the mother's serum. The absence of such a finding, however, does not exclude a possible diagnosis of congenital syphilis. Treponemal tests include the fluorescent treponemal antibody-absorption (FTA-ABS) test and microhemagglutination assay for *T. pallidum* antibody (MHA-TP). These tests are used to confirm the diagnosis of syphilis after a reactive nontreponemal test has been reported. They do not need to be performed in the neonatal period because no comparisons between maternal and infant results can be made; they are qualitative tests and are reported as being reactive or nonreactive. Because these tests detect IgG antibodies that are maternal in origin, all infants born to mothers with a reactive treponemal test result also have a reactive treponemal test. Polymerase chain reaction (PCR) has been used for detection of specific *T. pallidum* DNA in tissues and body fluids.

A practical approach to the evaluation and treatment of infants born to mothers with reactive serologic tests for syphilis is presented in Fig. 31-4. Testing of all pregnant women with syphilis for coinfection with the human immunodeficiency virus (HIV) is strongly recommended, as syphilis is a cofactor for transmission of HIV. All infants born to mothers with reactive serologic test results for syphilis should have a serum quantitative nontreponemal test performed and be carefully examined for physical signs of congenital syphilis. Infants who have (a) an abnormal physical examination that is consistent with congenital syphilis, (b) a serum quantitative nontreponemal serologic titer that is fourfold or greater than the mother's, (c) a positive dark-field or fluorescent antibody test result of body fluid, or (d) a combination of these signs should have a complete blood cell count (CBC) and platelet count performed, as well as CSF examination for cell count, protein content, and VDRL test. Other tests such as bone and chest roentgenography, liver function tests, cranial ultrasound, ophthalmologic examination, and auditory brainstem response, should be performed as clinically indicated. These infants are considered to have proved or highly probable disease; spirochetemia with invasion of the central nervous system is likely. Although these infants must receive a full course of penicillin therapy, which treats possible neurosyphilis, it is beneficial for follow-up purposes to establish central nervous system abnormalities at presentation. Nonetheless, the diagnosis of congenital neurosyphilis is difficult to establish. Diagnosis is based on CSF examination that shows a reactive result to the VDRL test, pleocytosis (greater than 25 leukocytes per microliter), and an elevated protein content (greater than 150 mg/dL). The presence of red blood cells in the CSF as a result of a traumatic lumbar puncture can produce a false-positive serologic reaction. Also, a reactive CSF VDRL test may be caused by passive transfer of nontreponemal IgG antibodies from serum into the CSF. Examination of the CSF for IgM reactivities to specific *T. pallidum* antigens and *T. pallidum* DNA by PCR may prove more useful for diagnosis of congenital neurosyphilis.

In infants who have a normal physical examination and a serum quantitative nontreponemal test result that is less than fourfold the maternal titer, further evaluation and treatment

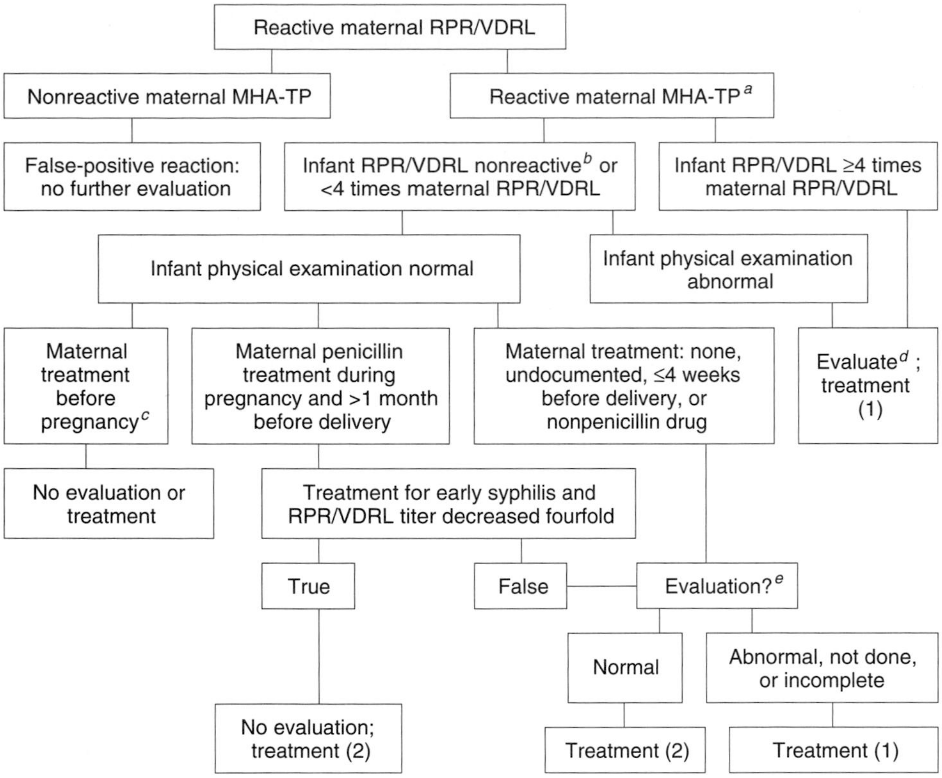

Figure 31-4. An approach to the evaluation and treatment of infants born to mothers with reactive serologic test results for syphilis. [a]Test for human immunodeficiency virus (HIV)-antibody. Infants of HIV-Ab positive mothers do not require different evaluation or treatment. [b]Infant's rapid plasma reagin test (RPR) may be nonreactive due to low maternal RPR titer or recent maternal infection. If the mother has untreated or inadequately treated syphilis and infant's physical exam is normal, some experts would not perform diagnostic evaluation but would treat the infant with a single intramuscular injection of benzathine penicillin (50,000 U/kg). [c]Women who maintain a VDRL titer of ≤1:2 (RPR ≤1:4) beyond 1 year after successful treatment are considered serofast. [d]Evaluation consists of complete blood cell count (CBC), platelet count; cerebrospinal fluid (CSF) examination for cell count, protein, and quantitative VDRL; other tests as clinically indicated (eye exam, long bone films; chest x-ray; liver function tests; cranial ultrasound; auditory brainstem response). [e]CBC, platelet count; CSF examination for cell count, protein, and quantitative VDRL; long bone films. Treatment: (1) Aqueous penicillin G, 50,000 U/kg intravenously every 12 hours (≤1 week of age) or every 8 hours (>1 week), or procaine penicillin G, 50,000 U/kg intramuscularly in a single daily dose for 10 days. (2) Benzathine penicillin G, 50,000 U/kg intramuscularly in one dose. MHA-TP, microhemagglutination assay for *Treponema pallidum* antibody.

depends on the maternal treatment history and stage of infection (Fig. 31-4). Whether to perform a complete evaluation (lumbar puncture, long bone radiography, and CBC and platelets) on the infant depends on the planned treatment. Such evaluation must be performed and be completely normal if a single intramuscular dose of benzathine penicillin G therapy is administered.

Infants with reactive serologic test results at delivery should have serial quantitative nontreponemal tests performed until the test results show nonreactivity. Similarly, infants who are seronegative but whose mothers acquired syphilis late in gestation should be followed with serial testing after penicillin therapy is instituted. In infants with congenital syphilis, nontreponemal serologic tests become nonreactive within 6 to 12 months after appropriate treatment. Uninfected infants usually become seronegative by 6 months of age. Infants with persistently low, stable titers of nontreponemal tests beyond 1 year of age may require retreatment. A reactive treponemal test beyond 18 months of age when the infant has lost all maternal antibody confirms the diagnosis of congenital syphilis. Infants with abnormal CSF findings should have a repeat lumbar puncture performed at 6 months after therapy. A reactive CSF VDRL test result or an abnormal protein content or cell count at that time is an indication for retreatment.

TREATMENT

Treatment at birth is required in the following situations: the infant has clinical, laboratory, radiographic, or a combination of the three findings consistent with a diagnosis of congenital syphilis (symptomatic); maternal treatment was inadequate or unknown; the mother was treated with drugs other than penicillin; the mother was treated within 4 weeks of delivery; maternal treatment cannot be fully evaluated because insufficient time has elapsed for nontreponemal test titer to decrease fourfold; the mother's sexual partner has not received treatment and the possibility exists of maternal reinfection; or adequate follow-up care of the infant is uncertain. Infants with proved or highly probable disease, or who have a normal physical examination but their evaluation is abnormal or incomplete, should be treated with either aqueous crystalline penicillin G (50,000 U/kg intravenously every 12 hours for the first week of life, followed by every 8 hours beyond 7 days of age) or aqueous procaine penicillin G (50,000 U/kg intramuscularly once daily) for 10 days. Infants who have a normal physical examination, CSF studies, CBC and platelet count, and long bone radiographs can be treated with a single intramuscular injection of benzathine penicillin G at a dose of 50,000 U/kg. If the risk of infection in these infants is significant and adequate follow-up cannot be ensured, the 10-day course of aqueous or procaine penicillin is recommended.

PREVENTION

Congenital syphilis is effectively prevented by prenatal serologic screening of mothers and penicillin treatment of infected women, their sexual partners, and their newborn infants. All pregnant women should have a nontreponemal serologic test for syphilis performed at the first prenatal visit in the first trimester with the test being repeated at 28 weeks' gestation and at delivery in areas with a high incidence of syphilis.

CHAPTER 32
Rubella

Adapted from Pablo J. Sánchez
and Jane D. Siegel

Rubella was first recognized in 1814 as a mild exanthematous disease. In 1941, an Australian ophthalmologist, Norman McAlister Gregg, made the association between congenital cataracts and a history of rubella early in pregnancy. His was the first description of the variety of defects now known as the *congenital rubella syndrome*. Isolation of the rubella virus in tissue culture in 1962 was soon followed by the development of live, attenuated vaccines. Since licensure of the vaccine in the United States in 1969, the total number of cases of rubella reported annually in the United States declined by 99% to 0.23 per 100,000 population in 1986. Outbreaks have occurred primarily in settings where unvaccinated young adults congregate with the highest risk being in specific racial and ethnic groups (e.g., Hispanics), immigration camps in border states, or in religious communities with low immunization acceptance (e.g., Amish).

PATHOGENESIS

Transplacental transmission of the rubella virus occurs during the viremic phase of primary maternal infection in the week before the onset of rash. Placental infection rates of 85% to 91% with fetal infection rates of 45% to 50% have been reported. In a 1982 prospective study of virologically confirmed rubella during pregnancy in England, Miller and colleagues found fetal infection rates of 90% when symptomatic maternal rubella occurred during the first 12 weeks of gestation, 25% to 30% during the second trimester, and 53% during the third trimester. Fetal viremia results in disseminated infection with persistence of the virus throughout fetal life and into postnatal life. Gestational age at the time of infection, the quantity of virus delivered to the fetus, the ability of the fetus to limit replication, and strain variation in virulence determine the risk for malformations. The incidence of anomalies according to gestational age when maternal infection occurs is as follows: weeks 1 to 4, 61%; weeks 5 to 8, 26%; weeks 9 to 12, 8%; weeks 13 to 16, 1% to 4%; weeks 17 to 20, 0.5% to 2%; and weeks 21 to 40, less than 1%. Rubella virus may be transmitted to the susceptible newborn in breast milk or by the respiratory route, but postnatal disease is usually not severe.

CLINICAL MANIFESTATIONS

Spontaneous abortion, stillbirths, and major organ defects are associated with congenital rubella infection. Maternal disease before implantation (just before and 3 weeks after the last menstrual period) may result in fetal infection. Although some investigators report no adverse effects associated with infection this early, an increased incidence of spontaneous abortion during this period is likely. Multiple-organ defects are most likely to result from maternal infection before completion of organogenesis in the first 12 weeks of gestation. The most commonly observed intrauterine defects are as follows:

- Auditory: Sensorineural hearing loss of varying degrees is present in nearly all patients. Deafness occurs in 50% of patients as one of several defects or as an isolated defect associated with infection beyond 12 weeks' gestation.
- Cardiac: Patent ductus arteriosus with or without pulmonary artery or pulmonic valvular stenosis, aortic stenosis, and ventricular septal defect
- Ophthalmologic: Cataract, pigmentary retinopathy, and microphthalmia
- Neurologic: Central auditory imperception, delayed development, intellectual deficits, microcephaly, and hypotonia
- Growth: Intrauterine and postnatal growth retardation

Clinical manifestations related to persistent infection that may be present at birth include hepatosplenomegaly, thrombocytopenia, hepatitis, jaundice, dermal erythropoiesis or "blueberry muffin spots," osteopathy with the characteristic "celery stalk" lesions, meningoencephalitis, interstitial pneumonitis, and myocarditis. Many infants with intrauterine infection have few or no clinical findings at birth but develop severe multisystem disease after a latent period of several months or years. The most notable manifestations of this late-onset rubella syndrome are a generalized interstitial pneumonitis associated with cough, tachypnea, and cyanosis, chronic rubelliform rash, chronic diarrhea, recurrent infections associated with defects of both the humoral and cell-mediated immune system, and progressive neurologic deterioration. Finally, endocrine abnormalities associated with autoantibody production may be observed. Insulin-dependent diabetes mellitus, hypothyroidism, and thyrotoxicosis manifest at several years of age in children with congenital rubella infection.

DIAGNOSIS

The diagnosis of congenital rubella infection is confirmed by isolation of the virus from the nasopharynx, urine, buffy coat, stool, cerebrospinal fluid, cataract, amniotic fluid, or chorionic villus samples. The lens is an excellent site for recovery of virus, especially considering that cataracts are removed in these infants within the first few weeks of life. Eighty percent of infected infants excrete the virus at birth and for as long as 1 year. Viral isolation is often impractical because the tissue culture cells required for isolation of the rubella virus are not usually available in routine virology laboratories. Therefore, serology is used most often for laboratory diagnosis of rubella. Demonstration of rubella-specific IgM antibody at birth and an increase in the infant's IgG titer over 3 to 6 months with stable or decreasing maternal IgG titers provides serologic confirmation of the diagnosis. Not all infants with congenital rubella infection have IgM present at birth; therefore, absent rubella-specific IgM does not exclude the diagnosis. Polymerase chain reaction (PCR) can be used for prenatal diagnosis by chorionic villus sampling and for postnatal diagnosis during infancy of congenitally acquired rubella.

The finding during pregnancy that a mother is immune to rubella is not sufficient to exclude the diagnosis because reinfection may occur, and maternal infection may have occurred before the screen. If the diagnosis of congenital rubella is suspected clinically when the mother is believed to have been immune, the infant should be screened with the rubella IgM ELISA, and viral cultures or PCR should be performed. The diagnosis of congenital rubella infection is eliminated if a women with a negative prenatal rubella screen is negative at the time of delivery.

PREVENTION

Active immunization with live, attenuated rubella virus vaccine is the most effective means of prevention of congenital rubella syndrome. The current vaccine in use is immunogenic in more than 95% of recipients older than 12 months and provides long-term protective immunity that is probably lifelong. The strategy of immunizing all children at 12 months is more efficacious for decreasing the incidence of congenital rubella syndrome than a selective strategy that calls for routine immunization of prepubescent girls and women of childbearing age only. Women who are identified during pregnancy as nonimmune should be immunized in the postpartum period. Vaccine virus shed by the mother does not cause disease in the neonate. Postpartum immunization is not a contraindication for breast-feeding.

Immunization with rubella vaccine is contraindicated during pregnancy, and it is recommended that a woman not conceive during the 3-month period after immunization. The theoretical maximum risk for the occurrence of congenital rubella syndrome after immunization is 1.2%, which is considerably less than the 20% to 50% risk associated with maternal infection with wild-type rubella virus during the first trimester of pregnancy and no greater than the 2% or 3% risk of major birth defects occurring by chance alone. Thus, although pregnancy remains a contraindication to rubella immunization, inadvertent administration of rubella vaccine during the first trimester of pregnancy should not be considered an indication to interrupt the pregnancy.

If a nonimmune pregnant woman is exposed to rubella during the first trimester of pregnancy, serial IgM and IgG rubella antibody studies should be performed to determine if infection has occurred. The risks of adverse effects on the fetus during the first 12 weeks of pregnancy must be explained to her. Immune globulin, 0.55 mL/kg administered intramuscularly within 72 hours of exposure, may prevent or modify infection in an exposed, susceptible person. Protection is not complete even in the absence of clinical disease in the mother because infants with congenital rubella have been delivered by women who received immune globulin shortly after exposure.

Infants with congenital rubella are considered contagious and are maintained in contact isolation for the first year of life unless repeated cultures of nasopharyngeal secretions and urine obtained after 3 months of age are negative. Only health care workers known to be seropositive should be permitted to care for such infants. Pregnant personnel and visitors who are not known to be immune should be restricted from contact with infants with congenital rubella. Rubella immunity should be documented in all health care workers and is required in many states. Vaccine is administered to those who do not have adequate documentation of immunity and is especially important for health care workers who have contact with pregnant women. Physicians are required to report all cases of congenital rubella to the local health department.

CHAPTER 33
Toxoplasmosis

Adapted from Jane D. Siegel
and Pablo J. Sánchez

Toxoplasma gondii is an intracellular parasite with a worldwide distribution. The cat family is the definitive host for this organism. Nonfeline mammals or birds ingest infective oocysts from contaminated soil. Tissue cysts then accumulate in the organs and skeletal muscle of these animals. The possible routes of transmission from animal to human are direct contact with cat feces, ingestion of undercooked meat containing infective cysts, and ingestion of fruits or vegetables that have been in contaminated soil. Infection may be passed from human to human by the transplacental route and, rarely, by transfusion of infected leukocytes or transplantation of infected organs or bone marrow. Transmission *does not* occur through contact with infected individuals. Most human infections are asymptomatic, and significant disease develops when reactivation occurs in association with suppression of the immune system. Toxoplasmosis is an important opportunistic infection in patients with human immunodeficiency virus (HIV) infection and acquired immunodeficiency syndrome (AIDS).

The prevalence of chronic or latent infection with *T. gondii* varies widely among different adult populations throughout the world. Seropositivity increases with age. In the United States, overall seropositivity of pregnant women is 32%, varying from 16% for the 15- to 19-year-old group to 50% for women 35 years of age or older. In contrast, the overall seropositivity rate for women in France is 87%, with variation only from 80% at 15 to 19 years to 96% at 35 years of age and older. On the basis of serologic screening, the incidence of congenital toxoplasmosis in the United States has been estimated to range from 1 in 1,000 to 1 in 12,000 live births as compared with a rate of 3 to 10 of 1,000 live births in Paris, Vienna, and the Netherlands.

PATHOGENESIS

Congenital *Toxoplasma* infection occurs during maternal parasitemia associated almost exclusively with primary infection or reactivation of latent infection in an immunocompromised pregnant woman. Transplacental transmission can occur from asymptomatic, as well as symptomatic maternal infection. No cases have been reported to occur in subsequent pregnancies of women who gave birth to congenitally infected children. Although the actual rate of fetal infection increases as pregnancy advances, the severity of clinical manifestations is greatest when maternal infection is acquired during the first trimester. Overall, the risk of transmission without treatment is 30% to 50%, with variations of 25% in the first trimester, 54% in the second trimester, and 65% in the third trimester. The risk of *severe manifestations* of infection decreases from 75% in the first trimester to 0% in the third trimester.

CLINICAL MANIFESTATIONS

Stillbirth and death in the early neonatal period are the most severe results of congenital infection. Most infants born with congenital toxoplasmosis are asymptomatic in the neonatal period with severe disease at birth in only 10% of infants. Long-term follow-up of untreated asymptomatic infants reveals chorioretinitis in as many as 85% and severe neurologic sequelae in 10% to 20%. The central nervous system is always involved in symptomatic infants. The prominence of neurologic abnormalities is indicative of toxoplasmosis. The classic triad of hydrocephalus, chorioretinitis, and intracranial calcifications can be accompanied by fever, maculopapular or petechial rash, hepatosplenomegaly, jaundice, anemia, convulsions, and abnormal cerebrospinal fluid (CSF) (xanthochromia and mononuclear pleocytosis). Markedly elevated protein concentrations (more than 1 g per 100 mL) in ventricular fluid and hydrocephalus may be explained by periaqueductal and periventricular vasculitis with necrosis that are specifically associated with toxoplasmosis. Intracranial calcifications are distributed diffusely throughout the brain in contrast to the periventricular pattern associated with cytomegalovirus. Severely affected infants may also have myocarditis, pneumonitis, thrombocytopenia, cataracts, microcephaly, and nephrotic syndrome. Sensorineural hearing loss has been reported in 15% to 26% of infants with congenital toxoplasmosis and occurs secondary to calcium deposits in the cochlea and tachyzoites in the middle ear, as well as from destruction of the auditory pathways in infected brain tissue.

DIAGNOSIS

Methods used to diagnose congenital toxoplasmosis include histopathologic examination of the placenta for visualization of tachyzoites and polymerase chain reaction (PCR) for detection of *Toxoplasma* DNA in amniotic fluid, placenta, CSF, and blood. Routine diagnosis is usually made serologically, although determination of the acuity of maternal infection and differentiation of maternal from infant antibody production may be problematic. *T. gondii*-specific IgG tests include the Sabin-Feldman dye test, which is considered the gold standard to which all newer tests are compared. This test is performed only in reference laboratories because of the requirement for viable *Toxoplasma* organisms. More readily available *Toxoplasma*-specific IgG tests include indirect immunofluorescent antibody test, direct agglutination test, and enzyme-linked immunosorbent assays (ELISAs). All of these tests compare favorably against the dye test and are reliable in identifying a seropositive individual or detecting seroconversion.

Because of problems with false-positive results obtained from commercial *Toxoplasma* IgM test kits, a Food and Drug Administration Public Health Advisory cautioned health care providers on reliance on these IgM kits to diagnose acute maternal *Toxoplasma* infection. Other tests that may aid in the diagnosis of congenital toxoplasmosis are the *Toxoplasma*-specific IgA ELISA and a *Toxoplasma*-specific IgE immunofiltration assay. Immunoblotting for detection of *Toxoplasma*-specific IgG, IgM, and IgA antibodies is performed only in research laboratories. The preferred reference laboratory for the performance of all specialized *Toxoplasma* serologic and PCR tests, other than the IgG assays, is the Toxoplasma Serology Laboratory in Palo Alto, California [tel. (415) 853-4828].

Acute maternal infection during pregnancy mandates fetal evaluation. Infection can be diagnosed during gestation using a combination of the following studies: culture specimens of amniotic fluid and fetal blood obtained by cordocentesis, presence of *Toxoplasma*-specific IgM and nonspecific markers of infection (leukocyte count and differential, platelet count, total IgM level, lactic dehydrogenase level, and 5-glutamyltransferase level) in fetal blood, and ultrasound examination of the fetal brain. Absence of IgM in fetal blood does not exclude the diagnosis of congenital infection because production of IgM may be delayed until after birth because of the immaturity of the immune system and possible inhibition of synthesis by maternal IgG. PCR performed on amniotic fluid, in addition to fetal ultrasound, has now supplanted cordocentesis for diagnosis of fetal infection.

After birth, serologic testing of both the mother and infant should be performed to evaluate differences in IgG production and presence of specific IgM antibody. In addition to a careful physical examination, evaluation of the infant consists of complete blood count and platelet counts, liver function tests, CSF evaluation including routine studies, as well as *Toxoplasma*-IgM test and PCR, ophthalmologic examination, and cranial ultrasound or computed tomography. Findings of a positive serum IgM ISAGA, serum IgA ELISA, CSF IgM ELISA, blood or CSF PCR, and increasing *Toxoplasma*-IgG titers during the first year of life are diagnostic of congenital toxoplasmosis. Low *Toxoplasma*-IgG titers and absent IgM antibody in an immunocompetent mother and infant suggest maternal infection before pregnancy and do not require continued follow-up. Because reactivation of past disease in HIV-infected women can lead to congenital infection, any positive maternal *Toxoplasma* titer should prompt neonatal serologic evaluation.

TREATMENT

In large studies of several hundred women with well-documented acute toxoplasmosis acquired during pregnancy, treatment with spiramycin during pregnancy for the prevention of severe fetal abnormalities has been shown to be efficacious. Spiramycin is a macrolide antibiotic that is active against *T. gondii* in animal experiments. It does not consistently cross the placenta; therefore, therapeutic benefits are attributed to its action within the placenta. Spiramycin is readily available in most countries, but in the United States, it must be obtained from the Food and Drug Administration by special request. A 3-week course of spiramycin (2–3 g/day in four divided doses) repeated at 2-week intervals until delivery resulted in significantly more normal children: 76% versus 44%, P less than .001. Spiramycin is recommended when the mother has acute toxoplasmosis during pregnancy but the fetal evaluation is normal. If the amniotic fluid PCR result is positive, the fetus has abnormalities consistent with congenital toxoplasmosis by ultrasound, or both, then the mother should receive pyrimethamine, sulfadiazine, and folinic acid (leucovorin).

All infected infants, even if completely asymptomatic, should receive therapy for toxoplasmosis. Antimicrobial therapy is beneficial against the proliferative forms of *T. gondii* and cure of disease is determined by the specific infecting strain and the time in the course of infection when therapy is initiated. Treatment trials are ongoing and drug regimens are being refined. Therefore, the National Collaborative Treatment Trial [Dr. Rima McLeod, University of Chicago, tel. (773) 834-4152] should be consulted for the currently recommended treatment regimen. The regimen described here is used at this time. The combination of pyrimethamine and sulfadiazine is preferred because of synergism against *Toxoplasma* organisms. Folinic acid, 10 mg three times weekly, is also administered because pyrimethamine is a potent folic acid antagonist. In the presence of active inflammation (e.g., active chorioretinitis that threatens vision, CSF protein greater than 1 g/dL), the addition of prednisone, 1 to 2 mg/kg/day in two divided doses may be beneficial. The prednisone is tapered after the active inflammation has resolved. In the United States, pyrimethamine, sulfadiazine, and folinic acid is continued for 1 year. In France, where spiramycin is readily available, after the first 6 months of treatment, 1 month of pyrimethamine and sulfadiazine is alternated with 1 month of spiramycin, 100 mg/kg/day in two divided doses, to complete the 12-month therapeutic course.

Asymptomatic infants born to mothers with primary infection during pregnancy, but in whom congenital infection has not been completely ruled out, should receive a 1-month course of pyrimethamine and sulfadiazine until further testing has been completed. No further therapy is indicated if congenital toxoplasmosis is not diagnosed. Spiramycin alone may be considered as initial therapy for infants whose mothers have serologic evidence of infection but the date of infection is unknown; therapy is discontinued when congenital infection is ruled out serologically.

Infants with congenital toxoplasmosis must be followed for many years to detect delayed appearance of chorioretinitis and central nervous system reactivation because tissue cysts persist for life at these sites. The extent of neurologic and developmental sequelae should also be evaluated. Evaluation of postnatal treatment of congenitally infected infants is difficult because of the variations in outcome of infection and disease associated with *Toxoplasma* infection. However, carefully performed longitudinal evaluations of infants and children with congenital toxoplasmosis have demonstrated clearly improved outcome when antimicrobial therapy was initiated early (less than 2.5 months of age) and continued for 1 year as compared with untreated historical patients. Of note, many of the treated infants with severe disease at birth (including hydrocephalus, microcephalus, intracranial calcification, and extensive macular destruction) had normal developmental, neurologic, and ophthalmologic findings on follow-up evaluations. Moreover, early and prolonged treatment may significantly decrease the incidence of sensorineural hearing loss.

PREVENTION

Prevention of primary infection during pregnancy is the most effective means of protecting the unborn infant. Several practices are recommended to prevent acquisition of infection by the susceptible pregnant woman. Meat should be frozen at –200°C or cooked at 60°C before eating. Hands and kitchen surfaces should be washed after handling uncooked meat, fruits, and vegetables. Fruits and vegetables should be washed before eating. Cat feces should be avoided and gloves should be worn when handling cat litter boxes. Cat litter boxes should be disinfected daily with boiling water left in place for 5 minutes. Boxes should be cleaned by someone other than the pregnant woman whenever possible. Gloves should be worn during gardening.

Serologic screening of women before pregnancy or early in pregnancy may be a cost-effective means of prevention in areas of the world with high rates of congenital toxoplasmosis. Although universal screening of pregnant women or their infants is not recommended in the United States at present, selective screening of pregnant women based on risk factor assessment should be performed because fetal and neonatal therapy is available and beneficial.

CHAPTER 34
Hepatitis B and C

Adapted from Pablo J. Sánchez and Jane D. Siegel

HEPATITIS B

Hepatitis B virus (HBV) is a double-shelled DNA virus. The inner core consists of hepatitis B core antigen, hepatitis B e antigen (HBeAg), DNA, and DNA polymerase. The outer shell is composed of hepatitis B surface antigen (HBsAg). In approximately 5% to 10% of adults with acute HBV hepatitis, a chronic HBsAg carrier state develops. HBeAg is found in the serum of some individuals who are HBsAg-positive and identifies an infected individual who is at increased risk of transmitting HBV. In the United States, 5% to 8% of the population have been infected with HBV, and 0.2% to 0.9% have chronic infection. In the absence of prophylaxis, 90% of infants delivered by women who are positive for HBsAg and HBeAg become infected. If the HBsAg-positive mother is HBeAg-negative or has antibody to HBeAg, only 25% or 12% of infants, respectively, become infected.

Vertical transmission of HBV occurs when the mother has acute hepatitis B during the third trimester or within the first 2 months postpartum, or if the mother is a chronic HBsAg carrier. Ninety-five percent of neonatal infections occur at the time of delivery from the infant's exposure to infected maternal blood or cervical and vaginal secretions. Approximately 5% of neonatal hepatitis B infections are transmitted transplacentally, presumably as a result of leakage of infected maternal blood into fetal circulation. HBV infection is not associated with congenital defects or fetal malformations. If perinatal infection does not occur, the infant may be at risk for subsequent infection from close contact with household members who are infected or are chronic carriers.

Neonatal infection is usually asymptomatic with only mild elevation of transaminase levels, although chronic hepatitis B with or without cirrhosis, chronic persistent hepatitis, and fatal fulminant hepatitis can occur. Infected infants usually do not become HBsAg-positive until several weeks after birth. Approximately 90% of infants infected perinatally become chronic HBV carriers, and one in four infants who become chronic carriers develops cirrhosis or hepatocellular carcinoma. Transmission from infants and young children occurs within households but is rare in childcare centers.

Effective prophylaxis of HBV infection has been possible since licensure of the first HBV vaccine in 1982. Recombinant vaccines are safe, highly immunogenic in neonates and have 90% to 95% efficacy. For discussion of the available vaccines and dosing, see the Immunizations chapter. The Centers for Disease Control and Prevention (CDC) recommend universal screening for HBsAg early in pregnancy. Testing should be repeated late in pregnancy for women who are negative initially and at high risk for HBV infection or who have had clinical hepatitis since screening was performed.

Perinatal transmission is prevented in greater than 90% of cases by simultaneous intramuscular administration of 0.5 mL of hepatitis B immune globulin (HBIG) and hepatitis B vaccine to both term and preterm infants of HBsAg-positive mothers as soon as possible but within 12 hours of delivery. In institutions with policies for universal immunization of infants at birth, HBsAg-positive women should still be identified before delivery because of the addition of HBIG to the immunoprophylaxis regimen for their infants. HBIG efficacy decreases markedly if treatment is delayed beyond 48 hours. HBV vaccine is administered intramuscularly at a separate site at birth (preferably) or within 7 days, and in infants with birth weight greater than or equal to 2 kg, administration is repeated at 1 to 2 months and 6 months after the first dose. In infants with birth weights less than 2 kg, the initial dose of hepatitis B vaccine does not count for the required three-dose schedule, and a follow-up dose should be given when the infant attains a weight of 2 kg, is 2 months of age, or is discharged (whichever is first). HBsAg may be detected for less than or equal to 1 week after a dose of vaccine. An HBsAg-positive result at any other time indicates a prophylaxis failure or *in utero* infection, and the infant should not receive additional doses of HBIG or vaccine. Testing for anti-HBs and HBsAg is recommended at 1 to 3 months after completion of the vaccine series. The presence of anti-HBs and absence of HBsAg indicates successful prophylaxis and immunization. Infants who are negative for anti-HBs and HBsAg should receive three additional doses of vaccine on a 0-, 1-, and 6-month schedule followed by retesting for anti-HBs 1 month after the third dose. Alternatively, additional doses of vaccine (one to three) can be administered and the infant can be tested for anti-HBs 1 month after each dose to see if subsequent doses are needed. Protection from immunization persists for at least 8 years. Infants delivered by HBsAg-positive women are bathed as soon as possible after delivery to remove all maternal blood and secretions. Intramuscular injections should be delayed until bathing is completed; if this is not possible, then meticulous cleaning of the site with alcohol is necessary. These infants require standard precautions. Infants who have received both active and passive prophylaxis may be breast-fed.

Both the American Academy of Pediatrics (AAP) and the CDC recommend universal immunization of all infants with HBV vaccine as the optimal strategy for prevention of HBV infections. For infants with birth weight greater than or equal to 2 kg and born to mothers who are negative for HBsAg, the first dose of HBV vaccine should be administered to newborns at or soon after birth, the second dose at greater than or equal to 1 month after the first dose, and the third dose at 6 to 18 months of age. The minimal interval between the second and third doses is 2 months, and the third dose should not be given before 6 months. For those infants who received their first dose at older than 2 months, the minimal interval between the first and third doses is 4 months. An alternative schedule of the three doses administered at 2, 4, and 6 to 18 months concurrently with other routine vaccines may be used for HBsAg-negative infants not vaccinated at birth.

Seroconversion rates in very low-birth-weight (VLBW) infants vaccinated shortly after birth are lower than those in older preterm infants and full-term infants vaccinated at birth. For this reason, for premature infants weighing less than 2 kg at birth and born to HBsAg-negative mothers, initiation of the vaccination series is delayed until hospital discharge if the infant weighs greater than or equal to 2 kg or until 2 months of age when other routine immunizations are given. The schedule for follow-up doses is the same as for other infants.

Infants with birth weight greater than or equal to 2 kg and born to mothers whose HBsAg status is unknown should receive the first dose of vaccine within 12 hours of birth. Blood should be drawn from the mother at delivery to determine her HBsAg status. If her HBsAg status is positive, then HBIG should be given as soon as possible, but no later than 1 week of age. If the infant's birth weight is less than 2 kg, then HBIG, in addition to vaccine, should be given within 12 hours of birth. This initial vaccine dose should not be counted as part of the three-dose schedule. The subsequent vaccine schedule is based on the mother's HBsAg status. If this remains unknown, then the infant should be treated as if the mother had been HBsAg-positive.

Infants suspected of having hepatitis B infection should be tested for HBsAg, and if positive, for HBeAg and anti-HBc IgM. The other antibody tests could be positive secondary to the presence of transplacentally acquired maternal antibody. Polymerase chain reaction (PCR) is also available to detect HBV DNA in serum.

DELTA HEPATITIS

Hepatitis D virus (delta virus) is an RNA virus with an internal protein antigen (delta antigen) coated with HBsAg. Because it requires HBV for replication, hepatitis D may occur as a coinfection with acute HBV hepatitis or as a superinfection of an HBsAg carrier. The route of transmission is similar to HBV. Hepatitis D is diagnosed by detection of delta antigen in serum during acute infection and by the appearance of delta antibody. Vertical transmission has been reported, but the risks to the infant are undefined. Infants who become HBsAg carriers as a result of perinatal infection are also at risk of delta infection. No product is available to prevent delta infection in HBsAg carriers either before or after exposure.

HEPATITIS C

Hepatitis C virus (HCV) is a single-stranded RNA virus. HCV is the leading cause of infectious chronic liver disease and the most common reason for liver transplantation in the United States. Chronic infection occurs in 85% of patients, and chronic hepatitis with persistent elevation of liver enzymes develops in approximately 70% of infected individuals. Chronic infection leads to cirrhosis in 20% and primary hepatocellular carcinoma in an estimated 1% to 5% within two decades of the onset of infection.

Seroepidemiologic studies show that approximately 1% of volunteer blood donors screen positive for anti-HCV antibody. Before 1986, receipt of multiple blood transfusions was the most frequent source of HCV infection with transfusion-associated hepatitis rates of 5% to 13%. New cases of posttransfusion hepatitis C have nearly disappeared since the introduction of multiantigen screening tests for antibody to HCV among blood donors in July 1992. Other modes of HCV transmission include organ transplantation, intravenous drug use, intranasal cocaine use, sexual activity, occupational injury with blood-contaminated needles, and perinatal exposure. Intrafamilial transmission has also been documented but is infrequent. The rate of seroconversion following exposure to blood from anti-HCV positive patients through accidental needlesticks or cuts with sharp instruments averages 1.8% (range, 0%–10%).

Perinatal transmission from HCV-infected mothers occurs in approximately 5% (range, 0%–25%) of their infants. No differences are apparent in infection rates between infants delivered vaginally and those born by cesarean section. HCV infection is not a contraindication for breast-feeding. Most perinatally acquired HCV infections are associated with elevated liver enzyme levels during the first year of life and progression to mild chronic liver disease throughout childhood. Infants born to HCV-antibody-positive mothers should be screened for anti-HCV with a second-generation enzyme immunoassay after 12 months of age. A PCR assay is available for detection of HCV RNA in blood. Infants who are infected perinatally should have annual screening of their liver enzymes even if they remain asymptomatic.

No chemoprophylaxis or immunoprophylaxis strategies with proven efficacy exist. Studies are ongoing to determine possible agents for postexposure prophylaxis or use in the HCV-exposed neonate.

Routine screening of pregnant women is not recommended.

CHAPTER 35
Neisseria gonorrhoeae

Adapted from Pablo J. Sánchez and Jane D. Siegel

The prevalence of gonococcal infection during pregnancy varies from 0.6% to 7.6%. The highest rates are found in single, low-income, nonwhite women younger than 30 years. Gonococcal infection during pregnancy has been associated with septic abortion, chorioamnionitis, premature rupture of membranes, delayed delivery after rupture of membranes, and premature delivery.

TRANSMISSION

Transmission of *Neisseria gonorrhoeae* to the newborn infant can occur *in utero* during delivery or after birth. *In utero* acquisition occurs via an ascending route after rupture of amniotic membranes. More commonly, neonatal infection occurs at delivery from passage through an infected birth canal. Approximately 30% of infants born vaginally to infected mothers become colonized with *N. gonorrhoeae*. Horizontal transmission via fomites and by nursery personnel has also been documented.

CLINICAL MANIFESTATIONS AND DIAGNOSIS

Conjunctivitis is the most frequently observed clinical manifestation of gonococcal infection in newborns. Gonococcal conjunctivitis typically appears 2 to 5 days after birth and produces an acute, purulent, bilateral conjunctivitis with lid edema and chemosis. If treatment is delayed, the cornea may ulcerate and scar resulting in loss of visual acuity. Ultimately, the eye may perforate resulting in panophthalmitis and loss of the eye. Presumptive diagnosis of gonococcal conjunctivitis may be made by Gram stain of the conjunctival exudate, which demonstrates gram-negative intracellular diplococci. Not only the conjunctiva, but also the pharynx, umbilicus, urethra, vagina, and rectum can serve as a focus of local or disseminated disease. Disseminated infection is usually manifested by septicemia, meningitis, or septic arthritis that typically involves multiple joints. Cutaneous gonococcal lesions in infants are rare, but gonococcal scalp abscess at the site of previous placement of a scalp electrode has been described.

TREATMENT

Infants with gonococcal ophthalmia should be hospitalized, placed on contact precautions for 24 hours after initiation of parenteral antibiotic therapy, and evaluated for signs of disseminated infection. Blood, cerebrospinal fluid, and localized sites should be cultured as clinically indicated. Tests for concomitant infection with *C. trachomatis* should also be performed. Because of the prevalence of both penicillinase-producing and chromosomally mediated resistant strains of *N. gonorrhoeae*, ceftriaxone administered intravenously or intramuscularly at a dosage of 25 to 50 mg/kg/day (maximum, 125 mg) is recommended for empiric therapy of nondisseminated disease. Alternatively, cefotaxime (100 mg/kg intravenously or intramuscularly) can be used and is preferred in the presence of significant jaundice. A single dose of either ceftriaxone or cefotaxime is sufficient for treatment of uncomplicated ophthalmia neonatorum. However, some experts prefer to continue antibiotics until blood and body fluid cultures, if obtained, are sterile at 48 hours. Hourly irrigation of the infected eye with saline until the purulent discharge resolves is an important part of effective therapy. Topical antibiotic treatment alone is inadequate and is unnecessary when the recommended parenteral antibiotic is given. Ceftriaxone (25–50 mg/kg intravenously or intramuscularly every day) or cefotaxime (50–100 mg/kg/day intravenously or intramuscularly in two divided doses) should be continued for 7 days in the presence of arthritis or septicemia and for 10 to 14 days in the presence of meningitis.

PREVENTION

Ophthalmic prophylaxis in the immediate postpartum period with either 1.0% silver nitrate, 0.5% erythromycin ointment, or 1.0% tetracycline ointment is effective in preventing gonococcal ophthalmia. Even with topical prophylaxis, some infants born to mothers with untreated gonococcal infection may develop gonococcal ophthalmia or disseminated disease. Therefore, these infants should receive a single intramuscular injection of ceftriaxone (25–50 mg/kg intravenously or intramuscularly; maximum, 125 mg). Alternatively, a single dose of cefotaxime (100 mg/kg intravenously or intramuscularly) can be given. The optimal preventive measure is diagnosis and treatment of maternal gonococcal infection before delivery. Gonococcal infections must be reported to the local health department so that contacts can be traced and treated.

SECTION H

Other Topics of Importance

CHAPTER 36

Neonatal Hyperbilirubinemia

Adapted from William J. Cashore

Jaundice is one of the most common conditions found in the newborn. Although most neonatal jaundice is benign, physicians caring for newborn infants must be alert for pathologic hyperbilirubinemia.

DEFINITION

The term *hyperbilirubinemia* implies an excessive level of serum bilirubin, potentially associated with a pathologic cause or outcome. The reason for physiologic hyperbilirubinemia is a developmental delay in the conjugation and excretion of bilirubin as the infant changes from dependence on maternal clearance to a self-contained enzymatic and excretory pathway for bilirubin conjugation and elimination.

In the first 3 to 4 postnatal days, normal infants have a physiologic increase in serum bilirubin from cord bilirubin levels of 1.5 mg/dL or less at birth to a mean value of 6.5 ± 2.5 mg/dL (mean ± SD) on the third or fourth postnatal day. A difference in mean serum bilirubin levels at this time exists between breast-fed infants (7.3 ± 3.9 mg/dL) and formula-fed infants (5.7 ± 3.3 mg/dL). This difference persists for the next several days, with clinically evident hyperbilirubinemia developing more frequently in breast-fed infants during the first week.

Although most newborns have hyperbilirubinemia by normal adult standards, physiologic jaundice is a benign and self-limited process resolving generally by the end of the first week. Virtually all newborns manifest a phase of physiologic jaundice; during this time, the serum bilirubin level generally increases to 6 and 8 mg/dL. This elevation, primarily due to limited bilirubin conjugation, results almost exclusively in an increase in the amount of unconjugated bilirubin (UCB).

Other potentially important factors in the genesis of physiologic jaundice (unconjugated hyperbilirubinemia) include the following:

- Persistent patency of the ductus venosus, which may divert blood flow away from the hepatic sinusoidal bed and, therefore, allow UCB to bypass the hepatocytes.
- Discontinuation of placental mechanisms for bilirubin removal and detoxification
- A greater rate of bilirubin production in the infant (6–8 mg/kg every 24 hours) than in the adult, secondary to a larger red blood cell mass and shortened red blood cell survival time
- Diminished binding of UCB to neonatal serum albumin
- Diminished levels of intracellular bilirubin binding (Y) protein

In addition, bilirubin appears to undergo a significant enterohepatic circulation in the newborn. Beta-glucuronidase activity, present in the neonatal intestine, hydrolyzes bilirubin diglucuronide into UCB, which is subsequently reabsorbed into the portal circulation. Thus, delayed passage of meconium can lead to an elevation in the serum bilirubin level. The pathways for production, distribution, excretion, and enterohepatic circulation are shown schematically in Fig. 36-1.

Some newborns with early onset jaundice, exaggerated levels, or an uncommonly long duration of hyperbilirubinemia may require medical attention. Maisels and Gifford found that 6.1% of 2,416 normal, asymptomatic, term infants had serum bilirubin concentrations greater than 12.9 mg/dL (9% for breast-fed infants and 2.2% for formula fed infants). A definite cause for this exaggerated hyperbilirubinemia was found in only 45% of the infants observed.

Visible cutaneous and scleral jaundice is usually noted only when the serum bilirubin level exceeds 7 to 8 mg/dL. The differential diagnosis of jaundice in these infants may be assisted

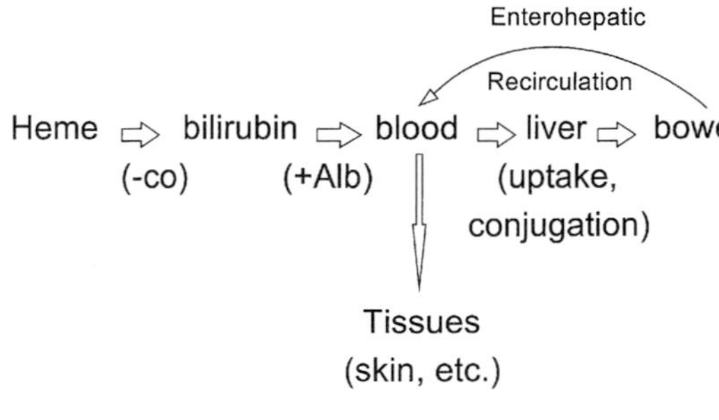

Figure 36-1. Bilirubin production and excretion. Heme oxygenase converts 1 mol of heme to 1 mol of biliverdin (not shown), then 1 mol of bilirubin is produced via biliverdin reductase. Bilirubin, bound to albumin in the blood and extracellular space, is transported to the hepatocytes for conjugation to monoglucuronides and diglucuronides and biliary excretion. Elevated plasma bilirubin levels are in equilibrium with the extracellular space, skin, and other tissues. Plasma bilirubin concentration increases if the rate of bilirubin production exceeds the rate of excretion and may remain elevated if excreted bilirubin is reabsorbed in the bowel and recirculated via the enterohepatic circulation. The enterohepatic circulation of bilirubin may be increased in some cases of breast-feeding jaundice and under some phototherapy conditions.

by noting the rapidity of onset, the presence of major or minor blood group incompatibility between the mother and her newborn, the presence of associated findings such as hematomas or evidence of infection, the method of feeding being used, and the duration and clinical course of jaundice beyond the third day. If visible jaundice in the range of 13 to 15 mg/dL is accepted as a working definition of exaggerated hyperbilirubinemia, approximately 3% of the newborn population will have jaundice in this range from detectable causes potentially requiring treatment and follow-up, whereas approximately 3% will represent the statistical upper limits of normal.

CAUSES OF HYPERBILIRUBINEMIA

Bilirubin is the breakdown product of heme, derived via heme oxygenase and biliverdin reductase with liberation of 1 mol of carbon monoxide for each mole of heme metabolized. Circulating bilirubin is transported on serum albumin to specific receptor proteins in the liver, and is then conjugated by uridine diphosphate-glucuronyl transferase (UDP transferase) to its water-soluble form, also called *conjugated* or *direct-reacting bilirubin.*

Bilirubin conjugates enter the small bowel via bile excretion and, in the course of normal metabolism, are oxidized further and excreted in the stool. Because the bowel does not function in fetal life, the hepatic conjugation and transport system is relatively inactive in the fetus, so that bilirubin produced from fetal red cells *in utero* mostly circulates in the unconjugated form. This unconjugated or indirect-reacting bilirubin is albumin-bound and relatively lipophilic and can be transferred across the placenta to the maternal circulation for conjugation and excretion by the maternal liver. At birth, this maternal excretory pathway is removed, and the development of normal conjugating capacity, canalicular transport, and metabolism and excretion of conjugated bilirubin in the small and large bowel require several days before this pathway becomes adequate for quantitative conjugation and excretion of bilirubin.

Delay in the conjugation and excretion of bilirubin appears to be highly individual, but some infants may have predisposing or contributing factors to delayed excretion. The most common underlying factor is immaturity. Breast-fed infants may have other factors that increase the concentration of UCB. These are generally considered to be a "suppression" in hepatic function mediated by substances in breast milk and an increased reabsorption of bilirubin from the small bowel or both. As noted previously, the mean bilirubin concentration is slightly higher, the duration of jaundice is somewhat longer, and the incidence of clinically detectable hyperbilirubinemia during the first week is more frequent in breast-fed than in formula-fed infants. In addition, approximately 2% of breast-fed infants have a prolonged (2- to 8-week) course of moderate unconjugated hyperbilirubinemia, usually in the range of 10 to 15 mg/dL, while they are feeding adequately on breast milk and have normal weight gain and no other abnormal clinical findings, this is referred to as breast milk jaundice. Possible contributing factors to breast-milk jaundice, proposed by some investigators but not confirmed by multiple independent studies, include high concentrations of lipase, beta-glucuronidase, or polyunsaturated fatty acids in breast milk. Multiple hormonal (such as 3a-,20b-pregnanediol) or enzymatic factors may be involved. Most patients with breast milk jaundice are asymptomatic and have only mild hyperbilirubinemia, and the majority respond, if any intervention is necessary, to temporary cessation of breast-feeding for 36 to 48 hours with a prompt decrease in the serum bilirubin level.

Infants who are not fed or have a high intestinal obstruction caused by conditions such as pyloric stenosis may have exaggerated jaundice as a result of the combined effects of lack of nutritional substrate for bilirubin conjugation, lack of peristalsis for the excretion of bilirubin in the stool, and consequent reabsorption of bilirubin from an obstructed or nonfunctioning bowel.

Crigler-Najjar syndrome (type I) is associated with extreme jaundice in the neonatal period; serum UCB concentrations may reach 15 to 35 mg/dL. This disorder is transmitted as an autosomal recessive trait, mapped to chromosome locus 2q37, and is caused by an absence of hepatic glucuronyl transferase activity. Kernicterus occurs frequently in patients with type I Crigler-Najjar syndrome. Phenobarbital does not increase bilirubin output or decrease serum bilirubin levels. This syndrome has generally been fatal, and attempts at treatment with long-term phototherapy and bilirubin-binding agents have been disappointing. Hepatic transplantation to provide the missing enzyme is curative and should be performed before irreversible neurologic damage occurs. Type II Crigler-Najjar syndrome is distinguished from type I by the fact that phenobarbital decreases the serum bilirubin level. The mutation, inherited at the same locus as for type I disease, may behave as autosomal recessive or dominant. The clinical course of type II is generally milder than that in type I disease.

Gilbert disease is characterized by a mild elevation in serum bilirubin levels, typically of 2 to 3 mg/dL. Liver function and histology are normal, except for minor changes noted on electron microscopy. The mutation is also on chromosome 2 with an estimated frequency of 2% to 6%. A single copy of the mutated gene acts in a partial dominant fashion, down-regulating glucuronide formation to approximately 15% of the normal level. No therapy is necessary, but glucuronidation and excretion can be induced with phenobarbital.

Hypothyroidism is a cause of persistent unconjugated hyperbilirubinemia, which may be the presenting sign of thyroid hormone deficiency. Because diagnosis is through assay of thyroxine (T_4) and thyroid-stimulating hormone levels, neonatal screening programs offer an early opportunity for detection of this disorder.

Lucey-Driscoll syndrome, which consists of severe neonatal hyperbilirubinemia and is capable of causing kernicterus, is thought to be caused by inhibition of glucuronyl transferase in the liver of the newborn by an unidentified factor present in maternal serum and urine. Drugs that can inhibit glucuronyl transferase or hepatic bilirubin uptake may cause an elevation in the serum UCB level.

Bilirubin production is increased by hemolysis or, much more rarely, by inefficient erythropoiesis. The principal causes of hemolysis in the newborn are antibody-mediated hemolytic anemias (e.g., Rh or ABO incompatibility); enclosed hemorrhage such as a cephalhematoma, skin bruising, or an intracranial hemorrhage; hemolysis resulting from bacterial endotoxin as in septicemia; or an abnormality of red cell structure (membrane) or metabolism such as G6PD deficiency.

The most common causes of hemolysis in term infants are isoantibody-mediated hemolytic anemias resulting from maternal-fetal ABO or Rh incompatibility. Although not all susceptible infants are affected, 25% of normal pregnancies are ABO incompatible and approximately 12% are Rh incompatible.

Neonatal polycythemia, as seen in infants of diabetic mothers, infants with adrenal hyperplasia, twin-to-twin transfusion, or aggressive "stripping" of the umbilical cord, when combined with shortened fetal red blood cell survival time, may result in the accumulation of an increased bilirubin load that must be excreted postnatally.

Extravasated blood such as that found in the presence of a cephalhematoma, extensive cutaneous bruising, or swallowed

TABLE 36-1. Differential Diagnosis of Neonatal Jaundice

Cause	Associated findings
Unconjugated (indirect) hyperbilirubinemia	
Hemolytic disease (isoimmune)	
ABO incompatibility	Positive Coombs antiglobulin test result (anti-A or anti-B); microspherocytes
Rh incompatibility	Maternal anti-Rh titer; positive Coombs test result; nucleated red blood cells
Other minor blood group incompatibility	Positive Coombs test result; red blood cell morphology variable
Structural or metabolic abnormalities of red blood cells*	
Hereditary spherocytosis	Family history; splenomegaly; microspherocytes
Glucose-6-phosphate dehydrogenase deficiency	Family history; recent exposure to an oxidant in food or drug; with or without splenomegaly
Hereditary defects in bilirubin conjugation	
Crigler-Najjar syndrome	Complete lack of glucuronyl transferase; severe, lifelong unconjugated hyperbilirubinemia
Gilbert disease (Arias syndrome)	Family history; partial defect of glucuronyl transferase; sometimes responds to phenobarbital
Bacterial sepsis	History and findings compatible with neonatal infection; often an increase in direct bilirubin as well
Breast-milk jaundice	Mild to moderate, but persistent, hyperbilirubinemia; usually improves when breast milk is discontinued
Physiologic jaundice	Usually mild to moderate; no predisposing factors; self-limited (duration less than 1 week)
Conjugated (direct) hyperbilirubinemia	
Congenital biliary atresia	Dilated intrahepatic ducts; no bile excretion
Extrahepatic biliary obstruction	Extrahepatic mass or cyst; dilated main or common bile ducts
Neonatal hepatitis	
Bacterial	Findings compatible with neonatal sepsis
Viral	Inflammatory changes; other systemic signs of a specific viral infection
Nonspecific	Inflammatory changes without a specific viral etiology
Inspissated bile syndrome	Persistent direct hyperbilirubinemia associated with isoimmune hemolytic disease
Postasphyxia	Compatible history, plus increased hepatocellular enzyme concentrations
$alpha_1$-Antitrypsin deficiency	Decreased, $alpha_1$-antitrypsin levels; recurrent or chronic lung disease
Neonatal hemosiderosis	Hemosiderin-filled macrophages on biopsy

*Only the two most common disorders are listed as examples.

maternal blood, can also present the neonatal liver with an increased bilirubin load. In small, premature infants, intracranial hemorrhage can contribute to increased bilirubin formation. Jaundice is generally evident by 3 to 5 days of postnatal life, because extravasated hemoglobin is metabolized slowly to bilirubin. Diagnosis is via inspection or, in the case of swallowed maternal blood, use of the Apt test.

The differential diagnosis of neonatal jaundice is summarized in Table 36-1.

BILIRUBIN TOXICITY

High circulating concentrations of bilirubin are toxic to the central nervous system, with the basal ganglia being the most vulnerable areas. The reason for the susceptibility of the basal ganglia to bilirubin toxicity is not known and the metabolic abnormalities underlying bilirubin toxicity in the central nervous system are not understood. Clinical manifestations of bilirubin toxicity most frequently involve the basal ganglia and cranial nerve nuclei. The most characteristic findings are opisthotonos, extensor rigidity, tremors, ataxic gait, oculomotor paralysis, and hearing loss. Fatal cases in the newborn period are often characterized by loss of the suck response and lethargy, followed by hyperirritability, then seizures and death. Neurologic damage in survivors corresponds to injury in the areas found to be stained in many autopsies. Intelligence and higher cortical functions are relatively spared, whereas ataxia, choreoathetosis, tremors, oculomotor palsy, and central hearing loss persist.

In general, the serum UCB concentrations that are associated with overt bilirubin encephalopathy (or *kernicterus,* the pathologic term for nuclear staining with bilirubin) are substantially higher than the indirect bilirubin levels normally seen among infants with hyperbilirubinemia in ordinary clinical practice. Bilirubin levels generally associated with clinical signs of kernicterus in term infants tend to be in the range of 25 to 30 mg/dL or even higher. In epidemiologic surveys of bilirubin encephalopathy associated with Rh hemolytic disease, basal ganglion staining or clinical signs of bilirubin encephalopathy were encountered occasionally when the serum indirect bilirubin level reached or slightly exceeded 20 mg/dL. In most proven cases, however, the serum bilirubin level was considerably higher, often approaching 30 mg/dL. On the other hand, there are well-documented patients with serum indirect bilirubin levels in the range of 30 to 35 mg/dL who did not experience serious long-term sequelae. Suffice to say, no precise bilirubin level has been established clearly at which either safety or permanent harm can be guaranteed.

Moderate hyperbilirubinemia in the range of 15 to 20 mg/dL poses little or no acute or long-term developmental risk for otherwise normal infants. Term infants with hyperbilirubinemia in this range show, at most, only subtle and short-term behavioral changes with no detectable long-term developmental or neurologic sequelae on follow-up.

In summary, uncontrolled levels of severe hyperbilirubinemia produce a characteristic pattern of damage in the basal ganglia manifested by basal ganglion staining at autopsy or by a subcortical neurologic deficit in survivors. In the range of 20 to 25 mg/dL of indirect bilirubin, some term infants show subtle but reversible sensory and behavioral changes of uncertain prognostic significance. Low bilirubin kernicterus in preterm infants or infants under metabolic stress remains a diagnostic and developmental puzzle.

DIAGNOSIS OF HYPERBILIRUBINEMIA

Determination of the serum bilirubin concentration is indicated only for visible jaundice in healthy term infants, unless prenatal or delivery room screening procedures reveal the presence of a hemolytic anemia with a positive Coombs test result. Daily inspection of the baby, undressed and in adequate light, allows early recognition of cutaneous or scleral jaundice in most cases. For nonwhite infants, part of the examination can include brief compression with the examiner's thumb of the skin over a firm surface such as the forehead, sternum, or upper thigh; briefly blanching the skin may help to reveal an underlying yellow color. Cutaneous jaundice progresses from the face downward in term infants. Scleral and facial jaundice becomes visible at bilirubin levels of 6 to 8 mg/dL, jaundice of the shoulders and trunk becomes apparent at 8 to 10 mg/dL, jaundice of the lower body is noticeable at 10 to 12 mg/dL, and generally distributed jaundice can be seen at 12 to 15 mg/dL. Visible jaundice on the first day is abnormal and requires evaluation and follow-up. In addition to a laboratory request for the measurement of total and direct (or conjugated) bilirubin, the clinical detection of hyperbilirubinemia should prompt a thorough examination of the infant's abdomen with palpation of the liver and spleen, and a review of the maternal and neonatal hospital records for evidence of blood group incompatibility, a positive antibody titer or Coombs test result, or a family history of neonatal or childhood jaundice in siblings or other relatives. All women who are receiving prenatal care or are admitted to a hospital for delivery should have their ABO and Rh status determined. If the mothers are Rh-negative, they should also have a titer for anti-Rh antibodies determined during the course of prenatal care. At the baby's birth, if the mother's blood type is group O, or if she is Rh-negative (with any major group), the jaundiced infant's major and minor blood groups should be determined in addition to a Coombs (direct antiglobulin) test. Although 25% of pregnancies are potentially ABO incompatible, only a minority (10%–15%) has hemolytic anemia as documented by a positive Coombs test result. In the absence of a positive antibody test result or dropping hematocrit, the diagnosis of ABO incompatible hemolytic anemia in the newborn would be difficult to confirm. If labs reveal the presence of a Coombs-positive hemolytic anemia, or if splenomegaly is present, then, in addition to serum bilirubin measurement, determination of hemoglobin, hematocrit, red cell indices, reticulocyte count, and red cell morphology should be undertaken. For the more common instance of benign, self-limited developmental hyperbilirubinemia, a complete blood count is not necessary unless strong reason exists to suspect hemolysis or infection as the source of hyperbilirubinemia.

The age at first presentation of clinical jaundice and the subsequent rate of increase in serum bilirubin levels sometimes allow the physician to infer the clinical course and probable outcome of an infant with hyperbilirubinemia. The rate of increase in the serum bilirubin level can be estimated by dividing the first serum bilirubin level by the patient's age at the time and by dividing all subsequent changes in bilirubin level by the change in age between determinations. This allows the physician to estimate whether the rate of increase is normal or abnormal, and whether the increase in bilirubin over time is sustained or declining. For example, the maximum rate of increase in bilirubin for otherwise normal infants with nonhemolytic hyperbilirubinemia is approximately 5 mg/dL/day, or 0.2 mg/dL/hour. Visible jaundice on the first day or a bilirubin concentration greater than 10 mg/dL within the second 24 hours, therefore, is outside the normal range for rate of increase in bilirubin and potentially results from a pathologic cause. Estimating the rate of increase during the interval between bilirubin determinations also allows the physician to estimate the change in bilirubin level that is likely to occur over the next 12- to 24-hour interval and to plan subsequent bilirubin determinations accordingly. In most cases, if an infant is jaundiced significantly (i.e., serum indirect bilirubin level greater than or equal to 10 mg/dL) at the first determination, and if the calculated rate of increase exceeds 0.2 mg/dL/hour, repeat determinations are indicated approximately every 12 hours until the serum bilirubin levels stabilize or a clear indication for treatment exists.

Physiologic jaundice and hemolytic hyperbilirubinemia are always predominantly of the indirect-reacting variety. Because obstructive liver disease from various causes may also present with hyperbilirubinemia in the newborn period, the initial evaluation of a jaundiced infant requires determination of the direct as well as the total serum bilirubin concentration. Direct bilirubin concentrations persistently higher than the range of 1.0 to 1.5 mg/dL should be regarded with suspicion, especially if the direct fraction continues to increase.

MANAGEMENT OF HYPERBILIRUBINEMIA

Table 36-2 outlines a suggested approach to the anticipatory management of neonatal jaundice. Most cases of physiologic hyperbilirubinemia can be managed with observation, serial bilirubin determinations, and reassurance. The benign and self-limited course of most cases of nonhemolytic hyperbilirubinemia makes it generally unnecessary to pursue sophisticated diagnostic studies in the first few days.

Hemolytic Hyperbilirubinemia: Rh Disease

Until recently, Rh isoimmunization was a common cause of neonatal hemolytic anemia and hyperbilirubinemia and was the underlying cause for most cases of kernicterus in term infants. Sixteen percent of North American women are Rh-negative, in most cases negative for the Rh D antigen. At delivery of her first Rh-positive child, or sometimes because of a placental hemorrhage or spontaneous abortion of an Rh-positive fetus, the Rh-negative mother receives a small transfusion of Rh-positive fetal cells. The maternal immune system then develops an

TABLE 36-2. Anticipatory Management of Neonatal Jaundice

1. Know maternal blood type
2. Know baby's blood type if mother is Rh-negative or group O
3. Identify jaundice (especially if early onset)
4. Identify risk factors present by
   a. Serum bilirubin
   and/or
   b. Coombs test result, hemoglobin, hematocrit, red blood cell indices and morphology
5. Observe, repeat, and discharge if jaundice is nonprogressive and no risk factor is present, *or,*
6. Start therapy as described below, if indicated by
   a. Approaching threshold
   or
   b. Risk factors present
7. Start phototherapy when unconjugated bilirubin is below expected exchange transfusion level
8. Exchange transfusion
   a. Early, if conditions are met
   b. Later, if phototherapy fails to control serum bilirubin

antibody response to the foreign Rh-positive red cell antigen. Later exposure to Rh-positive fetal cells increases the maternal IgG antibody titer against the cells of her fetus. Maternal anti-Rh IgG antibodies then recross the placenta to the fetal side, where they attack and destroy the Rh-positive fetal cells. As the maternal production of antibody increases, fetal cells are attacked and hemolyzed extravascularly, as well as intravascularly, as soon as they become sufficiently antigenic to be recognized by the circulating antibody. During the second half of a sensitized pregnancy, the fetus has a progressive hemolytic anemia and intrauterine hyperbilirubinemia. In the most severely sensitized cases, the intrauterine anemia becomes so profound that high-output cardiac failure, anasarca, and hydrops fetalis develop. Before effective prevention of Rh sensitization was possible, many of the most severe cases of hyperbilirubinemia and probably a majority of the neonatal cases of kernicterus were found among infants with Rh hemolytic disease. With proper maternal screening, all remaining cases of Rh sensitization should be detected prenatally and the pediatrician forewarned. The characteristic morphologic abnormality of the red cells in the newborn with Rh hemolytic disease is the presence of large numbers of nucleated red cells (erythroblasts); hence, the name *erythroblastosis fetalis*.

Management of the newborn with Rh hemolytic disease may serve as a model for aggressive intervention in severe cases of neonatal hyperbilirubinemia. Immediate correction of the circulating hemoglobin level by the transfusion of packed red cells is indicated if the hemoglobin concentration at birth is 10 mg/dL or less. The volume transfused, usually 25 to 50 mL/kg of packed red cells, is calculated to correct the newborn's hemoglobin level to the range of 11 to 13 g/dL. In addition, if the cord indirect bilirubin concentration exceeds 5 mg/dL, or if the immediate postnatal rate of increase is 1 mg/dL/hour or faster, a double volume exchange transfusion with whole blood should be performed as soon as possible. This procedure stabilizes the red cell mass by replacing most of the circulating red cells with Rh-negative cells that are compatible with the major blood groups and cannot be hemolyzed by the circulating antibody. Replacement of the plasma decreases the circulating antibody level somewhat, although much of the antibody accumulated over the weeks before birth is outside the vascular system and is not immediately accessible. The exchange of plasma also replaces jaundiced with nonjaundiced plasma and allows reequilibration of newly formed bilirubin into a nonjaundiced plasma compartment carrying fresh adult albumin that is not yet saturated with bilirubin. The initial exchange transfusion reduces the serum bilirubin concentration to approximately 50% of its preexchange level. Extravascular bilirubin equilibrates rapidly with the plasma causing a short-term 30% rebound increase in the plasma bilirubin level.

ABO Incompatibility

ABO hemolytic disease is more common than Rh hemolytic disease, but it is more benign. In nearly all cases, the mother's blood type is group O (the major blood type in 40% of the North American population) and the infant's blood type is group A or B. Prenatal detection of ABO incompatibility is not feasible and is not generally necessary. Instead of sensitization during pregnancy, preformed maternal anti-A or anti-B antibodies of the IgG class are transferred passively to the infant late in pregnancy or at parturition. Rapid early hemolysis of fetal cells occurs with splenic recognition and removal of antigen-antibody complexes. Because fetal red cells have only approximately 7,500 to 8,000 A or B antigen sites per cell (versus 15,000–20,000 in the adult), the fetal cells do not agglutinate, and they may not be destroyed completely. This decreased number of antigen–antibody sites on fetal cells may give a weakly positive or even a negative direct Coombs reaction. The antibody may be identified correctly by incubation of the neonatal serum with incompatible adult red cells and performance of an indirect Coombs test. Because not all ABO-incompatible pregnancies result in neonatal hemolysis, a positive Coombs test result (direct or indirect) is necessary to confirm the diagnosis.

ABO incompatibility seldom presents with severe jaundice or severe anemia at birth, but the rate of increase in bilirubin on the first postnatal day may lead to preparations for an exchange transfusion in some cases. If the initial rate of increase exceeds 1 mg/dL/hour, if the infant is significantly anemic (hemoglobin, 10 g/dL or less), or if the serum bilirubin level reaches the range of 15 to 20 mg/dL within the first 24 hours, a double volume exchange transfusion is indicated after the indirect bilirubin level has exceeded 15 mg/dL and before it exceeds 20 mg/dL. After the first postnatal day, the rate of red cell degradation and the subsequent rate of increase in the serum bilirubin level begin to diminish as the antigen-antibody complexes are cleared and the rate of hemolysis slows. This is often reflected in a rapid early increase in the serum bilirubin level to the range of 10 to 15 mg/dL or slightly higher, followed by a plateau at 15 to 20 mg/dL on the second hospital day. In this case, blood may be cross-matched and preparations made for an exchange transfusion, but the transfusion need not be done unless the hemolytic anemia becomes more severe or the serum bilirubin concentration exceeds 20 mg/dL.

As a general policy, exchange transfusion should be considered for any newborn with an indirect serum bilirubin level in the range of 20 to 25 mg/dL from any cause, if unresponsive to phototherapy. Sustained hyperbilirubinemia within this range may be potentially hazardous.

PHOTOTHERAPY

The systematic use of fluorescent light to lower serum bilirubin levels followed the observations of Cremer, Perryman, and Richards in 1958 that jaundice was less frequent in a well-lighted nursery in a new wing of their hospital than in a dimly lighted one in an older wing. The mechanism of phototherapy, once thought to be the degradation of bilirubin and excretion of its degradation products as smaller molecules, is now found to proceed through the light-induced formation of configurational and structural isomers of UCB. These isomeric forms of bilirubin are more water-soluble than the parent compound, bilirubin IX-a; therefore, they are transported through the liver more rapidly than the predominant form of UCB. The dose applied to the skin, ideally 5 to 10 $\mu W/cm^2/nm$ in the spectral range of 400 to 500 nm, rapidly converts UCB to its isomers in a dose-dependent fashion at the level of the skin. Doses of less than 3 to 4 $\mu W/cm^2/nm$ produce inefficient photoconversion, whereas the effectiveness of doses greater than 10 to 12 $\mu W/cm^2/nm$ is limited by a plateau in the photoconversion response and by practical limits on achieving higher light doses in the nursery setting. The photoconversion to isomers is rapid, followed by slower distribution of the isomers from the skin into the circulation and subsequent excretion of the isomers by the liver.

Current studies of the photoconversion and excretion process point to the conclusion that the excretion step of photoisomers via the liver may be rate-limiting for the dose response in newborns. In addition, once isomerized bilirubin reaches the bowel, it may reconvert to the normal form of UCB, because it is no longer exposed to light. Unless the photobilirubin that enters the small bowel is converted rapidly to other water-soluble products, or is excreted rapidly, some enterohepatic recirculation of photobilirubin via reconversion to bilirubin IX-a may occur. Therefore, even with rapid conversion of bilirubin to its photoproducts, a rapid decline in the serum bilirubin level may not always be seen. Rather, the bilirubin concentration in the plasma may be stabilized in equilibrium with its photoproducts, its rate of hepatic excretion, and its rate of recirculation from the bowel into the blood if, in the small bowel, it has merely entered a third space without being excreted. Perhaps, then, an apparent delay in serum bilirubin response to phototherapy is not surprising given the balance that must be achieved between the rates of bilirubin production, excretion, and reabsorption in a complex system.

OTHER THERAPEUTIC CONSIDERATIONS

Feeding promotes peristalsis and colonization of the bowel. Peristalsis increases the rate of bilirubin excretion as the stools change from meconium to transitional to the bilirubin-rich yellowish brown stools that are apparent at several days of life, whereas bowel colonization with normal flora promotes the enzymatic conversion of bilirubin to other bile products that cannot be reabsorbed or reconverted to UCB. Unfed or underfed newborns tend to have more persistent jaundice than do those who are fed adequately, so the underfed nursing infant may show improvement rather than worsening of jaundice with increased frequency of nursing and an increase in milk intake within the first few days.

Future therapy for unconjugated hyperbilirubinemia, both that seen in the neonate and that occurring in the older patient with Crigler-Najjar syndrome, may focus on the inhibition of bilirubin formation from its hemoglobin precursor. The synthetic heme analogue tin-protoporphyrin has been shown to inhibit competitively heme oxygenase, the rate-limiting enzyme in the degradation of hemoglobin to bilirubin. Experiments using animal models and some preliminary clinical studies have shown that administration of this agent results in decreased biliary excretion of bilirubin with concomitant increases in the excretion of heme pigment into bile. In addition, when it is given to neonatal animals or human newborns shortly after delivery, hyperbilirubinemia is prevented. Thus, with further development and documentation of its safety and efficacy, this approach may offer a specific therapy for unconjugated hyperbilirubinemia.

Management of Breast-Milk Jaundice

Most breast-fed infants have normal postnatal serum bilirubin levels that do not require any specific diagnostic or treatment measures. Early hyperbilirubinemia in breast-fed newborns may be associated with suboptimal feeding schedules and milk intake resulting in excessive weight loss, infrequent stools, and inadequate excretion of bilirubin. No fixed interval between birth and the first breast-feeding should be necessary if the mother and baby are in good condition immediately after delivery. During the first several days postpartum, nursing on demand or at intervals more frequent than every 4 hours may help to stimulate lactation, avert excessive weight loss, and aid the transition from meconium to normal stools.

Preterm infants of 35 to 37 weeks' gestation and weighing 2,500 to 3,000 g may appear healthy at birth but may not nurse as well as term infants and may still have immature liver function. This group includes some infants delivered by elective cesarean section before term with the smooth initiation of nursing complicated further by the mother's postoperative condition. Hepatic immaturity and inadequate intake may increase the likelihood of hyperbilirubinemia in such infants. Formula supplementation may be needed for adequate hydration and nutrition until lactation is well established, and phototherapy for hyperbilirubinemia in the range of 15 to 20 mg/dL may be used during the first several days until hepatic function matures and adequate excretion of bilirubin begins.

The discontinuation of breast-feeding in a well baby with persistent hyperbilirubinemia is largely a matter of clinical judgment. Many cases of breast-milk jaundice are mild enough to require no intervention except for bilirubin determinations once or twice in the first several weeks after discharge to follow the resolution of the problem. More severe cases, which often appear toward the end of the first week and then fail to resolve or progress to still higher levels of hyperbilirubinemia, may benefit from the therapeutic test of discontinuing breast-feeding for 36 to 48 hours. Hyperbilirubinemia caused by breast milk factors usually responds to the temporary cessation of nursing with a prompt decline of 2 to 4 mg/dL in the serum bilirubin level, after which nursing can usually be resumed with little or no further increase in bilirubin. In most cases, it appears that even temporary removal of the inhibiting factor allows an improvement in hepatic function and in the intestinal excretion of bilirubin. Only in rare cases is hyperbilirubinemia severe and persistent enough to require the complete discontinuation of breast-feeding.

Some authorities suggest that term breast-fed infants without other risk factors require no treatment until the serum indirect bilirubin exceeds 20 mg/dL, and that exchange transfusion is not indicated in these low-risk infants until the serum bilirubin level reaches or exceeds 25 mg/dL. Medical supervision and even daily follow-up of infants with borderline, but still increasing, bilirubin levels are important. Undetected, unsupervised hyperbilirubinemia in breast-fed infants thought to be at no risk may occasionally progress to levels of 25 to 30 mg/dL or greater. Besides the uncertain risk of later neurologic damage from prolonged, extremely high bilirubin levels, some unsupervised infants with extreme hyperbilirubinemia are later found to have risk factors that were not recognized at birth and may be at increased risk for the development of clinically evident bilirubin encephalopathy.

DIRECT (CONJUGATED) HYPERBILIRUBINEMIA

Obstructive hyperbilirubinemia resulting from intrinsic liver disease or a congenital hepatobiliary obstruction may first appear in the newborn. Early in the course, this condition may present with a predominantly indirect or unconjugated hyperbilirubinemia, but, in most cases, the direct or conjugated fraction of bilirubin quickly increases to levels in excess of 2 mg/dL and then remains elevated. Conjugated bilirubin appears to not be toxic to the central nervous system. Underlying causes may include infection, neonatal hepatitis, inspissation of bile, or congenital intrahepatic or extrahepatic biliary obstruction. Obstructive hyperbilirubinemia may present in the newborn period but generally persists well beyond neonatal life and has different implications for the child's health than does neonatal unconjugated hyperbilirubinemia.

CHAPTER 37
Congenital Malformation

Adapted from Robert J. Gorlin

FREQUENCY OF MAJOR AND MINOR ANOMALIES

A major malformation is usually defined as a structural abnormality that has surgical, medical, or cosmetic importance. Approximately 2% to 3% of infants of at least 20 weeks' gestational age have a major malformation (Table 37-1). Having a single major malformation is much more common than having multiple malformations.

Minor anomalies, which are much more common than major malformations, are defined as having no surgical or cosmetic significance and occur in fewer than 4% of all newborns of the same race and gender. Minor abnormal physical features that occur in more than 4% of infants are considered normal variations. The frequency of specific minor abnormal physical features varies among racial groups. For example, preauricular sinus and accessory nipples are more common among black than among white infants. Epicanthal folds are more common in white infants than black infants. Finding three or more minor anomalies should prompt a careful medical assessment for the presence of a major malformation, because such anomalies are present in approximately 20% of these infants. A few minor abnormal physical features are a significant physical finding that necessitates further diagnostic study.

RECOGNIZED ETIOLOGIES OF MALFORMATIONS

Malformations Caused by Multifactorial Inheritance

The most common malformations (e.g., heart defects and spina bifida) are attributed to multifactorial inheritance, a process in which mutant genes and environmental factors are involved. For all malformations attributed to multifactorial inheritance, the likelihood that a subsequent sibling (or the offspring of an affected parent) will be affected is ten to 20 times greater than the risk in the general population but less than in instances involving autosomal recessive and autosomal dominant genes with complete penetrance. As an example of an environmental factor, periconceptional supplementation with folic acid decreases the occurrence of spina bifida and heart defects. Studies have shown a strong interrelationship between maternal cigarette smoking, the presence of specific alleles of transforming growth factor-alpha, and the occurrence of orofacial clefts. New concepts, including uniparental disomy, mitochondrial inheritance, and somatic mosaicism, have been identified as potential etiologies. In addition, very small chromosome deletions can now be identified by the technique of fluorescent in situ hybridization such as the chromosome 22q11 deletion that is associated with several heart defects and the DiGeorge syndrome.

Malformations Caused by Teratogens

The teratogenic exposures during pregnancy that cause malformations include maternal conditions or diseases, maternal infections, drugs taken during pregnancy, exposures to heavy metals, and the prenatal diagnostic procedure chorionic villus sampling (Table 37-2). The first trimester of the pregnancy is the period of exposure most likely to produce malformations. The risk that the exposed fetus will be damaged is expressed relative to the frequency of similar problems in the general population. It ranges from an increase of at least ten- to 20-fold for the drugs isotretinoin (13-cis-retinoic acid) and valproic acid to two- to threefold for phenytoin and insulin-dependent diabetes mellitus. In general, the higher the exposure, the greater the risk of damage. Patterns of major and minor anomalies may exist with certain teratogens (thalidomide, phenytoin, isotretinoin) or maternal conditions (alcoholism and systemic lupus erythematosus). Some maternal conditions produce a variety of malformations involving several organ systems but no consistent pattern of abnormalities (maternal diabetes).

The mechanism of action is known for some teratogens. For example, the hypothyroidism produced by iodides and propylthiouracil is caused by interference with the synthesis of thyroid hormone.

Malformations Caused by Uterine Factors

The presumed uterine factors that cause fetal abnormalities are crowding, breech presentation, and vascular disruption. Breech presentation can cause hip dislocation and clubfoot deformity

TABLE 37-1. Congenital Malformations in Newborn Infants: Recognized Etiologies[a]

	Number[b]	Percent of total	Example
Genetic causes			
Chromosome abnormalities	157 (45)	10.1	Trisomies, deletions
Single mutant genes	48	3.1	Chondrodystrophies
Familial	225 (3)	14.5	Renal agenesis
Multifactorial inheritance	356 (23)	23.0	Anencephaly, some heart defects
Teratogens	49	3.2	Infants of diabetic mothers
Uterine factors	39 (5)	2.5	Breech presentation
Twinning	6 (2)	0.4	Acardia, conjoinings
Unknown cause	669 (24)	43.2	Gastroschisis
Subtotals	1,549 (102)	100.0	
Overall total births	69,227		

[a]Total frequency 2.2%.
[b]Parentheses indicate therapeutic abortions.
Reprinted with permission from Nelson K, Holmes L. Malformation due to presumed spontaneous mutations in newborn infants. *N Engl J Med* 1989;320:19.

TABLE 37-2. Recognized Human Teratogens

Drugs	**Maternal conditions**
Aminopterin/methotrexate (Amethopterin)	Alcohol use
Androgenic hormones	Insulin-dependent diabetes mellitus
Angiotensin-converting enzyme inhibitors	Iodide deficiency
Busulfan	Maternal phenylketonuria
Carbamazepine	Myasthenia gravis
Chlorobiphenyls	Smoking cigarettes or marijuana
Cocaine	Systemic lupus erythematosus
Cyclophosphamide	Vitamin A deficiency
Diethylstilbestrol	**Intrauterine infections**
Etretinate	Cytomegalovirus
Heroin/methadone	Herpes simplex
Iodide	Parvovirus
Isotretinoin (13-*cis*-retinoic acid)	Rubella
Lithium	Syphilis
Phenobarbital	Toxoplasmosis
Phenytoin	Varicella
Propylthiouracil	Venezuelan equine encephalitis virus
Prostaglandin	**Other exposures**
Tetracycline	Chorionic villus sampling
Thalidomide	Dilation and curettage
Trimethadione/paramethadione	Gasoline fumes (excessive)
Valproic acid	Heat
Warfarin	Hypoxia
Heavy metals	Methyl isocyanate
Lead	Methylene blue
Mercury	Toluene (excessive)
Radiation	Trauma, blunt
Cancer therapy	

because of continued fetal growth within the confines of the mother's pelvis. These are positional deformities, not structural abnormalities. Likewise, crowding in a septate uterus or in multiple gestations can produce positional deformities.

Vascular disruption is caused by a sequence of events that includes hypoxia, hemorrhage, and tissue loss. The result is referred to as amniotic band syndrome. Monozygous twins are more likely to have major malformations than are singletons. Some of these abnormalities (e.g., acardiac fetus, conjoined twins, and embolization of material from a deceased cotwin) occur only in monozygous twins. Other conditions such as cloacal exstrophy, are more common among twins than singletons.

CRANIOFACIAL DEFECTS

Cleft Lip and Cleft Palate

EPIDEMIOLOGY AND GENETICS

A combination of cleft lip and cleft palate is more common than an isolated occurrence of either. Cleft lip with cleft palate composes some 50% of the cases, with cleft lip and isolated cleft palate each constituting perhaps 25%, generally irrespective of race. Cleft lip with or without cleft palate occurs in approximately 1 per 1,000 white births (range, 0.8–1.6 per 1,000). Frequency is higher in Native Americans (3.5 per 1,000), Japanese (2.1 per 1,000), and Chinese (1.7 per 1,000); it is lower among blacks (0.3 per 1,000).

Isolated cleft lip may be unilateral (80%) or bilateral (20%). When unilateral, the cleft is more commonly located on the left side (approximately 70%), but it is no more extensive. Lips are cleft somewhat more frequently bilaterally (approximately 25%) when combined with cleft palate. The cleft lip and palate combination is more common in men than in women. Some 85% of cases of bilateral cleft lip and 70% of cases of unilateral cleft lip are associated with cleft palate. Cleft lip is not always complete (i.e., extending into the nostril). In approximately 10% of the cases, the cleft is associated with skin bridges or Simonart's bands.

Isolated cleft palate appears to be an entity separate from cleft lip with or without cleft palate. Numerous investigators have determined that siblings of patients with cleft lip with or without cleft palate have an increased frequency of the same anomaly but not of isolated cleft palate and vice versa. The incidence of isolated cleft palate among both whites and blacks appears to be 1 per 2,000 to 2,500 births. It occurs somewhat more often in girls, comprising some 60% of the cases. Although a 2:1 female-to-male predilection prevails for complete clefts of the hard and soft palate, the ratio approaches 1:1 for clefts of the soft palate only.

Recurrence data do not suggest a simple pattern of inheritance. This finding is bolstered by twin studies indicating the relative roles played by genetic and nongenetic influences. Among twins with cleft lip with or without cleft palate, concordance is far greater in monozygotic (35%) than in dizygotic (4.5%) twins. In twins with isolated cleft palate, concordance is not quite as great between the two groups (monozygotic, 26.0%; dizygotic, 5.8%). This finding suggests a stronger genetic basis for cleft lip with or without cleft palate than for isolated cleft palate. Both cleft lip with or without cleft palate and isolated cleft palate consist of three groups: sporadic (75%–80%), familial (10%–15%), and syndromal (1%–5%). Clefting is heterogeneous. Its variation and liability are probably determined by major genes, minor genes, environmental insults, and a developmental threshold.

RISK OF RECURRENCE

In most cases, the cleft is either isolated or associated with a constellation of anomalies that do not form a recognizable

TABLE 37-3. Facial Clefts: Risk of Recurrence

Parents	Siblings Normal	Siblings Affected	Cleft lip (palate) (%)	Cleft palate (%)
Normal	0	1	4.0	3.5
	1	1	4.0	3.0
	0	2	14.0	13.0
One affected	0	0	4.0	3.5
	0	1	12.0	10.0
	1	1	10.0	9.0
	0	2	25.0	24.0
Both affected	0	0	35.0	25.0
	0	1	45.0	35.0
	1	1	40.0	35.0
	0	2	50.0	45.0

Adapted from Tolarová M. Empirical recurrence risk figures for genetic counseling of clefts. *Acta Chir Plast (Praha)* 1972;14:234.

syndrome. Although more than 300 cleft syndromes or associations are recognized, they constitute a low percentage of cases. Efforts must be made to recognize a cleft syndrome, because the pattern of inheritance may be simple, and the genetic risk for future affected children may then be more precise. For example, a parent with or without a cleft and paramedian pits of the lower lip has a 50% chance of having a child with cleft lip or palate.

In the case of isolated clefts, the risk to a first-degree relative of an affected individual is 2% to 4%. This information applies only to risks for similar anomalies (i.e., a parent with isolated cleft palate has no greater risk of having a child with cleft lip with or without cleft palate than anyone else and vice versa). The risks increase as more individuals are affected. For example, if a parent and a child have clefts, the risk for a future affected sibling increases to approximately 10% to 12%. These and other situations are presented in detail in Table 37-3.

The severity of a facial cleft also affects recurrence risk in the offspring. For example, researchers have found that if a parent has isolated unilateral cleft lip, the recurrence risk is 2.5%. In the presence of unilateral cleft lip and palate, the risk increases to 4%, and the risk is more than 5.5% for bilateral cleft lip with cleft palate.

ASSOCIATED ANOMALIES

Cleft lip and palate often occur as isolated anomalies (i.e., thorough examinations conducted over several years have revealed no other primary abnormalities). When data are broken down according to subtype, isolated cleft palate (20%–50%) is generally acknowledged to be associated more often with other congenital anomalies than are either isolated cleft lip (7%–13%) or cleft lip with cleft palate (2%–11%). The frequency with which one or more malformations accompanies clefts of all types is almost 28%.

CARE OF THE INFANT WITH CLEFT LIP OR CLEFT PALATE

A cleft palate team—usually composed of a maxillofacial surgeon, audiologist, speech pathologist, prosthodontist, otolaryngologist, pedodontist, and geneticist—is extremely important in helping parents to understand the sequential approach to therapy for the many attendant problems.

Feeding usually requires considerable patience. Those with more severe clefts of the lip or palate should be fed in a sitting position to minimize fluid loss through the nose. Various techniques and equipment are used to feed infants with clefts, but no single method is optimal for all infants. Infants with cleft lip or cleft palate swallow normally but suck abnormally. A cleft in the lip or palate does not generally allow sufficient negative pressure. In the case of cleft lip only, breast-feeding or an artificial nipple with a large, soft base works well. For infants with cleft lip or palate, regular breast-feeding or normal bottle feeding is not often successful because they are unable to seal either their lips or their velopharynx. With cleft of the palate only, breast-feeding or normal bottle feeding can usually be carried out if the cleft is narrow or involves only the soft palate. Soft artificial nipples with large openings are more effective.

Regular bottle nipples do not work well for infants with wider palatal clefts or the Robin malformation sequence. Enlarging the nipple opening in association with a softer nipple with a large base and a long shaft often enables tongue movement to express a greater quantity of milk. One can also deliver milk directly into the mouth with a soft plastic bottle.

Children with cleft palate are prone to repeated infections of the middle ear and paranasal sinuses. The tonsils and adenoids enlarge, and chronic nasopharyngitis may lead to recurrent otitis media with resultant conductive hearing loss. Nasopharyngeal infection should be treated promptly with antibiotics. The tonsils and adenoids may play a vital role in allowing normal speech. Thus, tonsillectomy and adenoidectomy, especially in those with velopharyngeal insufficiency, may result in postoperative nasal speech.

Assessing auditory function in infants with cleft palates is important and may be carried out more accurately in infants or young children by auditory specialists.

SURGICAL REPAIR OF CLEFTS

Closure of the lip is usually carried out between the second and tenth week after birth depending on the infant's weight and state of health. The primary purpose is to create a seal to allow normal sucking. Various techniques have been used for repair of the lip depending on the degree and extent of defect. In those cases in which tissue in the two lip segments is insufficient to create an acceptable lip and nostril, the surgeon may have to move small flaps of tissue from other places in the upper or (occasionally) the lower lip. For bilateral cleft lip, surgery is more difficult. If the primary palate is not attached to the secondary palate, it requires repositioning. Usually, subsequent surgery is required to correct nasal alar form to compensate for uneven growth of tissue on the two sides of the lip or to evenly match the vermilion line on both sides. This secondary surgery is best performed during the teen years.

Surgical closure of the hard and soft palate is often performed at perhaps 18 to 24 months of age, but some surgeons prefer to wait longer. The object is to create airtight and fluid-tight closure of the cleft and to preserve the length and mobility of the soft palate, goals that often involve multiple surgical operations. If insufficient tissue is available for closure by any of the many techniques available, an obturator or speech bulb is made by the prosthodontist.

Craniosynostosis

Obliteration of sutures that takes place before or soon after birth inhibits the growth of adjacent bones perpendicular to the course of the obliterated suture. Consequently, skull diameter is reduced in this direction. Compensatory and abnormal growth, however, proceeds in directions permitted by open sutures and fontanelles (Fig. 37-1). If a single suture is involved, it is termed simple craniosynostosis; if multiple sutures are involved, it is called compound craniosynostosis. Early obliteration of the sagittal suture results in scaphocephaly (dolichocephaly; Fig. 37-2). The skull

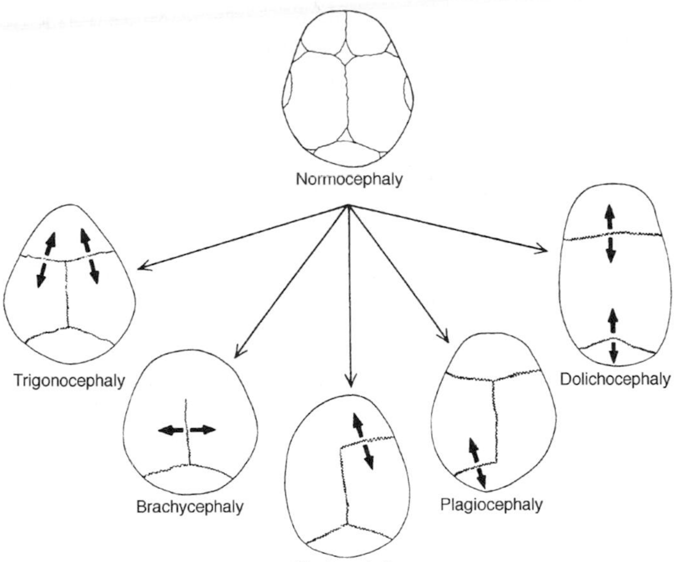

Figure 37-1. Craniosynostosis. Various skull shapes resulting from premature fusion of individual sutures or groups of sutures. (Courtesy of M. M. Cohen, Jr., Halifax, Nova Scotia, Canada.)

is long and narrow, and the parietal protuberances are absent. As the brain expands, the coronal and lambdoidal sutures are widened, and frontooccipital elongation takes place. In some cases, a bony crest is seen in place of the sagittal suture. In brachycephaly, the coronal sutures are fused prematurely resulting in a short, square-appearing cranial configuration (Fig. 37-3). Plagiocephaly refers to skewing of the skull due to premature unilateral fusion of a coronal or lambdoidal suture. Trigonocephaly describes a keel-shaped forehead due to premature fusion of the metopic suture. Acrocephaly (turricephaly) results from multiple suture closures. The highest point on the calvaria is usually near the anterior fontanelle, head form being short, high, and broad. Chiefly, the coronal suture is affected, although the sagittal and lambdoid sutures are frequently involved. If the anterior fontanelle and metopic suture remain open, the skull expands in abnormal directions resulting in steep frontal, parietal, and occipital bones and a high, broad, short skull. Often, digital impressions are evident.

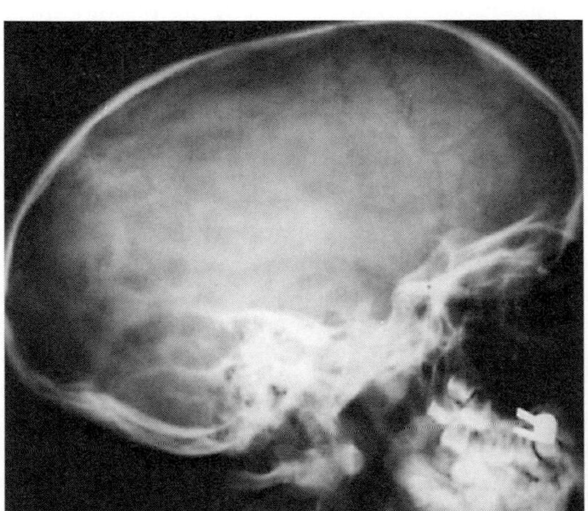

Figure 37-2. Scaphocephaly (dolichocephaly).

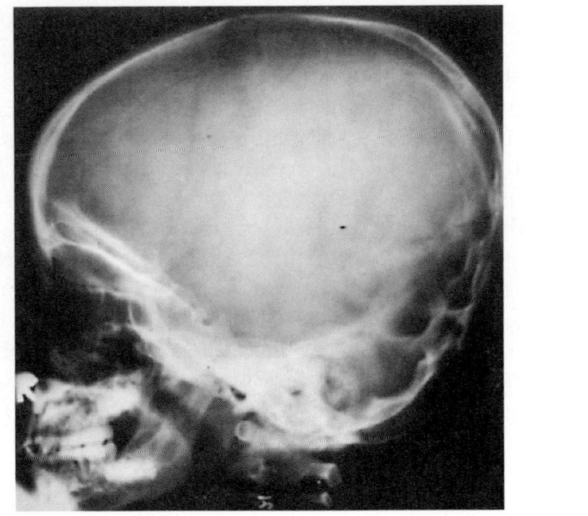

Figure 37-3. Brachycephaly.

Craniosynostosis may be primary, as in simple or compound premature fusion described earlier, or it may be secondary to a known disorder (e.g., thalassemia, hyperthyroidism, microcephaly, mucopolysaccharidoses, rickets). Little is known about pathogenesis. Transforming growth factor-beta (types 1, 2, and 3), insulin-like growth factor-1, and some fibroblast growth factors and receptors (1, 2, and 3) are expressed at the osteogenic fronts of developing calvarial sutures and play a role in early pathologic closure (i.e., craniosynostosis). Finally, craniosynostosis may be isolated or syndromic.

EPIDEMIOLOGY AND GENETICS

The frequency of simple or nonsyndromal craniosynostosis is approximately 0.34 to 0.40 per 1,000 newborns. Premature fusion of the sagittal suture is the most common type of simple synostosis constituting approximately 55% of cases. The male-to-female gender predilection is 3:1. Unilateral or bilateral coronal synostosis comprises approximately 20% to 25% of cases with a slight predilection for female infants. Metopic synostosis and lambdoidal synostosis each constitute a few percent. Involvement of two or more sutures comprises 15%.

Simple craniosynostosis is usually sporadic. Of patients with coronal synostosis, some 10% are familial; of patients with sagittal synostosis, some 2% are familial. Among those with familial occurrence, mutations in both fibroblast growth factor receptors 2 and 3 have been demonstrated. In some kindred, the same suture is subject to synostosis in affected individuals and, in others, different sutures are fused. Sagittal synostosis appears to be most consistent with multifactorial inheritance, the frequency in the general population being approximately 1 in 4,200 with a recurrence risk of approximately 1 in 64 siblings. Twin studies clearly indicated that single-gene inheritance does not play a large role in craniosynostosis because discordance is more frequent than is concordance in monozygotic twins.

TREATMENT IN INFANCY

Treatment of craniosynostosis in infancy is controversial. The craniosynostoses represent not only diverse groups; extreme variables are found within each group. Opinions regarding treatment vary from conservative observation until completion of facial growth to radical extensive surgical correction in the first months of life. Complications such as increasing intracranial pressure may mandate early treatment.

Some physicians recommend that patients with premature closure of cranial sutures should be treated surgically when younger than 2 years of age, as should those patients younger than 6 months with metopic suture closure. The operation performed most frequently for simple craniosynostosis is linear craniectomy parallel to the prematurely fused suture. Polyethylene film is inserted over the bony margins to delay secondary closure. Bilateral, premature closure of the coronal sutures is frequently accompanied by anomalies of the facial, orbital, and sphenoid bones, with downward displacement of the orbital roof and overgrowth of the lesser wing of the sphenoid, the orbits being markedly reduced in size, thus, causing exophthalmos. Maximum decompression of the cranial vault rather than orbital decompression is carried out. Canthorrhaphy is performed to avoid dryness of the cornea and prolapse of the globe. Complex plastic surgical treatment of severe facial deformities of craniofacial dysostoses has been described in detail by Tessier (1986). The optimal time for such operations is from 10 to 12 years of age.

Excellent results can be obtained from treating asymmetric synostosis at younger than 1 year of age by unilateral orbital repositioning and forehead remodeling. No further surgery is needed in more than 90% of patients. For bilateral or symmetric synostoses and mild upper-face deformity, orbital advancement and forehead reshaping carried out within the first year of life were less satisfactory, with some 50% of patients needing another major osteotomy. For those with moderate to severe symmetric synostoses (Crouzon disease and Apert syndrome), extensive facial reconstruction is performed between 7 and 14 years of age. Despite delayed and aggressive treatment, surgical outcome is less satisfactory.

CHAPTER 38
Renal and Genitourinary Diseases

Adapted from Billy S. Arant, Jr.

STRUCTURAL ABNORMALITIES OF THE NEONATAL KIDNEY AND URINARY TRACT

Failure in Morphogenesis

Developmental abnormalities of the kidney occur when metanephric induction fails, when normal differentiation and development fail after the metanephros is formed, or when the normal metanephros sustains an insult after nephrogenesis begins. Absence of nephrogenesis leads to renal agenesis, which can be unilateral or bilateral. If it is bilateral and associated with fetal compression, the criteria for Potter syndrome are fulfilled.

Obstructive Uropathy

The most common abdominal mass in the neonate is a hydronephrotic kidney. However, not every kidney thought to be obstructed *in utero* is enlarged at birth. Hydronephrosis occurs only when hydrostatic pressure in the collecting system is increased, and it implies that urine formation continued at least until just before discovery of the enlarged kidney. Normal renal function is not recovered when complete obstruction persists for more than a week. Moreover, the longer the obstruction continues, the less likely is the return of renal function.

The clinical problem associated most often with renal dysplasia in the neonate is obstructive uropathy, which occurs in 1 in 1,000 live births. Obstruction of the flow of urine can occur at any point along the urinary tract between the calyx and the urethral meatus; it can be partial or complete; and it can be transient, intermittent, or fixed. If, for example, the proximal ureter fails to canalize completely, ureteropelvic junction obstruction will result. This lesion is the most common form of obstructive uropathy; it may be partial or complete; and it is suggested or identified usually by routine ultrasonography in a fetus, during the evaluation of an abdominal mass or urinary tract infection in a neonate, and while investigating the complaint of intense flank pain after a large volume of fluid has been ingested by a child or adult. Surgical correction is not always indicated, because many uncomplicated lesions resolve spontaneously.

When mucosal folds obstruct the posterior urethra and limit the force or height of the urinary stream in male infants, the diagnosis of posterior urethral valves should be suspected and confirmed by voiding cystourethrography. Every male neonate should be screened for this obstructing lesion: At least one experienced observer should note the force or arc of the urinary stream during micturition. If this has not been recorded at the time of discharge from the nursery, parents should be instructed in how to make this observation and to report the finding to the pediatrician during the first week of life. The best treatment for posterior urethral valves is considered to be early intervention by initiating a well-planned approach for definitive care of the neonate at birth.

Prune-Belly Syndrome

Prune-belly syndrome is a condition in which the urinary tract findings are nearly identical to those for posterior urethral valves but for one important exception: No obstructing lesion can be found. Convincing evidence, however, implicates the developing prostate as obstructing the fetal urethra transiently. Another similarity between prune-belly syndrome and posterior urethral valves is that both can exhibit a variable degree of muscle tone in the abdominal wall. The classic presentation of prune-belly syndrome is a male neonate who is found to have complete absence of abdominal wall musculature, so that the outlines of bowel loops can be seen and the abdominal cavity can be examined easily by palpation. In addition, a paucity of smooth muscle is found in the ureters, the urinary bladder and, sometimes, the gastrointestinal tract. Clinical management of the neonate with prune-belly syndrome involves monitoring the urinary tract for relative obstruction to urinary flow and its major complication, infection; assessing GFR for subsequent comparison to identify change; establishing requirements for NaCl balance in an infant who will exhibit NaCl wasting and will fail to grow normally when replacement is inadequate; correcting the metabolic acidosis that develops because of decreased distal tubular secretion of hydrogen ion; and providing an activated form of vitamin D [1,25$(OH)_2$ vitamin D], because these infants, similar to those with other forms of primary uropathy, have hypocalcemia and renal osteodystrophy even when the GFR is nearly normal. Finally, appropriate counseling for the infant's parents is essential. Although renal function in the infant may seem normal at birth, end-stage renal disease develops in most patients before adolescence.

Renal Cystic Disease

Renal cystic disease occurs in many different forms and nearly defies meaningful classification, at least any that would explain cystogenesis for each type. For instance, a unilateral, single cyst may be discovered incidentally in a neonate with normal renal function. This cyst may persist unchanged throughout life and cause no problem for the individual, it may disappear altogether, or it may be the first of many more cysts to form over the next 30 to 40 years in both kidneys. When this diagnostic dilemma is encountered in a neonate, the patient can be observed serially to document changes in the cyst, in kidney function, and in blood pressure, as has been the practice until very recently. In the absence of a family history of polycystic kidney disease, this option should be exercised only after both parents have had ultrasonographic examination of their kidneys for the presence of cysts. The finding of cysts in other organs, particularly liver, lung, or pancreas, supports the diagnosis of autosomal recessive (infantile) polycystic kidney disease. One further clue to the latter condition is the ability to identify by ultrasonography early hepatic fibrosis in these patients. Although such fibrosis is not always present from birth, moderate to severe systemic hypertension develops in these patients within the first months of life, and so they should be monitored prospectively for this problem.

A multicystic kidney is usually unilateral, dysplastic, and nonfunctioning. Neonates who are found to have a multicystic kidney require only casual monitoring for the rare occurrence of enlargement or complicating infection; otherwise, these malformed kidneys should not be removed routinely. Physicians were once concerned that malignancy might develop in these kidneys, but long-term follow-up of these patients has identified no such added risk. A voiding cystourethrogram will identify another genitourinary abnormality, especially vesicoureteral reflux, in 30% to 40% of these infants.

A PROBLEM EFFECTING RENAL FUNCTION IN THE NEONATE

Nephrotoxic Drug Therapy

The nephrotoxic effects of antibiotics such as aminoglycosides, vancomycin, and amphotericin B occur with the same frequency in neonates as in older infants, children, and adults, even though they may not be recognized. For example, aminoglycoside therapy is prescribed for neonates in a higher dosage relative to body size than it is in adults. Moreover, therapy is adjusted according to arbitrarily chosen "effective" peak and trough plasma levels. Such levels can be misleading in the neonate because the drug is injected into the relatively larger volume of distribution. Therefore, more drug must be given to achieve the same peak plasma levels in neonates as compared to adults. Similarly, trough levels are determined by renal clearance of the circulating drug, and a much lower trough level will be observed in neonates than in adults. The decision to modify or discontinue nephrotoxic antibiotic therapy based only on an increase in plasma trough levels will come several days after glomerular filtration rate has decreased from the nephrotoxic effects of the drug. For aminoglycosides and vancomycin, the drug dose interval is every 18 to 24 hours in neonates younger than 34 weeks' conceptual age and every 12 hours in older infants. The same pattern of change in pharmacokinetics is characteristic of other drugs excreted by the kidney such as furosemide and indomethacin.

CHAPTER 39

Neonatal Endocrinology

Adapted from Elizabeth A. Catlin
and Mary M. Lee

HYPOGLYCEMIA

Hypoglycemia, defined as plasma glucose values of 40 mg/dL or less, is a common and typically transient problem in newborn infants. Maintaining neonatal plasma glucose concentrations greater than 50 mg/dL is a sensible and conservative therapeutic goal because fetal glucose levels are at least 40 mg/dL, and children and adults may have neuroglycopenic symptoms at glucose levels lower than this (as may neonates). Moreover, infants have an immature ketogenic capacity and are unable to generate ketones adequately as an alternative central nervous system fuel in response to hypoglycemia. Certain infants, including infants of diabetic mothers (IDMs), premature or growth-restricted infants, and neonates who are perinatally stressed, are especially prone to the development of transient neonatal hypoglycemia. Persistent neonatal hypoglycemia is less common and is caused by congenital hyperinsulinism, deficits in counterregulatory hormones, or metabolic disorders that affect fasting adaptation.

Hypoglycemia may develop in neonates with polycythemia-hyperviscosity. Some glucose is lost by metabolism to the greater red cell mass, less glucose is carried in a given volume of blood as a result of the diminished plasma fraction, and sludging may leave tissues poorly oxygenated and, thus, more dependent on glucose for anaerobic metabolism. A venous hematocrit higher than 65% defines polycythemia; with increasing hematocrit levels, an exponential rise in blood viscosity occurs. The hypoglycemia in these instances resolves with partial exchange transfusion to reduce the hematocrit.

Congenital hyperinsulinism is an unusual cause of hypoglycemia but is the most common etiology of persistent hypoglycemia in infancy, and the autosomal recessive form often presents in the neonatal period. Focal areas of beta-cell hyperplasia (adenomas) may also cause severe neonatal hyperinsulinemic hypoglycemia. Typically, affected infants have high glucose requirements and unstable hypoglycemia that is unrelated to feedings.

Neonates with the Beckwith-Wiedemann syndrome have macroglossia, visceromegaly, and omphalocele and are large for their gestational age. Nearly 50% of reported cases exhibit hyperinsulinemic hypoglycemia caused by islet cell hyperplasia. Hypoglycemia in such infants may be severe and long lasting, necessitating pharmacologic management of their hyperinsulinism, in addition to glucose supplementation.

Regarding diagnosis and therapy, clinicians must have a low threshold for suspecting hypoglycemia in neonates. Affected infants may be jittery or may manifest such nonspecific signs as apnea, seizures, poor feeding, or lethargy, but they may also be essentially asymptomatic. A careful pregnancy history and physical examination may reveal evidence of growth restriction, visceromegaly, or other clues to the etiology of the hypoglycemia. A plasma glucose level should be obtained; if capillary sampling is used, care must be taken to warm the heel adequately. If the glucose concentration is 40 mg/dL or less, treatment should be instituted. Stable and relatively mature babies may be treated safely with early enteral feedings and careful monitoring of subsequent plasma glucose values. If the Dextrostix reading is greater than 45 mg/dL, normal feeding can be started as soon as the infant's condition will permit; capillary glucose should be monitored by Dextrostix every 1 to 2 hours until it remains stably in the normal range. If the blood glucose level is less than 25 mg/dL, parenteral glucose supplementation is required; it may be initiated with a "mini-bolus" of 10% glucose, 2 to 3 mL/kg intravenously in water, followed by a constant infusion of 10% glucose delivered at a rate of 6 to 8 mg/kg/minute, which approximates the normal rate of glucose use. Glucose values must be monitored closely with titration of the infusate to maintain normoglycemia.

HYPERGLYCEMIA

Hyperglycemia in neonates is defined as random plasma glucose concentrations greater than 150 mg/dL. The incidence of hyperglycemia appears to have increased in association with the increased survival of very premature and high-risk infants. Overwhelming sepsis, surgical stress, hypoxia, respiratory distress syndrome, central nervous system insults (including intracranial hemorrhage), and treatment with methylxanthines are known to be associated with transient hyperglycemia. Stress-related hyperglycemia results, in part, from elevated catecholamine and cortisol levels. Pancreatic agenesis is a rare cause of neonatal glucose intolerance; these babies also exhibit significant intrauterine growth restriction. Neonatal diabetes, estimated to occur once in 500,000 births, has a highly variable course. Affected babies may have transient diabetes, with or without periods of remission, or permanent diabetes, and most are small for gestational age. The small size of these neonates, in contrast to the macrosomia of IDMs, is believed to reflect insulin's important role as an intrauterine growth hormone. In certain cases, however, intrauterine growth restriction is also speculated, in fact, to cause diabetes.

Plasma glucose levels greater than 150 mg/dL are hyperglycemic. If a neonate is receiving intravenous glucose-containing fluids, the glucose infusion rate in milligrams per kilogram per minute should be calculated and should be decreased by 1 to 2 mg/kg/minute every 3 to 4 hours, monitoring glucose levels 30 to 60 minutes after decreasing the infusion; hypotonic infusates should be avoided. Fluid balance, glycosuria, blood pressure, oxygenation, and perfusion should be checked carefully and, if sepsis is suspected, appropriate cultures should be obtained and antibiotics should be given.

HYPOCALCEMIA

Early hypocalcemia has been defined variously, often as a total serum calcium concentration of less than 8 mg/dL (2.0 mmol/L) in the full-term neonate or less than 7 mg/dL (1.75 mmol/L) in the premature neonate during the first several days with the nadir occurring between 24 and 48 hours of life. Parathyroid hormone release appears to increase after this hypocalcemic stimulus. Inasmuch as approximately 50% of the calcium in serum is bound loosely to protein and this inert fraction varies according to the protein concentration, pH, and other factors, a more helpful approach may be to think in terms of the biologically active ionized calcium concentration. Thus, values for ionized calcium of less than 1.0 mmol/L (4 mg/dL) are even more indicative of hypocalcemia. Premature neonates, babies with perinatal depression, and IDMs are particularly susceptible to early hypocalcemia; hypomagnesemia and hypocalcemia may coexist in the IDM. Late neonatal hypocalcemia occurs during the middle of or after the first week of life and is caused by hypoparathyroidism, hyperphosphatemia, and high-phosphate formula consumption (synonymous with late infantile tetany). Usually, congenital hypoparathyroidism is caused by agenesis or dysgenesis of the parathyroid glands and is often associated with the DiGeorge syndrome, now considered part of the chromosome 22-deletion syndrome. Hypomagnesemia may be seen in SGA babies, in neonates with hepatic disease or small-bowel resections and, very rarely, in infants with magnesium malabsorption. It may result in late hypocalcemia because of decreased parathyroid hormone (PTH) production, relative end-organ insensitivity to PTH, decreased exchange of magnesium for calcium at the bone surface, and decreased 25-hydroxylation of vitamin D.

Neonates with hypocalcemia may be completely asymptomatic or have seizures, tremors, tetany or lethargy, and poor feeding. Seizures associated with hypocalcemia are treated with intravenous 10% calcium gluconate, 1 to 2 mL/kg, given slowly over several minutes to avoid inducing bradycardia. Oral and intravenous calcium supplementation for early hypocalcemia may be achieved with elemental calcium, 75 mg/kg/day as an initial oral dose or 24 to 75 mg/kg/day parenterally, usually given for less than 3 days. The subacute and chronic conditions of late hypocalcemia are treated with calcitriol (1,25-dihydroxyvitamin D), starting with a dose of 0.125 μg once or twice daily and calcium supplementation. Parathyroid agenesis requires lifelong therapy to prevent hypocalcemia. During initiation of therapy, serum calcium and phosphorus should be monitored daily to maintain their concentrations in the low-normal range.

When hypocalcemia and hypomagnesemia coexist, the magnesium deficit should be corrected first with intravenous or intramuscular magnesium sulfate using 5 to 25 mg/kg of elemental magnesium given slowly over 10 minutes. Chronic therapy may be initiated with oral doses of elemental magnesium (as magnesium sulfate, gluconate, lactate, citrate, or glycerophosphate), 20 to 40 mg/kg/day.

HYPERCALCEMIA

Usually, hypercalcemia in neonates is the result of excessive calcium supplementation, especially in very premature newborns. Babies with Williams syndrome (idiopathic infantile hypercalcemia syndrome with elfin facies and supravalvular aortic stenosis) may have hypercalcemia and nephrocalcinosis, which typically resolves spontaneously by age 4 years. Primary hyperparathyroidism, although extremely rare, may also be seen in the neonatal period, with potentially very severe hypercalcemia.

Treatment of neonatal hypercalcemia should be prompt and includes hydration at one and a half to two times maintenance using 5% dextrose with 50% normal saline and potassium chloride (3 mEq/dL); furosemide given at 1 mg/kg per dose intravenously twice or three times daily to inhibit renal tubular calcium resorption; and phosphate supplementation to maintain normal serum phosphorus values. Vitamin D and calcium intake should be limited, and hydrocortisone may help to decrease intestinal absorption of calcium. Primary hyperparathyroidism often requires surgical resection of the parathyroid glands for definitive management.

DISORDERS OF GENITAL AMBIGUITY

One of the most important decisions clinicians make is announced in the delivery room: "It's a boy!" or "It's a girl!" This section deals with those rare situations in which this decision cannot be made with certainty. In this context, what must be remembered is that the potential for development of the structures by which we recognize maleness and femaleness is common to all zygotes, whether 46,XX or 46,XY. For example, should an accident render the gonads nonfunctional in an early embryo with a normal 46,XY constitution; at birth, the infant will be pronounced a girl without hesitation. On the other hand, female fetuses exposed to androgens, whether endogenous or environmental, will undergo virilization to an extent depending on the timing, duration, and severity of the exposure.

Clinical Characteristics

Different aspects of sexuality are considered in evaluating an infant with an intersex disorder. Genetic sex refers to the XX or XY sex chromosome constitution, and gonadal sex refers to whether testes or ovaries are present. Physical examination should address such questions as whether the infant has a "chromosomal look" with multiple dysmorphisms. Often, such an appearance is evident in the sex chromosome anomalies, especially the 45,X (Turner) and 45,X/46,XY (mixed gonadal dysgenesis) syndromes. It is even more pronounced in some of the anomalies of the autosomes—for example, in the genital hypoplasia (micropenis) of trisomy 21 or the chromosome 13q syndrome. Ascertainment of the position of the gonads is important. The female pseudohermaphrodite with congenital adrenocortical hyperplasia may exhibit full masculine development of the phallus with no hypospadias and a roomy, rugated, and often deeply pigmented scrotum, but this will always be empty (Fig. 39-1A). In contrast, male pseudohermaphrodites with decreased testosterone exposure in the third trimester such as infants with panhypopituitarism, GnRH deficiency, or a testosterone biosynthetic defect, will have a hypoplastic scrotum and small phallus (Fig. 39-1B).

Laboratory Evaluation

Laboratory studies are used in conjunction with radiologic imaging to complete the evaluation and to assist with gender assignment. In most instances, karyotyping is desirable. Screening for the congenital adrenal hyperplasias can be accomplished rapidly using the filter-paper assay for 17-hydroxyprogesterone in the states that include this assessment as part of the newborn screening program. Otherwise, blood should be obtained for adrenal steroids, testosterone, and gonadotropins. Electrolytes should be monitored if congenital adrenal hyperplasia is suspected. Testosterone steroid precursors and dihydrotestosterone levels are essential if a defect in the testosterone biosynthetic pathway is in question; making a definitive diagnosis may require a human chorionic gonadotropin stimulation test to test the pathway adequately.

A pediatric radiologist's help should be enlisted to ascertain the nature of the pelvic organs and adrenals by use of ultrasonography or retrograde injection of contrast materials. A pediatric surgeon should be involved to perform a cystoscopy to confirm the radiologic findings, to obtain the gonadal biopsy, and for expert guidance in considering the feasibility of surgical reconstruction to give the infant an appearance consonant with the gender assignment being considered.

Management

In patients who have diagnoses of partial gonadal dysgenesis or true hermaphroditism and are raised as boys, if the testis is left in place for testosterone synthesis (fertility being unlikely), the parents and, later, the children must be taught to examine the gonad regularly for tumors. Streak gonads, whether unilateral (the classic situation in partial gonadal dysgenesis) or bilateral, should always be removed when the karyotype contains a Y chromosome or fragment.

In infants who will be reared in the female gender role, any gonadal tissue should be removed that has the potential to secrete androgen under pituitary gonadotropin stimulation at adolescence. In some neonates, addressing the question of whether any such tissue exists is necessary. High levels of gonadotropins (luteinizing hormone and follicle-stimulating hormone (greater than 20 mIU/mL) with negligible serum concentrations of testosterone (less than 20 ng/dL) indicate a negative answer.

Skillful reconstruction of the genitalia to harmonize with the gender role selected for an affected infant is essential. For especially troubled parents, doing this even before the infant first goes home may constitute an emergency, at least in social terms. This case occurs most often with female pseudohermaphrodites who have undergone extensive virilization. The required procedures (perineoplasty and clitoral resection and recession with preservation of the glans and dorsal and ventral neurovascular

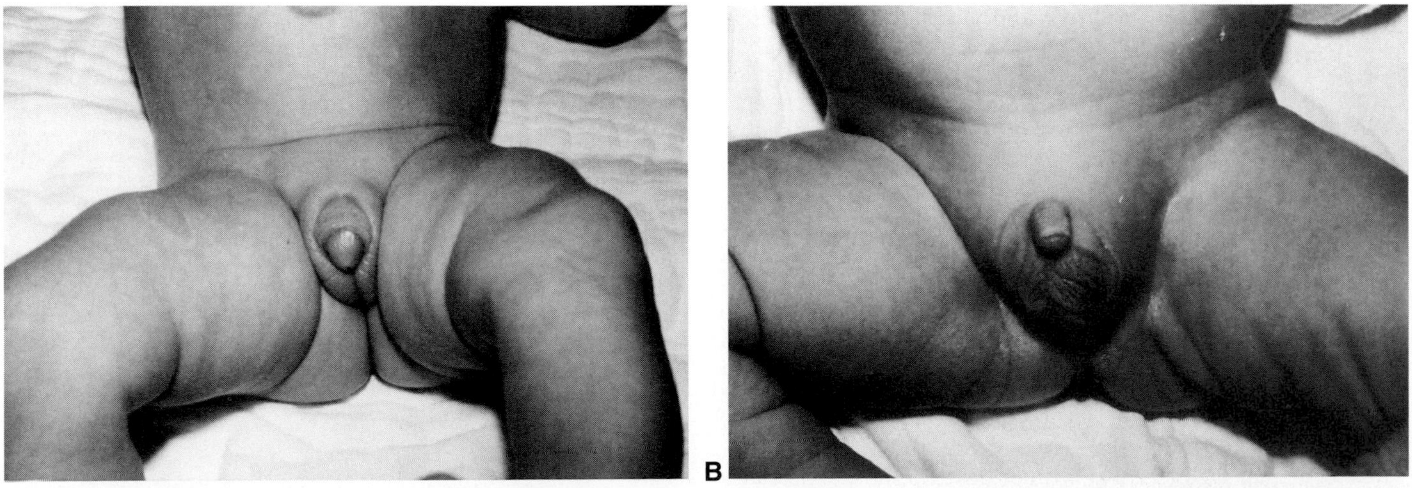

A B

Figure 39-1. Two infants with genital ambiguity. These two cases illustrate the difficulty of relying on examination of the external genitalia to determine genetic and gonadal sex. **A:** 46,XX virilized girl with congenital adrenal hyperplasia. The phallus is well developed with perineoscrotal hypospadias, and no gonads are palpable in the labioscrotal folds. **B:** 46,XY boy with microphallus and undescended testicles secondary to hypopituitarism. Normally, the phallus is formed with a penile urethral opening, but the phallus is small, and the scrotum is underdeveloped.

bundles) can be accomplished successfully in the neonatal period by a skilled pediatric surgeon. Vaginoplasty, especially when the opening of the vagina is "high" (i.e., into the posterior urethra), may be delayed until the child is near age 3 months.

In boys with micropenis, treatment with testosterone should not be delayed, because the responsiveness of the phallic tissue may diminish with age. Testosterone in one of the repository forms (testosterone cypionate or enanthate) can be given once a month, at 15 to 25 mg per dose intramuscularly for 3 to 6 months until satisfactory growth has been achieved. The aim of the surgeon attending to the staged procedures, which may include relief of chordee, repair of hypospadias, and placement of small-sized testicular prostheses (not currently available), should be to complete the work by the time the patient is 2 years old or shortly thereafter.

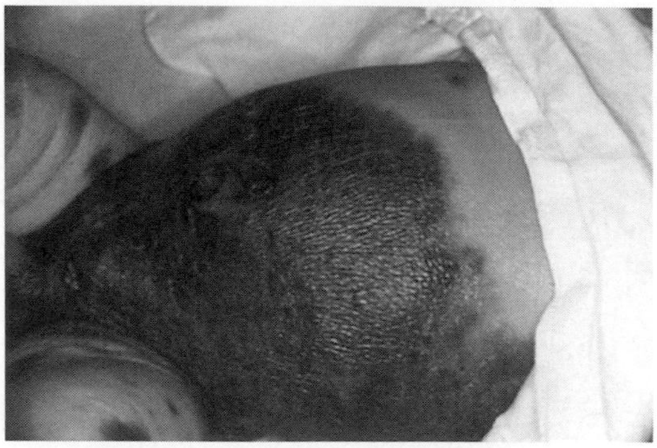

Figure 40-1. Giant congenital melanocytic nevus with atypical features including a scalloped border, irregular pigmentation, and variable thickness. (See Color Fig. 40-1.)

CHAPTER 40

Neonatal Dermatology

Adapted from Lynne J. Roberts
(This Chapter should be read in conjunction with Chapter 46, Pediatric Dermatology.)

BIRTHMARKS

Pigmented Lesions

CONGENITAL MELANOCYTIC NEVUS

Congenital melanocytic nevi (CMN) occur in up to 1% of all newborns and vary from a few millimeters to several centimeters or more in diameter. Giant CMN involving a major portion of the body have been referred to as "bathing trunk" or "garment" nevi. CMN may be flat or raised and range from pinkish tan to brown or black. They are significant because of their increased risk for development of malignant melanoma. The risk of malignancy in giant CMN is well documented and is at least 6.3% over a lifetime. Features that suggest development of melanoma in a CMN include change in color, irregular or scalloped border, change in size or thickness, and variation in color within the lesion, bleeding, or ulceration. CMN may have irregular borders and variation in color and thickness from the outset making it difficult to follow these lesions for early malignant changes (Fig. 40-1). All CMN with atypical or suspicious features should be excised regardless of size.

MASTOCYTOSIS

Mastocytosis should be considered in the differential diagnosis of pigmented lesions present at birth. Mast cell disease encompasses a spectrum from isolated cutaneous involvement to systemic disease. Cutaneous lesions, produced by local infiltration of the skin by mast cells, characteristically urticate with rubbing (Darier sign) because of mast cell degranulation and histamine release resulting in increased vascular permeability, edema, and wheal formation. If the edema is marked, blistering may occur. Mastocytomas are present at birth or develop shortly thereafter and appear as reddish brown or brown plaques or nodules. Single lesions are the rule, although occasionally two or three are present, typically involving the distal extremities, particularly the wrist. Most isolated mastocytomas resolve spontaneously after several years. The age of onset of the multiple red-brown, yellow, tan, or dark brown macules, papules, and plaques of generalized cutaneous mastocytosis (urticaria pigmentosa) ranges from birth to adulthood (Fig. 40-2). Most affected children have significant clearing or complete resolution of the cutaneous lesions by early adulthood. Systemic symptoms may occur because of release of histamine and other mediators from cutaneous lesions and include pruritus, flushing, hypotension, tachycardia, and, less often, diarrhea, dyspnea, and syncope. Systemic mastocytosis with mast cell infiltration of bone, liver, spleen, lymph nodes, skin, and gastrointestinal tract is rare in children.

NEVUS SEBACEOUS

Benign tumors of epidermis and epidermal appendages always present at birth; sebaceous nevi are characterized by a distinctive yellow-orange color because of the presence of a large number of sebaceous glands (Fig. 40-3). Initially, they are well circumscribed, hairless, and flat or slightly raised with a finely cobblestoned texture. At puberty, enlargement occurs as the sebaceous glands become active under androgenic influence. Small, isolated lesions of sebaceous nevi are not associated with other defects and are most commonly located on the scalp or face. An extensive linear sebaceous nevus on the head, neck, or trunk may be associated with congenital skeletal defects and CNS disease, including mental retardation and seizures, much like those seen in the epidermal nevus syndrome. A 15% to 20% risk exists for the development of a basal cell carcinoma, as well as other benign and malignant tumors within a sebaceous nevus, regardless of size; thus, excision before puberty is recommended.

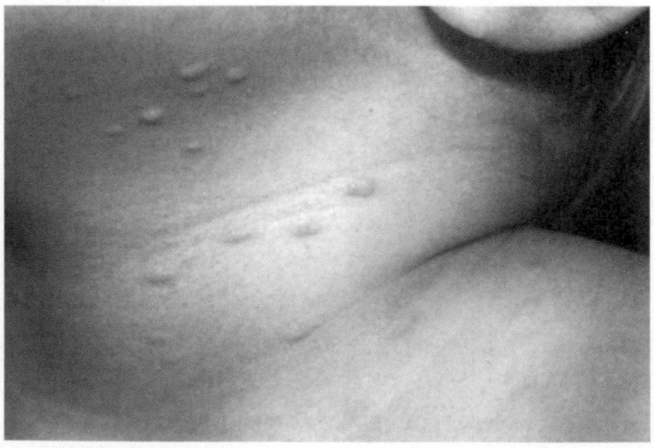

Figure 40-2. Multiple pinkish brown papules and nodules of generalized cutaneous mastocytosis. (See Color Fig. 40-2.)

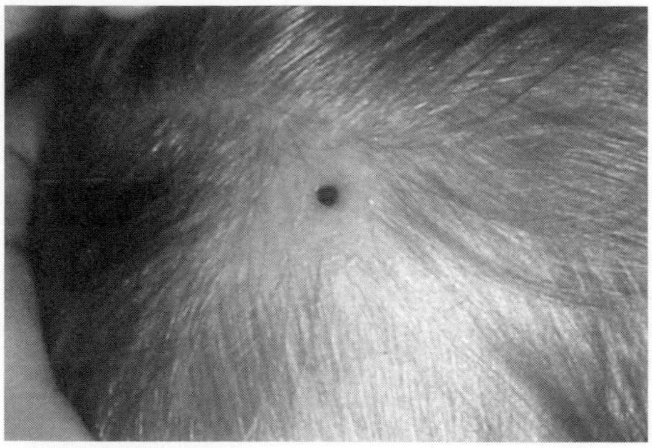

Figure 40-3. Striking yellow-orange, pebbly appearance of a typical nevus sebaceous on the scalp. Note the absence of hair within the lesion. The dark, crusted area is the site of a punch biopsy. (See Color Fig. 40-3.)

Hypopigmented Lesions

ASH LEAF SPOT

Hypopigmented, oval or leaf-shaped macules with smooth or jagged borders, ash leaf spots are the only cutaneous manifestation of tuberous sclerosis present at birth or in early infancy. Other skin lesions characteristic of this disorder develop later in childhood or in early adolescence including adenoma sebaceum (multiple facial angiofibromas), periungual fibromas, and shagreen patches. Ash leaf spots persist, and affected individuals may continue to develop new lesions during childhood. In fair-skinned infants, ash leaf spots are detected most easily with the aid of a Wood light.

Vascular Lesions

NORMAL VARIANTS

Cutis Marmorata

Cutis marmorata is the normal, reticulated, cyanotic mottling of the skin that is a physiologic response to chilling. This change is not normal if it persists after the infant is warmed. Persistent mottling or livedo reticularis implies an obstruction to blood flow such as hyperviscosity or vasculitis.

Harlequin Color Change

The harlequin color change is seen primarily in premature infants and is thought to be caused by immature vasomotor control. When the infant lies on his or her side, the lower half of the body becomes reddened and the upper half blanches. An episode may last for several seconds or minutes and resolves spontaneously when the infant is placed in a supine position.

CONGENITAL VASCULAR ABNORMALITIES

Congenital vascular abnormalities should be classified as malformations or hemangiomas (Table 40-1).

TABLE 40-1. Congenital Vascular Abnormalities

Hemangiomas
Capillary/superficial
Cavernous/deep
Mixed
Malformations
Nevus flammeus/salmon patch
Port wine stain
Cutis marmorata telangiectatica congenita
Angiokeratoma
Lymphangioma
Venous malformation
Arteriovenous malformation

Hemangiomas

True hemangiomas are produced by a proliferation of endothelial cells and have a proliferating phase and an involuting phase. Two types of congenital hemangiomas are recognized—capillary (superficial) and cavernous (deep). Both components may be present in one lesion. Capillary hemangiomas are characterized by proliferation of endothelial cells with relatively few capillary lumina. Cavernous hemangiomas are composed primarily of large, irregular vascular spaces without as much endothelial cell proliferation. Strawberry hemangiomas are of the capillary type but frequently have a cavernous component as well (Fig. 40-4). The fully developed, bright red, pebbly strawberry hemangioma may be present at birth or may be preceded by a flat or slightly raised area composed of telangiectatic vessels surrounded by an area of pallor or a solid red macule that begins to proliferate within a few weeks to produce the typical strawberry appearance. These early lesions are often mistaken for port wine stains (PWSs). The deeper location and less compact structure of cavernous hemangiomas give them a soft, compressible texture and a less distinct outline. The overlying skin may be normal or may have a bluish hue.

Parents frequently become alarmed when a hemangioma begins to grow, particularly if it becomes eroded or bleeds. The natural history of these lesions must be stressed, because more than 90% resolve spontaneously. Hemangiomas grow rapidly during the first 6 months of life with most reaching their maximal growth by 1 year. A general rule is that 50% resolve by 5 years of age, 70% by 7 years, and 90% by 9 years. Involution is heralded by a fading of the bright redness and the appearance of gray or white areas within the lesion. Indications for aggressive treatment include compromise of a vital function (sight, respiration, nutrition), high-output congestive heart failure, consumptive coagulopathy, and significant ulceration or deformity. A course of systemic corticosteroids is the treatment of choice with a starting dosage of 2 to 4 mg/kg/day followed by a tapering course over 2 to 4 months. Capillary hemangiomas are amenable to dye laser surgery. Intervention is most successful when laser surgery is begun before significant proliferation has occurred. Dye laser surgery can reduce or eradicate some proliferating and

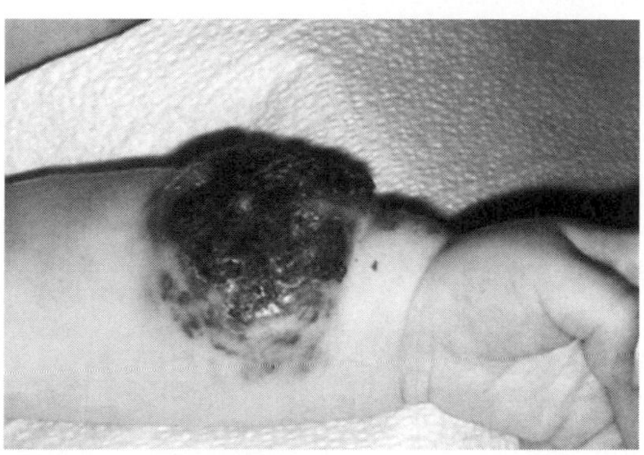

Figure 40-4. Large, mixed capillary and cavernous hemangioma on the left forearm with ulceration and crusting. The capillary component is superficial and bright red; the cavernous component is deeper and blue. (See Color Fig. 40-4.)

mature capillary hemangiomas but is not effective for cavernous hemangiomas. Alpha-interferon is sometimes used for the treatment of aggressive hemangiomas unresponsive to other therapeutic modalities. Kasabach-Merritt syndrome, in which platelets are trapped and coagulation factors are consumed locally within a vascular lesion, was originally associated with what were thought to be large hemangiomas. It has now been shown that the vascular lesions associated with this syndrome are tufted angiomas and spindle cell hemangioendotheliomas. This syndrome is manifested by an enlarging vascular lesion with surrounding ecchymoses and may develop into a full-blown disseminated intravascular coagulation-like picture with thrombocytopenia and a hemorrhagic diathesis.

MALFORMATIONS

Port Wine Stain

PWSs are pink to red vascular malformations present at birth, usually on the face. They are frequently unilateral. PWSs do not resolve, tend to darken and thicken with age, and many develop nodular angiomas. Soft tissue hypertrophy may produce deformity and dysfunction of the involved area. In addition to these medical indications for treatment, the psychological trauma of a large or disfiguring PWS should not be underestimated. Dye laser surgery has been shown to be a safe and effective method for removing PWSs with minimal risk for scarring. Several treatments of the entire PWS are necessary for optimal fading or resolution. Beginning laser surgery early in life reduces the number of treatments required for clearing and prevents progression of the PWS. By definition, the Sturge-Weber syndrome includes a facial PWS in the distribution of the ophthalmic branch of the trigeminal nerve, angiomatosis of the ipsilateral leptomeninges, and gyriform intracerebral calcifications. If the PWS occurs exclusively below the ophthalmic division, no CNS involvement occurs. The PWS may involve the trunk and extremities in addition to the face, but no correlation exists between the extent of the cutaneous involvement and the severity of the CNS vascular malformation. Other features of the Sturge-Weber syndrome include seizures (80%), mental retardation (60%), hemiplegia (30%), and glaucoma (45%). The highest risk for glaucoma is seen in those individuals with PWS involvement of both the ophthalmic and maxillary divisions of the trigeminal nerve. Studies suggest that all patients with a facial PWS in this distribution are at risk for glaucoma, regardless of the presence of Sturge-Weber syndrome. Therefore, any infant with a PWS involving the V1 or V2 divisions of the trigeminal nerve should be followed closely for evidence of glaucoma.

The Klippel-Trénaunay-Weber syndrome is characterized by a vascular malformation associated with localized overgrowth of bone and soft tissue of the involved extremity or portion of the trunk. The congenital vascular malformation may be of one or more types including a PWS, arteriovenous malformation, lymphangioma, or venous malformation. Hypertrophy of the limb or portion of the trunk may be present at birth or develop in infancy. In addition, superficial venous varicosities frequently develop within the affected area in childhood or adolescence. Treatment has been unsatisfactory.

VESICULOPUSTULAR AND BULLOUS DISORDERS

Vesicles and Pustules

MILIARIA

Resulting from the occlusion and rupture of sweat ducts in the skin, miliaria (heat rash) occurs in two forms: miliaria crystallina and miliaria rubra. If the ducts rupture superficially in the skin, small, clear vesicles form (miliaria crystallina); they are not associated with inflammation. These tiny, fragile, noninflammatory vesicles appear like dewdrops on the skin. In miliaria rubra, sweat ducts rupture more deeply within the skin and provoke an inflammatory response resulting in erythematous papules that may evolve into vesicles and pustules. Both types are seen most often on the face, upper trunk, neck, and other body-fold areas but may become widespread. Miliaria resolves spontaneously if the infant is kept cool and dry, and if topical creams or lotions, which aggravate the condition, are avoided.

ERYTHEMA TOXICUM

Erythema toxicum is a common eruption occurring in up to 50% of normal newborn infants. It may be present at birth but usually develops on day 2 or 3 of life and is characterized by large, splotchy areas of erythema studded with urticarial papules, vesicles, and pustules (Fig. 40-5). Lesions are found in greatest numbers on the trunk with fewer on the face and extremities. The palms and soles are not involved. The eruption lasts 7 to 14 days and resolves spontaneously without pigmentary change or scarring. The diagnosis can be confirmed with a Wright-stained smear of the pustule, which will reveal eosinophils with few or no polymorphonuclear cells and no organisms.

TRANSIENT NEONATAL PUSTULAR MELANOSIS

An eruption always present at the time of delivery, transient neonatal pustular melanosis is characterized by noninflammatory pustules. The pustules are fragile and rupture quickly, often resolving within 24 hours, leaving a hyperpigmented macule surrounded by a collarette scale (Fig. 40-6). Rarely, pigmented spots without pustules are noted at birth. The pigmented macules resemble freckles and may last for several weeks before resolving. The most common areas of involvement are the lower face, chin, neck, and extremities, although lesions may occur anywhere including the palms and soles. The incidence is much higher in blacks than whites. A Wright-stained smear of a pustule reveals polymorphonuclear cells with few or no eosinophils and no organisms.

INFANTILE ACROPUSTULOSIS

Infantile acropustulosis is a recently described syndrome of intensely pruritic 1- to 3-mm vesicles and pustules distributed primarily on the palms, soles, wrists, ankles, and backs of the hands and feet. The trunk and buttocks are less commonly affected. Onset is from birth to 1 year of age with spontaneous resolution within 2 or 3 years. Response to topical corticosteroids and antihistamines is poor, and intractable cases may be treated successfully with dapsone or sulfapyridine.

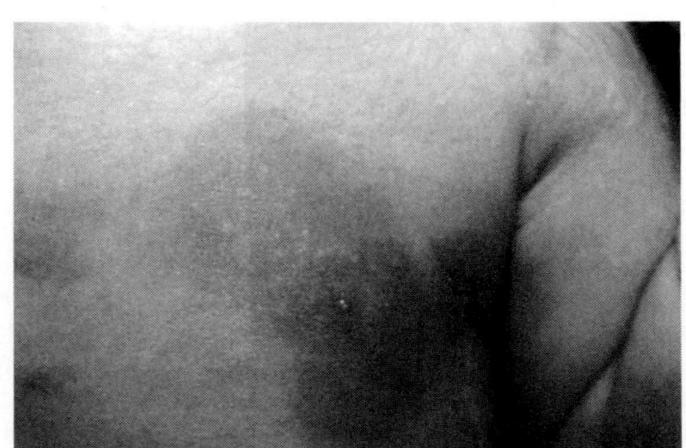

Figure 40-5. The hallmark splotchy erythema studded with small papules and pustules of erythema toxicum. (See Color Fig. 40-5.)

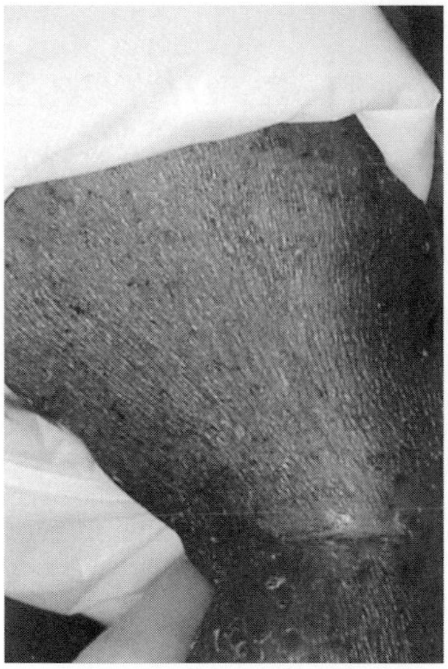

Figure 40-6. Hyperpigmented macules of transient neonatal pustular melanosis, many of which are surrounded by a collarette of scale that is the remnant of the roof of the preceding pustule. (See Color Fig. 40-6.)

CUTANEOUS CANDIDIASIS

In the newborn, cutaneous candidiasis exists in a congenital and a neonatal form. Neonatal candidiasis is manifested as oral thrush or diaper dermatitis and develops after the first week of life. Neonatal candidiasis is presumed to be acquired by the infant during passage through an infected birth canal. Congenital cutaneous candidiasis is an ascending, intrauterine infection. The eruption is noted at birth or within 12 hours after delivery and is characterized by erythematous macules and papules that evolve into vesicles and pustules scattered widely over the body including the palms and soles. Oral lesions are rare, and the diaper area is relatively spared. After several days, the eruption resolves with desquamation. The diagnosis is established by demonstrating pseudohyphae and budding yeast in a direct smear of the pustules. Most infants with congenital cutaneous candidiasis do not have systemic involvement and, therefore, do well with topical treatment alone. Conversely, systemic congenital candidiasis does not usually present with skin lesions and can lead to death *in utero* or in the immediate neonatal period. The most reliable indicators for predicting the outcome of congenital cutaneous candidiasis are the infant's birth weight and the presence of respiratory distress. Infants with birth weights of less than 1.5 kg or with early onset of respiratory distress are at risk for systemic disease including candida sepsis or pneumonia.

Bullae

The differential diagnosis of bullae in the newborn is presented in Table 40-2. Staphylococcal disease and impetigo are discussed in the infectious disease section. Epidermolysis bullosa and toxic epidermal necrolysis (TEN) are discussed in the dermatology section. Table 40-3 highlights the differences between TEN and staphylococcal-scalded skin.

TABLE 40-2. Differential Diagnosis of Bullae in the Newborn

Bullous impetigo
Staphylococcal scalded skin syndrome
Epidermolytic hyperkeratosis
Epidermolysis bullosa
Mastocytosis
Sucking blisters
Toxic epidermal necrolysis

TABLE 40-3. Differentiation of Staphylococcal Scalded Skin Syndrome and Toxic Epidermal Necrolysis

	Staphylococcal scalded skin syndrome	Toxic epidermal necrolysis
Etiology	Infectious; group II staphylococci	Immunologic; usually drug related
Morbidity/mortality	Low	High
Mucous membrane involvement	Rare	Frequent
Nikolsky sign	Present	Absent
Target lesions	Absent	Often present
Level of blister	Subcorneal	Subepidermal

EPIDERMOLYTIC HYPERKERATOSIS

An autosomal dominant form of ichthyosis with a 50% spontaneous mutation rate, epidermolytic hyperkeratosis is also referred to as *congenital bullous ichthyosiform erythroderma* because affected infants are born with widespread blistering and red, moist, denuded skin (Fig. 40-7). Within 1 to 2 weeks, generalized blistering resolves and the skin becomes dry, thick, and scaly. During infancy and childhood, crops of localized blisters may occur and heal without scarring. Ultimately, blisters are replaced by dark, foul-smelling, verrucous, hypertrophic lesions that are most pronounced in body-fold areas.

SUCKING BLISTERS

Vigorous sucking by the fetus *in utero* may produce isolated bullae 5 to 15 mm in diameter on the forearm, wrist, hand, fingers and, rarely, the toes. No treatment is necessary for these blisters because spontaneous resolution is the rule.

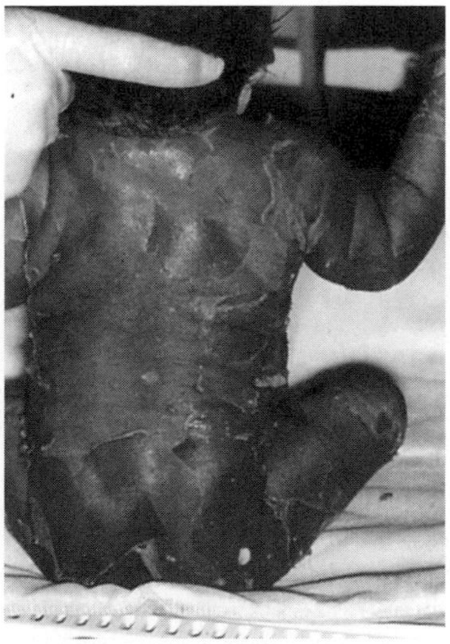

Figure 40-7. Newborn with widespread blistering of epidermolytic hyperkeratosis. (See Color Fig. 40-7.)

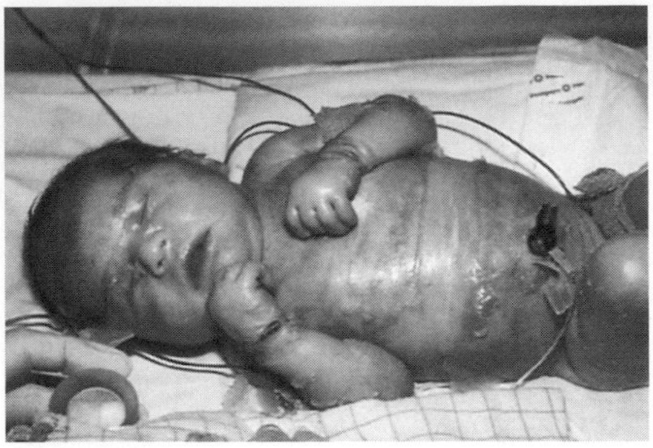

Figure 40-8. Collodion baby after partial shedding of the collodion membrane. The hands, arms, legs, and a portion of the abdomen are still encased in a tight, shiny membrane. (See Color Fig. 40-8.)

SCALING DISORDERS

Ichthyosis

Ichthyosis is classified into four major groups: autosomal dominant ichthyosis vulgaris, autosomal recessive lamellar ichthyosis/congenital ichthyosiform erythroderma, X-linked recessive ichthyosis, and autosomal dominant epidermolytic hyperkeratosis. Data suggest that lamellar ichthyosis and nonbullous congenital ichthyosiform erythroderma are separate and distinct disorders. Onset in the neonatal period may occur in all but ichthyosis vulgaris, in which symptoms develop later in childhood. Infants with epidermolytic hyperkeratosis are born with widespread blistering. The collodion baby may be the first manifestation of more than one type of ichthyosis, but most infants subsequently develop lamellar ichthyosis. Rarely, the skin remains normal in appearance after the collodion membrane is shed. Collodion babies are encased in a tight, shiny membrane that restricts movement and results in ectropion (Fig. 40-8). Fissuring and peeling begin shortly after birth, although complete shedding of the membrane may take weeks to months. Infants should be managed in an isolation incubator with careful temperature control and high humidity, which maximizes flexibility of the skin. Occlusive emollients should be avoided. The harlequin fetus is a severe form of congenital ichthyosis that probably represents a heterogeneous group of disorders. Affected infants are born with thick yellow skin that rapidly becomes criss-crossed by deep fissures with moist red bases (Fig. 40-9). Marked ectropion and eclabium are common, as are malformed hands, feet, and ears from restriction of normal development *in utero* by the inflexible skin. Survival beyond infancy is rare.

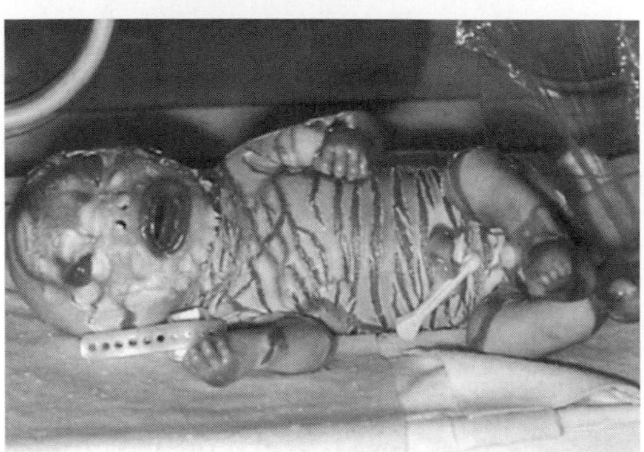

Figure 40-9. Harlequin fetus with thick yellow skin traversed by deep fissures, ectropion, eclabium, and mitten deformity of the hands and feet. (See Color Fig. 40-9.)

CHAPTER 41
Disorders of the Eye in the Newborn

Adapted from David S. Walton

VISUAL ANOMALIES

Disorders of vision are rarely detectable in the newborn period. Even anencephalic infants exhibit pupillary responses and blepharospasm in response to light. Visual behavior, however, develops rapidly, and its absence often becomes a cause for parental concern by 1 to 2 months of age. Parents' concern that their child "does not see" must never be disregarded. Blindness at birth is rare. Slow but normal development of vision must also be considered.

EYELID ANOMALIES

A common abnormality of the eyelid is ptosis (drooping eyelid), which is caused by weakness of muscles attached to the lid. This abnormality is usually an isolated defect, but it may be bilateral. Weakness of the levator palpebralis muscle is usually associated with an absent superior eyelid crease. Slight ptosis may be evidence of Horner's syndrome and might be associated with pupillary miosis and possible homolateral upper-extremity paralysis caused by a birth injury. Widening of the palpebral fissure may be the first evidence of a congenital facial nerve palsy or may be caused by proptosis. Proptosis in the newborn may be caused by a retrobulbar tumor or by hemorrhage associated with birth trauma. The eyelid margin position relative to the eye should be observed for evidence of an entropion that might put the lashes in harmful proximity to the cornea.

TEAR ANOMALIES

Normal tears for lubrication of the eye are present at birth. Excessive tears may suggest a common tear duct obstruction, and is usually noticed by parents promptly. The condition becomes complicated by a discharge early in its course.

DISORDERS OF EYE POSITION

An intermittent eye deviation in early life is common and is usually seen only during sleep or fatigue. A congenital esotropia is seen in approximately 1% of infants. Usually, the deviation is large and may be associated with impaired abduction of both eyes. A sixth nerve palsy may occur with birth, is usually unilateral, and often resolves spontaneously. A congenital fourth nerve paralysis can also occur and is frequently recognized early in life. Congenital third nerve palsies are rare; they cause ptosis, pupillary abnormalities, and external ophthalmoplegia often associated with an exotropia, and are frequently associated with other evidence of central nervous system defects such as hemiplegia.

Nystagmus is always an important sign of ocular disease. Tonic defects of eye position of supranuclear origin also occur. These defects are usually associated with tonic downgaze and may be transient.

ANTERIOR SEGMENT DEFECTS

Failure to carefully assess the anterior segment of the newborn may result in delayed diagnosis of significant ocular disease. Corneal opacification and enlargement are early signs of glaucoma or may be caused by congenital corneal defects. The possibility of birth trauma to the cornea must also be considered, particularly after a history of difficult delivery and forceps use. A small cornea may indicate microphthalmos and the presence of serious, more posterior defects such as a coloboma of the choroid, chorioretinitis, or cataract.

The irides are ordinarily similar in appearance. The pupils should be small, round, and similar in size. Coloboma of the iris, a congenital defect that gives the pupil a keyhole appearance, must be ruled out. Vascular congestion of the iris may be abnormal and suggestive of maternal cocaine use. A poor view of the iris can be caused by a neonatal hyphema (blood in the anterior chamber).

CATARACTS

The most common lens defect in the neonate is cataracts. This opacification of the lens may be unilateral or bilateral and is detectable with use of an ophthalmoscope or a hand-held slit beam and a magnification loupe. Cataracts may be anterior or posterior in the lens and may be partial or total. They may occur as an isolated defect or may be associated with other ocular or systemic abnormalities. Some cataracts are inherited, whereas others are sporadic. Autosomal dominant inheritance is common.

The diverse etiologies of congenital cataracts dictate the need for a careful and complete ocular and general examination of the young cataract patient to enable determination of the significance of the cataract abnormality.

The presence of bilateral cataracts in infancy may represent a significant impediment to the development of vision. Increased opacification, irregularity, posterior location, and largeness are features of a potentially more significant defect. The reader should be reminded that vision develops rapidly in early life and, if this process is impeded beyond a critical period of approximately 4 months after birth, the potential for the development of a high level of vision is forever lost. Therefore, the recognition of cataracts early in life is important. After cataracts are detected, prompt ophthalmologic evaluation is undertaken, during which the infant is considered for cataract removal. Both the ocular health and general health of the infant are considered in respect to determining his or her potential for improved vision by way of cataract extraction.

RETINAL HEMORRHAGES

Neonatal retinal hemorrhages are often present in the newborn and are seen less frequently when delivery is by cesarean section. Vitreous hemorrhage is far less common than is retinal hemorrhage. Visualization of retinal hemorrhages requires focusing the ophthalmoscope on the ocular fundus. Such hemorrhages are usually numerous, occupy the inner layers of the retina, and subside rapidly. Documenting their disappearance is important. Correspondingly, retinal hemorrhages seen later in the newborn (after 3 weeks of age) should, with great reservation, be interpreted as secondary to birth trauma. The probability of recent trauma, possibly caused by accident or by child abuse (shaken baby syndrome) must be considered, even in the absence of other immediate evidence of injury.

PART

III

General Pediatrics

SECTION

A

Ambulatory Pediatrics

1

Health Supervision

CHAPTER 42

Feeding the Healthy Child

Adapted from Laurence Finberg

BREAST-FEEDING IN INFANCY

From a nutritional standpoint, human milk provides a suitable caloric density, high-quality proteins in sufficient amount, adequate mineral content for cell and skeletal growth, with a low renal solute load affording plenty of water as protection from dehydration. These are not characteristics of other animal milks fed to human infants, because each milk is adapted to the needs of specific species.

Human milk also contains antibodies and macrophages that help to protect the infant from gastrointestinal pathogens and possibly other pathogens. Finally, psychological bonding takes place that helps ensure infant nurturing. The mother-infant dyad also ensures a proper caloric supply because vigorous sucking by the infant determines maternal milk production, which in turn leads to infant satiety and reduction in the vigor of sucking.

The technique of feeding is important for early success. Through the ages, such techniques were taught from generation to generation. In the United States, from 1920 to 1950, when breast-feeding was discouraged, one result was the lack of experienced relatives in the society when the desirability of breast-feeding was emphasized anew. Pediatricians should assist in this role.

An optimal time and place to start nursing is shortly after birth. Preferably, the Credé treatment to the eyes should be deferred until after the first suckling period. The mother should support her breast either with the thumb and forefinger above the areola with the other fingers below (scissor grip) or with all of the fingers under the breast with only the thumb above (palmer grip). The nipple should be placed squarely into the infant's mouth so that he or she may latch on securely with a tight seal. The infant should be allowed approximately 5 minutes on the first side and then given another 5 minutes or so on the other side. The first fluid received is colostrum, which has less nutrient but more immune factors than the milk that comes in a few days later. Once nursing has been established over the first 2 days, the act of suckling causes release of oxytocin in the mother producing the "let-down" phenomenon of spontaneous lactation. In time, this reflex occurs when the mother hears the infant cry or sees the infant receptive to feeding. The very occurrence of let-down signifies the establishment of a good early nursing relationship. Emptying of the breast by suckling or pumping stimulates prolactin release completing the mechanical and endocrine cycles.

Optimal technique is to nurse at the first breast for approximately 5 minutes and then to shift to the other so that both breasts are used at each feeding. At the next feeding, the baby should begin feeding on the alternate breast from that begun on the previous time. Usually, the infant nurses approximately eight times a day; it is wise to allow the infant's hunger to determine the schedule taking care not to let prolonged nursing on an empty breast cause soreness and inflammation.

Jaundice in excess of the usual neonatal physiologic bilirubin levels in plasma occurs in infants who are breast-fed because of either caloric deprivation or slow stool evacuation or both. Supplying supplemental glucose water feedings aggravates this increase. As the milk supply comes in and more rapid stooling begins, this breast-feeding phenomenon resolves. One must make sure that no concomitant pathologic cause for the jaundice exists. In approximately 0.5% of breast-fed infants, an increase in the unconjugated bilirubin level in plasma occurs between the fourth and ninth days of life, which is attributed to an inhibiting substance, possibly by a fatty acid in the milk suppressing glucuronidation in the infant liver. The bilirubin level decreases if breast-feeding is suspended, but this is rarely necessary because no consequence of this type of hyperbilirubinemia occurs. If uncertainty as to the cause of jaundice is present, one day of pumping the breast while giving formula to the infant will result in a significant decrease in bilirubin levels and then breast-feeding should be resumed.

If in the infant's first days of life, the mother, through inexperience or other problems, does not get the infant to suckle, starvation and water deprivation may occur leading to hypernatremic dehydration. Any low-volume output state results in an increased concentration of all of the solutes in the milk. Colostrum similarly has a higher concentration of minerals and protein while the volume is low. This increased concentration of sodium and chloride (usually up to 40–50 mEq/L) is not sufficient to cause hypernatremia if the volume is sufficient for the minimal water requirement. Thus, water deprivation, not increased solute, is causal and should be remedied by appropriate fluid therapy while an effort is made to increase milk production by the mother.

The breast-fed infant may exhibit a wide range of stooling patterns ranging from a stool with each feeding to as few as one every 2 days. The lack of foul odor to breast milk stools continues as long as no other food is supplemented.

Contraindications to breast-feeding are few. In general, the presence of chronic infection that is not quickly reversible (e.g., active pulmonary tuberculosis, human immunodeficiency virus) in the mother or the use of a few drugs is the only contraindication. The drugs mostly belong to the antineoplastic or antithyroid classes but include illicit drugs such as cocaine and heroin. References (*American Academy of Pediatrics Nutrition Handbook*) provide a more complete list. Obviously, drugs that suppress lactation such as bromcriptine are contraindicated for the mother. Virtually everything that appears in the maternal plasma or lipid tissue will appear in the milk. Water-soluble molecules will come from the plasma at plasma concentration (usually insignificant for an effect). Lipid-soluble molecules, however, may become concentrated in the milk with its high fat content.

The nutrient content of human milk serves the complete needs of the infant for the first 4 to 5 months of life with the exception of vitamin D. That substance, cholecalciferol, is produced in the skin from 7-dehydrocholesterol by the action of UV light. In modern urban environments in the temperate zone, the breast-fed infant should receive supplemented vitamin D in aqueous form, 400 units daily. The iron content of human milk is low but very well absorbed. Because the infant is born with excess hemoglobin in the blood for the oxygen environment outside the uterus, the excess iron produced as red blood cells break down is stored in the reticuloendothelial system. Rapid growth, with an increasing blood volume, reclaims this iron for optimal hemoglobin concentration in 3 to 4 months. The breast milk-derived iron adds another month or so. By 5 months, most infants require more iron than breast-feeding supplies for their increasing blood volume. At 5 months, swallowing may have matured sufficiently to accept the solid foods that should be offered to supply the needed iron.

FORMULA FEEDING

Although every effort should be made to encourage breast-feeding, such efforts should not include intimidation or provocation of guilt. The feeding of infant formula completely satisfies the nutritional needs of the infant for growth. Adequate affection and bonding are also easily achievable.

To make cow's milk suitable for infants, it must be modified. In the United States, a number of commercial infant formulas meet mandatory Food and Drug Administration specifications, which in turn are based on advice from the Committee on Nutrition of the American Academy of Pediatrics (AAP). Protein and lactose are extracted from cow's milk, the protein modified and reduced in amount, and both the protein and lactose returned to the formula. Vegetable fat is substituted for butter fat with some variance in composition by differing manufacturers. Vitamin and accessory substances are added, and the mineral composition is adjusted toward that of human milk. The addition of vitamin C, lacking in cow's milk, and the addition of vitamin D, not adequate in human milk, make the formula nutritionally complete obviating the need for supplementation. The addition of iron to the infant formula takes care of the need for the entire first year if fed for that period. The amount of iron present does not cause either diarrhea or constipation as has occasionally been alleged. The so-called low-iron formulas are never needed, and manufacturers should cease to offer them.

Soymilk products and special formulas are also available in which the protein is hydrolyzed to amino acids. The soy products use glucose and corn syrup for carbohydrate instead of lactose. They are often prescribed for milk intolerance or milk allergy, although such conditions are uncommon. If true allergy to cow's milk protein exists, then the hydrolysate mixtures, although expensive, are better, because soy protein is as likely to cause allergic reaction as cow's milk protein. Lactase deficiency in infancy is rare, although increasingly common with increasing age of more than 2 years in blacks, Asians, and some whites.

The prepared infant formulas are sold in three forms of decreasing expense: ready to feed, concentrated liquid requiring dilution with an equal amount of water, and powdered formula requiring mixing. Care must be taken with the latter two to keep the mixing accurate to provide neither overconcentrated nor dilute feedings. If the bottle is prepared fresh for each feeding, sterilization is not required. Partially consumed formula should not be kept longer than 1 hour. Unused formula may be stored in the refrigerator for up to approximately 8 hours. If longer storage is required for prepared formula, terminal sterilization (placing bottles in boiling water for 20 minutes) should be used.

SIX MONTHS TO 1 YEAR OF AGE

Between 6 months and 1 year of age, the baby's swallowing mechanisms have matured and he or she is ready for solid foods. Juices may be offered sooner, of course. For the breast-fed infant, foods containing iron such as fortified cereals or fruits, vegetables, and vegetable-meat mixtures, are important. Although cereal has become a traditional first solid, many infants accept the slightly sweet pureed vegetables or fruits more readily. Each new food should be introduced one at a time with a day or two between. After a few weeks, the diet can be quite varied with two to three solids (1 or 2 tablespoons each) offered two or three times daily. The same program should be offered to formula-fed infants. Unless an adverse reaction (uncommon) to a food occurs, the whole gamut of the diet, properly prepared (initially pureed, then increasingly textured as teeth appear) may be offered.

Toward the end of the first year is the customary weaning period from breast or bottle in present-day Western society, although other cultures wean infants earlier or much later. Breast-fed infants may usually be weaned directly to the cup if weaning occurs in this time period.

SECOND YEAR

During the second year of age, the period of very rapid growth has passed and the infant's previously robust appetite has slackened. Social interactions have also become complex, so that parents are often puzzled by periods of refusal of food. Such behavior is usual at this age and is interspersed with periods of eating more avidly. The weight gain during the year will be only 3 to 4 lbs (1.5–2.5 kg) while following the normal growth curve for length. Failure to follow the normal growth curve would be the only cause for nutritional concern.

TODDLER: 2 TO 5 YEARS OF AGE

During the toddler years, the diet enlarges to that of the adult range. Emphasis should be on variety with adequate protein, some of it from animal sources (milk, eggs, and meat including fish and poultry) and sufficient calories. Because of concern about the harmful effects of saturated fat in later years, many believe it prudent to restrict fat to not more than 30% of calories and saturated fat to 10% or less. Supplying low-fat milk and a minimum of butter and trans-fat margarines accomplishes this goal safely. If parents insist, for cultural or religious reasons, on a completely vegetarian diet, then vegetables, a grain (e.g., rice, corn), and a bean should be matched to offset the amino acid deficiency of each. So long as milk and eggs are included, such a diet is safe. The absence of all animal protein causes deficiency of vitamin B_{12} and, if the vegetables are not matched properly, to more serious malnutrition. Occasional binges on a single food occur from time to time in this age group and are usually self-limited and harmless.

SCHOOL-AGED: 6 TO 13 YEARS OF AGE

During the school-aged years, the diet assumes that of the adult in range, although sophistication in spicing is usually deferred in this age group. Good nutrition supports school performance. For inner-city children who may commonly experience food scarcity, the school breakfast program, as well as the school lunch program, should be encouraged. As the pubertal period approaches, the caloric consumption increases markedly.

ADOLESCENT YEARS

During adolescence, particular attention to iron and calcium intake, especially in girls, is important at this time of accelerated growth in general and of the skeleton in particular. Eating fast food becomes common and is not necessarily harmful if balanced with other items over intervals of a couple of weeks. Again, high fats, particularly saturated fat, should not exceed the previously advised limits, though occasional individual meals may do so. In many societies, the fascination with leanness in women has produced a special problem for adolescent girls that parents and physicians should recognize.

CHAPTER 43

Streams of Development: The Keys to Developmental Assessment

Adapted from Frederick B. Palmer and Arnold J. Capute

COGNITIVE ASSESSMENT

Language

The best single measure of cognitive development in infancy and childhood is language development. Traditional psychological testing relies heavily on language in its determination of an intelligence quotient, beginning in the preschool years and extending through school age and into adulthood. This is true as early as the third year of life, for which the Stanford-Binet Intelligence Test remains the most commonly used instrument. The Wechsler Scales, the most frequently used intelligence test in the school years and for adults, also emphasize use of language. Infant developmental scales such as the Bayley Scales of Infant Development and the Cattell Infant Intelligence Test make less use of language items as measures of developmental progress. However, infant language can be used as an objective tool for early assessment if professionals are familiar with language markers, their occurrence in the normal population, patterns of delay and deviance, and limitations in their use.

The pediatric assessment of early language relies almost entirely on milestones. These prelinguistic and linguistic milestones are related to later cognitive development, and recognition of early language delay is the most sensitive indicator of subsequent mental retardation or communication disorder. Subtle manifestations of language delay or deviancy indicate risk for school-aged learning disability and general academic underachievement.

The assessment of infant expressive language development begins in the prelinguistic phase with the sequential occurrence of cooing, babbling, indiscriminate "dada" and "mama," and the discriminate "dada" and "mama," followed by the child's first true word at approximately 1 year of age. With the development of words used spontaneously and with clear meaning, the child enters the linguistic phase. Between 12 and 24 months, an accelerating increase in vocabulary size occurs, which continues into and through the school years; it is easily measured up to approximately 2 years of age. Similarly, the increase in phrase length occurs with the sole use of single words to approximately 20 months of age, followed by development of two-word phrases, short sentences, and near-normal adult syntax by the late preschool years.

Receptive language development can be traced into the prelinguistic phase of the first several months of life. The earliest receptive language skills are neurosensory. They represent peripheral auditory functioning and the CNS response to sound. The normal newborn alerts to sound by crying, quieting, or otherwise changing state, and by startling, blinking, or by other recognizable responses. By 4 months of age, the child orients to voice by turning to the source of the sound.

Delay in achieving this 4-month skill of auditory orienting may indicate hearing loss, but it may also indicate CNS dysfunction as seen in mental retardation or communication disorders. It may indicate that the child's receptive language abilities are not yet at the 4-month level. By 9 months of age, the child should indicate his or her understanding of interactive gesture games by participating in them. He or she should follow a single-step command accompanied by gesture at 12 months and without gesture by 15 months. At 15 months, he or she should begin to point to body parts on request, and by 2 to 2.5 years of age, the child should be able to follow a series of two independent commands.

The pediatrician should be able to detect language delay associated with mild mental retardation or moderate communication disorders in children by the age of 2 years. To detect milder communication disorders and subtle delays in language, further assessment by a speech pathologist or psychologist is required, although atypical or deviant language development may have been noticed in the early months of life.

Infants with milder degrees of language impairment may not have overt delay. Their language abnormalities may be reflected as deviant or atypical attainment of milestones. For example, there may be a dissociation between receptive language development and expressive language development, with language understanding at a significantly higher level than language expression, a rather common finding in preschoolers with communication disorders. Another common, but less easily recognized, phenomenon is a better single-word vocabulary than connected language ability. The child may have an age-appropriate expressive vocabulary, but he or she is unable to put these words together into phrases and sentences at the similar developmental level suggested by vocabulary size. This can be manifested as an uncoupling of the milestones that normally occur together such as two-word phrases and a 25-word vocabulary or two- to three-word sentences and a 50-word vocabulary.

Similar deviant phenomena are seen in receptive language development. A preschooler may have a large single-word receptive vocabulary (e.g., can point to named pictures), but does not understand connected language (e.g., cannot follow commands) at the same developmental level. This phenomenon is especially important to recognize. If parents and educational personnel assume the relatively good vocabulary skills are representative of ability in connected language, they can overestimate the child's capacity and create unrealistic expectations and treatment goals for the child.

Echolalia, repetition of words and phrases without understanding, is normally seen in infants younger than 30 months. It may be seen in preschoolers with language disorders with good rote memory skills but poor language comprehension. If prominent, it suggests receptive language skills below the level of 30 months. Recognition of such deviancy is key in early detection of milder disorders. It should prompt a complete evaluation by a speech and language pathologist or psychologist.

TABLE 43-1. Visuomotor Skills with Pencil and Paper

Skill	Age
Simple marks	12 mo
Scribble in imitation	15 mo
Scribble spontaneously	18 mo
Stroke	24 mo
Horizontal and vertical strokes	27 mo
Circle in imitation	30 mo
Copy circle	36 mo
Copy cross	42 mo
Copy square	4 yr
Copy triangle	5 yr
Copy Union Jack	5–6 yr
Copy horizontal diamond	6 yr
Copy vertical diamond	7 yr
Copy Greek cross	8 yr
Copy cylinder	9 yr
Copy cube	12 yr

Visuomotor Skills

Visuomotor or problem-solving skills make up the other major cognitive stream of development. The purpose for assessing this stream is to quantify the cognitive components of visual and fine motor manipulative tasks. A task may not be achieved because of factors other than cognitive delay. These include visual impairment, gross or fine motor liability, or refusal. However, adequate cognitive abilities frequently overcome mild or moderate upper extremity motor limitations.

The earliest visuomotor tasks are assessable in the first 3 months of life. The visual neurosensory skills include visual fixation before 1 month of age and the development of visual tracking skills and the blink response to visual threat at 3 to 4 months. By this age, basic visual fixation and tracking skills approach full maturity. At the same time, the infant is gradually coming out of the neonatal flexor habitus (with suppression of primitive reflexes) and, by 3 months of age, he or she should be able to bring his or her hands to midline and be relatively unfisted. With development of visual tracking abilities and early upper extremity control, eye, head, and upper extremity movements can be used in combination. This represents the beginning of assessable fine motor problem-solving skills beginning with the ability to reach, attain, and transfer objects from hand to hand by 5 months of age.

During subsequent months, the infant's abilities become more sophisticated, and the examination draws heavily on tasks demanding the manipulation of blocks, pegboards, form boards, and pencil and paper. Like language development, as the child enters the preschool years, visuomotor abilities become increasingly complex and require the evaluation of a psychologist to describe and quantify. Commonly used infant and preschool psychometric tests include the Bayley Scales of Infant Development, Cattell Infant Intelligence Scale, Stanford-Binet Intelligence Scale, McCarthy Scales of Children's Abilities, and the Wechsler Preschool and Primary Scale of Intelligence.

Although an infant or child may possess the motor ability to carry out certain visuomotor functions, these skills cannot be accomplished unless the necessary cognitive ability exists. This can be exemplified by the 9-month cognitive skill of examining a bell. If the infant is at the 9-month visuomotor level, examination of the bell and manipulation of the clapper are accomplished. If the infant is functioning below this cognitive level, this problem-solving activity is not carried out; the child ignores the bell, mouths it, or pushes it aside.

A valuable sequence of visuomotor pencil and paper tasks are listed in Table 43-1. These tasks range from 12-month random marking through the traditional copying of the Gesell figures and provide information up to a mental age of 12 years. This sequence of tasks should be a component of any visuomotor assessment.

Unlike language milestones, visuomotor tasks do not lend themselves to parental questioning about previously attained skills. The pediatrician is usually limited to determining a current visuomotor age and developmental quotient. Contrasting the rate of visuomotor development with the rate of language development allows the pediatrician to differentiate global mental retardation from a communication disorder. In the former, broad cognitive delay is manifested in language and visuomotor skills. In language disorders, relative preservation of visuomotor abilities occurs with significantly greater delay observed in language skills (i.e., language/visuomotor dissociation). Before the developmental diagnosis of mental retardation can be made, assessment of language and problem-solving skills must be accomplished.

MOTOR ASSESSMENT

Motor, particularly gross motor, development is the stream most familiar to parents and physicians. Motor development is the key to early detection of many disabilities. Significant early motor delay and abnormalities of the neuromotor examination are the hallmarks of cerebral palsy. Most infants with moderate or severe cerebral palsy can be identified in the first 6 to 8 months of life by recognition of delay, abnormalities on examination, and perhaps accompanying risk factors.

No useful quantitative association exists between the rates of motor and language development. The degree of motor delay cannot be used to predict the degree of cognitive delay. However, a clear qualitative association exists; infants with motor delay are likely to have other nonmotor developmental abnormalities including mental retardation and communicative disorders. Mild motor delay is often the first developmental concern expressed for an infant who is ultimately diagnosed as moderately mentally retarded. Table 43-2 lists the mean age of motor milestone attainment.

TABLE 43-2. Mean Age of Motor Milestone Attainment

Milestone	Mean age (mo)	Standard deviation
Roll prone to supine	3.6	1.4
Roll supine to prone	4.8	1.4
Sit tripod	5.3	1.0
Sit unsupported	6.3	1.2
Creep	6.7	1.5
Crawl	7.8	1.7
Pull to stand	8.1	1.6
Cruise	8.8	1.7
Walk	11.7	1.9
Walk backward	14.3	2.4
Run	14.8	2.7

The evolution of primitive reflex activity during the first year of life offers a key to early recognition of CNS abnormality. Primitive reflexes are subcortical whole-body motor responses, which develop during gestation, are elicitable at birth, and are generally suppressed during the first 6 months of life with CNS maturation. Abnormally intense primitive reflexes or reflexes that are not suppressed as expected during the first 6 months are signs of neurologic dysfunction. This finding, combined with significant motor delay, suggests cerebral palsy. With minimal or no delay, the primitive reflex abnormalities still reflect CNS dysfunction; abnormalities in other developmental streams should be pursued. Examples of clinically meaningful abnormalities in primitive reflexes are shown in Table 43-3. Asymmetries in primitive reflex activity such as asymmetric grasps, toe standing, or shoulder retraction, are also clinical signs of abnormality.

ACTIVITIES OF DAILY LIVING

Assessment of self-help abilities or activities of daily living provides useful information. These skills of self-feeding, dressing, and related activities provide information on how the infant integrates the developmental streams into basic daily functioning. Most activities of daily living require a minimal level of motor, language, problem-solving, and attentional maturity to be accomplished. Any problems with attaining these skills further clarify the level of competence in individual streams. For example, the mental age for toileting independently is usually approximately 18 months. A child with mental retardation who is toilet trained by 36 months has a cognitive age of at least 18 months. However, failure to achieve toileting independence does not mean the child does not have the cognitive level of 18 months; it may suggest motor, problem-solving, attentional, or language deficiencies or a lack of opportunity.

TABLE 43-3. Clinically Recognizable Abnormalities in Primitive Reflexes

Primitive reflex	Abnormality
Moro	Moro at any age associated with opisthotonos; visible Moro after 4 months
Asymmetric tonic neck reflex	An obligatory response from which the infant cannot free himself or herself; visible response after 6 months of age
Tonic labyrinthine in supine position	Persistent neck and trunk arching with the child in supine position at any age; visible arching or shoulder retraction after 6 months of age

SOCIAL DEVELOPMENT

Social development, like activities of daily living, should be seen as an amalgamation of development in multiple streams, particularly language. Although environmental influences are important, social dysfunction may be a symptom of neurodevelopmental abnormality. For example, the child who prefers playing with younger children may do so because his or her communicative abilities are at that level. Certain traditional social milestones such as play skills, domestic mimicry, parallel play at 24 months, and associative group play at 42 months, are best used as markers of language development.

CHAPTER 44
Immunization

Adapted from Neal A. Halsey
and Edwin J. Asturias

ROUTINE IMMUNIZATION SCHEDULE

The American Academy of Pediatrics (AAP), the American Academy of Family Physicians, and the Advisory Committee on Immunization Practices (ACIP) of the Centers for Disease Control and Prevention (CDC) jointly prepare an updated immunization schedule every January, which is published in *Pediatrics, Morbidity and Mortality Weekly Report, and Family Physician* (Fig. 44-1). Readers are encouraged to obtain updated schedules every year and familiarize themselves with the changes. Specific information regarding each vaccine and details regarding the immunization process are available in the *Red Book* (Report of the Committee on Infectious Diseases), which is published every 3 years (1997, 2000, 2003, etc.).

SPECIFIC IMMUNIZING AGENTS

Hepatitis B Vaccine

Hepatitis B vaccines currently available in the United States are made by recombinant technology in yeast. All of the vaccines are highly (more than 95%) effective at inducing immunity and protection against the chronic carrier state and other related diseases. In the United States and more than 70 other countries, hepatitis B vaccine is recommended for routine administration to all infants. Catch-up immunization is indicated for all children through 18 years of age. Preference is given for starting immunization at birth, with the second dose administered 1 or 2 months later; the third dose is given at least 2 months after the first dose, but preferably at 6 months of age. Hepatitis B vaccine alone has been shown to be highly effective in reducing the risk of maternal infant transmission from chronic carrier mothers. However, additional administration of hepatitis B immune globulin shortly after birth further reduces the risk of transmission to approximately 5%. In developing countries where the cost of hepatitis B immune globulin is prohibitive, routine immunization with

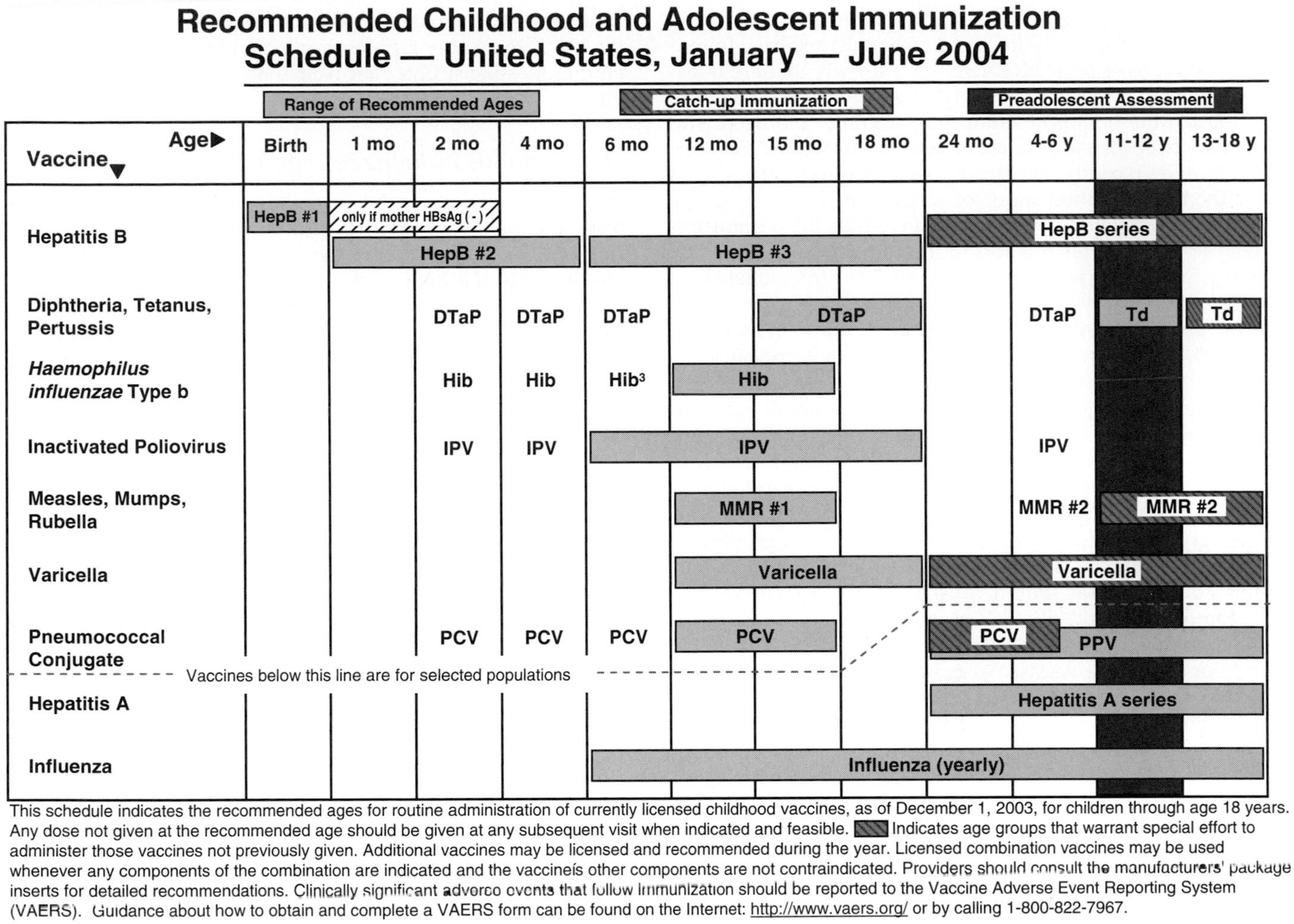

Recommended Childhood and Adolescent Immunization Schedule — United States, January — June 2004
Range of Recommended Ages
Catch-up Immunization
Preadolescent Assessment
Age▶
Vaccine▼
Birth
1 mo
2 mo
4 mo
6 mo
12 mo
15 mo
18 mo
24 mo
4-6 y
11-12 y
13-18 y
Hepatitis B
HepB #1
only if mother HBsAg (-)
HepB #2
HepB #3
HepB series
Diphtheria, Tetanus, Pertussis
DTaP
DTaP
DTaP
DTaP
DTaP
Td
Td
Haemophilus influenzae Type b
Hib
Hib
Hib3
Hib
Inactivated Poliovirus
IPV
IPV
IPV
IPV
Measles, Mumps, Rubella
MMR #1
MMR #2
MMR #2
Varicella
Varicella
Varicella
Pneumococcal Conjugate
PCV
PCV
PCV
PCV
PCV
PPV
Vaccines below this line are for selected populations
Hepatitis A
Hepatitis A series
Influenza
Influenza (yearly)
This schedule indicates the recommended ages for routine administration of currently licensed childhood vaccines, as of December 1, 2003, for children through age 18 years. Any dose not given at the recommended age should be given at any subsequent visit when indicated and feasible. Indicates age groups that warrant special effort to administer those vaccines not previously given. Additional vaccines may be licensed and recommended during the year. Licensed combination vaccines may be used whenever any components of the combination are indicated and the vaccineís other components are not contraindicated. Providers should consult the manufacturers' package inserts for detailed recommendations. Clinically significant adverse events that follow immunization should be reported to the Vaccine Adverse Event Reporting System (VAERS). Guidance about how to obtain and complete a VAERS form can be found on the Internet: http://www.vaers.org/ or by calling 1-800-822-7967.

Figure 44-1. Recommended childhood immunization schedule, United States, January to June 2004. Approved by the Advisory Committee on Immunization Practices (ACIP), the American Academy of Pediatrics (AAP), and the American Academy of Family Physicians (AAFP).

vaccine alone is the usual practice. Immunization schedules for older children and adults are usually at time 0, 1 to 2 months later, and 4 to 6 months after the first dose. Immunization at intervals up to 1 year between doses have been shown to be highly effective in simplifying the catch-up immunization of older children who are routinely seen only at annual intervals. Routine administration of hepatitis B vaccine to all children, adolescents, and high-risk adults has contributed to the marked decline in the incidence of hepatitis B in the United States. The target is elimination of transmission, but this will take 20 to 40 years because of the large number of chronic carriers in this country.

Diphtheria and Tetanus Toxoids and Pertussis Vaccine

Combined diphtheria and tetanus toxoids and pertussis vaccine (DTaP or DTP) is recommended for routine administration at 2, 4, 6, 12 to 18 months and 4 to 6 years of age. Although whole cell pertussis vaccine is still an acceptable alternative in the United States, acellular pertussis vaccines are associated with lower rates of fever, local redness and swelling, grand mal seizures, hypertensive hyporesponsive episodes, malaise, and decreased appetite. Therefore, DTaP is now routinely used for most children. DTaP combined with Hib conjugate vaccines are available for administration of the fourth and fifth doses in children.

Diphtheria and tetanus toxoids are highly effective, and their routine use has led to almost complete elimination of diphtheria and tetanus in the United States. Only a few cases of diphtheria occur each year in the United States, most in inadequately immunized immigrants. Toxin-producing *Corynebacterium diphtheriae* have been eliminated in most areas of the United States, but isolates were obtained in South Dakota in a population that was previously known to have circulation of the organism. These data indicate the continued circulation of toxin-producing strains and emphasize the need for complete and timely immunization of all children. Immunity from diphtheria and tetanus toxoids wanes with time. Booster doses are recommended at 11 to 12 years of age with a preparation containing a reduced concentration of diphtheria toxoid to reduce the risk of local adverse events. Although tetanus toxoid alone is available, it is not recommended for use because of the need to maintain diphtheria immunity. Most tetanus cases occurring in the United States have occurred in individuals 40 or 50 years and older who were never completely immunized in infancy or who had received no booster doses beyond early childhood. The majority of cases have occurred in individuals who had fewer than three doses for primary immunization.

The occasional cases of neonatal tetanus that occur in this country have usually occurred in infants born to women who were pregnant when they entered the United States or became pregnant shortly after entering the United States. In many developing countries, only 25% to 50% women of childbearing age have been adequately immunized against tetanus. Immunized women have protective levels of antibody that are transmitted across the placenta and protect the infant against tetanus, even though the umbilical stump may become colonized with tetanus spores because of unclean deliveries. Pediatricians caring for families recently immigrating to the United States should verify the immunization status of women of childbearing age and ensure complete immunization including the administration of two doses of tetanus toxoid in pregnancy (separated by at least 1 month) for women with uncertain or inadequate past immunization records.

DTaP preparations licensed in the United States have induced 72% to 90% efficacy in clinical trials conducted in European studies. Although whole cell DTP preparations have been considered interchangeable in the past, some uncertainty exists as to the interchangeability of DTaP products because of the varying concentrations of different antigens and different methods of preparation. Therefore, the AAP and ACIP have recommended that, when feasible, the same DTaP preparations should be used for the primary series. However, if the preparation used previously is unknown or unavailable at the time a child presents for immunization, then any DTaP should be used to ensure timely completion of immunization. All DTaP preparations contain pertussis toxoid, which is believed to be the most important antigen for prevention of serious disease. Also, studies have demonstrated that two doses of some DTaP preparations produce high levels of protection.

Because pertussis in infants younger than 6 months is a severe and life-threatening illness, extra efforts are being made to find a way to prevent transmission of *Bordetella pertussis* from adolescents and adults to young infants. Studies are under way to evaluate the safety and effectiveness of acellular pertussis preparations administered to adolescents or young adults, because immunity wanes after either immunization or natural infection. If the vaccine is shown to be effective, then a special formulation of diphtheria toxoid and acellular pertussis should become available and be recommended for routine use in adolescents and young adults. This additional dose of vaccine could reduce the likelihood of transmitting *B. pertussis* to young infants.

Poliomyelitis Immunization

Both inactivated (IPV) and live OPV are available for use in the United States. IPV was licensed in 1955, and widespread use led to a rapid termination of the large-scale epidemics that were affecting 30,000 to 50,000 children every year in the United States. The original IPV was of lower potency than the current enhanced potency IPV, which became available in 1987. OPV became the standard vaccine for immunizing infants in 1962 and was responsible for the complete elimination of wild type polio in the United States since 1979. OPV causes vaccine-associated paralytic polio in the recipient or a contact at a rate of approximately 1 in 780,000 children who receive their first dose of vaccine. The risk after subsequent doses is much lower, so the overall risk is approximately 1 per 2.5 million doses of vaccine administered. To prevent vaccine-associated paralytic polio, advisory committees have recommended that children in the United States receive IPV at all four visits. The enhanced-potency IPV has been shown to be highly effective at inducing individual protection and partial intestinal immunity, which has been sufficient to protect communities in several European countries against epidemics of poliomyelitis. Global efforts to eradicate polio from the world are underway. In developing countries, OPV will continue to be used until certification of the eradication of wild type viruses. Immunization with IPV in developed countries will probably continue for 1 to 2 years after OPV is terminated to ensure protection of all infants against potential recirculation of vaccine-associated viruses.

Haemophilus influenzae Type b Vaccine

Hib vaccine consists of the outer polysaccharide coat from type b strains of *H. influenzae*, which is chemically linked to protein carriers. The conjugation of the polysaccharide to a protein alters the way the host immune system processes the antigen. Plain polysaccharide was ineffective in children younger than 18 months, but the conjugated polysaccharide vaccines have been highly effective in infants beginning at 6 weeks of age. Four polysaccharide conjugate vaccines are available.

The three vaccines approved for primary immunization of infants are considered equivalent and interchangeable. PRP-OMP (polyribosylribitol phosphate conjugated to the outer membrane protein of *Neisseria meningitidis*) has been successfully combined with hepatitis B vaccine and can be administered in a two-dose series rather than a three-dose primary series. A single dose of this vaccine induces protection rapidly and, therefore, is preferred in settings where a high incidence of invasive Hib disease occurs in young infants such as the Native American population. PRP-T (PRP conjugated to tetanus toxoid) and HbOC (PRP conjugated to a mutant diphtheria toxoid) have been successfully combined with whole cell DTP preparations, and one preparation of PRP-T combined with DTaP is available for administration on the fourth and fifth doses but not for primary immunization of infants.

Measles, Mumps, and Rubella Vaccine

MMR is routinely administered at 12 to 15 months of age, and a second dose is given at 4 to 6 years of age. The second dose can be administered at any time, as long as at least 1 month has elapsed after the first dose. The first dose of measles vaccine may be given as early as 6 months of age in settings where a measles outbreak occurs in the community. If this occurs, then a dose of MMR is given at the usual 12 to 15 months of age and a third dose at 4 to 6 years of age. The response to measles vaccine at less than 12 months of age is suboptimal because of interference by passively acquired maternal antibodies that disappear at a variable and unpredictable rate. Some infants receive little or no antibodies from their mothers and respond adequately as early as 6 months of age. Others receive much higher concentrations of maternal antibody and still have trace amounts of passive antibody to blunt the replication of the live virus vaccine as late as 12 months of age. Advisory committees now recommend that all children in elementary, middle, and high school should receive two doses of MMR. A second dose is needed to ensure close to 100% immunity, because the first dose of each vaccine induces protection in approximately 95% of vaccinees. The very high infectivity of measles has resulted in continuing outbreaks of disease despite populations in which 98% to 100% of children have received one dose of vaccine. Intensive efforts have been made to ensure that all children receive measles-containing vaccines at the recommended age. This enhanced program has resulted in a marked diminution in the transmission of measles in the United States to an all time low of 135 cases in 1997 and fewer than 100 cases through the first 9 months of 1998.

Approximately 5% to 15% of children receiving the first dose of MMR develop fever of 39.4°C or higher, a rash lasting 1 to 3 days, or both. Other complications include rare cases of transient thrombocytopenia, and encephalitis occurs in less than 1 per million vaccinees. The rates of adverse events are lower in children receiving the second dose of vaccine, because only approximately 5% are susceptible. Hypersensitivity reactions have been demonstrated to be caused by allergy to the gelatin stabilizer or neomycin. Studies have demonstrated that skin testing for egg allergy or with the vaccine was not predictive of which children would develop allergic reactions to the vaccine. Current guidelines call for routine administration of MMR to children, even if they have severe egg hypersensitivity, because no significant amount of egg protein is present in these vaccines.

Children who have received blood or blood products, including IGIV, need to be assessed individually to determine the length of time after blood product administration that vaccines can be effectively administered. Administration of washed red blood cells delivers only a small amount of passive antibody, and virtually no delay in administration of measles vaccine is necessary. However, children who receive large doses (1,600–2,000 mg/kg) of IGIV need to have immunization deferred for 11 months. Specific guidelines can be found in the references from the AAP and the CDC listed at the end of this chapter. Measles and other live virus vaccines should not be administered to children with underlying immune deficiency. An exception is children who have asymptomatic human immunodeficiency virus (HIV) infection and whose CD4 counts reveal that they are not severely immunocompromised. Children who have received high doses ($\geq$2 mg/kg/day) of corticosteroids for 2 or more weeks should wait at least 1 month before measles-containing vaccines are administered.

Varicella Vaccine

Varicella vaccine became available in 1995 and is recommended for universal immunization of all children 12 months to 18 years of age who have not had chickenpox. A single dose is considered sufficient for children through 12 years of age, but two doses are recommended for children 13 years and older. One dose provides approximately 95% protection against severe disease and 70% to 80% protection against any illness. Children who have developed signs of varicella after close exposures (usually in households) have modified or very mild cases, with an average of only 40 small skin lesions, many of them papules rather than vesicles. Some physicians and parents have been apprehensive about accepting the vaccine because of concern about long-term protection, and they point out that subclinical boosts in immunity from exposure to varicella may have occurred. The vaccine has been shown to induce long-lasting immunity in Japan, where it has been in use for more than 20 years. In the United States, studies of children followed up to 10 years have shown lasting protection. Advisory committees have not recommended a second dose of vaccine, in part, because of the relatively high cost of the vaccine. In time, perhaps with other manufacturers entering the market, a second dose of vaccine may be administered, which would help allay concerns regarding the breakthrough cases that do occur. All parents should be strongly encouraged to vaccinate their children. Approximately 100 deaths per year occur from varicella in the United States, almost all of which could be prevented if immunization was universal. More than 80% of the children dying from varicella have no underlying immune deficiency disorders or other factors that would allow for prediction for severe disease. Varicella vaccine may be administered simultaneously with MMR at separate sites. Efforts are under way to produce a combination MMR-V vaccine, which would reduce the number of injections needed, and such a combination would be the key to routine administration of the second dose.

Side effects from the varicella vaccine include the development of mild vaccine-associated macular, papular, or vesicular rash in 7% to 8% of children and adolescents. The median number of skin lesions is less than five in most studies, and most of the lesions were macular or papular resembling mosquito bites. In approximately 4% of cases, one or two varicella-like lesions developed at the site of injection, presumably from tracking of the virus along the needle. Rare cases of zoster have occurred in vaccinated children, and the vaccine virus has been isolated from a zoster lesion on at least one occasion indicating the potential for persistence of the vaccine virus, as well as wild type virus in the dorsal route ganglion. However, the rate of zoster developing after vaccination appears to be much lower than after administration of wild type virus. Thus, the vaccine protects against zoster, as well as wild type disease. Formulations of varicella vaccine must be stored at –15°C or colder. Efforts are under way to improve the stabilizers so that the vaccine can be kept at routine refrigerator temperatures. Children 13 years and older should receive two doses of vaccine, and all health care workers should be immunized. As noted previously, children with underlying immune-compromising conditions should not receive the vaccine. These children should receive varicella-zoster immunoglobulin after exposures, and extra efforts should be made to ensure that all household contacts are immune through immunization or a past history of natural disease to prevent the introduction of varicella into the household.

Meningococcal Vaccine

A vaccine is available to protect against *Neisseria meningitidis* types A, C, Y, and W135. This vaccine is not administered routinely to children because the risk of infection is very small. However, the American College Health Association recommends the vaccine for those college students who will be living in a dormitory setting. Meningococcal vaccine is effective only in children 2 years and older, and the highest risk is in those younger than 2 years of age. Efforts are under way to produce conjugate meningococcal vaccines that might be effective as early as 6 to 8 weeks of age.

Pneumococcal Vaccine

Two licensed pneumococcal vaccines are available. A seven-valent conjugate vaccine (*Prevnar*) was approved by the FDA in 2000. The vaccine contains seven pneumococcal serotypes that account for the majority of invasive disease (bacteremia, meningitis, pneumonia) in the United States. The conjugate vaccine is recommended for all children younger then 24 months and the schedule of administration is the same as the Hib vaccine (2, 4, 6, 12–15 months). Children 24 to 59 months who have high-risk medical conditions such as sickle cell disease, asplenia, nephrotic syndrome or chronic renal failure, immunosuppression, HIV infection, leaks of cerebrospinal fluid, and children with chronic cardiovascular or pulmonary disease should receive two doses of the conjugate pneumococcal vaccine 6 to 8 weeks apart.

The second pneumococcal vaccine contains polysaccharides from 23 pneumococcal serotypes. The vaccine is approved for use only at 2 years or older. The 23 antigens will not provide complete protection against all pneumococcal infections because more than 80 serotypes of pneumococcus exist. However, the 23 antigens come from the most common pneumococcal serotypes, which together are responsible for approximately 80% of all invasive infections in children. The vaccine is recommended for children who are at increased risk at developing severe complications from *Streptococcus pneumoniae* infections (see above) even if they have received the conjugate vaccine. Revaccination 3 to 5 years after the first dose is recommended for children 10 years of age or younger who are at high risk of severe disease including those with sickle cell disease, asplenia, nephrotic syndrome, renal failure or transplantation, and HIV infection or malignancy.

Influenza Vaccine

Currently, only inactivated influenza vaccines are available, but a cold-adapted, live, intranasal vaccine is being investigated. Both vaccines effectively prevent severe disease caused by influenza in children depending on the ability of vaccine manufacturers to match the current circulating influenza strains. The overall efficacy for inactivated influenza vaccines has been 70% to 80% for prevention of influenza-related illness. These studies have been conducted primarily in older adults for whom the vaccine is recommended routinely. However, these individuals have decreased responses to vaccines of all types, and the true efficacy in younger children is probably higher if the match is correct. Inactivated influenza vaccine is recommended on an annual basis for children at increased risk of complications from influenza. For children 6 months to 12 years of age, only the split virus vaccine is recommended because of lower rates of adverse events. Whole virus vaccines are effective and associated with no increased risk of adverse events in children who are older than 12 years. The first year that children younger than 9 years receive influenza vaccine, they should receive two doses (Table 44-1) at least 1 month apart. Subsequently, a single dose administered every year just before the influenza season (usually in October or early November) is indicated. Children for whom the vaccine is routinely recommended include those with chronic pulmonary disease such as asthma, significant cardiac disease, immunosuppressive disorders or therapy, HIV infection, sickle cell anemia or other hemoglobinopathies, and children who require long-term aspirin therapy for treatment of rheumatoid arthritis or Kawasaki disease. The groups of children receiving aspirin therapy may be at increased risk for development of Reye syndrome after wild type influenza infection. Advisory groups recommend that other children who are potentially at increased risk of complications may also benefit from vaccination including those with diabetes mellitus, chronic renal disease, chronic metabolic disease, or any other condition that may compromise children. In addition, the ACIP has recommended that women who will be in the third trimester of pregnancy during the influenza season should be immunized. Also, household and other close contacts of high-risk patients should be immunized to decrease the risk of introduction of wild type influenza into the home. The AAP has indicated that vaccination should be considered for individuals whose group activities could be significantly disrupted by outbreaks of influenza including students, athletes, and those living in residential institutions. In addition, the AAP has recently recommended that all healthy children 6 months to 2 years be immunized. Their risk of influenza-related morbidity and hospitalization is similar to the adult population in which routine immunization is already indicated (age greater than 55). Finally, pediatricians are advised that any healthy child or adolescent who requests immunization should be immunized.

Influenza vaccine is associated with low-grade fever and malaise in a very small percentage of children, usually 6 to 24 hours after vaccination. In children 13 years of age and older, approximately 10% develop local reactions. Studies in adults have indicated a small increased risk of Guillain-Barré syndrome, approximately 1 to 2 per million vaccinees. The data are from adults only because insufficient numbers of children have been immunized to determine accurately if any increase in risk exists. The risks of serious consequences from influenza are several hundred-fold higher, and this observation has not changed the recommendations for use of this vaccine.

Hepatitis A

Two hepatitis A vaccines are available in the United States. Both are inactivated subcomponent viral vaccines. The antigen content is determined by two methods that are not directly comparable (Table 44-2). Both vaccines are administered in a two-dose series separated by 6 months. Both vaccines are approved only for use in children 2 years and older, and available evidence indicates that the two-dose series should produce long-lasting immunity. Side effects are relatively mild and consist primarily of pain at the injection site. Children who should receive hepatitis A vaccine include those traveling to countries where increased risks of hepatitis A exist (most developing countries). Consideration needs to be taken with regard to the length of time that children will be traveling and the conditions under which they will be living and selecting foods. Most experts recommend vaccine rather than passive antibody even for short-term stays because long-term protection is desirable. Children who reside in high-risk communities, including Native American, native Alaskan, and other communities with periodic epidemics, should receive the vaccine routinely beginning at 2 years of age. Patients with underlying chronic liver disease, including those with hepatitis C or chronic hepatitis B infection, should be immunized. Men who have sex with men, users of illicit drugs, and workers in high-risk settings (i.e., handlers of nonhuman primates) should be immunized. The available data do not reveal an increased risk of hepatitis A for children attending day care or for hospital or other medical personnel. The effectiveness of the vaccine after

TABLE 44-1. Schedule for Influenza Immunization[a]

Age	Recommended vaccine[b]	Dose (mL)[c]	Number of doses
6–35 mo	Split virus only	0.25	1–2[d]
3–8 yr	Split virus only	0.5	1–2[d]
9–12 yr	Split virus only	0.5	1
>12 yr	Whole or split virus	0.5	1

[a]Vaccine is administered intramuscularly.
[b]Split-virus vaccine may be termed *split, subvirion,* or *purified surface-antigen* vaccine.
[c]Dosages are those recommended in recent years. Physicians should refer to the product circular each year to ensure that the appropriate dosage is given.
[d]Two doses administered at least 1 month apart are recommended for children who are receiving influenza vaccine for the first time.

TABLE 44-2. Hepatitis A Vaccine Doses[a]

Age (yr)	Vaccine	Antigen dose	Volume per dose (mL)
2–18	Havrix (SmithKline Beecham)	720 EL.U.[b]	0.5
	Vaqta (Merck)	25 U[c]	0.5
19 and older	Havrix (SmithKline Beecham)	1,440 EL.U.	1.0
	Vaqta (Merck)	50 U	1.0

[a]Both vaccines are administered in a 0, 6 to 12 month schedule.
[b]EL.U. indicates enzyme-linked immunoassay units.
[c]Antigen units (each unit is equivalent to approximately 1 mg of viral protein).

exposure is unknown, but studies are under way to evaluate its effectiveness at controlling outbreaks.

CONTRAINDICATIONS TO IMMUNIZATIONS

In general, there are few absolute contraindications to receiving any vaccine for the first time or subsequent doses in a series. The following general rules apply to all vaccines.

Immediate Hypersensitivity Reactions

Anaphylaxis after a previous dose of the indicated vaccine or a vaccine component, dilutent, or preservative is a contraindication to giving subsequent doses. Vaccines produced in chick embryo tissue culture, including measles and mumps vaccine, contain insignificant amounts of egg protein, and skin testing before administering these vaccines is no longer indicated for children with true egg hypersensitivity. However, inactivated influenza and yellow fever vaccines are produced in eggs, and true hypersensitivity to egg protein is a contraindication to these vaccines. Some hypersensitivity reactions to vaccines are caused by the stabilizers such as the gel stabilizer in measles vaccines.

Encephalopathy or Encephalitis

Encephalopathy or encephalitis after DTP or DTaP administration is a contraindication to receipt of subsequent doses.

Immune Deficiency Disorder

Patients with immune deficiency disorders should not generally receive live viral or bacterial vaccines. In the absence of an effective host immune system, the live viral or bacterial agents can replicate unchecked and cause serious systemic disease. For example, the risk of vaccine-associated paralysis after OPV is increased by at least 1,000-fold in persons with agammaglobulinemia. Some exceptions may be made after consultation with experts in immunology or infectious diseases. New techniques have led to the diagnosis of mild immune deficiency disorders affecting selected aspects of the immune system that are not involved in controlling replicating viral agents.

Pregnancy and Live Vaccines

Pregnancy is a contraindication for administering live vaccines. However, having a pregnant woman in the household is not a contraindication to administering OPV, MMR, or varicella vaccines. The MMR vaccine viruses are not transmitted from the vaccinated child to household contacts. Although one instance of varicella vaccine virus transmission from a child to his pregnant mother has been documented, no evidence of infection was observed after an elective abortion for other reasons. Some experts have advised waiting until the second trimester to immunize children with varicella vaccine if a susceptible pregnant woman is in the household.

Noncontraindications and Misconceptions

Children with mild upper respiratory infections or gastroenteritis can receive routine immunizations. Vaccines should be administered to these children, especially in circumstances in which uncertainty exists regarding return for completion of the immunization series. The presence of mild illnesses has not interfered with the immune response to vaccines, although there are insufficient data to know if gastroenteritis is associated with a reduced response to rotavirus vaccine. Low-grade fever (less than 39%) is not a contraindication to immunization. If children have other manifestations of illness or the etiology of the fever is undetermined, however, a febrile response to the vaccine could be confused with signs of progression or exacerbation of the intercurrent illness. A judgment should be made regarding the feasibility of the child's returning within a few days to be immunized if uncertainty exists regarding the etiology of the concurrent illness.

CHAPTER 45

Injury Prevention and Control

Adapted from Modena Hoover Wilson

MOTOR VEHICLE-RELATED INJURIES

Not surprisingly, most children and adolescents who die of transportation-related injuries were motor vehicle occupants. Pedestrians struck by motor vehicles in traffic make up the second largest group. A significant number of deaths is also attributed to motorcycle and bicycle incidents. Because of their impressive numbers and severity, prevention of motor vehicle occupant deaths has served as the flagship effort of the field of injury control, but the protection of child passengers needs continuing attention. Of particular concern are the injuries related to the improper use and placement of car safety seats.

Injuries from motor vehicle crashes are a leading cause of death well into adulthood, and they are an important cause of permanent disability. Among the pediatric age groups, adolescents are at highest risk for motor vehicle-related injury, but the number of deaths related to motor vehicles far exceeds those caused by any other source of unintentional injury throughout the pediatric age span. The male-to-female ratio, which portrays an increased risk for male subjects at every age after 1 year, is especially high during adolescence. The fatality rate for motor vehicle injury is particularly high for unrestrained infants involved in crashes. For children aged 5 to 9 years, the number of pedestrian deaths approaches the number of motor vehicle occupant deaths. For all other age groups except the very elderly, motor vehicle occupant injuries far outstrip pedestrian injuries as a cause of death.

Motor Vehicle Occupants

INCIDENCE

Motor vehicle occupant fatalities are more common during warm months, at night, and on weekends. Direct frontal impacts account for the largest group of the fatal crashes; side impacts comprise the second-largest group. Single-vehicle crashes produce a higher death rate than do multiple-vehicle crashes. Occupants who are ejected from a vehicle in a crash or at the time of a sudden stop are particularly likely to sustain severe or fatal injury. Occupants of smaller, lighter vehicles are at increased risk in both single- and multiple-vehicle crashes, even in crashes with other vehicles of the same size. Urban roads are associated with lower death rates per passenger mile than are rural roads and limited-access roads with lower death rates than uncontrolled-access roads. Probably because of superior engineering and the separation of opposing traffic, the crash rate per passenger mile is low on the interstate system. However, when crashes do occur, they tend to be severe because of high vehicle speed.

In a substantial but decreasing proportion of crashes with fatalities, a driver's blood alcohol is found to be elevated. Elevated blood alcohol is more often found with nighttime crashes and with young and middle-aged male drivers.

Motor vehicle occupant death rates have been declining since the 1960s, a fortunate fact attributed to changes in roads and vehicles, as well as to seat belts, car safety seats, and, more recently, airbags.

Approximately 5,000 children and adolescents younger than 20 years were killed as motor vehicle occupants in the United States in 1993. Injury and death rates peak during adolescence for both girls and boys, although adolescents travel fewer car miles than adults. Male teenage drivers have higher fatal crash rates than any other group.

PREVENTION

Motor vehicle occupant injuries can be reduced by preventing crashes or by reducing the forces that impinge on the body during crashes. In addition to modifying vehicles and reducing speed, forces can be reduced by spreading them over a wider area of the body and by increasing the distance over which the body decelerates. This is accomplished by restraint systems and airbags. Measures of specific interest to health professionals caring for children include counseling and advocacy issues.

COUNSELING POINTS

Injury can be prevented by the use of appropriate restraint systems for age and size. Parents of very small premature infants, children with severe developmental disabilities, and children in casts that preclude using a standard safety seat need special guidance. Counseling should include information about the correct use of car safety seats. The American Academy of Pediatrics (AAP) publishes a "Family Guide to Car Seats" each year with support from the National Highway Traffic Safety Administration. Because infants restrained in car safety seats in the front passenger seats of automobiles with passenger-side airbags and young children out of position in the front seat have been killed when airbags deployed, it is particularly important to counsel families that infants and young children should always ride properly restrained in the back seat.

Parents should be encouraged to make the transition from safety seats to the three-point seat belt system, to continue to insist on the use of seat belts through adolescence and into adulthood, and to set the standard by using their own seat belts. The advantage of airbags plus seat belts for adolescents and adults should be stressed. Drinking and driving should be discouraged, and parents should be encouraged to provide adolescents with a safe ride home.

ADVOCACY ISSUES

Advocacy issues include the provision of restraint devices for children with special needs, extending persons and vehicles covered under state safety seat and seat belt laws, enforcement of safety seat and seat belt laws, increasing the minimum licensing age or the provisional licensing period or extending the curfew (i.e., limitation on nighttime driving) associated with provisional licenses, and maintaining lower speed limits.

Pedestrians

INCIDENCE

The second-largest category of vehicle-related deaths is that of persons on foot killed by motor vehicles. In such crashes, the pedestrian is completely unshielded and is at great disadvantage. The severity of the injuries that result from a motor vehicle striking a pedestrian is well illustrated by the high death-to-injury ratio. Of every 1,000 pedestrians injured, 52 die, whereas "only" 27 deaths occur for every 1,000 motorcyclists injured in crashes with other motor vehicles and 12 deaths for every 1,000 persons injured as motor vehicle occupants. The overall trend in pedestrian death rates has been downward despite the fact that little evidence exists that effective countermeasures for pedestrian injury are known. Improvement in the childhood pedestrian injury rate may be related more to declining rates of walking rather than to injury prevention campaigns or counseling.

The highest pedestrian death rates are experienced by the elderly, but peaks are also seen in childhood and adolescence. During the pediatric years, the death rates are highest for those between 5 and 14 years, and boys are more likely to die, with the gender differential appearing by the second year of life. Pedestrian deaths are an urban disease with two-thirds of the deaths and even more of the injuries occurring in urban areas. Although less frequent than urban pedestrian injury events, rural events are much more likely to result in death, probably because of higher vehicle speeds.

Only 20% of adult pedestrian deaths occur at intersections, and even fewer pediatric deaths occur there. Most occur when children run into the street in the middle of a block or attempt to cross between intersections. Some deaths occur when motor vehicles invade the pedestrian's space on a sidewalk or median strip. Allowing motorists to make a right turn after stopping at a red light has increased pedestrian injuries in urban areas, because as drivers look left for oncoming traffic, they do not always see approaching pedestrians. Although most pedestrian injuries and deaths do occur in traffic, during the first few years of life a sizable proportion of pedestrian deaths occur in nontraffic areas (e.g., driveways, lanes), often with the driver backing over a toddler playing in the area. Nontraffic pedestrian deaths are particularly high in rural areas.

Pedestrian injuries peak at approximately 4 p.m., but the peak time of fatal injury is approximately 1 hour after sunset, but that time changes with the seasons. Adult pedestrians believe that motorists can see them from a much greater distance than is possible. Children are probably even more likely to misjudge the ability of the driver to see and to stop, and they may not consider the possibility at all.

Most often, the front of a motor vehicle strikes the pedestrian, but children are also killed when they run into the side of the moving vehicle, are struck by the vehicle's protruding hardware (e.g., mirror), or are run over by the rear wheels of a truck or bus. More pedestrians are killed walking along a roadway in the same direction as traffic than against traffic.

The weight of the vehicle and the speed at which it is traveling are important determinants of the severity of injury. The death-to-injury ratio is approximately three times higher for heavy trucks than for cars, and it increases as the posted speed limit increases.

PREVENTION

Wherever and whenever possible, motor vehicle traffic and pedestrians should be physically separated with barriers or space, or they should not be using the same space at the same time. Anything that decreases the number of vehicles and vehicular speed will benefit pedestrians. Young children cannot be trusted near traffic. They must have fixed barriers between them and traffic or continuous supervision from an adult. Children younger than 7 years should cross streets only with assistance, and for a few years after that age, children are still too young to cross unassisted where traffic volume is high because they have difficulty judging speed and distance. Ideally, incursions into the street should only be made at intersections and in accordance with traffic rules. Adults must set a good example. Children playing and in groups often forget all about traffic, and yet many children must cope with traffic and street crossings as they make their way to school. They should demonstrate their knowledge of, and adherence to, safe pedestrian practices before they make that journey unassisted. The parent should plan a route that avoids heavy, high-speed traffic and walking in the street. That being said, it must also be admitted that programs to train children to avoid pedestrian injury have not been widely evaluated and, where they have, the results have not been encouraging.

COUNSELING POINTS

Counseling might include advice on street-crossing timing and training, using barriers between play areas and traffic, planning the route to school, and avoiding walking in or along streets or roads, especially at night.

ADVOCACY ISSUES

Advocacy issues include the development of safe, attractive off-street play areas, diverting traffic from residential areas and around schools, loading and unloading school buses and cars away from traffic, building convenient walkways where pedestrian traffic is heavy or making other modifications of high-risk sites, using and constructing sidewalks, slowing motor vehicle speeds in residential areas, and prohibiting parking where children are likely to cross. Extension of daylight savings time later into the fall would likely decrease pedestrian injuries.

Motorcycles and Other Motorized Vehicles

INCIDENCE

The rate of injuries associated with vehicles that travel at high rates of speed, especially on roads and highways, and provide no external protection for riders is high. Although children and adolescents may be physically capable of operating vehicles such as motorcycles, minibikes, mopeds, trail bikes, all-terrain vehicles, and snowmobiles, the risk under many conditions, including off-road driving, is excessive. Use by children and young adolescents should be strongly discouraged.

A peak in motorcycle deaths occurred in the early 1980s. Subsequently, the number of registered motorcycles and the number of motorcyclist deaths declined. Nevertheless, motorcycles claim the lives of 200 to 300 adolescents a year.

Compared with passenger cars, motorcycles are extremely dangerous: The per mile death rate is 15 times higher, the number of deaths per registered vehicle is three times higher, and the death-to-injury ratio is twice as high. The disparity between death rates by gender is extreme, with rates for young men ten times those of female riders. Fifteen male motorcycle drivers die for every female driver, but more female than male subjects die as motorcycle passengers. Collisions with other motor vehicles account for slightly more than one-half of the deaths. Crashes and injuries increase with increasing vehicle power. Alcohol abuse plays a part, particularly in nighttime, single-vehicle crashes. Helmets clearly decrease severe injury and death rates among motorcyclists. Deaths decrease when laws requiring riders to wear helmets are in place, although perfect compliance with the laws does not occur.

Minibikes, minicycles, and trail bikes are all motorized two-wheeled cycles that range from little more than a bicycle to almost a motorcycle. They vary in speed and other capabilities. Because they are marketed for off-road use, they do not fall under federal safety standards for road vehicles or the usual licensing procedures for vehicle and driver. The size and marketing of many off-road vehicles are clearly targeted at children and adolescents.

Although minibikes may be considered the most benign because of their low horsepower, they carry an injury per vehicle rate four times that of bicycles. Trail bikes, which are more powerful, account for 33,000 injuries a year, more than one-third to children younger than 14 years. Although trail bikes are not intended for the roadway, many injury-producing crashes occur there and involve other motor vehicles.

In 1986, almost 30,000 children between 5 and 14 years of age were injured riding all-terrain vehicles (ATVs). ATVs come in three- or four-wheel versions and are marketed for use on rugged terrain. The three-wheeled version is notably unstable with overturns on slopes leading to catastrophic injury. A ban on the sale of three-wheeled ATVs in the United States became effective in December 1987, but many are still in use. Manufacturers have agreed that high-powered ATVs should not be marketed to children younger than 16 years, but dealer compliance is thought to be less than perfect. High speeds; lack of differential on the rear wheels, which makes turning difficult, especially for children; and vehicle weight all contribute to the high risk.

Snowmobiles, capable of reaching high speeds, also take a heavy toll among the pediatric age groups. Of the 12,000 to 13,000 injuries in 1 year, almost 20% were to children 14 years or younger, with persons between 15 and 24 years of age incurring almost one-half of all injuries. Given the seasonal and regional limitations on snowmobile use, the injury rate appears quite high. Although some states require registration of snowmobiles, few put restrictions on driver age. Head injuries from crashes and rollovers cause most of the deaths, but drowning is also important because snowmobiles are often operated over frozen bodies of water. The low profile of the snowmobile may make it especially difficult for motorists to see when operated on or near the roadway.

PREVENTION

The vehicles discussed in this section, especially the heavy and powerful ones, carry a very high injury risk. They are not toys. Operation of motorized vehicles by persons under the legal driving age should be strongly discouraged. Careful instruction by an experienced and mature operator should precede operation at any age, and helmets and protective clothing should be worn. Adults should be discouraged from carrying children as passengers on these vehicles, but if they do, they should be experienced drivers, sober, and willing to drive slowly.

COUNSELING POINTS

Counseling, although unstudied for this subject, might include information about avoiding motorcycles and off-road vehicles for children younger than driving age, discouraging the use of motorcycles and off-road vehicles by adolescents because of the high rate of serious injury, using helmets and other protective clothing for operators and passengers, and avoiding use of off-road vehicles on public roads because other motor vehicles may be encountered.

ADVOCACY ISSUES
Advocacy issues include regulating the marketing and sales of the products to children, licensing of operators and minimum age requirements, prohibiting the use of off-road vehicles on public roads, and enforcement of helmet laws.

Bicycles

INCIDENCE
Children and adolescents are disproportionately represented among the bicyclists killed in the United States. The death rate is highest for children between the ages of 10 and 14 years. Bicyclist deaths account for approximately 15% of all transportation-related deaths during those years. Nine of ten bicycling deaths involve collision of the bicyclist with a motor vehicle, and most involve head or neck injury. Male riders have higher injury rates and much higher death rates than female riders.

Most injuries and deaths occur during warm months and in the afternoon or early evening. The weekend is not a particularly vulnerable time, as it is for other motor vehicle deaths, probably because alcohol abuse does not play as large a part. Rates also vary less with urbanization, socioeconomic status, and region.

Children are often seriously injured when they ride out of a driveway, side street, or alley into the path of a motor vehicle. Cyclist error can be identified as a precipitating factor in many crashes, although this is unlikely to be the most fruitful area for prevention. Collisions during street riding occur most often at intersections or when the cyclist is riding against traffic.

Although collisions with motor vehicles are more likely to result in severe injury or death, falls from bicycles are much more common with some resulting in serious head injuries or fractures of the extremities. The quality of the riding surface affects the likelihood of a fall. Also contributing to injury are mechanical failure, clothing entanglement, stunt riding, and double riding. Infants and young children carried on the back of an adult's bicycle are a special case of double riding. The extra weight of the passenger makes the bicycle more difficult to maneuver and to stop. Without a special carrier that shields and restrains the child, the child may fall from the bicycle or get feet or legs caught in bicycle spokes. The infant passenger is vulnerable during any crash.

The pressure of the handlebars or seat can cause neuropathy or perineal irritation. Falls on the top bar of the boy's-style bike cause straddle injuries, and abdominal injuries result from falls on the handlebars.

PREVENTION
Whenever and wherever possible, bicyclists, especially child bicyclists, should be separated from motor vehicle traffic. All cyclists should wear helmets, because most serious injuries and deaths are caused by head injury. Helmets can reduce the likelihood of brain injury in a crash or fall by as much as 88%.

COUNSELING POINTS
Counseling should include, as the highest priority, the proven strategy of always wearing a helmet. Additional counseling points might include carrying infants in a special protective seat, preventing young children from riding in the street or on the road, stressing the importance to older children and adolescents of obeying traffic rules when riding on the road, avoiding riding after dark, using lights and reflective clothing, and buying a bike of the correct size.

ADVOCACY ISSUES
Advocacy issues include bicycle helmet laws, separating bicycle and motor vehicle traffic, decreasing the speed of motor vehicles on shared roadways, and improving the riding surface.

INJURIES NOT INVOLVING MOTOR VEHICLES

Drowning

INCIDENCE
Drowning (i.e., death from submersion) is second only to transportation injuries as a cause of unintentional injury death for children and adolescents accounting for approximately 1,500 deaths each year. Drowning death rates peak at 1 to 2 years of age and rise again in older adolescence. The increased drowning risk experienced by boys is apparent at a very early age, but it becomes even more exaggerated in adolescence when male drowning death rates are almost ten times higher than rates for girls of the same age.

Most toddler and preschooler drownings occur when a briefly unattended child falls into a body of water. One-third of these drownings, approximately 250 each year, take place in swimming pools, often at home. The increasing popularity of home whirlpools, hot tubs, and spas is providing a new place for young children to drown. Infants and toddlers can drown in any amount of water that is sufficiently deep to cover the nose and mouth; diaper pail, toilet bowl, large bucket, and bathtub drownings occur. Older children, adolescents, and adults also inadvertently fall into water and drown, and approximately one-third of unintentional drowning deaths occur that way. Only one-fourth of the drowning victims were swimming before death. Of those, most were not swimming in designated areas but in unsupervised rivers, creeks, or quarries. Drowning while scuba diving, skin diving, or surfing make up only a small fraction of all cases. Most boating-related drownings are associated with small recreational boats. Drowning follows a boat's capsize or a fall overboard. Personal flotation devices were not often available or were not in use.

Drownings are more likely to occur on weekends and during the warm months. Alcohol is involved in many adolescent drownings. The number of boating drownings has decreased modestly and other drownings more dramatically, with the largest decrease for those between 5 and 19 years of age. Although drowning deaths among adolescents are declining, those deaths among toddlers have changed little despite considerable understanding of how they occur.

Water is associated with additional injury hazards. For instance, diving where the water depth is inadequate accounts for approximately 700 spinal cord injuries a year, a significant proportion of all such injuries. Body surfing is also associated with spinal cord injuries. Hair can become trapped or body parts affixed by the suction developed by improperly grated pool and spa drains resulting in submersion injury.

PREVENTION
Home water hazards should be eliminated. An adult should never leave the room with an infant in the bathtub, not even for a few seconds. Children should not play in or near water without supervision. Wherever possible, fixed physical barriers should prevent young children from accessing water hazards. Particularly important is the requirement for unbreachable fencing around all four sides of swimming pools. For home pools, this separates the pool from the house and yard. Swimming and boating should be permitted only in designated areas, after adequate training, and with supervision by an adult who has not

been drinking alcohol. All persons in boats should wear personal flotation devices.

COUNSELING POINTS

Counseling includes advice on adult monitoring of infants and young children during bathing, maintaining constant visual contact by an adult of young children in and around water, isolation fencing of pools, decreasing water hazards in a young child's environment, discouraging swimming lessons for infants because of the risk of water intoxication and hypothermia, swimming and boating in designated areas only, wearing personal flotation devices, avoiding use of alcohol during water-related recreation, and cardiopulmonary resuscitation training for pool owners.

ADVOCACY ISSUES

Advocacy issues include requiring four-sided pool fencing, draining or fencing quarries and other sites where water may pool over hidden hazards, decreasing alcohol consumption during water-related activities, and enforcing requirements for use of personal flotation devices.

Fires and Burns

INCIDENCE

Fires and burns cause more than 1,000 child and adolescent deaths each year. House fires cause most injuries. Most persons who die in house fires die of smoke inhalation and are dead before rescue and medical attention arrive. House fire death rates are highest for young children and the elderly. Both groups are disadvantaged in at least two ways. They are less able to escape after fire breaks out, and they have high fatality rates with burn injury. Although male subjects have higher fire and burn death rates, the disparity between the genders is not so great as for some other kinds of injuries.

Only approximately 10% of house fires are attributed to children playing with matches or other ignition sources. Cigarettes are a much more common cause. Typically, a cigarette falls onto upholstery or a bed during the evening hours and smolders there until conflagration breaks out in the early morning hours while the residents sleep. Heating equipment (e.g., portable heaters, chimney fires, wood sparks) is the next most prominent cause of residential fires. Improperly installed or maintained heaters also cause deaths from carbon monoxide poisoning. Approximately 5% of fire fatalities occur in fires attributed to arson.

Racial differences in death rates are particularly pronounced for young children with black and Native American death rates at least twice as high as for whites. These rates are partially explained by socioeconomic differences, because the disparity decreases in high-income areas. Death rates are lower for blacks and whites in areas with higher per capita income. House fires occur more commonly in the winter and on the weekend, the latter perhaps reflecting a period of increased alcohol use.

Although house fire death rates had been increasing, that trend reversed in the early 1980s, and childhood deaths from other thermal injuries have decreased even more. Clothing ignition burns, although second to house fires as a cause of death in the fires and burns category and once relatively common for young girls, account for only approximately 4% of all burn deaths and are now rare in children. Gasoline and automotive burns are important in adolescence. Although decreasing, fire and burn injury is still of marked significance because of the proportion of injury fatalities for which it is responsible and because of the terrible toll of pain, prolonged medical treatment, and permanent disfigurement it exacts.

Scald and contact burns are an important cause of injury morbidity in childhood. Hot liquids, often coffee or the liquid spilled from a cooking pot, cause most childhood burn hospitalizations. Another major source of scald burns is hot water from the tap. Burns from contact with a hot object, including the iron, stove, oven, hot comb, grill, cooking pot, heater grate, lighted cigarette, and fireworks, are common in childhood. Although occasionally severe or permanently damaging, these burns usually affect a more limited skin area and are, therefore, more easily treated than scalds. Burns to the face, eyes, hands, and genitals are particularly likely to result in long-term developmental problems.

Some contact burns and hot water scalds are inflicted by the caregiver or result from willful neglect. Often, however, the circumstances of injury remain in doubt. Some prevention strategies may protect without regard to intent. If water from the tap is not hot enough to burn infant skin, the injury would be prevented no matter what the intent.

PREVENTION

The greatest gains in preventing fire and burn injuries can be made by the elimination and early detection of house fires. Working smoke detectors should be on every floor of every home. Self-extinguishing cigarettes, child-resistant cigarette lighters, and elimination of substandard heating and wiring are all helpful. Although it has a smaller effect on mortality statistics, decreasing hot water temperature can decrease morbidity, as can measures that redesign products (e.g., wide-based cups, coffee pots that do not tip) to reduce other sources of scald and contact burns.

The severity of burns can be decreased by immediately cooling the burned skin by immersing it in cool water or applying a cool wet pack.

COUNSELING POINTS

Counseling includes advice on having working smoke detectors on every floor of the home, turning down the hot water heater so that tap water is not more than 120°F to 125°F, avoiding cigarette-initiated fires, planning escape routes in case of fire, placing home fire extinguishers near locations where fires are likely to start (e.g., kitchen), keeping ignition sources away from children, using safe home heating, avoiding private use of fireworks, learning "drop and roll" in case of clothing ignition, and cooling a burn.

ADVOCACY ISSUES

Advocacy issues include smoke detector requirements, fire-safe cigarettes, childproof cigarette lighters, automatic sprinkler systems in new buildings, building codes that prevent house fire deaths, and firework bans except for community displays.

Asphyxiation

INCIDENCE

A major cause of injury death during infancy is asphyxiation by choking or by mechanical suffocation. Choking on food or other items kills more than 100 children each year. Child fatalities are concentrated among children younger than 4 years with the peak occurring in the first year. Round, firm food products (e.g., pieces of hot dog, candy, nuts, raw vegetables, grapes) are the most common airway-blocking agents in early childhood. In addition, small objects like round or pliable toys (e.g., small balls, uninflated balloons), soda pop tops, safety pins, coins, and pieces of makeshift pacifiers, bottle nipples, or plastic-lined disposable diapers can also choke young children. Older children and adults usually choke on meat.

Asphyxiation can occur when the child is trapped in an airtight space or when the child's airway is constricted from the outside, as in hanging. Crib strangulations occur when the baby's relatively small body slips between the bars and the head, too large to follow, is trapped. Current Consumer Product Safety Commission (CPSC) regulations for slat spacing for new cribs ($2^3/_8$ in. or less) prevent such events, but old cribs must be checked.

Children are also asphyxiated in inadvertent hangings in drapery, pacifier, clothing, or toy cords; when lids fall on them as they peer inside a toy chest; when they are trapped between frame and mattress of a bed or in the folds of a mesh playpen; when nose and mouth are covered in a soft basket, pillow, beanbag, or waterbed; when, unattended, they slip out of a high chair; inside plastic bags; in old refrigerators; in excavations that collapse; or when inadvertently covered by materials such as grain in the farm environment. The likely events vary with age.

Part of the apparent decrease in asphyxiation deaths among babies since the 1960s is an artifact of coding changes for sudden infant death syndrome (SIDS), but a decrease has also been noted in the 1- to 4-year age group, reflecting, in part, a decrease in refrigerator entrapments after changes in design and disposal of these appliances.

PREVENTION

Parents can be taught what to do if a child chokes and can be cautioned about household choking and suffocation hazards such as foods that may block the airway of a young child and unsafe crib designs. The most promising prevention strategies, however, are probably those strategies that involve redesign and regulation of hazardous products.

COUNSELING POINTS

Counseling includes advice on avoiding foods and nonfood objects on which infants and toddlers are likely to choke; avoiding cords in children's clothing or environments in which they may hang; purchasing age-appropriate toys so that toys for young children do not have small parts; ensuring a safe sleeping environment for infants (e.g., crib slat space no more than $2^3/_8$ in.; no soft enveloping surfaces); avoiding entrapment hazards; explaining the danger of earthen caves, tunnels, and excavations; and knowing rescue techniques for choking.

ADVOCACY ISSUES

Advocacy issues include regulation of hazardous toys and children's furniture, building and playground codes and regulations, clothing designs that eliminate cords, and fencing of construction sites and excavations.

Unintentional Firearm Injuries

INCIDENCE

Children in the United States have a uniquely high risk of being shot. As with burn injuries, intent is not always easy to judge. Guns in this culture are widely available and over all age groups are responsible for 2% of all unintentional injury deaths, approximately two-thirds of homicides, and more than one-half of suicides. Children can be the victims of all three. Unintentional shootings kill several hundred and severely injure many additional children and adolescents each year. Even more children and adolescents are murdered with guns. Suicide, most often accomplished with a gun, is the third leading cause of death in male adolescents, exceeded only by unintentional injuries and homicide. Nonwhite adolescent boys are more likely to be murdered with a gun than to die in any other way.

No other type of injury shows such a strong inverse association with socioeconomic status. Rates for unintentional firearm deaths are ten times higher in low-income areas than in high-income areas and are highest in rural and remote areas. Boys and men are at highest risk, with a male-to-female ratio of 6:1 for unintentional shootings.

Boys between the ages of 13 and 17 years have the highest rates of unintentional shooting deaths. The most common scenario for unintentional shootings is for one child to shoot another at home with a gun kept by an adult, ostensibly for the family's safety. Although unintentional firearm deaths have been decreasing, suicides and homicides have increased for adolescents and children, respectively. The presence of a gun in the home increases the risk of adolescent suicide.

Although some fiercely assert the right of the individual to keep a gun for protection, the fact remains that a gun in the home is much more likely to kill a family member than an intruder. Children cannot be trusted to handle a gun safely, even though they quickly acquire the mechanical skill and strength to fire one. No amount of exhortation is enough to ensure that they will not make a deadly error. What effect television or toy gun play has on the number of gun injuries in this country is not clear. Nonpowder firearms, often provided to children as toys, are clearly associated with high injury rates.

PREVENTION

Children should never have access to firearms. If parents choose to own guns, the unloaded guns should be locked away and kept in a separate location from ammunition. If parents allow older children to learn to shoot, such training should be under the strictest supervision.

COUNSELING POINTS

Counseling includes advice about the danger of guns in the home, safe storage of firearms, removal of firearms from the homes of suicidal adolescents, and the danger of nonpowder firearms as toys.

ADVOCACY ISSUES

Advocacy issues include laws that prohibit access to firearms by minors and control the manufacture, sale, and use of handguns. The sale and use of nonpowder firearms should also be addressed.

Acute Poisoning

INCIDENCE

Most deaths from acute poisoning are among adults. Two pediatric age groups incur most of the childhood poisoning events: children between the ages of 1 and 4 years (fewer than 100 deaths per year) and adolescents between the ages of 13 and 19 (approximately 150 unintentional deaths per year). For every death, more than 20 hospitalizations occur. Centers belonging to the American Association of Poison Control Centers, which cover 60% of the U.S. population, record more than 800,000 calls a year about children and adolescents. More than one-half of all calls to poison centers concern children, but children younger than 5 years comprise only 1% of poisoning fatalities. Most fatalities among the young are secondary to ingested drugs: aspirin, antidepressants, and cardiovascular drugs. Petroleum products make up the second-largest category in the youngest age group. Caustics, although much less frequently involved, remain a source of particularly damaging ingestions.

A satisfying decrease in the number of early childhood poisoning deaths has occurred, partially because of the vigorous efforts of many health care professionals and a combination of strategies. The sharpest decline followed the introduction of child-resistant packaging in 1970, after legislation required that toxic substances accessible to children be sold in containers difficult for a young child to open. Effort is required to sustain and extend this success, and acute poisoning still results in many hospital admissions and emergency department visits for children. Adolescent intentional poisoning deaths (i.e., suicides) have not decreased but are covered in Chapter 59.

Children and adolescents are not exempt from carbon monoxide poisoning from car exhaust and faulty heating systems. For all ages taken together, carbon monoxide from motor vehicle exhaust is the most common agent in poisoning deaths. Many unintentional deaths result from motor vehicle exhaust each year. Deaths peak in adolescence for girls and women and early adulthood for boys and men. Rates are higher in low-income and rural areas and during the coldest months. Suicidal deaths from carbon monoxide are much more common than unintentional deaths.

PREVENTION

The key to preventing unintentional and intentional poisonings is to prevent access to lethal quantities of chemicals. This can be done in several ways, but the more automatic the approach (i.e., the less it depends on a caregiver's watchfulness), the better.

COUNSELING POINTS

Counseling includes advice on keeping medications in a locked cabinet, buying medications in modest amounts and in child-resistant packages, safe storage of poisonous substances, knowing when and how to call the Poison Control Center, keeping syrup of ipecac in the home for use as a postingestion emetic when recommended by a physician or Poison Control Center, maintaining the home heating system and car exhaust system, and eliminating hazardous chemicals (e.g., kerosene, caustics) from the home environment.

ADVOCACY ISSUES

Advocacy issues include maintaining and extending requirements for child-resistant packaging, continuing the practice of packaging antipyretics for children in sublethal total doses, and supporting regionalized Poison Control Centers.

Falls

INCIDENCE

Approximately 13,000 deaths are attributed to falls each year, but most of these occur among adults and partly reflect the high injury and fatality rates in the elderly. In 1993, more than 200 children and adolescents suffered fatal falls. The highest pediatric fall death rates are in the very early years and during adolescence. Most fatal falls in these age groups are from extreme heights.

Falls are the most common cause of nonfatal injury. Every year, 1 in 20 persons receive medical care for injuries sustained in a fall. Falls are the leading cause of unintentional injury emergency department visits for children and a prominent cause of hospitalization. Falls are an important cause of brain injury.

Falls can occur on the same level (e.g., slipping while walking on an icy sidewalk), from one surface to another (e.g., off a bed or changing table to the floor, down stairs), from a vehicle (e.g., a car, pickup truck, bike), or from a height (e.g., out of an upper-story window, off the slide).

Falls are common at all ages, but the peak incidence of medically treated falls is 1 year of age. In contrast to the figure of 1 in 20 for the whole population, each year, 1 in 10 children between the ages of 1 and 3 years receives emergency treatment for a fall. Of these, approximately one-eighth fell down stairs, and stair-related falls constitute approximately one-fourth of hospital series. Most of the other hospitalized children fell from one surface to another.

Little variation is seen between high- and low-income areas or between urban and rural areas in overall morbidity and mortality from falls, but the specific events vary. Illustrating the special risks of the environment and the success of intervention is the decrease in fatal falls of children from New York City high-rise apartment windows after the Board of Health's program to install guards on the windows of apartments with young children.

Several risk situations have been implied by the examples used here, and no list can be exhaustive, but several additional common or severe types of falls should be mentioned. Most injuries that occur on playgrounds result from falls. Baby walkers appear to be associated with a very high risk, particularly because of their propensity for being ridden down unguarded stairways, and they cannot be recommended as safe. Falls from vehicles (e.g., from the back of a pickup truck) and falls that occur while playing on roofs, in trees, on bridges, or other elevated structures affect older children and adolescents and are likely to be severe. Falls associated with recreation are common in childhood and adolescence (e.g., from a skateboard, bicycle, horse, or playground equipment). Work-related falls such as from scaffolding or ladders, also occur in adolescence. The health provider must remember that many inflicted injuries are falsely attributed to falls.

The forces that cause injury in a fall depend on velocity at impact, which is determined by the height of the fall and the stopping distance. A fall from a greater height is more serious. Although not so intuitively obvious, it is better to stop slowly (i.e., to decelerate over a greater distance). The compressibility of the surface and of the presenting body part are important. Contrast the head of a toddler landing on cement with the buttocks landing on a thick carpet; the laws of physics and clinical experience predict much less damage in the latter situation. Surfaces that allow increased distance for deceleration are referred to as "forgiving" and are greatly preferred where children are likely to fall.

PREVENTION

Environmental redesign has much to offer in protecting all segments of the population from falls. Falls from a height should be prevented by barriers. Where falls are predictable, forgiving surfaces should be in place to cushion the child who falls.

COUNSELING POINTS

Counseling includes advice on choosing not to use a baby walker, timing of the move from crib to a low bed, guarding stairways with special gates in homes with toddlers, using restraining belts on baby furniture (e.g., high chairs, changing tables) and constant attendance of babies on high surfaces, installing screens that cannot be pushed out by a child or window guards on all open windows above the first story, choosing safe home playground equipment and installing it over a forgiving surface, using protective equipment and helmets where appropriate for recreational activities, using side rails on bunk beds, and not allowing children to ride in a vehicle in which they cannot ride restrained (e.g., the back of a pickup truck).

ADVOCACY ISSUES

Advocacy issues include the design and regulation of baby walkers, the design and use of furniture for children, window guard regulations, code specifications of guard rails small children cannot climb over or fall through, playground design and regulations, provision of forgiving surfaces where children are likely to fall, and building codes that reduce falls on steps.

ANTICIPATORY GUIDANCE

Health care providers cannot ignore in their professional encounters with children and adolescents the primary cause of morbidity and mortality. Discussion of every possible event and safety measure, however, would overwhelm both practitioner and patient. Although specific research on the subject has not been done, injury control experts think it is doubtful that counseling on more than three or four issues at a single visit can be effective. Issues must be chosen for emphasis. When the practitioner follows a child through time, advice can be staged in an age-appropriate schedule (Table 45-1).

ADVOCACY

Clinicians can be pivotal in the community approach to injury control by providing consultation, urging design changes, testifying for legislation, informing regulations, and ensuring that the trauma system serves children well. Many of the gains recorded in injury control have resulted from such open advocacy on the part of health care workers.

TABLE 45-1. Age-Appropriate Injury Prevention Topics and Advice

Age	Advice for prevention
0 to <1 yr	
Car crashes, falls, choking, suffocation, fires, burns, drowning, poisoning	Use a safe car seat correctly. Never leave infants alone on high places. Avoid baby walkers. Keep small objects, hard foods, and harmful substances out of reach. Never leave a child alone in or near water, hot liquids, or any heat source. Install a smoke detector. Have syrup of ipecac in the home. Write Poison Control Center number on the home phone. Know how to save a choking child. Lower hot water heater to 120–125°F.
1–2 yr	
Poisoning, falls, choking, fires, burns, drowning, car crashes	Use safety caps on medications. Store all toxic household products and medicines out of reach. Use window screens that cannot push out and gates. Keep toddler in an enclosed space and closely supervised when outdoors. Keep electrical cords and handles of pots and pans on stove out of reach, and keep hot foods away from edge of table. Never leave child in a tub or pool. Use toddler car seat. Eliminate or safely store firearms.

(continued)

TABLE 45-1. *(Continued)*

Age	Advice for prevention
2–4 yr	
Falls, fires, burns, poisoning, drowning, car crashes, pedestrian injury	Keep doors to dangerous areas locked. Use screens, guards, and gates. Keep firearms locked up. Teach children about watching for cars in driveways and streets and danger of following ball into street, but continue to supervise. Keep medicines, knives, electrical equipment, and matches out of reach. Arrange group swimming lessons after 3 years of age. Never leave child in a tub or pool. Use toddler car seat and then belt-positioning booster seat. Continue to keep syrup of ipecac in the home. Teach children to avoid unknown animals.
5–9 yr	
Car crashes, pedestrian injury, bicycle injury, drowning firearms, burns	Teach pedestrian, motor vehicle, and bicycle safety. Use seat belts and bicycle helmets. Do not allow bicycling on roadway before 10 years of age. Continue swimming classes. Supervise around water. Keep firearms locked up. Avoid off-road motor vehicle use. Supervise use of matches.
10–15 yr	
Car crashes, pedestrian injury, bicycle injury, firearms, drowning, burns, falls	Continue rules of bicycle, pedestrian, and motor vehicle safety, with good examples set by adults. Insist no seat belts and bicycle helmets. Discourage night bicycle riding and riding of off-road and other motorized vehicles. Discourage nonpowder firearms. Provide safe facilities for recreation and social activities. Stress the buddy system in all sports. Prohibit unsupervised swimming or boating. Discourage alcohol use. Eliminate or safely store firearms.
16–19 yr	
Car crashes, drowning, pedestrian injury, other motorized vehicles, firearms, suicide, homicide	Provide appropriate driver's education. Insist on seat belt use. Insist on helmets for bicycling and for riding other motorized vehicles. Prohibit driving or swimming when under the influence of alcohol or other drugs. Prohibit firearms except under the most stringent safety and training conditions.

Adapted from McIntire MS, ed. *Injury control for children and youth,* 2nd ed. Elk Grove Village, IL. American Academy of Pediatrics, 1987.

2a
Common Ambulatory Issues—General Topics

CHAPTER 46

Pediatric Dermatology

Adapted from Walter W. Tunnessen, Jr. and Daniel P. Krowchuk

SKIN LESIONS IN THE NEONATAL PERIOD

(This section should be read in conjunction with Chapter 40, Neonatal Dermatology.)

Pigmented Macular Lesions

MONGOLIAN SPOT

Mongolian spot is an unfortunate name for this common, benign skin discoloration. Present at birth, mongolian spots are blue-gray or blue-green and represent areas of dermal melanocytosis. They occur most frequently in the lumbosacral area (Fig. 46-1) and over the shoulders. Occasionally, they are found on the anterior trunk and extremities; only rarely are they seen on the face. The occurrence of mongolian spots is related to the degree of natural pigment. The more pigment infants have, the more likely they are to have these spots. More than 90% of blacks and Asians have mongolian spots, whereas fewer than 10% of whites have them. Infants of Hispanic and Mediterranean heritage are more likely to have the spots than are infants of northern European ancestry.

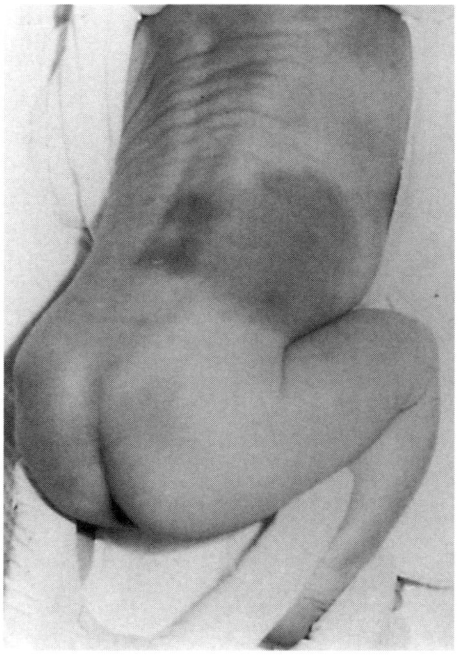

Figure 46-1. The blue-gray hyperpigmentation of mongolian spots is most common over the buttocks and back.

Although these lesions tend to disappear with time (usually by the ages of 4–5 years), the color change persists in 5% of children. Because mongolian spots have been mistaken for bruises associated with child abuse, educating parents and nursery or day-care workers regarding the congenital nature of the patches is important. The cause of these collections of melanocytes deep in the dermis is unknown. Because the spots are benign, no therapy is necessary. Malignant degeneration has not been reported.

CAFÉ AU LAIT SPOTS

Café au lait spots are macules of various shapes and sizes. Their color ranges from light to dark brown, the pigmentation is even throughout, and the margins are sharply defined. In a cohort of 4,641 newborns, 1.9% of black and 0.3% of white infants had at least one of these lesions. Black infants were more likely to have more than one lesion: Some 0.6% had two, and 0.2% had three or more. None of the white infants had more than one lesion. Multiple café au lait spots are associated with neurofibromatosis; they can also be seen in other syndromes (see Changes in Pigmentation, later in this chapter.)

Macular Vascular Birthmarks

FLAME NEVI

Flame nevi are the most common vascular lesions in infancy seen in almost one-half of all newborns. These dull-pink macules composed of distended dermal capillaries are most prevalent over the eyelids and forehead. Almost all infants with lesions on the face also have lesions on the nape of the neck and on the occiput. Facial lesions tend to fade with time, generally within the first years of life. Neck lesions, however, are likely to persist. The macules are often called salmon patches, stork bites, or angel kisses. During crying, older infants and children may demonstrate flushing in areas of previous lesions that have faded.

Hypopigmented Macules

Hypopigmented macules are present in 0.4% to 0.6% of newborn infants. Although the great majority of newborns with these macules are normal, the macules or patches of depigmented skin in such newborns may signify the presence of underlying problems. Small hypopigmented macules are an early cutaneous sign of tuberous sclerosis, an autosomal dominant inherited condition associated with seizures and mental retardation, among other things. Large patches or swirls of depigmentation may indicate the presence of Ito syndrome, a neurocutaneous disorder that affects various bodily systems including the central nervous system (CNS) and the bones. Infants who have piebaldism and who usually have depigmentation of the skin of the forehead and other areas may also have associated abnormalities including deafness. Most hypopigmented lesions probably represent a simple absence of pigment, known as a nevus depigmentosus.

Papules and Vesicles

MILIA

Multiple 1- to 2-mm yellowish white cystic lesions, known as milia, occur in some 40% of newborns. These lesions are found most commonly over the cheeks, forehead, nose, and nasolabial folds. Much less commonly, they may be found on the trunk or extremities. Histologically, the cysts are composed of keratin and are similar to Epstein pearls, the whitish papules noted on the palates of many newborns. Treatment is unnecessary; the cysts disappear in the first few weeks of life.

SEBACEOUS GLAND HYPERTROPHY

Stimulation of the sebaceous glands (which lie at the base of the pilosebaceous units) by maternal hormones often leads to the appearance of tiny, yellowish to flesh-colored papules over the face and, less commonly, at other sites on full-term newborns. Because the source of the stimulation is removed with birth, the appearance of these papules is transient, and clearing occurs in a few weeks. No therapy is necessary.

NEONATAL ACNE

Comedones (plugged pilosebaceous units), erythematous papules, and pustules—all resembling the acne of adolescence—may occur in the neonatal period, generally at 2 to 4 weeks of life. Male infants are affected primarily, and the lesions generally occur on the cheeks and are almost never seen on the chest and back. Hormonal stimulation of the sebaceous glands is thought to be responsible for the appearance of the lesions. Generally, the eruption disappears in weeks or months, and no therapy is required. Occasionally, in severe or prolonged cases, a mild keratolytic agent such as 2.5% benzoyl peroxide, can be prescribed. Pustules suggesting neonatal acne may be caused by Malassezia furfur yeast. A potassium hydroxide scraping may differentiate yeast from acne.

Bullous Lesions

EPIDERMOLYSIS BULLOSA CONGENITA

Newborns affected by the group of hereditary disorders that cause fragile skin often have bullae or erosions as a result of the trauma associated with birth or minimal trauma induced by handling and care after birth. These disorders are discussed more completely later in this chapter (see Vesicular and Bullous Eruptions).

CONGENITAL SYPHILIS

Bullae are an unusual presentation of congenital syphilis (Fig. 46-2). Most common on the extremities, they rupture rapidly leaving a raw, oozing surface. Ovoid, macular, slightly scaly, salmon-colored lesions are much more common; they generally appear between the age of 2 and 6 weeks (Fig. 46-3).

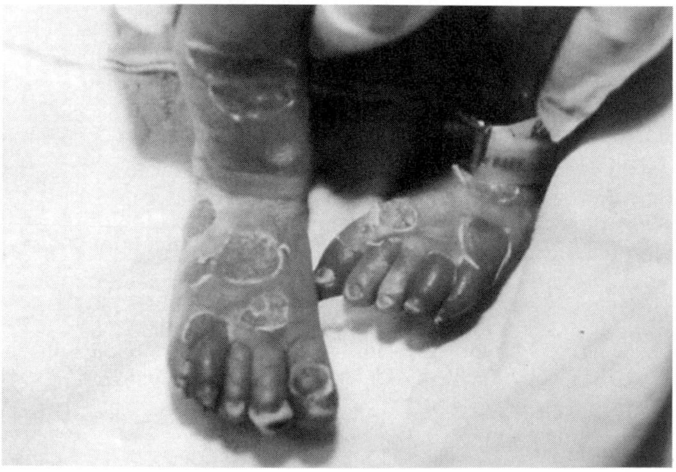

Figure 46-2. Pemphigus syphiliticus, a widely disseminated vesiculobullous eruption in an infant with early congenital syphilis. (Courtesy of Charles Ginsburg, M.D.) (See Color Fig. 46-2.)

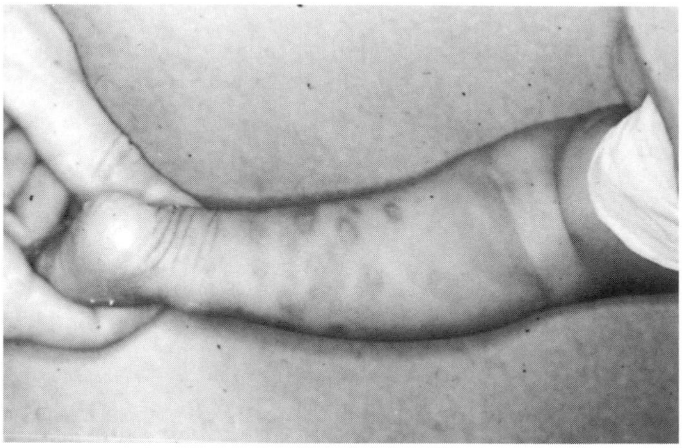

Figure 46-3. Ovoid, brownish lesions with a fine scale on the leg of a neonate with congenital syphilis.

Purpuric Lesions

CONGENITAL RUBELLA

Purpuric lesions of infants infected with rubella virus *in utero* are caused most commonly by thrombocytopenia. On occasion, the purpuric lesions take on an infiltrative or nodular quality producing a blueberry-muffin appearance (Fig. 46-4). The lesions are actually areas of extramedullary hematopoiesis rather than true cutaneous hemorrhage.

CONGENITAL CYTOMEGALOVIRUS INFECTION

Petechial lesions in conjunction with intrauterine growth retardation, hepatosplenomegaly, and hyperbilirubinemia should always raise the question of congenital infections. Cytomegalovirus is the most prevalent of these infections. Most of the purpuric lesions are the result of thrombocytopenia. Blueberry muffin-like lesions (Fig. 46-5) have also been documented.

Lumps and Indurations

SUBCUTANEOUS FAT NECROSIS

Irregular lumps and bumps may occur in the subcutaneous tissue of neonates, probably as a result of pressure or trauma

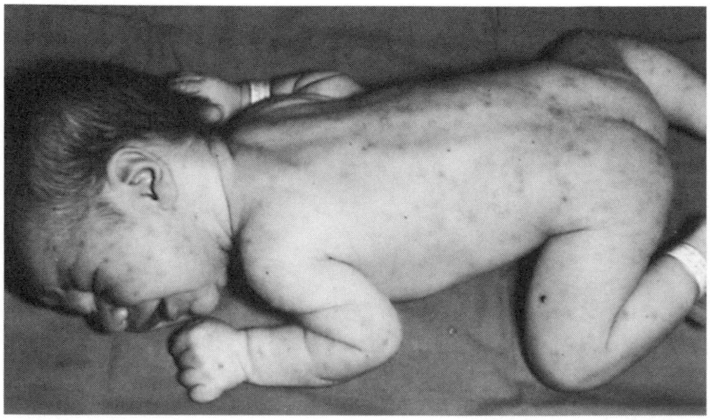

Figure 46-4. Diffuse, purplish papules and nodules create a blueberry-muffin appearance in an infant with congenital rubella.

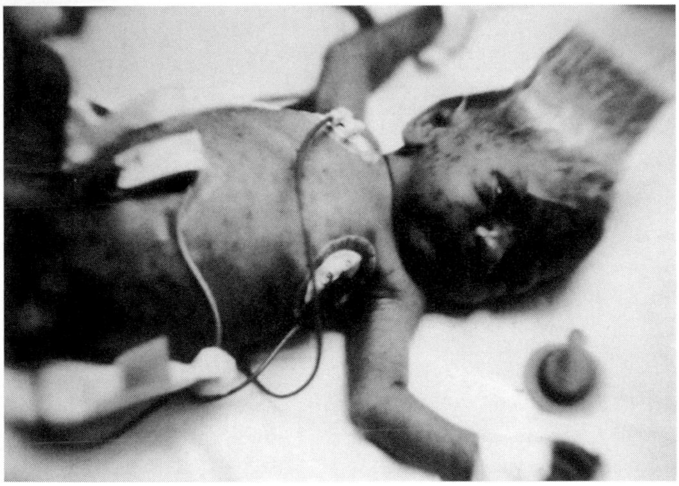

Figure 46-5. So-called blueberry-muffin spots. Extramedullary dermal erythropoiesis is observed in the most severely affected infants with congenital cytomegalovirus infection and congenital rubella. (See color Fig. 46-5.)

associated with the birth process. The areas most commonly affected are the cheeks, buttocks, back, arms, and thighs. The areas are irregular, hard, erythematous or violaceous, and they seem nontender. The size of the lumps varies. Occasionally, the lesions may become calcified, but generally they resolve spontaneously in 1 to 2 months without scarring. Some infants may develop symptomatic hypercalcemia. These lesions occur much less commonly later in life. No therapy is necessary.

PAPULAR DISORDERS

Warts

Warts are among the most common skin lesions affecting children; they are also among the most frustrating, because treating and controlling them is often difficult. Warts are caused by infections with human papillomaviruses, DNA viruses of which at least 70 different types have been described. Each type of human papillomavirus can usually be related to a specific clinical presentation of the wart. The highest incidence of these infections occurs in the second decade of life. Untreated warts generally have a life span of a few months to 5 years or more. Some two-thirds disappear within 2 years, but self-inoculation and spread to other persons may occur.

VERRUCAE VULGARIS

The common wart is recognized by most laypersons without difficulty. The surface of the wart is rough, sometimes lumpy, and usually flesh-colored. Occasional lesions, particularly those on the face and scalp, may be linear or have finger-like projections. The lesions are usually round, and tiny dark specks can frequently be seen through the surface. These dots are often termed the seed of the wart, but they merely represent thrombosed capillaries in the warty tissue.

PLANTAR WARTS

When warts occur on the plantar surface, pressure forces their growth inward resulting in deep, painful lesions. Plantar warts may be single, scattered, or grouped together in clusters. The black specks of thrombosed capillaries help to distinguish warts from corns, which are localized areas of hyperkeratosis over pressure points.

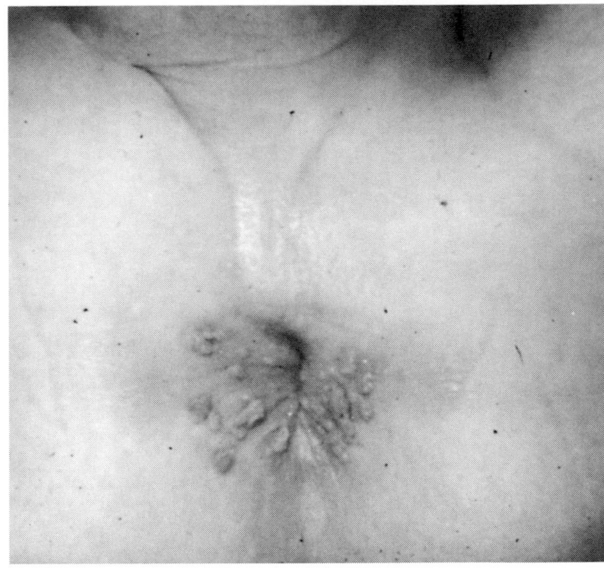

Figure 46-6. Flesh-colored papules of condylomata acuminata in the anal verge.

CONDYLOMATA ACUMINATA

Genital warts tend to be soft, flesh-colored to slightly pigmented, and papular or pedunculated (Fig. 46-6). The occurrence of genital warts in children should always raise the suspicion of sexual abuse; viral typing by molecular hybridization examinations has revealed that these lesions are of the same type as those affecting adults. In children younger than 2 years, the condition may simply be the result of the child having passed through a birth canal infected with papillomavirus. Some estimate that one-third or fewer of the venereal warts seen in children are the result of sexual abuse.

TREATMENT OF WARTS

When multiple therapies are recommended for a disorder, treatment is unlikely to yield excellent results. Such is the case with warts. Some clinicians use benign neglect, because warts have a finite life span. Parents and older children often desire treatment, so primary-care physicians should be able to make some recommendations. For common warts, keratolytic agents such as salicylic and lactic acids in flexible collodion, offer painless and effective, albeit slow-acting, therapy. Extremely important is soaking the warts in warm water for 10 to 20 minutes before "sanding" down the lesions with a pumice stone or an emery board and applying the keratolytic agent daily. Covering the wart with tape also seems to increase the effectiveness of the treatment. The application of liquid nitrogen and use of electrocautery are similarly effective, but these treatments are painful, particularly for small children. Plantar warts can be treated with higher-potency keratolytic agents that are applied after soaking and "sanding down." In resistant warts, cantharidin, a blistering agent, can be applied carefully to enhance removal.

Flat warts are tiny and scattered over wider areas. Retinoic acid A or salicylic acid may be applied lightly on a daily basis over the areas involved. Genital warts often respond to the weekly application of podophyllin in a tincture of benzoin base, which is washed off after 3 to 4 hours. Removal by laser therapy may be necessary.

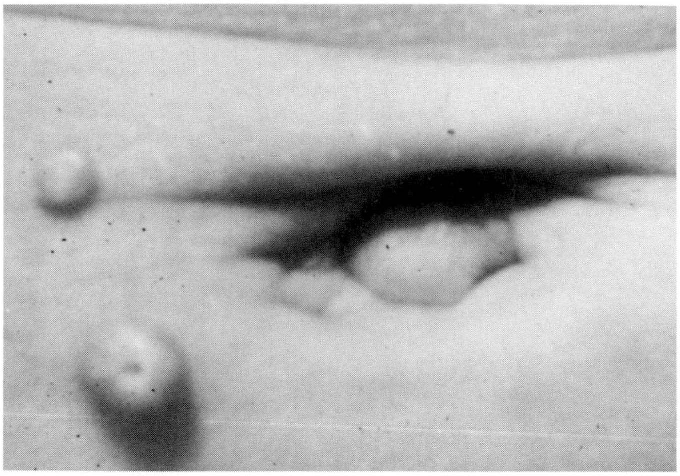

Figure 46-7. Pearly molluscum contagiosum papules on the abdomen. Note the central umbilication of the larger lesion.

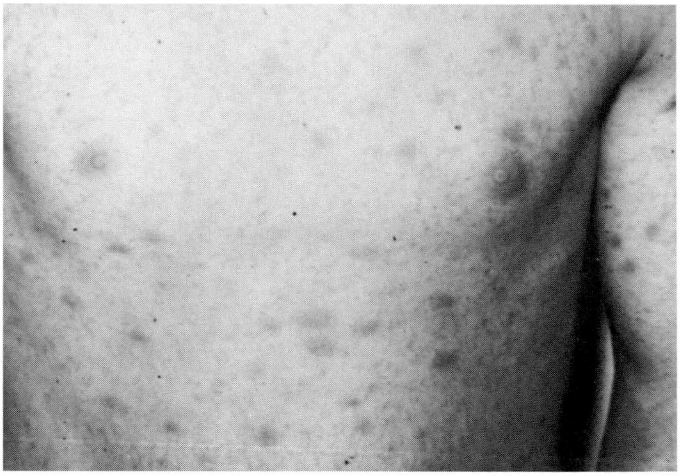

Figure 46-8. Pityriasis rosea. The diffuse erythematous papules may obscure the classic lesions, which are scattered, ovoid, pink plaques.

The success of the various therapies is said to be 70%. Therefore, more than one therapeutic approach may be necessary for each wart.

Molluscum Contagiosum

Lesions of molluscum contagiosum, caused by a DNA poxvirus, are described best as pearly papules. Their size may vary from that of a pinhead to more than 1 cm in diameter. The top of the lesion is almost translucent, often revealing a whitish core known as the molluscum body. Larger lesions may have a central umbilication (Fig. 46-7). The number of papules present may vary from few to hundreds. Spread by autoinoculation is common; other members of the family can become infected through contact with the affected person. The diagnosis may not be readily apparent on the basis of clinical examination alone; it may require opening of a lesion with a large-bore needle and extraction of the molluscum body.

Although some physicians recommend no treatment, the lesions have a life span of months to years, and parents frequently insist that something be done. In the presence of only a few lesions, they can be picked off or excised with a curet. Cantharidin, applied carefully in small amounts to each lesion, is effective in causing blistering and extrusion of the central core. This potent medication should be applied only by physicians or other trained personnel. Liquid nitrogen and podophyllin have also been used. Individuals with atopic dermatitis are prone to the development of widespread lesions.

Pityriasis Rosea

Although pityriasis rosea does not seem to fit neatly into the category of papular lesions, it is a papulosquamous disorder consisting of oval lesions composed of tiny papules with a fine scale. At times, individual papular lesions may be prominent. The presence of myriad individual papules occasionally confuses the diagnosis by rendering the ovoid lesions less noticeable (Fig. 46-8). The cause of pityriasis rosea is unknown but is believed by many to be viral. The disorder occurs most commonly in teenagers and young adults but has been described in infants. Recurrent episodes are not rare, and small epidemics have been reported among individuals in close contact.

The name pityriasis rosea means "rose-colored scale." The herald patch is a single, papular, erythematous lesion that enlarges over 1 to 2 days. It may precede the appearance of the more extensive rash, or it may not appear at all; its reported prevalence has varied in different series from 12% to 94%. At times, this raised lesion may be mistaken for tinea corporis. The interval between the appearance of the herald patch and the more generalized eruption is 1 to 2 weeks.

The typical ovoid lesions of pityriasis rosea have their longest axis along skin tension lines; thus, their distribution on the patient's back gives the appearance of the boughs of a pine tree. Often, viewing the child's rash from across the room is helpful for seeing the characteristic pattern. Individual lesions may have a pinkish to brownish color. Most lesions are covered by a fine, wrinkled scale.

The lengthy course of this disorder should be emphasized to the patient or the parents. The eruption itself develops over a 2-week period, persists for 2 weeks, then fades over another 2 weeks. This pattern varies greatly, however, and rashes lasting 3 to 4 months are not unusual. The lesions are generally distributed on the trunk, but a "reverse" distribution can also be seen, more commonly in black skin, with lesions appearing primarily on the face and proximal extremities. Occasionally, the lesions may have urticarial, bullous, or even purpuric tendencies. Pruritus is one of the most annoying features of pityriasis rosea occurring in up to one-half of the cases. Treatment with an emollient containing menthol and phenol is helpful. No therapy will shorten the course of the eruption.

The differential diagnosis includes dry nummular eczema and nummular dry skin. Because secondary syphilis can have a similar appearance, a serologic test for syphilis should be considered if the patient is in a sexually active age group. The histologic appearance of a skin biopsy specimen of pityriasis rosea lesions is nonspecific.

Keratosis Pilaris

Keratosis pilaris is a common, benign skin condition that usually goes unnoticed, unless it involves the face. The scattered follicular papules with an adherent scale are distributed most commonly on the extensor surfaces of the upper arms and thighs. The lesions are not grouped, are occasionally erythematous, and give the appearance of gooseflesh. They appear most commonly in the second decade of life and, when present on the face, can be mistaken for early comedonal acne. The cause of the follicular keratinous plugs is unknown, but they are most prone to appear in individuals with atopic dermatitis or ichthyosis. For patients who are distressed by the appearance of the lesions, mild keratolytics (emollients with 6%–12% lactic acid) can be used to reduce their prominence. On the face, retinoic acid may prove to be the most effective therapy.

Id Reaction

Dermatophyte infections, particularly tinea capitis, may be associated with the presence of myriad tiny flesh-colored papules, especially over the face, neck, and shoulders. The scalp infection may be subtle. The id reaction is more common after systemic antifungal therapy is begun. The id should not be mistaken for a drug reaction. The presence of papules, vesicles, and other lesions of the palms and fingers may suggest an id reaction caused by tinea pedis. Appropriate antifungal treatment of the site of infection will result in resolution of these papules.

Lichen Nitidus

The tiny papules in lichen nitidus are also flesh-colored, but their surface is smooth and shiny. They do not form the patterns seen in lichen spinulosus, although the areas of skin involved do have multiple lesions. The trunk, genitalia, abdomen, and forearms are affected most frequently. Linear lesions at sites of trauma, known as the *Koebner phenomenon*, are common. The cause is unknown, and the pinhead- to pinpoint-sized lesions have a variable course lasting months to years.

Lichen Planus

The papules in lichen planus, a disorder found mostly in adults, are characteristically polygonal. When the lesions are examined closely, the flat-topped papules seem to form rectangles, squares, and other shapes (Fig. 46-9). The classic lesions are violaceous and occur most frequently on the wrists and extensor surfaces of the forearms. They may coalesce to form plaques. Significant scaling of the lesions may occur on the lower extremities. Oral lesions, consisting of tiny white papules in lacy patterns, may occur on the buccal mucosa. Nail changes, including roughening of the nail surface or total dystrophy, are not common in children with lichen planus.

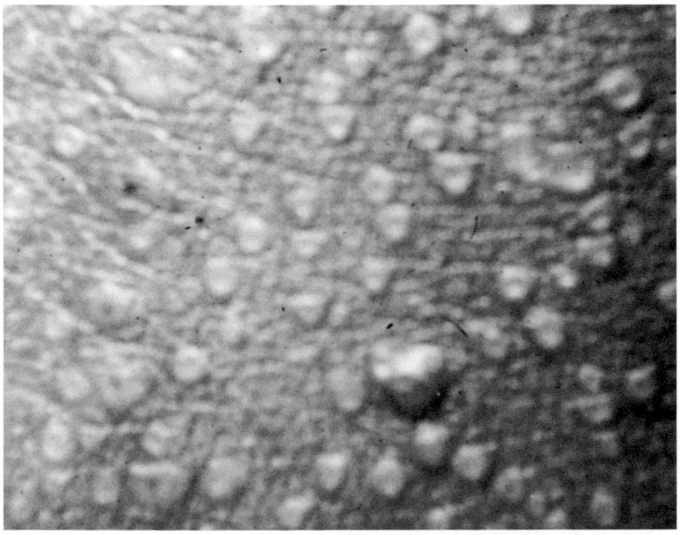

Figure 46-9. The classic papules of lichen planus are not only flat-topped, but also polygonal.

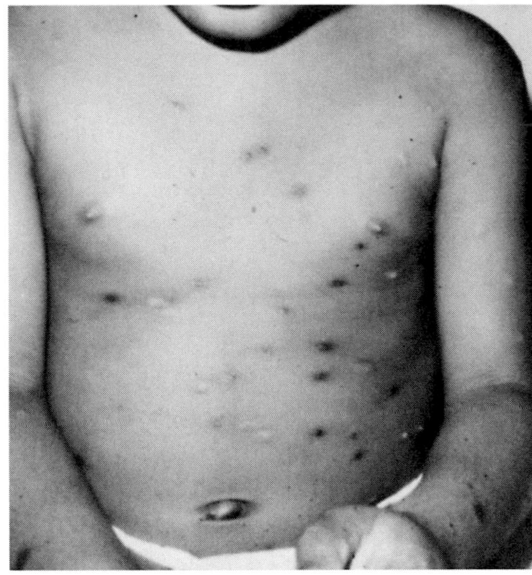

Figure 46-10. Papular urticaria. Old, hyperpigmented lesions and recent, erythematous papules with central puncta from flea bites.

Lichen planus is intensely pruritic. Excoriations can lead to secondary infection and to the occurrence of lesions in lines of trauma. The cause of the eruption is unknown, and the lesions persist for 8 to 18 months. Therapy is nonspecific, consisting of antihistamines for the pruritus and emollients for the associated dryness.

Red Papules

PAPULAR URTICARIA

Papular urticaria is a common, intensely pruritic disorder caused by hypersensitivity to insect bites. The fresh lesions are papules with an erythematous flare capped by a central punctum at the site of the bite (Fig. 46-10). Lesions generally appear in crops, particularly on exposed skin surfaces. Most cases occur in the late spring and summer, but household exposure to fleas from animals can cause problems any time of year. Not all lesions have a central punctum. Linear or irregular clusters may be related to localized reactions caused by immunoglobulins and complement released into surrounding vessels.

Fleas are the most common cause of papular urticaria. Mosquitoes and other biting insects may also produce the lesions. Secondary infections from excoriations are extremely common and, in some children, the wheals may progress to bullae. Treatment success depends on eliminating the biting insects from the child's environment and preventing insect bites. Permethrin applied to clothing may inhibit bites. Topical antipruritic agents may be of some help. Secondary infections also need to be treated. This severe reaction to the bites lasts 1 to 2 years.

GIANOTTI-CROSTI SYNDROME

Gianotti-Crosti syndrome, also known as papular acrodermatitis of childhood (PAC), has a distinctive clinical picture because of the predominant location of the erythematous papules on the face and extremities (Fig. 46-11). First described in Italy in 1955, it has received increasing attention throughout the world in association with a number of viruses. The papules are generally larger in infants (up to 5 mm) than in older children (2–3 mm);

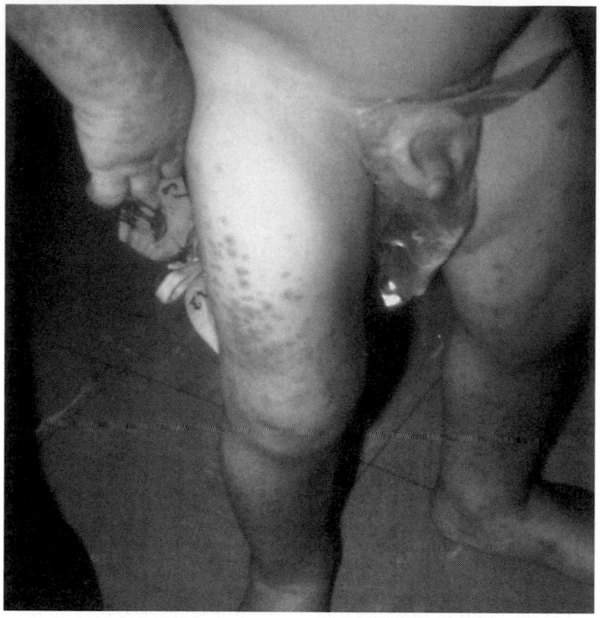

Figure 46-11. Diffuse reddish papules are present over the arms and legs, whereas the trunk is spared, in a patient with papular acrodermatitis of childhood.

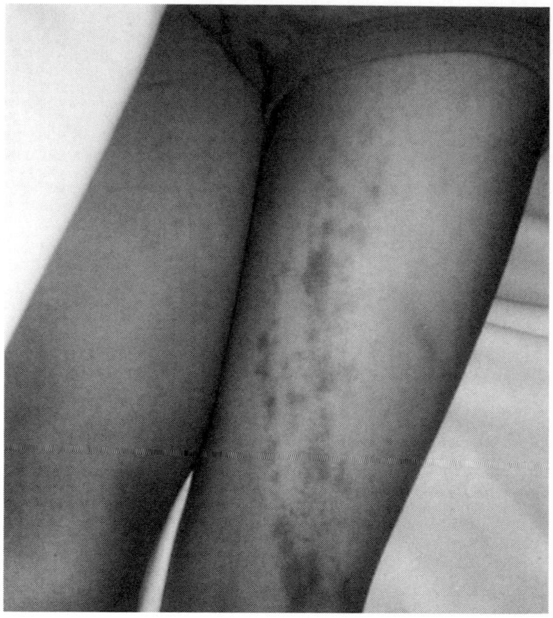

Figure 46-12. Linear arrangement of confluent papules in lichen striatus.

they tend to be of similar size, usually appear rapidly, and may be associated with pruritus. One of the features of this exanthem that is most distressing to parents is its long duration, often 3 to 5 weeks.

Discussion in the literature addresses the cause of PAC and the need to differentiate it from another, similar rash. Some feel that PAC is a distinct syndrome, often associated with hepatitis B surface antigenemia (HB_sAg; subtype ayw). Affected children have hepatosplenomegaly, lymphadenopathy, and laboratory evidence of hepatitis. The lesions are said to be nonpruritic and, occasionally, purpuric. This association is rarely found in the United States, but it is prevalent in Italy and Japan.

Those who believe PAC to be part of a distinct syndrome refer to similar rashes associated with other viruses as papular or papulovesicular acral-located syndromes (PAS). In PAS, pruritus is common, hepatomegaly is uncommon, and HB_sAg is always lacking. Occasionally, juicy papules may have a vesicular appearance. PAS also has a prolonged course. Viruses found in association with PAS include Epstein-Barr virus, parainfluenza virus, coxsackievirus A16, cytomegalovirus, poliomyelitis virus, and respiratory syncytial virus.

Regardless of whether PAC and PAS are classified singly or together, their association with HB_sAg should be recognized, particularly in certain countries. The exanthem is much more common than is generally recognized. The distinctive distribution and duration of the papules should help in making the clinical diagnosis. The rash is regarded best as a self-limited cutaneous response to a viral infection.

Linear Papules

LICHEN STRIATUS

Lichen striatus, a self-limited eruption most common in children, is characterized by the rapid development of multiple tiny, discrete papules arranged in a linear, band-like pattern over an extremity (Fig. 46-12). The bands may be 1 cm to several centimeters in width, irregular or fairly uniform, and continuous or interrupted; they occur most commonly on the upper extremities. The papules may be scaly and are generally flesh-colored, although in black individuals, a hypopigmented discoloration may be prominent. The cause of this distinctive lesion is unknown. It tends to have a duration of a few weeks to as long as a year. Topical steroids and keratolytics may hasten its resolution. Linear epidermal nevi, linear psoriasis, and linear lichen planus are included in the differential diagnosis.

INCONTINENTIA PIGMENTI

Incontinentia pigmenti is a neurocutaneous disorder characterized by a rash that may progress through four distinct stages. The first, which is usually present at birth, consists of papules and vesicles distributed linearly (Fig. 46-13). These lesions, which may fade in weeks or months, are often followed by the second

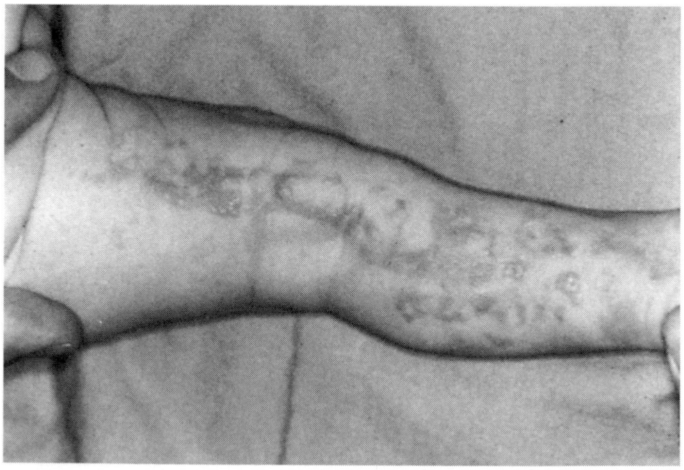

Figure 46-13. Papulovesicular lesions of incontinentia pigmenti in a linear distribution on the flexor surface of one leg.

stage: linear verrucous lesions. These wart-like lesions also fade gradually after several months. The pigmented stage follows, although not necessarily in skin affected by previous lesions. The pigment usually appears as large patches, bands, or swirls; eventually, it may disappear. The final stage is seen in some adult women and consists of subtle, hypopigmented, atrophic patches of skin, especially on the lower extremities.

Incontinentia pigmenti is inherited as an X-linked dominant trait that is lethal to male fetuses *in utero*. A family history is present in more than one-half of the cases. Eighty percent of affected infants have associated systemic anomalies including alopecia, dental and eye anomalies, seizures, mental retardation, and skeletal deformities.

NODULAR DISORDERS

Red Nodules

PYOGENIC GRANULOMAS

Pyogenic granulomas are benign vascular proliferations arising from the connective tissue of skin or mucous membranes. They are usually precipitated by trauma and infection, although the mechanism for growth stimulation is not known. The lesions grow rapidly, may be papular or nodular, and are often pedunculated. They are usually solitary and dark red to purple, with a surface that is generally moist, crusted, or eroded and that may bleed easily when traumatized (Fig. 46-14). The best-known pyogenic granuloma is the fleshy tumor associated with ingrown toenails.

The differential diagnosis of pyogenic granuloma includes warts, molluscum contagiosum, and superficial hemangiomas. The best treatment is excision and electrodesiccation of the base of the lesion to prevent recurrence.

ERYTHEMA NODOSUM

The lesions of erythema nodosum are fairly distinctive. The presentation is usually one of painful, erythematous, warm nodules on the pretibial surfaces. The number of nodules may vary from one to many. Their bright-red color changes in a few days to brown-red or purple and later to yellow-green, as seen with a bruise. Lesions may occur on other body sites including the arms and face. Erythema nodosum is a hypersensitivity reaction pattern triggered by various infections, drugs, and other conditions. It is not a disease entity in itself but requires evaluation to uncover the underlying cause.

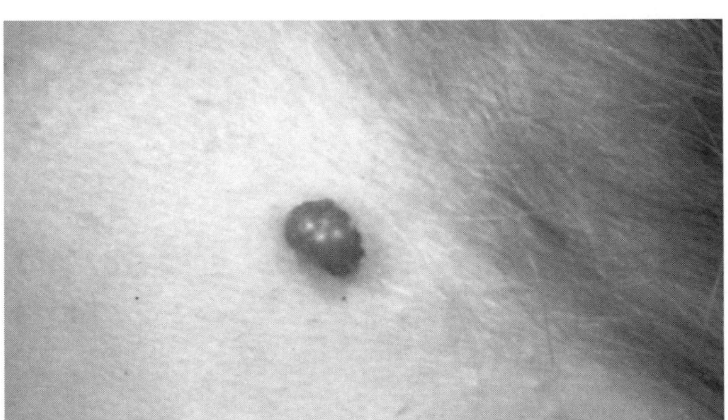

Figure 46-14. This pyogenic granuloma of the forehead is red, pedunculated, and moist.

The most common precipitating agent in erythema nodosum in children in the United States is a preceding streptococcal infection. In the past, tuberculosis was the foremost cause. Other, less common precipitants include cat-scratch disease, Yersinia, histoplasmosis, coccidioidomycosis, and leptospirosis. An association with inflammatory bowel disease and sarcoidosis has been noted with increasing frequency. Drugs most frequently incriminated include sulfonamides, diphenylhydantoin, and contraceptive agents. Chronic or recurrent episodes suggest more serious systemic disorders such as a collagen vascular disease, lymphoma, or inflammatory bowel disease.

The lesions of erythema nodosum may initially be confused with areas of cellulitis, insect bites, or bruises. Arthralgias occur in some cases, and arthritis may be present suggesting rheumatic disorders. Biopsy samples of lesions reveal intense inflammation deep in the dermis and subcutaneous tissues with involvement of arteries and veins. Most patients respond to bed rest, and the episodes resolve in 2 to 3 weeks. The trigger for this delayed cell-mediated hypersensitivity reaction may not be found.

Skin-Colored Nodules

DERMOID CYSTS

The small, firm, smooth intracutaneous or subcutaneous nodules characteristic of dermoid cysts occur most frequently on the head and neck. Congenital lesions formed from embryonic ectoderm are lined by stratified squamous epithelium. Almost 40% are periorbital, and some 30% occur in the eyebrows. The lesions are usually solitary and asymptomatic, and they are managed by surgical excision.

EPIDERMAL CYSTS

Most epidermal cysts occur after puberty. Clinically, they appear as discrete, enlarging, raised, somewhat compressible nodules of variable size. The margins may be irregular. The overlying skin is normal. Epidermal cysts occur most frequently on the face, scalp, and back, and they seem to be a result of the proliferation of surface epidermal cells within the dermis. Trauma may be responsible for some of these lesions.

LIPOMAS

The subcutaneous tumors typical of lipomas are spongy and are often lobulated. They occur most frequently in the subcutaneous tissue of the back and abdominal wall. The overlying skin is unaffected and not attached to these lesions, which are nontender and slow-growing and may be solitary or multiple. Lipomas may be part of Gardner syndrome (other features of which include polyposis of the colon, epidermal cysts of the skin, and multiple osteomas), have an accompanying macrocephaly, and occur as isolated events or as an autosomal dominantly inherited disorder.

Pigmented Nodules

MAST CELL DISEASE

Lesions composed of infiltrates of mast cells may occur in a number of shapes and forms. In infants and young children, solitary mastocytomas are most common. The typical picture is one of a raised brown or tan plaque, often with an orange-peel surface, that has recurrent flares of erythema or that develops vesicles, bullae, or (sometimes) crusting resembling an infectious process (Fig. 46-15). Occasionally, the bullae take on a hemorrhagic appearance. Irritation of the lesion may cause the release of histamine; which, in turn, may stimulate facial flushing and colic.

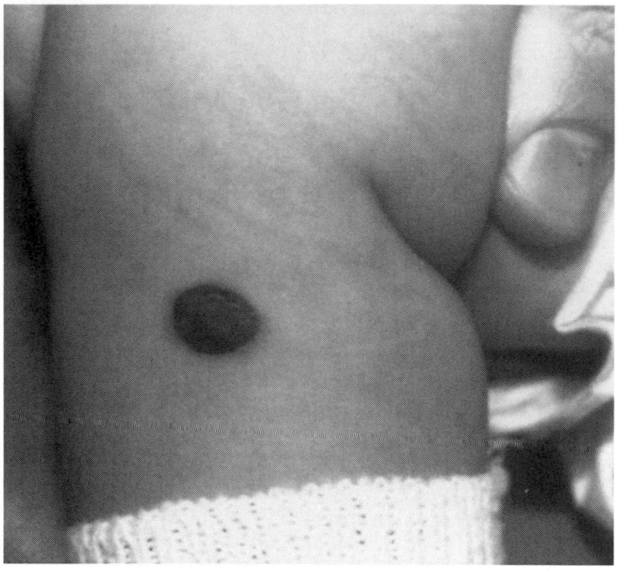

Figure 46-15. A brownish mastocytoma on the lower leg of an infant.

The most common form of mast cell disease in childhood is urticaria pigmentosa. The lesions, which are macular or slightly elevated papules and nodules that occur primarily on the trunk, may number from a few to hundreds and often appear in the first few months of life, although they can occur at any time (Fig. 46-16). The most helpful clue to diagnosis is the appearance of an erythematous or urticarial flare after vigorous rubbing of the lesion (Darier sign). In some cases, systemic symptoms including diarrhea and GI bleeding may be prominent.

Mast cell disease in children is generally benign. The younger the child's age at the lesions' appearance, the more likely is their resolution. Isolated mastocytomas are usually gone by the time affected children are 10 years old, and one-half of all cases of urticaria pigmentosa that develop early in childhood are resolved by the late teenage years.

VESICULAR AND BULLOUS ERUPTIONS

(Herpes Simplex, Zoster, and Varicella are discussed in the Infectious Diseases section.)

Disorders with Linear Vesicles (*Rhus* Dermatitis)

Vesicles that occur in lines are characteristic of allergic contact dermatitis that, in the United States, is caused most commonly by poison ivy or poison oak (Fig. 46-17). The eruption is a delayed-contact hypersensitivity reaction to a sap-like material that is known as urushiol and is present in the plants. Trauma to the leaves of the plants releases this material, which can be transferred to the skin. The rapidity of reaction to contact depends on the affected individual's sensitivity to the toxin and on the amount deposited on the skin. Pruritic papules and vesicles may appear in a few hours in areas of heavy contamination or over a few days on skin areas where contact was minimal. The development of new lesions over a few days' time has fueled the false notion that the vesicular fluid itself spreads the lesions.

Poison ivy most frequently occurs in the summer, but it can occur at any time of year. Dried leaves, stems, and roots may release the toxic material. Burning vines may release into the air particles that affect very sensitive individuals. If done early enough, scrubbing of areas known to have come in contact with these plants can prevent the development of lesions. The urushiols are bound rapidly to the skin on contact, however.

The classic lesions of Rhus dermatitis are vesicles arranged in lines, but linear and nonlinear erythematous papules can be found as well. Children's faces may be edematous and erythematous resembling the manifestations of angioneurotic edema. To establish the diagnosis, the arms, legs, and neck should be examined carefully for the presence of linear lesions.

The treatment of Rhus dermatitis is symptomatic. Wet compresses and calamine lotion assist in drying the lesions, and antihistamines may help to relieve the pruritus. Topical steroids are probably of little benefit in extensive cases. Oral steroids such as

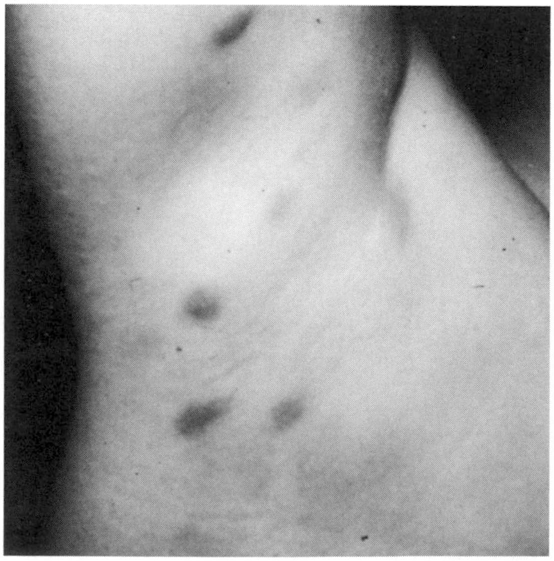

Figure 46-16. Multiple pigmented nodules of urticaria pigmentosa in the axilla. Rubbing causes an erythematous flare and swelling.

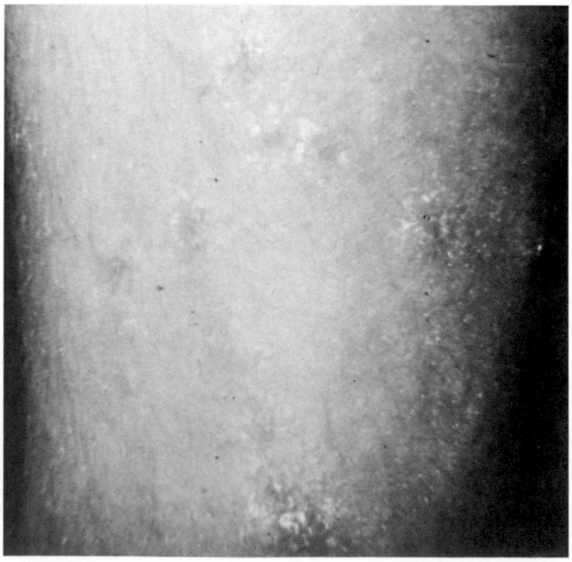

Figure 46-17. Rhus dermatitis caused by poison ivy is characterized by linear papules, vesicles, and bullae.

prednisone (1–2 mg/kg/day) in decreasing doses over a 2-week period are indicated. As in any other pruritic disorder, care must be taken to prevent or (if prevention is not possible) recognize secondary skin infection.

Vesicular Lesions with Typical Distributions

HAND-FOOT-AND-MOUTH DISEASE

The characteristic feature of hand-foot-and-mouth disease is the distribution of the vesicular eruption as per the name. This viral exanthem occurs most often in the summer months, often in miniepidemics. The most frequent site of lesions is the mouth, where the vesicular tops are eroded rapidly leaving ulcers. The exanthem on the hands and feet is vesicular, but the vesicles often have a curious linear or arcuate shape (Fig. 46-18). The rash may appear maculopapular at the outset. Occasionally, the buttocks may be involved. Coxsackievirus A16 is associated most frequently with this disease with occasional coxsackievirus A5 and A10 infections.

The primary disorder to differentiate from hand-foot-and-mouth disease is primary herpes gingivostomatitis. Treatment is symptomatic, and the course of the illness is usually benign.

TINEA PEDIS

Athlete's foot is not common before puberty. The presence of erythema and scaling in the interdigital webs of the toes, particularly the third and fourth and fourth and fifth, should always suggest this diagnosis, particularly in adolescents and adults. The lesions may appear vesicular or bullous as well. An id reaction on the palms or fingers resulting in lesions that vary from plaques to vesicles to other types of lesions may be associated with tinea pedis. The presence of any lesion on the hands should prompt an examination of the feet for tinea pedis. Treatment can usually be accomplished with a topical antifungal agent. After clearing, the feet should be washed and dried carefully, and an antifungal powder should be applied daily.

DYSHIDROTIC ECZEMA

Dyshidrotic eczema is a poorly understood but relatively common vesicular eruption that appears most often on the hands and feet. The lesions are deep-seated vesicles that give the involved areas an appearance akin to that of tapioca. Pruritus associated with the vesicles is usually pronounced. If they are excoriated and ruptured, the lesions may be erythematous and crusted. Vesicles may also coalesce to form bullae. Despite the name of the condition, the eccrine apparatus is not affected.

Although its cause is not clear, dyshidrotic eczema tends to occur in individuals with a personal or family history of atopy. Contact dermatitis and id reactions of tinea pedis, in addition to primary tinea infections, must be considered in the differential diagnosis. Treatment includes the application of compresses and a fluorinated topical steroid.

Bullous Lesions

BULLOUS IMPETIGO

The classic lesions of bullous impetigo, a staphylococcal infection, are bullae filled with cloudy fluid and surrounded by a thin margin of erythema. Characteristically, many of the bullae have ruptured leaving dried-up lesions scattered in contiguous areas (Fig. 46-19). The lesions most recently ruptured have an erythematous, shiny base resembling lacquered paint, whereas older lesions are completely dry and nonerythematous, a collarette of scale being the only remnant. In infants and toddlers, the diaper area is affected most frequently. *Staphylococcus aureus* is the organism responsible for this infection with the exfoliative toxin released locally by this bacteria causing production of the bullae.

The lesions are highly contagious and may spread both cutaneously and systemically. For that reason, parenteral, rather than topical, antibiotics are required for treatment.

STAPHYLOCOCCAL SCALDED-SKIN SYNDROME

Some *S. aureus* produce an exfoliative toxin, usually phage group II, type 70 or 71. Infections with these phage-producing strains may often be subtle, but they produce a striking picture befitting the name. The entire skin surface may be erythematous, and

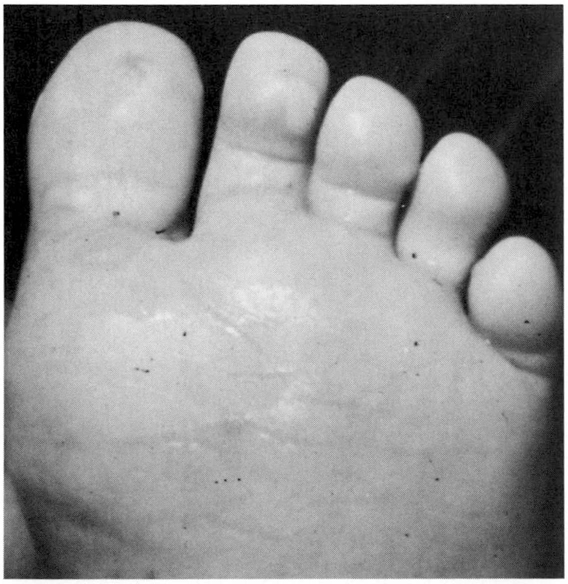

Figure 46-18. In hand-foot-and-mouth disease, vesicles are present on the hands and feet, as well as in the mouth. Note the linear configuration of these vesicles.

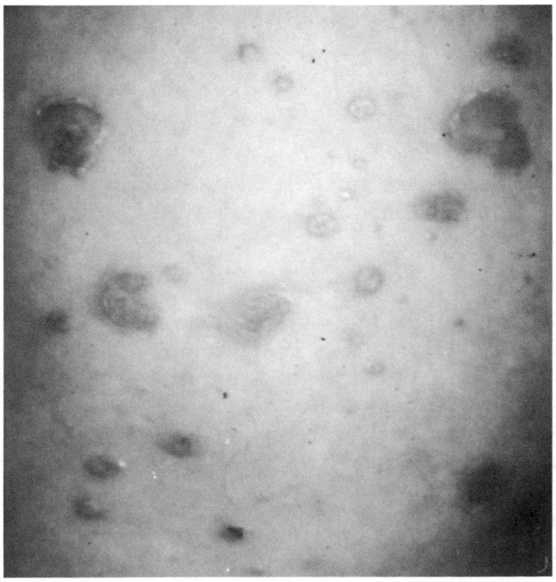

Figure 46-19. Fresh and ruptured bullous lesions of staphylococcal impetigo complicating varicella.

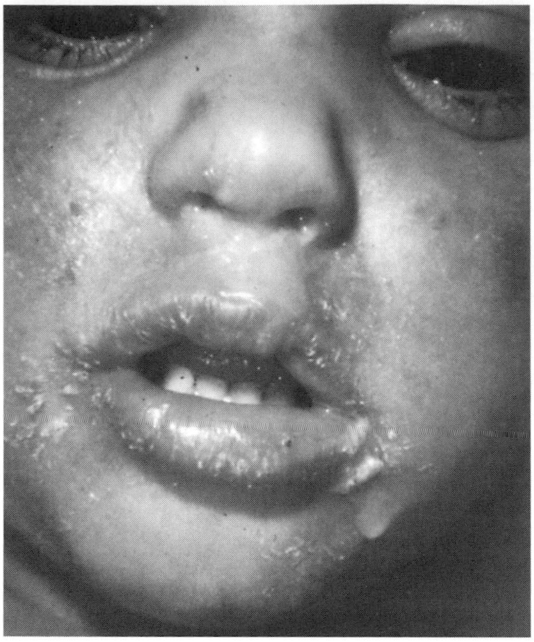

Figure 46-20. The purulent nasal discharge is the likely site of infection in this child with staphylococcal scalded-skin syndrome. Note the early perioral scaling.

bullae may appear in areas of trauma or in areas that are rubbed or simply touched. The separation of skin at sites of trauma is known as Nikolsky sign. Affected children experience extreme pain. A characteristic feature is crusting in a radial pattern (sunburst) around the mouth, nose, and eyes (Fig. 46-20). The mucous membranes are not involved, which may help to distinguish this illness from Stevens-Johnson syndrome.

The skin separation in staphylococcal scalded-skin syndrome is intraepidermal rather than deeper, at the epidermal basement membrane, as occurs in toxic epidermal necrolysis. In the latter disorder, mucous membranes are usually involved, and no sunburst of crusting occurs around the mouth and eyes. With or without antibiotic treatment, improvement occurs within 3 to 5 days. Antibiotic therapy should be used to prevent recurrences of the problem. Occasionally, dehydration is a major complication because of the loss of cutaneous covering.

URTICARIA PIGMENTOSA

Urticaria pigmentosa is manifested most frequently by the presence of small, pigmented macules and papules on the skin, their number varying from a few to hundreds. Vigorous rubbing of the lesions causes histamine to be released from the mast cells present in large numbers in the macules, which, in turn, causes the lesions to swell and develop an erythematous flare (Darier sign). In early childhood, these lesions may form vesicles or bullae. In bullous mastocytosis, an unusual form of mast cell disease, recurrent bullae appear on normal-appearing skin devoid of pigmented macules or nodules. The lesions are generally fairly pruritic. Secondary skin infections are common. The disease usually remits by early adolescence.

EPIDERMOLYSIS BULLOSA

The skin disorders listed as epidermolysis bullosa are a mixed group of hereditary, mechanobullous diseases. Eighteen hereditary types have been described. Their characteristic feature is the development, in response to trauma, of vesicles, bullae, or erosions. A wide spectrum of degree of skin fragility and involvement characterizes this group.

The autosomal dominant form of nonscarring epidermolysis bullosa simplex may be present at birth and may involve the mucous membranes and the rest of the skin. Although this form tends to be milder than some of the other types, it may be severe in newborns. Lesions develop over traumatized areas in most children, especially the hands, feet, extremities, and trunk. The disorder generally improves with time, although it worsens in warm weather.

An interesting form of epidermolysis bullosa simplex is the localized type (Weber-Cockayne syndrome) that is confined to the hands and feet. This disorder is also inherited in an autosomal dominant fashion and may be confused with friction blisters unless a careful family history is obtained.

Junctional epidermolysis bullosa, an autosomal recessive disorder, may present at birth or shortly thereafter. Although this type may seem benign at first, it is often progressive. Death is common, although it may occur after weeks or years later. Large granulomatous ulcers usually appear in the perioral area (Fig. 46-21). The nails are lost, and teeth are dysplastic. Mucous membranes are frequently involved early in the course of the disease, and strictures of the esophagus can develop. Scarring may be present. Complications include anemia from chronic blood loss and secondary infections.

The most severe and devastating form of epidermolysis bullosa is the autosomal recessive dystrophic type. The bullae and erosions are usually present at birth, and the entire skin surface may be affected at different times by minor trauma. Scarring, milia formation, and nail loss are prominent features. Oral involvement leads to scarring with the tongue bound down, and swallowing is affected by esophageal strictures. The hands and feet become mitten-like, and contractures develop in the large

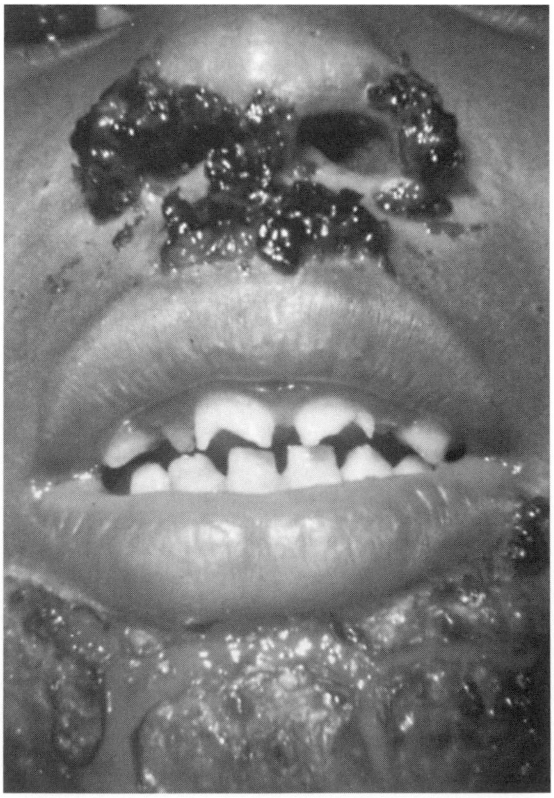

Figure 46-21. In junctional epidermolysis bullosa, erosions with hemorrhagic crusting are typical in the perioral area.

joints. The prognosis is poor, even with the best of parental care. Secondary skin infections, anemia, growth retardation, amyloidosis, and skin cancer are complications.

The pathogenesis of these disorders seems to differ with each type, as does the depth of the blister formation. Treatment consists of careful attention to the skin to prevent friction and to maintain cleanliness, treating secondary infection and anemia, and maintaining adequate nutrition.

VESICULOPUSTULAR LESIONS

Impetigo

Bacterial infections of the skin are the most common dermatologic condition for which children are brought to physicians. Superficial infections account for the great majority of these infections, and impetigo is the most common pyoderma. The prevalence of impetigo varies with the season of the year occurring most often in the warm summer months among individuals who practice poor hygiene and live in crowded conditions. Previously, impetigo was divided into two types, each with a typical clinical picture and different bacterial etiology. However, an increasing number of studies have found that *S. aureus* is the primary agent responsible for most impetigo, whether the lesion is golden crusted (the type formerly caused by group A beta-hemolytic streptococci) or bullous (the type that has always been staphylococcal in origin).

The crusted lesions of impetigo have little surrounding erythema, but local lymphadenopathy is common (Fig. 46-22). The lesions tend to spread locally, and scratching, particularly of insect bites, may result in widespread lesions. Family members are often infected as well. Any area of the body may be involved, and any break in the skin (e.g., abrasions, excoriations, lacerations, burns) may provide access.

When group A beta-hemolytic streptococci were the most common bacteria responsible for impetigo, secondary nonsuppurative complications such as poststreptococcal glomerulonephritis, were common in some areas of the United States and other countries. Acute rheumatic fever, however, has never been reported to follow impetigo.

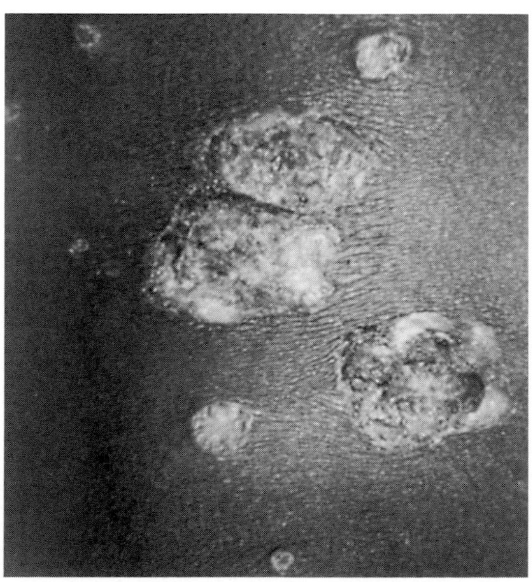

Figure 46-22. Crusted lesions of superficial pyoderma in a perioral distribution.

When impetigo is widespread, usually systemic therapy is indicated. Until reports of a change in the bacterial cause of impetigo appeared, crusted lesions were treated with penicillin, and bullous impetigo was treated with an antistaphylococcic antibiotic. The present trend is to treat all impetigo as if the infection were caused by *S. aureus*. Mupirocin, a topical antibiotic cream, may be used effectively when the lesions are not widespread.

Folliculitis and Furunculosis

Infections of the hair follicle unit are caused most frequently by *S. aureus*. Folliculitis is a superficial infection; a small rim of erythema surrounds the hair follicle, which is topped by a small, yellowish pustule. Furuncles are deeper infections with a larger rim of erythema, more swelling and, often, a cavity of pus in the center.

Common sites for these infections include the scalp in children who have their hair pulled tightly, the buttocks in infants wearing occlusive diapers, the beard area in some teenagers, and areas of the skin that are rubbed by padding in athletes. Often, folliculitis can be treated successfully with topical antibiotics and washing, but furunculosis usually requires the addition of systemic antistaphylococcic antibiotics.

A gram-negative folliculitis may occur in teenagers who have acne and are treated with systemic antibiotics. Hot tub or whirlpool folliculitis is characterized by the appearance of erythematous macules, papules, or pustules 8 to 48 hours after immersion in these tubs. The lesions are most likely to occur under swimsuits. Usually, the bacterial agent responsible is *Pseudomonas aeruginosa;* because the infection is superficial, normally no treatment is required.

Candidiasis

Yeast infections are caused most commonly by *Candida albicans,* a dimorphic fungus that occurs in both budding and mycelial phases. *Candida* thrives in warm, moist places; the diaper area of infants, the atmosphere of which can be likened to that of a tropical rain forest, is an ideal site for proliferation (Fig. 46-23). Characteristically, the inguinal creases are involved in candidal infections, which produce a confluent erythema, often with maceration and fissuring. The earliest lesions of *Candida* are small vesicopustules on an erythematous base. The lesions enlarge and tend to become confluent. Their roofs are then lost rapidly

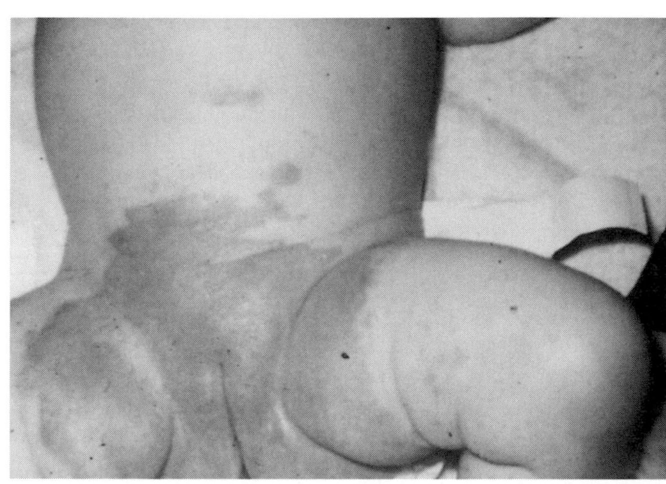

Figure 46-23. Candidal infection is characterized by involvement of the inguinal creases and satellite pustules.

leaving the red base. Other common sites of candidal infection include the axillae, the neck in young infants, and the corners of the mouth.

Infants commonly have "thrush," which appears as adherent, cheesy plaques of candidal infection in the mouth. Infection of the nails and paronychia may also develop in young children who suck their fingers or in individuals who immerse their hands in water for extended periods on a regular basis. Outside the neonatal period, overt candidal infections are uncommon. The presence of *Candida* might suggest the presence of diabetes mellitus, hypoparathyroidism, Addison disease, an altered immunologic response to infection, acquired immunodeficiency syndrome, or malignancy.

Usually, cutaneous infection with *Candida* can be treated effectively with drying and the application of an anticandidal agent such as nystatin and ketoconazole.

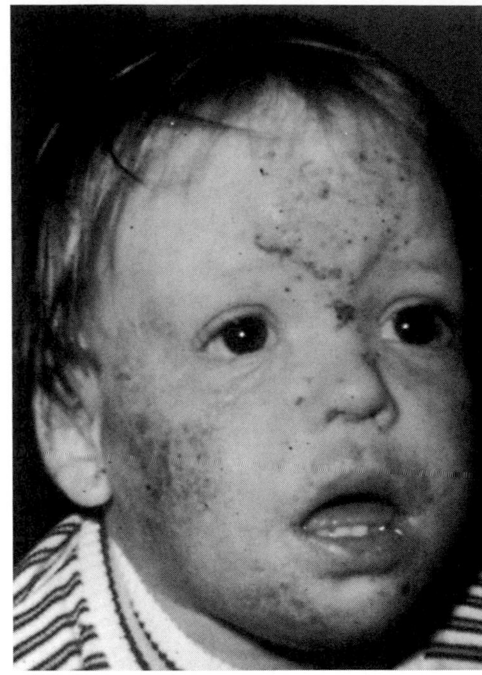

Figure 46-24. Typical morphology and facial distribution of infantile atopic dermatitis.

SCALING AND DRY LESIONS

Atopic Dermatitis

Atopic dermatitis, a common skin condition better known among laypersons as *eczema*, seems to be increasing in frequency. In northern Europe, 15% to 20% of the population may be affected. Its cause is unknown but seems to be multifactorial; heredity plays a role modified by environmental factors. The basic problem seems to be a sensitivity of the skin to numerous stimuli, all of which produce pruritus. An apt description of atopic dermatitis is "an itch that rashes." If the itch can be controlled, usually the rash will not develop.

Atopic dermatitis is rare in infants younger than 2 months old, primarily because the "itch-scratch" mechanism does not mature until approximately 3 months of age. Onset of the rash occurs before the age of 1 year in 60% to 80% of affected children and before the age of 5 years in 90%. The rash of atopic dermatitis most often appears as dry patches, but sometimes it is eczematoid (weeping), particularly on the cheeks and the extensor surfaces of the arms and legs (Fig. 46-24). Dry patches may occur on much of the body surface. Lesions may become hyperpigmented, especially in black individuals, from the scratching and rubbing. In toddlers, the rash characteristically appears in the popliteal and antecubital fossae, although other areas are also involved. In adults, the periorbital and neck areas are often affected. Generally, the skin of most patients is dry, and the decreased humidity of the environment that is associated with heating in the winter commonly accentuates the problem.

In addition to appearing dry and somewhat scaly, the skin of individuals with atopic dermatitis is thickened or has undergone lichenification (Fig. 46-25), and normal skin markings are accentuated (Fig. 46-26). Scratching commonly results in secondary infections, particularly with staphylococci. The presence of infection, which may be occult, often leads to accentuation of the pruritus with a resultant flare in the rash.

The major and minor criteria used to diagnose atopic dermatitis are listed in Table 46-1. Because this disorder is chronic and relapsing, treatment involves a great deal of teaching and explaining to parents and children and of prescribing of medications. Given that ichthyosis commonly accompanies atopic dermatitis, other medications may be necessary to give the skin a relatively normal texture and appearance.

Factors that may precipitate pruritus in atopic skin include soaps; sweating and (conversely) exposure to cool air; certain materials, especially wool and synthetic fibers; and stress. Well-controlled studies have demonstrated food sensitivity in as many

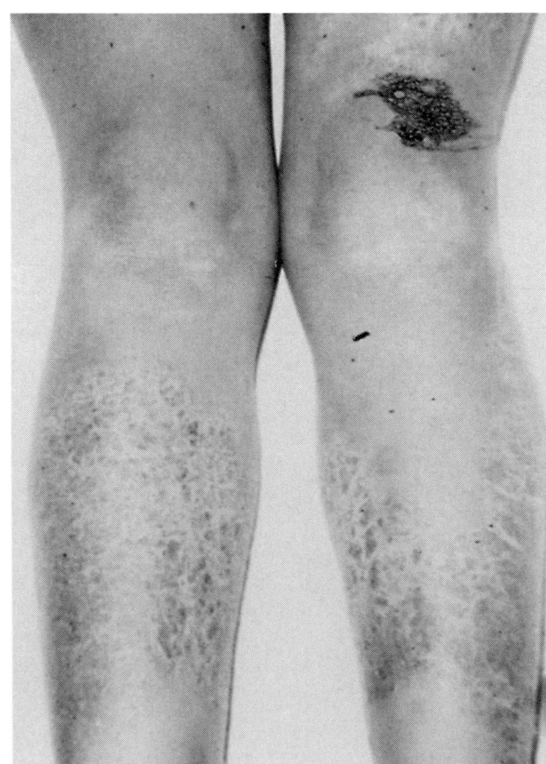

Figure 46-25. Lichenous plaques of atopic dermatitis involving both lower legs.

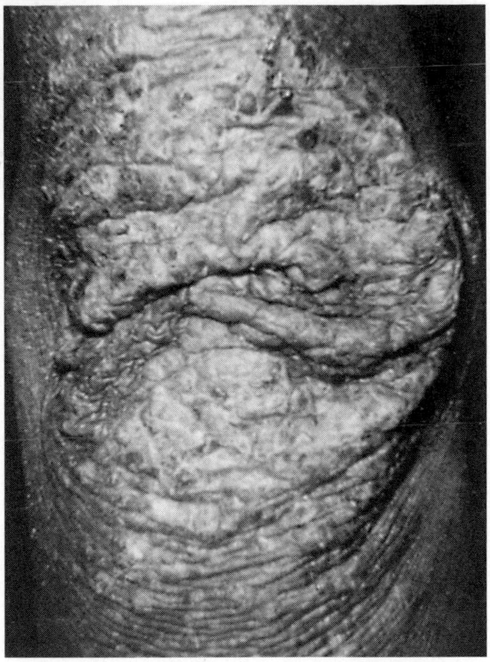

Figure 46-26. Dramatic lichenification from chronic scratching in atopic dermatitis.

as 5% of affected children. The foods most frequently implicated are eggs, milk, wheat, peanuts, soybeans, and chicken. The role of inhalants (pollen, mold, and dust mites) is not clear.

Atopic skin is almost always colonized by *S. aureus*, and infections are common, often leading to exacerbation of the rash. The role of *S. aureus* in exacerbation may be seen in direct biological action or in indirect damage mediated by the immune and inflammatory systems.

TABLE 46-1. Diagnostic Criteria for Atopic Dermatitis

Major criteria (3 of 4 required)
Pruritus
Typical morphology and distribution
Adults: flexural lichenification or linearity
Children and infants: facial, extensor
Chronic or relapsing dermatitis
Personal or family history of atopy
Minor criteria (3 or more required)
Xerosis
Ichthyosis/keratosis pilaris/palmar hyperlinearity
Type I skin test reactivity
Elevated serum IgE
Tendency to skin infection
Hand or foot dermatitis
Conjunctivitis
Keratoconus
Orbital darkening
Facial pallor or erythema
Pityriasis alba
Itch when sweating
Intolerance to wool and lipid solvents
Perifollicular accentuation
Food intolerance
Course influenced by environmental or emotional factors
White dermographism or delayed blanch

Modified from Hanifin JM, Rajka G. Diagnostic features of atopic dermatitis. *Acta Derm Venereol Suppl (Stockh)* 1980;92:44.

Atopic skin is also prone to viral infections; herpes simplex may spread rapidly and extensively over the entire skin surface resulting in severe disease and even death. Molluscum contagiosum can also be extensive on atopic skin. Interestingly, atopic children are less prone than normal children to contact dermatitis.

Of children with atopic dermatitis, 50% to 80% progress to allergic rhinitis or asthma. Although the skin of the majority of children improves by adulthood, it tends to remain "sensitive," especially to winter dryness and soaps, throughout their lives.

The keys to treatment, in addition to education, are avoidance of precipitants (particularly drying soaps), use of emollients to keep the skin moist, and application of corticosteroids to reduce the inflammation and pruritus. Ointments are better lubricating agents than creams. Nonfluorinated steroids should be used to circumvent adrenal suppression and skin atrophy, which may occur with stronger medications. Topical fluorinated steroids should be applied only to the most severely affected areas for the shortest possible time, and they should never be used on the face or perineum. Hydrocortisone may be added to an emollient to produce a 1% concentration. A potent oral antipruritic agent such as hydroxyzine, should be prescribed in doses large enough to reduce the pruritus, which results in the itch-scratch-itch cycle. A large dose at bedtime will help to reduce scratching during sleep.

For any suspicion of possible secondary bacterial infection, an antistaphylococcic antibiotic should be administered by mouth. In severe cases of recalcitrant atopic dermatitis, children may need to receive daily doses of antibiotics. As the rash improves, the frequency of application of steroid medications and the use of antipruritic agents may be reduced. Emollients, however, must often be continued, particularly after bathing.

Atopic dermatitis may be confused with seborrheic dermatitis in young infants or with "dandruff" in older children and adults. Scabies, which is also characterized by pruritus, should be differentiated easily from atopic dermatitis by the presence and distribution of the papulovesicular lesions and the short duration of the skin condition. In addition, allergic or contact dermatitis usually has a shorter course than does atopic dermatitis.

Seborrheic Dermatitis

Seborrheic dermatitis is a common skin condition with a predilection for two pediatric age groups, infants and adolescents. In infants between 2 and 10 weeks of age, seborrheic dermatitis generally begins on the scalp producing a greasy, yellowish scale. The base may or may not be erythematous. Commonly, the scaling extends down the forehead to involve the eyebrows, nose, and ears. In black individuals, significant hypopigmentation may accompany the rash (Fig. 46-27). The scale may be barely perceptible, and generally the rash is not pruritic. The diaper area may also be involved; this area, which is usually infected with *Candida*, exhibits an erythematous, diffuse rash involving the creases. Without treatment, seborrheic dermatitis clears by 8 to 12 months of age. Intertriginous areas must be treated with a mild steroid combined with an anticandidal agent. Continued dandruff of the scalp should suggest other disorders including tinea capitis, atopic dermatitis and, rarely, histiocytosis X.

In adolescents, the scaling occurs most commonly on the scalp, eyebrows, eyelashes, nasolabial folds, postauricular crease, and presternal and interscapular regions. Usually, a mild tar-based or ketoconazole shampoo keeps the scalp involvement under control. Other areas of the skin respond to 2% ketoconazole cream or 1% hydrocortisone cream.

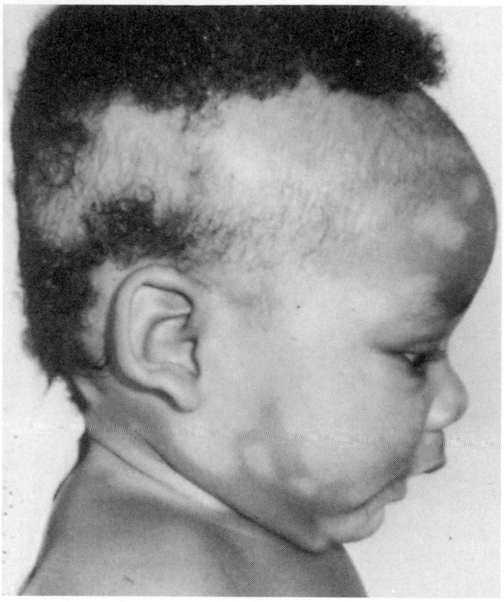

Figure 46-27. Note the facial hypopigmentation and scalp hair loss without prominent scaling in this child with seborrheic dermatitis.

The etiology of seborrheic dermatitis is not clear; the histopathology is nonspecific. The idea that the condition has something to do with sebaceous glands is supported by development of the dermatitis in areas with the highest density of these glands. The appearance of seborrheic dermatitis in infants probably reflects the effect of transmitted maternal sex hormones on these glands; reappearance of the condition during puberty occurs with the resurgence of sex hormones.

Psoriasis

The fact that psoriasis often has its onset in childhood is not commonly known. Some estimate that 10% of cases begin before the patient is 10 years old and that 35% begin by age 20. The cause of the condition is not known, although hereditary factors clearly play a role. Trauma to the skin is a common precipitant in susceptible individuals.

Usually, the clinical lesions are distinctive, with well-demarcated, erythematous papules or plaques covered with a silvery scale. The scale tends to build up in layers, and its removal may cause a bleeding point (Auspitz sign). The papules enlarge to form plaques. Usually, the distribution is symmetric with plaques commonly appearing over the knees and elbows because they are sites of repeated trauma. The Koebner phenomenon (i.e., the appearance of rash at sites of physical, thermal, or mechanical trauma) is often evident. Frequently, the scalp shows a thick, adherent scale; often the nails demonstrate punctate stippling or pitting or become discolored and crumbly, and the palms and soles may show scaling and fissuring.

A variety of inciting factors, in addition to trauma, have been associated with the appearance of psoriatic lesions. An interesting factor in children is the development of guttate psoriasis, a condition characterized by multiple, small, teardrop-like lesions associated with group A beta-hemolytic streptococcal infection (Fig. 46-28). Other agents implicated are sunburn, drug eruptions, and viral infections. The histologic picture is one of hyperproliferation of the epidermis.

The course of psoriasis is unpredictable. Treatment consists of the application of a good lubricant. Other therapies include

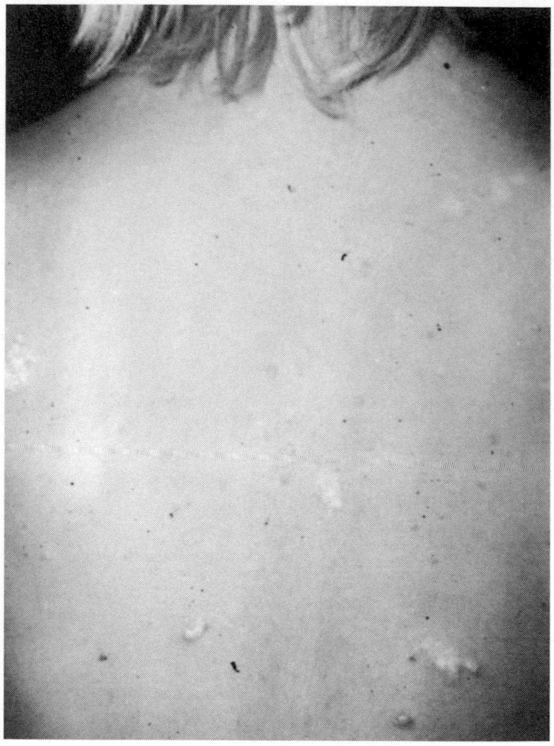

Figure 46-28. The sudden widespread appearance of small, scaly plaques is characteristic of guttate psoriasis.

the application of an appropriate topical corticosteroid, tar, or calcipotriene. Exposure to sunlight, with care taken not to burn the skin, is often beneficial. Oral psoralens combined with ultraviolet light and methotrexate therapy are rarely indicated for use in children.

The differential diagnosis in childhood includes such uncommon disorders as pityriasis rubra pilaris, parapsoriasis, and lichen planus. Occasionally, atopic dermatitis may be confused with psoriasis, but psoriasis is not pruritic. Pityriasis rosea, tinea corporis, and seborrheic dermatitis may also mimic psoriasis.

Nummular Eczema

As the name denotes, nummular eczema is characterized by the presence of coin-shaped plaques of eczema. The lesions of this poorly understood disorder may be "dry" (i.e., covered with dry scales) or "wet" (i.e., composed of papules and vesicles with a scale that gives a wet appearance to the base). They are discrete, often on an erythematous base, and may be hyperpigmented or may have undergone lichenification. Pruritus is variable. Lesions appear most commonly on the extensor surfaces of the arms and legs and on the dorsa of the fingers and hands.

An association seems to exist between a dry environment and appearance of the lesions. Frequent bathing with drying soaps aggravates the rash. Other stimuli may also precipitate or contribute to the rash. Nummular eczema is not thought to be related to atopic dermatitis. Treatment consists of decreased bathing, frequent application of emollients, and (occasionally for recalcitrant lesions) the use of topical corticosteroids. The differential diagnosis includes allergic contact dermatitis, atopic dermatitis, psoriasis, tinea corporis, and impetigo.

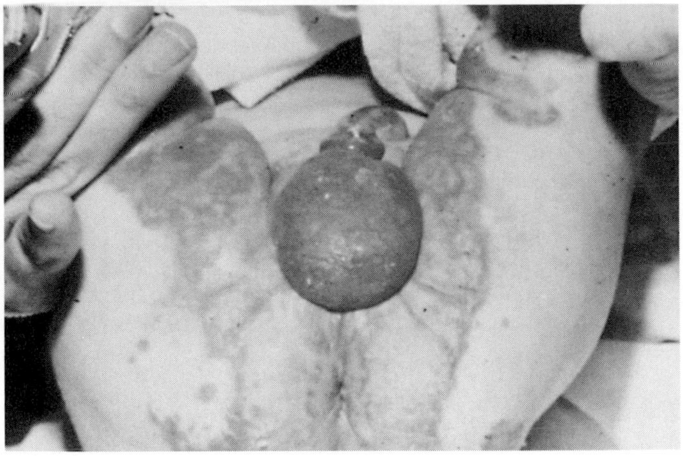

Figure 46-29. Erythematous, scaling, well-demarcated perianal dermatitis in an infant with acrodermatitis enteropathica.

Acrodermatitis Enteropathica

Although the early lesions of acrodermatitis enteropathica are vesicles, bullae, and pustules, the primary clinical appearance is usually one of dry, scaly, or crusted lesions with sharply marginated borders (Fig. 46-29). The lesions begin around the body orifices (i.e., mouth, eyes, perianal areas). The vesicles rupture rapidly revealing a moist, red base, and then dry and become plaque-like. Lesions develop on the hands and feet as well and, with time, other areas of the body similarly may be involved.

Acrodermatitis enteropathica was a cruel and devastating illness until zinc deficiency was discovered to be its cause in the early 1970s. Affected children respond readily to oral zinc supplementation. The dermatitis has its onset between a few weeks and 20 months of age, and it is often accompanied by alopecia and diarrhea. Affected infants are irritable and listless and fail to thrive. Secondary skin infections are common.

Patients receiving total parenteral nutrition are prone to zinc deficiency if they do not receive adequate zinc supplementation. In young infants receiving total parenteral nutrition, a recalcitrant diaper rash should always suggest this possibility. Zinc deficiency was thought to be rare in breast-fed infants; however, the number of cases associated with low levels of zinc in maternal milk has increased.

DISORDERS INVOLVING ABNORMAL SKIN TEXTURE

Sclerosis

MORPHEA

Although most physicians have read about progressive systemic sclerosis, few seem to have heard of morphea, also known as *localized scleroderma*. Morphea is much more common than progressive systemic sclerosis, and generally its outcome is excellent. The lesions consist of well-demarcated patches of sclerosis of the skin. The patches may be singular, multiple, or linear, and they occur in various patterns and locations. The skin feels indurated to the touch and exhibits loss of its normal elasticity. The skin appendages are also lost. A slight depression or atrophy of the area may be noted with some loss of skin color. Areas of increased pigmentation are occasionally intermixed (Fig. 46-30).

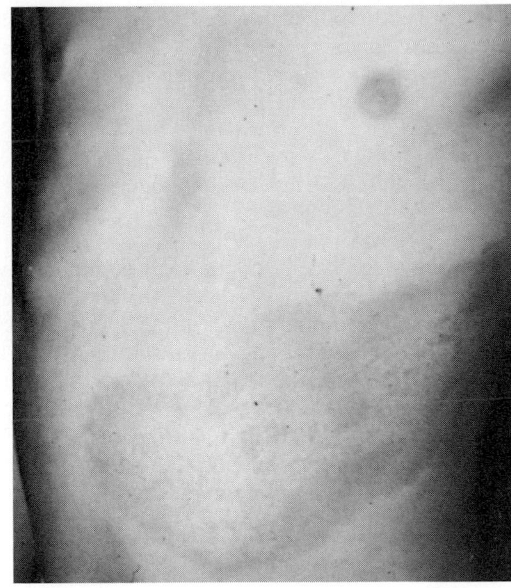

Figure 46-30. An irregularly pigmented patch of morphea on the abdomen. The skin has lost its elasticity and feels firm.

Lesions may appear waxy, ivory to yellow, and plaque-like, and they may have violaceous borders.

Morphea comes in many varieties. Large-patch, guttate (small, scattered lesions), and linear forms occur. The linear form may affect underlying subcutaneous tissue, muscle, and bone resulting in significant shortening and deformity of an extremity. Facial lesions, known as *coup de sabre*, usually appear on the forehead and scalp just lateral to the midline and may cause significant cosmetic deformity.

The cause of morphea is unknown. The histologic picture is indistinguishable from that of progressive systemic sclerosis, but systemic involvement in the two disorders is quite different. Arthralgias are common, and sometimes polyarthritis is found in morphea, but the progressive involvement of other organs does not occur. The relationship to progressive systemic sclerosis is still controversial. The lesions of morphea develop insidiously and remain for many years, although most show a tendency to resolve spontaneously within 3 to 5 years. No effective therapy for the disorder is known. Importantly, morphea should not be confused with progressive systemic sclerosis.

LICHEN SCLEROSUS ET ATROPHICUS

The characteristic features of lichen sclerosus et atrophicus are patches of atrophy and whitening of the skin. The initial lesions begin as papules, which become white, enlarged, and, as dermal sclerosis occurs, appear to be depressed below the surface of normal skin. The surface is white and thin, almost resembling cigarette paper. The most common site of involvement in female subjects is the perineum, where the lesions encircle the vulva and anus in an hourglass shape. Pain and pruritus of the area lead to excoriation and secondary infection. Occasionally, patients develop erosions or purpuric areas that may be mistaken for sexual abuse. Vaginal discharges are a frequent accompaniment. In male subjects, the foreskin may be involved creating a phimosis.

The cause of lichen sclerosus et atrophicus is not known, although some believe that hormonal factors play a role. Female subjects are affected ten times as often as male subjects. Three-fourths of children have symptomatic improvement in 3 to 5 years. Although no curative therapy appears to be available, the application of a low-potency topical corticosteroid often improves symptoms. Some success with testosterone cream has been reported in adults; however, this agent should not be used in children due to the potential for virilization.

Depressed Lesions

STRIAE

As linear, shallow depressions of the skin commonly seen in adolescents, striae occur in areas where the skin has been subjected to stretching. Common sites include the shoulders, abdomen, hips, buttocks, thighs, and breasts. Initially, the lesions may appear red or red-blue, but they become white with time. The cause is not understood, but lesions are more likely to occur in individuals who are receiving systemic steroids. Topical steroids may cause similar lesions. Striae may appear after severe illness such as infections or oncologic therapy or after excessive weight loss or gain. No effective therapy is available for the lesions.

CORTICOSTEROID ATROPHY

Depressions in the skin may develop at sites of intramuscular injections of steroids, particularly triamcinolone acetonide or diacetate, or after the prolonged application of a potent topical corticosteroid. The dermis and subcutaneous fat demonstrate local atrophy. In most cases, the tissues regenerate. The overlying skin appears normal.

CHANGES IN PIGMENTATION

Dark Lesions

NEVI

Acquired Melanocytic Nevi

The common mole may appear at any time after birth with peaks in appearance occurring between the ages of 2 and 3 years and again between 11 and 18 years. The average number of nevi in white adults is approximately 40, but the range is large. Black individuals have many fewer lesions. Moles are divided into three clinical types, differentiation of which may not be easy. In the junctional nevus, which occurs predominantly in children, all the nevus cells are contained within the epidermis. The lesions are macular or only slightly raised and are smooth and hairless. Compound nevi have nevus cells both at the dermal-epidermal junction and lying free within the dermis. The lesions are raised and smooth-bordered and often contain hair. Intradermal nevi have their nevus cells entirely in the dermis. They are raised, dome-shaped, smooth-bordered, and even in pigmentation.

The appearance of nevi varies considerably and ranges from deeply pigmented to colorless. Acquired nevi do not have to be removed routinely, unless they develop worrisome signs of change suggestive of melanoma. Although malignant change is uncommon in children, melanomas may develop at any age. Features that should suggest further evaluation include rapid enlargement or darkening with the development of irregular borders; the appearance of whitish, fibrotic areas, or nevi with various shades of pink or blue; spontaneous bleeding or ulceration; and the development of satellite lesions or palpable regional lymph nodes. The lifetime risk of developing cutaneous melanoma is 0.6% in whites and perhaps 0.06% in blacks.

Dysplastic Nevi

Attention has been drawn to the propensity of melanoma to develop in certain families. Members of these families seem to have an abnormally large number of acquired pigmented lesions, many of which are termed *dysplastic.* The dysplastic lesions are larger (5–12 mm) than common nevi, have macular and papular components, and are characterized by irregular and ill-defined borders. Often their color is variegated, tan to dark brown, sometimes with a pink background. Dysplastic nevi begin in adolescence and continue to appear into adulthood. The risk for melanoma development among affected persons is 10% over their lifetime; the risk approaches 100% in melanoma-prone families.

Halo Nevi

Nevi occasionally develop a hypopigmented ring around them and, over time, disappear (Fig. 46-31). Such halo nevi represent an apparent immunologic attack by the body against its own nevocytic cells. Some one-fourth of individuals with halo nevi also have areas of vitiligo. Halo nevi are almost always benign, although the associated color change frequently precipitates parental concern.

Benign Juvenile Melanoma

The name *benign juvenile melanoma* is misleading, because melanoma has a decidedly negative connotation, and these nevi are benign. This lesion is best called a *Spitz nevus,* after the person who first described it. Spitz nevi occur most commonly in young children at approximately age 3 years and in adolescents. Usually, they are solitary, occurring most commonly on the cheeks. The typical lesion is dome-shaped, has a smooth surface and distinct border, is hairless, and is pinkish (Fig. 46-32). Spitz nevi tend to grow rapidly over a 3- to 12-month period. Usually, they are removed because of concern about a true melanoma or for cosmetic reasons.

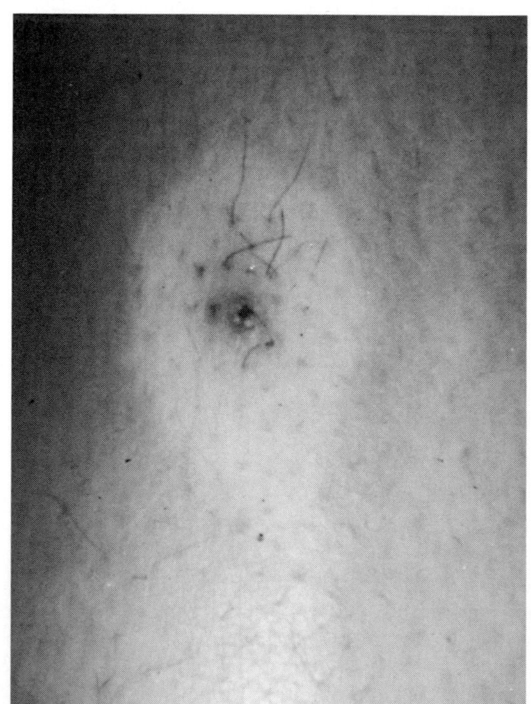

Figure 46-31. Depigmentation of the central nevus and surrounding skin in a halo nevus.

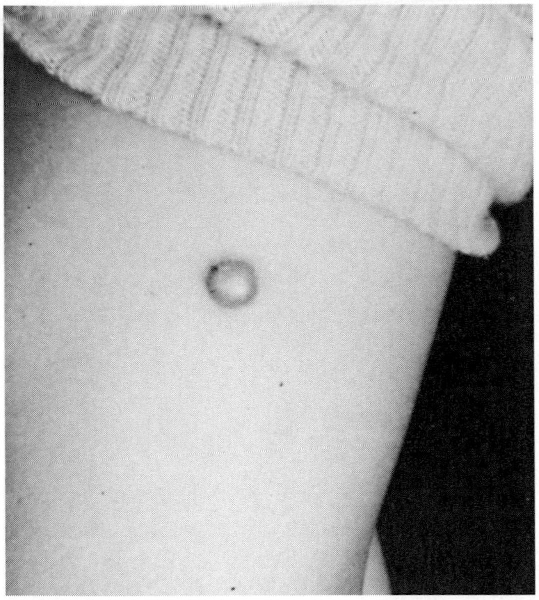

Figure 46-32. A well-circumscribed, pigmented spindle cell or Spitz nevus in a typical location, the upper arm.

Blue Nevi

The blue nevus is a benign lesion that may also be mistaken for a melanoma. Blue nevi are usually solitary, blue to blue-black, and generally less than 15 mm in diameter. They tend to occur most frequently on the hands, feet, buttocks, and face. No malignant changes have been reported.

LENTIGINES

Unlike freckles, lentigines develop not only on sun-exposed skin, but also on unexposed areas. They are small (0.2–1.0 cm), discrete, dark brown to black, round to oval macules. Lentigines may be present at birth, but usually they develop in early infancy and increase in number with age.

A number of different disorders have been associated with lentigines. The Peutz-Jeghers syndrome features multiple lentigines, usually in a perioral distribution, in association with intestinal polyposis. The LEOPARD syndrome is an acronym for the association of *l*entigines with *e*lectrocardiographic abnormalities, *o*cular hypertelorism, *p*ulmonic stenosis, *a*bnormalities of the genitalia, *r*etardation of growth, and *d*eafness.

POSTINFLAMMATORY HYPERPIGMENTATION

Darkening of the skin at sites of preceding inflammation or irritation is a common phenomenon, especially in black individuals. The pathophysiology of the deposition of melanin is unclear. Commonly, varicella produces macular, round remnants of previous infection, and children with atopic dermatitis often have significant pigmentation in the areas that have undergone lichenification. Generally, the pigmentation fades with time.

PHYTOPHOTODERMATITIS

A macular hyperpigmentation, phytophotodermatitis is caused by an increased sunburn response after contact with photosensitizers present in certain plants. Crushing of these plants releases furocoumarins, the photobiologically active portion of which—psoralen—induces cross-linking of DNA strands on exposure to ultraviolet light. Lime juice, particularly from lime skin, is a relatively common culprit. Other plants producing a similar effect include lemon, celery, parsnip, and fig. The hyperpigmented areas may assume unusual shapes depending on the type of exposure. Rarely, the lesions may appear erythematous or vesicular. These lesions have been confused with bruises caused by child abuse.

FIXED DRUG ERUPTION

A fixed drug eruption is a localized drug reaction characterized by the appearance of a purple to red plaque with clearly demarcated borders. Often the plaque is singular and occasionally is urticarial, nodular, or eczematous. Lesions heal over 10 to 14 days leaving hyperpigmentation. Common drugs responsible for these lesions include salicylates, tetracyclines, barbiturates, sulfonamides, and phenolphthalein (present in many laxatives). The reason for such localized reactions from systemically administered drugs is unknown. Each time the drug is given, the eruption recurs in the same spot.

ACANTHOSIS NIGRICANS

Acanthosis nigricans is manifested characteristically by the appearance of a hyperpigmented, somewhat velvety thickening of the skin. The most common sites of involvement are the nape and sides of the neck, the axillae, and the groin. Although acanthosis nigricans may be associated with an internal malignant tumor in adults, this association is extremely rare in children. The problem most commonly connected with the disorder is obesity. In some cases in which the disease onset is early in life, a familial association may be found. The presence of acanthosis nigricans should alert one to the possible coexistence of endocrinologic abnormalities including hyperandrogenism, obesity, insulin resistance, and diabetes mellitus. No effective therapy is available for the lesions.

Yellow Skin

CAROTENODERMA

Carotenoderma is a common yellowish to orange skin discoloration caused by the ingestion of excessive amounts of carotene-containing foods. Occasionally, carotenoderma is associated with hypothyroidism, diabetes mellitus, or nephrosis. Foods commonly connected with the disorder are carrots, squash, and other yellow vegetables. The areas most often involved are the face, palms, and soles. The disorder is asymptomatic and noninjurious; the main reason for concern is its possible confusion with jaundice. The sclerae are not yellow in carotenoderma.

LYCOPENEMIA

Less well recognized than carotenoderma is lycopenemia, an orange-yellow discoloration of the skin associated with high levels of lycopene, the red carotenoid of tomatoes. No therapy is necessary.

Light-Colored Lesions

PITYRIASIS ALBA

Patches of pityriasis alba are slightly hypopigmented and somewhat ill-defined; often, they have a fine, adherent scale. They are asymptomatic, are round to oval, and occur most frequently on the face, neck, upper trunk, and proximal extremities. Although its cause is unknown, the condition likely represents postinflammatory hypopigmentation occurring in children with atopic dermatitis. Often, lesions become apparent after sun exposure when the contrast between normal and affected skin is enhanced. Most lesions resolve spontaneously, although some believe that mild

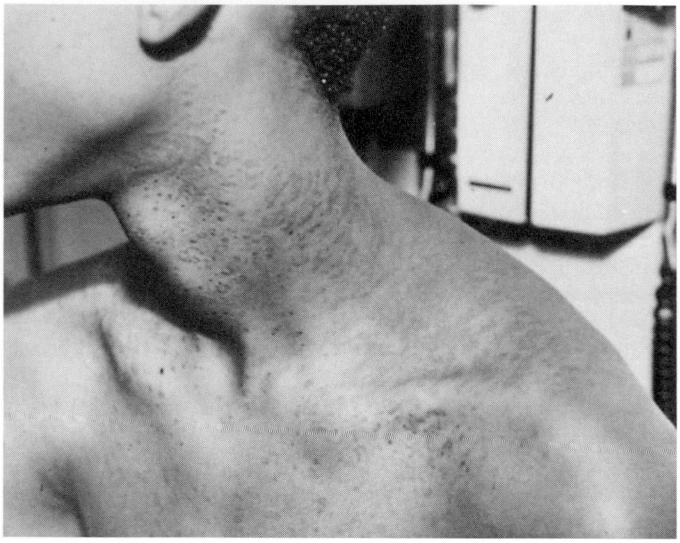

Figure 46-33. Hyperpigmented, minimally raised tinea versicolor lesions on the neck, shoulders, and trunk.

topical steroids and emollients hasten the return of pigment. Included in the differential diagnosis are tinea corporis, tinea versicolor, and vitiligo.

POSTINFLAMMATORY HYPOPIGMENTATION

Areas of decreased pigmentation may occur in traumatized skin. These areas regain their normal coloration more rapidly than those areas with postinflammatory hyperpigmentation because of the superficial nature of the problem.

TINEA VERSICOLOR

Hyperpigmented or hypopigmented macules and patches, often ovoid or round and exhibiting a fine scale, are typical of tinea versicolor (Fig. 46-33). The lesions appear most commonly over the trunk and neck, most often in adolescents and young adults. The rash may be asymptomatic or may be associated with mild pruritus; the cosmetic appearance prompts the medical visit. *P. orbiculare,* a yeast-like organism, is responsible for the discoloration. The diagnosis can be confirmed easily by microscopical examination of the scale dissolved in potassium hydroxide for the classic spaghetti-and-meatball appearance of the hyphae and spores. Usually, Wood's light examination reveals a golden fluorescence, unless the patient has bathed in the previous 6 to 12 hours. The superficial infection tends to persist, and eradication is difficult. Commonly, selenium sulfide lotion, 2.5%, applied to affected areas of the skin is used. The medication may be applied for 10 to 15 minutes and then washed off in a regimen of nightly treatment for 7 nights. Alternatively, an 8- to 12-hour treatment may be used once each week for 4 weeks. Ketoconazole, 400 mg orally, in a single dose has also proved effective. Regardless of the initial therapy selected, an 8- to 12-hour application of selenium sulfide performed bimonthly is recommended to prevent recurrences.

VITILIGO

The lesions of vitiligo are depigmented and, therefore, are much lighter than those of the disorders listed earlier. This disorder destroys many (or all) of the pigment cells in the skin. The cause of vitiligo is unknown. It is probably not an autoimmune disorder, as once suspected, although individuals with autoimmune disorders are more prone than normal to this disorder. It is more common than most people suspect; as many as 2% of the general population may have vitiligo, and 50% of those have the problem before age 20 years.

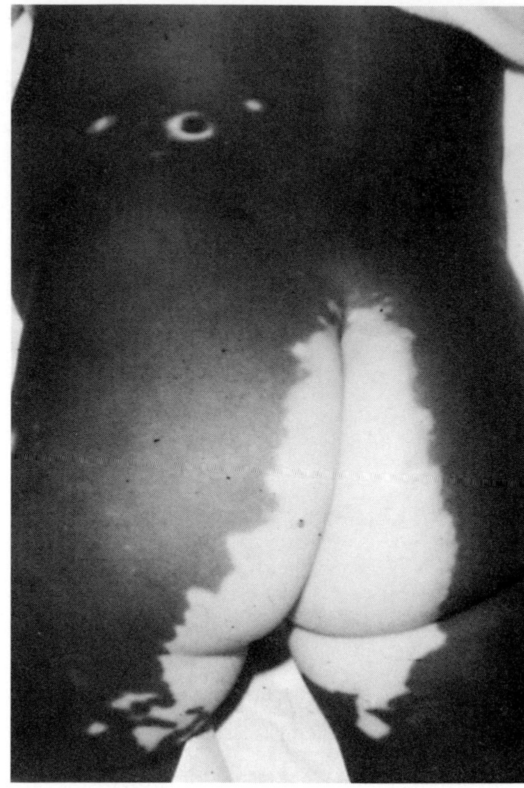

Figure 46-34. In vitiligo, depigmentation with distinct borders frequently involves the perineum.

Usually, the lesions are bilateral and symmetric, commonly appearing around body orifices (Fig. 46-34). The most frequent sites of involvement are the face, backs of the hands and wrists, umbilicus, and genitalia. Halo nevi are common in individuals with vitiligo. Topical steroids result in the return of normal color to the skin in approximately 20% of treated patients. Treatment with psoralens and ultraviolet A light should be reserved for older children. Care must be taken to protect the depigmented skin from sunburn.

ALBINISM

At least seven types of oculocutaneous albinism have been described. The hypopigmentation is present at birth. Melanocytes are present in the skin but fail to produce melanin. In white individuals, the skin appears milk-white, and the hair appears white to yellow. The pupils are pink, and severe photophobia is typical. Affected black individuals may have white or tan skin, blond to red hair, and blue to hazel irises. Most oculocutaneous albinism is inherited as an autosomal recessive disorder.

PRURITIC LESIONS

Contact Dermatitis

In allergic contact dermatitis, in contrast to primary irritant contact dermatitis, pruritus is a prominent feature. *Rhus* dermatitis, which includes poison ivy, is the most frequently recognized disorder of the allergic contact group. The characteristic feature of this eruption is the appearance of vesicles and vesicular papules in a linear distribution. The rash may be localized with groups of erythematous papules and vesicles, may have widely scattered lesions or, on occasion, may be limited to the face, which appears swollen. A history of contact with eruption-producing plants is helpful to the diagnosis. The linear vesicles (or papules, if the lesions are early) may be subtle. Often, pruritus is severe. Contrary to common belief, the vesicular fluid does not spread the rash. The rapidity of appearance of the rash depends on the affected person's degree of sensitivity to the toxin and the amount of toxin reaching the skin. In sensitive individuals, areas of significant exposure may show a rash within hours, whereas areas of minimal toxin exposure may not show a rash for days. (Lesions might not develop in less sensitive individuals until several days or a week later.)

Rhus dermatitis should not be confused with atopic dermatitis, which is a chronic disorder. Usually, atopic dermatitis begins in early childhood and has a morphology and distribution much different from those of poison ivy. In addition, individuals with atopic dermatitis do not usually react to exposure to poison ivy.

Other contact rashes may create problems in diagnosis. Some are localized to areas that indicate the underlying problem. Contact dermatitis from metal, for example, develops in areas where metal comes in contact with the skin (e.g., on fingers with rings, wrists with watches, the neck with necklaces, earlobes with earrings). Occasionally, cosmetics produce less obvious rashes. Eyelid dermatitis from fingernail polish is common.

Foot dermatitis in children is often mistaken for tinea pedis; however, this infection is uncommon in prepubertal children. If the rash involves the dorsum of the foot, an allergic contact dermatitis is likely. The reactions are caused primarily by rubber antioxidants and potassium dichromate leather-tanning agents. If the dermatitis appears on the weight-bearing surface, contact dermatitis can usually be ruled out. A more likely diagnosis is juvenile plantar dermatosis, believed by many to be a unique presentation of atopic dermatitis.

Treatment of contact dermatitis involves removal of the cause of the outbreak. A topical steroid may aid in relieving the pruritus and inflammation. Oral antihistamines may be needed in extensive cases. Oral steroids, which are sometimes indicated in severe cases of contact dermatitis, should be given in decreasing doses over a 10- to 14-day course.

Pediculosis

The human louse has a "field day" with children. *Pediculosis humanus capitis* is an extremely common problem, and eradicating it is difficult, despite the best efforts of schools, health agencies, and physicians. The human head louse is an obligate human parasite; it cannot survive away from its host for more than 10 days in the adult form or more than 3 weeks as a fertile egg. The insect, which is 2 to 4 mm in length and ivory-colored, is rarely seen. Nits, the egg sacs of lice, are the usual sign of infestation. Firmly cemented to the hair shaft, usually within 1 cm of the scalp, they resemble dandruff but cannot be picked off easily.

Usually, *P. humanus capitis* results in pruritus of the scalp. Common accompaniments to the scratching are folliculitis and impetigo. The lice are spread easily through close contact, toilet articles such as combs and brushes, and clothing, especially hats. Treatment may be difficult, especially in young children, who may be reinfested by lice from playmates. Permethrin is the standard form of therapy. Treating other family members and close contacts is important as well. Black individuals are rarely infested with head lice; the reason for their resistance is not known.

Pediculosis humanus corporis is a much less common problem in the United States. These lice live in the seams of clothing and feed on the skin, producing small, red papules and wheals. Ridding the clothing of the lice requires sterilization or at least running a hot iron over the seams.

Usually, pubic lice are acquired through contact during sexual intercourse; thus, sexual abuse must be considered in a finding of pubic lice in a child. Although the lice usually cling to pubic hair, in young children they may attach to body hair. Nits may be found in the eyelashes as well. The primary symptom is pruritus, and excoriations are common in heavy infestations. The nits on hair shafts are seen more commonly than the louse itself, which is broader and shorter than head and body lice. Sometimes infestation is manifested by the appearance of bluish gray, faint purpuric lesions. Known as *maculae ceruleae* or *taches bleuâtres,* these spots are sites of feeding by the louse. Treatment consists of an application of permethrin or lindane to affected areas. If the eyelashes are involved, petrolatum, applied twice daily for 7 days, may prove effective.

Scabies

Epidemics of scabies seem to occur in 30-year cycles. A peak in cases occurred in the United States in the 1970s, but the infestation is still prevalent. The culprit, *S. scabiei,* is a 0.2- to 0.4-mm female mite that burrows into the stratum corneum where it deposits eggs and excrement. The clinical picture, which usually develops 4 to 6 weeks after infestation, is thought to be the result of sensitization to the mite and its products. A person can have mites on the body and transmit them to others without having symptoms and signs of the disorder.

Usually, the pruritus of scabies is intense and unremitting. A characteristic feature is that it seems worse at night, perhaps as a result of a rise in skin surface temperature and increased activity of the scabies mites. The lesions of scabies are papules, tiny vesicles, and pustules. Most are excoriated and, in longstanding cases, lichenification may be extensive. Burrows (i.e., linear tracks) are not commonly seen in children. Usually, the distribution of lesions is located from the neck down, although young infants and children can have scalp and even facial involvement. Characteristically, the lesions are most intense on the hands, particularly in the webs of the fingers in older children and adults and on the palms and soles in infants; on the wrists; in the axillae; on the belt line; on the gluteal cleft; and around the nipples and genitalia in adults and older children. Scabies in babies can produce nodular-vesicular lesions on the palms and soles that mimic pyoderma. Secondary infections occur frequently.

Although the clinical picture may be typical of scabies, an attempt to identify the mite in a scraping from one of the lesions is always prudent. A simple technique is to choose a nonexcoriated, fresh vesicle or papule, place a drop of immersion oil on it, scrape it with a scalpel blade to open it, collect the oil from the skin, place the oil on a glass slide with a coverslip on top, and look for the mite, eggs, or feces.

Usually, treatment of scabies can be accomplished effectively by the application of 5% permethrin cream to the entire body surface including the head in infants. The permethrin cream should remain on for 8 to 14 hours and then should be washed off. Usually, one treatment is effective, although some prefer a second application 10 to 14 days later. Lindane, applied as a 1% concentration, is also effective and should remain on the skin for 6 to 8 hours. Regardless of the treatment used, the pruritus may take a week or more to resolve after treatment. All family members must be treated at the same time. Failure to treat close contacts such as baby-sitters, grandparents, and aunts and uncles, often results in reinfection. Many contacts may be infested despite a seeming absence of lesions.

The use of lindane on children has been the subject of much concern and debate. A review of reported cases of toxicity, however, has shown the preparation to be safe if it is not ingested or used inappropriately. Nevertheless, lindane is best avoided in infants and young children. Lindane is not recommended for use on pregnant women. Ten percent crotamiton is much less effective. Two applications, 24 hours apart, are recommended before the agent is washed off 48 hours later. Benzoyl benzoate, 12.5% to 25.0%, is effective, but obtaining it is difficult. A 6% to 10% precipitate of sulfur in petrolatum is rarely used because of its unpleasant odor. Clothing worn and bedding used by the family before treatment should be washed or stored for 72 hours before reuse to prevent reinfestation by mites.

Scabies can affect families at all socioeconomic levels. Its presence denotes contact with a source. Generally, although the contact requires intimate exposure, epidemics can occur in hospital settings, where nurses and physicians care for children and adults with undiagnosed scabies. Simple hand washing after patient contact prevents infection of health care providers.

Insect Bites

The pruritic, erythematous papules of insect bites, particularly fleabites, are commonly grouped together. A central punctum on top of the papule or wheal is strong evidence that the papule is the result of a bite.

DIFFUSE ERYTHEMA

Scarlet Fever

In the past, scarlet fever was manifested by a finely papular rash on an erythematous background that felt like sandpaper to the touch. However, the disease seems to have become much milder. Although still common, it is not frequently diagnosed because typical features are lacking. The slapped-cheek appearance is not common. Pastia lines (i.e., the erythematous accentuation of flexural creases), circumoral pallor, and even severe pharyngitis are seen infrequently. Most cases feature a fine, rough, papular rash predominantly over the bridge of the nose and face, shoulders, and upper chest. In fair-skinned individuals, the erythematous base may be present.

The rash of scarlet fever is produced by sensitization to those strains of group A beta-hemolytic streptococci that produce an erythrogenic toxin. Because prior exposure to the toxin is required, this disorder is rarely seen in children younger than 2 years. The incubation period is only 24 to 48 hours. Parents must be warned that their child's hands and feet may exhibit significant sheets of desquamation in 7 to 14 days.

Toxic Epidermal Necrolysis

At one time, the staphylococcal scalded-skin syndrome was included under the category of toxic epidermal necrolysis (TEN). It became apparent, however, that the disorders were dissimilar in many respects. TEN is usually the result of a reaction to a medication, particularly penicillins, sulfonamides, or barbiturates. Early signs of this disorder include malaise, fever, inflammation of the eyelids and mucous membranes (including the genitalia), and a generalized painful erythema. Flaccid blisters may develop, areas of skin may become denuded, and a maculopapular morbilliform rash may be present. The site of skin separation on performance of a biopsy is subepidermal.

Children with TEN usually appear ill. Involvement of the mucous membranes may make the oral intake of food or medications difficult. Supportive care is the primary therapy available. TEN may be categorized with the group of disorders that includes erythema multiforme and Stevens-Johnson syndrome.

PHOTOSENSITIVITY DISORDERS

Sunburn

The erythema resulting from damage to the skin by ultraviolet radiation is known as *sunburn*. Although, in our society, such damage to the skin is considered cosmetically pleasing and even a sign of good health; it is actually additive over the years producing an appearance of premature aging and acting as a carcinogen. The relationship between the increasing incidence of malignant melanoma and sun exposure is alarming. Part of the role of physicians caring for children should be early education of parents and children about care and protection of the skin.

Variations in skin types are easily recognized by laypersons. A classification system has been devised that grades the likelihood of irritation and resulting complications occurring from ultraviolet light exposure. Individuals with class I skin always burn and never tan; they generally have red hair and freckles and are of Celtic origin. Those with class II skin always burn, tanning only minimally; they are fair-skinned, fair-haired, blue-eyed whites. Individuals with class III skin burn moderately and tan gradually; they are generally darker-skinned whites. Persons with class IV skin, who are usually of Mediterranean background, burn minimally and tan well. Individuals with class V skin rarely burn and tan profusely; examples are Middle Eastern whites and Mexicans. Finally, persons with class VI skin (i.e., blacks) almost never burn and are deeply pigmented. This classification system can be used to counsel patients about the dangers of sun exposure and to advise them regarding the use of sun-protection agents such as sunscreens. Potent sunscreens contain active ingredients that absorb, reflect, or scatter light. Once sunburn has occurred, no effective therapy exists. For mild burns, an emollient and oral nonsteroidal antiinflammatory agent may provide relief. For moderate to severe burns, cold, wet compresses may be used to relieve the burning and tenderness. Simple sunburn needs to be separated from the disorders discussed next, which represent pathologic reactions to sunlight.

Drug Photosensitivity

Drug reactions to light have been divided into two types, toxic and allergic. Toxicity reactions occur after a single exposure and appear to be an exaggerated sunburn. Immediate reactions may occur with sulfonamides, phenothiazines, griseofulvin, and some tetracyclines. Delayed phototoxicity may follow the systemic administration of furocoumarins or psoralens. Most photoallergic reactions occur after topical contact with chemical agents. Early signs are pruritus and eczema, which appear within 24 hours after chemical and light exposure. Drugs in this category include sulfonamides, griseofulvin, hydrocortisone, benzocaine, coal tar, and phenothiazines. In reactions caused by the combination of drugs and light, the distribution of the rash, which is confined to sun-exposed areas, is an important diagnostic clue. Treatment consists primarily of removal of the offending agent and of the sun exposure.

Polymorphous Light Eruption

As the name implies, the clinical presentation of polymorphous light eruption is variable. The lesions, which represent a reaction to ultraviolet B light, range from small papules and vesicles to plaques. They may appear eczematous and are often pruritic, thus causing confusion with atopic dermatitis. At times, large nodules may appear in areas of light exposure. The eruption generally occurs within several hours to several days of exposure. Polymorphous light eruption may be confused with atopic dermatitis. A high incidence of this malady is found in North and Latin American Indians and in persons of Finnish descent; American Indians are most likely to experience onset of the disease in childhood. Topical or systemic steroids may provide relief for acute lesions, but sun protection is the ultimate therapy. In some cases, prolonged treatment with antimalarial agents may be necessary.

ANNULAR LESIONS

Tinea Corporis

Superficial fungal infections are probably the most readily identified annular lesions of the skin. The ring-like lesions are recognized by most laypersons, although not all ringed lesions are tinea. Because the infection of nonhairy areas of the skin by dermatophytes is limited to the epidermis, only the most superficial layers of the skin are involved. The rings are generally erythematous. As the inflammation spreads, the active infection in the center of the lesions is destroyed, and this area clears, frequently resulting in the picture of an advancing border with central clearing. The border is generally scaly and slightly elevated, and, on close inspection, may contain microvesicles and pustules (Fig. 46-35). The lesions, which may be single or multiple, are not always round. Bizarre shapes and, occasionally, a coalescence of lesions may be noted, and borders may not be continuous. Target-like lesions may occur as a result of reinfection or failure of clearing of the central part of the lesion. Tinea corporis is usually asymptomatic, although pruritus may be present.

The organism responsible for most cases of tinea corporis is *Trichophyton tonsurans*. *Microsporum canis*, *Microsporum audouinii*, and *Trichophyton mentagrophytes* infections are also seen. The diagnosis may be confirmed by potassium hydroxide preparations. Because tinea corporis occurs on nonhairy skin, the lesions do not fluoresce with a Wood's lamp. The three lesions most frequently confused with tinea corporis are granuloma annulare, the herald spots of pityriasis rosea, and dry nummular eczema. Treatment consists of application of one of the topical antifungal agents such as clotrimazole, haloprogin, or miconazole. Application twice daily for 2 to 3 weeks or until the lesion clears is recommended.

Granuloma Annulare

The uninitiated almost always mistake granuloma annulare for tinea corporis. Granuloma annulare is an inflammatory disorder characterized by the eruption of papules, which may be superficial or subcutaneous, in a ringed arrangement. The initial papule enlarges outward and the center clears, sometimes seeming depressed (Fig. 46-36). The key to differentiation from tinea corporis is close inspection of the borders: In granuloma annulare, the surface of the lesion is devoid of scale, vesicles, or pustules; skin markings are normal. In tinea, the border of the lesion is scaly, often with microvesicles and pustules, and the color of the lesions varies from skin tone to erythematous. The lesions of granuloma annulare are asymptomatic, being neither pruritic nor tender.

The cause of granuloma annulare is unknown. Some believe that it represents a delayed type of hypersensitivity. Most lesions resolve spontaneously within 2 years, but some may last for decades. In adults, an association with diabetes mellitus has been reported, but this has not been noted in children. Nearly one-half of all individuals with granuloma annulare have a single lesion. The lesions most frequently appear on the distal extremities. Deep-seated lesions can appear to be attached to the periosteum of bone, particularly the tibia. On biopsy samples, these lesions resemble rheumatoid nodules, but no association is made with connective tissue diseases. Because the nodules regress in 6 weeks to 6 months, treatment is not generally required.

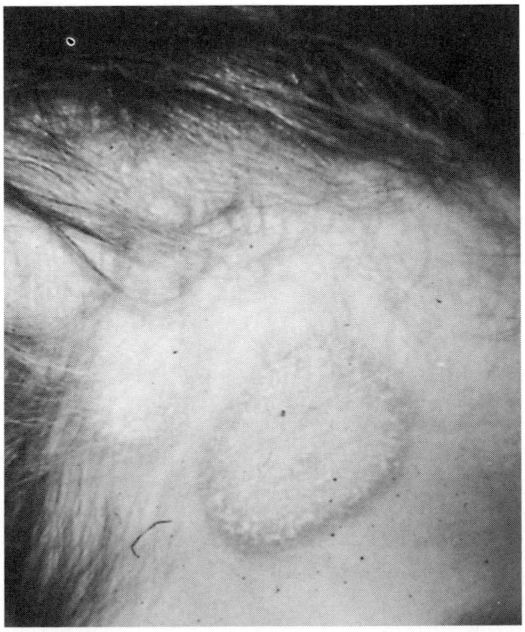

Figure 46-35. Annular lesion of tinea corporis with a raised border and scaling on the forehead.

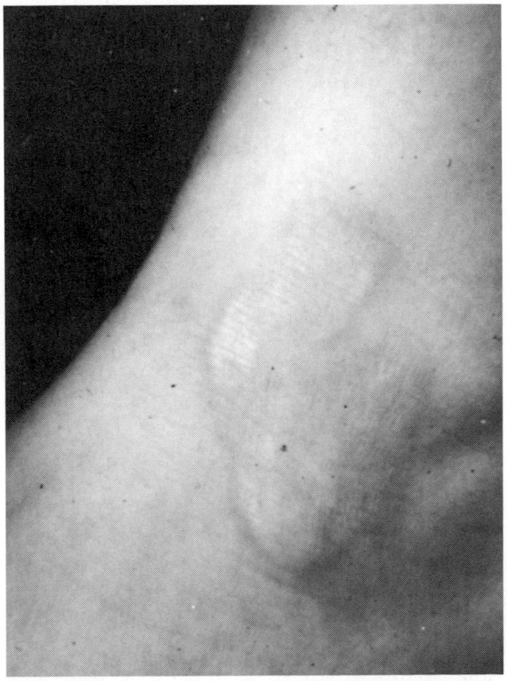

Figure 46-36. A granuloma annulare lesion on the ankle. Note the lack of epidermal involvement.

Urticaria

Hives, or wheals, are common in both children and adults. The lesions represent a localized vasodilation and transudation of fluid from capillaries and small blood vessels. Hives are transient lasting less than 24 hours. They are erythematous papules and plaques that may be round or oval or form rings or arcs. Stasis of blood in the center of lesions frequently creates an appearance of purpura. Pruritus is a common feature.

Urticaria is a manifestation of the release of mediators from cutaneous mast cells, which increase vascular permeability. Histamine, kinins, and prostaglandins are among the mediators released. Urticaria may be caused by drugs, foods, inhalant allergies, infections, and arthropod bites and stings. Other agents include contactants, internal diseases, psychogenic factors, genetic abnormalities, and physical agents. Given the wide variety of possible agents, pinpointing the cause of urticaria is often difficult.

Infections that may cause urticaria include those with group A beta-hemolytic streptococci, hepatitis virus, and Epstein-Barr virus. Physical agents that may result in urticaria include heat, cold, pressure, light, water, and vibration. Cholinergic urticaria is a fairly distinctive form manifested by the appearance of 2- to 3-mm papules surrounded by large erythematous flares. These flares are very pruritic and follow the onset of perspiration.

Uncovering the cause of chronic urticaria, defined as urticaria of at least 6 weeks' duration, is particularly difficult. In most series, the cause of the problem has been uncovered in fewer than 20% of the cases. The presence of urticarial lesions that persist for more than 24 hours should raise the suspicion of urticarial vasculitis. A skin biopsy of one of the lesions will be diagnostic.

Treatment of urticaria depends on the extent and severity of the condition. Acute episodes that threaten vital functions should be treated with epinephrine, as well as with antihistamines. Systemic steroids are indicated occasionally. Usually, an antihistamine alone is satisfactory therapy until the problem resolves.

Erythema Multiforme

The target-like lesions of erythema multiforme evolve over a period of 1 week and should not be confused with the lesions of urticaria, which occasionally resemble targets because of their bluish centers. The primary lesion of erythema multiforme is a dull red macule or wheal in the center of which is a papule or vesicle. The macule becomes papular and then plaque-like, and the center forms concentric rings of color. The center may blister and appear purpuric or even necrotic.

Erythema multiforme is a nonspecific hypersensitivity reaction that can be divided into two types, minor and major, depending on the extent and severity of the lesions. The minor form is often preceded by an upper respiratory infection. Herpes simplex recurrences are responsible most often for recurrent erythema multiforme. Other infections implicated include infectious mononucleosis, *Yersinia* infection, tuberculosis, and histoplasmosis. The underlying cause is not usually defined, however.

Erythema multiforme major is a much more serious disorder. Mucous membrane involvement is significant, and erosive lesions on mucous membrane surfaces may lead to dehydration if the patient fails to take in adequate fluids. Eye involvement may lead to blindness. Large areas of the cutaneous surface may become denuded. Affected children appear ill and experience fever, prostration, and myalgias. Mycoplasma pneumoniae infections have rarely been implicated in erythema multiforme major. However, the condition is usually drug-related. The drugs most frequently associated with this reaction are sulfonamides, penicillins, and phenytoin. The reaction follows drug therapy by 1 to 3 weeks allowing time for the antigenic stimulus to cause the host immune response. The course of the illness is prolonged; Stevens-Johnson syndrome, which is the most severe form and often exhibits severe mucocutaneous involvement, lasts for weeks. Although therapy is mainly supportive, hospitalization is recommended. The skin is handled best as if it were burned, with the healing lesions being treated with wet compresses, whirlpool baths, and ointments. Ophthalmologic consultation is important because of the high incidence of corneal involvement with consequent scarring. The use of systemic steroids remains controversial.

Erythema Marginatum

The clinical appearance of the skin lesions occasionally seen in acute rheumatic fever is not pathognomonic. Erythema marginatum begins as erythematous blotches or papules that spread peripherally. The borders may form annular, sometimes polycyclic or serpiginous lesions. The margins are sharp, and the lesions advance and change shape rapidly. Dull red, pink, or violaceous, the lesions may resemble urticaria, but they are not pruritic. Their rapid change distinguishes them from erythema multiforme.

Erythema marginatum occurs in approximately 10% of patients with acute rheumatic fever. The rash is not specific for acute rheumatic fever, however, having also been reported in patients with juvenile rheumatoid arthritis. It occurs most commonly on the trunk and inner aspects of the upper arms and thighs. A skin biopsy of the lesion may be helpful in establishing an early diagnosis of acute rheumatic fever.

Erythema Migrans

The rash of erythema migrans takes two general forms. One is an expanding red patch in which are varying intensities of redness; the other is a central red patch surrounded by normal-appearing skin that is, in turn, surrounded by an expanding red band producing a target or ring-within-a-ring configuration. The lesions are usually flat or slightly elevated. The eruptions tend to be asymptomatic, but burning, pruritus, or pain may be present. In three-fourths of the patients, a single lesion begins 1 to 3 weeks after a bite from a tick. The spirochete *Borrelia burgdorferi*, which is responsible for the rash and its progression to Lyme disease, is usually transmitted by the deer tick, *Ixodes scapularis (dammini)*.

DISORDERS OF THE SCALP

Scaling

TINEA CAPITIS

Dermatophyte infections should be ruled out whenever scaling of the scalp is found (Fig. 46-37). During the last few decades, *T. tonsurans* has replaced Microsporum species as the most common fungus responsible for tinea capitis. With this change has come an alteration in the appearance of the scalp infection. *Trichophyton* infections are manifested by a variety of lesions; the most common of these, and the one that is mistaken frequently for other conditions, particularly seborrheic dermatitis, involves scalp scaling without significant hair loss. Patches of hair loss, pustules, and boggy masses are other types of presentation and are discussed later in this section.

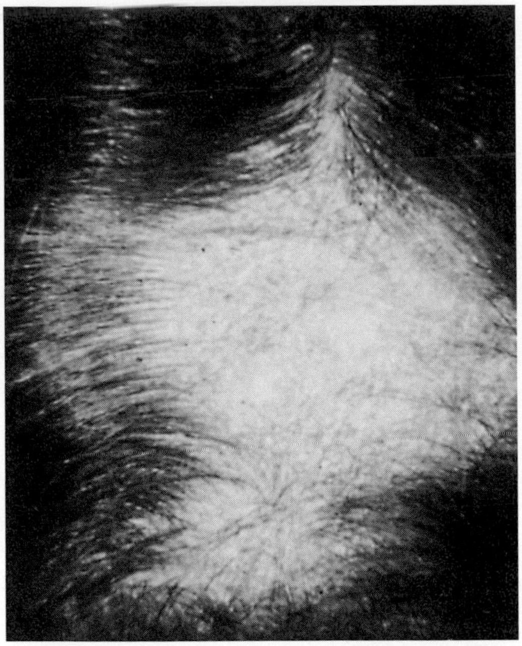

Figure 46-37. Scaling and hair loss in the classic form of tinea capitis.

In the past, the Wood's lamp was used frequently as a reliable screen for tinea capitis. *Microsporum* species invaded the outside of the hair shaft (ectothrix) producing by-products of infection that fluoresced with ultraviolet light. In contrast, *Trichophyton* infections grow within the hair shaft itself (endothrix) and do not fluoresce. In addition, with *Trichophyton* infections, the hair becomes fragile and tends to break off near the scalp resulting in so-called black-dot alopecia.

Tinea capitis is transmitted easily among children and is the most common fungal infection occurring before puberty. After puberty, tinea capitis is much less common, for reasons that are not clear. The infection can also be transmitted by animals, although this mode of transmission has decreased in frequency.

A 10% potassium hydroxide preparation may be used to demonstrate the hyphae and spores causing tinea capitis. The diagnosis is established most easily by the examination of broken hairs, which are most likely to be infected. If the diagnosis is in doubt, a culture of hair and scale may be placed on Sabouraud medium to grow the fungus. Office culture bottles that are inexpensive and easy to read are available for this test.

Given that the infection invades the hair shaft, topical antifungal therapy is not effective. Systemic antifungal agents such as griseofulvin, 15 to 20 mg/kg/day, given once daily with a meal for 6 to 8 weeks, are effective in eradicating this infection. Care must be taken to examine other household members for similar infection. Selenium sulfide solution, 2.5%, used as a shampoo twice weekly, will decrease the shedding of live fungi.

TINEA AMIANTACEA

The thick, adherent scaling of tinea amiantacea is usually mistaken for tinea capitis. The scales are silvery and tend to overlap, often trapping hair and, thereby, causing thinning of the scalp hair. Despite its name, tinea amiantacea is not caused by a fungal infection. The etiology is not clear, although some suspect a relationship to psoriasis. Aggressive applications of scale-softening agents, similar to those used in psoriasis of the scalp, are often helpful.

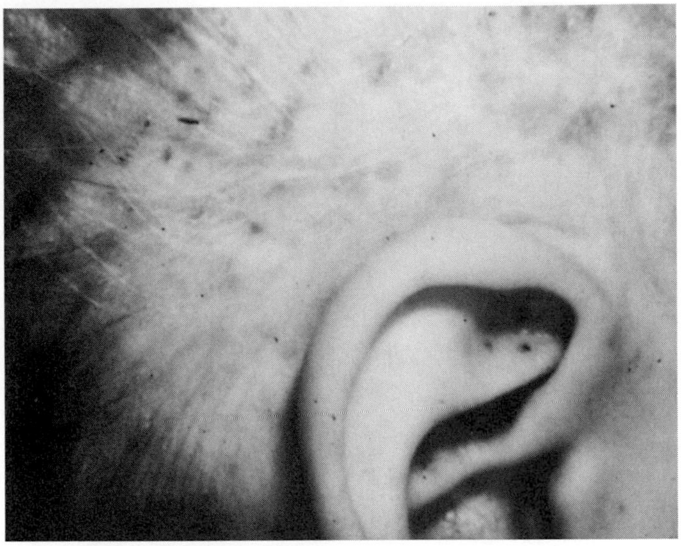

Figure 46-38. Seborrhea-like scaling of the scalp with underlying petechiae in a patient with histiocytosis X.

HISTIOCYTOSIS X

Histiocytosis X is frequently manifested by a scaly, erythematous dermatitis of the scalp and retroauricular areas. The scaling may be mistaken for seborrheic dermatitis until other systemic features appear. A clue to the diagnosis is the presence of petechiae underlying the scale (Fig. 46-38). Other areas of the body may exhibit a variety of lesions including vesicular pustules, discrete erythematous papules, hemorrhagic crusted papules, and ulcerations in creases. This diagnosis should always be considered in any recalcitrant scaling eruption of the scalp.

Pustules

TINEA CAPITIS

As noted previously, tinea capitis can take on many disguises in the scalp. Scattered pustules are one of the various manifestations of dermatophyte infection. The most impressive, however, is the *kerion*—a boggy, indurated, raised mass on the scalp, the surface of which has no hair and is studded with pustules (Fig. 46-39). On first glance, the kerion resembles a bacterial abscess. Incision and drainage of the mass, however, is unsuccessful; as implied by the name, which means "honeycomb," the kerion is made up of channels rather than a cavity.

A kerion is a hypersensitivity reaction to an infecting dermatophyte, usually *T. tonsurans*. The lesions may be single or multiple and often appear over a short period. Although a superficial culture frequently yields bacteria (often staphylococci), treatment need not include antibiotics. Most cases respond to a 6- to 8-week course of oral griseofulvin. Large lesions shrink rapidly with a tapering course of oral prednisone over a 2-week period. Although lost hair will not have grown back by the time the lesion resolves, it almost always regrows eventually.

TRACTION FOLLICULITIS

Prolonged or excessive traction on hair from tight braiding may result not only in hair breakage and loss, but also in the development of pustules at the borders of the areas of pulled hair. Resolution of the problem can usually be accomplished by removal of the traction. Occasionally, a secondary bacterial infection, most commonly staphylococcal in origin, may become established in

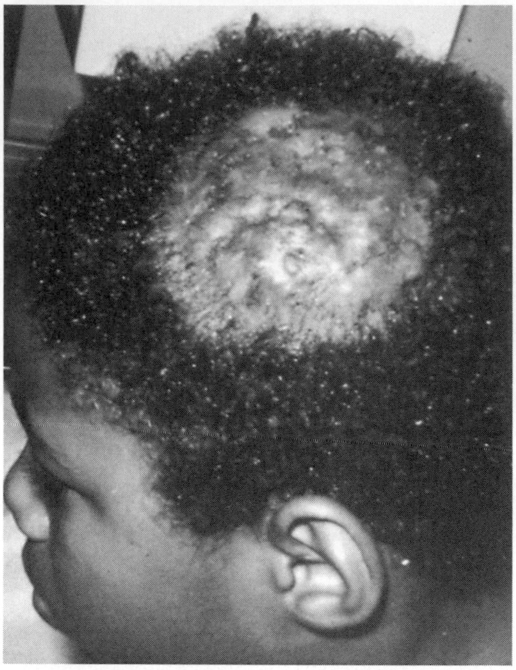

Figure 46-39. This boggy, oozing mass with pustules and hair loss is a kerion, one of the many varieties of tinea capitis.

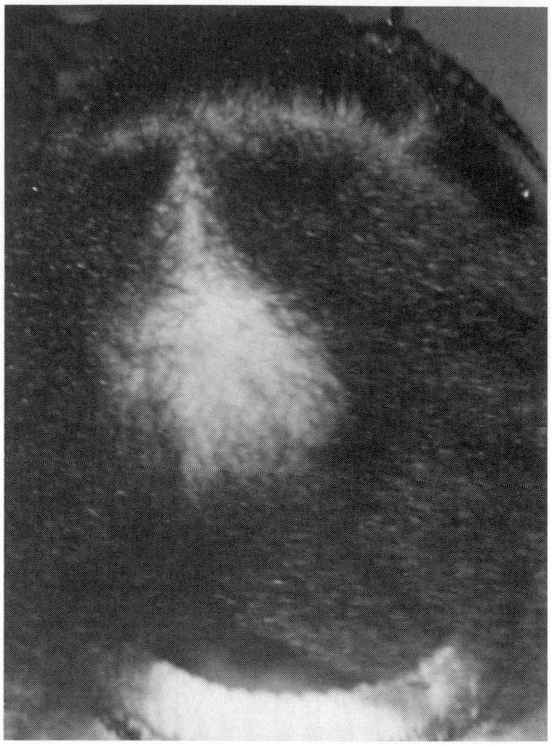

Figure 46-40. Traction alopecia over the midline of the occiput as a result of braiding.

the hair follicles that were damaged by the pulling. Treatment with topical or systemic antibiotics may be indicated.

Hair Loss

ALOPECIA AREATA

The hallmark of alopecia areata is the appearance of well-circumscribed, round or oval patches of complete or relatively complete hair loss. The scalp appears normal without scale or scarring. The lesions tend to appear rapidly and may be single or multiple. Hair at the periphery of the lesions can be pulled out easily. Alopecia totalis is total loss of scalp hair; alopecia universalis is the complete loss of body hair.

Alopecia areata is much more common than most physicians realize. In reviews of dermatology clinics, as many as 2% of new patients have been found to have this disorder. The cause is not known, although an autoimmune phenomenon is suspected. Psychiatric disturbances used to be considered the underlying cause.

Alopecia areata rarely occurs in patients younger than 4 years, but almost one-half of the cases appear in those younger than 20 years. The course is totally unpredictable. Factors associated with a poor prognosis for eventual recovery include extensive alopecia in areas other than the scalp; occurrence in association with atopic dermatitis; the presence of nail changes such as pitting; prepubertal onset; and ophiasis, the loss of hair in a swath above and behind the ears and across the occiput. The prognosis is good for most older children and adults. However, hair may regrow in some places only to be lost in others. Regrown hair is often light or even white.

The treatment of alopecia areata is disappointing. A wide variety of therapeutic techniques have been tried with little sustained effect. Hair regrown during a course of systemic steroids is lost again when the steroids are discontinued. Therefore, these agents should not be used. Local injections of triamcinolone into the scalp usually result in hair regrowth in injected areas, but the procedure is painful and the regrowth is temporary. Topical irritants of various types were in vogue for some time but are rarely effective. The key to treatment is careful, empathetic education of the patient and the parents. Support groups of similarly affected patients are increasingly common in large communities and offer a great deal of help to both patients and parents. Artificial hairpieces may help some patients to maintain a positive body image.

TRACTION ALOPECIA

The hair loss in traction alopecia is secondary to prolonged tension on the hair shaft, usually from braiding of the hair. Traction most commonly produces hair loss at the margins of the scalp or as oval or linear areas in part lines (Fig. 46-40). Permanent hair loss may result if pressure is maintained for a long time.

PRESSURE ALOPECIA

Pressure alopecia is most common in young infants who lie supine and rub their occiputs on the bedding. Such hair loss occasionally indicates a lack of stimulation by the parents. Persistent rubbing of the scalp by any means may result in hair breakage and loss.

TRICHOTILLOMANIA

Hair loss as a result of trichotillomania, the pulling out of one's own hair, often assumes bizarre shapes and irregular patterns (Fig. 46-41). The hair loss in this condition is never complete. A key feature distinguishing this from other forms of alopecia is the lack of scalp lesions and the presence of broken hairs of different lengths within the lesions. Body hair from other areas may also be lost, especially from the eyebrows or eyelashes. Rarely will a child admit to hair pulling, and rarely will the parents have noticed such behavior.

In young children, hair pulling usually represents a fairly benign reaction to stress. Over time, most children discontinue the

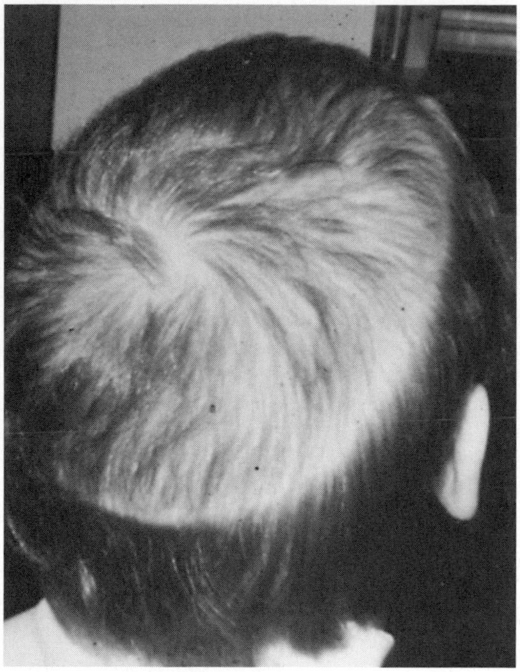

Figure 46-41. Alopecia with various hair lengths in an unusual configuration is characteristic of trichotillomania.

habit spontaneously. A short haircut and grease applied to the hair may help discourage the activity. In older children and adolescents, trichotillomania may reflect a more serious psychologic problem. An attempt should be made to uncover the cause of the stress. Open discussion with the child and the parents may lead to resolution of the problem.

TELOGEN EFFLUVIUM

The hair loss in telogen effluvium is diffuse and rarely involves more than 50% of the scalp hair. Postnatal and postpartum alopecias affect almost all infants and many of their mothers. The hair loss is actually an acceleration of the normal physiologic process of aging of the hair. Some 85% to 90% of hair on the scalp is in the anagen (or growing) phase, which generally lasts for 3 to 7 years. The remainder is primarily in the telogen (or resting) state, which lasts for 3 to 6 months and is followed by shedding. The shedding of 50 to 100 hairs from the scalp each day is normal. In telogen effluvium, many of the hairs in the anagen phase are thrown suddenly into the telogen stage. Inciting factors include febrile illnesses, drug reactions, and severe stress. Hair loss begins 4 to 16 weeks after the inciting event; the hair returns to normal by 5 to 6 months. The diagnosis may be confirmed by pulling out a few hairs and examining the roots for the appearance of hair in the anagen or telogen phase. In telogen effluvium, the number of hairs in the telogen phase is unusually high.

NAIL INFECTIONS

Tinea Unguium

Chronic fungal infections of the nail, also known as onychomycosis, are caused most often by *Trichophyton rubrum, T. mentagrophytes,* and *Epidermophyton floccosum*. These infections are not seen commonly in young children but may appear in adolescents. The infection usually begins at the distal nail edge as an opaque white or silvery patch that later turns yellow or brown. Debris tends to accumulate underneath the nail plate. Treatment of this condition is frustrating and prolonged. Oral griseofulvin may have to be taken for 6 months, and the cure rate is only 50%. In adults, terbinafine has proven more effective than griseofulvin for the treatment of tinea unguium.

CANDIDAL INFECTIONS

Infections with *Candida* are seen most often in young children who suck their fingers or in adults whose occupations require repeated immersion of the hands in water. The key to diagnosis is the appearance of a swollen, erythematous, and slightly tender area of skin adjacent to the involved nail. The nail itself is discolored, often greenish, and separates from the nail plate. The edges of the nail are eroded. Treatment consists of removal of the source of continued wetness, as well as application of a topical anticandidal agent to the infected nail.

DISORDERS INVOLVING BLOOD VESSELS

Spider Angioma

Prepubertal children commonly have tiny erythematous macules or papules on the face, hands, and arms that blanch with pressure. These lesions generally represent benign telangiectases, in contrast to those associated with liver disease, pregnancy, or estrogen therapy. Some of the lesions, particularly on the face, may develop thin branches that radiate from the central punctum resulting in the name *spider angioma*. Sometimes, the radiation of fine vessels produces a noticeable lesion.

Most spider angiomas do not regress with age. If cosmetically indicated or desired, careful microcoagulation of the central vessel with electrocautery, freezing, or the pulsed laser may result in eradication of the lesion.

Ataxia-Telangiectasia

The appearance of fine telangiectases, usually first on the bulbar conjunctivae, may be a clue to the cause of a child's ataxia, which has usually appeared much earlier. The telangiectases generally develop between 3 and 5 years of age and become increasingly extensive over time. This disorder is inherited as an autosomal recessive trait. Affected children face a relentless downhill course with recurrent sinopulmonary infections and progressive CNS involvement. Death usually occurs during the second decade of life.

DIAPER DERMATITIS

Almost all children who wear diapers have a rash in the covered area at some point. In most cases, the irritation is minimal and can be treated effectively with any of a host of available creams, ointments, or powders. As many as 10% of children, however, have a problem rash that leads the caregiver to consult with a physician. Diaper dermatitis is not a life-threatening condition, but it may produce discomfort for the infant and it certainly causes anxiety for the parents.

The etiology of diaper dermatitis is multifactorial. The rash itself may take on a number of forms and must be differentiated from a variety of other conditions. The basic problem is the diaper. If infants did not wear diapers, no diaper rashes would occur; in countries where diapers are not worn, diaper dermatitis is nonexistent. Diapers protect us and the environment from the urine and stools of infants. As barriers, however, they also impede the evaporation of moisture from the skin. The stratum corneum becomes edematous and increasingly susceptible to friction from the diaper itself. Friction leads to maceration, which allows other irritants, bacteria, and fungi (especially *Candida*) to gain a foothold and create even more inflammation.

Ammonia was once considered to play a major role in diaper dermatitis. Bacteria that are capable of producing ammonia from urea are present in the perineal area of most infants. Although ammonia itself will not initiate diaper dermatitis, the rise in pH that accompanies its production activates enzymes in stool that act as irritants. In contrast, *Candida* may be able to initiate an inflammatory response in the skin and produce a diaper dermatitis.

Diaper dermatitis can be grouped into two major categories: primary irritant and candidal. *Primary irritant diaper dermatitis,* also called *generic diaper dermatitis,* is characterized by varying degrees of erythema and papules, often with a shiny, glazed surface. The creases tend to be spared; primarily involved are the convex surfaces, which are directly in contact with the diaper itself. *Tidemark dermatitis* is the name given to the form that features chafing from the recurrent wet-dry effect of urine contact. Nodules and ulcerations of the convex surfaces occur only rarely, usually as a result of prolonged contact of the skin with soiled diapers.

Candidal diaper dermatitis, caused by infection with the yeast *C. albicans,* is characterized by the appearance of the rash in the inguinal and other creases with erythema, superficial erosions, and numerous bright-red satellite pustules. Infantile seborrheic dermatitis may also produce a diaper dermatitis involving the inguinal creases; however, although seborrhea may play a role, treatment should be aimed at eradicating the secondary *Candida* infection that is usually present.

The treatment of diaper dermatitis would be easier if diapers could be removed during the treatment period. Realities of daily life and societal pressures make the removal of diapers difficult for any length of time. Nevertheless, in recalcitrant cases, that may be the recommended treatment. Wet diapers should always be removed quickly. The perineum should then be washed gently with mild cleansing agents, these agents should be rinsed off thoroughly, and the whole area should be dried completely before putting on a new diaper. In primary irritant dermatitis, a number of soothing ointments, most of which contain zinc oxide, are available to protect the skin and decrease friction from diapers. Persistence of any diaper dermatitis for more than 48 to 72 hours indicates possible secondary infection with *Candida;* in such cases, an antifungal agent specific for this yeast should be used. Treatment of candidal diaper dermatitis requires use of the preceding measures, as well as application of an antifungal agent and a mild hydrocortisone cream to treat the inflammation. In some cases, prudence might dictate the use of a separate antifungal agent and hydrocortisone product to be applied alternately every 2 hours with each diaper change.

Talcs and cornstarch may be used to protect the skin and absorb excess fluid. Parents must be warned that talc can be inhaled by the infant, however, resulting in respiratory problems. Cornstarch does not enhance candidal growth, contrary to common belief.

Whether cloth or disposable diapers are less likely to result in dermatitis is a moot concern. Some infants seem to react to the detergents used to clean cloth diapers. The plastic covering on disposable diapers may cause irritation of the skin. The elastic bands in disposable diapers and plastic covers for cloth diapers may result in contact dermatitis in susceptible infants. Disposable diapers with absorbent gels will hold a greater amount of fluid and pull it away from the skin.

Although most diaper dermatitis is the result of primary irritant dermatitis or *Candida,* other disorders may also cause rashes in the diaper area. Impetigo, a bacterial infection, is common in the diaper area. Bullous impetigo, characterized by blisters that rupture rapidly and leave moist areas of erythema or dried lesions with collarettes of scale, is the most frequent bacterial infection found in the diaper region. This infection is caused by *S. aureus* and, therefore, is treated best with oral antistaphylococcal antibiotics. Folliculitis and furunculosis may occur, particularly on the buttocks. Recurrent staphylococcal furuncles generally resolve once the child no longer wears diapers. Tinea corporis occasionally masquerades as diaper dermatitis. An advancing border of microvesicles, crusting, and erythema is usually present. The lesions may not be as clearly ring-like as they are on other body areas.

Psoriasis may also occur in the diaper area, because the skin at this site is subjected to repeated irritation. Because of the moisture produced by diapers, the thick, silvery, adherent scale typical of psoriasis may not be clearly evident. Allergic contact dermatitis may also mimic diaper dermatitis. Parents may apply to the skin of the perineum a variety of ointments and creams that contain sensitizing agents, only to create a worsening dermatitis. The clinician must obtain a complete list of all medicaments used in this area.

Herpes simplex infections can usually be distinguished readily by the presence of grouped vesicles but, occasionally, larger areas of erosion may simulate diaper dermatitis. Acrodermatitis enteropathica typically produces vesiculation and erosions around the mouth and nose, in the perineum, and on the acral surfaces (i.e., hands and feet). Affected infants are irritable, usually suffer diarrhea and failure to thrive, and lose their hair. Infants with histiocytosis X may have an erythematous, papular or nodular and, occasionally, ulcerative rash in the diaper area, particularly in the inguinal creases. The rash may mimic a candidal infection but does not respond to appropriate treatment for such an infection. The scalp may be affected with a scaly rash, frequently with underlying petechiae. Scabies may result in a diaper dermatitis, but the infestation has signs of involvement in other areas as well, and, therefore, its diagnosis is not difficult. Finally, child abuse or neglect must be considered in cases of suspicious lesions of the perineum or severe, unattended diaper dermatitis.

A discussion of diaper dermatitis is not complete without mention of granuloma gluteale infantum. This rare but worrisome-looking disorder is characterized by red-purple nodules occurring in any portion of the diaper area, most commonly on the abdomen and upper thighs. The lesions are asymptomatic and are firm or soft and elastic. They usually develop in children who have had preceding irritant dermatitis. Although the cause is not known, many cases seem to occur in children who were previously treated with moderate- to intermediate-potency topical steroids. The lesions sometimes suggest lymphomatous nodules.

ACNE

Pathogenesis

The pathogenesis of acne is not clearly understood. Many factors seem to contribute to development of the lesions. Development of acne starts in the sebaceous gland, a large, multilobular gland that empties into a relatively long canal containing a vellus hair, the follicle for which lies at its base. The concentration of sebaceous follicles is highest on the face, chest, and back, areas that commonly develop acneiform lesions. At puberty, the sebaceous glands are stimulated by androgens to increase in size and lipid production resulting in an increase in the oiliness of the skin.

Dihydrotestosterone, a product of testosterone, is the most potent androgen end-organ effector. Dihydrotestosterone is formed primarily in cells located within the sebaceous glands. An important event along the path to acne is obstruction of the sebaceous follicle unit. For some reason, sebum and keratin from the shedding of cells lining the follicle stick together to form plugs. The plugs, called *comedones*, are invaded by bacteria, especially *Propionibacterium acnes.* The primary role of bacteria in the pathogenesis of acne may be the production of lipases, which hydrolyze the triglycerides of sebum into free fatty acids and other extracellular products, which, in turn, stimulate an inflammatory response (chemotaxis) leading to the rupture of the pilosebaceous unit. The presence of lipids outside the sebaceous follicle causes a further inflammatory response and the production of the papular pustules of acne. All these factors act in concert to produce the lesions of acne.

Acne vulgaris, or common acne, begins with the appearance of comedones, usually in early adolescence (Fig. 46-42). Blackheads, or open comedones, represent sebaceous follicles whose orifices at the skin surface are patulous. The blackhead is not composed of dirt, contrary to popular belief; rather, it represents discoloration of the sebaceous plug by melanin. Blackheads are unsightly, but they are not typical precursors of inflammatory lesions.

The closed comedo, or whitehead, is more likely to become inflamed. In these lesions, the opening of the sebaceous follicle is tiny, and a plug of sebum pushes the skin up in a small mound. Rupture of the follicular wall is likely to cause the lesion to become inflammatory and to produce papulopustules in an attempt to clean up the "oil spill." Generally, the follicular wall reforms; the neutrophils, macrophages, and other debris from the inflammation are expelled or cleared; and the lesion eventually recedes.

Deeper lesions, or nodules, may develop when the products of inflammation take longer to clear and fibrous tissue is laid down. Scars may result from the formation of this fibrous tissue. Nodules of inflammation may coalesce to form large lakes of pus resulting in cystic lesions, which heal slowly, frequently become reinflamed, and may form sinus tracts. In acne conglobata, a severe, disfiguring form of acne generally occurring in male adolescents, a maze of channels may form in the dermis; the skin surface is distorted by large, purplish mounds and by myriad pustules and blackheads (Fig. 46-43).

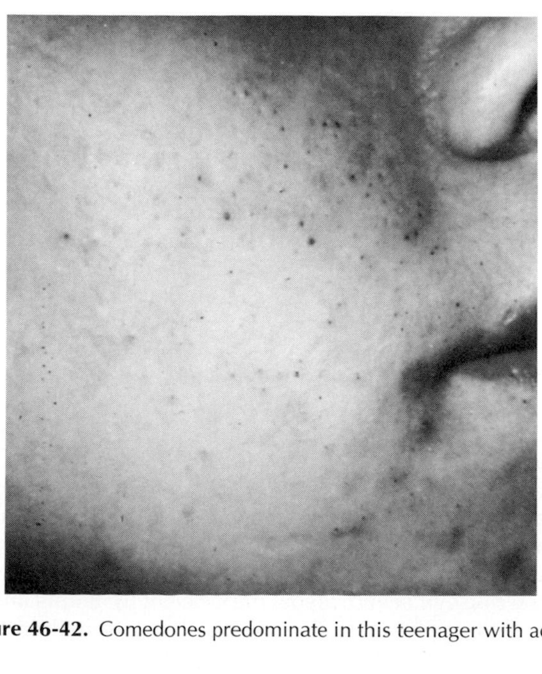

Figure 46-42. Comedones predominate in this teenager with acne.

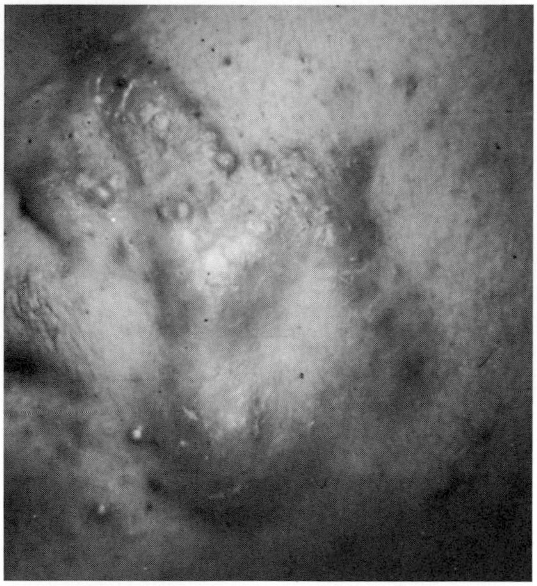

Figure 46-43. Large cysts and pustules are characteristic of acne conglobata, a severe form of acne.

Treatment

The treatment of acne begins with education. The adolescent should be aided in understanding, insofar as is possible, the pathogenesis of the problem. Old myths should be discarded, particularly the relationship between "junk" food and acne. The patient must be instructed that the medications used to treat acne take time to work and sometimes must be changed or combined.

The most commonly used medication is benzoyl peroxide, which appears to have three modes of activity: a sebostatic effect, mild comedolytic activity, and a strong inhibitory effect on bacteria. Most over-the-counter acne medications contain benzoyl peroxide. Unfortunately, the adolescent does not usually read the directions carefully, uses too much or too strong a concentration, and gives up after a short time because of irritation from the medication or lack of rapid response.

Tretinoin, a metabolite of vitamin A, is another excellent topical medication for acne. In addition to having a strong comedolytic effect, this medication increases superficial blood flow, enhancing clearing of existing lesions. A new synthetic topical retinoid, adapalene, appears comparable in efficacy to tretinoin.

Antibiotics have long played a role in acne therapy. Tetracycline and erythromycin reduce the surface concentration of bacteria and, equally important, decrease the surface content of free fatty acids. Their primary beneficial effect may be their ability to depress the chemotaxis of leukocytes, thereby, reducing the pustular inflammatory response to follicular injury. Topical antibiotics, including erythromycin and clindamycin, are also useful in treating inflammatory acne. Formulations containing both erythromycin and benzoyl peroxide offer greater efficacy than either agent used alone. Azelaic acid is a recent addition to the armamentarium of acne therapy that possesses both antibacterial and comedolytic activity.

A key to success in treating acne is development of a partnership with the patient. Most physicians should be able to treat the great majority of their acne-afflicted patients. Failure of therapy is generally the result of a lack of understanding of the disorder. Adolescents expect overnight cures and must be made to understand that often 4 to 6 weeks will pass before treatment effects much change.

Topical medications are often used only on papulopustules. They should be used on the entire surface involved in acne, however, to keep all sebaceous follicles open. Care should be taken not to apply too much of the topical medication. That a little bit is good does not mean that a lot is better; excessive application leads to dryness and irritation of the skin, which often causes the patient to discontinue use of the medication.

In 1982, a derivative of vitamin A, isotretinoin, was approved by the U.S. Food and Drug Administration for oral use in cases of severe cystic acne. It has proved to be a highly effective agent. Unfortunately, it is expensive and has many annoying side effects, and its long-term effects are unknown. It also is a highly teratogenic agent. Therefore, isotretinoin is best prescribed only by those experienced in its use.

Gail Demmler, M.D., contributed to the sections on warts and molluscum contagiosum.

CHAPTER 47
Eye Problems

Adapted from Elias I. Traboulsi and Irene H. Maumenee

OPTHALMOLOGIC EXAMINATION

All infants should be examined by 6 months of age for fixation preference, ocular alignment, and eye disease. Vision screening should begin by the age of 3 years. Visual acuity can be assessed in the pediatrician's office with Allen cards or Sheridan-Gardiner cards for children 3 to 5 years of age, and with Snellen acuity charts for older children who know the alphabet well. The E chart may also be used. In preverbal or retarded children, symmetry of visual acuity between the two eyes can be determined by the pattern of fixation. Vision is recorded as being central or eccentric, steady or interrupted by abnormal or involuntary movements, and maintained or preferred to one eye or the other.

The primary health care provider can check ocular alignment using the cover test, the cover-uncover test, or the Hirschberg corneal light reflex test. The light reflexes should be symmetrically located in both corneas. The cover and cover-uncover tests are based on the observation that children with strabismus use one eye for fixation, whereas the other eye is deviated. When the fixating eye is covered, the deviated eye moves in or out to pick up fixation. If the eye moves from the nasal side to the temporal side, it is esotropic; if it moves from the temporal side toward the nose, it is exotropic. Pupillary responses are checked with a bright light source, and the direct (i.e., stimulated pupil constricts) and consensual (i.e., other pupil constricts when light is shined in one eye) light reflexes are recorded. An afferent pupillary defect during the swinging light test (i.e., pupil dilates instead of constricting as light is moved from the other eye back to the one with the dilating pupil) usually indicates an optic nerve problem such as atrophy or neuritis on the side of the afferent defect.

Direct ophthalmoscopy can be used to check for the presence of cataracts or other ocular media opacities. A plus-ten diopter lens is dialed into the ophthalmoscope, and the ophthalmoscope light is shined into the pupil from a distance of approximately 1 m while the observer is looking into the ophthalmoscope; cataracts appear as black shadows over a red background. Direct ophthalmoscopy allows examination of the disc, macula, and blood vessels in the posterior pole area.

Children with strabismus or those with evident or suspected ocular abnormalities should be seen immediately by an ophthalmologist, as should infants with suspected impaired vision. Children with syndromes or diseases known to involve the eye, those with a family history of early onset of ocular disease, or those with developmental delay or suspicion of visual handicap should be examined immediately. Ocular handicaps need to be ruled out in children with scholastic failure or learning disabilities.

COMMON EYE PROBLEMS

Errors of Refraction

The most common cause of poor vision in childhood and adolescence is an error of refraction, the presence of which can be determined accurately by retinoscopy. The indications for prescribing glasses in children include significant visual impairment that interferes with the child's activity, the presence of asthenopia (ocular strain), strabismus, anisometropia (unequal error of refraction between the two eyes), or high astigmatism. The latter three conditions all predispose to amblyopia.

Visual Impairment

The pediatrician or ophthalmologist may be faced with the very delicate situation in which parents observe poor visual responsiveness in their baby; the situation is even more complex in the case of a concomitant developmental delay or associated systemic disease. Before any statement is made about the infant's visual status or prognosis, a pediatric ophthalmologist should be consulted to perform a thorough evaluation. The clinical assessment includes observation of the infant's general responsiveness to visual stimuli, recording abnormal ocular movements, and documentation of wandering conjugate eye movements, which in blind children are usually horizontal and roving, with or without tonic spasms and vertical jerky movements. Strabismus may or may not be present, and pupillary responses to a bright light stimulus may be reduced from normal levels. A careful search for organic eye disease and developmental anomalies is made, and refraction is tested. Optokinetic testing and cortical visual-evoked responses are helpful in documenting the presence of vision. Electroretinography should be performed for children in whom blindness is strongly suspected but who have a normal ocular examination. This test allows the detection of Leber congenital amaurosis, an autosomal recessive retinal dystrophy in which fundus changes may be absent or minimal.

Unilateral vision loss is more difficult to detect. Affected infants or children usually present with strabismus or leukocoria, or the condition may be discovered on routine examination. Causes of unilateral blindness include unilateral high errors of refraction, various congenital abnormalities of the eye, trauma, and, rarely, retinoblastoma. All efforts should be made to uncover the cause of severe visual impairment in infants and children so that appropriate therapy can be instituted early and prognosis and genetic counseling can be offered in cases of inherited diseases with ocular involvement.

Obstruction of the Lacrimal System

The majority (61%) of lacrimal drainage obstructions in children is developmental; others are caused by infections (24%), trauma (12%), and dysfunction (3%). Infants with lacrimal obstruction present with a wet-eyed appearance, persistent or intermittent tearing, and various degrees of mucopurulent discharge over the medial canthal area and lids. Pressure over the lacrimal sac area expresses whitish material from the lacrimal puncti. Superimposed dacryocystitis may exist, and dacryocystoceles or fistulas may develop.

Most obstructions (90%) resolve spontaneously by 18 months of age, and lid hygiene alone is the indicated treatment in most cases. Fingertip or cotton-tip applicator massage over the lacrimal sac area, with massage directed inferiorly while the upper end of the lacrimal system is blocked, may be tried for a short period of time; this results in increased pressure inside the system, possibly causing the distal membrane to rupture into the nose. Chronic antibiotic therapy should be avoided. Some pediatric ophthalmologists prefer early probing after a short trial of conservative management for 2 to 4 weeks; this results in early patency of the system and avoids potential infections and continuous cosmetic annoyance. The surgery is successful in more than 90% of patients. If it fails, it may be repeated with or without silicone intubation of the lacrimal system. Silicone stents are left in place for 3 to 6 months. If probing and silicone intubation fail to maintain a patent system, a dacryocystorhinostomy is performed. This procedure provides direct drainage of tears from the lacrimal sac into the nose. Dacryocystitis should be treated with systemic antibiotics and may resolve only after nasolacrimal probing.

Infections

CONGENITAL INFECTIONS

The growing fetus acquires toxoplasmosis transplacentally in the third trimester of gestation from the often clinically healthy mother. At birth, affected infants have hydrocephalus, although intracranial calcifications may not yet be seen. Prematurity, low birth weight, microcephaly, and failure to thrive are frequent. The typical ocular lesions are large, healed chorioretinal scars with pigmented borders, usually in the macular area. Chorioretinal scars may be unilateral or bilateral. Occasionally, a newborn exhibits active lesions. Areas of active retinitis have a whitish, fluffy appearance and are associated with vitreous inflammatory cells. Strabismus and nystagmus may develop later. The diagnosis is made on clinical grounds and is confirmed serologically through complement fixation, indirect hemagglutination, and fluorescent-tagged antibody determinations.

Toxoplasma retinitis in older children, mostly around puberty, is usually caused by reactivation of dormant organism at the edges of old congenital scarring. Growing evidence suggests that primary infection from the ingestion of organisms in raw meat can lead to retinitis. The condition may be associated with various degrees of vitreous and anterior segment inflammation. Small peripheral lesions without vitreous inflammation can be observed. Larger lesions warrant antimicrobial therapy; sulfadiazine, pyrimethamine, clindamycin, and tetracycline have been used in various combinations. There is no strong evidence that antimicrobial therapy decreases the incidence of recurrences.

One of the main features of rubella embryopathy is the accompanying ophthalmopathy. Cataracts develop in more than one-half of patients with ocular rubella and are most likely to follow maternal infection between the second and eleventh weeks of gestation. The cataracts have a distinctive appearance with a dense central opacity surrounded by a rim of more normal, although liquefied, cortex and a normal capsule. The lens may be swollen, and a total cataract may develop. Corneal clouding caused by glaucoma should be differentiated from corneal clouding caused by corneal involvement by the virus. Microphthalmos or microcornea may occur because of interference of the virus with normal ocular development. Oculomotor disorders such as strabismus, nystagmus, and ocular torticollis, occur in 20% of children with congenital rubella syndrome.

Most cytomegalovirus infections at birth are clinically insignificant. Symptomatic babies are usually quite ill with hepatosplenomegaly, jaundice, petechiae, microcephaly, intracranial calcification, optic atrophy, and retinitis. Mortality is high. Long-term effects of congenital infection are deafness and slow development. The typical ocular feature is a retinitis similar to that of adults with hemorrhages and exudates usually along blood vessels. Ocular disease is seen in 20% of symptomatic newborns that have other affected organs and occurs only if the infection is intrauterine. Associated ocular abnormalities include anophthalmia, optic nerve hypoplasia and colobomas, Peter's anomaly, and iridocyclitis. Cytomegalovirus retinitis has been observed in infants with acquired immunodeficiency syndrome and may lead to blindness if the macula is involved.

Congenital syphilis is rare in developed countries because of the widespread use of antibiotics, screening for the disease before marriage, and maternal screening at the onset of pregnancy. Infants with congenital syphilis have fever, skin rash, pneumonitis, and hepatosplenomegaly. Active choroiditis may be seen, but most affected babies have only peripheral pigmentary changes. Active keratitis is rare.

Neonatal herpes simplex virus ocular infection is transmitted to the newborn in the mother's infected birth canal during delivery, or shortly before, through ruptured membranes. Twenty percent of neonates with herpes simplex virus infection have ocular involvement, which can take the form, in order of decreasing frequency, of conjunctivitis, keratitis, retinitis, cataracts, and microphthalmia. Most cases are associated with cutaneous herpetic vesicles. Neonatal herpes simplex virus conjunctivitis and keratitis are seen in the first 2 weeks and must be differentiated from other causes of ophthalmia neonatorum. Cataracts associated with neonatal herpes simplex virus infection may be unilateral or bilateral. They may be secondary to uveitis or to direct viral invasion of the lens. Retinitis is usually diagnosed between 3 weeks and 3 months of age but may be detected earlier. Retinal findings range in severity from small peripheral chorioretinal scars to blinding necrotizing retinitis. Active retinitis is marked by patches of yellow-white intraretinal exudates, intraretinal hemorrhages, vascular sheathing, vitritis, and anterior chamber pleocytosis. Retinal detachment may occur in severe cases.

OPHTHALMIA NEONATORUM

Conjunctivitis is the most common ocular disease of newborns occurring in 1.6% to 12.0% of neonates. The cause and incidence of neonatal conjunctivitis have been altered by the routine use of silver nitrate and antibiotic prophylaxis. Silver nitrate is effective in preventing gonococcal conjunctivitis, but it has no effect on Chlamydia trachomatis. The 1980s were marked by a dramatic increase in the prevalence of chlamydial neonatal conjunctivitis caused by maternal genital chlamydial disease. The use of 1% tetracycline ointment or erythromycin ointment, instead of silver nitrate drops, has reduced the incidence of gonococcal and chlamydial ophthalmia neonatorum. Direct immunofluorescent monoclonal antibody staining has proved useful in the diagnosis of neonatal chlamydial conjunctivitis. Other causal agents in ophthalmia neonatorum include Staphylococcus aureus, Haemophilus influenzae, Streptococcus pneumoniae, Escherichia coli, Proteus mirabilis, Klebsiella pneumoniae, Branhamella catarrhalis, Neisseria gonorrhoeae, Pseudomonas aeruginosa, Staphylococcus epidermidis, Streptococcus viridans, and coxsackievirus A9.

The external appearance of the eye is generally the same regardless of the causative agent. In addition to swelling of the lids and conjunctiva, profuse and sometimes bloody discharge is present, especially if pseudomembranes are formed. The timing of the infection in relation to birth is helpful, although not diagnostic, in the determination of the causative agent. Chemical and mechanical conjunctivitis occur in the first day of life and are caused by birth trauma and manipulation or by silver nitrate prophylaxis itself. Gonococcal conjunctivitis, which is acquired in the birth canal, usually becomes manifest between days 2 and 4. The remaining organisms cause conjunctivitis at various intervals after birth. Pseudomonas conjunctivitis is particularly aggressive and may be complicated by corneal ulceration and blindness. It is acquired in the hospital and should be suspected in infants on mechanical ventilation with other foci of Pseudomonas infection. Treatment consists of frequent instillation of fortified topical aminoglycoside eye drops and systemic aminoglycosides if other foci of infection are present. Gonococcal conjunctivitis and chlamydial conjunctivitis require systemic and topical antibiotic therapy.

An infant suspected of having conjunctivitis should be isolated immediately. If the infant is in the nursery, strict handwashing precautions should be observed. If the mother is found to be free of gonorrhea, the nursery staff should be checked for the disease, which may be transmitted through hand contact. Conjunctival scrapings for Gram and Giemsa stains and for a direct immunofluorescent monoclonal antibody stain for Chlamydia should be obtained. Aerobic, anaerobic, and chlamydial cultures should all be done. Therapy is initiated based on the results of the staining with definitive culture pending. Patients suspected of having chlamydial disease should be given oral erythromycin ethylsuccinate, 50 mg/kg/day in four divided doses, for 2 weeks. If erythromycin fails to clear chlamydial conjunctivitis, a 2-week course of oral trimethoprim-sulfamethoxazole and a concurrent 1-week course of topical tetracycline usually result in the eradication of the infection. If gonococcal conjunctivitis is suspected, the infant is admitted to the hospital and started on intravenous aqueous penicillin G potassium, 50,000 U/kg/day (20,000 U/kg/day if the infant is premature) in four divided doses, and saline lavage of the eyes. Parents and their sexual partners should be treated for chlamydial and gonococcal infection in the usual manner. Gram-negative bacilli indicate treatment with gentamycin sulfate ophthalmic ointment, using one application four times per day for 1 week. If gram-positive cocci or inflammatory cells without organisms are found, erythromycin ophthalmic ointment should be given four times per day for 1 week.

Bacteria may be cultured from the conjunctivae of infants with chlamydial conjunctivitis. The child with recurrent conjunctivitis should be suspected of having nasolacrimal duct obstruction, and patency of the lacrimal system should be tested. The management of obstruction of the lacrimal system was discussed earlier in this chapter (see Obstruction of the Lacrimal System).

HORDEOLUM AND CHALAZION

A hordeolum results from acute infection of the meibomian glands that are located in the tarsal plates in the lid and that secrete the mucinous component of the tear film. A hordeolum is characterized by swelling, redness, and pain near the lid margin.

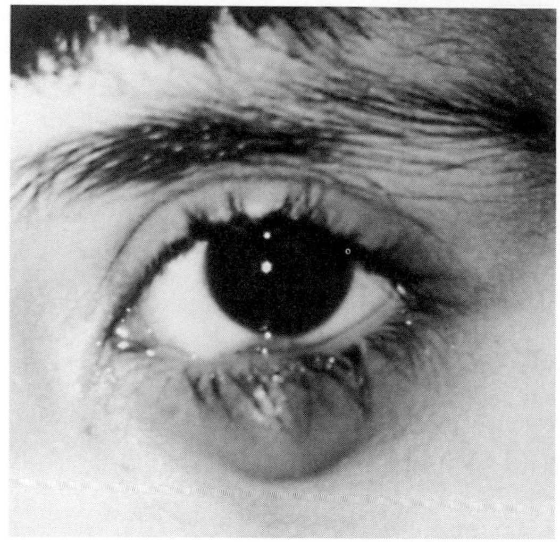

Figure 47-1. An unusually large chalazion of the lower lid. Chalazia are usually much smaller than hordeola and can be detected by palpation.

The inflammatory process leads to the formation of a small abscess that points and ruptures to the outside within a few days. Treatment consists of the frequent application of warm water compresses and the application of antibiotic ointment three to four times per day.

Granulomatous inflammation of the meibomian glands leads to the formation of chalazia that appear as small bumps within the lid tissues over the tarsal plates (Fig. 47-1). Treatment consisting of warm compresses and combination antibiotic-corticosteroid ointment should be tried for 2 to 4 weeks. If the chalazion fails to resolve and is cosmetically blemishing, it can be excised through a conjunctival approach. Intralesional Celestone (betamethasone) injections have been tried with some success.

CONJUNCTIVITIS

In bacterial conjunctivitis, conjunctival hyperemia is marked, and a moderate-to-copious purulent discharge occurs. The patient is usually in pain and has a foreign body sensation in the eye. Vision, pupillary reflexes, intraocular pressure, and corneal clarity are all normal. Staphylococcal blepharitis or chronic infection or inflammation at the lid margins is a common associated finding. Cultures may be obtained, and bilateral antibiotic eye drops or ointment should be started. Ten percent sulfacetamide or erythromycin is a good initial choice; this may be changed later depending on the results of culture and antimicrobial sensitivity. Antibiotics may prevent recurrences and shorten the course of the disease somewhat, but bacterial conjunctivitis usually improves within 4 to 5 days, irrespective of treatment.

Viral conjunctivitis may lead to a mild purulent discharge, but tearing and lid swelling, with or without preauricular lymphadenopathy, are the prominent features. Photophobia and blepharospasm with squeezing of the lids, usually in response to light, occur if the cornea is involved. Adenoviruses are common causative agents. Primary herpetic conjunctivitis is not easily recognized unless it is accompanied by herpetic lesions on the lids. Treatment of viral conjunctivitis (except for herpes simplex type 1) is symptomatic; mild corticosteroid drops may be given if inflammation and swelling are severe. Cold compresses and lubricants can be used.

The hallmark of allergic conjunctivitis is itching. There is usually a stringy mucoid discharge. Allergic conjunctivitis may be seasonal or be associated with hay fever. The patient frequently has a history of allergic disorders. Mild vasoconstrictor, decongestant drops are usually sufficient to improve symptoms in mild cases; mild corticosteroid drops may be necessary in more severe cases. In vernal conjunctivitis, a seasonal, rather severe allergic ocular condition characterized by large palpebral conjunctival papillae and perilimbal infiltrates, 4% cromolyn sodium drops have decreased recurrence rates and shortened the course of the disease if administered frequently and prophylactically. Several new agents are available for the treatment of ocular allergy and include the antihistamines Patanol and Livostin and the mast cell stabilizer Alomide.

The classic example of a chemical conjunctivitis is the one induced by silver nitrate prophylaxis or Credé procedure in newborns. Any chemical that reaches the ocular surface is potentially toxic. The most serious of the chemical conjunctivitides are those caused by alkali. Many common household detergents are strong alkali that can cause serious ocular injuries if they come in contact with the eye. An ophthalmologist should be immediately consulted in case of suspected ocular alkali burns. Pending the ophthalmologist's arrival, topical anesthetic drops should be instilled and the eye copiously irrigated for as long as possible with at least 2 L of normal saline solution or until a litmus paper test reveals a normal pH. Any debris or foreign bodies should be washed out of the conjunctival fornices. Because the bulk of the ocular damage occurs within the first few minutes of exposure, irrigation should be done immediately. The ophthalmologist treats the patient for the ocular surface, cornea, and lid problems that are produced by these potentially severe injuries.

KERATITIS AND CORNEAL ULCERS

Bacterial keratitis and corneal ulceration are unusual in the absence of trauma or use of contact lenses. The conjunctiva is hyperemic, and a central or peripheral corneal epithelial defect with surrounding infiltration is present. There is usually an anterior chamber cellular reaction with or without hypopyon formation. When a bacterial ulcer is suspected, scrapings of the ulcer margins should be obtained for Gram stain, and routine cultures should be taken. Patients are started on hourly eyedrops of fortified topical gentamycin (15 mg/mL) and cefazolin (50 mg/mL). The most common organisms to spread after trauma are staphylococci. For wearers of soft contact lenses with rapidly progressing central corneal ulceration and melting, *P. aeruginosa* should be considered as the causative agent until proved otherwise. Antibiotic treatment should be modified according to results of cultures and antimicrobial sensitivities.

Herpes simplex keratitis is one of the leading causes of vision loss in young adults. Primary infection occurs in childhood in the form of a conjunctivitis or keratoconjunctivitis with or without the formation of classic epithelial dendritic lesions. After the primary infection, the virus remains latent in the trigeminal or other ganglia. In recurrences, the virus travels to the cornea by way of the sensory nerves causing dendritic or geographic lesions. Treatment in such cases consists of debridement of the ulcer margin and frequent administration of topical antiviral agents such as idoxuridine, adenosine arabinoside, or trifluorothymidine until healing occurs. The use of oral acyclovir in primary herpetic keratoconjunctivitis is controversial.

Strabismus and Amblyopia

The pediatrician often has reason to suspect ocular misalignment in an infant or child. Pseudostrabismus is the false impression of ocular misalignment as a result of a prominence of epicanthal folds or variations in orbital alignment in a young child. Pseudostrabismus may simulate esotropia (inward deviation of an eye) or, less frequently, exotropia (outward deviation of an eye). Well-centered corneal light reflexes in both eyes and normal fixation patterns are usually sufficient to rule out true strabismus. Parents can be reassured that epicanthal folds will decrease as the child grows and the nasal bridge becomes more prominent, pulling the skin away from the globe and uncovering more of the sclera. A positive family history of strabismus should raise suspicion of true strabismus, in which case a detailed ophthalmologic assessment is always mandatory. Some common forms of strabismus are briefly described here.

Phorias are misalignments of the visual axes that are kept latent by fusional mechanisms and can be elicited by disruption of fusion, as produced by the cover-uncover and alternate cover tests. A phoria may become a tropia, or constant deviation, when a child is ill or tired. Exophoria or esophoria is recognized depending on the direction of drift of the covered eye.

An intermittent tropia exists if ocular misalignment occurs spontaneously and alternates with longer periods of good ocular alignment and fusion. Intermittent tropias occur when the deviation exceeds fusional capabilities, especially when the child is tired. In a tropia, one eye is constantly deviated whereas the other eye is used for fixation. In alternating tropias, vision is equal in the two eyes, and either one deviates when the other is fixating. In constant tropias, one eye is always in the abnormal position, and a strong fixation preference exists for the other eye. Strabismic amblyopia develops with constant tropias in very young children.

Amblyopia is vision loss caused not by an organic ocular or visual pathway lesion but, rather, by disuse of one eye and predominant use of the other. The mechanism of vision loss is thought to be of central nervous system origin. This process is reversible in younger children, and one major aim of strabismus treatment is the prevention or reversal of amblyopia, in addition to the restoration of good ocular alignment and of binocular vision. Amblyopia therapy consists of patching the better eye to allow stimulation of the central visual centers from the deviated eye. The younger the child, the faster and more dramatic is the response to short periods of occlusion therapy. Longer periods of patching are required in older children. There is some debate about the upper age limit at which amblyopia is still reversible; it may be approximately 10 years of age. Pharmacologic penalization using atropine cycloplegia of the better seeing eye may be used as an alternative to part-time occlusion. Pharmacologic penalization is especially useful in patients whose vision in the amblyopic eye is only slightly reduced.

Congenital or infantile esotropia is not present at birth but is diagnosed in the first 6 months of life. The angle of ocular deviation is usually large with little refractive error. Associated conditions include overacting inferior oblique muscles and dissociated vertical deviations, which may manifest later in childhood despite initial surgical therapy and good ocular alignment (Fig. 47-2). Surgery should be performed before 2 years of age and, preferably, near 6 months of age, if binocular vision is to be achieved. Frequently, a positive family history is found for this likely autosomal recessive disease with high gene frequency.

Accommodative esotropia becomes evident in the first few years of life. It is caused by accommodative efforts made in response to a relatively large degree of hyperopia. Therapy consists of use of corrective glasses and surgery for any residual deviation.

Exophoria is an intermittent outward deviation of either eye that may become evident when the affected child is tired or ill. Exophoric patients often squint in the sunlight. Treatment consists of the correction of any error of refraction and close follow-up. There is no associated amblyopia. Surgery is indicated only if fusion breaks down and an intermittent exotropia is present more than 50% of the time.

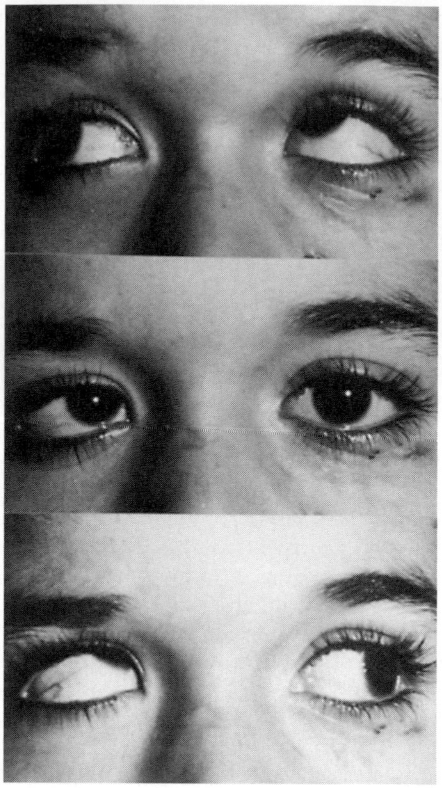

Figure 47-2. Right esotropia with overaction of the inferior oblique muscles. Notice the elevation of the adducted eye (toward the nose) in right and left gazes, indicating overaction of the inferior oblique muscles.

Duane syndrome type I is characterized by esotropia, limited abduction of the eye, and retraction of the globe with palpebral fissure narrowing on attempted adduction. In Duane type II, adduction of the involved eye is limited, and type III is characterized by limited adduction and abduction. Some patients with Duane type I have ipsilateral hearing loss. Others have associated Goldenhar syndrome or radial ray skeletal defects. Some cases have occurred in patients with the fetal alcohol syndrome. Duane syndrome type I results from innervation of the lateral rectus muscle from the oculomotor nerve and absence of the sixth nerve nucleus; this leads to cocontraction of the medial and lateral rectus muscles on attempted adduction.

Möbius syndrome is characterized by unilateral or bilateral sixth and seventh nerve palsies. Affected children usually demonstrate esotropia and an expressionless face. Babies with this condition have difficulties breast-feeding and sucking their bottles. Associated anomalies include the Poland anomaly (absence of the pectoralis muscle and radial defects) and terminal limb defects.

Third-nerve palsies are most commonly caused by trauma or increased intracranial pressure, and they may be complete or incomplete. Other causes include inflammation, infectious and parainfectious processes, vascular lesions, tumors, and degenerative and demyelinating disease involving the nerve. Diabetes is not a cause of third-nerve palsy in the pediatric population. Associated neurologic defects are good clues to the location of the lesion causing the nerve palsy. Like third-nerve palsies, fourth-nerve palsies are commonly caused by trauma or tumor, but many are idiopathic and present at birth. Examination of photographs from when the child was younger reveal the characteristic head tilt and provide a good clue to the chronic and benign nature of congenital fourth-nerve palsies. Surgery is indicated to relieve the torticollis that may lead to chronic neck pain and scoliosis.

Sixth-nerve palsies are common in children. They may indicate neurologic disease but many are transitory and benign and follow viral infections. A sixth-nerve palsy may be the result of increased intracranial pressure from hydrocephalus, tumor, intracranial hemorrhage, or cerebral edema. It may be caused by trauma, inflammatory conditions such as meningitis, and degenerative or demyelinating conditions. Benign sixth-nerve palsy in children develops 1 to 3 weeks after a febrile illness and usually subsides within 6 months. The child with cranial nerve palsy should undergo a complete neurologic evaluation including computed tomography or magnetic resonance imaging of the head. A history of recent viral disease should be obtained, and the child should receive care from an ophthalmologist and a neurologist.

Nystagmus refers to rhythmic oscillations of the eyes that occur independently of normal movements. In pendular nystagmus, the velocity of movement is equal in the two directions. In contrast, jerk nystagmus has slow and fast components. The different kinds of nystagmus are named according to the refixation and the direction in which the nystagmus occurs (e.g., in right-beating jerk nystagmus, the fast refixation component is to the right). In conjugate nystagmus, binocular oscillations are in phase, unlike disjugate or dissociated nystagmus, which can be monocular or binocular with a slow component that is out of phase. Latent nystagmus is elicited by interruption of binocular vision such as occlusion of one eye. Congenital nystagmus is present at birth and may be associated with abnormal head movements and positions. Visual acuity is usually decreased. Albinism is probably the most common cause of nystagmus in childhood. Tyrosinase-positive oculocutaneous albinism may be difficult to diagnose except by using the slit lamp. Retroillumination reveals total iris transillumination in patients with any type of albinism. In addition, patients with albinism have foveal hypoplasia and misrouting of optic nerve fibers.

Spasmus nutans is characterized by small-amplitude and very fast velocity nystagmus accompanied by head nodding and sometimes torticollis. Spasmus nutans starts between 4 and 12 months of age and usually subsides spontaneously after 3 years of age. Intracranial tumors have rarely been associated with this type of nystagmus. Neuroimaging studies are indicated. Any child with abnormal eye movements should be promptly evaluated by an ophthalmologist.

Cataracts

Cataracts are opacities of the crystalline lens. Hereditary cataracts are most often transmitted in an autosomal dominant fashion. Developmental cataracts may be associated with chromosomal abnormalities, intrauterine infections, and certain metabolic diseases. Ocular disorders associated with cataracts include chronic uveitis, retinal detachment, microphthalmos, Peters anomaly, and aniridia. Ocular trauma may result in the development of lens opacities. Chronic corticosteroid and other drug ingestion may lead to the development of cataracts, as may exposure to therapeutic irradiation for the treatment of orbital or ocular tumors.

Bilateral complete cataracts should be extracted early, and visual prognosis is generally good if there is no other ocular disease. In the case of congenital cataracts, surgery is generally done as early as 2 weeks to 1 month of age to avoid severe sensory amblyopia. The infant is fitted with a contact lens soon after surgery, and in the case of a unilateral cataract, the normal eye is patched for an increasing number of hours each day through middle childhood to treat amblyopia. Frequent refractions and changes of contact lens power are needed, and parents should be aware of the importance of perseverance if good visual results are to be obtained. Conservative management of partial cataracts includes the use of mydriatics if the opacity is central, and patching of the uninvolved eye for the treatment and prevention of amblyopia. During the 1990s, use of intraocular lenses has increased for the optical correction of aphakia in children older than age 2 years and occasionally in younger infants. Experience with these devices indicates an acceptable level of safety.

Ptosis

Congenital ptosis, the most common cause of upper-lid drooping in children and young adults, is caused by faulty development of the levator palpebrae muscle. Most cases are unilateral, and the degree of severity varies. Superior rectus palsy may coexist. Familial cases are inherited as an autosomal dominant trait, and a dominant syndrome of congenital ptosis, phimosis, and epicanthus inversus exists. Infants with severe ptosis usually assume a chin-up head posture and look with both eyes in downgaze. Amblyopia is uncommon, and cosmetic surgery is usually delayed until the child attends school. Exceptions include instances in which the lid covers the pupil and the child develops a habitual chin posture, then gives it up for monocular vision and is at high risk for amblyopia.

Acquired ptosis in childhood demands special attention because it usually indicates potentially serious neurologic disease. Paralytic ptosis is seen in third-nerve palsy, and the differential diagnosis of acquired paralytic ptosis is the same as that of acquired third-nerve palsy. Neuromuscular ptosis is seen in myasthenia gravis and in myopathies such as myotonic dystrophy and congenital myotonia. Lid trauma can result in transient or permanent ptosis. Inflammation, swelling, scar tissue, and tumors of the lids can lead to acquired ptosis.

Pseudoptosis may be caused by hypotropia of the ipsilateral eye or lid retraction or proptosis of the contralateral eye.

In Horner syndrome, sympathetic denervation leads to mild ptosis, miosis, and anhydrosis of the ipsilateral face. Heterochromia, with a lighter iris on the affected side, may be present in congenital Horner syndrome. Ptosis is caused by denervation of Müller muscle, which is supplied by the sympathetic nerves and inserts on the upper tarsal plate.

Infantile Glaucoma

Primary infantile glaucoma, with an incidence of approximately 1 in 100,000 births, is caused by an abnormal development of the trabecular meshwork (i.e., trabeculodysgenesis) resulting in reduced outflow of aqueous humor from the developing eye and increased intraocular pressure. Symptoms and signs include corneal enlargement and clouding, tearing, photophobia, and blepharospasm. Intraocular pressure measurements vary from 20 to 50 mm Hg or more. Corneal diameter is usually enlarged but may be normal early. Corneal epithelial edema and stromal clouding result from failure of the endothelial cell pump, which normally dehydrates the cornea. Horizontal breaks in Descemet's membrane (i.e., Haab striae) are diagnostic. The corneal enlargement in congenital glaucoma should be differentiated from megalocornea.

The treatment of infantile glaucoma is surgical. Goniotomy and trabeculotomy open the Schlemm canal to the anterior chamber. In trabeculotomy, the approach is through a sclerotomy site, but in goniotomy, it is through a directed incision at the opposite limbus by way of the anterior chamber. Multiple surgeries may be necessary to achieve optimal control of the intraocular pressure, but results appear to be equal for the two approaches. Oral acetazolamide (10–15 mg/kg/day) and topical timolol maleate (0.25%) or other drops may be given while the child awaits surgery. Optic nerve cupping is reversible in infants after normalization of intraocular pressure. High myopia and astigmatism are generally present because of ocular axial elongation and corneal deformity. Any error of refraction should be corrected postoperatively to prevent anisometropic amblyopia.

Infantile glaucoma is associated with several other conditions including anterior segment dysgenesis, congenital rubella, neurofibromatosis 1, mucopolysaccharidosis I, Lowe oculocerebrorenal syndrome, Sturge-Weber syndrome, and several chromosomal abnormalities. In diseases manifested by microspherophakic or dislocated lenses such as Weill-Marchesani syndrome, homocystinuria, and Marfan syndrome, pupillary block by the dislocated lens and secondary glaucoma may develop. Other causes of secondary glaucoma in children include trauma, inflammation, retinopathy of prematurity (ROP) with secondary angle-closure glaucoma, lens-induced glaucoma, corticosteroid-induced glaucoma, and glaucoma secondary to intraocular tumors such as retinoblastoma, juvenile xanthogranuloma, and medulloepithelioma.

Uveitis

The uveal tract comprises the iris, ciliary body, and choroid. Iritis, cyclitis, iridocyclitis, choroiditis, and panuveitis refer to inflammation of the different parts of the uveal tract singly or in combination. Iritis produces exudation of protein into the anterior chamber with the production of flare or diffraction of a light beam. Inflammatory cells, seen floating in the anterior chamber, can form keratic precipitates on the posterior surface of the cornea.

Inflammation of the posterior uveal tract produces a cellular reaction in the anterior or posterior vitreous. Prolonged inflammation results in peripheral anterior synechiae (adhesions between the peripheral iris and cornea) or posterior synechiae (adhesions between the iris and the lens). Cataracts may develop. Choroiditis may spread to overlying retina producing a chorioretinitis. Active chorioretinal lesions are white; inactive lesions or chorioretinal scars have black areas of hyperpigmentation and white areas of scarring. A particular complication of chronic uveitis in children is the deposition of calcium in a band-shaped pattern in the superficial layers of the cornea, mostly in the interpalpebral fissure area, producing band keratopathy. This complication is seen predominantly in conjunction with juvenile rheumatoid arthritis.

Children with uveitis may complain of pain, photophobia, lacrimation, and blepharospasm, and if they are old enough, they may notice disturbances in vision. Other children may be completely asymptomatic.

The most common cause of posterior uveitis in children is toxoplasmosis. Anterior uveitis is seen in juvenile rheumatoid arthritis, Still disease, herpes simplex, and sarcoidosis. Many cases are of undetermined cause. Because symptoms may be lacking altogether in children with juvenile rheumatoid arthritis and uveitis, frequent routine examinations are indicated to rule out asymptomatic inflammation. These examinations are done at intervals of 2 to 4 months, especially in subtypes of juvenile rheumatoid arthritis, where uveitis is more commonly present. Untreated uveitis results in adhesions between the iris and lens (posterior synechiae), cataracts, glaucoma, and cystoid macular edema. Approximately 15% to 25% of cases of uveitis in children are of the peripheral variety, also called pars planitis. This disease is usually bilateral and can start as early as 7 years of age. Its onset is insidious; redness, photophobia, and tearing are usually absent. Progressive visual impairment occurs secondary to macular edema and posterior subcapsular cataracts. Characteristic "snowball" inflammatory deposits may be seen in the pars plana area, but they are not a universal finding. The cause of this disease is unknown. Therapy consists of administration of topical and systemic corticosteroids. The disease runs a variable course with exacerbations and remissions over several years. Other causes of uveitis in children include sarcoidosis, syphilis, tuberculosis, sympathetic ophthalmia, Behçet disease, Vogt-Koyanagi-Harada disease, histoplasmosis, and ankylosing spondylitis.

Trauma can induce an iridocyclitis, with cells and flare in the anterior chamber and symptoms of pain, photophobia, lacrimation, and blepharospasm. Treatment consists of administration of cycloplegic drops with or without mild corticosteroid drops for a few days.

TUMORS

Capillary Hemangioma

Capillary hemangiomas of infancy are vascular orbital tumors composed of proliferating capillaries. The bulk of the tumor consists of proliferating plump endothelial cells. More than 90% of these tumors have a visible superficial component allowing diagnosis on the basis of clinical inspection alone. A bluish discoloration of the overlying skin, a tangled vascular mass, or the classic strawberry mark may be seen. The tumor swells when the child cries. One-third of tumors are present at birth, and 95% are diagnosed by 6 months of age. The lesion continues to grow after birth but eventually regresses spontaneously. Regression is complete in approximately 75% of patients by 7 or 8 years of age. Girls are affected more frequently than boys.

Local complications include ptosis (Fig. 47-3), occlusion of the visual axis, ulceration and bleeding from the tumor surface, and infection. One rare complication in large hemangiomas is platelet sequestration. Amblyopia may result from occlusion of the eye by the tumor and the droopy lid. The tumor may also compress the globe and lead to high degrees of astigmatism, anisometropia, and amblyopia. One-fourth of patients have one or more cutaneous capillary hemangiomas elsewhere on their body.

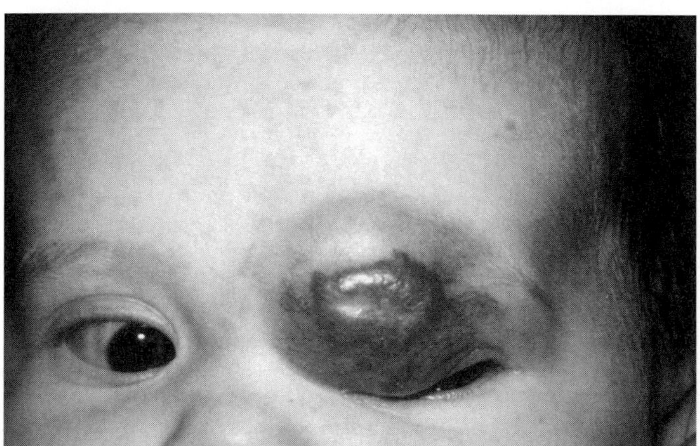

Figure 47-3. Capillary hemangioma of the left upper lid causing an S-shaped deformity and occluding the visual axis. The patient also had significant astigmatism, presumably from compression of the globe by the tumor.

Treatment consists of observation if the visual axis is clear and there is no astigmatism. Systemic corticosteroids and intralesional injections of Celestone are the mainstay of therapy in vision-threatening capillary hemangioma. One or more injections induce rapid regression of the tumors in most cases. Other modes of therapy include surgery and low-dose radiotherapy, but these are not commonly used.

Idiopathic Inflammatory Pseudotumor

The diagnosis of idiopathic orbital pseudotumor requires exclusion of several inflammatory, tumorous, infectious, and traumatic orbital conditions that may have an inflammatory component. These latter disorders include Graves disease, systemic vasculitis, Wegener granulomatosis, juvenile xanthogranuloma, sinus histiocytosis with massive lymphadenopathy, angioneurotic edema, bacterial orbital cellulitis, mucocele, orbital mucormycosis, parasitic infestations, trauma with retained foreign body, inflammatory reactions around primary benign tumors, and malignant orbital tumors. Approximately 5% of patients with idiopathic inflammatory pseudotumor are in the pediatric age group, and only 2% of biopsied orbital masses in children fall into this disease category.

Pain differentiates this condition from other orbital mass lesions that cause proptosis. Most cases are unilateral. Bilateral cases are likely to be associated with a poorer prognosis or with the subsequent diagnosis of systemic disease such as Wegener granulomatosis. Iritis occurs in approximately 25% of cases. The erythrocyte sedimentation rate and eosinophil count may be elevated.

Pathologically, there is a localized or diffuse aggregation of inflammatory cells that may form well-defined lymphoid follicles. There may be an aggregation of plasma cells, lymphocytes, or eosinophils, and a granulomatous inflammatory response. In some cases, proliferation of connective tissue predominates, whereas in others, the inflammatory infiltrate is predominantly perivascular. Ultrasonography and computed tomography are helpful in diagnosing idiopathic inflammatory pseudotumor if components of inflammatory edema and an inflammatory mass lesion can be identified. A trial of systemic corticosteroids is often used to confirm the diagnosis and initiate treatment. Response to treatment may be dramatic, and approximately 75% of patients respond well to this modality. Low-dose irradiation has been used in refractory cases.

Retinoblastoma

Retinoblastoma is discussed in Chapter 173, and the discussion here is restricted to some general diagnostic considerations. The average age at diagnosis is approximately 1 year for bilateral disease and 2 years for unilateral disease. Disease in infants with a positive family history is discovered earlier because of examination shortly after birth. The most common manifestation of retinoblastoma is a white reflex from the pupil (i.e., leukocoria), most often observed by parents when the child is looking in a direction that puts the tumor in the path of the incident light. Other manifestations include convergent or divergent strabismus, pseudohypopyon, hyphema, periorbital swelling, and red eye.

Accurate and prompt diagnosis is invaluable if adequate therapy is to be instituted and enucleation for simulating conditions is to be avoided. Pediatricians should suspect the tumor in any patient with leukocoria, especially if any other family member has had an eye enucleated in infancy or childhood. Strabismus is the next most common sign of retinoblastoma, and a search for retinal pathology or tumor should be routinely carried out in infants and children with ocular misalignment.

Age at presentation, sex, laterality of ocular involvement, and family history are good clues to the differential diagnosis of retinoblastoma, because the various simulating conditions appear in characteristic age groups and may show male predominance or predominantly uniocular or binocular involvement. More than 90% of retinoblastomas can be diagnosed easily by ophthalmologists using indirect ophthalmoscopy and ultrasonography or computed tomography.

EMERGENT EYE PROBLEMS

Battered Child

The ophthalmologic manifestations of physical child abuse have received much attention in the literature, as have the social and medical manifestations. The spectrum of ocular problems seen in battered children is broad, and findings may be caused by delayed complications of acute injuries. The incidence of ocular involvement in abused children is approximately 30% to 40%. Most commonly, intraocular hemorrhages are seen in the retina (Fig. 47-4), vitreous, or anterior chamber. Less common findings include periorbital edema and ecchymosis, retinal detachment or dialysis, cataracts, chorioretinal atrophy, subluxated lenses, traumatic mydriasis, papilledema, subconjunctival hemorrhage, esotropia, corneal opacity, and optic atrophy. Bleeding into the optic nerve sheath may be the only finding in shaken babies. A detailed ophthalmologic examination should be part of the routine evaluation of children suspected of being physically abused.

Trauma

Contusions to the eyeball may result in subconjunctival hemorrhage, hyphema, iritis, iridodialysis and iris sphincter tears, subluxated lenses that may become cataractous, angle recession with delayed glaucoma, ghost cell glaucoma, vitreous hemorrhage, retinal and choroidal tears, detachment and rupture, and optic nerve injury with edema or avulsion. Penetrating injuries to the globe may produce corneal lacerations, corneoscleral lacerations, scleral lacerations, or double-penetrating injuries. An intraocular foreign body may be retained. Lid lacerations may involve the lacrimal drainage system and may result in traumatic ptosis. Extraocular muscles may become entrapped in blow-out orbital fractures leading to restrictive strabismus.

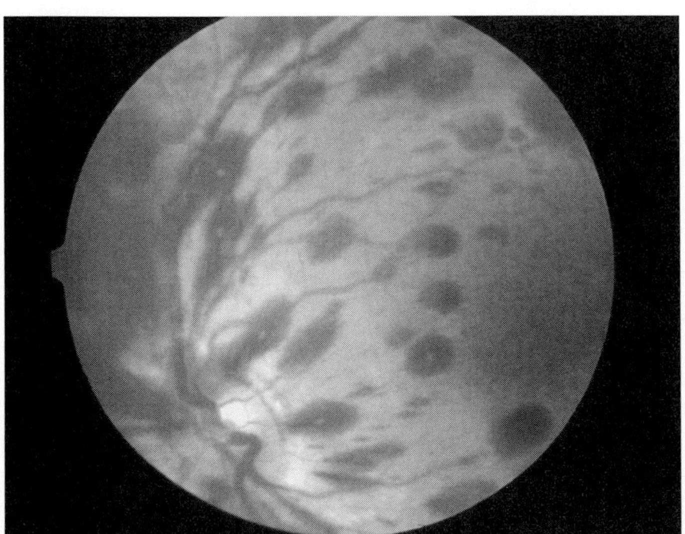

Figure 47-4. Numerous retinal hemorrhages in an abused infant. (Courtesy of Dr. F. James Ellis.)

A detailed ophthalmologic examination by an ophthalmologist is mandatory in all cases of periocular and ocular injuries, and all of the described complications are looked for so the appropriate management plan can be instituted. Patients with suspected penetrating ocular injuries should have a protective metallic shield placed over their eyes, and no attempts should be made to open the lids forcefully; especially in the case of a young child, opening of the lids may need to be done with the patient under anesthesia. Tetanus immunization should be given, as in any penetrating injury.

Sports and work-related ocular injuries are receiving increased attention. The use of protective eyegear in athletic activities should be encouraged, especially in one-eyed children and children with compromised ocular function, a predisposition to retinal detachment, or subluxated lenses.

Optic Neuritis

In children, optic neuritis is usually a manifestation of systemic or neurologic disease. Two forms are recognized: retrobulbar, in which the optic nerve head appears normal, and papillitis, in which the nerve head is swollen with nerve fiber layer hemorrhages. In contrast to papilledema, visual acuity is decreased in optic neuritis, and there is abnormal color perception, an afferent pupillary defect, and always a central scotoma. Pain on moving the eye may or may not be present. If the retina is inflamed, the condition is called neuroretinitis. In children, optic neuritis may occur as a complication of the encephalomyelitis that follows an exanthem, or it may develop as part of acute meningitis. Multiple sclerosis may develop years later. A number of toxins (including lead) and drugs (including ethambutol and isoniazid) can cause optic neuritis. An ophthalmologist should be consulted in the case of any child with optic neuritis.

Papilledema

Papilledema is optic disc swelling caused by increased intracranial pressure (Fig. 47-5). Several stages are differentiated ophthalmoscopically. In the early stages, hyperemia and blurring of the disc margins with mild disc swelling are seen. In fully developed papilledema, there is more disc swelling, venous engorgement, splinter hemorrhages at the disc margins, and various amounts of exudate in the macular area. The chronic stage is characterized by persistence of disc elevation, resolution of hemorrhages, and the appearance of grayish exudates on the surface of the rounded disc. In the late stage, postpapilledema atrophy is present, in which the disc becomes flat and atrophic and retinal vessels are attenuated.

Papilledema in children may be accompanied by headaches and nausea that are caused by increased intracranial pressure. Vision is usually unimpaired, and visual fields show only an enlarged blind spot. There is no color vision defect and usually no afferent pupillary defect.

Chronic papilledema may be associated with visual field and acuity loss. Causes of papilledema include intracranial tumors such as infratentorial lesions, subdural hematomas, brain abscesses, arteriovenous malformations, subarachnoid hemorrhage, and meningoencephalitis; rarely, papilledema is caused

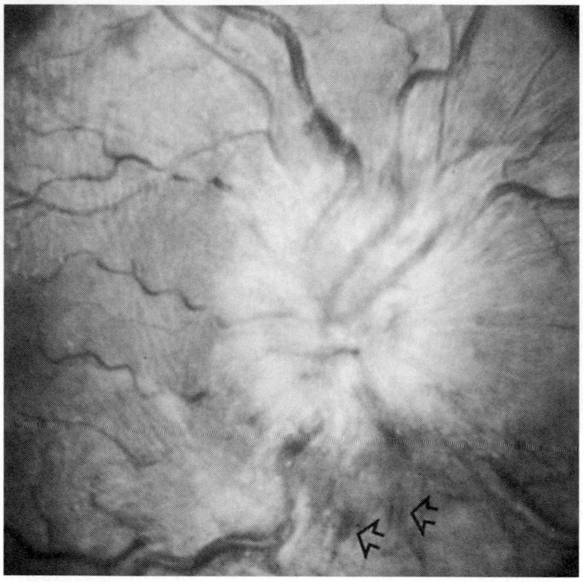

Figure 47-5. Papilledema. Notice the elevated disc, folds in the peripapillary retina, and the flame-shaped hemorrhages (*arrows*).

by a spinal cord tumor. Optic disc swelling is seen in the mucopolysaccharidoses, the craniostenoses, juvenile diabetes, and rarely, Guillain-Barré syndrome.

Papilledema in benign intracranial hypertension (i.e., pseudotumor cerebri) is associated with increased intracranial pressure, normal or small ventricles, and normal cerebrospinal fluid. Symptoms of this condition include headache, disturbances of visual acuity, diplopia, nausea, dizziness, alterations of consciousness, and tinnitus. Pseudotumor cerebri is an isolated phenomenon in 50% of cases but may be associated with obstruction of cerebral venous drainage, endocrine and metabolic dysfunction, ingestion of certain drugs and toxins, and several systemic illnesses. Although this condition was considered benign by many, progressive visual field and acuity loss may result. Patients with intractable headaches or those with evidence of optic neuropathy have been treated with various degrees of success by repeated lumbar punctures with acetazolamide, corticosteroids, ventriculoperitoneal shunting, and optic nerve sheath decompression.

Retinal Detachment

Retinal detachment is rare in the pediatric population. Hereditary conditions featuring vitreoretinal degeneration and high myopia are associated with early onset of retinal detachment in some cases. These conditions include familial high myopia, the Stickler syndrome, Kniest dysplasia, spondyloepiphyseal dysplasia congenita, Ehlers-Danlos syndrome, and Marfan syndrome. Retinal detachment may complicate congenital ocular abnormalities such as the morning glory disc anomaly, optic pits, and chorioretinal colobomas.

Symptoms of retinal detachment include sudden onset of floaters, flashes of light, and the appearance of a black veil in parts of the visual field. Early diagnosis and surgical correction are imperative, and patients with predisposing conditions should be examined at frequent intervals. Retinal breaks may be treated prophylactically. All children with signs or symptoms consistent with retinal detachment should be referred to an ophthalmologist.

Orbital and Periorbital Cellulitis

Adapted from Elias I. Traboulsi, Irene H. Maumenee, and Ellen R. Wald

Periorbital and orbital cellulitis are bacterial infections of the eyelids and orbital area. In preseptal or periorbital cellulitis, the infection remains anterior to the orbital septum, a fibrous structure located in the lids and separating the orbit proper from the subcutaneous lid structures. In orbital cellulitis, the infection involves the orbit proper and may affect all orbital structures including extraocular muscles, sensory and motor nerves, and the optic nerve. The two types may coexist, and one may lead to the other.

Bacterial organisms may gain access to the preseptal or orbital space through the lid skin secondary to insect bites, pustules, or trauma. They may also gain access through adjacent infected paranasal sinuses, upper respiratory tract, or teeth. *S. aureus* is the most common cause of disease acquired through the lids. Other causative organisms are *Streptococcus pyogenes, Peptostreptococcus, Bacteroides,* and others. *H. influenzae* gains access to the orbit from upper respiratory tract infections, bacteremia, or sinusitis. Children younger than 5 years are immunologically most susceptible to *H. influenzae,* especially to the b serotype (HiB). However, after the introduction of the conjugated HiB vaccine, there has been a dramatic decline in invasive disease due to this organism.

Clinical Characteristics

Children with orbital complications as a result of acute sinusitis typically present with a swollen eye. A classification useful in establishing the severity of the orbital cellulitis is shown in Table 47-1. Clinical establishment of the severity of the cellulitis

TABLE 47-1. Clinical Staging of Orbital Cellulitis

Stage	Clinical features
I. Inflammatory edema	Inflammatory edema, beginning in medial aspect of upper or lower eyelid; nontender erythema may be prominent; no induration, visual impairment, or limitation of extraocular movement
II. Subperiosteal abscess	Abscess beneath the periosteum of the ethmoid or frontal bone; proptosis down and out, varying degrees of chemosis, and limitation of extraocular movement
III. Orbital abscess	Abscess within the fat or muscle cone in the posterior orbit; severe chemosis and proptosis; complete ophthalmoplegia and moderate to severe vision loss (globe displaced forward or down and out)
IV. Orbital cellulitis	Edema of orbital contents with varying degrees of proptosis, chemosis, limitation of extraocular movement, or vision loss
V. Cavernous sinus thrombophlebitis	Proptosis, globe fixation, severe loss of visual acuity, prostration, signs of meningitis; progresses to proptosis, chemosis, and vision loss in contralateral eye

Modified from Chandler JR, Langenbrunner DJ, Stevens ER. The pathogenesis of orbital complications in acute sinusitis. *Laryngoscope* 1970;80:1414.

is essential so that appropriate decisions can be made regarding specific therapy and the need for surgical drainage. With early involvement (stage I), the inflammatory edema is confined to the medial aspect of the upper or lower eyelid. Gradual onset of lid swelling, minimal skin discoloration, and low-grade or no fever are present. No proptosis, visual impairment, or limitation of extraocular movement is observed. This condition is not an actual infection of the orbit but, rather, swelling caused by impedance of the local venous drainage. As such, it must be distinguished from a much more virulent form of periorbital or so-called preseptal cellulitis caused by bacteremic infection with either *H. influenzae* type b or *S. pneumoniae*. Both "inflammatory edema" and preseptal cellulitis involve tissues anterior to the orbital contents. Other entities to distinguish from inflammatory edema include an infected periorbital or blepharal laceration, insect bite, contact allergy, conjunctivitis, dacryocystitis, and eczematoid dermatitis.

When proptosis and ophthalmoplegia are present, stages II to V of orbital complications must be considered (Table 47-1). When infection tracks backward into the cavernous sinus, affected patients will have signs of meningitis, focal or generalized seizures, deterioration of consciousness and, usually, involvement of the opposite eye by way of the circumfundibular communicating conduits between the two cavernous sinuses.

When eye swelling is the result of inflammatory edema, plain-film radiography of the sinuses will disclose partial or complete opacification, mucous membrane thickening, or an air–fluid level. Most commonly, the ethmoid and maxillary sinuses are involved together but, in patients with a history of chronic sinus disease, pansinusitis is the usual finding. In early and late stages, the orbit, the paranasal sinuses, and the intracranial dural venous sinuses can be studied simultaneously with contrast-enhanced CT. Thin CT cuts of the orbit, using the multiplanar imaging technique, are also helpful in detecting and defining the extent of subperiosteal and orbital abscesses.

Treatment and Outcome

Occasionally, children with stage I disease can be treated carefully as outpatients by the usual regimen for acute sinusitis, provided their parents are cooperative and can return for reevaluation readily. The antimicrobial agent selected must provide an antibacterial spectrum that includes beta-lactamase-producing *H. influenzae* and *M. catarrhalis*, as well as *S. pneumoniae*. Careful follow-up is essential to detect progression of infection and the need for hospitalization. If the infection has progressed beyond stage I, hospitalization and intravenous antibiotics are mandatory. The choice of antibiotics is guided by knowledge of the usual bacteriology of acute sinusitis. Cefuroxime, 150 mg/kg/day intravenously in three divided doses, or cefotaxime, 200 mg/kg/day in three to four divided doses, is an appropriate selection. Ampicillin-sulbactam (Unasyn), 200 mg/kg/day intravenously in four divided doses, is likewise, a reasonable combination. Once periorbital induration and redness decrease, oral antibiotics can be substituted for intravenous therapy for an additional 7–10 days. Some authors recommend 2 weeks of intravenous antibiotic therapy before changing to oral antibiotics. Blood and sinus aspirates should be obtained and cultured aerobically and anaerobically; appropriate antimicrobial agents should be added if unsuspected organisms are isolated or observed on Gram staining of purulent material obtained from the sinus cavity or orbit. Surgical drainage is required for a subperiosteal or an orbital abscess, but orbital cellulitis may respond to antimicrobial agents without surgical intervention. Usually, the prognosis for patients with stage I and stage II disease is excellent if diagnosis and appropriate therapy are carried out promptly, but residual loss of vision as a result of infection of the optic nerve may complicate orbital abscesses. Severe neurologic sequelae or death may follow cavernous sinus thrombophlebitis.

CHAPTER 48
Oral Problems

Adapted from Katherine S. Kula
and J. Timothy Wright

PRIMARY DENTITION

The dental stage in which only primary teeth are present is called primary dentition. Twenty primary teeth normally erupt between the ages of approximately 4 and 30 months. The timing of eruption varies among ethnic and racial groups (e.g., American blacks tend to have an earlier eruption and exfoliation pattern than American whites). Eruption is usually symmetric from side to side. Eruption tends to occur slightly earlier in the mandibular arch than in the maxillary arch. The sequence of eruption is usually the central incisor, lateral incisor, first molar, canine, and second molar. All primary teeth are usually into occlusion by the age of 3 years.

PERMANENT DENTITION

Permanent dentition is the stage that follows replacement of the last remaining primary tooth with a permanent tooth. Depending on the eruption sequence, the second and third permanent molars may not yet be erupted. However, the second molar should erupt within a year. The third molar varies in its eruption time but is not expected to erupt before the age of 17 years. The normal complement of permanent teeth is 32, with 16 in the maxilla and 16 in the mandible.

Occasionally, a permanent tooth erupts before exfoliation of the primary tooth (Fig. 48-1). This does not present a problem if the primary tooth is mobile; the permanent tooth usually moves into proper position within the arch. However, the child should be encouraged to extract the primary tooth as soon as possible. If the primary tooth is firmly attached, the child should be referred to a dentist for evaluation of the primary tooth, because it may prevent the permanent tooth from coming into good arch alignment.

CONGENITAL ANOMALIES

Natal and Neonatal Teeth

Premature eruption of primary teeth occurs in the United States in approximately 1 in 2,000 to 3,500 live births. Teeth present at birth are called natal teeth; teeth that erupt within 30 days after birth are called neonatal teeth (Fig. 48-2). Natal and neonatal teeth are usually part of the normal complement of primary teeth and may result from vertical displacement of the tooth follicle. Neonatal teeth erupt most frequently in the area of the mandibular central incisor. Crown and root formation is incomplete, and the teeth are frequently mobile making aspiration of

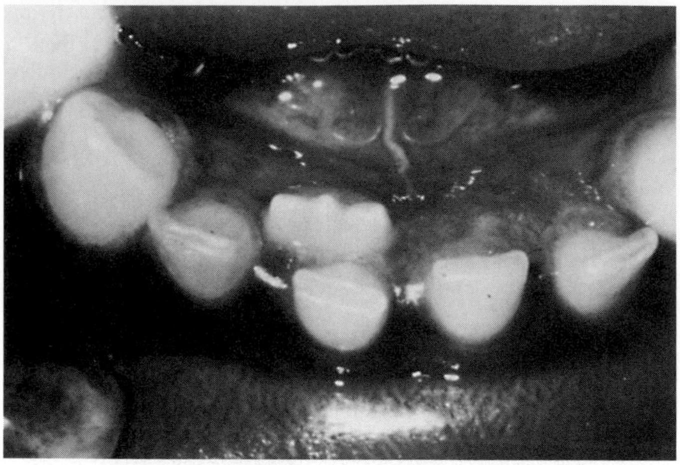

Figure 48-1. Double row of teeth in which a permanent incisor has erupted before primary tooth exfoliation. (Courtesy of Dr. Mark Wagner, University of Maryland Dental School.)

tooth shells a risk. Breast-feeding may produce maternal discomfort. Extraction is recommended if these teeth are excessively mobile or cause lesions; otherwise, they should be allowed to remain.

Cysts

Newborn infants may exhibit several types of dental cysts related to vestigial embryonic structures. Two cysts, Epstein pearls and Bohn nodules, occur in approximately 80% of newborns. Epstein pearls are white-yellow cysts occurring along the median palatal raphes or at the junction of the hard and soft palates. They result from remnants of epithelial tissue entrapped during palatal fusion.

Bohn nodules are white-yellow cysts occurring along the lateral aspects of the alveolar ridges and along the periphery of the palate. They may develop from heterotrophic salivary gland tissue or from remnants of the dental lamina. No treatment is necessary.

Dental lamina cysts, named after their potential source, are fluid-filled cystic formations found on the crest of the alveolar ridges. In most cases, they are asymptomatic and regress spontaneously; however, if they interfere with eating, surgical intervention may be indicated.

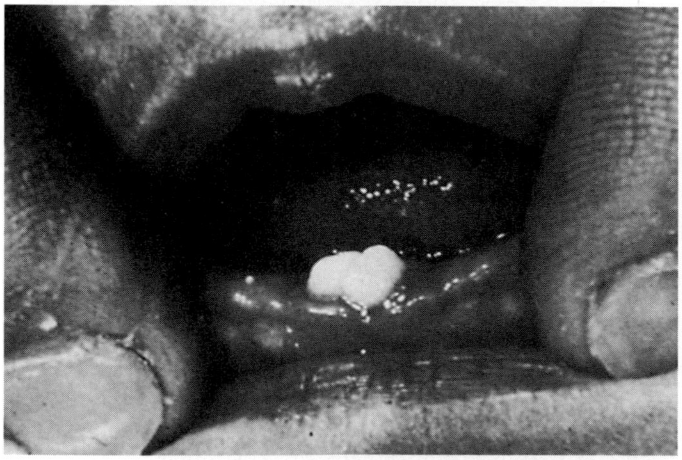

Figure 48-2. Neonatal teeth. (Courtesy of Dr. Mark Wagner, University of Maryland Dental School.)

ORAL ULCERS

Aphthous ulcers are painful, yellowish depressions of necrotic tissue surrounded by erythema. Usually fewer than six lesions occur during an outbreak. These ulcers range in size from a few millimeters to 1 cm in diameter and occur only on buccal or labial mucosa and other unbound oral tissue. Their onset may occur in childhood, and each recurrence may last as long as 14 days. Recurrent aphthous ulcers appear to be familial. Some investigators suggest that the causative factor is Streptococcus sanguis; others suggest autoimmune factors; deficiencies of vitamin B_{12}, folate, iron, and zinc; and gluten sensitivity. Cases of aphthous ulcers in which scarring occurs are called periadenitis mucosa necrotica recurrens. These lesions may persist for as long as 6 weeks and occur so frequently that the patient is rarely free of aphthae. Treatment for aphthous ulcers is usually empiric; however, for children older than 8 years, a tetracycline mouth rinse (125 mg/5 mL) used four times daily produces good results and prevents secondary infection. Corticosteroid treatment can be helpful and should be considered in severe debilitating cases of major recurrent aphthous.

Traumatic ulcers, which occur relatively frequently, are associated with a history of trauma such as tooth brushing, or with an obvious associative factor such as a fractured tooth. Saltwater rinses or correction of the causative factor is usually adequate treatment. Viscous benzocaine should be used with caution because of the potential for seizures in patients who use it excessively.

Oral mucositis is one of the major oral complications of cancer treatment and can be caused by head or neck irradiation or by chemotherapy. The mucositis produced by head or neck irradiation is painful at rest and particularly when eating hard or spicy foods. Chemotherapeutic treatment of leukemia produces stomatitis more frequently than chemotherapy for solid tumors because of the higher doses of drugs and greater immunologic suppression. Interference with DNA, RNA, or protein synthesis by the drugs results in a thinning of the oral mucosa, which may ulcerate and allow life-threatening bacterial, fungal, or viral infections to occur. Because indigenous oral flora are associated with many of these infections, cancer patients must establish and maintain good oral hygiene.

A high proportion of mucositis in immunologically suppressed patients is associated with herpes simplex virus (HSV). Diagnosis based on clinical impressions is inadequate and must be based on viral cultures or immunologic test results. Prophylactic regimens are suggested if a patient is seropositive for HSV. Mouthwashes such as chlorhexidine and allopurinol may reduce the severity of mucositis.

Before cancer treatment, all patients should have dental examinations to identify and remove or minimize potential sources of irritation and infection including orthodontic and prosthetic appliances and broken restorations and teeth.

ERUPTION CYSTS

A swelling on the gingiva of a young patient with an edentulous area where teeth are expected to erupt may be an eruption cyst. Occasionally, blood fills the cystic area making the swelling appear bluish like a hematoma; this kind of cyst is called an eruption hematoma. Observation alone is usually the treatment of choice. However, simple incision into the crestal portion of the swelling may be necessary.

MUCOCELES

Mucoceles (i.e., mucous retention cysts) appear primarily on the lower lip but may occur elsewhere in the mouth. Superficial mucoceles are usually translucent and round, and deeper ones appear blue and manifest swelling, particularly if traumatized frequently. Mucoceles are generally painful and tend to recur even when ruptured. The treatment of choice is simple excision.

Ranulas are large mucoceles that occur under the tongue. They are usually unilateral, painless, and soft and may appear bluish. Continued growth of a ranula may cause respiratory distress. The treatment of choice is marsupialization. Recurrence requires excision of the lesion and the adjacent salivary gland.

INFECTIONS

Oral candidiasis (i.e., thrush) may appear anywhere on the soft tissue of the mouth. It ranges in appearance from mild erythema to small, white plaques to an extensively white mouth. The plaques are easily removed leaving a raw-appearing surface. Severe ulcerative or necrotic lesions indicate invasive infection of underlying tissues and are, therefore, associated with a poorer prognosis than superficial lesions. Newborns can be infected during passage through the vagina of a mother with a *Candida albicans* infection, and infants can contract it from mothers with breast infections. Persons with angular cheilosis of the commissures of the mouth, which appears as a symmetric cracking of tissue, are susceptible to Candida infection.

Immunosuppressed patients and patients on long-term, broad-spectrum antibiotics and oral contraceptives are susceptible to infection. Nystatin is used successfully in the treatment of infants. For older patients, removal of the primary problem, in addition to nystatin rinses, is necessary. Chlortrimazole troches are recommended.

Herpetic gingivostomatitis is an HSV infection in which the primary attack is characterized by fever, malaise, dysphagia, sialorrhea, pain, and lymphadenitis. Vesicles may occur on the lips and throughout the entire mouth. They usually rupture within 24 hours leaving shallow yellow ulcers surrounded by erythema. Onset is usually in early childhood. Recurrent infections produce small vesicles or ulcers surrounded by erythema on tissue bound to bone (e.g., attached gingiva and palate). Exfoliative cytology within 4 days of lesion formation is diagnostic. Treatment is primarily palliative and includes administration of nonacidic fluids. Prevention of dehydration is important. Lesions heal within 7 to 14 days.

Geographic tongue represents a benign reduction in the filiform papillae in patches that may migrate periodically. The cause is unknown, but psychosomatic factors have been suggested.

The effects of teething on infants remain in question. Although teething disturbances such as diarrhea, drooling, and fever have been reported, the association may not be causative. The 2-year period during which the primary teeth are erupting happens to be a period during which a child's immunologic capabilities are relatively low and infections are frequent. Hard or cold teething rings have variable effects depending on the child. Acetaminophen liquid may help relieve an irritable child.

DENTAL CARIES

Caries increases with age as more permanent teeth erupt into the mouth. The average child between the age of 5 and 9 years has approximately three decayed, missing, or filled teeth as a result of dental caries. The rate of attack on permanent teeth appears to be the greatest during adolescence when the posterior teeth with the most grooves and fissures erupt. Approximately 20% of all children have eight or more permanent teeth with caries.

Dental caries results over time from a multifactorial interaction among a susceptible tooth (i.e., host), microorganisms, and a cariogenic diet. A tenacious deposit of plaque, which is composed of salivary glycoproteins, bacteria, and bacterial products, forms on the teeth. Cariogenic bacteria metabolize dietary carbohydrates, particularly sucrose, and produce acids such as lactic acid, which demineralize enamel and dentin. Streptococcus mutans and lactobacilli are the major bacteria in the caries process.

Frequent contacts with food, particularly food that is sticky and contains sucrose, expose teeth to prolonged decreases in the pH of the plaque and potentially long demineralization times. Physical or chemical disruption of plaque such as occurs with tooth brushing, flossing, or use of chlorhexidine rinses, minimizes the colonization of the cariogenic bacteria and the decrease in plaque pH. Dental grooves and fissures, fluoride and carbonate ions, and salivary flow influence the susceptibility of teeth to dental caries.

Although numerous methods are used to detect caries for research projects, clinically, a clinician should be able to visualize white-spot lesions and cavitations on the exposed surfaces of the teeth. Caries may attack any surface of a tooth, however, the most susceptible surfaces appear to be those with pits or fissures. These areas may become carious within 6 to 12 months after eruption of the tooth. The smooth (i.e., interproximal, buccal, lingual) surfaces of the teeth usually develop caries more slowly than the pits and fissures. A patient is considered to have rampant caries if the caries occurs in typically less susceptible areas such as between the lower incisors and on the lingual surfaces of the mandibular molars.

Dental caries still in the white-spot stages with clinically intact surfaces can remain static or be remineralized by a decrease in the factors that contribute to demineralization or an increase in the factors that contribute to remineralization. This can be accomplished to varying degrees, depending on the extent of compliance by the patient, but it usually requires a multifactorial approach. Dental caries is best controlled through increased frequency of exposure to topical fluoride through fluoridated water, toothpastes, rinses, or gels; diet, with the emphasis on decreasing the number of sweets contacting the teeth throughout the day; and increased oral hygiene. Caries on the buccal and lingual surfaces is more easily controlled in this manner than interproximal caries or caries in the pits and fissures, because the former is detected visually at early, surface stages when it is most accessible to fluorides and plaque removal. Caries in the pits and fissures is less accessible to such treatment and, therefore, not as easily controlled.

Dental caries in pits and fissures can be minimized by the placement of sealant materials that adhere to the surface of the enamel, by the creation of micropores in the enamel surface into which tags of sealant physically lock, or by chelation. These materials are most effective when introduced as soon as possible after eruption of a susceptible tooth. Sealants stop incipient caries and significantly reduce the number of vital bacteria in a groove. The effectiveness of sealants is related to their retention, which depends on patient cooperation, saliva control, and the eruptive status of the tooth.

Caries frequently progresses through the enamel as a wedge-shaped lesion that spreads laterally at the dentinoenamel interface when it reaches the dentin and undermines the enamel. By the time the enamel surface fractures under masticatory forces (e.g., chewing on ice), the lesion is usually large and may have progressed as far as the pulp. As caries progresses toward the pulp, inflammation may cause the pulp to form more dentin, which acts as a barrier to the carious process. However, if demineralization is taking place faster than dentin formation, caries may proceed into the pulp causing more inflammation. The edema that occurs within the closed pulp chamber may cause dental pain.

Progressive caries may lead to infectious complications such as cellulitis and abscess formation. If the infection involves the submandibular, sublingual, and submental spaces, elevation of the tongue and floor of the mouth may obstruct the patient's airway. Trismus (i.e., inability to open the mouth) may occur. High fever, malaise, and lethargy are frequently associated with acute dental infection. The patient may not eat properly as a result of pain on mastication or sensitivity to hot or cold.

Children exhibiting pain and swelling caused by a dental abscess should be referred immediately to a dentist for extraction or pulpal treatment to save the tooth. The patient should be placed on antibiotics for 7 to 10 days. The antibiotic of choice is penicillin; erythromycin is the second choice. Recalcitrant infections should be cultured for antibiotic sensitivity. Analgesics may be given for pain, but aspirin should be avoided in case tooth extraction is required.

Nursing Caries

Dental caries can be particularly destructive in children older than 1 year who continue to nurse (Fig. 48-3). Frequent contact with liquids from the bottle throughout the day and particularly during sleep, when the salivary flow rate is minimal, exposes the child to multiple and prolonged decreases in salivary pH. Because the salivary flow rate is minimal during sleep, a child who nurses just before or periodically during sleep is particularly susceptible to caries. Decalcification is rapid in the newly erupting and partially mineralized primary teeth, and pulpal involvement occurs rapidly because the primary tooth enamel is relatively thin.

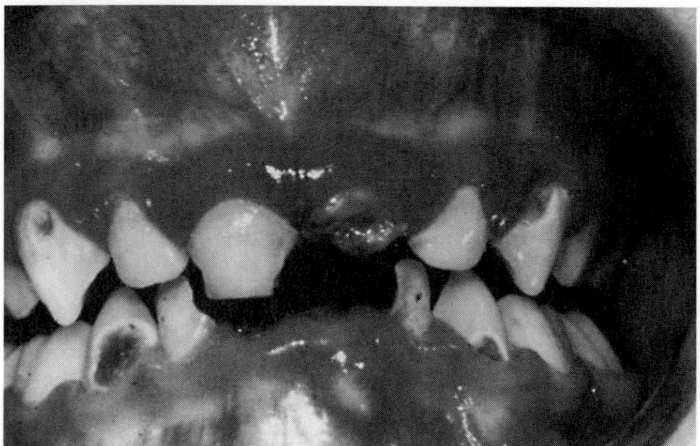

Figure 48-3. Nursing caries.

Continued and frequent breast-feeding is also implicated as a causal factor in nursing caries. Mothers should be informed that nursing on demand past the age of 1 year can result in dental caries. Sweetened pacifiers are also sources of dental caries. The number of teeth and severity of caries involved in nursing caries probably depend on the eruption sequence of the primary teeth, the length of time nursing continues, the frequency of nursing throughout the day, the types of fluids given in the bottle, and whether nursing occurs just before or periodically during sleep.

Nursing caries begins as a white-spot lesion, usually on the buccal or lingual side of the tooth. The white-spot lesion is not likely to appear at the gingival border of the tooth, because primary teeth are continuing to erupt in the infant. Depending on the rate of demineralization, the lesion may cavitate and proceed to the pulp. If the rate of demineralization is rapid, the root of the tooth may not develop fully before the tooth abscesses. If this occurs, the tooth must usually be extracted.

The maxillary incisors are most frequently and extensively involved with the primary molars being the next most frequently and severely involved. The mandibular incisors are not as commonly involved, although they erupt at approximately the same time as the maxillary incisors. The position of the tongue during nursing and the saliva released from under the tongue may protect the mandibular incisors. Mandibular incisor involvement usually indicates frequent and probably continued nursing; in the case of patients who have continued to nurse until 4 years of age, the destruction can be devastating.

In particularly advanced cases, extraction of primary incisors has been necessary at 14 months of age. Early extraction of primary incisors before eruption of the canines (at approximately 18 months) may result in loss of arch space and create future orthodontic problems; extraction of primary incisors at a later age does not usually compromise arch space.

Water is the only safe fluid in a baby bottle for children older than 1 year. Sugar water, commercial sodas, sweetened tea, fruit juices, fruit drinks, and milk contribute to nursing caries.

If nursing caries is identified, the parent should be informed of the cause and of the potential results of lack of treatment and should be referred to a dentist who treats young children. Parents should be told to completely discontinue bottle feedings or, if necessary, to gradually dilute the contents with water until the child is taking only water in the bottle or discontinues use of the bottle completely. Although not all children who nurse for prolonged periods develop dental caries, it is currently not possible to determine which children will have problems.

A complete diet history should be obtained from the parents to determine whether the total diet is adequate. A child who is ingesting only the contents of the bottle may be malnourished. Extensive nutritional counseling may be required. Other members of the family should be involved if they provide care for the child.

Although most children with nursing caries do well with simple ambulatory dental care, some require sedation or general anesthesia. The treatment approach depends on the extent of disease, the extent of patient and parent cooperation, and the existence of compromising medical conditions.

Restorative procedures and tooth extraction for nursing caries are often carried out in same-day surgery units, although some patients may require overnight hospitalization because of medical problems. If the cost of same-day surgery or overnight hospital care is prohibitive for the parents, the procedures may be carried out in the dentist's office with sedation. Office treatment with sedation may be used in cases in which treatment is not extensive, the patient is amenable to ambulatory care, and parent cooperation is good.

GINGIVITIS

Gingivitis, the most common periodontal disease, is an inflammation of the gingival tissues usually caused by a bacterial infection. The amount of edema and the tendency for gingival bleeding increases with the severity of the gingivitis. The factor most commonly associated with gingivitis is poor oral hygiene, but other factors such as mouth breathing, fractured or decayed teeth, and use of birth control pills, may contribute to an increased inflammatory response.

Bacterial colonization of the teeth and gingiva is normal. The pathogenicity of the organisms in the dental plaque is the key determinant in gingivitis. As gingivitis progresses, the bacterial population within dental plaque exhibits a characteristic shift from low to high numbers of organisms, from gram-positive cocci to rods and gram-negative anaerobes, filamentous organisms, and spirochetes. No conclusive evidence exists that gingivitis in children develops into periodontitis, a more progressive form of periodontal disease that involves loss of alveolar bone.

In most cases, a professional dental cleaning followed by good home care, including tooth brushing and flossing, decreases the incidence and severity of gingivitis. In some cases, restoration of fractured or carious teeth decreases the severity of localized inflammation.

A physician should recognize that the inflammation, bleeding, and openings through the epithelial layers around the tooth associated with gingivitis can contribute to profound systemic problems in compromised patients. In hemophiliacs who do not practice good oral hygiene, areas around the teeth may bleed spontaneously or with eating. Ulcerated gingiva is a source of bacterial infection in children who are susceptible to subacute bacterial endocarditis infection, children who are immunosuppressed, and children with uncontrolled diabetes mellitus, kidney disease, or transplanted organs. Children with leukemia who are undergoing chemotherapy are at risk for septicemia if they develop pericoronitis or periodontitis.

Fibrotic hyperplastic gingiva often occurs in children receiving phenytoin (Dilantin) for seizure control. Careful titration of the dosage of Dilantin and excellent oral hygiene may control the severity of the gingival overgrowth. However, surgical removal of the overgrowth may be required in some cases.

TRAUMA

Crown Fracture

Crown fractures are diverse in nature and degree of severity, as shown in Figure 48-4. Fracture of the enamel can be incomplete, such that no structure is lost but fine cracks, called crazings, are visible. Crazing alone usually requires no treatment, but if the fracture is complete but limited to the enamel only, smoothing of sharp tooth edges may be indicated as an emergency measure. Incomplete and complete enamel fractures have excellent prognoses.

Fractures extending into the dentin require immediate coverage to protect the exposed odontoblastic processes. The use of a calcium hydroxide dressing under the coverage may stimulate the pulp to produce more dentin as protection and acts as palliative treatment for the increased sensitivity to hot or cold. The prognosis is not as good as with crazings or enamel fractures.

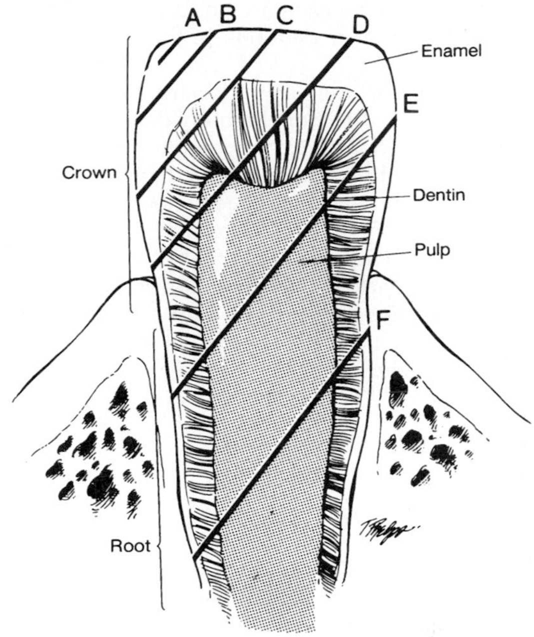

Figure 48-4. Diagram of various tooth fractures. **A:** Crazing; **B:** enamel fracture; **C:** dentin and enamel fracture; **D:** fracture into pulp; **E:** crown-root fracture; **F:** root fracture.

As many as 7% of teeth with dentin fractures become necrotic. If the teeth are treated within 24 hours, the prognosis is improved. The prognosis is worse as the amount of dentin exposure increases.

Fractures extending into the pulp require immediate pulpal therapy. Depending on the amount and time of pulpal exposure, a calcium hydroxide dressing and coverage should be placed on the tooth, or the pulp should be extirpated and a root canal started. Recently erupted permanent teeth with incomplete roots require additional treatment to stimulate root completion or closure before definitive pulpal treatment. Primary teeth can be treated similar to permanent teeth. Cooperation of the patient and root length are two major factors in the decision to save primary teeth; extraction is often the treatment of choice. Lack of treatment inevitably results in necrosis with possible abscessing and loss of the tooth. The prognosis for teeth with pulp exposure depends on the type of treatment and the amount of time elapsed before treatment.

Color is a good criterion for determining the extent of crown fracture. Enamel is relatively white, dentin is more yellow, and pulp is red. Therefore, an enamel fracture alone should be white, a fracture into dentin should exhibit yellow surrounded by white, and a fracture into the pulp should appear as red surrounded by yellow and white.

Approximately 20% to 65% of reported dental trauma is crown fracture without pulp exposure; approximately 5% to 8% is crown fracture with pulp exposure. Immediate dental referral is the treatment of choice.

Root Fracture

Root fractures, which involve dentin, cementum, and pulp, constitute approximately 0.5% to 7.0% of traumatic injuries to the permanent dentition and approximately 2% to 4% of traumatic injuries to the primary dentition. Root fractures are relatively uncommon in primary or permanent incisors with incomplete root formation. They occur predominantly in the permanent maxillary central incisor area in persons between 11 and 20 years of age and in the primary dentition in those between 3 and 4 years.

Clinical findings include a slightly extruded tooth frequently displaced in a lingual direction. Mobility depends on the site of the fracture. The child may express symptoms of sensitivity on occlusion. Radiographs are necessary for diagnosis. Other dental injuries (e.g., alveolar fracture) frequently occur simultaneously.

Pulpal necrosis occurs in approximately 20% to 45% of teeth with root fractures. The type of dental treatment indicated depends on numerous factors. If the tooth can be retained, splinting is necessary. Dislocated permanent teeth that are not splinted are at the highest risk for necrosis. The patient should be referred to a dentist immediately.

Crown-Root Fracture

Crown-root fractures extend from the crown into the root. The portions of the tooth may be visibly distinct, or a fragment may be missing. Depending on the direction of the fracture and soft tissue attachment, the extent of the fracture may not be visible. Crown-root fractures are reported in as many as 5% of trauma cases. For primary teeth, extraction is usually the treatment of choice. Permanent teeth can be salvaged if the fracture occurs less than one-third of the root length from the crown.

Concussion

The supporting structures of a tooth can be traumatized without clinically apparent mobility or displacement. The child may exhibit transient sensitivity to percussion or occlusion. The treatment of choice is relief of occlusion.

Subluxation

Subluxation of a tooth may cause bleeding and mobility of the tooth as a result of injury to the periodontal fibers. Displacement of the tooth is not usually apparent. Approximately 15% to 20% of reported trauma cases exhibit concussion or subluxation. The treatment is similar to that for concussion.

Displacement

Displacements with or without alveolar fractures include intrusive, extrusive, or lateral movement of the tooth. An injured tooth may undergo more than one movement, as may adjacent teeth.

Pulpal necrosis occurs with the highest frequency in cases of intrusion and extrusion, respectively. Intrusion forces the tooth apically into the alveolar bone. Clinically, the crown of the intruded tooth appears shorter than those of the adjacent teeth. Bleeding may be apparent.

Trauma to the primary teeth may cause injury to the underlying permanent teeth, which may be in various stages of development. The extent of injury to the permanent teeth may include one or all of the following: discoloration, malformation, hypomineralization, and eruption problems.

An intruded primary tooth may be allowed to reerupt by itself over a few months if it appears that it will cause no additional damage to the permanent tooth. A displaced primary tooth with an exposed root should be extracted. Intruded permanent teeth may require repositioning and splinting if it appears that the tooth will not erupt at all or will not erupt into an ideal position. Orthodontic repositioning of the teeth may be required if immediate ideal positioning is not possible.

An extruded tooth is usually longer than the crowns of the adjacent teeth. Treatment of extruded permanent teeth involves immediate intrusive force followed by splinting. The physician should force the tooth into the socket, have the child bite on gauze, and then immediately refer the child to a dentist. If the teeth cannot be repositioned fully into the sockets, the child should simply be referred immediately to a dentist. Local anesthesia may be required for the child to accept treatment. Extruded primary teeth should be extracted.

Avulsion

Avulsion is the total displacement of a tooth from its socket. The frequency of avulsion caused by trauma ranges from 7% to 15% in the primary dentition and from 0.5% to 15.0% in the permanent dentition. The maxillary central incisors are avulsed most frequently because of their single conical tapering roots and their potential prominence.

A bleeding hole appears where a tooth should appear. However, the clinician should never assume that a tooth has been totally avulsed unless a radiograph shows no evidence of tooth structure or the child presents the entire tooth. Partial avulsion or total intrusion can occur.

In the case of avulsed permanent teeth, treatment should be instituted as soon as possible. The parent or guardian should quickly wash the tooth in saliva or saline solution and reinsert the tooth as closely as possible into the alveolus. If the tooth cannot be reimplanted by the parent or physician immediately, it could be stored in the buccal vestibule of an adult's or the child's mouth, depending on the child's age and cooperation. An alternate storage medium is saline solution. Keeping the tooth moist is of greatest concern. The child should be seen by a dentist immediately. Splinting and possibly root canal therapy is required.

The prognosis depends on the time elapsed between avulsion and treatment, and the conditions under which the tooth has been stored. Root resorption is the most common complication after reimplantation. Root resorption increases in frequency from 10% when the tooth is implanted within 30 minutes of avulsion to 95% when reimplantation has not occurred within 2 hours. Reimplantation of primary teeth is not indicated because of potential damage to the underlying permanent teeth.

OCCLUSION

Occlusion refers to the manner in which the teeth fit together when biting and in the variety of tooth contacts that occur during mastication, swallowing, clenching, grinding, and other normal and abnormal mandibular movements. Occlusion is affected by the relative positions of the skeletal bases, by the position of the alveolar bone on the base, and by the relative positions of the teeth within the alveolar bone.

In dentistry, every bite that differs from ideal occlusion is considered malocclusion. Malocclusion can be caused by skeletal or dental imbalance or by a combination of the two. Various degrees of malocclusion occur. Some malocclusion is considered within the normal range and is compatible with good dental health and function.

The significance of malocclusion is that it can interfere with chewing coarse or tough foods. It may not be aesthetically appealing, an important factor that causes psychological problems for some children. Malocclusion can cause trauma of soft tissues so severe that the tissue is stripped from the bone around teeth and the teeth are lost. Some malocclusions can be corrected with early growth modification and some at a later age with orthodontics alone. Some malocclusions are so severe that orthognathic surgery is required in addition to orthodontics.

Evaluation of Occlusion

Teeth in the maxillary arch should encompass those in the mandibular arch by approximately one-half of a tooth width. A cross-bite exists if one or more maxillary teeth lie inside the mandibular teeth or completely outside the lower teeth (Fig. 48-5). Cross-bites can be the result of dental positioning or skeletal discrepancies in the maxilla or the mandible. Small dental or skeletal discrepancies can cause the cusp tips of the teeth of both arches to meet and deflect to one side resulting in a functional unilateral cross-bite. Small discrepancies are often difficult to detect and require more analysis than large discrepancies. However, large discrepancies can result in noticeable facial asymmetry. Many patients with a unilateral cross-bite also exhibit facial asymmetry. Cross-bites should be corrected as soon as possible to prevent increased asymmetry with age.

The vertical relation between the permanent front teeth (i.e., overbite) is considered ideal when the maxillary incisors cover no more than 1 to 2 mm (approximately 20%) of the mandibular incisors. An overbite is considered deep if 50% of the mandibular incisors are covered; it is considered serious if more than 80% of the mandibular incisors are covered.

A vertical open bite exists when the maxillary incisors do not touch the opposing incisors. The severity of the open bite can vary in the vertical height and in the number of teeth involved. Some children have an open bite that extends to their molars. For these children, chewing such as biting through a sandwich, can be a problem.

Determining the anteroposterior relation of the maxillary teeth to the mandibular teeth is difficult for the average nondental clinician. The key to screening a patient for gross malocclusion problems is that the profile frequently reflects the relation of the maxilla to the mandible. The maxilla and the mandible are the skeletal bases holding the teeth, but the teeth may not be ideally positioned on their bases, and the profile can be used to screen for gross malocclusion problems only.

A young child normally has a slightly convex facial profile that becomes straighter with growth of the mandible. Teenagers who have a maxilla and a mandible that are in good relation to each other tend to have straight profiles. A profile that is definitely convex indicates that the maxilla is too far forward compared with the mandible. This situation can be the result of growth problems in the maxilla only, the mandible only, or a combination of both. If the profile tends to be concave, the maxilla is not adequately forward, the mandible is too far forward, or a combination of both. Orthodontic referral is recommended for patients with convex or concave faces. Early intervention in the growth processes of the maxilla or mandible may prevent future surgical procedures to position the jaws better. However, mandibular growth can be difficult to predict. Mandibular growth can continue into adulthood requiring surgery to correct the facial deformity and malocclusion it can cause.

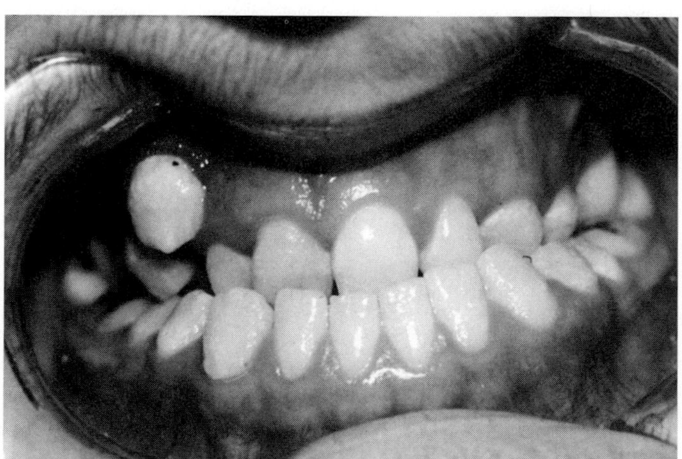

Figure 48-5. Anterior and posterior cross-bites. The permanent canine is crowded out of the arch.

HABITS

Digit Sucking

Digit sucking, which usually begins during the first year of life or before weaning, is the most common oral habit. Although the habit usually diminishes in frequency with age, some adults continue to suck. A wide range exists in the reported prevalence reaching a level as high as 86% of children between 1 and 10 years of age.

Digit sucking is a dental and social concern when it detrimentally affects occlusion. Many children discontinue the habit early or do not suck frequently or with great intensity. However, when the habit is frequent and intense, a greater chance exists that significant dental and skeletal deformities will be present. The deformities include anterior open bite, flaring maxillary incisors, retruded and crowded mandibular incisors, increased overjet, posterior cross-bite, anteriorly displaced maxilla, and retruded mandible.

The critical age at which digit sucking should be stopped to minimize the effect on the permanent dentition is controversial. Treatment is often recommended at 4 or 5 years of age. However, many open bites self-correct if a child stops sucking before eruption of the maxillary permanent anterior teeth. Self-correction of the malocclusion depends on its severity, the flaccidity of the perioral soft tissue, and the presence of other oral habits such as tongue position, mouth breathing, and lip habits. Severe oral problems require early intervention.

Digit sucking may involve the thumb or one or more fingers. A variety of positions for the digits are assumed during sucking and appear to cause different occlusal changes. For example, a child who sucks only a digit on one side may exhibit a one-sided open bite. In contrast, a two-thumb sucker usually exhibits a wide and more symmetric open bite.

A simple explanation of the effects of the habit on the teeth may help some children. Before deciding on any definitive treatment, however, the physician should determine the child's desire to stop. If the child is motivated, positive reinforcement programs with the parents' cooperation can be established. A reward system or a reminder such as an adhesive bandage on the digit, can be used. If the habit is too deeply established to stop by positive reinforcement alone, the dentist can insert an intraoral habit appliance to serve as a reminder. This is usually effective. Additional orthodontics may be required in some children.

If the child is not motivated to stop the habit, appliances should not be used. The child may continue to suck, embedding the appliance into the soft tissue or causing orthopedic movement of the maxilla or intrusion of abutment teeth. Alternatively, the child may cause tissue damage by removing the fixed appliance. Counseling should be suggested to determine the reason for the child's lack of motivation.

Pacifier Sucking

Prolonged and intense sucking of a pacifier can cause malocclusions similar to those produced by digit sucking. The problems are usually minimal and tend to self-correct after the habit is discontinued.

Pacifiers are used to satisfy an infant's nonnutritive sucking needs and delay an infant's feeding time when nursing or bottle-feeding is inconvenient. Prevalence studies report that as many as 45% of infants use pacifiers. The habit is discontinued in most children by 3 years of age, but it should be discontinued by 1 year. The simplest form of treatment is to discard the pacifier so that the child cannot find it. Parents should be cautioned not to dip pacifiers in honey or other sweet liquids, a practice associated with rampant caries.

Bruxism

Bruxism refers to the grinding of the teeth. The maxillary and mandibular teeth normally contact only during chewing and swallowing. During most of the day, they assume a rest position in which as much as 5 mm of interocclusal space exists between the two arches. However, some children clench or grind their teeth.

The clinical signs vary from small wear facets to extensive wear of the teeth. The abrasion appears to stimulate the odontoblasts within the pulp to form additional (sclerotic) dentin to protect the pulp. In some cases, the rate of abrasion is so great that the pulp can be seen through clear sclerotic dentin. In severe cases, the rate of abrasion exceeds the rate of dentin formation exposing the pulp and resulting in a dental abscess. Bruxism can contribute to fracture of the teeth, muscle fatigue, and temporomandibular joint dysfunction and discomfort.

Bruxism is usually a subconscious activity and may occur during waking or sleeping periods. Parents usually report that the child grits his or her teeth together, particularly at night. Children with neurologic disorders are reported to brux with the same intensity day and night.

Bruxism has been attributed to numerous factors including occlusal interferences, psychological stress, iron-deficiency anemia, anal pruritus caused by pinworms, and neurologic disorders. Identification of the underlying cause is the primary factor in managing bruxism. Eliminating occlusal problems by reshaping the teeth solves or minimizes some problems. Occasionally, cross-bites are observed, in which case, orthodontic treatment is indicated. If psychological stress is contributing to the bruxism, parental and child counseling and psychiatric referral may be necessary. Bite guards can provide palliative treatment when worn at night and, if necessary, during the day.

PARENTAL COUNSELING AND REFERRAL

A physician should inform parents about the importance of good dental care to the overall health and future dentition of their children. Nursing by bottle should be discouraged when the child is able to take fluids by cup, typically, 12 to 18 months of age, and the child should never go to bed with a bottle filled with anything but water. A well-balanced diet containing few refined carbohydrates, particularly sticky sugars, should be emphasized. Between-meal snacks should consist of cheeses, fresh fruits and vegetables, and other nonsweet foods.

The importance of good oral hygiene should be stressed, and parents should be advised that they should clean their children's teeth because young children are not generally capable of cleaning their teeth adequately. Children's teeth should be cleaned after breakfast and at night before sleep. Tooth cleaning should be started with the eruption of the first primary tooth, when it can be accomplished with a soft gauze or cloth. A small, soft toothbrush can be used when the child is older and accepts it. Parents do not need to floss their children's teeth until tight contacts exist between adjacent teeth. The lack of fine motor skills prevents most children from learning to floss their own teeth adequately until approximately 8 to 10 years of age. Waxed and unwaxed floss are equally effective in removing plaque.

Children should be referred by 1 year of age to a dentist who is concerned about primary prevention. This is particularly important for children who have medical, physical, or mental handicaps. The focus should be on preventing dental disease. Physicians are strongly encouraged to refer to dentists willing to work with young children.

The physician should inform parents of the importance of fluoride in controlling dental caries. Water fluoridation is the most effective and economic means of controlling caries and does not generally require patient compliance. In areas that have suboptimal fluoride concentrations in the drinking water (less than 0.7 ppm), fluoride supplements should be prescribed after 6 months of age. Children should use fluoride toothpastes that are approved by the American Dental Association. Toddlers should use no more than required to color the bristle tips of the toothbrush.

CHAPTER 49
Failure to Thrive

Adapted from Rebecca T. Kirkland

Failure to thrive is a sign that describes a particular problem rather than a diagnosis. The term is used to describe instances of growth failure or, more specifically, failure to gain weight in childhood, although in more severe cases, linear growth and head circumference may be affected. It differs from other causes of poor weight gain or growth failure because of its lack of obvious organic etiology. Failure to thrive is attributed to a child, usually younger than 2 years, whose weight is below the fifth percentile for age on more than one occasion or whose weight is less than 80% of the ideal weight for that age, using the standard growth charts of the National Center for Health Statistics (NCHS).

Failure to thrive is a problem common in pediatric practice and accounts for 1% to 5% of all referrals to children's hospitals or tertiary-care centers. In a rural primary-care setting, 10% of children in the first year of life have had failure to thrive. Failure to thrive occurs more frequently among children living in poverty.

ORGANIC VERSUS NONORGANIC ETIOLOGIES

The distinction between organic causes of failure to thrive and nonorganic or psychosocial etiologies has limited usefulness. In the child with congenital heart disease or other chronic disease, the nonorganic or environmental factors may also contribute to the failure to thrive and should not be overlooked. Likewise, the child within an emotionally disturbed family may also have an organic problem. One-third to more than one-half of cases of failure to thrive investigated in tertiary-care settings and almost all the cases in primary-care settings have nonorganic etiologies. Approximately one-fourth of all cases have involved a combination of organic and psychosocial factors.

APPROACH TO THE SIGNS AND SYMPTOMS

History

The pediatric history of the patient who fails to thrive should include an elicitation of symptoms suggesting organic diseases. A detailed environmental assessment is essential. Adverse psychosocial circumstances are known to have an association with diminished weight gain and growth in infancy.

A detailed nutritional and feeding history includes information related to duration of feeding time, quantity of food consumed, and breast-feeding in the breast-fed infant. Deficient calorie intake caused by increased losses of nutrients in the stool (malnutrition or diarrhea), vomiting or regurgitation, or impaired utilization can be clarified. A history of food preferences may indicate avoidance of foods with certain textures, suggesting an underlying dysfunction, or elimination of specific foods from the diet without adequate explanation (e.g., the child with inflammatory bowel disease may avoid foods that cause abdominal discomfort without verbalizing that those foods cause pain). A history of excessive low-calorie liquid or fruit juice ingestion may indicate inappropriate nutrient intake with losses caused by fructose and sorbitol malabsorption. A report of food allergies may lead to inappropriate restriction of nutrient. If a psychosocial problem is suspected, caution should be used when interpreting a dietary history, because parental guilt may result in inaccuracies.

The psychosocial history should include an assessment of the true caretakers and family composition (absent parents), employment status, financial state, degree of social isolation (absence of a telephone or of nearby neighbors), and family stress. Poverty indicators, including eligibility for the Supplemental Food Program for Women, Infants, and Children (WIC), should be sought. The history should include whether adequate food is available in the home or whether the caregiver runs out of food on occasion. Maternal factors relating to the pregnancy such as planned or unplanned pregnancy, young maternal age, use of medications for illness, substance abuse, physical or mental illness, postpartum depression, or inadequate breast milk, may be significant. A maternal history of being abused as a child or of eating disorders may be significant. Assessment should be made of levels of knowledge about parenting and how to provide an adequate diet. Predisposing factors in the infant are low birth weight, intrauterine growth retardation, perinatal stress, prematurity, chronic disease, and frequency of intercurrent illness such as diarrhea, vomiting, or otitis media. In the dynamic interaction between the parent and the child, factors in the child such as being "difficult" or chronically ill or giving diminished feedback may contribute to the overall problem. Questions regarding the child's sleep pattern, other behaviors, and the amount of time spent alone may be helpful.

Family members' heights and weights, their history of illness, and any developmental delay in family members that may contribute to slow growth or constitutional short stature should be included in the assessment. Support systems available to the family and frequency of changes of home address should be examined. Initially, parents may avoid mentioning psychosocial problems such as marital discord or spousal abuse; discussions of such issues should take place during several visits. These conversations should be conducted in a nonthreatening manner demonstrating concern and compassion.

Simple Observation

The infant's behavior can give valuable clues regarding his or her ability to interact appropriately for age. Behavioral features suggestive of psychosocial or environmental deprivation may include avoidance of eye contact, absence of smiling or vocalization, and a lack of interest in the environment. The negative response of the child to cuddling, and an inability to be comforted, may indicate a problem. The child may exhibit repetitive motions such as head-banging or self-stimulatory activity such as anogenital manipulation, or may be relatively immobile with infantile posturing. The infant may be withdrawn and socially unresponsive, even to the mother, and actually may look away from her. Some infants inappropriately seek affection from strangers. Historically, these behaviors have been described in institutionalized infants who lack care and affection. Some infants are described as irritable secondary to malnutrition.

Observing the mother feeding the child may be helpful. Does she cuddle the infant or merely "prop" the bottle? Does she allow sufficient time for feeding? The parents' level of concern may be inappropriate if they are eager to relinquish the child to the health team quickly. Observing the parents' interactions with each other indicates whether they are supportive of each other. Observing the child feeding can indicate oral motor or swallowing difficulties. Prolonged duration of feedings and intolerance for foods of certain textures may suggest a mild neurologic dysfunction. The setting for eating may not be optimal for the child who is easily distracted. Feeding the child in front of the television set may be distracting.

Physical Examination

Accurate assessment of the child's height, weight, and head circumference is essential. In the child younger than 2 years, the recumbent length rather than the standing height should be obtained carefully. This figure, along with weight and head circumference, should be plotted on the NCHS growth charts and related to previous measurements. Attention to the percentile curves of length, weight, and head circumference may give valuable clues as to the etiology of failure to thrive. When all measurements are below the fifth percentile, the incidence of organic disease has been noted to be 70%. Gastrointestinal disorders are more common when only the weight is below the fifth percentile. The single assessment of height and weight may have limited usefulness without an indication of whether the child's pattern is deviating from the percentile or how far below the curve the measurement may be. In intrauterine growth retardation, the child is initially small for height and weight; weight gain and growth velocity may be adequate, yet continue to be below the fifth percentile. Also, 5% of the normal population has had growth patterns at or below the fifth percentile (constitutional short stature). Therefore, determining the median age for the child's length (height or length age) and the median age for the child's weight (weight age) may be useful.

The complete developmental assessment is important. Careful evaluation should be made for dysmorphic features (clinical or genetic syndromes) and for signs of neurologic or central nervous system (hypotonia or spasticity), pulmonary, cardiac, or gastrointestinal (swallowing difficulties, gastroesophageal reflux) disorders. Isolated defects in the soft or hard palate may indicate a feeding problem.

Signs of neglect may be indicated by a diaper rash, impetigo, flat occiput, poor hygiene, protuberant abdomen, lack of appropriate behavior, and inappropriate infantile postures. Child abuse may result in bruises and fresh lesions or healed, unexplained scars. Notation of drooling and bowel habits is essential.

Some of the many possible causes of failure to thrive are listed in Table 49-1.

TABLE 49-1. Causes of Failure to Thrive

Inadequate caloric intake			Inadequate calorie absorption: no weight gain during refeeding; increased losses	Increased calorie requirements
Weight gain during refeeding	**No weight gain during refeeding**	**Inadequate appetite or inability to eat large amounts**		
Inappropriate feeding technique Disturbed mother-child relationship* Inappropriate nutrient intake (excess fruit juice consumption, factitious food allergy, inadequate quantity of food, inappropriate food for age, neglect)	Psychosocial problems* Maternal-infant dysfunction, economic deprivation Mechanical problems (adenoidal hypertrophy, dental lesions, vascular slings) Insufficient lactation in mother Cleft palate Nasal obstruction Sucking or swallowing dysfunction (CNS, neuromuscular, esophageal motility problems) Regurgitation (gastroesophageal reflux) Malformation Congenital syndromes (alcohol, phenytoin, drugs) Genetic syndromes (Turner)	Psychosocial problems (apathy)* Cardiopulmonary disease Hypotonia (muscle weakness) Anorexia of chronic infection (chronic sinusitis) or immune deficiency diseases (human immunodeficiency virus infection or acquired immunodeficiency disease) Endocrine disorders (hypothyroidism, diabetes insipidus) CNS tumors Genetic syndromes Metabolic conditions (lead toxicity, iron deficiency, zinc deficiency) Anemia Chronic constipation Disturbance in appetite and satiety	Psychosocial problems (refeeding diarrhea, intercurrent illnesses, hepatitis, rumination, regurgitation)* Malabsorption: diarrhea (lactose intolerance, cystic fibrosis, cardiac disease, malrotation, inflammatory bowel disease, milk allergy, parasites, celiac disease) Vomiting, spitting up, or diarrhea (gastroenteritis) Intestinal tract obstruction (pyloric stenosis, hernia, malrotation, intussusception, chalasia) Biliary atresia or cirrhosis CNS problems: increased intracranial pressure (subdural hematoma) Chronic metabolic problems (hypercalcemia, storage diseases, and inborn errors of metabolism such as galactosemia, methylmalonic acidemia, renal tubular acidosis, diabetes mellitus, adrenal insufficiency)	Hyperthyroidism Cerebral palsy Malignancy Chronic systemic disease (juvenile rheumatoid arthritis) Chronic systemic infection (urinary tract infection, tuberculosis, toxoplasmosis) Chronic respiratory insufficiency (bronchopulmonary dysplasia) Congenital or acquired heart disease Anemia Toxins (lead)

CNS, central nervous system.
*Environmental causes are the most common source of problems.

MANAGEMENT

Laboratory Investigation and Evaluation

A careful history and physical examination of the child with failure to thrive may suggest clues to organic disease in the child who is found to have an organic diagnosis. The search for organic disease should be guided by the signs and symptoms found in the initial examination. If the history includes enrollment in day care, recent travel, or living in a homeless shelter, enteric pathogens should be considered. Laboratory studies not suggested on the basis of the initial examination are rarely helpful. Simple routine testing, including hematocrit, urinalysis and culture of urine, blood urea nitrogen, calcium, electrolyte levels, human immunodeficiency virus enzyme-linked immunosorbent assay, and Mantoux tuberculin skin testing, is appropriate. Additional testing, radiography, and imaging may be indicated specifically by the clinical examination.

Hospitalization may not be helpful or necessary unless the child is seriously ill or is at risk of physical or sexual abuse, or parental concern and anxiety warrant it. Separation of the child from the family by hospitalization may promote anxiety and anorexia in the child and cause a delay in feeding and supporting the child within his or her environment. Psychosocial factors should also be examined in children with organic problems.

In the past, hospitalization was considered essential to demonstrate rapid weight gain in the child with failure to thrive to distinguish between organic and nonorganic etiologies. Although immediate, rapid weight gain suggests evidence for a nonorganic cause of failure to thrive, however, failure to gain weight does not rule out the nonorganic etiology. Children in whom the initial history and physical examination suggest an organic basis for failure to thrive can either be admitted to an acute-care hospital or be evaluated as outpatients, if indicated. The child who has no evidence of organic disease or who may have a combination of organic and psychosocial problems can be evaluated and supported in either outpatient or inpatient settings.

Effective evaluation, whether inpatient or outpatient, requires involvement of the parents from the beginning, along with the support provided by an interdisciplinary program. In addition to the pediatrician, the program may involve social workers, nurses, developmental specialists, nutritionists, child-life workers, psychiatrists, and workers from social and educational services in the community. The low self-esteem that many parents have, suggests that the health care providers should not focus blame but should work with the strengths of the family to encourage development of a nurturing environment.

Nutrition and Growth Recovery

An aggressive approach to nutritional therapy is suggested. Supernormal calorie intake may be required to achieve catch-up growth, but frequently this increased intake is achieved by the child's own demands after entering the recovery phase. The following points may be used as a guide:

- Feeding and appropriate nutritional intake should be based on age and weight.
- In the nutritionally deprived child, feeding should be allowed to proceed ad libitum as the child demands.
- After a child goes into the recovery phase, the ad libitum intake frequently achieves 150% of the daily requirement or greater.
- During the catch-up growth phase, existing stores of vitamins may not be sufficient. A multivitamin preparation including iron and zinc is recommended.
- The child should be the guide as to when to increase the intake. This guideline applies to the child who is nutritionally deprived as a primary problem with no other abnormalities and who can take food by mouth.

The primary goal for improved nutrition must be accompanied by addressing the psychosocial difficulties. Hospital volunteers, when available, may provide valuable role modeling, support, and aid in feeding. Home visitation may be helpful. Eligibility for WIC, food stamps, and Temporary Assistance for Needy Families (formerly Aid for Families with Dependent Children) should be considered and facilitated.

If weight gain does not occur in 4 to 6 weeks, the oral feedings should be supplemented with feeding by nasogastric tube. Assessment of feeding and occupational therapy to improve sucking and swallowing may be needed. After weight gain has been demonstrated in 4 to 6 months, oral feedings can be resumed. If weight gain is inadequate, gastrostomy tube placement may be appropriate.

During nutritional recovery, some children may experience the symptoms of a nutritional recovery syndrome, including sweatiness, hepatomegaly (caused by increased glycogen deposition in the liver), widening of the sutures (the brain growth is greater than the growth of the skull in infants with open sutures), and fidgeting or a mild hyperactivity.

FOLLOW-UP AND PROGNOSIS

Close follow-up and frequent contact with the health care team are essential for reinforcing nutritional recommendations and psychosocial support. Involvement with the family by community social service workers, visiting nurses, and nutritionists is important. Although the prognosis with respect to weight gain and growth is good, one-fourth to one-half of infants with failure to thrive remain small. The possibility that calorie deprivation in infancy produces severe, irreversible developmental deficits is the reason why treatment should begin expeditiously. Cognitive function is below normal in one-half of the children with failure to thrive, and a high frequency of behavior problems and learning difficulties is found on follow-up. Whether these findings are a direct result of the failure to thrive or of the contribution of continued adverse social circumstances is not known. The families need education and community services to help them cope and to provide a nurturing environment for the children.

2b
Common Ambulatory Issues—Adolescent Issues

CHAPTER 50
Adolescent Drug Abuse

Adapted from Hoover Adger

DEFINITIONS

Alcohol and other drug (AOD) abuse is diagnosed according to the presence of one or more of a distinct and specific set of behaviors occurring within a 12-month period. The characteristic pattern includes recurrent substance use that results in failure to fulfill major role obligations at home, school, or work; use in physically hazardous situations; and recurrent AOD-related legal problems or continued use despite persistent social or interpersonal problems caused or exacerbated by use. Another distinct and specific set of behaviors is used to define dependence. Dependence is distinguished from abuse more than by simply being a continuum of severity. Substance dependence is characterized by loss of control over use, compulsion, and AOD use that continues despite the presence of persistent or recurrent adverse consequences related to use. The use of progressively larger amounts or over longer periods than intended, and the development of tolerance (decreased effect from similar amounts of the substance or increased amount needed for similar effect) are characteristic features. Preoccupation with activities necessary to get or maintain a steady supply of drugs is common. Dependence can (but does not necessarily) include a characteristic physiologic withdrawal syndrome after interruption of use. Although no single criterion is required to make the diagnosis of dependence, these features paint a graphic picture of an individual who has lost the ability to control his or her use of AOD and whose use continues despite persistent consequences that are either caused or exacerbated by AOD use. Important prognostic reasons exist to distinguish between use, abuse, and dependence. Dependence reliably predicts more severe medical sequelae, poorer treatment outcome, higher relapse rates, and worse overall prognosis.

EPIDEMIOLOGY

Alcohol

Despite a minimum legal drinking age of 21, alcohol is the drug most often used by young people. The 1996 National Household Survey on Drug Abuse (NHSDA) found that past-month use of alcohol was reported by 18.6% of 12- to 17-year-old adolescents. Overall, the use of alcohol has remained at a high level and has changed little since the early 1990s. However, the 1997 Monitoring the Future (MTF) survey reported a gradual upward drift in the proportion of students who say they have been drunk frequently (20 or more times in the past month). The MTF study also showed that binge drinking increased slightly in the 1990s (defined as having five or more drinks in a row). In 1997, 15%, 25%, and 31% of eighth, tenth, and twelfth graders, respectively, reported binge drinking.

Although alcohol is a legal drug that many adults use without negative consequences, it holds unique dangers for underage drinkers. The younger the onset of drinking, the greater the chances of developing a clinically defined alcohol use disorder. One study found that young people who begin drinking before age 15 are four times more likely to become alcohol dependent and twice as likely to abuse alcohol than individuals who start drinking at age 21.

Drinking by young people correlates with increases in other high-risk behavior including unsafe sexual practices. Drinking greatly increases the risk of being involved in a motor vehicle crash. More than 2,300 youths aged 15 to 20 died in alcohol-related crashes in 1996, 33.6% of total traffic fatalities in this age group. A survey focusing on alcohol-related problems experienced by high school seniors and dropouts revealed that within the preceding year, approximately 80% reported getting drunk, binge drinking, or drinking and driving. More than one-half said that drinking had caused them to feel sick, miss school or work, get arrested, or be involved in an automobile accident. Alcohol use among adolescents has also been closely linked to increased risk for suicide. According to one study, 37% of eighth graders who drank heavily reported attempting suicide, compared with 11% who did not drink.

Tobacco

Cigarette smoking constitutes one of the single largest long-term threats to the health and well-being of adolescents. The 1996 NHSDA found that an estimated 18% of youths aged 12 to 17 were smokers in 1996. According to the MTF, after 6 years of steady increase, cigarette smoking among eighth and tenth graders has leveled off. In 1997, 9% of eighth graders reported smoking on a daily basis; 3.5% smoked one-half a pack or more per day. Among twelfth graders, smoking continued on the upward trend that began in 1992, with 25% being daily smokers.

Tobacco use, particularly among youth, has been shown to be correlated with the later onset of illegal drug use. Most smokers start between 10 and 18 years of age. Approximately 4.5 million American children younger than 18 now smoke, and every day another 3,000 adolescents become regular smokers. Seventy percent of adolescent smokers say they would not have started if they could choose again. Unfortunately, one-third of these new smokers will eventually die of tobacco-related diseases.

Marijuana

Marijuana continues to be the illegal drug most frequently used by young people. Furthermore, adolescents are beginning to smoke marijuana at a younger age with the average age of first use now being 14.4 years. The 1997 MTF study shows that among high school seniors, 49.6% reported using marijuana at least once in their lives. By comparison, the figure was 32.6% for seniors in 1992 and 41.7% in 1995. After 6 years of steady increase, current marijuana use decreased in 1997 among eighth graders from 11.3% in 1996 to 10.2%. Further, there was evidence of a deceleration in the rate of increase among tenth and twelfth graders. The 1996 NHSDA found that current marijuana use among 12- to 17-year-old adolescents was 7.1%. Similar to figures from the MTF study, NHSDA findings suggest an end to the trend that resulted in a doubling of marijuana use between 1992 and 1995.

Cocaine

The use of powder and crack cocaine has increased steadily among youth during the 1990s. The 1997 MTF survey found that the proportion of students reporting use of powder cocaine in the past year was 2.2%, 4.1%, and 5% in grades 8, 10, and 12, respectively. This rate represents a leveling off in eighth-grade use and no change in tenth and twelfth grades. Among eighth graders, perceived risk also stabilized in 1997, and disapproval of use increased, both after an earlier erosion in these attitudes. The 1996 NHSDA found current use among 12- to 17-year-old youths to be 0.6%, twice the rate of 1992, yet substantially lower than the 1.9% reported in 1985. However, young people are still experimenting with cocaine, underscoring the need for effective prevention. This need is further substantiated by the finding of a steady decline in the mean age of first use.

Heroin

Although quite low, rates of heroin use among teenagers increased significantly among eighth, tenth, and twelfth graders during the 1990s. Many communities throughout the country are experiencing an increase in heroin-related overdoses and deaths in adolescents and young adults. The 1997 MTF showed that use among eighth graders either equaled or exceeded the rates seen in tenth and twelfth graders, which is of great concern. The report also discovered that more young people perceive heroin as dangerous; 56.7% of twelfth graders thought that trying heroin was a "great risk," the highest percentage recorded in 23 years. The 1996 NHSDA found that the mean age of initiation declined from 27.3 years in 1988 to 19.3 in 1995. The widespread availability of high-purity and low-cost heroin and the ability to snort or smoke heroin, instead of injecting it, have undoubtedly played a major role in the increasing use of this drug.

Methamphetamine

Methamphetamine is by far the most prevalent synthetic controlled substance clandestinely manufactured in the United States. Methamphetamine is also imported from Mexico and is cheaper than cocaine in many markets. Methamphetamine, known as "ice," is often smoked or burned in rock form, but instead of an effect of 20 to 30 minutes' duration as with cocaine, the effects of methamphetamine last 6 to 8 hours. Methamphetamine use, which had been increasing since 1992, leveled off in 1997; 2.3% of twelfth graders reported use of methamphetamine in the past year.

Other Substances

The 1996 NHSDA reported no significant change in the prevalence of inhalants, hallucinogens (such as LSD and PCP), or psychotherapeutics (tranquilizers, sedatives, analgesics, or stimulants) used for nonmedical purposes between 1995 and 1996. Rates for both hallucinogens and inhalants remained well below 1% in 1996. However, the number of initiates to hallucinogen use, 1.2 million in 1995, has doubled since 1991. Additionally, current use of stimulants (a category that includes methamphetamine) declined among eighth and tenth graders and increased among twelfth graders.

The 1997 MTF reports that inhalant use is most common in the eighth grade, where 5.6% of children used it on a past-month basis and 11.8% did so on a past-year basis. Inhalants can be deadly, even with first-time use, and often represent the initial experience with psychoactive substances. Polydrug use among young people continues to be the dominant trend. The indiscriminant mixing and use of hallucinogenic or sedative drugs such as ketamine, LSD, and methylene dioxymethamphetamine (also known as ecstasy) continues to be reported throughout the country—and, unfortunately, the age of initiation of use continues to decline.

PROGRESSION OF ALCOHOL AND OTHER DRUG USE

Not all children and adolescents who use AOD become problem users. Although risk factors may help identify those who are most vulnerable, it does not mean that any individual who exhibits them inevitably develops problems. For some, experimental or casual use progresses to heavy use and dependency. For others, even experimental or casual use leads to unfavorable outcomes. For this reason, it is helpful to look at AOD use and abuse on a continuum. Death can be an unfortunate outcome of use at any point on the continuum.

The use of a psychoactive substance such as beer or marijuana, at the experimentation and learning stage generally occurs within the context of initial curiosity and is often in response to peer pressure. Hence, the experiential learning encompasses several facets. First is the knowledge that psychoactive substances result in a welcome or perhaps unwelcome mood swing. In addition, it may be appreciated that these mood swings or feelings can be reliably produced and even controlled to some extent by modulation of the amount, quality, or variations of the substance used. Often at this stage, little behavioral change occurs and an absence of discernible consequences exists.

Through experience, some adolescents learn to anticipate and welcome the mood swing. For most, these experiences occur within the context of social functions in which it is perceived as fun, socially rewarding, and without untoward effects. For some at this stage, the euphoric feelings gained through the use of various substances seem to provide an answer by helping the adolescent to cope, relieving feelings of anxiety, or perhaps by providing a desired change in social or peer group status. At this point, there may be a change in peer group, new friends, and the beginning of deterioration in school and other life areas as substance use escalates.

Progression to the next stage involves a movement from anticipation to preoccupation. Drug use at this stage takes on a different relationship as the motivations and role of increasing substance use assume more of a primary role in the life of the individual. Often, problems with family, school, or the law become evident. Polydrug use becomes more frequent, and friends who do not also use drugs become scarce.

The final stage in the progression, dependence, is characterized by loss of control, compulsion, and evidence of dysfunction. The behavior of the chemically dependent adolescent shows a development of primary relationships with mood-altering drugs. Values, habits, and relationships that had been primary appear to no longer exist.

RISK AND PROTECTIVE FACTORS

Individuals who have been identified as particularly at risk for development of alcohol and other drug problems include children from families in which alcoholism or drug abuse is present. In addition, the following adolescents are at increased risk: those who experience significant problems in behavior such as aggressiveness and rebellious deviancy; those with difficulties in cognition such as learning disabilities or attention deficit disorders; those with problems in psychological well-being such as depression, isolation, and low self-esteem; and those with impaired familial functioning such as neglect, abuse, loss, and lack of close relationships. Protective factors include parental involvement and monitoring; success in school; strong bonds with family, school, and religious organizations; and knowledge of the dangers posed by drug use. Promising prevention approaches focus on minimizing the risk factors and maximizing the protective factors.

EVALUATION AND TREATMENT

Diagnosing substance abuse rests on the realization that all children and adolescents are at risk, but that some are at substantially more risk than others. Sources of diagnostic information might include history and mental status examination, physical examination, self-report questionnaires, structured interview and standardized tests, and laboratory screening. Although an in-depth assessment and actual diagnosis may be beyond the time limitations and skills of many practitioners, several approaches to office screening and assessment of adolescent substance abuse provide guidance for a meaningful role for the pediatrician.

Substance abuse should be included in the primary differential diagnosis whenever behavioral, familial, psychosocial, or related medical problems occur. As part of the routine health examination, all adolescents should be questioned about the use of cigarettes, alcohol, and other drugs. In addition, there should be an assessment of risk by reviewing risk factors and behaviors with adolescents and their parents.

The actual treatment of adolescents with chemical dependence is beyond the scope of most pediatricians. Even without special expertise in this area, however, most clinicians should be able to perform an initial assessment of an adolescent's use of drugs and to determine indications for further assessment and intervention. The primary tasks of the evaluation are to determine if the use of mood-altering chemicals is associated with identifiable consequences and if such use is causing behavioral impairment. A general assessment of psychosocial functioning can provide a basis for determining whether behavioral dysfunction exists. Information should be gathered specifically about family relationships, peer relationships, school performance and attendance, recreational and leisure activities, employment, vocational aspirations, frequency of conflicts with parents, and legal difficulties. Often, use patterns of peers and self-perceptions of the adolescent regarding his or her own use and whether or not it is a problem provide additional useful information.

A number of treatment alternatives are available for the chemically dependent adolescent. Short-term inpatient treatment, residential care, and outpatient care span the spectrum from traditional office-based care to intensive and structured day programs. In most treatment programs, treatment begins with the interruption of use, requires continued abstinence from drugs, and sets the development of a drug-free lifestyle as a goal. Because of the wide variety of settings and a number of different approaches to the treatment of adolescents, the clinician should be aware of resources in the community and become familiar with the philosophies of the agencies that render services. With this information, the physician can better assume a responsible role in intervention and assisting the family find appropriate treatment resources.

CHAPTER 51
Menstrual Disorders

Adapted from Michele Diane Wilson

AMENORRHEA

Amenorrhea, the absence of menses, is a symptom that generally brings teenagers in for evaluation. The patient may be a young woman who has not experienced menarche, which is called primary amenorrhea. In other cases, the patient has previously menstruated but experiences an interval without menses, which is called secondary amenorrhea.

Primary amenorrhea is usually defined as the absence of menses by age 16 years in the presence of normal secondary sex characteristics, by age 14 years without any pubertal development, or by 4 years after the onset of pubertal development. Secondary amenorrhea is defined as the absence of menses for 6 months or the length of three cycles after establishment of regular cycles. For both primary and secondary amenorrhea, the defined periods without menses are useful as guidelines and should be applied with flexibility.

Differential Diagnosis of Amenorrhea

HYPOTHALAMUS

Constitutional delay in puberty is a common reason for primary amenorrhea. Individuals who enter puberty at a late age typically progress normally. Family history of late puberty may be elicited. Kallmann syndrome is characterized by primary amenorrhea and anosmia.

Any chronic illness, particularly those that interfere with normal growth and nutrition, can affect the hypothalamic-pituitary axis resulting in amenorrhea. Thus, patients with inflammatory bowel disease, cystic fibrosis, and chronic renal failure often suffer from amenorrhea. Weight loss in patients with eating disorders can result in primary or secondary amenorrhea. Women who engage in strenuous exercise may experience amenorrhea. Stress such as that experienced when moving away to college or traveling, may result in missed menses. Medications, including contraceptives and other drugs, can alter menstrual function.

Polycystic ovary syndrome, thought to be a hypothalamic disorder, represents a spectrum of disorders variably manifested by amenorrhea or oligomenorrhea, hirsutism, obesity, and acne.

PITUITARY

Pituitary tumors, including adenomas with elevated prolactin levels, can result in menstrual irregularities after initiation of menses. Patients may complain of headaches and galactorrhea.

OVARIES

Gonadal dysgenesis [Turner syndrome (45,XO) or mosaicism] is the most common reason for primary amenorrhea. Patients often lack secondary sex characteristics. Clues to the diagnosis include short stature, a history of lymphedema at birth, webbed neck, shield chest, and widely spaced nipples. History of exposure to viral, toxic, radioactive, or chemotherapeutic agents suggests the possibility of premature ovarian failure.

UTERUS

Congenital anomalies of the uterus that present with primary amenorrhea, despite normal secondary sex characteristics, include Mayer-Rokitansky-Küster-Hauser syndrome and testicular feminization. Uterine synechiae (Asherman syndrome) can cause secondary amenorrhea. Pregnancy is the most common etiology of secondary amenorrhea and an infrequent cause of primary amenorrhea.

VAGINA

Congenital malformations of the vagina such as agenesis, septum formation, or imperforate hymen are manifested as outflow disorders. Women develop normally but do not have menses. Patients with imperforate hymen may have cyclic pain because menstrual blood accumulates in the uterus.

Other Endocrine Disorders

Hyperthyroidism or hypothyroidism may result in amenorrhea. Adrenal disorders can cause amenorrhea and virilization.

Evaluation of the Adolescent with Amenorrhea

A careful, complete history and physical examination direct the assessment and help prevent unnecessary diagnostic testing. Information regarding the young woman's growth, age of onset of pubertal development and subsequent progression, lymphedema at birth, and family history of age of onset of puberty guide the evaluation. It is important to ask about any changes in weight or diet, participation in competitive athletics, and recent stress. A complete review of systems may suggest the possibility of a previously undetected chronic illness. Specifically, one should ask about gastrointestinal symptoms suggestive of inflammatory bowel disease and symptoms of excessive or diminished thyroid activity. Severe headaches suggest the possibility of an intracranial tumor. The adolescent must be questioned privately regarding sexual activity, use of prescription medications, and use of illicit drugs. A young woman may not reliably provide information regarding sexual activity; therefore, a urine pregnancy test should be obtained.

A complete physical examination is indicated. Short stature is suggestive of Turner syndrome. Weight loss may indicate an eating disorder or undiagnosed chronic illness. It is important to examine for hirsutism and other signs of virilization. Careful ophthalmologic examination with attention to signs of papilledema or visual field defect is indicated. The extent of breast, axillary hair, and pubic hair development should be assessed. The breasts should be examined for galactorrhea, and the thyroid gland should be palpated. When the cause of amenorrhea cannot be made by the history and physical examination, a pelvic examination is indicated. It is important to look for clitoromegaly. Although a speculum examination need not be performed on all individuals, the patency of the vaginal orifice should be assessed. Additionally, the cervix and uterus should be palpated by either vaginal or rectal examination. Enlargement of the uterus suggests pregnancy.

When the history and physical examination are completed, possible causes are identified. If pubertal development has not started but the uterus is present and the outflow tract is patent, prepubertal levels of estrogen may be present, caused by lack of hypothalamic or pituitary stimulation, or the ovary may be unable to respond to stimulation. Measurement of follicle-stimulating hormone (FSH) levels is suggested. If FSH levels are high, gonadal dysgenesis (Turner syndrome), mosaicism, or a nonfunctioning X chromosome are likely causes for amenorrhea. On the other hand, if the uterus is absent but development is normal, the patient may have congenital absence of the uterus or testicular feminization. The evaluation of patients who have a uterus and normal development is similar to that of patients with secondary amenorrhea. A karyotype is indicated for patients who have not experienced pubertal development and do not have a uterus.

When evaluating secondary amenorrhea, a pregnancy test should be performed first before an extensive evaluation. If the young woman is not pregnant, the progesterone challenge test is a useful diagnostic tool. If withdrawal bleeding ensues, evidence exists that estrogen had primed the uterus and the anatomy of the lower reproductive tract is intact. Diagnostic possibilities, therefore, include polycystic ovarian syndrome, as well as hypothalamic and pituitary disorders. If withdrawal bleeding does not occur, serum FSH and luteinizing hormone can be obtained. High levels indicate ovarian failure, and low or normal levels implicate hypothalamic or pituitary disorders.

ABNORMAL UTERINE BLEEDING

Abnormal uterine bleeding is a common problem among adolescents. Commonly accepted definitions of excessive bleeding include bleeding that lasts 8 days or longer, use of ten or more sanitary pads per day, or frequency of bleeding more often than every 21 days. In the absence of one of the previously mentioned criteria, abnormal bleeding exists if bleeding is associated with a decrease in hemoglobin.

Differential Diagnosis

The most common reason for abnormal menstrual bleeding in adolescents is anovulation or dysfunctional uterine bleeding. Before making the diagnosis of dysfunctional uterine bleeding, organic lesions must be ruled out.

Pregnancy and its complications (ectopic pregnancy; threatened, incomplete, or spontaneous abortion) are causes for abnormal bleeding. Infectious processes such as endometritis or acute salpingitis may cause bleeding. Trauma from rape or coitus may result in bleeding. Foreign bodies, often retained tampons, may present with bleeding. Blood dyscrasias may result in severe bleeding that necessitates hospitalization. Tumors of the reproductive system such as vaginal or uterine polyps, fibroids, and, rarely, malignancies, must be in the differential diagnosis. Chronic or systemic illnesses, including thyroid disorders and medications or drug abuse, can cause abnormal menstrual bleeding.

Evaluation

The severity of the blood loss must be assessed and its cause determined. A menstrual history including the age of menarche and the usual pattern of menses is critical information. Sexual activity should be discussed to assess risk of pregnancy and infection. It is important to ask about trauma and to examine for evidence of a bleeding disorder.

By physical examination, either pallor or orthostatic changes in pulse and blood pressure suggest severe blood loss. Signs of thyroid, liver, renal, or coagulation disorder should be sought on examination. In a teenager who has mild bleeding without anemia, is not sexually active, and has experienced menarche within 2 years, a pelvic examination can be deferred. By contrast, a pelvic examination is indicated in the patient who has been sexually active, has severe bleeding with anemia, or has pain. The pelvic examination is done to detect abnormalities of the vagina, cervix, or uterus by localizing the site of bleeding; to obtain cultures; to look for a foreign body or tumors; and to assess for pregnancy or tenderness (as evidence of infection).

The extent of laboratory evaluation is determined by the extent of bleeding. A low hemoglobin, hematocrit, or both confirms the severity of blood loss. A sensitive pregnancy test should be done to rule out pregnancy. An elevated white blood count or erythrocyte sedimentation rate suggests infection. When a bleeding disorder is being considered, clotting studies should be obtained. Thyroid function tests are indicated when blood loss is severe.

Treatment

Therapy for most causes of abnormal uterine bleeding is directed toward the underlying condition. If the bleeding is anovulatory and mild with a stable hematocrit, reassurance and careful monitoring of subsequent menstrual pattern are indicated. Iron supplementation may be needed. When bleeding is more severe and anemia exists, therapy with progesterone supplementation stabilizes the endometrial lining and usually stops the bleeding. Various regimens use either progestins alone or oral contraceptives (estrogen and progestin). Either regimen is effective. Therapy should continue for several months to build up the endometrial lining. Iron supplementation is also indicated.

DYSMENORRHEA

Definition

The term dysmenorrhea is derived from the Greek and means "difficult monthly flow." Symptoms generally occur a few hours before or simultaneously with the appearance of menses. Pain is typically most severe on the first day and usually resolves by the third day of menses. Women describe crampy, colicky, suprapubic pain that may be accompanied by other complaints. The most common associated symptoms include nausea, vomiting, diarrhea, and lower back pain. Less frequently, patients suffer from dizziness, syncope, and headaches.

Differential Diagnosis

Primary and secondary causes of dysmenorrhea must be distinguished from one another. Primary dysmenorrhea is more prevalent and refers to the occurrence of painful menses without pelvic pathology, whereas secondary dysmenorrhea indicates that an identifiable organic disorder exists.

Primary Dysmenorrhea

Primary dysmenorrhea has its peak onset 6 to 18 months after menarche, which corresponds to the onset of ovulatory menstrual cycles. Levels of prostaglandins are linked to severity of dysmenorrhea. Therapies with prostaglandin inhibitors are effective.

Secondary Dysmenorrhea

Secondary dysmenorrhea refers to pain that is the result of a pathologic process. Congenital anomalies of the reproductive tract may cause dysmenorrhea coincident with menarche. Uterine malformations, including a bicornuate uterus with a blind horn, may cause dysmenorrhea. The pelvic examination may reveal a midline mass. Ultrasound confirms the diagnosis. Polyps or fibroids may cause menstrual discomfort. Endometriosis, previously believed to occur only in older women, is increasingly recognized in adolescents. In a surgical series of 282 teenage women who had laparoscopy because of chronic pelvic pain, endometriosis was found in 45% of the patients. The diagnosis of endometriosis should be considered in any patient whose symptoms are severe and unresponsive to conventional therapy. A young woman who is sexually active and experiences dysmenorrhea of recent onset or increased severity may have acute salpingitis. A patient who has previously experienced a pelvic infection may suffer from dysmenorrhea and chronic pelvic pain as a consequence. A sexually active teenager may experience painful vaginal bleeding as the result of pregnancy including threatened, missed, or incomplete abortion. Patients with an ectopic pregnancy complain of severe lower abdominal pain, vaginal bleeding, and an abnormal menstrual history. Thus, the diagnosis of pregnancy should be considered in the evaluation of dysmenorrhea.

Assessment of the Patient with Dysmenorrhea

A complete physical examination with careful abdominal palpation should be performed. A pelvic examination is indicated at the initial evaluation if the patient is sexually active or the pain is severe. Any sexually active patient should have cervical cultures obtained for gonorrhea and chlamydia. On bimanual palpation, any uterine enlargement or masses consistent with pregnancy, uterine malformations, or fibroids should be noted. An adnexal mass suggests the possibility of an ectopic pregnancy. The cul-de-sac should be carefully palpated for the nodularity suggestive of endometriosis.

Laboratory Evaluation

The extent of laboratory evaluation is dictated by history and physical findings. When the diagnosis of a congenital anomaly is entertained, pelvic ultrasound or magnetic resonance imaging studies may be helpful. If pain is severe and unresponsive to medical management, diagnostic laparoscopy to rule out endometriosis may be indicated.

Treatment

Treatment for secondary dysmenorrhea is directed toward correction of the underlying problem. Various treatment modalities are advocated for primary dysmenorrhea. Nonsteroidal antiinflammatory agents are effective. For sexually active individuals, oral contraceptives protect against pregnancy and successfully treat primary dysmenorrhea in 80% to 90% of cases.

Dysmenorrhea is common among adolescents. Evaluation of the patient with dysmenorrhea includes a careful search for pathologic etiologies. Most individuals with primary dysmenorrhea respond well to nonsteroidal antiinflammatory agents or oral contraceptives.

CHAPTER 52
Adolescent Pregnancy and Contraception

Adapted from Michele Diane Wilson

ADOLESCENT SEXUAL ACTIVITY AND PREGNANCY RATES

Since the 1970s, the rates of sexual activity have increased among teenagers in the United States. The 1995 National Survey of Family Growth found that 50% of women aged 15 to 19 years had had intercourse. Two-thirds of young men have experienced coitus by age 17. The United States has one of the highest teenage pregnancy rates among the developed countries. The high rates of pregnancy in the United States compared with other countries do not appear to reflect a greater rate of sexual intercourse but, rather, the lack of use or inadequate use of contraception by teenagers. Overall, more than 85% of teenagers delay seeking professional advice regarding contraception or sexually transmitted disease (STD) protection until after engaging in sexual intercourse. On average, adolescent women delay 11.5 months from the time they initiate sexual intercourse until they go to a clinic for family planning. It is estimated that one in eight teenaged girls in the United States becomes pregnant. The pregnancy rate among teenagers has not changed dramatically during the past 20 years. Although the rates of sexual activity have increased, the proportion of teenagers using contraception has also increased. In 1996, the total number of births to teenaged mothers was 494,272; the birth rate for teenagers was 54.7 births per 1,000 women aged 15 to 19 years.

DIAGNOSIS OF PREGNANCY

It is important to maintain a high index of suspicion for pregnancy when providing health care to adolescents. Young women should be questioned in private regarding sexual activity and use of contraception. The diagnosis of pregnancy may be entertained immediately because of the chief complaint or may not be suspected until much later in the evaluation. Adolescents may present requesting pregnancy tests. In other cases, pregnancy is uncovered only after a lengthy evaluation, especially if patients do not reveal pertinent information. The most common diagnosis among adolescent patients who present with secondary amenorrhea is pregnancy. Other symptoms that suggest the possibility of pregnancy include nausea, fatigue, dizziness, syncope, urinary frequency, weight gain, breast tenderness, and nipple sensitivity.

The physical examination can support the diagnosis of pregnancy. On abdominal examination, a midline lower abdominal mass may be palpable after the first trimester of pregnancy. On pelvic examination, the cervix acquires a cyanotic appearance and softens. The uterine size should be assessed to estimate the length of gestation. At 12 weeks' gestation, the uterus is palpable at the symphysis pubis; at 20 weeks' gestation, the uterus is palpable at the umbilicus.

Laboratory confirmation of pregnancy can be made with either urine or blood measurement of human chorionic gonadotropins. Immunometric tests are most commonly used in the ambulatory setting because they are accurate, sensitive, and easy to perform. Pregnancy can be diagnosed as early as 7 days after implantation.

COUNSELING ISSUES

Once pregnancy has been diagnosed, adolescents need to be informed and counseled about their options. If personal reasons prevent practitioners from doing the counseling, referral of patients for services elsewhere is suggested. Whenever possible, parents should be involved to provide support to their teenagers. Pregnancy options include continuing the pregnancy to term and either keeping the baby or placing the baby for adoption or, if the pregnancy is diagnosed early, obtaining an abortion.

ADOLESCENT CONTRACEPTION

Oral Contraceptives

Oral contraceptives are the most popular form of contraception during adolescence. Oral contraceptives are very effective and safe for teenagers. Combined oral contraceptive pills are prepared from a combination of estrogen (ethinyl estradiol and, less commonly, mestranol) and progestin (synthetic progesterone). The various progestin components of oral contraceptives include norethindrone, levonorgestrel, norgestrel, ethynodiol diacetate, norgestimate, and desogestrel.

Oral contraceptives have several mechanisms of action. They suppress ovulation; they alter the cervical mucus, rendering it impermeable to sperm; and they thin the endometrial lining making it inhospitable to implantation.

Oral contraceptives have advantages that make them particularly well suited for teenagers. They are extremely effective with 3.0 pregnancies per year occurring among 100 women aged 15 to 44 years of age. Among teenaged users, the failure rates may be as high as 18%. Because a daily pill is ingested, use is not directly related to the act of coitus. Furthermore, many women experience noncontraceptive benefits from the pills. Specifically, acne, dysmenorrhea, irregular menses, benign breast disease, rheumatoid arthritis, iron deficiency anemia, and ovarian cysts are less common in oral contraceptive users compared with nonusers. Risk of ovarian and uterine cancer is significantly reduced in users. The relationship between oral contraception and cervical cancer is unclear.

Oral contraceptives do not provide protection against STDs or human immunodeficiency virus (HIV) infection. Thus, adolescents should be counseled to use oral contraceptives in conjunction with condoms.

In general, oral contraceptives are extremely safe for teenagers. Mortality among women younger than age 20 years using any method of contraception is significantly less than rates for women carrying a pregnancy to term. Young, healthy women rarely have serious medical complications from oral contraceptive use.

Conditions that contraindicate prescribing oral contraceptives include thrombophlebitis or thromboembolic disease (or a history of either) and cerebrovascular or coronary artery disease. Cholestatic jaundice of pregnancy or jaundice with prior pill use, hepatic adenomas, or carcinoma are contraindications. Known or suspected estrogen-dependent neoplasia, carcinoma of the endometrium, and known or suspected carcinoma of the breast are also absolute contraindications. Known or suspected pregnancy is a contraindication to oral contraceptive use.

Individuals may have other medical problems that make oral contraceptive use more risky. Such conditions include severe headaches, particularly vascular or migraine headaches that begin after oral contraceptive use; hypertension; acute mononucleosis; or elective major surgery or immobilization planned in the following 4 weeks. Abnormal vaginal bleeding should be evaluated before initiating oral contraceptive use. Other conditions that make oral contraceptive use less than ideal include diabetes mellitus, prediabetes or a strong family history of diabetes, sickle cell disease, active gallbladder disease, Gilbert disease, or completion of a term pregnancy within the past 2 weeks. Teenagers who want to use oral contraceptives and smoke cigarettes require counseling regarding cessation of cigarette smoking, because smoking increases the risk of pill-associated thromboembolic disorders.

Minor side effects include symptoms that, although not dangerous, may bother patients and may, therefore, result in discontinuation of oral contraceptive use. Common complaints include gastrointestinal disturbance. Frequently, patients experience nausea and, occasionally, vomiting during the initial months of oral contraceptive use. Taking the medication with meals, especially in the evening, usually alleviates this condition. Patients can be reassured that gastrointestinal problems generally resolve within the first few months of therapy.

Adolescents commonly experience either spotting or breakthrough bleeding in the first few months of oral contraceptive use. This problem can often be corrected by consistent time of medication ingestion. If irregular bleeding persists and is bothersome, selection of a pill with higher progestational activity usually corrects the condition. Breast tenderness is a common side effect. Expecting common problems and providing anticipatory guidance reassure patients and may prevent unnecessary discontinuation of therapy.

Many preparations of combined oral contraceptives with varying compositions are available. These oral contraceptive programs consist of 21 pills with hormones followed by 7 pills with an inert substance (pill-free), during which time menses is expected. Fixed-dose combination preparations contain a constant dose of estrogen and progestin for 21 days. Multiphasic pills provide varying doses of progestin, estrogen, or both during the cycle in either a biphasic or triphasic manner. Biphasic pills have two phases of hormonal treatment; triphasic pills have three phases of hormonal preparations. The ideal choice for adolescents beginning therapy is a low-dose combined oral contraceptive that has 35 mg or less of estrogen coupled with a low-dose progestin to minimize side effects of weight gain, acne, and menstrual problems. These pills offer excellent protection against pregnancy while minimizing significant side effects.

In contrast to the combined oral contraceptive, the minipill or progestin-only pill contains only synthetic progesterone. Progestin-only pills are best suited for women who cannot use estrogen. The minipill is less effective than the combined pill. It offers the advantage of inducing fewer metabolic alterations and, thus, it may be useful for women with diabetes mellitus, hypertension, or sickle cell disease, for whom concerns about thromboembolic disorders are great. Menstrual irregularities occur in one-third to one-half of patients, however. This side effect, coupled with a higher failure rate, limits the usefulness of progestin-only pills in most teenagers.

Injectable Depot Medroxyprogesterone Acetate

Depot medroxyprogesterone acetate (DMPA) is a long-acting, highly effective progestin-only contraceptive that was approved by the U.S. Food and Drug Administration in 1992. It has become one of the most commonly chosen methods among adolescents. DMPA is administered intramuscularly in a single injection of 150 mg every 3 months. The mechanism of action is inhibition of ovulation and thickening of the cervical mucus. It is highly effective with a failure rate of less than 0.3%. It can be used in individuals who cannot use estrogens. Contraindications to use of DMPA are similar to those of subdermal implants.

Side effects include menstrual irregularities. When patients initiate DMPA use, spotting and breakthrough bleeding are common. Irregular menstrual bleeding can be managed with nonsteroidal antiinflammatory drugs or addition of estrogen formulation. After 1 year of use, one-half of DMPA users have amenorrhea. Weight gain averages 2.3 kg in the first year of use. Headaches, acne, hair growth or loss, mood changes (depression or nervousness), libido change, and abdominal pain may occur. Loss of bone density is a concern for teenagers using DMPA. In addition, return to normal fertility may be delayed for up to 2 years after discontinuing DMPA.

Adolescents who are appropriate candidates for DMPA and select it receive their initial injection within 5 days of the onset of a normal menstrual period after documentation of a negative pregnancy test result. Subsequent injections are given every 3 months. Despite its low failure rate, pregnancies do occur. Furthermore, when injections are late, pregnancy may be more likely to result. As with other hormonal contraceptives, condoms should also be used to prevent STDs.

Emergency Postcoital Contraception

Emergency postcoital contraception is the use of contraception after unprotected intercourse has occurred. The most commonly used method is known as the Yuzpe regimen, in which oral contraceptive pills are given. The morning-after pill is two doses of combined oral contraceptives taken 12 hours apart and within 72 hours of unprotected intercourse. Postcoital contraception prevents 60% to 75% of pregnancies that would have occurred without its use.

Emergency postcoital contraception is contraindicated in individuals who cannot take oral contraceptives. Side effects include nausea or vomiting. If the patient vomits within 3 hours after a dose, an additional dose of pills is recommended. Antinausea medication can be prescribed.

Three weeks after treatment, the patient should return for a pregnancy test if normal menses has not occurred.

Barrier Methods

The commonly recommended barrier devices include condoms, diaphragms, and vaginal spermicides. Barrier methods, especially condoms, deserve increasing attention because of their role in preventing the spread of STDs, including HIV infection, among sexually active teenagers.

Male Condom

The male condom is the second most frequently used method of contraception during adolescence. Data collected from the 1992 Centers for Disease Control and Prevention (CDC) national school-based Youth Risk Behavior Survey showed that 49% of men and 40% of women reported using a condom at last coitus. The overall trend has been an increase in condom use among teenagers in the past few decades. Condoms have a failure rate of approximately 30% in adolescent users. When used with spermicide, their effectiveness increases. They are extraordinarily safe without any major medical risks. Latex condoms effectively decrease the transmission of STDs and HIV when used correctly and consistently. Condoms are easily available at low cost without prescription. Condoms provide a unique opportunity to involve male adolescents in contraceptive decision making because they are the only available male-initiated, reversible method of birth control. In view of the current epidemic of STDs, particularly AIDS, all sexually active young people should receive instruction and encouragement for condom use even if they use another method of contraception. STD prevention is an important reason for male teenagers to use condoms. It is important to stress the need for consistent and correct use of condoms. Adolescents need to know that they should use latex condoms rather than natural membrane condoms because only latex products have been shown to reduce the transmission of STDs. Patients may cite diminished sensation as a disadvantage to condom use. Occasionally, an allergy to latex or foam is encountered. Condoms may tear. A great deal of motivation is required, because the condom must be available and used consistently to be effective. New male polyurethane condoms are indicated for individuals with latex allergy. They are thinner than latex condoms and, therefore, may be more desirable.

Female Condom

Female condoms are prelubricated, polyurethane sheaths that cover the external genitalia, as well as the vagina. STD protection is one of the advantages. High cost and difficulty of use are disadvantages to use.

Diaphragm

The diaphragm is chosen by only a small number of adolescents. It is a dome-shaped rubber cup that acts as a physical barrier to conception, while jelly or cream applied to it provides spermicidal properties. Diaphragms provide some protection against STDs. Health care providers require specific skills to fit diaphragms. Additionally, patients must feel comfortable with its insertion and removal. Diaphragms must be available and inserted before intercourse to be reliable. The reported failure rates among teenaged users have ranged from 10% to 35%. Allergies to materials and a few cases of toxic shock syndrome have occurred with diaphragm use. The risk of cystitis is increased among diaphragm users.

Vaginal Spermicides

Vaginal spermicides contain spermicidal agents, either nonoxynol-9 or oxtoxynol-9, coupled with an inert substance (i.e., foam, cream, or suppository). Vaginal spermicides can be purchased without prescriptions. Spermicides are inserted vaginally within 1 hour before intercourse. When used alone, vaginal spermicides have a failure rate of 29% to 35% among teenagers. Therefore, it is recommended that spermicides be used with condoms. Nonoxynol-9 has antibacterial and antiviral properties that may help protect against STDs.

Intrauterine Device

The intrauterine device (IUD) is a plastic contraceptive device that is inserted into the uterus. IUDs require minimal patient motivation after insertion. Despite its low failure rate of 2% to 6%, IUDs are rarely ideal for teenagers because of considerable risk of ascending pelvic infection, ectopic pregnancy, and infertility.

Periodic Abstinence

Periodic abstinence, often known as natural family planning, encompasses several techniques that require recognition of the fertile period in the menstrual cycle and a willingness to practice abstinence during that time. Methods include the calendar method,

Billings method (recognition of symptoms of ovulation), and basal body temperature measurement. Periodic abstinence has a very high failure rate among teenagers; pregnancy occurs in 25% to 34% of teenaged users. Natural family planning provides no STD protection. These methods are most effective for patients with regular menstrual cycles coupled with high motivation and body awareness. Thus, they are not generally recommended for teenagers.

Coitus Interruptus

Coitus interruptus, or withdrawal before ejaculation, is used by many teenagers. This method offers the advantage of easy availability without advance planning. Disadvantages include its failure rate of 18% in adult women, potential interference with intercourse, and lack of STD protection.

Noncoital Sex

Noncoital sex refers to sex without intercourse. Adolescents should know that if ejaculation occurs close to the vagina, pregnancy can occur.

Abstinence

Abstinence is frequently used without seeking medical advice. It offers the clear advantage of preventing pregnancies and STDs. Adolescents who practice abstinence may benefit from health care providers' support and encouragement regarding their decision to postpone sexual activity.

Evaluation for Contraception

Before initiating contraception, it is important to obtain a careful history and physical examination to define medical and behavioral factors relevant to contraceptive choices. Health care practitioners must determine whether conditions exist that preclude use of a particular method. A complete gynecologic history should be obtained including age of menarche, recent menstrual pattern, and symptoms of dysmenorrhea. Although it is preferable for young women to experience regular menses for 1 to 2 years before initiating hormonal contraceptives, no evidence exists that long-term fertility is compromised by early oral contraceptive use. Thus, the desired establishment of regular menses is not absolute and may be waived if no other suitable method exists for patients who are sexually active.

Prior use of contraception and the reason for discontinuation helps in making future recommendations. Obtaining a sexual history is critical. Those young women or men who have not yet engaged in sexual intercourse but are feeling peer pressure might need reassurance regarding choosing abstinence rather than contraception. Young persons who engage in infrequent intercourse may select a barrier method. All individuals should be counseled regarding risks for STDs and the need for condom use.

A complete physical examination is recommended for young women beginning contraceptive use. Particular attention is paid to blood pressure, cardiovascular system, thyroid, and breast. Skin should be inspected for xanthomas, chloasma, jaundice, or scleral icterus. Extent of pubertal development should be assessed, because hormonal contraceptives are recommended only for those young women who are at Tanner sexual maturity rating stage 4 or 5. Abdominal examination is done to evaluate for liver enlargement or tenderness. Because fear of pelvic examinations may deter young women from seeking contraception, many health care providers will defer the pelvic examination when initiating oral contraceptive use in healthy young women. When doing pelvic examinations, yearly Papanicolaou smears, as well as screening cultures for STD pathogens including gonorrhea and chlamydia, are recommended. Syphilis serology should be obtained in the sexually active individual. When a positive family history for hyperlipidemia or early cardiovascular disease is elicited, some clinicians recommend that a serum lipid profile be obtained.

CHAPTER 53
Sexually Transmitted Diseases

Adapted from Hoover Adger

GONOCOCCAL INFECTIONS

Gonorrhea is caused by the gram-negative diplococcus *N. gonorrhoeae.* In the United States, an estimated 600,000 new infections with *N. gonorrhoeae* occur each year. Of the total reported cases, approximately 30% occur in individuals between ages 15 and 19 years, and approximately two-thirds of cases occur in those aged 15 to 24.

Clinical Characteristics

The clinical spectrum of diseases associated with *N. gonorrhoeae* is fairly broad. In men, gonorrhea is frequently a cause of urethritis. Complications due to direct extension to other sites are unusual in men; however, epididymitis, prostatitis, and seminal vesiculitis can occur. In addition to experiencing localized infection of the cervix, urethra, and Bartholin's or Skene's glands, affected women frequently sustain an extension to the upper genital tract structures causing endometritis, salpingitis, parametritis, and perihepatitis (commonly known as *Fitz-Hugh–Curtis syndrome*). Extragenital mucosal infections in men and women due to *N. gonorrhoeae* are manifested commonly as proctitis and pharyngitis. Rare occurrences in both genders include meningitis, endocarditis, arthritis, and dermatitis.

Anorectal infections due to gonorrhea are common in women and in men practicing anal intercourse. Even in the absence of rectal contact, 40% to 60% of women with cervical gonorrhea have been shown to also have the organism isolated from the rectum. The majority of women with rectal gonorrhea are asymptomatic. Usually, those men or women who have symptoms complain of perianal irritation, painful defecation, constipation, blood or mucus in the stool, or tenesmus. Frequently, in men who engage in anal receptive intercourse, other pathogens are associated with proctitis including *C. trachomatis,* herpesvirus, syphilis, *Campylobacter, Shigella,* or other ectoparasites.

Disseminated gonorrhea, or the arthritis-dermatitis syndrome, occurs primarily in women and is present in fewer than 1% of all patients with gonorrhea. Dissemination occurs as a result of hematogenous extension of the gonococcus from the site of entry. Frequently, it is seen after menstruation. Patients may note the presence of myalgia, headache, malaise, fever, or anorexia initially, but the clinical manifestations that are noted most frequently include the characteristic hemorrhagic- or necrotic-appearing skin lesions, arthralgias, tenosynovitis, and monoarticular or oligoarticular arthritis. The joints most frequently affected include the knees, elbows, ankles, wrists, and small joints of the hands or feet.

Frequently, patients with disseminated gonococcal infection are colonized with strains that cause asymptomatic mucosal infection. These particular strains differ by having specific nutritional requirements, and usually they are exquisitely sensitive to penicillin. Often, recovering the organism from such nonmucosal sites as blood, synovial fluid, or skin lesions is difficult. Blood cultures early in the course are positive in only 10% to 30% of cases. Frequently, Gram stains of synovial fluid contain an increased number of leukocytes but are positive for gram-negative diplococci in only 10% to 30% of cases, and fluid is culture-positive in fewer than 30% of cases. Although the definitive diagnosis of disseminated gonococcal infection is made by recovery of the organism from the blood, synovial fluid, skin lesions, or cerebrospinal fluid in the case of meningitis, it is most often based on the typical clinical manifestations, the recovery of the organism from a mucosal site, and the appropriate response to therapy. Hence, culturing the cervix, urethra, pharynx, and rectum before treatment is important.

Diagnostic Tests

The *in vitro* isolation of *N. gonorrhoeae* on selective media carried out in a 5%- to 10%-carbon dioxide environment is still the gold standard by which all other methods are measured. However, new technology using nucleic acid amplification may be as sensitive as, if not more sensitive than, traditional culture techniques and is becoming more readily available.

A Gram stain of a smear of urogenital secretions has been used for the diagnosis of gonococcal infection of the male urethra and the female cervix for more than 75 years. In men with a urethral discharge, the Gram stain has a sensitivity and specificity almost equal to that of culture. Hence, in men who experience a urethral discharge, the demonstration of the typical gram-negative diplococci within polymorphonuclear leukocytes is sufficient for the diagnosis. In men without a discharge, the Gram stain, although somewhat less sensitive, remains a very specific test. A Gram stain of secretions from the cervix is less sensitive and, therefore, not as reliable for the diagnosis of gonococcal infection in women. In experienced hands, however, it remains a specific test and is helpful in identifying gonococcal or nongonococcal cervicitis.

Treatment

Treatment regimens recommended for uncomplicated gonococcal infections include cefixime, 400 mg orally in a single dose; ceftriaxone, 125 mg given intramuscularly; ciprofloxacin, 500 mg orally; or ofloxacin, 400 mg orally. Each of these regimens should be followed by azithromycin, 1 g orally, or doxycycline, 100 mg twice daily for 7 days. Patients who are unable to tolerate cephalosporins or quinolones can be treated alternatively with spectinomycin, 2 g intramuscularly.

Adolescents who have had recent exposure to gonorrhea should be cultured and treated as if they have infection. Patients who have uncomplicated gonorrhea and who are treated with any of the recommended regimens do not need a follow-up test of cure. However, those who have symptoms that persist after treatment should be evaluated by culture, and any gonococci isolated should be tested for antimicrobial susceptibility. Also important is that all teenagers with gonorrhea have a serologic test for syphilis performed at the time of diagnosis. Additionally recommended is that all patients with gonorrhea be offered confidential counseling and testing for the human immunodeficiency virus (HIV).

In cases with complicated gonococcal infections such as disseminated gonorrhea, the usual recommendation is for hospitalization and treatment with intramuscular or intravenous ceftriaxone or an acceptable substitute. Acceptable treatment regimens can be found in the frequently updated *Sexually Transmitted Disease Treatment Guidelines* published by the Centers for Disease Control and Prevention (CDC).

CHLAMYDIAL INFECTIONS

C. trachomatis is the sexually transmitted agent most commonly isolated today. It is most prevalent in the age group 15 to 19. From 1987 through 1996, reported cases of chlamydia increased from 48 to 195 cases per 100,000 persons. This trend reflects increased screening, recognition of asymptomatic infections, improved reporting, and the continuing high burden of disease. *C. trachomatis* has been isolated from 10% to 26% of female adolescents in teenage clinics and is much more prevalent than is gonococcal infection in most studies.

The risk factors noted most frequently for infection with *C. trachomatis* include young age, history of multiple sexual partners, the presence of other sexually transmitted diseases (STDs), the use of oral contraceptives, the use of a nonbarrier method or no method of contraception, and an abnormal Papanicolaou smear. Young adolescents appear to be at particular risk for acquisition of chlamydia. One explanation for this finding may be the presence of ectopy or ectopic columnar epithelium, which is often present on the exposed surface of the immature adolescent cervix and which is particularly susceptible to invasion by chlamydiae.

Clinical Characteristics

The clinical presentation associated with chlamydial genital tract infections is fairly similar to that of gonococcal infection. Infections commonly associated with *C. trachomatis* include acute urethral syndrome, bartholinitis, cervicitis, salpingitis, nongonococcal urethritis, epididymitis, proctitis, conjunctivitis, and Reiter syndrome.

Chlamydial infection in women may be associated with mucopurulent cervicitis or urethritis, but it is frequently asymptomatic. Ascending infection may occur leading to salpingitis and perihepatitis (Fitz-Hugh–Curtis syndrome). Chlamydial salpingitis is frequently subclinical and has been implicated as a significant cause of involuntary infertility.

Currently, nongonococcal urethritis (NGU) is recognized as the most common form of urethritis in men. *C. trachomatis* is the most common identifiable cause of NGU, responsible for 30% to 60% of cases depending on the population studied. In addition, *C. trachomatis* is the most common cause of epididymitis and is a common cause of prostatitis in men younger than 35 years.

Infants born to women with cervical chlamydial infection are at significant risk for the development of chlamydial infection. Approximately 60% to 70% of infants exposed to chlamydiae during passage through an infected birth canal become infected. The approximate risk of developing conjunctivitis is 30% to 40%; pneumonia, 10% to 20%; and asymptomatic nasopharyngeal infection, 20%.

Because of the extremely high prevalence and the very real potential for serious morbidity among infected individuals, all sexually active teenagers with genital tract symptoms should be evaluated for *C. trachomatis* infection. Testing for chlamydia in sexually active women should be as routine as are Papanicolaou smears and gonococcal cultures. Routine culture of male adolescents is impractical in most settings. However, the examination of a first-voided urine specimen may be a helpful adjunct in the identification of asymptomatic men with chlamydial urethritis.

Diagnostic Tests

Tissue culture techniques are the most sensitive and specific methods and are the preferred method of detection. Two rapid diagnostic nonculture methods currently available and proven to be very helpful are Microtrak, which depends on direct fluorescent staining of chlamydial elementary bodies, and Chlamydiazyme, an enzyme-linked immunosorbent assay (ELISA). The immunofluorescent antibody technique is fairly sensitive among symptomatic patients but may be less sensitive in detecting asymptomatic, but infected, individuals. The ELISA technique appears to be relatively sensitive but may have more false-positives associated with it. New nucleic acid amplification tests enable detection of *C. trachomatis* and *N. gonorrhoeae* from directly obtained specimens or from first-voided urine. In some settings, these tests are more sensitive than are traditional culture techniques.

Treatment

Treatment regimens for chlamydial disease include azithromycin (1 g orally as a single dose), doxycycline (100 mg twice daily for at least 7 days), or erythromycin (500 mg four times daily for 7 days) or ofloxacin (300 mg twice daily for 7 days), as an alternative. Treatment of genital infections in children who weigh less than 45 kg is erythromycin, 50 mg/kg/day for 10 to 14 days. Children who are older than 8 years can be treated with azithromycin or doxycycline. The recommended therapy for chlamydial conjunctivitis or pneumonia is oral erythromycin, 50 mg/kg/day for 10 to 14 days.

SYPHILIS

Syphilis is caused by the spirochete *Treponema pallidum. T. pallidum* is a pathogen only in humans and is transmitted from infected individuals through close intimate contact. In 1996, more than 11,000 cases of primary and secondary syphilis were reported in the United States.

Clinical Characteristics

Usually, the initial lesion of primary syphilis—the *chancre*—develops 14 to 21 days after the initial infection. However, the incubation period can vary from 10 to 90 days. Usually, the primary lesion appears as a small, solitary, round or elongated, indurated ulcer with a clean base. The chancre does not usually cause pain and, if located in an inconspicuous site, may go unnoticed. The lesions vary in size from 3 to 4 mm or 1 to 2 cm. Usually, regional lymphadenopathy accompanies the chancre. The chancre usually remains stable in appearance for several weeks and, if untreated, slowly resolves.

Secondary syphilis is heralded by the presence of a generalized macular or maculopapular eruption that, at times, can also be nodulopapular in appearance and is not usually associated with pruritus. Usually, the rash of secondary syphilis is concentrated on the trunk, but the characteristic lesions can frequently be found on the face, palms, and soles. The rash may be accompanied by fever or malaise. Other clinical signs of secondary syphilis include the presence of flat moist papules in the anal or genital region (called *condyloma lata*), small patches of alopecia in the scalp, and loss of the lateral eyebrows.

When the symptoms and signs of secondary syphilis disappear, the disease is termed *latent syphilis*. Patients with latent syphilis have no signs or symptoms but may still be infectious, if untreated, for a period of several years. Approximately one-third of those with latent syphilis progress to late syphilis if untreated; this condition may occur within 2 to 30 years after the original infection. The clinical manifestations are highly variable and take the form of benign late syphilis in approximately 50%, cardiovascular syphilis in nearly 30%, and neurosyphilis in close to 20%.

Diagnosis

The best method for verifying the diagnosis of primary syphilis is dark-field microscopical examination and direct fluorescent antibody tests of exudate or tissue from the lesion. If results are positive, this test is all that is required to establish the diagnosis of primary syphilis. When dark-field examination is not available, the diagnosis is usually based on the standard serologic tests: the VDRL test and rapid protein reagin (RPR), which are used for screening. A fourfold change in titer, equivalent to a change of two dilutions (e.g., from 1:16 to 1:4 or from 1:8 to 1:32), is usually considered necessary to demonstrate a clinically significant difference. Because these two nontreponemal tests are nonspecific, a positive result should be confirmed by the highly specific fluorescent treponemal antibody (FTA) test. Approximately 90% of patients with primary syphilis have a positive FTA, whereas only 80% have a positive VDRL or RPR. The difficulty in using the FTA in the diagnosis of early syphilis is that, once it is positive, this test often remains positive over the life of the individual. Thus, it does not rule out a positive test as a result of prior infection. In contrast, although it may be negative in individuals early in the course of the disease, the VDRL test often has a titer that correlates well with activity of the disease and, therefore, can be used as a baseline for follow-up.

The diagnosis of secondary syphilis is much easier, because the RPR or VDRL is positive in 99% of cases. False-positive results do occur, but they are found in only 2% of tests confirmed by FTA.

Treatment

The choice of treatment for primary, secondary, or latent syphilis of less than 1 year's duration is benzathine penicillin G, 2.4 million units intramuscularly at one visit. Patients who are allergic to penicillin should be treated with doxycycline, 100 mg twice a day, or tetracycline, 500 mg four times daily for 14 days. All patients should be encouraged to return for repeat VDRL tests at 3, 6, and 12 months after treatment. All patients with syphilis should be counseled concerning the risks of HIV and should be encouraged to be tested for HIV antibody.

The optimal treatment regimen for syphilis of more than 1 year's duration has not been as well established. In general, with the exception of neurosyphilis, suggested treatment is benzathine penicillin G, 2.4 million units intramuscularly each week for 3 successive weeks; or doxycycline, 100 mg twice daily; or tetracycline, 500 mg four times daily for 30 days in those who are allergic to penicillin.

HERPES SIMPLEX VIRUS INFECTIONS

Infections due to herpes simplex virus (HSV) have become increasingly more common in the United States. The spectrum of clinical manifestations associated with this organism includes primary and recurrent genital herpes, pharyngitis, urethritis, cervicitis, proctitis, neonatal HSV infections, and the possible association with cervical carcinoma.

Primary genital herpes may be caused by either type 1 or type 2 HSV. In the United States, 70% to 90% of primary genital infections are caused by HSV-2, although the two types are clinically indistinguishable. Primary HSV infections may or may not produce clinically apparent symptoms. In general, however, first episodes of genital herpes are more likely than are recurrent episodes to be associated with systemic signs and symptoms, with more severe and prolonged symptoms, and with increased and prolonged viral shedding. Commonly, patients experience central nervous system involvement during a primary HSV infection. Aseptic meningitis, autonomic dysfunction resulting in hyperesthesia or anesthesia, transverse myelitis, and encephalitis are frequently documented. Dissemination with viremia and widespread involvement can occur but is rare.

Usually, the clinical diagnosis of genital herpes is made by recognition of the characteristic lesions of grouped vesicles on an erythematous base. Both primary and recurrent HSV infections are accompanied by tender lymphadenopathy. Usually, the inguinal nodes are mildly tender on palpation, nonfixed, and only slightly firm.

Several methods are available for documentation of the organism including isolation by tissue culture, detection of viral antigen by direct fluorescent assay (ELISA), cytologic examination of clinical specimens, or serology. Diagnosis should be confirmed by culture if an alternate initial method of detection is used.

Oral acyclovir is the preferred treatment in most episodes of symptomatic HSV disease. Topical therapy is substantially less effective than oral therapy, and its use is discouraged. Systemic acyclovir provides partial control of the symptoms and signs of HSV infections when used to treat first clinical episodes, or recurrent episodes, or when used as daily suppressive therapy. Systemic therapy prevents new lesion formation and, because of the high incidence of urethral, cervical, and oral infections, oral acyclovir is preferable in first-episode infections. All patients who have first-episode genital HSV and present with active lesions should be treated. The currently recommended therapy is acyclovir, 400 mg three times daily or 200 mg five times daily for 7 to 10 days; or famciclovir, 250 three times daily; or valacyclovir, 1 g twice daily for the same period. Patients should be counseled to understand that sexual transmission of HSV can occur during asymptomatic periods.

Most patients with first-episode genital HSV infection will have recurrent episodes of genital lesions. Episodic or suppressive antiviral therapy might shorten the duration of lesions or ameliorate recurrences. Because many patients benefit from antiviral therapy, options for episodic or suppressive treatment should be discussed with all patients. If episodic treatment is chosen, patients should be provided with antiviral therapy or a prescription for the medication, so that treatment can be initiated at the first signs of prodrome or genital lesion. Daily suppressive therapy reduces the frequency of genital herpes recurrences by more than 75% among patients who have frequent recurrences. Suppressive treatment reduces, but does not eliminate, asymptomatic viral shedding. Hence, the extent to which suppressive therapy may prevent HSV transmission is not known.

HUMAN PAPILLOMAVIRUS INFECTION

Genital warts are an STD caused by human papillomavirus (HPV). Genital wart virus infections appear to be increasing in prevalence and are rapidly becoming one of the most common STDs diagnosed. To date, more than 50 HPV types have been characterized. Acute infections may be asymptomatic or may produce exophytic or flat condylomas; chronic persistent infections may result in intraepithelial neoplasia or squamous cell carcinoma. HPV types 6 and 11 are the viral types associated most commonly with exophytic warts.

Genital warts are transmitted through close intimate contact including sexual intercourse. It is unclear whether transmission rates differ for HPV types, and indirect transmission through fomites has never been demonstrated convincingly.

The association of HPV and genital malignancy is an area of active study. HPV types 16 and 18 are the most frequent types found in malignancies, and types 10, 11, 33, and 35 are found in a small percentage of cases. However, HPV types 16 and 18 cause only a small percentage of genital warts; the most common cause of warts, type 6, is rarely found in genital malignancies. Hence, despite the strong association of HPV and genital malignancy, the precise role of HPV remains uncertain. Several methods for the diagnosis of HPV infection are available and range from simple visual inspection to colposcopy, cytology, histology, antigen detection, and molecular DNA hybridization.

Traditionally, the standard treatment of genital warts has been based on the ablation of grossly visible warty tissue. Although treatment can induce wart-free periods in most patients, no evidence indicates that currently available treatments eradicate or affect the natural history of HPV infection. The removal of warts may or may not decrease infectivity. If left untreated, visible warts may resolve on their own, may remain unchanged, or may increase in size or number. No evidence indicates that treatment of visible warts affects the development of cervical cancer.

The available treatments for visible genital warts include patient-applied therapies (podofilox, 0.5% solution or gel, and imiquimod, 5% cream) and provider-administered therapies [i.e., cryotherapy, podophyllin resin, trichloroacetic acid (TCA), bichloroacetic acid, interferon, and surgery]. None of the available treatments is superior to other treatments, and no single treatment is ideal for all patients. In general, warts located on moist surfaces or on intertriginous areas respond better to topical treatment (e.g., TCA, podophyllin, podofilox, and imiquimod) than do warts on drier surfaces.

For women who have exophytic cervical warts, high-grade squamous intraepithelial lesions should be excluded before treatment is started. Women should be counseled regarding the need for regular Papanicolaou smears as recommended for patients without genital warts; however, the presence of genital warts is not an indication for cervical colposcopy.

SPECIFIC SEXUALLY TRANSMITTED DISEASE SYNDROMES

Vaginitis

The three most common types of vaginitis are bacterial vaginosis (formerly called *nonspecific* or *Gardnerella vaginalis vaginitis*), *Trichomonas vaginalis* vaginitis, and candidal vaginitis. Adolescents presenting with the complaint of a vaginal discharge often have a specific etiology for their symptoms. Careful evaluation should include measurement of vaginal fluid pH, examination of vaginal fluid saline and KOH preparations, endocervical culture, antigen detection tests or nucleic acid amplification tests for *C. trachomatis* and *N. gonorrhoeae*, a Gram-stained smear of endocervical secretions, and a Papanicolaou smear.

Bacterial vaginosis is the most common cause of an abnormal vaginal discharge. Several anaerobic bacteria, in addition to

G. vaginalis, are thought to be involved in this complex syndrome. This complex alteration of the vaginal flora appears to be closely linked to sexual activity, but no specific etiologic organism has been defined. The diagnosis is based on the finding of a homogenous discharge, a vaginal fluid pH greater than 4.5, a positive whiff test (fishy odor when KOH is added to vaginal fluid), and clue cells on the examination of a wet preparation of vaginal secretions. When a Gram stain is used, determining the relative concentration of the bacterial morphotypes characteristic of the altered flora of bacterial vaginosis is an acceptable laboratory method for diagnosis. Metronidazole, 500 mg twice daily for 7 days; or clindamycin cream 2%, one applicator at bedtime for 7 days; or metronidazole gel 0.75%, one applicator twice a day for 5 days, are the treatments of choice. An alternative choice is metronidazole, 2 g orally in a single dose.

T. vaginalis vaginitis is characterized by a malodorous vaginal discharge that is homogenous and classically described as yellow-green, frothy, and possessing a vaginal fluid pH greater than 4.5. The vagina and cervix may be erythematous and, occasionally, punctate hemorrhages or strawberry spots are seen on the cervix. On examination of the saline wet preparation, flagellated organisms and polymorphonuclear leukocytes are seen. The only effective treatment for *Trichomonas* vaginitis is oral metronidazole. A single 2-g dose appears to be as effective as the 7-day treatment regimen and is the preferred regimen for most adolescents.

The characteristic findings of candidal vaginitis include vaginal and vulvar erythema, vulvar edema, pruritus, and the presence of a thick, cottage cheese-like discharge. The diagnosis can be confirmed by the microscopical finding of yeast forms on a KOH preparation or by culture. Predisposing factors include diabetes, recent use of antibiotics, immunosuppressive therapy, obesity, or use of oral contraceptives. Usually, treatment with one of a number of intravaginal or oral antifungal agents results in relief of symptoms.

Pelvic Inflammatory Disease

Pelvic inflammatory disease (PID) is the syndrome resulting from the ascending spread of microorganisms from the vagina and cervix to the endometrium, the fallopian tubes, and the contiguous upper genital tract structures. It is a disease primarily of young women, with adolescents aged 15 to 19 constituting the group at highest risk when rates are adjusted for age. Although rates for women in other age groups show declines, rates for adolescents appear to be increasing.

Although the microbiological etiology of pelvic inflammatory disease has been found to be polymicrobial in nature, *C. trachomatis, N. gonorrhoeae,* and a variety of anaerobic bacteria (*Peptostreptococcus, Peptococcus, Bacteroides*) are the organisms identified most commonly from tubal cultures. Mycoplasmas, *Ureaplasma urealyticum,* and facultative bacteria (most frequently *G. vaginalis, Streptococcus* species, *Escherichia coli,* and *Haemophilus influenzae*) also have been isolated from tubal cultures.

Frequently, PID poses a difficult diagnostic problem and may be confused with appendicitis, pyelonephritis, and a host of other gynecologic problems such as ruptured ovarian cyst, ectopic pregnancy, and septic abortion. The diagnosis is particularly difficult in adolescents who have milder PID and in whom chlamydia is more likely to be the causative agent. The suggested minimum criteria for the diagnosis of PID include the following: (a) lower abdominal tenderness, (b) cervical motion tenderness, and (c) adnexal tenderness. Additional criteria to support the diagnosis of PID include temperature of at least 38°C, abnormal cervical or vaginal discharge, elevated erythrocyte sedimentation rate or C-reactive protein, and documentation of cervical infection with *N. gonorrhoeae* or *C. trachomatis.*

The goal of treatment is the prevention of infertility and the chronic residua of infection. To be effective, treatment should be instituted early and should cover the polymicrobial spectrum of the disease. Often, the most difficult therapeutic decision for the physician is whether to hospitalize adolescents with PID or to treat them as outpatients. No currently available data compare the efficacy of parenteral with oral therapy or inpatient therapy with outpatient therapy. The decision as to whether hospitalization is necessary should be based on clinical assessment and on the discretion of the health care provider. Current recommendations for hospitalization are based on observational data and theoretic concerns and include inability to exclude a surgical emergency such as appendicitis; pregnancy; failure to respond to oral antimicrobial therapy; inability to tolerate an outpatient oral regimen; severe illness, nausea and vomiting, or high fever; tuboovarian abscess; and immunodeficiency. Although several treatment regimens are suggested, intravenous cefotetan or cefoxitin and doxycycline is favored by most individuals because of its excellent coverage for *N. gonorrhoeae, C. trachomatis,* and the anaerobic organisms.

Suggested oral regimens for treatment on an ambulatory basis include ofloxacin, 400 mg twice daily, plus metronidazole, 500 mg twice daily for 14 days, or an intramuscular or parenteral dose of a cephalosporin plus doxycycline, 100 mg twice daily for 14 days. Individuals who do not respond to oral therapy within 72 hours should be reevaluated to confirm the diagnosis and should be administered parenteral therapy on either an inpatient or outpatient basis. In addition, partner treatment should always be a part of the therapeutic approach.

At least one-fourth of women with acute PID experience one or more serious long-term sequelae. Involuntary infertility due to tubal occlusion is experienced by approximately 20% of young women after one episode of PID. Other sequelae include an increased risk of ectopic pregnancy, chronic pelvic pain, dyspareunia, pelvic adhesions, pyosalpinx, and the development of inflammatory masses. The prevention of the sequelae through prompt and accurate diagnosis coupled with effective treatment should be a primary goal in the approach to adolescents with this disease.

2c
Common Ambulatory Issues—Developmental and Psychological Issues

CHAPTER 54
School Difficulties and Attention Deficit Hyperactivity Disorder (ADHD)

Adapted from Stewart H. Mostofsky and Martha B. Denckla

CHILDREN WHO HAVE UNEXPECTED READING DIFFICULTY

In some children who present with a complaint of difficulty with reading, the problem can be attributed to an isolated reading disability (RD), more commonly termed dyslexia in the medical and psychological professions. Developmental dyslexia is defined as a chronic disorder characterized by difficulty with acquisition and use of written language that is unexpected on the basis of normal general development and overall cognitive aptitude. Theoretically, other exclusions include emotional problems, educational deprivation, and sensory impairment. Outside the scope of this discussion is that dyslexia is a lifelong disorder; residual effects, particularly slow reading, are observed in adults with the disorder.

Pure dyslexia is more the exception than the rule; most children with dyslexia have deficits not limited to written language. Almost universally, dyslexia is viewed as a specific disorder of the phonologic subdivision of the language system. The border between deficits in reading and deficits in broader aspect of language can be fuzzy, and most children with dyslexia have a broader language deficit that involves aspects of both spoken and written language.

Most public school systems define an RD on the basis of discrepancy criteria (a discrepancy between full-scale intelligence quotient and performance on tests of reading achievement) rather than by the appearance of a subtle neurocognitive deficit in phonologic awareness. Under Public Law 94-142 (the Education for All Handicapped Children Act) passed in 1975, public school systems are required to provide services for children with handicapping conditions including learning disabilities. However, often children with dyslexia have difficulty with broader aspects of language, which can adversely affect intelligence quotient scores (particularly the verbal subtests). This outcome can create difficulty for dyslexic children in meeting the discrepancy criteria adopted by most public school systems. The underlying language deficits in such children lower both aptitude and achievement precluding a discrepancy.

The etiology of developmental dyslexia is presumed to be congenital. Certain genetic and fetal developmental factors are theorized as possible contributors to the development of brain differences that result in ineffective performance of reading and other language-based tasks. Investigations have elicited genetic contributions to dyslexia. Family studies reveal that in individuals with dyslexia, the risk of giving birth to a male child with the disorder is estimated to be 35% to 45%, whereas familial risk in female individuals is estimated to be 17% to 18%; both are elevated as compared to the risk in the general population of 5% to 10%. The chance of a sibling being affected is approximately 40%; the chance of a parent is 27% to 49%. Other work (that includes twin studies) has suggested heritability for single-word reading and phonologic decoding. Linkage studies have implicated possible loci on chromosomes 6 and 15.

CHILDREN WHO HAVE DIFFICULTY IN STAYING ON TASK

Pediatricians must respond to another very common school-related problem found in children: difficulty in staying on task. Often, this difficulty is associated with symptoms of impulsivity and hyperactivity. Frequently, these symptoms will be due to attention-deficit hyperactivity disorder (ADHD), however, differential diagnoses, including language and learning disabilities and psychiatric disorders, must be considered. Very often, the issue occurs "in addition to" rather than "instead of" ADHD, as is commonly true for language-based disabilities.

Public awareness of ADHD has been increased; however, the symptoms that comprise the disorder have been recognized under a variety of names (minimal brain dysfunction, hyperkinetic disorder, attention deficit disorder) for more than 30 years. ADHD is common, affecting 3% to 5% of elementary school-aged children, leaving little doubt about its impact on school functioning across a large population of children. Studies have revealed a higher incidence of ADHD in boys than in girls with a ratio of approximately 3:1; however, gender-biased diagnostic criteria may account for the size, if not the direction, of the ratio.

ADHD is characterized by symptoms of hyperactivity, impulsivity, and a decreased ability to maintain on-task behavior, particularly during nonpreferred tasks. Currently, the *Diagnostic and Statistical Manual of Mental Disorders,* Fourth Edition (*DSM-IV*) uses the term attention-deficit hyperactivity disorder and includes three subtypes: "predominantly inattentive," "predominantly hyperactive-impulsive," and a "combined type." By definition, signs must be observed before age 7 years. The forms can change over the lifespan: One individual can have the hyperactive-impulsive type as a preschooler, have the full syndrome until middle school, and exhibit the inattentive type thereafter.

Often, children with the inattentive form of the disorder will present with isolated complaints of school difficulty. In children with the hyperactive-impulsive or combined forms of the disorder, signs are typically recognizable at an early age and often include both behavioral and academic difficulties. In the inattentive form, signs may not be evident until affected children enter school and begin engaging in nonpreferred activities that require a much greater ability to inhibit off-task behavior. With persistent, focused questioning, however, clinicians can often find a history of off-task behavior during the preschool years. (As is the case for dyslexia, importantly, ADHD is no longer a diagnosis restricted to childhood. Of those patients, in whom the diagnosis is made in childhood, 30% to 50% continue to have residual ADHD in adult life; adults—often parents of those children referred for ADHD—have presented with signs consistent with ADHD.)

As with dyslexia, ADHD is often associated with comorbid conditions. What is more, these comorbid conditions are often part of the differential diagnosis that must be considered in the evaluation of children who present with difficulty in staying on task. As mentioned, ADHD is often associated with dyslexia and other language-based learning disabilities. These disorders must also be considered in the differential diagnosis, as problems in staying on task can result from difficulty in understanding verbal and written instructions. In addition, psychiatric disorders such as oppositional defiant disorder, conduct disorder, anxiety disorders, and mood disorders (including depression) are common comorbidities that must also be considered as possible causes or contributors to difficulty in staying on task.

EVALUATING CHILDREN WHO HAVE SCHOOL DIFFICULTIES

In children with "pure" dyslexia, a history should reveal difficulties specific to tasks involving reading, spelling, and the academic language arts. Developmentally, problems begin to emerge in preschool and kindergarten when affected children are asked to begin naming written letters or to associate the letters with their assigned sounds (the most basic reading task) or such children are unable to read words by first grade. Sometimes a useful history of speech quirks may be elicited (for example, "It's a froggy day," or "The Madonna is also called the Merchant Mary"). However, it takes a sophisticated parent or teacher to report these malapropisms as anything but cute when elicited. Most of these children go on to read; however, typically they remain slow readers throughout their lives. The disorder brings a continuing impact on any academic task involving reading and written language output; as such children grow older, they experience increased frustration and school failure.

As discussed, dyslexia is a restricted type of language-based disorder (restricted to the phonologic portion of the language domain). Clinically, the division between pure dyslexia and a broader language disorder is often unclear, and most children with dyslexia have a history of difficulty with other aspects of language tasks (semantics, syntax). Children presenting with difficulty in reading may reveal a history of delay in acquisition of early language milestones. Often, children with language-based disabilities have problems with finding the correct sounds (to form words) in expressing ideas resulting in imprecise and circumlocutory speech. In contrast to having difficulties with one or more aspects of language, such children often demonstrate a history of strong visuospatial abilities.

The observation of letter reversal in reading is the best known and most misunderstood feature of dyslexia. Despite the common perception that these reversals (most commonly b and d) are due to difficulties with visuospatial processing, research has demonstrated clearly that such reversals are secondary to errors in phonologic awareness. More likely, reversals of b and d are due to the fact that they sound the same and that the oral movements used to produce the sounds are very similar, rather than because they a mirror images of each another.

ADHD is a diagnosis by history; in children presenting with school difficulties, the use of multiple techniques for obtaining a history, including clinical interview and rating scales or questionnaires, is critical for accurate diagnosis. The diagnosis of ADHD requires that difficulties be present in at least two settings; it is important that historical information be obtained from multiple sources that should, at the very least, include parents and teachers. Available school records, including teacher observations, are an important source of information and should be reviewed.

Typically, history reveals problems with maintaining on-task behavior and impulsivity associated with inhibitory insufficiencies. In young children, difficulty in maintaining on-task behavior tends to manifest as hyperactivity and difficulty in sitting still; older children present more commonly with problems in focusing on schoolwork. Gender also accounts for differences in phenotype, with boys more commonly showing hyperactivity and impulsivity and girls demonstrating lack of focus, although possibly "motor mouth" hyperactivity and impulsive interruptive speech is more common in younger girls but does not reach the threshold for hyperactivity or impulsivity on existing rating scales. Signs of inattentiveness and disinhibition are subject to situational variation and often depend on interest in a given task; nonpreferred tasks require greater inhibition of off-task behavior and result in greater appearance of inattentiveness. Independent of interest in task, variability in task performance is a nearly consistent feature of the disorder.

An important aspect of understanding the impact of ADHD on school performance is realizing that individuals with the disorder often have difficulties in planning, organizing, and generating strategies for future actions (often collectively termed executive functions in neuropsychology). The histories of children with ADHD are typically filled with anecdotes about disorganization and poor time management; book bags, desks, and lockers are often in a state of chaos; homework assignments are left at home; books are left at school; and lateness is the rule rather than the exception. These issues assume greater importance as affected children reach the upper elementary grades, when longer-term assignments are introduced, and they reach serious proportions when self-management is assumed to be the norm (in the early teenage years).

General physical examination should be conducted with a focus on particular features. Dysmorphic features can be suggestive of genetic disorders associated with learning disabilities such as Turner syndrome, fragile X syndrome (particularly in girls), and Klinefelter syndrome. The skin should be examined for stigmata suggestive of neurocutaneous disorders such as tuberous sclerosis and neurofibromatosis, which can be associated with learning disabilities.

A critical component of the examination of any child presenting with school difficulty is a neurocognitive evaluation, which is performed by an individual (e.g., a psychologist) whose expertise is administering and interpreting neurocognitive tests in children. In children presenting with school difficulties, neurocognitive testing should include language-based tests. In children with dyslexia, testing typically reveals variable degrees of language inefficiency with dramatic deficits on tests of phonologic awareness (including rhyming and phoneme segmentation) and decoding (reading of nonsense words, pronounceable pseudowords, often called word attack).

Many children with dyslexia have strong visuospatial abilities; testing this and other visual perceptual aspects of cognition is important. This assessment helps to establish cognitive strengths important for self-esteem and to make recommendations for techniques to accommodate areas of weakness. No diagnostic test can measure ADHD; however, tests of response preparation, inhibition, and organization such as computerized go–no-go tests, complex figure copying, and visual search, are important in detecting deficits in response consistency, inhibition, and approach to task and can be supportive of the diagnosis that is made by history.

TREATING CHILDREN WHO PRESENT WITH SCHOOL DIFFICULTIES

The approach to the treatment of children presenting with school difficulties is multimodal, involving integration of various components that include academic interventions and accommodations, speech-language therapy, behavior modification and other mental health intervention, and pharmacotherapy. The combination of these interventions is aimed at achieving three goals: (a) providing the best possible academic environment in which children can learn (academic interventions and accommodations), (b) relieving symptoms that may create more difficulty for children to function in the school environment (pharmacotherapy), and (c) remedying conditions that may be contributing to or exacerbated by children's school difficulties (e.g., with speech-language therapy and behavior modification and other mental health interventions).

The treatment of children with dyslexia is focused on academic interventions and accommodations and, for broader and deeper language issues, speech-language therapy; at this time, no known medications address dyslexia or other learning disabilities. Recommendations regarding educational interventions are, in part, based on age. In younger children (elementary school), emphasis should be placed on remedial therapies that address the underlying deficit in phonologic awareness and go on to use a phonics-based approach to reading instruction. Once affected children become efficient in reading using phonics, care should be taken to advance them into using the more rapid whole-word reading. Otherwise, such children are in danger of "getting stuck on phonics," which could significantly impair reading speed. Some children are so deficient in phonologic skills that a balanced, multifactorial approach must be used from early in the remedial process, and professionals should be monitored for their possible perseveration on exclusively phonics-based methods.

Older children and adolescents are better served by use of accommodations to work around the difficulty with reading (Table 54-1). Emphasis should be placed on the use of visual cues to help with learning; often, the visual-perceptual system is a strength in affected children. Slow reading should be accepted as a residual problem, and accommodations should include untimed tests and reductions in the amount of required reading. Videotapes or book audiotapes can be used as adjuncts to texts. Other accommodations include use of computers with spelling checkers, tutors to help in reviewing the content of written material (including spelling), and the use of oral presentations or visual displays (on science or history topics) in place of written tests.

For children with ADHD, treatment involves the use of behavior modification techniques to improve on-task performance maintenance, the use of medications that boost inhibitory control to decrease off-task behavior, and the use of academic accommodations to help create an academic environment in which children are better able to learn.

Behavior modification is based on techniques of operant conditioning that stress positive reinforcement to alter behavior. The optimal approach is to have a behavioral psychologist involved who would work not only with affected children, but also with parents, teachers, and other supervisory adults. Consistency is extremely important, and psychologists can help in setting up a coordinated program in which caregivers provide preestablished responses to both positive and negative behavior. Importantly, for children with ADHD, consequences should be immediate and consistent, and praise and reward for good behavior and performance should be emphasized.

For children with ADHD, academic accommodations are important for providing a school setting in which the greatest amount of learning can take place (Table 54-2). Teachers should attempt to provide as much structure and routine as possible. Classrooms should be small, and affected children should be given preferential seating toward the front of the classroom. Frequent changes of teachers during the day should be avoided. Studies consistently reveal that individuals with ADHD are slow in responding; thus, untimed tests are an essential accommodation, as is limiting the length of homework assignments. Attempts should also be made at helping to provide organization by using a combination of techniques including keeping an extra set of textbooks at home and using a daily assignment notebook that allows teachers to communicate directly with parents regarding homework assignments. Alternately, if tactfully arranged, a buddy system can be useful, designating a classmate who helps with providing a copy of the assignments and books needed.

Much interest in or controversy about ADHD is prompted by the most commonly known aspect of its treatment: stimulant medication, often methylphenidate, (Ritalin) or Dextroamphetamine (Dexedrine). Long-acting preparations of methylphidate (Concerta) and Dexadrine (Adderall) are available and allow convenient once-daily dosing. The newest agent available is atomoxetine (Strattera) classified as a non-stimulant allowing practitioners to write refills. Although a multimodal approach to ADHD is recommended (combining a stimulant with home and school behavioral management plans, as discussed), the highly publicized stimulant therapy is frequently the first and sole treatment. The stimulants are reported to be effective in at least 70% of individuals with ADHD, although part of the problem is that many conditions

TABLE 54-1. Some Recommended Academic Accommodations for Children with Reading Disability (Dyslexia)

Classroom and course work
Untimed or extended-time tests
Customized tests to circumvent word retrieval problems
Permission to give oral reports and demonstrations or to create illustrative displays
Reduction in amount of required reading
Instruction and therapy
Use of visual cues and reinforcement
Use of videos and books on tape as adjuncts to texts
Use of computers with word-processing and spelling- and grammar-checking programs
Subject-matter (reading) tutoring (type and intensity individualized)
Speech-language therapy, if indicated

TABLE 54-2. Recommended Academic Accommodations for Children with Attention-Deficit Hyperactivity Disorder

Classroom and course work
Small class size
Seating that, in context, best accommodates either nondisruptive out-of-seat restlessness or need to keep classmates "out of sight, out of mind," avoiding frequent changes of classes and teachers
Stimulating course work (intrinsically motivating)
Structured course work and classroom setting (explicitly organized, broken into steps that can be reinforced positively)
Untimed or extended-time tests
Instruction and therapy
Organizational coaching (help with "how" and "when")
Parent-teacher training in behavior modification, skewed toward the positive ("Catch them being good")

other than ADHD (and normal status as well) can show improvement with stimulant administration. Dose-response relationships may vary with age, intelligence, and the nature of the targeted behavior. Although a clear neurotransmitter mechanism remains undefined, the stimulants are thought to affect dopaminergic or noradrenergic motor inhibitory control systems in the brain, thereby reducing impulsive and off-task behavior and potentiating delays between stimuli and responses.

Fears surrounding adverse effects of stimulants include possible stunted growth after chronic childhood administration and triggering tics or even Tourette syndrome. Several longitudinal studies have failed to produce evidence of stunted growth in stimulant-treated ADHD with some articles suggesting that shorter-than-expected stature may be associated with the disorder itself. The relationship of stimulants to tics raises more complex issues; transient tics (not full-blown Tourette syndrome) can be elicited as a side effect usually subsiding after cessation of treatment. When Tourette syndrome makes its appearance while an affected child is taking stimulants, this development would have likely occurred later, absent the stimulants. That is because more than one-half of those with Tourette syndrome also have ADHD and initially present clinically with symptoms and signs of ADHD.

The other side effects of stimulants are appetite suppression, insomnia, rebound exacerbations of symptoms and signs, and manifestations of "bad mood." Frequently, these side effects are manageable by means of altering dosage or the timing of the doses. Remarkably, the sole nonbrain-mediated side effect (liver toxicity) is reported only with pemoline, the least prescribed of the stimulants.

CHAPTER 55
Pervasive Developmental Disorder and Autistic Disorder

Adapted from James C. Harris

In 1980, the term pervasive developmental disorder (PDD) was introduced into the child psychiatric classification to describe children whose developmental difficulties cross multiple developmental lines. This category has been substantially expanded from one specific disorder in the original 1980 classification, autistic disorder, to the inclusion of several other conditions in the *Diagnostic and Statistical Manual of Mental Disorders,* Fourth Edition (*DSM-IV*). The conditions described as PDD in both the International Classification of Diseases, Tenth Edition (*ICD-10*), and in *DSM-IV* are autistic disorder, Rett syndrome, childhood disintegrative disorder, Asperger syndrome, and unspecified forms of PDD.

The syndrome of autistic disorder, in which social, language, and cognitive deficits are apparent, is the prototype of a PDD. The relationship between cognitive and language deficits and social abnormalities has been a focus of research. Diagnostic criteria for autistic disorder have been introduced that focus on qualitative impairments in social interactions and in interpersonal communication, along with a stereotyped restricted pattern of interests and activities. These abnormalities affect functioning in all situations and, in most instances, are present from infancy onward. The disorder is most commonly recognized in the second year of life but may be recognized up to approximately 30 months of age. The disorder is defined in terms of behavior that is deviant in relation to the child's mental age. The majority of children with this disorder have mental subnormality as a feature of their PDD. Efforts are ongoing to identify additional subgroups within this category.

DIAGNOSTIC ISSUES

Autistic disorder is seen as the most severe form of PDD. Impaired development is manifest before 2.5 years of age with characteristic abnormal functioning in social interactions, communication, and restricted, repetitive behavior. When the full autistic syndrome is not present, the term PDD not otherwise specified (atypical autism) is used in *DSM-IV*. It may be atypical in regard to the age of onset or in not meeting the full diagnostic criteria. Asperger syndrome should be considered in children with no general delay or retardation in language or cognitive development who show qualitative abnormality in social interaction and demonstrate restricted, stereotyped interests. If the child has a period of normal development followed by a loss of previously acquired developmental skills (including social, communicative, and behavioral functions) that persists over time, the diagnosis childhood disintegrative disorder may be used. Overall, the younger the child, the more severe the handicap and the more problems are associated with it.

Associated with PDD are abnormalities in cognitive skills. The specific skill profile is usually uneven regardless of the level of intelligence. In most cases, an association with mental retardation exists, most commonly in the moderate range (IQ 35–49). Abnormalities of posture and motor behavior may occur including repetitive jumping, arm flapping when excited, walking on tiptoe, and unusual hand or body postures. Motor coordination is variable. Responses to sensory input may be unusual (e.g., insensitivity or excessive sensitivity to pain, cold, or heat; covering the ears in response to some sounds; or resistance to being touched and preoccupations with perceptual sensations such as lights or odors). There may also be associated abnormalities in eating, drinking, or sleeping, with diet restricted to a few foods, excessive fluid intake, or recurrent waking at night. Feeling states are difficult to identify in most of the younger children. Lack of fear of realistic dangers is of particular concern. One may see fluctuations in mood for no reason, but absence of emotional reactions is far more common. Self-injury may occur with head-banging or self-biting.

ETIOLOGY

Autistic disorder has been associated with some genetic syndromes such as phenylketonuria and tuberous sclerosis complex. The disorder occurs in boys three to four times more often than in girls. An increased prevalence has been shown in siblings of autistic children of whom approximately 2% are affected with the full syndrome. The general population risk is 2 to 5 per 10,000. There is a 50-fold increase for siblings. The disorder has also been found more frequently in same-sex twins: four of 11 twin pairs who were monozygotic were concordant for the disorder, but it occurred in none of ten dizygotic twin pairs. An increased association of organic brain dysfunction was noted in the affected twin suggesting the possibility that genetic factors and postpartum stress may interact. Whether it is autistic disorder per se or a cognitive profile related to learning problems and inherited social cognitive deficits is unclear, however, because the prevalence of learning disability is also increased in siblings.

TREATMENT

Treatment in autistic disorder requires clarification of the diagnosis and the development of an individual treatment plan. Children with autistic disorder have an abnormality in their development that involves socialization, language, and cognition. The children are both delayed and deviant in each of these areas. Most children with autistic disorder (75%) test in the mentally retarded range on psychological assessments as well; they have an uneven pattern of cognitive abilities, with enhanced factual memory and visuospatial and puzzle-solving abilities, but deficits in symbolic operations, conceptual understanding, and abstract abilities. Language is delayed, and some children do not acquire speech. When language does develop, its development is abnormal, particularly because the children fail to use language for the purpose of social communication in a normal socially reciprocal fashion characteristic for their age. Using stereotyped phrases and echoing back words are common problems. Finally, socialization itself is deviant, and early milestones in initiating social interaction (e.g., reaching to be picked up, developing selective attachments, nodding yes and shaking one's head no, recognizing the meaning of others' facial expressions, using the eyes to communicate needs, and gesturing to share the reference with others) are delayed or abnormal. As the child with autistic disorder gets older, he or she may want to have friendships but often does not know how to go about establishing them.

Treatment is further complicated by the child's rigidity and inflexibility in learning new skills. Skills are often learned concretely; therefore, generalizing to new situations is difficult. Applying knowledge to new situations is problematic, and a fear of change may be expressed with a preference for maintaining routines. Play is not imaginative, particularly at the younger ages. Objects are lined up and placed in patterns rather than used in an imaginative way. When imaginative activities do develop, they tend to be stereotyped, and specific rituals may be seen that have a strong compulsive or persevering quality. Object attachment is deviant in that attachment may be to objects such as stones, belts, or cans rather than soft toys. Additionally, treatment of associated overactivity, behavioral disruption, tantrums, aggressiveness, and self-injury is required. Some children develop phobias and fears or have difficulty with sleep and with developing toileting routines. Each of these areas needs to be addressed in any treatment plan.

The overall goals of treatment are to foster normal development and promote specific language development, social interaction, and learning. Treatment requires the establishment of active meaningful experiences, which involves planned periods of interaction, simplified communication, selection of specific learning tasks, and direct teaching. Individual therapy has the psychoeducational goal to help the child understand social interactions and make appropriate adaptations. Family treatment is needed to help the family understand the nature of the disorder and to resolve guilt. Behavioral approaches are directed toward particular target symptoms such as aggression or self-injury.

CHAPTER 56
Development and Disorders of Speech, Language, and Hearing

Adapted from Beth M. Ansel, Rebecca M. Landa, and Lynn E. Luethke

HEARING

Despite the complexity of the auditory system, clinicians can characterize and classify most hearing loss in a fairly straightforward manner. Hearing function can be assessed using electrophysiologic means [e.g., otoacoustic emissions (OAE), auditory brainstem responses (ABR), tympanometry] or behavioral means (e.g., pure tone threshold and speech-understanding measures). Newborns and infants who are younger than approximately 6 months and are suspected of having a hearing loss can be assessed using a combination of electrophysiologic measures. Infants and toddlers who are not yet capable of participating in more traditional behavioral tasks (e.g., "raise your finger when you hear a tone") can be assessed using visual reinforcement audiometry or electrophysiologic measures. Typically, behavioral audiograms can be obtained in children older than approximately age 3 years, but this varies with the developmental level and the level of cooperation of the individual children and the skill of the clinician. A clinician specifically trained in the assessment of hearing in infants and children (i.e., an audiologist or pediatric audiologist) is an essential member of the team charged with the correct diagnosis and characterization of childhood hearing loss.

Usually, hearing loss is described according to type and degree. Type of hearing loss is referenced to the part of the auditory system affected. Thus, disorders of the outer ear (e.g., atresia, otitis externa) and of the middle ear (e.g., otitis media, cholesteatoma) are referred to as conductive disorders because they impede the conduction of sound; disorders of the cochlea (e.g., damage from infection, noise, drugs; genetic defects) are termed sensory or sensorineural, because they involve the sensory and neural interface in the cochlea; and disruptions of the auditory nerve (e.g., acoustic neuroma) or other parts of the central auditory nervous system are called retrocochlear pathologies. A combination of conductive and sensorineural hearing loss is called a mixed loss. Central auditory processing disorders presumably arise from disruptions of the central auditory nervous system, but precise etiologies are rarely known. Occasionally, children feign hearing loss; this practice is termed *pseudohypacusis*. Typically, the type of hearing loss is determined by a combination of physical examination (e.g., otoscopy) and one or more of the electrophysiologic and behavioral measures already briefly outlined.

Degree of hearing loss derives from behavioral or electrophysiologic measures of hearing threshold at various frequencies. The traditional pure-tone audiogram plots hearing thresholds for each ear separately as a function of hearing level (in decibels) and signal frequency (in Hertz). In Fig. 56-1, the right ear exhibits a mild hearing loss in the low frequencies and a moderate hearing loss in the middle and high frequencies; the left ear shows a severe hearing loss in all frequencies. The ABR and OAE can provide some threshold information and are good

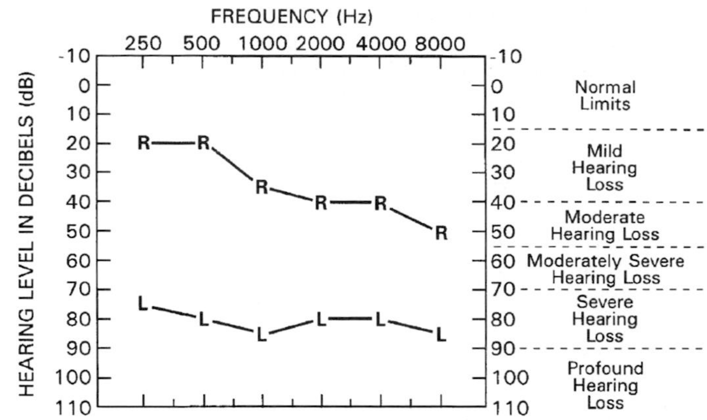

Figure 56-1. Audiogram depicting a mild hearing loss for the low frequencies and a moderate loss for the middle to higher frequencies for the right ear (R), and a severe hearing loss for all frequencies for the left ear (L). Commonly used qualitative descriptors of degree of hearing loss given on right side of figure (e.g., normal limits, profound hearing loss).

localizers of pathology, but they are less frequency-specific than most behavioral measures. Tympanometry is a good indicator of middle-ear status. Diagnosing and characterizing hearing loss in children is best approached using a battery of tests and collaboration between medical and audiologic practitioners.

The type and degree of hearing loss determine the course of action to be taken. Conductive hearing loss (e.g., otitis media) is often amenable to medical treatment; when it is not (e.g., in malformations of the middle ear), hearing aids or other amplification devices are usually very useful in providing adequate auditory input for normal speech and language development and function. Controversy still exists regarding the effects of relatively mild conductive hearing losses such as those related to otitis media commonly seen in preschool children. However, even mild speech or language delays from other causes are likely compounded by the fluctuating hearing that accompanies recurrent otitis media. Thus, this condition should receive close medical attention and audiologic monitoring. Usually, sensorineural hearing loss is not amenable to medical treatment, often the etiology is unknown, and it usually requires some form of aural rehabilitation. Approaches to intervention for children with sensorineural hearing loss vary with the severity of the hearing loss. In general, children with mild to moderate hearing loss (and no other complications) can function fairly well with appropriately fit amplification combined with support services from a speech-language pathologist and educational audiologist, as appropriate.

Children with more severe forms of hearing loss usually require more intensive support services to function well in regular classroom settings and to develop optimal speech, language, and auditory function. Parents of children with profound forms of hearing loss (or deafness) should be offered a variety of options including the use of sign language, oral-aural training, vibrotactile devices, a cochlear implant, or some combination of these approaches. Availability and quality of services and medical options for these children vary widely across geographic regions. Children with central auditory processing disorders often have serious problems with speech and language acquisition and subsequent educational problems that require specialized intervention.

The early identification of children with hearing impairment is an important public health objective with as many as 33 children per day born with significant hearing impairment in the United States. Technological advances have allowed for accurate and efficient means of screening hearing in neonates using two different physiologic measures (ABR and OAE). Tremendous growth has taken place in universal newborn hearing screening programs over the last few years. Most states now mandate universal newborn hearing screening. As neonatal hearing screening is implemented throughout the United States, issues regarding the adequacy of the available diagnostic and intervention strategies have become increasingly urgent. The critical questions of when to intervene and which intervention strategy to use have yet to be determined. Evidence clearly shows that normal human infants begin the speech and language acquisition process early in the neonatal period. Perturbations in that normal process produce lasting deficits. Therefore, early identification and intervention may prevent serious long-term language delays.

SPEECH

Table 56-1 lists the possible manifestations of speech disorders. A speech-language pathologist in the community or school system is invaluable when considering the evaluation and treatment of a child with speech delay. This section will highlight problems related to articulation and fluency.

Articulation

Many articulation problems are associated with obvious structural anomalies (e.g., cleft palate, macroglossia, severe malocclusion, significant ankylosis of the tongue). Additionally, they may result from such neurologic impairment as the dysarthrias or from sensory deficits such as in hearing impairment during infancy and childhood or in hearing loss caused by serious otitis media or ossicular chain deformity. In some instances, no obvious etiologic factor accounts for an articulatory disturbance. Such articulation problems have been regarded as functional and

TABLE 56-1. Possible Manifestations of Speech Disorders

Disorders of respiration
Insufficient respiratory support for speech
Abnormal breath pattern: clavicular breathing, forced inspiration and expiration, audible inspiration
Disorders of phonation
Abnormalities in loudness: monoloudness, excess loudness variation, inappropriate loudness
Abnormalities in pitch: pitch breaks, monopitch, inappropriate pitch
Abnormalities in voice quality: breathy, harsh, hoarse, strained-strangled, tremor, voice stoppages, aphonia
Disorders of resonance
Hypernasality
Hyponasality
Nasal emission
Vowel distortion
Disorders of articulation
Distortion of speech sound
Omission of speech sounds
Imprecision of speech sounds
Inconsistent speech errors
Disorders of prosody
Abnormalities in rate of speech: short rushes of speech, variable rate, increase in rate of sound segments, increase in overall rate
Abnormalities in rhythm of speech: excessive and equal stress, reduced stress, prolonged intervals, inappropriate silences
Prolongation of speech sounds (phonemes)
Repetition of speech sounds (phonemes)

are estimated to account for 75% to 80% of all speech problems in children.

Articulation problems occur among boys more frequently than among girls and among younger children more frequently than among older children. Prevalence is estimated at 10% in children in kindergarten and first grade with a gradual decline thereafter. However, the data regarding prevalence vary widely according to the source and method of detection. Approximately 4% of 11-year-olds and 1% of 17-year-olds continue to show articulation problems.

Traditionally, an articulation error has been defined as an omission, substitution, distortion, or addition of a sound or sounds. The degree of severity of the articulation disorder depends on the perceived interaction of these types of errors and on the frequency with which an error is used. Evaluation of the disorder must consider the number of errors, frequency or consistency of errors, type or patterns of errors, ability to imitate sounds and to produce the same sounds spontaneously, contextual effects, and the relation between articulation and language function.

Current therapeutic methods afford a good prognosis for normal speech production. However, for children with a severe communicative disorder resulting from a severe neuromotor speech disturbance, supplemental communication systems may be required. The selection of an optimal system is a complex matter requiring the cooperation of speech-language pathologists, physical and occupational therapists, special education instructors, and psychologists.

Fluency

Fluency disorders are a special case of prosody disruption usually termed stuttering. In stuttering, the speaker experiences blocks that are significant disruptions in the flow of speech. The speaker may react to these blocks by struggling to overcome them, producing secondary reactions involving movements of other parts of the body, not just the articulators.

Many children exhibit periods of disrupted fluency, most commonly from ages 2 to 5 years. Because the disorder is frequently episodic in preschool years, the parent may be advised that the child will "outgrow it." Such advice runs the risk of overlooking an incipient problem and of withholding treatment when it could be most successful. The longer the dysfluency exists, the more difficult it is to change it; secondary characteristics complicate the disorder. The earlier in the development of symptoms that intervention is begun, the greater the likelihood that treatment will be successful. Concerned parents should not be counseled to ignore the child's dysfluent speech but should be referred to a speech and language pathologist for evaluation, counseling, and possible treatment.

When severe stuttering occurs frequently, the family and physician may have little difficulty in recognizing that a disorder exists. More advanced stutterers show, by their struggle or avoidance reactions and emotionality, that they are aware of having a serious fluency problem. However, the differential diagnosis between stuttering and normal dysfluency is more difficult in young children. The following symptoms are guidelines to assist the physician in determining when a referral is appropriate:

- The child is aware that a problem exists.
- The child shows marked tension and audible or visible signs of struggle when speaking.
- The child's speech pattern commands attention from listeners and interferes with communication.
- The child's speech is characterized by sound prolongations, syllable or word repetitions, or silent pauses within word boundaries, before speech attempt, or after the dysfluency.
- The child exhibits episodes of more than two sound repetitions per word or more than two word repetitions per 100 words.
- The child avoids certain words or sounds.
- The parent speaks for the child if a communicative difficulty is evident.
- The child is frequently interrupted by a parent.
- Parents are concerned about the way the child speaks and about the child's reaction to the dysfluencies.

Environmental variables affecting fluency are primarily social, interactive variables. Communicative stress is perhaps the most important. Usually, stutterers can speak to animals or young children with relative ease. They may have most difficulty when they must compete with others to be heard or when they have to speak in front of a large group. The cause of stuttering is unknown, but electrophysiologic and behavioral studies have the potential to increase our understanding of the disorder. Studies of intermittent stuttering as a sequel to neurologic insult should be taken into account. Although numerous approaches to treatment have proved fairly successful, they are not based on a clear understanding of the nature of the disorder. Most agree that the disorder is multifaceted and that an eclectic treatment approach is more successful than one based on a narrow set of beliefs.

LANGUAGE

Like speech, language is a multidimensional phenomenon. It may be conceptualized as four interdependent (yet theoretically distinct) subsystems: phonology, grammar (i.e., morphology and syntax), semantics, and pragmatics. Phonology pertains to the sound system of the language. Table 56-2 lists the possible manifestations of language disorders.

In the course of children's acquisition of communication skills, a disruption may occur in the development of one or more of the language subsystems. This disruption may occur as delayed or deviant development of communication skills or can result from an acquired neurologic insult such as a closed-head injury or stroke. In delayed development, children exhibit communication behavior that is typical for normally developing children of a younger chronologic age, and skills are acquired in a normal sequence at a slower-than-normal rate across all four major language subsystems. In deviant development, children exhibit communication behaviors not observed in normal children or acquire skills in an abnormal sequence. Children may exhibit delays that are more severe in some subsystems than in others. In these children, language subsystems are developing heterochronously, a pattern of development that is deviant.

Some causes of developmental language disorders are hearing impairment, mental retardation, infantile autism, and social and emotional anomalies. In most cases, the cause is unknown, and no clear neuroanatomic or neurophysiologic basis can be identified. A genetic etiology is suspected for subgroups of children with language impairments, particularly those with hearing impairment, specific language impairment, and autism. Regardless of etiology, children with language disorders require assessment of processes related to speech, language, and hearing. Early identification permits early intervention, which is necessary for optimal outcome.

Moderate to severe developmental language disorders are found in at least 6% of preschool children. As in the case of speech disorders, language disorders are more likely to occur in boys

TABLE 56-2. Possible Manifestations of Language Disorders

Disorders of grammar
Inconsistent, inappropriate, or no use of some grammatical markers (e.g., past tense-*ed*)
Inappropriate arrangement of words in a sentence
Limited variety of grammatical forms in the sentences produced
Use of stereotyped phrases that result in limited flexibility of expression and may result in socially inappropriate message expression (e.g., being too blunt)
Failure to produce or comprehend grammatically complex sentences
Difficulty with recognizing grammatical errors produced by self or others
Disorders of semantics
May have developed an inappropriate definition of a word, may use words inappropriately
Difficulty with comprehending words that have multiple meanings or abstract meanings and that require simultaneous consideration of multiple referents
May produce odd word combinations; failure to recognize inappropriate word combinations or to understand another's message
Difficulty with integrating information in a conversation or story
Difficulty with inferring information that is not explicitly expressed
Literal interpretation of expressions (e.g., sarcasm, jokes, figures of speech)
Word-finding problems
Difficulty with producing a well-organized story portraying main events instead of insignificant details
Limited variety of meaningful relationships expressed (e.g., possession, location)
Disorders of pragmatics
Limited variety of communication intentions expressed
Difficulty with expressing and understanding indirect messages
Monopolizing conversation
Reticence or unelaborated responses
Poor strategies for topic initiation, maintenance, elaboration, or termination
Often abrupt topic changes or tangents
Difficulty with assessing the listener's informational needs (e.g., provides insufficient background information)
Difficulty with recognizing and repairing misunderstandings

than in girls, and the incidence declines with age. Most children with psychiatric disorders have concomitant language disorders. Academic learning problems are likely to occur in children who are first identified as language-impaired. Importantly, language problems should be identified as early as possible. Current assessment tools and understanding of brain, language, social, and cognitive development permit identification of communication disorders as early as the first year of life.

Usually, the cause of children's acquired language disorders is known. For example, language disorders are common sequelae to stroke, viral encephalitis, gunshot wounds, or closed-head injury. The onset age is thought to be a more important variable influencing recovery than the extent or site of the lesion. In younger children, the greater plasticity of the central nervous system may favor the reacquisition or recovery of speech and language. Recovery may take place over 2 years or even longer. Acquired language disorder (i.e., aphasia) is frequently a concomitant of seizure disorder and may improve as seizures are brought under control, most remarkably in children who have Landau-Kleffner syndrome and are treated successfully with steroids. Aphasia may persist in children with focal lesions. In children with closed-head injuries, speech and phonatory disturbances are almost always found in the early stages of recovery, and difficulties in word finding and discourse (conversation and storytelling) often persist.

Despite a relatively good prognosis for speech and language recovery in children sustaining neural insults, later academic difficulties are common. Typically, longitudinal studies of these children demonstrate poor academic records. Academic failures in reading, spelling, and mathematics are often recorded after recovery of spoken language. These learning problems may be related to persistent generalized impairment in complex integrative linguistic processes that are necessary for acquisition of many academic skills.

CHAPTER 57
Mental Retardation

Adapted from Pasquale J. Accardo and Arnold J. Capute

DEFINITION AND CLASSIFICATION

The definition of mental retardation has three components: some degree of cognitive delay, impaired adaptive behavior, and onset before 18 years of age. Cognitive delay is delineated by the IQ with the levels of mental retardation roughly correlating with the number of standard deviations below the mean (Fig. 57-1). The single most important qualification for a diagnosis of mental retardation is a validly obtained IQ score of more than two standard deviations below the population mean for the test. Subject to various qualifications, the specific IQ score is the deciding basis for developmental diagnosis, biomedical assessment, parent counseling, educational habilitation, vocational rehabilitation, and disability determination. For using and interpreting the test instruments, the IQ cutoffs for the different levels of retardation (e.g., 70, 50, 35, 20) are more accurately viewed

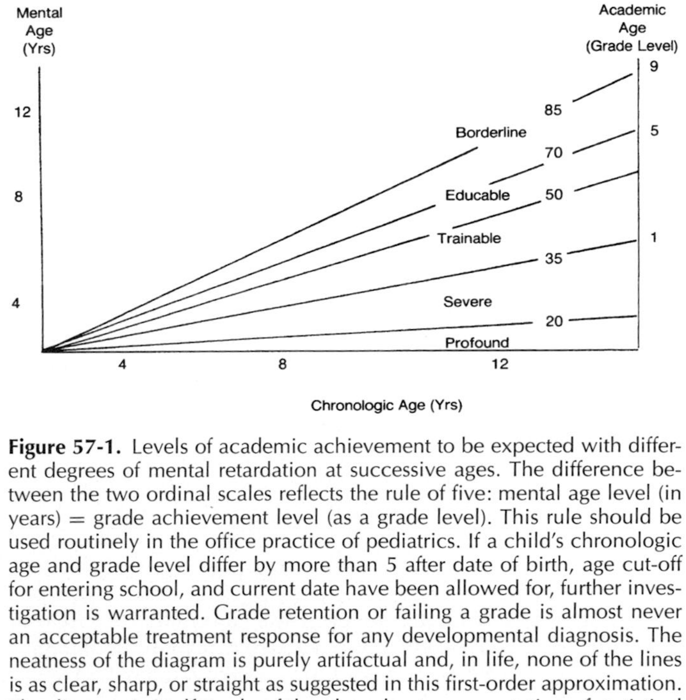

Figure 57-1. Levels of academic achievement to be expected with different degrees of mental retardation at successive ages. The difference between the two ordinal scales reflects the rule of five: mental age level (in years) = grade achievement level (as a grade level). This rule should be used routinely in the office practice of pediatrics. If a child's chronologic age and grade level differ by more than 5 after date of birth, age cut-off for entering school, and current date have been allowed for, further investigation is warranted. Grade retention or failing a grade is almost never an acceptable treatment response for any developmental diagnosis. The neatness of the diagram is purely artifactual and, in life, none of the lines is as clear, sharp, or straight as suggested in this first-order approximation. The diagram is itself a rule of thumb and not a presentation of statistical data.

as ranges (e.g., 65–75, 45–55, 30–40, 15–25). For understanding adaptive behavior requirements, it allows a higher degree of correlation with cognitive level. The Vineland Adaptive Behavior Scales can aid clinical judgment of self-help and socialization skills.

PREVALENCE

Despite continued medical advances in prenatal maternal care and prenatal and perinatal treatment of the fetus and newborn, the overall incidence of mental retardation has remained remarkably stable at approximately 3% of the population. More than 80% of all persons with mental retardation are in the mildly retarded range, and twice as many male as female patients exist. Atypical children with the developmental pattern of borderline intelligence and superimposed language disorders or other deviance or dissociation can be misclassified as mentally retarded. Careful attention to the discrepancies between the different streams of development should allow the correct reclassification of these children and a lowering of the incidence of mild mental retardation.

SCREENING AND EARLY DIAGNOSIS

The first step in the pediatric assessment of mental retardation is to define the child at risk. Genetic, familial, prenatal, perinatal, and postnatal factors that can affect the developmental rate should be documented. However, the at-risk categorization remains distinct from a developmental diagnosis. Most children at risk progress normally, but many not at risk exhibit severe delays. Many older children with confirmed developmental diagnoses were never at risk. Children at risk should have their development monitored more closely with early signs and symptoms of brain dysfunction being weighted more heavily. The treatment of undiagnosed children categorized as at risk remains problematic.

With few exceptions, motor development does not mirror cognitive development. Significant mental retardation is compatible with normal motor milestones. However, cerebral palsy is associated with mental retardation in 50% to 75% of patients, and severe mental retardation often exhibits some degree of motor dysfunction such as transient hypotonia, visual motor organization problems, clumsiness, tremor, and ataxia. Some mental retardation syndromes exhibit motor deterioration over time, as occurs early in Rett syndrome and late in mental retardation with autistic features.

The most sensitive early marker for mental retardation is language development. Prelinguistic vocalizations in the first year of life show a clear pattern of delay even in mild mental retardation (Table 57-1). However, a significant disorder of language or a learning disability may also present with distortion of early language milestones, and these indications must be supplemented by an assessment of problem-solving skills. The evaluation can range from an observational description of type of play (i.e., 0–3 months, visual tracking; 3–6 months, reach, grasp, mouthing; 6–9 months, grasp, transfer, bang; 9–12 months, voluntary casting and release) to the use of formal assessment instruments such as the Bayley Scales of Infant Development and the Cattell Infant Intelligence Scale.

A child with an overall developmental quotient of less than 80 should be followed closely; persistence of a developmental quotient of less than 80 should lead to formal evaluation. A child with a developmental quotient of less than 60 should receive a comprehensive biomedical and psychological assessment. This recommendation is a logical implication of the two-group theory of retardation in which organic brain pathology, identifiable causes, and other medical complications increase dramatically as the general cognitive level decreases to less than an IQ of 50. The milder the retardation, the later it comes to the pediatrician's attention. The preschool child with mental retardation often presents with language delay and the younger school-aged child with grade retention.

TABLE 57-1. Clinical Linguistic and Auditory Milestones Scale*

Age (mo)	Expressive milestone	Receptive milestone
1		Alerts, soothes
2		Social smile
3	Coos	
4	Laughs	Orients to voice
5	"Ah goo," raspberry	Orients (I)
6	Babbles	
7		Orients (II)
8	"Dada" (inappropriately); "Mama" (inappropriately)	
9	Gesture	Orients (III)
10	"Dada" (appropriately); "Mama" (appropriately)	Understands "no"
11	One word	
12	Two words	One-step command with gesture
14	Three words, immature jargoning	
16	Four to six words	One-step command without gesture
18	Mature jargoning, seven to ten words	Points to one picture, points to body parts
21	20 words, two-word phrases	Points to two pictures
24	50 words, two-word sentences	Two-step commands
30	Pronouns, repeats two digits	Concept of one, points to seven pictures
36	250 words, three-word sentence, repeats three digits, personal pronouns	Two prepositional commands

*The Clinical Linguistic and Auditory Milestones Scale is an infant language assessment intended for office use by the practicing pediatrician.

Certain neurobehavioral symptoms and parental concerns can suggest severe cognitive impairment in infancy, especially if accompanied by CNS irritability and other signs of neurologic disorganization. To various degrees, these behaviors can be considered early nonspecific markers for mental retardation and other neurodevelopmental disorders: failure to thrive, prolonged colic, arching, standoffishness and lack of cuddliness, and suspected deafness or blindness. These markers are not to be interpreted in isolation but rather against the background of risk factors and the pattern of milestones yielded by the streams of development as discussed previously. Careful clinical analysis can often derive these behaviors from a preexisting substrate of delay, dissociation, and deviance.

MEDICAL EVALUATION

The pediatric assessment of the mentally retarded child consists of a careful history to obtain information about familial,

TABLE 57-2. Sample Tests to Be Considered in the Assessment of the Child with Mental Retardation

Amino acids
Metabolic screening
Chromosome studies
Karyotype
Banding
Fragile X (chromosome)
Fragile X (DNA)
Skull radiographic films
Computed tomography scan of the head
Magnetic resonance imaging of the head
Electroencephalography
Evoked potentials, auditory and visual
Thyroid function tests
Fibroblast cultures
Titers for infectious agents

None of these procedures is routine. For specific indications, consultations with genetics, neurology, ophthalmology, and dermatology specialists may provide further diagnostic leads.

genetic, prenatal, perinatal, and postnatal influences on development; a detailed listing of developmental milestones reinforced by records, baby books, photographs, and home movies or videotapes, if appropriate; a neurodevelopmental assessment of the child's abilities that includes a formal psychometric evaluation by a competent child psychologist skilled in testing handicapped children; and a physical examination that focuses on neurologic correlates of organic brain dysfunction and the minor malformations associated with specific syndromes or that nonspecifically reflect prenatal causes. The goals of this pediatric assessment are to measure functional level; determine the time of onset, duration, and impact of adverse biomedical influences on brain development; delineate associated dysfunctions or other organ system malformations needing treatment; and identify syndromes of genetic importance. Degenerative or progressive conditions can often be ruled out by a careful developmental milestone history.

As in other pediatric problem areas associated with many different causes, a shotgun approach to biomedical diagnosis is not warranted. Leads from the history and physical examination should be carefully followed, but no routine workup occurs. Table 57-2 provides a list of diagnostic tests that can be considered. Appropriate consultations should be sought, but the family's energies and resources should not be squandered in pursuit of mythic comprehensiveness. In the earliest stages of the diagnostic process, the family is exquisitely vulnerable to overstated claims by physicians, psychologists, educators, and other involved professions. The eventual failure of implied promises can have serious long-term negative effects on the child with mental retardation, the parents' marriage, and the siblings.

TREATMENT AND OUTCOME

The pediatric follow-up of the child with mental retardation depends on the nature of the underlying cause and the specific neurobehavioral pattern of cognitive deficits. For example, with an incidence of 14 in 10,000 live births, approximately 35% of children with Down syndrome have congenital heart disease, 20% develop thyroid dysfunction, 15% have cervical spine instability, and 80% have conductive hearing loss with a higher-than-normal incidence of cataracts, strabismus, congenital duodenal atresia, Hirschsprung disease, leukemia, and seizures. A complex, structured, multidisciplinary follow-up procedure is indicated with the frequency of visits determined, in part, by the specific organ systems involved. In contrast, what may be the second most common (10 in 10,000 live births) genetic contribution to severe mental retardation, the fragile X syndrome, has fairly subtle phenotypic features without any commonly associated organ system malformations. As an X-linked disorder, it contributes to the marked excess of retarded boys over retarded girls.

In the absence of seizures and major organ system malformations, most of the treatment of mental retardation is carried out through the educational system, parent support groups, and other community-based resources. Progressing at a steady rate, the mildly retarded child eventually achieves a sixth-grade academic level and is capable of economic independence (Fig. 57-1). The moderately retarded child does not attain a fourth-grade academic level with its attendant functional literacy but is capable of sheltered workshop employment and group home living. A new emphasis on independent living and supported employment is beginning to change these oversimplified patterns.

The education of severe and profoundly retarded children focuses on self-help skills; some can use group home settings, and others require more institutional residential placements. A few profoundly retarded adults do not speak and cannot be toilet trained (i.e., functional age less than 18 months).

Regardless of the predicted long-term outcome and placement, the optimal environment for the young child with mental retardation is with his or her family. Parents of children with mental retardation should be advised early to specify guardianship arrangements in their wills and to finalize legal certification of permanent minority status by middle adolescence.

CHAPTER 58

Depression in Childhood and Adolescence

Adapted from James C. Harris

EPIDEMIOLOGY

More than 40% of adolescents interviewed by a psychiatrist reported complaints of misery and sadness. Furthermore, 20% had feelings of self-depreciation, and 7% to 8% had suicidal thoughts. In prepuberty, depressive feelings are much less common. Symptoms were equally divided between boys and girls in prepuberty, but with the onset of puberty, the prevalence increased in girls. In one study, major depressive disorder was found to be rare in 10- to 11-year-old children with a rate of 3 per 2,000. When the same group was assessed 4 years later, however, the rate had increased threefold suggesting a potential role of physiologic changes at puberty in the onset of major depression.

Other authors have identified a prevalence of 1.8% of major depressive illness and a 2.5% prevalence of dysthymic disorder (discussed later in this chapter) in an epidemiologic population survey of 9-year-old children. In adolescence, those authors found a prevalence of 4.7% of major depression and 3.3% of dysthymic disorder, which is similar to the adult prevalence.

PHYSICAL COMPLAINTS

Depression presents as a biopsychosocial illness. It is a disorder of mood with symptoms related to neuroendocrine and autonomic dysfunction along with specific cognitive problems in self-perception. Problems in falling asleep and remaining asleep, anorexia and weight loss, abdominal pain, chest pain, headache, and constipation are associated somatic symptoms. Depression in the parent or child may lead to increased office visits and increased hospitalization for diagnostic evaluations for ill-defined complaints. How the child presents is influenced by the parent-child relationship; in making the diagnosis, the words that the child has learned to use to describe emotional states must be considered. If the child does not recognize the bodily experience of their feelings, his or her vague complaints of not feeling good may be misunderstood. An emotionally healthy child is active, feels good, and has fun in his or her activities.

The child may also have learned to use physical complaints to get attention when experiencing depressed feelings in a household where emotional expression is discouraged, or the child may have modeled his or her symptoms on a parent's complaints. These patterns may continue in adulthood, so they are best dealt with directly in childhood. Somatic symptoms and vague complaints may be the child's way of expressing the dysphoric feelings associated with grief and minor or major depression.

Complaints of sleep and eating problems are characteristic of depression. In addition, studies of hospitalized children have found headache, fatigue, muscle pain, recurrent vomiting, and abdominal pain to be physical symptoms associated with depression; gastrointestinal symptoms were found to be the most characteristic. Separation anxiety symptoms often accompany depressive symptoms and are classically associated with physical complaints on school mornings. Abdominal pain is often associated with separation anxiety, which may accompany depression. Chest pain is also associated with depression. In one study, 13 of 100 children seen in a cardiac clinic had depressive symptoms; the chest pain had no associated cardiac diagnosis in this population.

Children with severe burns, trauma, or chronic illness are another group at risk for depressive symptoms. Restricted physical activity, sensory isolation, repeated treatment intervention, and sudden and severe loss of health may be factors in their apathy, regression, and withdrawal. Children with chronic handicaps may also be symptomatic. Twenty of 100 handicapped children reporting for orthopedic hospitalization had depressive symptoms.

Although the focus is generally on the child's complaint, attention must also be paid to the parent's problems. In one study, children with recurrent abdominal pain were not different from a control group in degree of depressive symptomatology; however, 25% of the mothers were mildly to moderately depressed.

ASSESSMENT

It is ordinarily the parents who request help for their distressed or dysfunctional child. Depression can present as a symptom, syndrome, or disorder. As a symptom, it is the expected emotional response to stressful situations; as a syndrome or disorder, it represents an abnormally persistent dysphoric mood. It is essential to differentiate between transient mood changes, which may be normal reactions to stressors, and the despair, irritability, and loss of interest and pleasure that signify depression.

TABLE 58-1. Diagnostic Criteria for Major Depressive Episode

A. Five (or more) of the following symptoms have been present during the same 2-week period and represent a change from previous functioning; at least one of the symptoms is either (1) depressed mood or (2) loss of interest or pleasure. Note: Symptoms that are clearly due to a general medical conditions or mood-incongruent delusions or hallucinations should not be included.
   1. Depressed mood most of the day, nearly every day, as indicated by either subjective report (e.g., feels sad or empty) or observation made by others (e.g., appears tearful). Note: In children and adolescents, can be irritable mood
   2. Markedly diminished interest or pleasure in all, or almost all, activities most of the day, nearly every day (as indicated by either subjective account or observation made by others)
   3. Significant weight loss when not eating or weight gain (e.g., a change of more than 5 percent of body weight in a month), or decrease or increase in appetite nearly every day. Note: In children, consider failure to make expected weight gains
   4. Insomnia or hypersomnia nearly every day
   5. Psychomotor agitation or retardation nearly every day (observable by others, not merely subjective feelings of restlessness or being slowed down)
   6. Fatigue or loss of energy nearly every day
   7. Feelings of worthlessness or excessive or inappropriate guilt (which may be delusional) nearly every day (not merely self-reproach or guilt about being sick)
   8. Diminished ability to think or concentrate, or indecisiveness, nearly every day (either by subjective account or as observed by others)
   9. Recurrent thoughts of death (not just fear of dying), recurrent suicidal ideation without a specific plan, or a suicide attempt or a specific plan for committing suicide

B. The symptoms do not meet criteria for a mixed episode (manic episode and depressive episode).

C. The symptoms cause clinically significant distress or impairment in social, occupational, or other important areas of functioning.

D. The symptoms are not due to the direct physiologic effects of a substance (e.g., a drug of abuse, a medication) or a general medical condition (e.g., hypothyroidism).

E. The symptoms are not better accounted for by bereavement (i.e., after the loss of a loved one); the symptoms perist for longer than 2 months or are characterized by marked functional impairment, morbid preoccupation with worthlessness, suicidal ideation, psychotic symptoms, or psychomotor retardation.

Reprinted with permission from American Psychiatric Association. *Diagnostic and statistical manual of mental disorders,* 4th ed. Washington, DC: American Psychiatric Association, 1994.

From a diagnostic perspective, the current classification of psychiatric diagnoses lists several emotional disturbances of increasing severity. These range from uncomplicated bereavement and adjustment reaction with depressed or anxious mood to dysthymic disorder and major depression. An adjustment disorder with depressive symptoms following either acute or chronic stress is the most common diagnosis; the next most common is dysthymic disorder. In dysthymic disorder, symptoms have less intensity, are of shorter duration, and occur intermittently, in contrast to a major depressive disorder, which is accompanied by more severe physical symptoms, alterations in perception, and cognitive status. Tables 58-1 and 58-2 list the diagnostic criteria for major depression and dysthymic disorder, respectively.

TREATMENT

Depression may have no specific identifiable single cause; environmental, familial, and physical factors all contribute.

TABLE 58-2. Diagnostic Criteria for Dysthymic Disorder

A. Depressed mood for most of the day, for more days than not, as indicated either by subjective account or observation by others, for at least 2 years. Note: In children and adolescents, mood can be irritable and duration must be at least 1 year.
B. Presence, while depressed, of two (or more) of the following:
  1. Poor appetite or overeating
  2. Insomnia or hypersomnia
  3. Low energy or fatigue
  4. Low self-esteem
  5. Poor concentration or difficulty making decisions
  6. Feelings of hopelessness
C. During the 2-year period (1 year for children or adolescents) of the disturbance, the person has never been without the symptoms in criteria A and B for more than 2 months at a time.
D. No major depressive episode has been present during the first 2 years of the disturbance (1 year for children and adolescents); that is, the disturbance is not better accounted for by chronic major depressive disorder, or major depressive disorder, in partial remission. Note: There may have been a previous major depressive episode provided there was a full remission (no significant signs or symptoms for 2 months) before development of the dysthymic disorder. In addition, after the initial 2 years (1 year in children or adolescents) of dysthymic disorder, there may be superimposed episodes of major depressive disorder, in which case both diagnoses may be given when the criteria are met for a major depressive episode.
E. There has never been a manic episode, a mixed manic/depressive episode, or a hypomanic episode, and criteria have never been met for cyclothymic disorder.
F. The disturbance does not occur exclusively during the course of a chronic psychotic disorder such as schizophrenia or delusional disorder.
G. The symptoms are not due to the direct physiologic effects of a substance (e.g., a drug of abuse, a medication) or a general medical condition (e.g., hypothyroidism).
H. The symptoms cause clinically significant distress or impairment in social, occupational, or other important areas of functioning.

Specify if:
  Early onset: if onset is before age 21 years
  Late onset: if onset is age 21 years or older
Specify (for most recent 2 years of dysthymic disorder):
  With atypical features

Reprinted with permission from American Psychiatric Association. *Diagnostic and statistical manual of mental disorders,* 4th ed. Washington, DC: American Psychiatric Association, 1994.

Therefore, comprehensive treatment requires multiple therapeutic modalities. Preventive approaches include anticipatory guidance before considering hospitalization and dealing with stressful life crises such as an impending death in the family. When the stress has already occurred, preventive intervention programs using individual and family approaches to help deal with the effect of the loss have the goal of preventing complications and progression to a depressive disorder. The convening of a support group is of considerable importance at the time of bereavement. One investigation found a preventive intervention program of three to six child-oriented bereavement counseling sessions led to fewer behavioral problems, fewer sleep problems, and less depressed mood in children at a 1-year follow-up. Children who received the intervention talked more about the deceased parent. Attending the funeral of the deceased also resulted in improvement in the child's behavior.

Early detection and referral for treatment of suspected cases of depression in children and adolescents is important. When a case is diagnosed, reducing disability and helping the child to achieve maximal function are the primary goals. An educational aspect to treatment involves working with family members. Also, an interpersonal treatment helps the child to deal with the consequences of the depressive illness on his or her interpersonal relationships with others. Loss of peer relations and secondary family problems are common complications. Prevention or amelioration of poor performance at school, poor social skills, social withdrawal, somatic concerns, and suicide are all targets for intervention and rehabilitation. Early diagnosis may prevent unnecessary medical evaluations. Psychotherapeutic modalities include crisis management, parental counseling, and individual, group, or family therapy.

In the major depressive disorder in which weight loss, sleep disturbance, and cognitive changes are severe, pharmacotherapy with antidepressants is frequently used; definitive studies on the effectiveness of these drugs are now in progress. Serotonin reuptake inhibitors, tricyclic antidepressants, and antidepressants with effects on more than one neurotransmitter system such as venlafaxine, are available. Because a risk of self-poisoning exists, knowledge of drug overdose toxicity, especially for the tricyclic antidepressant group of medications, is essential. A baseline electrocardiogram provides the most sensitive index for assessing later tricyclic toxicity. Antidepressant dosage should not be increased if the resting heart rate exceeds 130 beats per minute (bpm) or the PR interval is greater than 0.21 ms, QRS interval is greater than 130% of baseline, systolic blood pressure is greater than 145, or diastolic blood pressure is greater than 95 mm Hg. Tricyclic antidepressants should not be used in children with cardiac conduction defects. Because oral dosage is not well correlated with blood level, plasma levels, when available, it must be routinely measured at least 8 hours after a dose.

The most convincing argument for pharmacotherapy is the chronicity and long duration of a major depressive disorder and the depth and extent of psychosocial impairment. However, pharmacotherapy alone does not ameliorate interpersonal problems with parents and peers; psychotherapy is indicated for these symptoms. A parent's depressive disorder must be considered and recognized, because the parent's symptoms may influence personality development and increase the likelihood of symptom expression in the child.

CHAPTER 59
Suicide

Adapted from James C. Harris

EPIDEMIOLOGY

Childhood suicide is described as a self-inflicted death occurring before the fifteenth birthday. It is the only psychiatric condition that is subject to documentation by age, gender, and method in all developed countries. At all ages, the rate in whites is greater than that in nonwhites. In the male population, completed suicides are more common than in the female population, although attempts are more common in the female population. The rate in 10- to 14-year-olds has been stable for some years; the increases are found primarily in the 15- to 18-year-old age group. The incidence of suicide among this latter group has increased from perhaps 6 per 100,000 in 1965 to 17.8 per 100,000 in 1992. Some 4% of high-school students have made a suicide attempt in the last year, and 8% have attempted suicide in their lifetime. Estimates hold that only one in eight suicide attempts comes to medical attention.

Some have suggested that the increase in suicide in the United States for the 15- to 19-year-old group may be explained largely by the availability of firearms. The most common means for completed suicide is a firearm, followed in descending order of incidence by hanging or suffocation, self-poisoning, and the use of gas. In England, government control of gas in the home led to a significant reduction in suicide, and the control of availability of firearms has often been suggested to bring about a similar effect in the United States.

Suicide attempts occur three times more often in girls than in boys during the adolescent years. Young men often use firearms, jump from heights, or inhale carbon monoxide, whereas young women more often use self-poisoning. Often, the word overdose is used in emergency room settings to describe such behavior, but the more appropriate designation is self-poisoning.

ETIOLOGY

An important etiology of suicide in adolescents is affective disorder. This condition may be primary, as a response to severe stress, or it may be secondary to another preexisting illness. It is the most significant diagnosis related to completed suicide, and increased risk occurs during the depressed phase or episode. When those with affective disorders are in remission from their depression, the risk of suicide is not increased statistically. The greatest risk occurs during the first year after the diagnosis of the depression.

Two other conditions are associated with completed suicide: drug abuse (particularly alcoholism) and schizophrenia. Suicide associated with schizophrenia is less common than that associated with an affective disorder. For a schizophrenic individual, the history of a previous attempt, the presence of an associated depressive syndrome, or self-destructive hallucinations increase the risk.

In contrast to completed suicide, attempted suicide is more common in individuals who have a hysterical personality style or antisocial personality traits. These personality traits, complicated by the use of drugs, increase the risk for an attempt. An additional risk factor is a family history of suicide. This may be related to the modeling that can occur from knowing that another family member has completed suicide. A genetic factor may also contribute to the more severe forms of affective disorder.

TREATMENT OF UNDERLYING ILLNESS

Because nothing guarantees that suicidal intent will not recur, treating the underlying illness is essential. If that illness is a major affective disorder, antidepressants may be used, prescribed always with the awareness of the risk of overdose or self-poisoning with these agents. Because most individuals communicate their distress, attending to their distress is the most essential intervention.

Profiles of both completed and attempted suicide must be kept in mind. Completed suicides are associated with depressive disorder and schizophrenia. The act is planned carefully, and the method chosen is effective, with plans to be carried out in isolation, often with provisions to prevent interruption of the attempt. The plan is to die. In contrast, those who attempt suicide are more often women than men, they are less likely to be suffering from a major psychiatric illness, and they act impulsively. Often, the means chosen is not thought out carefully and is not rapidly effective. Generally, caution is not taken to prevent rescue, and the act may be carried out in the presence of others, or a means to notify others about the individual's despair may be available. The plan is not to die, but to escape a stressful situation. However, an attempted suicide should not be viewed as a failed suicide, because it might have led to death. The closer the individual's behavior to the pattern of completed suicide, the more concern is indicated. The usual attempt, however, may be a wish to affect another person by the behavior. Consequently, it occurs in a social context and may represent a request for help. The distress is misdirected: The behavior is an act of desperation.

Assessment should be conducted as soon as the child or adolescent can participate in an interview after the appropriate emergency measures. This assessment should take place before discharge from the emergency room or hospital. Ideally, the interview involves a psychiatrist who can help in assessing the risk of recurrence and in other forms of intervention. Both the young person and family members are interviewed. The preferable approach is interviewing the adolescent first, then the parents, and finally the family together. Table 59-1 lists questions to be asked in assessing the risks for suicide.

The first issue to be addressed in the assessment is whether treatment should occur on an inpatient or outpatient basis. Inpatient treatment is essential in the presence of major risk factors (i.e., a serious life-threatening event that was planned and carried out in isolation by a depressed child or adolescent) and of precipitating circumstances: an unsettled and poor support system, continuing suicidal thoughts, and an attitude of hopelessness. Each of these circumstances must be taken into account in developing a treatment plan, which includes treatment of the underlying psychiatric disorder, family intervention in regard to family treatment and psychosocial support, crisis intervention focusing on dealing with precipitating circumstances, and appropriate educational programming.

Ordinarily, the person attempting suicide is admitted to a hospital psychiatric unit for major psychiatric conditions or to a pediatric floor for medical treatment before psychiatric admission. Individual psychotherapy, family therapy, or both may be needed during admission. The impact of a suicide attempt on peers in the neighborhood and at the child's school is another important consideration in community treatment; several instances of multiple suicides in one school have occurred.

TABLE 59-1. Assessment for Suicide Risks

1. Establish details of the attempt with specific emphasis on the means used (e.g., self-poisoning, strangulation, self-inflicted wound).
2. What is the expressed intention about death in regard to the attempt?
3. Was anyone informed before or after initiation of the attempt?
4. What were the circumstances that are said to have precipitated the attempt?
5. In what way has the attempt altered these circumstances?
6. Does the child or adolescent have current suicidal intentions and express an attitude of hopelessness?
7. What is the current mental status, with an emphasis on affective symptomatology?
8. Was a history of emotional or behavioral difficulties exhibited in previous weeks or months?
9. Has a physician or a community agency been involved?
10. What is the current support system: friends, family, teachers, religious groups, and other community contacts? How can a confiding relationship be established and a support system be convened?

SECTION

B

Emergency Pediatrics

CHAPTER 60

Selected Topics in Emergency Medicine

Adapted from Paula J. Schweich
and William T. Zempsky

FOREIGN-BODY ASPIRATION

Foreign-body aspiration is a significant health hazard in young children, particularly those between ages 6 months and 3 years. Most foreign bodies that children aspirate are small and, rather than lodging in the trachea and causing acute obstruction, pass through the trachea to lodge in a main stem bronchus. These small foreign bodies, usually composed of organic matter, are not immediately life-threatening.

Evaluation

Frequently, the diagnosis of foreign-body aspiration is missed, as children often present with no known history of aspiration with only subtle signs and symptoms. The diagnosis requires a high index of suspicion and should be considered in any child with unexplained pulmonary complaints. A history of sudden onset of coughing while eating or playing with small objects is helpful but not always obtainable. With delayed diagnosis, affected children may present with recurrent attacks of wheezing diagnosed as asthma, pneumonia, or bronchiectasis.

In most children, a history of sudden onset of coughing with acute respiratory distress or subsequent coughing, wheezing, or stridor suggests the diagnosis of foreign-body aspiration. The clinical symptoms depend on the location of the foreign body (Table 60-1). The most frequent physical findings are wheezing, decreased air movement, and rhonchi, all localized over the lung with the involved airway.

In children with foreign-body aspiration, the chest radiographs range from diagnostic to totally unremarkable. The appropriate views include inspiratory and expiratory or bilateral decubitus chest radiographs. Persistent air trapping on an expiratory or lateral decubitus radiograph may be found. Persistent atelectasis or infiltration are other common findings. The foreign body itself is rarely opaque and, therefore, is rarely visible on the radiograph. If initial films appear equivocal or normal and aspiration is still suspected, fluoroscopy should be performed. Often, the difference in chest wall expansion that may occur with foreign-body aspiration is detected by fluoroscopy.

TABLE 60-1. Foreign-Body Aspiration

Location of foreign body	Common signs and symptoms
Trachea	
Total obstruction	Acute asphyxia, marked retractions
High partial obstruction	Decreased air entry, inspiratory and expiratory stridor, retractions
Low partial obstruction	Expiratory wheezing, inspiratory stridor
Main stem bronchus	Cough, expiratory wheezing, blood-tinged sputum[a]
Lobar or segmental bronchus	Decreased breath sounds[b]; wheezing, rhonchi

[a]Usually a later finding.
[b]Localized to area of lung related to affected bronchus.
Adapted from Cotton E, Yasuda K. Foreign body aspiration. *Pediatr Clin North Am* 1984;31:937.

Management

If the child presents to the ED with no air movement, the Heimlich maneuver (for children older than 1) or back blows (for children younger than 1) are administered. Children with asphyxiating foreign-body aspiration require immediate rigid bronchoscopy for foreign-body removal. Most aspirations, however, are not life-threatening, and a thorough history and physical examination can be obtained.

If suspicion of foreign-body aspiration is supported by physical examination or radiographs, bronchoscopy is the treatment of choice for foreign-body removal. On radiographic evidence of a radiopaque foreign body or on other strong evidence of a foreign-body aspiration such as unilaterally decreased breath sounds or obstructive emphysema, rigid bronchoscopy should be performed for foreign-body removal. If the evidence for an aspiration is less convincing, flexible bronchoscopy can be performed first to confirm the diagnosis; then, rigid bronchoscopy can be performed if a foreign body is found. Using flexible bronchoscopy first avoids the risks and expense of general anesthesia in those patients without an aspiration. The degree of urgency depends on the location of the foreign body and the degree of respiratory distress.

ANAPHYLAXIS

Anaphylaxis is an extreme systemic allergic reaction. It is the clinical manifestation of a type I hypersensitivity reaction mediated by immunoglobulin E (IgE) or IgG. It is caused by hypersensitivity to a foreign substance and usually occurs within a few hours of oral or parenteral exposure to the antigen. Histamine is an important major early mediator; other secondary mediators contribute to the reaction. The onset is unpredictable, and the organ systems involved, symptoms, and severity vary.

Common causes of anaphylactic reactions include Hymenoptera stings, primarily bees and wasps; drugs such as penicillins and local anesthetics; foods such as nuts, seafood, and eggs; iodinated contrast media for radiologic studies; blood products; hormones such as insulin; and latex.

Anaphylaxis may progress slowly or rapidly. Most commonly, manifestations are limited to the first few hours after exposure to the allergen; however, the initial reaction may be delayed for hours or may recur up to 72 hours after initial recovery. Urticaria may be localized to the exposed area or may be generalized; often, it is accompanied by angioedema, a swelling of the lower dermis and subcutaneous tissues. Cardiovascular collapse is the most common life-threatening event.

Evaluation

In evaluating anaphylaxis, an affected patient's history focuses on the time immediately preceding the reaction in an effort to determine exposure to an antigen. The physical examination focuses on vital signs; airway, including swelling and bronchospasm; circulation, including heart rate and rhythm; skin changes such as urticaria and angioedema; and central nervous system changes. In the presence of clinical signs of respiratory distress such as voice change or dyspnea, difficulty in swallowing, or circulatory collapse, treatment must proceed immediately.

Treatment

Treatment begins with support of the airway, circulation, and cardiac rhythm. Epinephrine, given subcutaneously or intramuscularly, is the drug of choice in most systemic reactions (0.01 mL/kg of 1:1,000 concentration; maximum, 0.4 mL). This dose can be repeated as often as every 5 minutes if necessary. Antihistamine such as diphenhydramine, should also be given, but it plays a secondary role in treatment. Intravenous epinephrine (0.1 mL/kg; 1:10,000 solution) should be used only in severe cases in monitored patients.

Many patients, including those with a history of asthma, will develop bronchospasm during anaphylaxis. This condition is treated with oxygen, subcutaneous or intramuscular epinephrine, a nebulized bronchodilator (e.g., albuterol), and steroids. If severe airway obstruction cannot be relieved, intubation or tracheotomy may be necessary.

Anaphylaxis may include vasodilation and a rapid decrease in plasma volume requiring intravenous fluid boluses for support of blood pressure. Oxygen should be given, and ventilation should be supported as necessary. Colloid or crystalloid infusion such as lactated Ringer's solution or normal saline, is given in boluses of 20 mL/kg of body weight and is repeated as often as necessary. If an affected patient remains hypotensive, the Trendelenburg position and a 1:10,000 epinephrine infusion, starting at 0.1 μg/kg/minute, may be used. Occasionally, other vasopressors may be necessary for severe hypotension.

Generalized cutaneous reactions such as urticaria or angioedema, may be treated with intravenous, intramuscular, or oral diphenhydramine at the dose of 1 mg/kg administered every 4 to 6 hours. In patients with persistent allergic urticaria, intravenous cimetidine (5 mg/kg; maximum, 300 mg) may be beneficial.

The acute symptoms of anaphylaxis should subside within 1 to 2 hours. If symptoms persist, intravenous methylprednisolone followed by prednisone for 2 to 3 days should be administered. After initial treatment, the patient should be observed for several hours to ensure that a late response does not occur.

After treatment of the acute reaction, careful follow-up is essential. If at all possible, the cause of the reaction should be determined. Affected patients should see their doctor for possible allergy testing, counseling about allergens, and preventive therapy.

FEVER IN YOUNG INFANTS

Fever is a common complaint of patients in a pediatric ED. It can signify a range of illness from minor viral processes to serious bacterial infection. The average normal core temperature of a young infant is 37.5° ± 0.3°C with fever defined as a temperature in excess of 38.0°C. This temperature can be influenced by illness, age, metabolic rate, environmental temperature, and excessive bundling.

The standard method of determining the core temperature in an infant is rectal measurement. As compared to rectal measurements, axillary methods detect fever in approximately one-half of febrile infants, and often skin measurements are also inaccurate. The tympanic thermometer has limited use in infants; it is not reliable in detecting the presence and height of fever.

Infants with elevated temperature have an increased risk for serious bacterial infection (SBI), including bacteremia, meningitis, urinary tract infection, gastroenteritis, pneumonia, and bone and soft tissue infections. Very young infants have immature immune systems and also may not be able to localize infection well increasing the risk for SBI. The risk of SBI in infants who are younger than 3 months and have temperature in excess of 38.0°C is between 5% and 10%.

Young infants with infection from herpes simplex virus type 2 may also present with fever. Infected mothers are asymptomatic at delivery in up to 75% of cases. Primary infection has a 30% transmission rate to the baby; recurrent infection has a 3% transmission rate. In the presence of a positive maternal history for infection or any lesions on the child, appropriate cultures should be obtained and treatment should be started with intravenous acyclovir.

Evaluation

The dilemma in evaluation and treatment of infants with fever stems from the difficulty in determining those infants who are at highest risk for SBI. Even the best clinical judgment is limited, as well-appearing infants may have SBI. In large studies, more than 10% of infants with bacteremia look well to the examining physician. Many signs and symptoms of illness in these infants are subtle such as decreased eye contact or alertness, poor feeding, mild tachypnea, or increased sleeping.

The traditional workup and treatment for affected febrile infants includes a chest radiograph; blood for complete blood cell count and culture; urine for urinalysis and culture; spinal fluid for chemistries, cell counts, and culture; and admission for intravenous antibiotics until cultures are negative. This traditional conservative approach has been challenged by many researchers and clinicians.

Another approach has been developed for infants who fit into a "low-risk" category for SBI. The criteria to define "low risk," termed the Rochester criteria, apply to term, well-appearing infants who have been previously healthy, have received no recent antibiotics, and have no focal bacterial infection on physical examination (except otitis media). The criteria include the following laboratory test results: peripheral white blood cell count between 5,000 and 15,000 cells per cubic millimeter; band count less than 1,500 cells per cubic millimeter; urinalysis with fewer than ten white blood cells per high-power field on a spun urine; and fewer than five white blood cells per high-power field on stool (if diarrhea). Some experts also recommend studying the cerebrospinal fluid (CSF) in such infants, especially if antibiotic treatment is planned. The negative predictive value for SBI in these infants is 99%. Growing evidence suggests that hospitalization or antibiotics may not be necessary in such low-risk infants avoiding the risk of iatrogenic complications (including infiltrated intravenous lines, contaminated cultures, and drug reactions) and the high cost of hospitalization. The options for these low-risk infants include hospitalization without antibiotic treatment, home observation with intramuscular ceftriaxone, or home observation without antibiotic treatment. If home observation is planned, crucial factors are having a reliable caregiver to observe an affected child, a telephone at home, transportation, and the ability to return for follow-up care within 24 hours.

Guidelines

Guidelines were developed for the management of febrile infants aged 28 to 90 days. As with any guidelines, they allow great flexibility for options, taking into account the experience of the treating physician, the place of evaluation (ED versus office), the reliability of the caregivers, and the parental preference after a discussion of risks and benefits of the treatment options. No universal consensus exists for the evaluation and treatment of these young infants.

The minimum evaluation includes a very careful history and physical examination, a complete blood count and urinalysis, and application of the Rochester criteria. Infants who are ill-appearing or do not meet the Rochester criteria should have a complete evaluation (see the foregoing) including CSF analysis. A chest radiograph is only necessary for respiratory signs or symptoms. Affected infants are admitted for parenteral antibiotics pending culture results. If such children appear to have a specific problem such as potential respiratory syncytial viral illness, they may only need a focused evaluation and treatment rather than a full workup.

If affected infants are well-appearing and meet the Rochester criteria, they may qualify for outpatient management. One option is to obtain urine and blood cultures, to perform a lumbar puncture to rule out meningitis (including culture), to treat them with intramuscular ceftriaxone (50 mg/kg), and to arrange for follow-up in 24 hours. If an involved physician is comfortable in observing such patients without antibiotic treatment and if follow-up is assured, an affected child can be managed at home after obtaining a urine culture. Some physicians would also obtain a blood culture or a lumbar puncture. Affected children should be reevaluated in 24 hours, or sooner, in the presence of any new concerns by the caregiver.

On follow-up, in the event of a positive blood culture or a positive urine culture in affected children who are still febrile, they are admitted to a hospital for intravenous antibiotics after a full sepsis evaluation. If the urine culture is positive and such children appear well and are afebrile, they can be treated with outpatient antibiotics.

Although the original Rochester criteria applied to infants younger than 60 days, considerable controversy still surrounds management of febrile infants younger than 30 days. Even though most studies do not find a significantly increased risk of SBI in these infants as compared to those aged 30 to 60 days, most physicians are uncomfortable with outpatient management of such infants. Most physicians would perform a complete workup, including CSF, and would admit them for intravenous antibiotics.

Many physicians are more comfortable with outpatient observation without antibiotics in infants aged 60 to 90 days. These infants are treated, as in the foregoing guidelines, with more physicians choosing fewer tests and simple observation.

CHEST PAIN

Chest pain is a common complaint of children in the ED, a condition affecting a wide range of patients but exhibiting no gender predominance. This complaint elicits particular anxiety in children and their parents, who often equate chest pain with cardiac disease. However, cardiac disease is rare in such patients, and usually the origin of the pain is benign. Children younger than 12 account for approximately one-half of children with chest pain and are more likely to have a cardiorespiratory cause of pain such as pneumonia, cough, asthma, or cardiac disease; adolescent patients are more likely to have psychogenic causes. All patients deserve to be evaluated carefully and thoroughly.

Etiology

The causes of chest pain in children are listed in Table 60-2. An organic cause is found more often with acute onset of pain, abnormal findings on physical examination, pain that awakens a child from sleep, or fever. Nonorganic causes are found more often with a family history of heart disease or chest pain (raising concerns in a child or the family) or a history of chronic chest pain in the child. A large prospective study from an inner-city pediatric ED evaluated more than 400 patients with chest pain. The most common diagnosis in the study (21%) was "idiopathic."

TABLE 60-2. Possible Causes of Chest Pain

Idiopathic
Musculoskeletal
Chest wall strain
Trauma
Rib fracture
Costochondritis
Respiratory
Severe cough
Asthma
Pneumonia
Pneumothorax
Pulmonary embolus
Psychological
Anxiety
Conversion disorder
Depression
Cardiac
Coronary artery disease (ischemia)
Dysrthythmias (supraventricular tachycardia, ventricular tachycardia)
Structural abnormalities
Infection (pericarditis, myocarditis)
Gastrointestinal
Reflux esophagitis
Esophageal foreign body
Miscellaneous
Sickle cell anemia
Abdominal aortic aneurysm
Shingles
Cocaine ingestion
Breast tenderness

History

Getting as much information as possible is important regarding the character of the chest pain. Considerations include the frequency and severity of the pain, whether it interrupts daily activity such as school attendance, and whether it wakes an affected patient at night. Constant or severe pain will be more distressing to such children but may not imply a serious etiology. The location of the pain is only occasionally helpful in the diagnosis such as burning pain in esophagitis.

Patients with chronic chest pain are unlikely to exhibit a serious organic cause. However, acute pain is more likely to be organic (though not necessarily serious).

As regards precipitating factors, pain induced by exercise is more likely to have a cardiac or respiratory origin. Asthma is a common cause of exercise-induced chest pain. Other important historical precipitating factors include trauma, muscle strain, and foreign-body ingestion. Any current psychological stresses should also be investigated.

A history should evaluate for more serious associated symptoms such as palpitations, syncope, or fever. Chest pain may be part of an underlying illness such as asthma or pneumonia. If cough is present, its character, chronicity, and timing should be investigated.

The examiner should ascertain whether any previous factors in an affected patient predispose to chest pain. These factors include trauma, asthma, heart disease, Kawasaki disease, collagen vascular disorders, sickle cell disease, chronic anemia, diabetes mellitus, cigarette smoking, and shingles.

Substance abuse is an equally important consideration. An examiner should determine whether an affected child has any history of substance abuse, in particular, the possibility of cocaine ingestion.

Rare disorders such as hypertrophic obstructive cardiomyopathy, are familial. Most children with a family history of heart disease or chest pain, however, are more likely to exhibit a nonorganic cause of chest pain.

Physical Examination

A strong correlation exists between an abnormal physical examination and the presence of organic disease. The physical examination starts with assessment for any acute emergency and follows with a system-by-system approach. For severe distress, immediate treatment is begun.

Patients with pain from psychogenic causes may be in acute distress with hyperventilation or may be calm, rendering the anxiety and stress less apparent. Hyperventilating patients do not demonstrate cyanosis or accessory muscle use.

After a general examination, the investigation should focus on the chest examination. A respiratory etiology should evince some respiratory signs or symptoms such as cough, respiratory distress, decreased breath sounds, rales, wheezes, or tachypnea.

Chest wall tenderness is the most common finding in children experiencing chest pain and may be indicative of trauma or costochondritis. Costochondritis produces tenderness over the costochondral junctions, it may be sharp or radiating or unilateral or bilateral, and it may last for months. It can be exacerbated by deep breathing, activity, or change in position. Inspection and palpation of the chest wall may reveal evidence of trauma such as bruising.

If an affected child exhibits respiratory distress, fever, stabbing chest pain, and a cardiac examination with friction rub, distant heart tones, and neck vein distention, pericarditis is the likely diagnosis. The symptoms of myocarditis are more subtle with mild pain, fever, muffled heart tones, tachycardia and, possibly, orthostatic changes. The heart would appear enlarged on a chest radiograph.

Cocaine use should be considered in adolescents who present with anxiety, severe chest pain, hypertension, and tachycardia.

Laboratory Tests

Generally, laboratory studies are not helpful in establishing a specific diagnosis but may confirm what is suspected from a history and a physical examination. Certain findings in the history and physical examination warrant further studies: history of acute onset of pain or pain on exertion; history of heart disease or related serious medical conditions; history of drug use; serious associated symptoms such as syncope, shortness of breath, or palpitations; foreign-body ingestion; fever; or history of trauma. Further studies should also be obtained for abnormal findings on the examination such as respiratory distress, subcutaneous air, or other heart or lung abnormalities.

In the event of severe respiratory distress, an arterial blood gas analysis and a chest radiograph should be obtained. A chest radiograph is also indicated in children with fever or abnormal breath sounds. An electrocardiogram (ECG) is indicated on any evidence of cardiac involvement such as severe tachycardia, palpitations, arrhythmia, murmur, or rub. A screen for toxicology may be indicated in adolescents with acute chest pain, hypertension, and tachycardia, looking for the possibility of cocaine ingestion. Patients with unexplained syncope need referral for a Holter monitor to detect arrhythmias and structural heart disease. A complete blood count and a sedimentation rate test have very limited value except for suspected infection or collagen vascular disease.

Not every patient presenting with chest pain requires a chest radiograph and ECG. If affected patients have chronic chest pain and a normal history and physical examination, they only need reassurance and follow-up care.

Treatment

Children with chest pain and severe distress need immediate treatment, possibly including blood gas analysis, to determine respiratory status, chest radiograph, ECG, and administration of oxygen. However, the majority of patients will need no immediate therapy.

Children with specific disorders are treated appropriately. For pneumonia, antibiotics and close follow-up are appropriate. For an esophageal foreign body, the appropriate specialist should be consulted. If esophagitis is suspected, a trial of antacids is initiated. If the final assessment is musculoskeletal pain, analgesics and rest are recommended. If pain is thought to be psychogenic or idiopathic, reassurance is given, and appropriate follow-up is arranged.

For concern about cardiac disease, the patient should be referred to a cardiologist. Included are patients with known cardiac disease and patients with new findings suspicious for cardiac disease such as chest pain with exertion or accompanied by syncope, dizziness, or palpitations.

All patients should be offered follow-up if symptoms persist. A study of patients receiving long-term follow-up for chest pain showed that finding serious disease over time is unlikely if it is not found initially.

PAIN AND SEDATION

Assessment

A number of methods can be used to assess pain in infants and children. Physiologic parameters such as heart rate, blood pressure, and respiratory rate, can be used. A number of scales such as the "faces pain scale" or a visual analog scale, rely on patient self-report to determine the level of pain in a patient. Other behavioral scales such as the Children's Hospital of Eastern Ontario Pain Scale or the Observational Scale of Behavioral Distress, use observed pain behaviors to determine a pain or anxiety score for individual patients. Some pain scales allow evaluation of even our youngest patients. To use these scales, practitioners must believe that affected patients have pain. Multiple studies have confirmed that even the smallest infants experience and remember pain.

Management

The type of pain management used should be individualized to patients and their pathologic condition and to the level of pain experienced by them. Patients with a minor injury or medical illness may be treated with oral analgesics such as acetaminophen, ibuprofen, or acetaminophen with codeine. Patients who present with conditions amenable to these medications should be treated while in the ED, just as antipyretics are given to patients with fever.

Usually, patients in severe pain require parenterally delivered narcotics to achieve pain relief. The intravenous route allows for rapid drug delivery and allows for a medication to be titrated to effect. In the ED, morphine is the standard opioid for the management of severe pain, whether the pain derives from a femur fracture or from a vasoocclusive crisis in patients with sickle cell disease. Initially, morphine should be delivered at a dose of 0.1 mg/kg in opioid-naive patients, although significantly more may be necessary in patients with recurrent acute pain (Table 60-3). In either class of patients, the dose should be titrated to relieve their pain. Fentanyl is a short-acting synthetic opioid that can be used for treating pain or as part of a regimen for treating procedural pain such as fracture reduction or burn débridement. The advantages of fentanyl include its rapid onset (3–5 minutes) and its short duration of action (20–40 minutes). Fentanyl is also available for delivery in a transmucosal oralet form that obviates the need for intravenous placement in some patients. However, this form of fentanyl has been associated with a particularly high incidence of vomiting, which may limit its use for procedural pain management and sedation.

TABLE 60-3. Agents Administered to Manage Pain with Suggested Initial Dose

Drug	Dose	Use
Morphine	0.1 mg/kg IV	Severe pain (vasoocclusive episode, fracture)
Fentanyl	1–3 μg/kg IV	Pain, painful procedure (fracture reduction, burn débridement)
Ketamine	0.5–2.0 mg/kg IV 2–4 mg/kg IM	Procedural pain, sedation (fracture reduction, laceration repair)
Nitrous oxide	50%	Procedural pain, sedation (laceration repair, fracture reduction)
Toradol	1 mg/kg IV	Pain (migraine headache, vasoocclusive episode)
Midazolam	0.1–0.2 mg/kg IV 0.25–0.75 mg/kg PO	Anxiolytic for painful procedures (laceration repair with local anesthetic, fracture reduction with fentanylketamine)
Pentobarbital	1–3 mg/kg	Painless procedures (CT scan)
Chloral hydrate	50–100 mg/kg PO or PR	Painless procedures (CT scan)

CT, computed tomography; IM, intramuscular; IV, intravenous; PO, *per os;* PR, per rectum.

Side effects of opioids include nausea, vomiting, respiratory depression, hypotension, and urinary retention. Naloxone, an opioid antagonist, should be on hand for the reversal of severe opioid side effects.

Toradol is a parenteral nonsteroidal antiinflammatory drug useful in the treatment of pain associated with vasoocclusive episodes and migraine headaches, conditions in which narcotic medication may be undesirable. It can also be used as an adjunct to opiates in other painful conditions.

Ketamine is a dissociative anesthetic that will produce a trance-like state in many patients. It can be used for management of procedural pain and sedation in the ED (Table 60-3). It is especially useful for complex laceration repair or fracture reduction. Side effects of ketamine include bad dreams and hallucinations, which can be reduced by the concurrent use of a benzodiazepine. Hypersalivation should be treated with a concurrent dose of atropine or glycopyrrolate. Other rare side effects include laryngospasm, hypertension, and increased intracranial pressure.

Nitrous oxide can be used for management of procedural pain and sedation. It produces an amnestic and dissociative effect. Nitrous oxide is used in a 50:50 mixture with oxygen for analgesia during laceration repair, fracture reduction, and burn débridement. Its advantages include rapid onset and offset. Vomiting can occur and can lead to aspiration in sedated patients. A scavenging system should be in place to prevent health care workers from exposure to the gas. Nitrous oxide is not universally effective, so other methods of analgesia may be necessary.

Midazolam is a short-acting benzodiazepine that provides sedation but not analgesia for many pediatric procedures (Table 60-3). It can be used alone or in conjunction with opioids or ketamine for conscious or deep sedation before a procedure such as lumbar puncture or fracture reduction. It can also be used for radiologic procedures such as CT scan. Midazolam can be given orally for sedation and anxiolysis before wound repair and other minor procedures. Onset of sedation with orally administered midazolam is 20 to 30 minutes. This agent must be used in conjunction with systemic analgesia or local anesthesia for painful procedures.

Pentobarbital is a barbiturate that can provide effective sedation for such nonpainful procedures as radiologic imaging.

Chloral hydrate can be given orally or rectally for sedation. Choral hydrate produces unconsciousness; patients should be monitored closely. The prolonged sedation achieved with chloral hydrate may limit its usefulness in the emergency setting.

Appropriate monitoring is essential for those patients receiving parenteral pain medications or sedation. Monitoring should include pulse oximetry at a minimum but may also include cardiorespiratory monitoring and intermittent blood pressure evaluation. The American Academy of Pediatrics (AAP) guidelines for sedation should be followed whenever possible.

In some cases, behavioral or mind-body methods can be used to alleviate pain. These techniques can be complex hypnotic or imagery techniques or simple distraction techniques such as bubble blowing. Often, these techniques of pain control can be used in conjunction with pharmacologic relief.

Local Anesthetics

Often, local anesthesia is necessary before wound repair, incision and drainage, lumbar puncture, and intravenous cannulation in the ED. Lidocaine is the local anesthetic used most commonly. A 1% solution (10 mg/mL) is infiltrated locally to provide anesthesia. Lidocaine with epinephrine can also be used for areas that are not end organs or mucous membranes. Techniques to minimize the pain of lidocaine infiltration include slow infiltration, buffering with sodium bicarbonate, injection of the solution into the open wound instead of through the epidermis, and warming the lidocaine solution to body temperature before infiltration.

TAC (tetracaine, 0.5%; adrenaline, 1:2,000; and cocaine, 11.8%) is an effective solution for topical anesthesia before wound closure. Because of concerns of toxicity and cost, TAC has been replaced by LET (lidocaine, 4%; epinephrine, 1:2,000; and tetracaine, 0.5%). LET is used as a solution or is mixed with cellulose to form a gel applied to the wound for 20 to 30 minutes to allow for anesthesia. LET is effective in 90% of facial lacerations. The efficacy is considerably less in extremity lacerations; thus, supplemental lidocaine should be used for patients with those lacerations.

EMLA cream is a combination of lidocaine (2.5%) and prilocaine (2.5%); it provides transdermal anesthesia before painful procedures such as intravenous catheter placement, lumbar puncture, and drainage of abscesses. EMLA takes at least 1 hour of application to be effective, which limits its use in the ED.

Numby Stuff delivers lidocaine via transdermal iontophoresis. Iontophoresis is the delivery of charged molecules into biological tissue under the influence of electric current. Lidocaine, which is positively charged, can be transported actively into the skin under the influence of a positive electrical current. In 7 to 12 minutes, this method can provide effective local anesthesia before painful procedures such as intravenous line placement and lumbar puncture. Iontophoretic dose is a product of current and time and is measured in milliampere minutes. A dose of 30 to 40 milliampere minutes is required to provide dermal anesthesia.

Vapocoolant sprays such as ethyl chloride, or a similar product, Fluori-methane (dichlorodifluoromethane-trichloromonofluoromethane), can be sprayed onto the skin just before injection. The chemical is then allowed to evaporate for a few seconds, the skin is cooled, and the injection is given.

BURNS

Burn injuries are classified as thermal (i.e., flame, scald, contact, inhalation), electrical, or chemical, including battery burns. Most burned children are younger than 5 years (average, 2.5 years). Eighty-five percent of these injuries are scalds from hot tap water or from liquids spilled from cooking pots. Flame, electrical, and chemical burns are less common. Most burn deaths are caused by burns sustained in house fires, in which young children are at greatest risk. Usually, death is caused by smoke inhalation rather than by surface burns.

Initial Emergency Treatment

The emergency management of burn patients starts with removal of their clothing and assessment of airway, breathing, and circulation. Hot or smoldering clothing will continue to burn an affected patient, and synthetic fabrics melt to become hot plastic, possibly extending injury. Upper airway edema from smoke-inhalation burns or soft tissue edema of the neck and face may compromise airway patency and breathing. Respiratory status must be evaluated quickly, and oxygen must be applied. Intravenous access is established for inhalation injury or if more than 10% to 15% of the body surface area is burned. For chemical injury, copious irrigation with water should begin as soon as possible. Initially, small burns can be covered with cool, saline-soaked dressings; large burned areas should be covered with clean bed sheets.

History

A detailed history of a burn injury (i.e., environment of burn, materials burned, clothing worn) and an affected child's medical history, including status of tetanus immunization, are essential for care. For example, if a burn injury included a fall, explosion, or child abuse, other serious injuries may be involved. If an affected child was in a fire in an enclosed space, smoke inhalation must be considered. If the burn was electrical, extensive damage may exist below the surface of the skin.

Physical Examination

After any resuscitative or emergency management, a complete physical examination is performed. The depth and extent of the burn injury, presence or absence of smoke-inhalation injury, hydration status, associated injuries, and neurologic examination determine the management plan.

Assessment of depth of burn injury is explained in Table 60-4. First-degree burns are not included in calculations of burn size. The extent of the burn can be estimated roughly using the "rule of nines" (Fig. 60-1). A helpful rule for estimating the extent of scattered, irregular burns is that one surface of the patient's palm represents approximately 1% of body surface area.

Laboratory Studies

Laboratory and other studies to be considered in significantly burned patients are complete blood count; type and crossmatch of blood; carboxyhemoglobin, cyanide, and lactate levels; electrolytes; blood urea nitrogen, creatinine, albumin, and total protein; prothrombin time; arterial blood gas; chest radiography; and radiography of associated injuries.

TABLE 60-4. Assessment of Depth of Burn

Characteristic	First-degree	Second-degree	Third-degree
Example of injury	Sunburn	Very deep sunburn, scalds	Fire, prolonged exposure to hot liquids, electricity
Thickness	Superficial epithelium	Partial thickness: destruction into but not through epidermis	Full thickness: destruction of skin into hypodermis, death of all skin appendages, involves subcutaneous tissue
Appearance	Erythema	Blisters, peeling epidermis, swelling; white or red, mottled; weepy, wet*	Translucent, mottled, waxy white*; leathery, usually dry
Sensation	Painful	Painfully hypersensitive to air currents	Painless

*Second- and third-degree burns initially may appear similar.

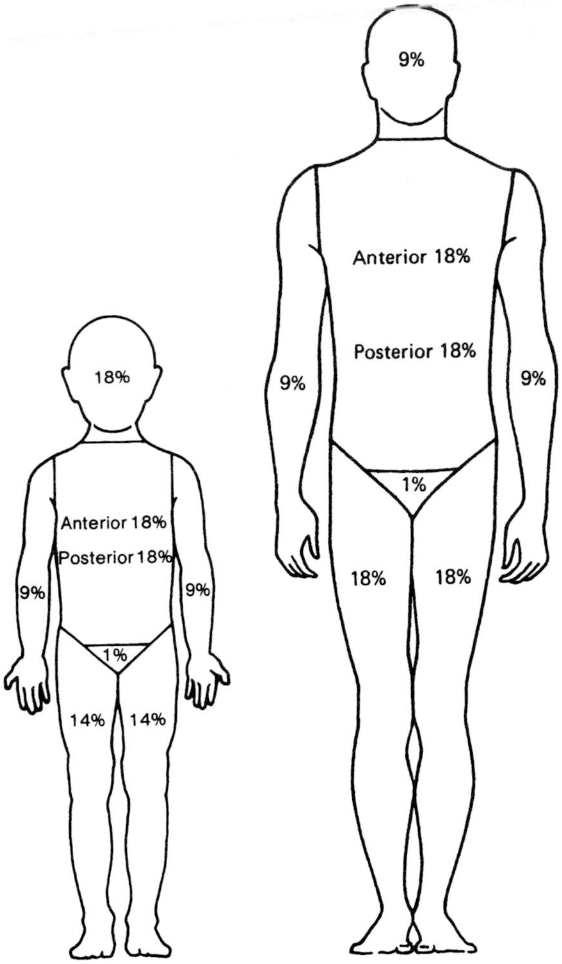

Figure 60-1. Rule of nines for child (*left*) and adult (*right*). (Adapted from Scherer JC. *Introductory medical-surgical nursing,* 4th ed. Philadelphia: Lippincott, 1986:687.)

Definitive Treatment

AIRWAY MANAGEMENT

Patients with inhalation injury have a marked increase in morbidity and mortality. The upper airway is extremely susceptible to swelling and obstruction from exposure to hot, moist air or toxic gases. Direct thermal injury from hot air is unlikely, unless the heat is conveyed by steam. The subglottic airway is protected from direct injury by the larynx. Inhalation injury can damage the lower respiratory tract resulting in pulmonary edema, aspiration pneumonia, and pneumonitis.

Often, diagnosis of airway or pulmonary injury is difficult because affected patients may initially show little or no respiratory distress. With a history of fire in an enclosed space or presence of facial burns, singed nasal hairs, carbonaceous sputum, or inflammatory changes in the pharynx, such patients are at risk for respiratory injury. Because children's airways are narrow and they have small respiratory reserve and high metabolic demands, they should be intubated prophylactically if airway or pulmonary injury is suspected. For any stridor, tracheal noise, or hypoxemia, intubation is an emergency. Humidified 100% oxygen must be applied. Positive-pressure ventilation may be necessary later to prevent pulmonary edema.

Acute asphyxia occurs in humans in an enclosed space in which oxygen is consumed by a fire. Inhalation of carbon monoxide seriously impairs oxygen delivery to the tissues, because carbon monoxide binds to hemoglobin with 200 to 300 times the affinity of oxygen and shifts the oxyhemoglobin dissociation curve to the left causing more tissue hypoxia. Oxygen saturation may seem normal in carbon monoxide poisoning because it measures saturation of hemoglobin by both oxygen and carbon monoxide. Arterial blood gas measurement also may not be helpful to measure Po_2, because the oxygen saturation is calculated from the measured dissolved oxygen and, therefore, may seem normal even with significant carbon monoxide poisoning.

Measurement of the carboxyhemoglobin level from either an arterial or venous sample is performed early in patients involved in an enclosed-space fire. Symptoms of mild intoxication such as impaired judgment, headache, and decreased fine-motor skills, may begin at a carboxyhemoglobin level as low as 5% in a nonsmoker. At a level of 20% carboxyhemoglobin, most patients suffer from mild dyspnea and confusion; higher levels produce lethargy, nausea, tachycardia, and coordination problems. At levels of 60% carboxyhemoglobin, patients are at risk for convulsions, coma, and death. Treatment is removal from the "contaminated" environment and administration of 100% oxygen. The half-life of carboxyhemoglobin decreases from approximately 4 hours in room air to less than 1 hour in 100% oxygen. Treatment with hyperbaric oxygen decreases the half-life even further, and it can be helpful in severely toxic patients.

In the first 36 hours after an inhalation injury, acute pulmonary insufficiency can result from several elements in a fire. Most of the damage is caused by toxic gases such as aldehydes, oxides of sulfur and nitrogen, and hydrochloric acid released from combustion. These agents cause atelectasis, pulmonary edema, and direct parenchymal damage.

Cyanide toxicity from incomplete combustion of plastics and acrylics may contribute to affected children's depressed mental state, metabolic acidosis, or shock. For a child obtunded with metabolic acidosis resulting from burns in an enclosed space, cyanide and lactate levels should be measured.

Chest radiographs obtained shortly after a burn injury are not sensitive in determining the presence of acute lung injury; they may show no evidence of inhalation injury for up to 36 hours. Radiographs should be obtained only on evidence of respiratory symptoms.

Affected patients are placed on high-flow humidified oxygen to reverse hypoxemia, to displace carbon monoxide from hemoglobin, and to reduce pulmonary hypertension in pulmonary edema. After initial airway management, affected patients are observed for pulmonary edema and (later) bronchopneumonia. Generally, care is supportive; prophylactic antibiotics and steroids have not proved beneficial. Bronchodilators such as inhaled albuterol, may help for bronchospasm.

FLUID MANAGEMENT

Usually, an affected alert child with less than 10% full-thickness or 15% partial-thickness burns and no hypoxia or gastric distention can be hydrated orally. Otherwise, at least one large-bore intravenous line must be inserted. Upper-extremity placement is preferable to that in the lower extremity because of a lower incidence of infection and phlebitis in the upper extremities. Careful aseptic technique is crucial and, although the intravenous line can be placed through burned skin, placement in an unburned area is preferable.

During the first 24 to 48 hours, shock may be associated with loss of intravascular volume into a burned area. Water, sodium,

TABLE 60-5. Fluid Requirements of Burn Patients During the First 24 Hours After a Burn[a]

By weight[b]	3–4 mL/kg/% BSA burn + maintenance (per weight per 24 hr)
By BSA[c]	5,000 mL/m² burned area + 2,000 mL/m² BSA/24 hr (maintenance)

BSA, body surface area.
[a]One-half of the estimated fluid is given during the first 8 hours after injury, and the rest is administered during the next 16 hours.
[b]From the Committee on Trauma, American College of Surgeons. Advanced trauma life support course: instruction manual, 1989.
[c]From Carvajal HF. A physiologic approach to fluid therapy in severely burned children. *Surg Gynecol Obstet* 1980;150:379.

and protein are lost and should be replaced. Multiple resuscitation formulas have been used with success during the initial 48 hours after beginning treatment. Table 60-5 shows two formulas for volume replacement, one based on weight and one based on body surface area (BSA). In each formula, the maintenance fluids are calculated separately. In children, the ratio of BSA to weight will change with growth. A formula based on weight underestimates the fluid for a small child with a large BSA-weight ratio and overestimates the fluid for a larger child with a smaller BSA-weight ratio. A formula based on BSA is more effective in pediatric patients with extensive burns and is the method of choice. However, any formula, whether based on weight or BSA, provides only an estimate of required fluids. An essential factor is to monitor hydration status and to adjust the fluids accordingly by following the general appearance and sensorium, vital signs, weight, urine output and specific gravity, capillary refill, serum osmolality, electrolytes, and acid–base status.

Although some investigators have recommended hypertonic salt solutions, the most common resuscitation fluid used is isotonic crystalloid such as lactated Ringer's solution or 5% dextrose in normal saline. For more than a 20% BSA burn, adding colloid to the rehydrating solution may help, because intravascular protein loss results from increased vascular permeability. This protein loss is most marked in the first 6 to 8 hours after a burn, and 12.5 g of human serum albumin is added to each liter of fluid for the first 24 hours.

SUPPORTIVE CARE

Because burn patients have an elevated metabolic rate resulting in increased oxygen consumption, increased urinary nitrogen excretion, and fat breakdown, minimizing any extra metabolic work is essential. Continuing care involves keeping the room temperature stable at 28°C to 33°C, minimizing pain, and supplying adequate calories. Pain control is essential and opiates such as morphine and the fentanyl oralet are good choices. Anxiety associated with dressing changes can be treated with hydroxyzine or a benzodiazapine.

All patients with significant burns should have a Foley catheter (for monitoring urine output) and a nasogastric tube (to prevent acute gastric dilation). A physiologic ileus may last 1 or 2 days in a patient with burns of more than 20% of BSA.

WOUND CARE

Cool, wet compresses are applied to small burns but should be avoided on large areas to prevent hypothermia. The burned area is cleaned with a dilute antiseptic soap solution, and broken blisters are débrided. Intact blisters are left intact.

The burn surface is a warm, moist, protein-rich environment, and colonization with fungi and bacteria is a constant source of infection. Meticulous wound cleansing and dressing minimize colonization and infection. With full-thickness burns, later skin grafts survive better on wounds with lower bacterial colony counts. Topical antimicrobial agents are used to limit bacterial proliferation. Silver sulfadiazine (Silvadene) is the antimicrobial agent used most commonly, because it suppresses bacterial growth but does not prevent healing. It is not used on the face. Nystatin can be added to reduce fungal colonization. Tetanus prophylaxis is given if indicated by the history.

Children cared for as outpatients should be bathed once a day, after which Silvadene should be applied. On small burns, bacitracin ointment is a good alternative. Gauze is placed over the cream or ointment. A burned extremity should be elevated to avoid swelling. Broad-spectrum antibiotics are contraindicated. Daily follow-up care is necessary until clean healing is ensured.

CRITERIA FOR HOSPITALIZATION

Table 60-6 lists criteria for hospital admission of burn patients. If a specialized burn center is available, a burned child should be admitted there.

Special Burns

Usually, chemical burns are caused by acids or alkalis. Alkali burns penetrate deeply and are generally more serious than are acid burns. The severity of a chemical burn is influenced by the amount and concentration of the agent and by the duration of the contact. Treatment involves extensive irrigation for at least 20 minutes with large amounts of a neutral solution such as water or normal saline. If the eyes are involved, irrigation should continue while an ophthalmologist is consulted.

Electrical burns range from a lip commissure wound from biting an electrical wire to electrocution from a lightning bolt. Frequently, lip commissure burns are more serious than they appear and often involve deeper tissues including the lingual artery. As current passes through the body, it may destroy muscles, nerves, and vessels. If an extensive burn is suspected, an affected patient must be observed with ECG monitoring and should receive intravenous fluids and general supportive care.

Prevention

The key to decreasing morbidity and mortality from burn injuries, as in all accidents, is prevention. Burn deaths, caused mostly by house fires, can be prevented by extensive education of parents and children, increased adult supervision of children, and increased use of smoke detectors and sprinklers. Many hot water scald burns can be prevented if water heaters are turned down to 120°F. Children can help themselves in fires if they are taught to drop and roll if they are on fire and to crawl under smoke. Many electrical injuries in the home can be prevented by plastic outlet protectors.

TABLE 60-6. Criteria for Admission of Burn Victims

More than 10% body surface area of full-thickness burn
More than 15% body surface area of partial-thickness burn
Serious burns of hands, feet, perineal area, face, joints
Inhalation injury
Other significant injuries or medical problems
Chemical or electrical burns
Suspected child abuse

WOUND CARE

Examination

The initial examination includes the extent and severity of the visible lesion, where it is located, and the pulse and sensation distal to the injury. Any obvious associated injuries to nerves, muscles, tendons, vessels, or bones at the wound site or elsewhere should be sought.

Anesthesia and Sedation

In young children, especially those younger than 3 years, restraint and sedation may be necessary for proper examination and repair of a wound. An affected child can be wrapped in a sheet or placed on a papoose board for restraint. A variety of available sedatives and analgesics can decrease the anxiety and discomfort associated with wound repair in young children. Sedatives, analgesics, and their doses are listed in Table 60-3.

The wound and surrounding area should be washed gently with soap and water or dilute iodine solution before injection of local anesthetic. Buffered lidocaine (1:10 mixture of sodium bicarbonate and lidocaine) or bupivacaine (0.25% or 0.50%) is injected slowly through the wound margins with a small-gauge needle (27-gauge; Table 60-7). Bupivacaine allows longer duration of anesthesia. If the wound is in a highly vascular area (excluding the digits, nose, ears, or genitalia), lidocaine with epinephrine can be used. Topical anesthesia with lidocaine, epinephrine, and tetracaine (LET) is an excellent alternative for head and face lacerations in children. Topical anesthetics must be kept away from the eyes and mouth. Fingers and toes are anesthetized most easily with a digital block.

Decontamination

For minimizing wound infection, removal of contaminating bacteria, devitalized tissue, and any foreign bodies is crucial. When it is anesthetized, the wound can be irrigated using a large blunt needle and a 20- to 30-mL syringe. The volume used depends on the suspected contamination of the wound. Normal saline is an effective irrigant. A 1% povidone-iodine solution does not have any significant benefit over saline. Detergent-containing products can cause local tissue injury and should not be used for irrigation. Wounds may also be scrubbed with a soft brush to remove any gross contamination. After irrigation, any devitalized tissue must be débrided, and irregular edges should be excised.

TABLE 60-7. Local Anesthetics

Drug	Dose	Use
Lidocaine	4 mg/kg (maximum) 7 mg/kg (maximum with epinephrine)	Wound anesthesia, local dermal anesthesia
Bupivacaine	2 mg/kg (maximum)	Peripheral nerve blocks; prolonged anesthesia
LET	3 mL	Wound anesthesia
EMLA*	2.5–5.0 g	Local dermal anesthesia
Numby Stuff	30–40 milliampere minutes	Local dermal anesthesia

LET, *l*idocaine, 4%; *e*pinephrine, 1:2,000; and *t*etracaine, 0.5%.
*EMLA consists of lidocaine (2.5%) and prilocaine (2.5%).

The wound should be explored carefully for injuries to deep tissues and structures, for joint penetration, and for foreign bodies. Foreign bodies are more likely in wounds with a mechanism of injury suggesting foreign body, severe pain, joint tenderness, or signs of infection. Examining a wound correctly requires proper hemostasis, a cooperative or properly restrained and sedated patient, and a direct and close light source. After inspection, the wound should be probed using a blunt instrument. If in doubt about the presence of a foreign body, particularly glass, metal, or gravel, appropriate radiographs should be obtained. Ultrasonography may also be used in certain circumstances. If a foreign body is found in a wound and is not removed easily, appropriate consultation is obtained.

Wound Repair

Most lacerations can be approximated with simple interrupted skin sutures using nonabsorbable suture material such as mild chromic gut, to avoid the necessity of removing the sutures. Sutures should be placed just tightly enough to approximate and evert the edges; the ensuing wound edema after the closure may cause ischemia if the sutures are too tight.

Subcutaneous sutures with an absorbable suture material such as Vicryl or chromic gut, are placed for a deep wound or significant tension. Extensive wounds to the face, hand, perineum, or genitals or a wound in combination with a fracture should be seen in consultation with a surgeon.

"Dirty" wounds such as animal bites and deep punctures, should not be sutured immediately; delayed primary closure may be possible after 4 or 5 days. Surgical tape may be used in wounds partially through the dermis if no stress is evident on the edges; this tape is not to be used over joints or on any area in which wound edges will be pulled apart.

A dressing is applied to absorb blood and to protect, compress, and immobilize the area. The first layer of the dressing should be nonadherent, with an absorbent material overlying it, wrapped with a bulky immobilizing dressing. Extremities should be elevated and ice should be applied during the first 24 hours.

Topical antibiotic ointment (bacitracin or neosporin) should be applied to the wound for 2 days after repair. Most patients do not need systemic antibiotics. If the wound is more than 18 hours old before treatment or shows signs of infection, antibiotics should be prescribed for a short course. Affected patients are seen again in 24 to 48 hours to allow checking the wound for healing and signs of infection. Sutures are removed from the face in 3 to 5 days, from the scalp in 7 days, from the extremities in 7 to 10 days, and from the joints in 10 to 14 days.

BITES

Human and nonhuman animal bites are common among children. More than one-half of such bites are minor, but certain initially innocuous-appearing bites can lead to serious infectious complications. Most often, animal bites affect the extremities; however, nearly two-thirds of bites to children younger than age 4 involve the head and neck. Dog bites account for approximately 90% of nonhuman bites that require medical attention, and cat bites account for almost 10%, with rodent and rabbit bites composing the remainder. Factors that increase the risk of infection include poor local wound care, location on the hand or over a joint, puncture or crush injury, treatment delay of more than 12 hours, and patient immunosuppression.

Most wounds are colonized by mixed aerobic and anaerobic organisms obtained from the skin of the victim and the oral cavity of the biter. An average infected bite wound yields three to five organisms on culture with the highest estimate of organisms emanating from human bites. The most common aerobic organisms found in infected dog bite wounds are *Staphylococcus* species, *Streptococcus* species, and *Corynebacterium* species. *Pasteurella multocida*, the most common aerobic pathogen in cat bite infections, is also found commonly in dog bites. Clinical infection with *P. multocida* is characterized by rapid development of an intense inflammatory response with significant pain and swelling within 24 to 48 hours. The most common anaerobes in dog and cat bite infections are *Bacteroides fragilis, Prevotella, Porphyromonas, Peptostreptococcus*, and *Fusobacterium* species. Approximately 50% of the wounds have at least one organism with beta-lactamase activity. The predominant aerobic organisms isolated from human bites are alpha- and beta-hemolytic streptococci, *S. aureus, Staphylococcus epidermidis, Corynebacterium* species, and *Eikenella corrodens*. *S. aureus* produces severe bite wound infections and often produces beta-lactamase. The anaerobic bacteria isolated most frequently are similar to those in dog and cat bite infections.

Management

Cleansing, irrigation, and careful débridement reduce the incidence of infection. The area around the wound should be cleansed with povidone-iodine solution, which has a wide antibacterial and antiviral spectrum. This treatment is followed by forceful irrigation with normal saline through a 19-gauge needle attached to a large syringe. This high-pressure irrigation is more effective in reducing bacterial counts than is soaking. After local anesthesia, all visible devitalized tissue is débrided, and the wound is checked for foreign matter and injuries to tendons, joints, and bones. Irrigation is repeated. If fracture or foreign body is suspected, radiographs are obtained.

Closure of bite wounds is controversial. If a wound is uninfected and is examined within 24 hours of injury, it can usually be closed primarily. Primary closure does not increase the incidence of infection unless closure is more than 24 hours old or the wound is clinically infected, is a hand wound, or is a deep puncture wound. All wounds that are infected or are more than 24 hours old initially are left open. These wounds can heal by granulation or delayed primary closure.

Human and cat wounds in high-risk locations can be packed with gauze soaked in an antibacterial agent and can be sutured in 4 to 7 days in the absence of signs of infection. If the bite is small and in a cosmetically acceptable area, it is left to heal by granulation and secondary intention. Wound cultures for aerobic and anaerobic organisms should be obtained only if the wound appears infected. The face is an area of rich vascularity with decreased risk of infection. Most bites to the face are closed in a single layer to minimize scarring.

Use of prophylactic antibiotics is a complex and controversial issue for which no large prospective randomized studies have provided substantiation. Prophylactic antibiotics are probably useful for patients with wounds at high risk for infection. These wounds include bites to the hand, bites more than 8 hours old, deep puncture wounds or severe injuries, and most cat bites. Minor bite wounds have a low risk of infection and generally do not require prophylaxis. If an antibiotic is used for prophylaxis, a 3- to 5-day course of amoxicillin with clavulanate potassium (Augmentin) or cefuroxime covers all the common organisms. Erythromycin can be used for patients with penicillin allergy. Additional therapy of infected wounds is guided by Gram stain and culture results.

After initial care, most children with bite wounds can be managed as outpatients with careful follow-up. Affected patients are asked to return within 48 hours for a check of the wound, at which time, any infection should be apparent with redness, swelling, tenderness, or drainage. Initial cultures of wounds do not predict subsequent infection.

Larger injured areas on extremities and wounds over joints are immobilized and elevated. Tetanus toxoid is given if indicated, and rabies prophylaxis is considered depending on the animal species and area. In the United States, the animals infected most commonly with rabies are skunks, raccoons, and bats; but other animals, including dogs and cats, may be infected. A final decision about whether to treat a potentially exposed patient can be made in conjunction with a local health department. Treatment consists of thorough local wound care (irrigation with iodine solution and débridement) and passive and active immunoprophylaxis. Human rabies immune globulin is given as soon as possible to cover the time during which the patient has insufficient active antibody production. One-half the dose of 20 IU/kg is given into the wound, and one-half is given as an intramuscular injection. At the same time, active immunization is begun with human diploid cell vaccine; 1 mL is given intramuscularly on days 1, 3, 7, 14, and 28. If the offending animal is found to be uninfected, treatment is stopped.

Bite wounds that have a high incidence of complications and should be seen by a consultant include nonsuperficial or hand wounds older than 8 hours, wounds with extensive infections, severe disfigurement or tissue loss potentially requiring grafting, and wounds suggesting the possibility of tendon, joint, or cartilage injury. Most patients affected thus require hospital admission. Patients with systemic signs of infection or failure of outpatient management should be admitted for intravenous antibiotics.

CHAPTER 61
General Principles of Poisoning

Adapted from James D. Fortenberry and M. Michele Mariscalco

GENERAL MANAGEMENT OF POISONING

The diagnosis of poisoning may not be obvious. Diagnosis can be difficult; often, it is not considered because of purposeful falsification by older patients or because young or confused patients are unable to provide an adequate history. Poisoning should be strongly considered in children who exhibit acutely developed disturbed consciousness, abnormal behavior, seizures, coma, respiratory distress, shock, arrhythmias, metabolic acidosis, severe vomiting and diarrhea, or other puzzling multisystem disorders. Underlying drug or ethanol intoxication should be considered in adolescent and adult victims of accidental trauma.

During stabilization, information should be obtained from family members, friends, or paramedics who have transported the patient to the hospital about the possible agent, the mode of intoxication, the maximum potential dose, and the time since exposure. If poisoning is suspected but the history is not confirmatory, information regarding the different drugs in the home should be obtained by inquiring about illnesses of the patient and other family members.

TABLE 61-1. Toxidromes: Prominent Clinical Findings as an Aid to Diagnosis of the Unknown Ingestion

Drug involved	Clinical manifestations
Anticholinergics (atropine, scopolamine, tricyclic antidepressants, phenothiazines, antihistamines, mushrooms)	Agitation, hallucinations, coma, extrapyramidal movements, mydriasis, dry mouth, tachycardia, arrhythmias, hypotension, decreased bowel sounds, urinary retention; flushed, warm, dry skin
Cholinergics (organophosphates and carbamate insecticides	Salivation, lacrimation, urination, defection, nausea and vomiting, sweating, meiosis, bronchorrhea, rales and wheezes, weakness, paralysis, confusion and coma, muscle fasciculations
Opiates	Slow respirations, bradycardia, hypotension, hypothermia, coma, meiosis, pulmonary, edema, seizures
Sedatives and hypnotics	Coma, hypothermia, central nervous system depression, slow respirations, hypotension, tachycardia
Tricyclic antidepressants	Coma, convulsions, arrhythmias, anticholinergic manifestations
Salicylates	Vomiting, hyperpnea, fever, lethargy, coma
Phenothiazines	Hypotension, tachycardia, torsion of head and neck, oculogyric crisis, trismus, ataxia, anticholinergic manifestations
Sympathomimetics (amphetamines, phenylpropanolamine, ephedrine, caffeine, cocaine, aminophylline)	Tachycardia, arrhythmias, psychosis, hallucinations, delirium, nausea, vomiting, abdominal pain, piloerection
Alcohols, glycols (methanol, ethylene glycol; also salicylates, paraldehyde, toluene)	Elevated anion gap, metabolic acidosis

Reprinted with permission from Mofenson NC, Greensher J. The unknown poison. *Pediatrics* 1974;54:337.

The physical examination may be particularly helpful in the case of a questionable exposure to a toxic agent. Specific physical findings may suggest a diagnosis (Table 61-1). However, children who arrive in the emergency department with a diagnosis of poisoning are frequently asymptomatic.

Routine laboratory tests may play an important role in the diagnosis and management of poisoned patients. Decreased hemoglobin saturation with a normal or increased P_aO_2 is found in patients with carbon monoxide poisoning or in methemoglobinemia. Metabolic acidosis with an increased anion gap suggests ingestion of methanol, ethylene glycol, paraldehyde, toluene, iron, isoniazid, or salicylates. An elevated measured serum osmolarity compared with a calculated osmolarity indicates the presence of low-molecular-weight and osmotically active compounds such as methanol, ethanol, isopropyl alcohol, mannitol, and ethylene glycol. Hypoglycemia may affect patients intoxicated by ethanol, methanol, isopropyl alcohol, isoniazid, acetaminophen, salicylates, and oral hypoglycemic agents. Pregnancy testing should be obtained in pubertal females as a possible etiology for intentional ingestion.

Toxicology testing may be helpful in confirming the clinical diagnosis of drug intoxication. However, identifying all available drugs with a high degree of specificity and sensitivity is impossible because of time limitations. Instead, a drug screen is performed. Because drug screens vary among institutions, the physician should know exactly which drugs can be detected. Generally, toxicology screening tests detect a wide range of narcotics, analgesics, barbiturates, antidepressants, tranquilizers, sedative-hypnotics, and various other drugs and abused substances. Ethylene glycol, lithium, iron, cyanide, lead, and other heavy metals are agents that are not usually included in drug screening tests. Some centers have access to rapid comprehensive drug screening by high-performance liquid chromatography methodology. In general, the history and physical examination are more important in acute management of drug overdose than is a comprehensive drug screen. Positive drug screen findings merely confirm exposure to that substance, and such an exposure should not be assumed to be responsible for the clinical findings of the moment.

Treatment

The three goals of treatment are preventing further drug absorption, providing antidotal therapy, and hastening the elimination of an absorbed poison. Several methods may be used to terminate the patient's exposure to a toxic substance or to mitigate its effects. For respiratory exposure, removal of the victim from the toxic environment is usually all that is necessary with careful observation for latent effects of exposures to pulmonary irritants. Involved eyes should be washed with water for at least 10 to 15 minutes. For dermal exposure, the skin should be flushed immediately with water and then should be washed with copious amounts of water and soap. All contaminated clothing should be removed.

Gastrointestinal Decontamination

The American Academy of Pediatrics (AAP) used to recommend that parents keep a 1-oz. bottle of ipecac (an emetic) in the home in case of an ingestion, only to be used on the advice of a physician or poison control center. However, recent evidence suggests that any small benefit incurred from inducing emesis is outweighed by the potential harm to the poisoned child. Therefore, ipecac is no longer recommended as a home treatment strategy for ingestions. The first thing a parent should do when faced with a stable child who has ingested a potentially toxic substance is to call their local poison control center.

Gastric lavage may be more effective than ipecac for removing toxins but is probably beneficial only within the first hour after ingestion and with drugs that delay gastric emptying such as narcotics or TCAs. Lavage is contraindicated in alkali ingestions because of the increased risk for esophageal perforation. It should be used cautiously in patients at risk for developing mental status changes, and endotracheal intubation should be performed first to protect children with absent or compromised airway reflexes. Given the uncertain benefits of gastric lavage, patients who are otherwise asymptomatic should not be sedated and intubated for the sole purpose of performing lavage. Lavage should be performed with an affected patient in a left-side-down, head-down position and is accomplished best with use of a large orogastric hose. A 28 Fr. (9-mm) Ewald tube is the smallest that can be used effectively, because pills and fragments may not pass through smaller bores. This problem limits the benefits of lavage

TABLE 61-2. Toxins Not Effectively Adsorbed by Activated Charcoal

Ethanol
Methanol
Hydrocarbons
Cyanide
Iron
Ethylene glycol
Acids
Alkalis
Lithium

in small children. A 36 Fr. (12-mm) tube is optimal for adolescents and adults. The most significant retrieval may result from aspirating gastric contents before instilling lavage fluid. Warm physiologic saline should be used in aliquots of 10 mL/kg in pediatric patients (200–400 mL in adolescents) and should be continued until the lavage return is clear.

Activated charcoal effectively minimizes gastrointestinal absorption of toxins by adsorbing them onto its large surface area. The use of activated charcoal has risen significantly, as studies have demonstrated that activated charcoal produces better toxin recovery and fewer complications, than emesis or gastric lavage techniques. It should be considered as the primary means of gastrointestinal decontamination in most ingestions, with the exception of a few compounds in which its use is not effective or recommended (Table 61-2). Activated charcoal is most effective if administered during the first several hours after ingestion. Approximately 5 to 10 g of charcoal is required for each gram of drug ingested. Treatment for ingestions of unknown amounts of toxin should be achieved by standard charcoal doses of 1 g/kg (50–100 g for adolescents). The initial dose of charcoal should be given with a cathartic such as sorbitol, to minimize constipation. Commercial preparations containing both medications are available.

Activated charcoal is odorless and tasteless, but its appearance often renders oral acceptance difficult. Nasogastric tube administration should be performed without delay if an affected child refuses oral intake. Charcoal aspiration can occur, causing bronchospasm and pneumonitis, and emphasizes the need for adequate airway protection before administration in the obtunded patient.

Activated charcoal in multiple doses increases the serum clearance of certain medications. Multiple-dose activated charcoal uses "gastrointestinal dialysis" to adsorb drugs available across the gastrointestinal mucosa and to take advantage of enterohepatic recirculation of certain medications. This method has proved effective in oral and intravenous theophylline overdoses and is beneficial for other selected compounds (Table 61-3). A standard dose of activated charcoal should be given initially; then 0.5 g/kg should be administered orally every 4 hours until serum drug levels are nontoxic or clinical symptoms of ingestion have resolved. Some patients tolerate repeated doses poorly. The histamine$_2$-receptor antagonists such as ranitidine, may decrease vomiting, and administering charcoal as a continuous drip in saline through a syringe pump can be helpful.

TABLE 61-3. Toxins with Improved Clearance by Multiple-Dose, Activated Charcoal

Theophylline or aminophylline
Phenobarbital
Carbamazepine
Benzodiazepines
Salicylates
Tricyclic antidepressants
Phenothiazines
Phenytoin

MANAGEMENT OF SPECIFIC TOXINS

Iron Ingestion

Ingested iron increases capillary permeability, intravascular permeability, and vasodilation on overwhelming the intestinal barrier and entering the circulation. When available, free iron exceeds circulating transferrin-binding levels, and toxicity of the liver and other parenchymal organs ensues. Classically, iron intoxication follows four clinical stages, although the presence, duration, and order of these stages may vary. The typical initial phase, occurring shortly after ingestion, is produced by direct effects on gastric and ileal mucosa to induce abdominal pain and vomiting. Gastrointestinal hemorrhage may occur. Fever, leukocytosis, and hyperglycemia are associated findings. In severe intoxications, shock and encephalopathy may occur in this early stage. In the second phase, a deceptively stable period of ameliorated symptoms and subtle physical findings may follow for 6 to 72 hours. However, some patients advance to a third phase with return of gastrointestinal symptoms, metabolic acidosis, coagulopathy and overt shock, and liver dysfunction, rarely progressing to hepatic necrosis. Survivors may develop a fourth phase of gastrointestinal scarring and acute obstruction 4 to 6 weeks after ingestion.

Prediction of potential iron toxicity determines treatment. Estimation of the total dose ingested is helpful but often unreliable. A conservative estimate of 60 mg/kg elemental iron warrants physician evaluation. Serum iron levels should be obtained 2 to 4 hours after ingestion; after 6 hours, the liver has cleared most free iron, and levels may be misleading. Mild toxicity may occur with iron levels of 100 to 300 μg/dL, and moderate toxicity occurs at levels of 300 to 500 μg/dL. Generally, severe toxicity is associated with serum iron levels greater than 500 μg/dL. Empiric deferoxamine challenge with 40 mg/kg (maximum dose, 1 g) administered intramuscularly can be used to demonstrate excess circulating free iron, which is chelated and excreted in the urine with a classic pink-orange "vin rose" color. Significant symptoms should encourage aggressive treatment, and abdominal radiographs should be obtained to look for tablet concretions.

Gastric emptying procedures, including lavage with bicarbonate and deferoxamine, have been attempted but have not been shown to be effective. Activated charcoal does not adsorb iron and is not recommended. Whole-bowel irrigation has been used to hasten the gastrointestinal passage of undissolved iron tablets. Deferoxamine, an avid iron chelator, should be initiated in cases of moderate or severe iron poisoning (serum iron level greater than 500 μg/dL, or greater than 350 μg/dL with significant symptoms). Doses may be given intramuscularly or as a continuous intravenous infusion (15 mg/kg/hour). Adverse effects from deferoxamine are unusual, but hypotension or pulmonary edema may occur with high doses or rapid infusion rates. The end point for discontinuing deferoxamine is uncertain, but use should be considered for 8 to 12 hours with moderate toxicity and for 24 hours with severe toxicity. Close monitoring and supportive therapy for shock are essential.

Organophosphate Poisoning

Organophosphate poisoning is a leading cause of nonpharmaceutical ingestion fatality in children. Such organophosphates as parathion, malathion, and diazinon are common components of agricultural and domestic insecticides. They are absorbed across skin and mucous membranes by means of ingestion and inhalation, and they bind irreversibly to neuronal and erythrocyte cholinesterase and to liver pseudocholinesterase. This process results in failure to terminate the effects of acetylcholine centrally at cortical, respiratory, and cardiac centers and peripherally at nicotinic and muscarinic receptor sites. Symptoms include muscle fasciculations, weakness, paralysis (i.e., nicotinic effect), miosis, salivation, lacrimation, diarrhea, bradycardia (i.e., muscarinic effect), obtundation, seizures, and apnea (i.e., central effect). Symptoms are evidence for more than 50% reduction in enzyme activity. The onset of symptoms may be immediate or delayed for up to 24 hours.

Measurement of decreased serum pseudocholinesterase and erythrocyte cholinesterase confirms the diagnosis, but treatment should be based on suspicion with these symptoms, even without documented organophosphate exposure. Gastric emptying by lavage should be considered with adequate airway protection. Atropine given in high doses (0.05 mg/kg) antagonizes central and muscarinic effects, but it does not decrease muscle weakness and paralysis induced by nicotinic blockade. Repeated doses are given until cholinergic signs resolve. A continuous infusion may be necessary, because recrudescence can occur for at least 24 hours. The patient should be monitored for anticholinergic toxicity. Pralidoxime is a cholinesterase-reactivating oxime indicated for patients with significant muscle weakness, particularly those requiring mechanical ventilation for respiratory muscle dysfunction. Pralidoxime should be initiated early owing to rapid development of resistance by organophosphate-cholinesterase complexes, and doses may have to be repeated over the first 24 hours of treatment.

Hydrocarbon Ingestion

Usually, hydrocarbon ingestion involves common household products, most commonly furniture polish or gasoline. Substances with low viscosity and high volatility such as gasoline and kerosene, present the greatest risk for aspiration, which is the major danger from hydrocarbon ingestion. Determination of the exact formulation ingested is important, because some mixtures may include aromatic compounds such as benzene, that produce central nervous system toxicity. Fluorinated hydrocarbons such as Freon contained in aerosol propellants of various products, can induce seizures and cardiac dysrhythmias if inhaled. Children rapidly develop coughing, gagging, choking, and vomiting, which limit the volume of ingestion but may increase the likelihood of aspiration. Typically, dyspnea, cyanosis, and respiratory failure ensue over the first 24 hours. Roentgenographic changes are seen in most cases within 12 hours after exposure, and patients with these changes are almost always symptomatic on initial presentation.

Management of hydrocarbon ingestion is primarily symptomatic. Gastric emptying procedures should be used only in ingestions of aromatic substances, if the hydrocarbon is mixed with another toxin, or in very high-volume ingestions; otherwise, the risk of aspiration may increase. Activated charcoal is ineffective in hydrocarbon ingestion. Patients with asymptomatic ingestion should be observed for approximately 6 hours and can be discharged if no symptoms or hypoxemia develop. Symptomatic patients should be hospitalized for observation, pulse oximetry monitoring, and serial roentgenograms. Neither prophylactic antibiotics nor corticosteroids have proved beneficial and may increase the risk for superinfection. Patients who develop respiratory failure require intubation and mechanical ventilation, often needing high levels of positive end-expiratory pressure for adequate oxygen delivery.

Tricyclic Antidepressant Ingestion

Ingestion of tricyclic antidepressants (TCAs), including imipramine, amitriptyline, and the secondary amine desipramine, has been a major cause of ingestion-related fatalities and is responsible for up to 25% of all serious overdoses in children and adults and up to 20% of pediatric deaths. TCAs have very narrow therapeutic windows; therapeutic imipramine doses are 1 to 3 mg/kg, whereas 10 to 20 mg/kg produces moderate to severe toxicity, and 30 to 40 mg/kg may be fatal. TCAs block presynaptic uptake of neurotransmitters norepinephrine and serotonin. In addition, TCAs block sympathetic alpha-adrenergic receptor and parasympathetic muscarinic (cholinergic) receptor response, thus, producing a variety of hemodynamic effects in toxic doses. TCA absorption may be delayed owing to its anticholinergic effects. TCAs have quinidine-like activity at therapeutic doses, prolonging conduction times that predispose to wide-complex tachycardias at toxic levels. Decreased cardiac conduction rate, as seen by widened QRS interval (greater than 100 ms) is a helpful clinical correlate of severe toxicity but may be normal in children even in the presence of serious overdose. TCA toxicity should be suspected in patients presenting with signs of anticholinergic poisoning, coma, or hypotension.

Most TCA ingestions that require treatment will necessitate intensive care monitoring owing to the potential for respiratory difficulties, life-threatening arrhythmias and hypotension, and seizures. No specific antidotes are yet available, although specific Fab fragment antibodies are in development. Use of flumazenil specifically should be avoided. General therapeutic measures include gastric decontamination and use of multiple-dose activated charcoal. Hemoperfusion and dialysis are ineffective removal techniques. Strict attention should be paid to monitoring vital signs and to intervening early with an artificial airway and mechanical ventilation. Induction of alkalemia has been shown to be one of the best specific TCA therapies due to its potential stabilization of cardiac membranes and consequent reduction of arrhythmias. Hypotension can occur from alpha-adrenergic blockade and is treated with fluids and alpha agonist vasopressors as needed. Both arrhythmias and seizures can occur, and treatment is often difficult. Pseudoseizures (myoclonus, tremor, chorea) can occur in up to 50% of patients with TCA overdose and must be differentiated from true seizure activity. Metabolic acidosis and hypokalemia are also seen in the first 24 hours.

Newer antidepressant formulations include the serotonin reuptake inhibitors such as fluoxetine (Prozac) and sertraline (Zoloft). This class has proved safer in overdose than TCAs with less potential central nervous system and cardiovascular toxicity.

CHAPTER 62

Acetaminophen Overdose

Adapted from M. Michele Mariscalco

With the concern about the role of salicylate in the pathogenesis of Reye syndrome, acetaminophen has become the most widely used medication for relief of pain and fever in infants and children. Although it has a large therapeutic index, acetaminophen has recognized toxic effects, primarily hepatic, when administered in single doses exceeding 150 mg/kg for children or 7.5 g for adults. Children younger than 6 years and adolescents are the two groups most often associated with single-dose toxicity. However, acetaminophen overdose has been increasingly recognized to be associated with multiple dosing with therapeutic intent that occurs in children younger than 10 years. The single-dose ingestion by children younger than 6 years is usually less than that by adolescents. In the adolescent group, the overdose is either a suicide attempt or a manipulative episode. Handfuls of tablets are typically consumed. In overdose associated with therapeutic intent, multiple (three or more) excessive doses of acetaminophen are consumed before significant hepatic injury develops.

PHARMACOLOGY

Approximately 94% of the drug is metabolized to the glucuronide or sulfate conjugate; 2% is excreted unchanged in the urine. Neither the conjugated forms nor the unchanged forms are hepatotoxic. The remaining 4% is metabolized through the cytochrome P-450 mixed-function oxidase system. Acetaminophen conjugates with glutathione to produce mercapturic acid, which is excreted in the urine. With a significant overdose, the P-450 mixed-function oxidase becomes the major system for metabolizing acetaminophen. When the liver glutathione stores are sufficiently depleted, usually to approximately 70% of normal, which can occur with an acute or chronic overdose, the highly reactive and toxic intermediate metabolite, N-acetyl-p-benzoquinone-imine (NAPQI) is produced. NAPQI is very short lived. It attaches to the hepatic cell membrane and injures the lipid bilayer if not neutralized by an antioxidant. Hepatic glutathione appears to be the primary antioxidant that conjugates and neutralizes NAPQI. Organ systems other than the liver are rarely affected immediately after overdose, although isolated case reports describe acute nephrotoxicity and altered mental status. Rarely, a renal defect occurs without concomitant hepatic damage. Elevation of pancreatic enzyme levels has been reported in as many as 22% of unselected patients.

CLINICAL COURSE

The clinical course of acetaminophen toxicity has four stages. In the first stage (i.e., first 24 hours), adult and adolescent patients develop nausea, vomiting, diaphoresis, and general malaise. Children younger than 6 years show little diaphoresis and vomit earlier. They develop vomiting regardless of the acetaminophen level and have no symptoms, unless the blood level is in the toxic range. Symptoms usually develop within 14 hours in patients with toxic levels of acetaminophen. Evidence of liver injury as reflected by elevations in AST and ALT may appear as early as 8 hours after overdose, and more than one-half of all patients with liver injury develop some elevation within 24 hours. Lethargy is rarely seen during this stage. If lethargy develops, some other agent should be considered in addition to, or instead of, the acetaminophen. During the second stage (i.e., second 24 hours), most patients begin to feel better. If no treatment was received or treatment was unsuccessful, the levels of AST, ALT, or both increase. Patients who have elevations of AST or ALT levels greater than 1,000 IU/L commonly demonstrate other evidence of liver dysfunction by 24 to 72 hours after overdose including elevations in prothrombin time and bilirubin.

During the third stage, from 48 to 96 hours after ingestion, transaminase levels as high as 50,000 IU/L may be seen in patients with severe acetaminophen overdoses. Examination of the liver at this point demonstrates centrilobular necrosis. In the final stage, within 14 days of ingestion, hepatic abnormalities should return to normal. Follow-up evaluations of patients who experienced significant hepatotoxicity and survived reveal no sequelae clinically or on hepatic biopsy. Patients who ultimately die or require liver transplantation progress to hepatic necrosis including jaundice, coagulation defects, hepatorenal syndrome, and hepatic encephalopathy.

TREATMENT

Treatment consists of an initial evaluation to determine respiratory and cardiovascular status. For adolescents, the history should be interpreted with caution because studies have shown it is impossible to differentiate potentially toxic from nontoxic overdoses based on patient history. Plasma levels should be tested no sooner than 4 hours after ingestion. A significant change in sensorium necessitates investigation into ingestion of other substances.

If the ingestion has occurred recently (within 4–6 hours), initial therapy is directed at decreasing absorption of acetaminophen. Activated charcoal effectively absorbs acetaminophen if administered within the first 4 to 6 hours after ingestion. Gastric lavage is rarely indicated for isolated acetaminophen overdose. Acetaminophen ingestion is frequently associated with polypharmacy overdose. As activated charcoal may absorb these other medications, activated charcoal should be administered after 6 hours if polypharmacy is suspected. Activated charcoal can absorb NAC and reduce peak serum NAC levels. Past guidelines for gastrointestinal decontamination after acetaminophen overdose recommended that activated charcoal be lavaged from the stomach before administration of NAC, that NAC be alternated with activated charcoal, or that the loading dose of NAC be increased. None of these interventions appears to be necessary. Laboratory evaluation on arrival at a health care facility includes an acetaminophen level obtained 4 or more hours after ingestion, baseline AST level, ALT level, bilirubin level, prothrombin time, creatinine level, pregnancy test for women of childbearing age, and toxicologic screen. Because aspirin is a frequent coingestant, a salicylate level should be considered.

Crucial to making appropriate management decisions about patients who have ingested a single overdose of acetaminophen is determination of the time elapsed since ingestion (Fig. 62-1). For a patient who has ingested a potentially toxic amount (7.5 g in an adult or 150 mg/kg in a child), from whom an acetaminophen level cannot be obtained within 8 hours after the ingestion, a loading dose of NAC should be administered immediately. If the acetaminophen level is found to be in the nontoxic range, no further doses of NAC are needed; otherwise a complete course of NAC should be given. NAC should be administered as late as 24 hours after ingestion. For nonpregnant patients who present less than 8 hours after overdose, the decision to initiate NAC

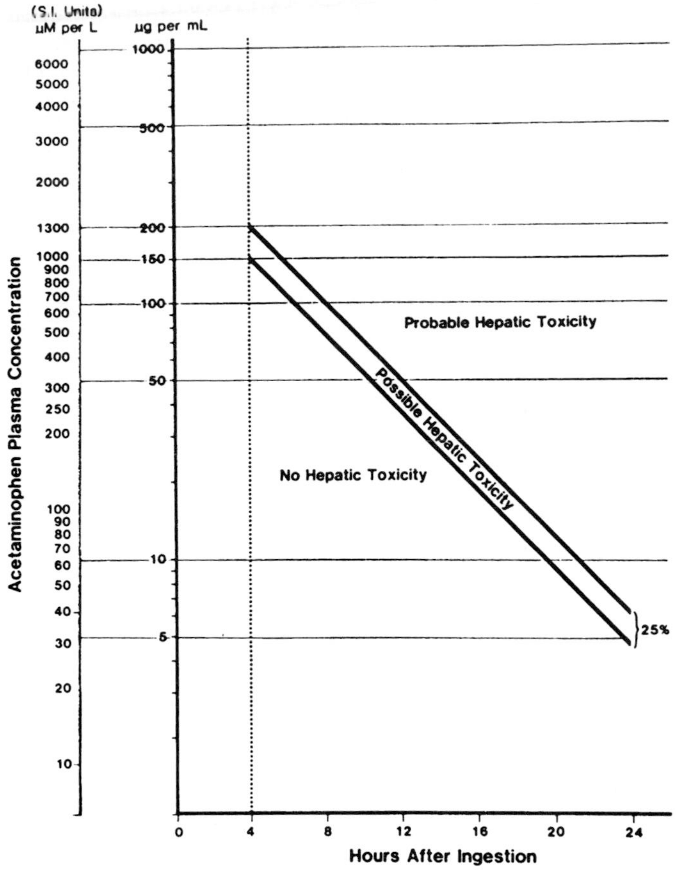

Figure 62-1. Semilogarithmic plot of plasma acetaminophen levels over time. Levels drawn less than 4 hours after ingestion may not represent peak levels. The lower solid line 25% below the standard nomogram is included to allow for possible errors in acetaminophen plasma assays and estimated time from ingestion of an overdose. (Reprinted with permission from Rumack BH, Matthew H. Acetaminophen poisoning and toxicity. *Pediatrics* 1975;55:871.)

therapy may be delayed until an acetaminophen level is available and it is determined whether the patient has a toxic level. A pregnant woman should be administered a loading dose of NAC as soon as possible, regardless of time since overdose, because a potential exists for fetal toxicity after maternal overdose, and fetal wastage has been correlated with treatment delay. If the acetaminophen level is then found to be nontoxic, further doses of NAC are unnecessary. Additionally, late administration of NAC is beneficial to patients with fulminant hepatic failure. Although late administration does not improve the biochemical markers of liver function, it has been shown to improve survival and decrease the incidence of cerebral edema.

In the patient who ingested an unknown quantity of acetaminophen, the plasma level is determined not earlier than 4 hours after ingestion (Fig. 62-1). Second and third levels are of interest, but they are not used to determine whether treatment should continue. NAC (Mucomyst) is administered orally in a final concentration of 5% (weight/volume). The initial oral dose is 140 mg/kg with subsequent doses at 4-hour intervals of 70 mg/kg for an additional 17 doses. The dose must be repeated if the patient vomits within 1 hour of administration. Aggressive antiemetic therapy is critical to successful treatment with oral preparations of NAC. These drugs include metoclopramide (0.5–1.0 mg/kg intravenously). Diphenhydramine should be considered for coadministration to decrease the risk of metoclopramide-induced dystonic reaction. If emesis persists, ondansetron (0.15 mg/kg intravenously) or droperidol (0.05–0.06 mg/kg per dose) may be useful. If emesis still persists, insertion of a nasogastric tube or duodenal tube and drip of the NAC over 30 minutes should be instituted. In the patient with persistent vomiting, intravenous administration of NAC should be considered. At present, intravenous NAC is available only as an investigational drug. In an open-label trial in children, a 52-hour course of intravenous NAC was as effective as 72 hours of oral NAC. Intravenous administration of oral NAC has been studied and found to have anaphylactoid-type reactions similar to the intravenous preparation. It is recommended that oral NAC not be used intravenously without an institutional protocol in place.

Although children younger than 6 years are unlikely to experience toxic effects, the recommendation is that any patient with a plasma acetaminophen level in the toxic range should be treated. A child accidentally consuming small amounts of children's acetaminophen can be managed safely at home if follow-up care is ensured.

OVERDOSE WITH THERAPEUTIC INTENT

A profile of 47 children who developed hepatotoxicity after sustained supratherapeutic acetaminophen administration was reported. Of note, 47% involved children younger than 2 years, 88% had received acetaminophen for 1 to 5 days, and six (15%) had received daily doses ranging from 50 to 75 mg/kg/day. Fifty-two percent had been given adult-strength acetaminophen. In those patients in whom a serum acetaminophen concentration was available and the last dose of acetaminophen could be discerned with accuracy, 73% had serum concentrations that were in the potentially toxic range. In marked contrast to children with acute intoxication, of whom more than 99% recover without sequelae, 54% of the patients died. Three potential therapeutic variables could contribute to iatrogenic therapeutic acetaminophen poisoning in infants and children: (a) confusion by the caretaker in the interpretation of dosing information; (b) administration of adult-strength preparations; and (c) observation that pediatric-strength preparations are not working and, therefore, stronger adult preparations are administered to improve the desired effect. In addition, changes in the induction of P-450 enzymes by foodstuffs or drugs (i.e., ethanol, phenobarbital) or decreases in glutathione availability (fasting and repeated acetaminophen administration) may contribute to the toxicity.

CHAPTER 63
Lead Poisoning

Adapted from J. Julian Chisolm, Jr.

The lead content of food and air has decreased drastically since the early 1980s causing a dramatic reduction in blood lead levels. After the almost complete removal of lead additives from gasoline, air lead levels decreased from 1.5 to less than 0.2 $\mu g/m^3$, even in congested cities. This reduction and the systematic elimination of domestically produced food cans with lead-soldered seams diminished food lead in young children to 1 $\mu g/kg/day$ by 1991. Lead in drinking water may be associated with significant overexposure in some areas of the country in which drinking water is acidic, plumbosolvent, and conveyed in lead pipes or in copper pipes with lead-soldered joints. This problem can often be managed in public water supplies by neutralizing the water. After the substantial reductions in the lead content of food, drinking water, and air, lead in interior household dust and old residential paints currently constitutes the major source of overexposure to lead among children in the United States, and this will continue to be the major source for the foreseeable future. High numbers of children, particularly black children, live in the oldest housing and have the lowest income, which is also where the highest blood and environmental lead levels are found.

Exterior surface soil lead and interior paint contribute significantly to interior household dust lead. A major pathway of lead into the bodies of children is the hand-to-mouth route. More severe degrees of poisoning are generally associated with repetitive ingestion (i.e., pica) of lead paint debris.

TOXICITY

The main toxic effects of lead occur in the central and peripheral nervous systems, erythroid cells, bone marrow, and kidney. The developing nervous system is the system most sensitive to the toxic effects of lead in fetuses and young children. Reversible abnormal thyroid function and cardiac conduction have been reported in severe cases. Lead causes partial inhibition in the biosynthesis of heme at several enzymatic steps. Basophilic stippling is an inconstant finding in peripheral blood, but it is a relatively constant finding in bone marrow normoblasts in severe cases. As the concentration of lead in blood increases to more than 50 to 60 μg/dL of whole blood, hemoglobin decreases. Lead causes a mild, well-compensated hemolytic normocytic anemia that can be differentiated morphologically from the hypochromic microcytic anemia of iron deficiency.

Lead interferes with normal cellular calcium metabolism with a resultant intracellular buildup of calcium. Severe acute lead poisoning (i.e., blood lead level greater than 150 μg/dL of whole blood) can cause the Fanconi syndrome (i.e., generalized renal aminoaciduria, melituria, hyperphosphaturia in the presence of hypophosphatemia) as a result of acute proximal renal tubular injury. Lead nephropathy, which is characterized by hyperuricemia with or without gout, has been reported as a late sequela of chronic plumbism in Australian children. Acute lead encephalopathy in the very young is characterized by massive cerebral edema caused primarily by a generalized increase in vascular permeability. Neuronal destruction also occurs.

PATIENT EVALUATION

Clinical Diagnosis

Before the onset of acute encephalopathy, symptoms are subtle and nonspecific, and physical examination generally reveals little or nothing. Burton lines are rare, seen only in severe cases in which dental caries exist. Plumbism should be included in the differential diagnosis of anemia; seizure disorders; severe behavioral disorders; mental retardation; colicky abdominal pain; and the arthralgia, bone pain, and cerebral and abdominal crises of sickle cell disease. Isolated seizures and self-limited episodes of vomiting during the recent past may represent episodes of unrecognized clinical plumbism, especially if the child lives in or visits old houses, if the parent is unavailable for much of the time, or if a history of excessive hand-to-mouth activity is obtained. Recent changes of address, recent renovations in the home, and particularly time spent unsupervised or with baby-sitters and relatives should be ascertained. Persistent hand-to-mouth activity is associated with such histories. This information is essential in planning the appropriate management for each patient. Emphasis must be placed on environmental sampling for sources of lead and laboratory data. Whenever an index case is found, all housemates should have a blood lead test, and the possibility of uncommon sources should be ascertained.

Screening

The Centers for Disease and Prevention (CDC) considers all venous blood lead levels equal to or greater than 10 μg/dL of whole blood to be levels of concern. Until the high-risk areas are determined within any given state, all children should receive a blood lead test. Where the previously recommended questionnaire (Table 63-1) is used, any children in whom the answer is "yes" or "don't know" should receive a blood lead test. The questionnaire is now considered supplementary, because it has been demonstrated that it is quite insensitive and does not discriminate well among affected and unaffected children. The questionnaire's chief value may be the detection of children with elevated blood lead concentrations from sources other than old dilapidated housing.

Classification of children (Table 63-2) is based on a confirmed venous blood lead concentration equal to or greater than 20 μg/dL of whole blood. Although venous blood lead tests are preferable, capillary test results placing the child in classes I and IIA need not be confirmed. No unanimity of opinion exists regarding the use of chelating agents. In some programs, it is instituted at a blood lead level equal to or greater than 40 μg/dL of whole blood and, in most programs, when the blood lead level reaches a level equal to or greater than 45 μg/dL of whole blood. Physicians generally agree that chelation therapy should be instituted immediately if the blood lead level is equal to or greater than 70 μg/dL of whole blood, because the onset of serious symptoms is unpredictable at these higher levels.

Among children residing in older housing with deteriorating lead-based paint, blood lead concentration increases most rapidly between 6 and 12 months of age and tends to reach a peak at 18 to 24 months. Therefore, the first screening test is

TABLE 63-1. Assessing the Risk of High-Dose Exposure to Lead: Basic Personal-Risk Questionnaire

1. Does your child live in or regularly visit a house that was built before 1950? This could include a day-care center, preschool, baby-sitter, or relative.	Yes	Don't know	No
2. Does your child live in or regularly visit a house built before 1978 with recent or ongoing renovations or remodeling or repainting (within the past 6 months)?	Yes	Don't know	No
3. Does your child have a brother, sister, housemate, or playmate who has been treated for lead poisoning or is being followed for a blood lead level equal to or greater than 15 μg/dL?	Yes	Don't know	No
4. Additional questions may be added at the state level to reflect possible exposure to local conditions such as a battery recycling plant, lead smelter, or other industry likely to release lead.			

Adapted from Centers for Disease Control and Prevention. *Screening young children for lead; guidance for state and local public health officials.* Atlanta: Centers for Disease Control and Prevention, November 1997.

TABLE 63-2. Classification of Children According to Blood Lead Concentration

Blood lead levels (μg/dL)*	Comments
<10	Reassess or rescreen in 1 year. No additional action necessary unless exposure sources change; immediately retest after change.
10–14	Provide family lead education. Provide follow-up testing.
15–19	Provide family lead education. Provide follow-up testing. Refer to social services. Initiate professional environmental cleanup. If blood lead levels persist (i.e., 2 venous blood lead levels in this range at least 3 months apart), reclean.
20–44	Refer to clinical center specializing in lead poisoning where available. Provide case management. Provide both clinical and environmental management. Ensure lead hazard control.
45–69	Within 48 hours, begin coordination of care (case management), clinical management (described in text), environmental investigation, and lead hazard control. Consider chelation therapy.
≥70	Hospitalize child and begin medical treatment immediately. Begin coordination of care (case management), clinical management (described in text), environmental investigation, and lead hazard control immediately.

*Based on confirmatory venous blood lead level.
Adapted from Centers for Disease Control and Prevention. *Screening young children for lead; guidance for state and local public health officials.* Atlanta: Centers for Disease Control and Prevention, November 1997.

recommended to be given at 9 to 12 months of age and again at 24 months of age.

THERAPY

The cornerstone of treatment is prompt separation of the child from the sources of lead, followed by careful reduction of lead hazards in the home or preferably removal to a lead-safe dwelling as documented by interior dust lead measurements. The local health agency is usually responsible for identifying and supervising the removal of lead hazards. Children and pregnant women, because of the sensitivity of the fetus to lead, must remain out of the home day and night until the abatement of lead paint hazards has been completed and the dwelling completely vacuumed with a HEPA vacuum, scrubbed with detergents two or three times, and vacuumed with a HEPA vacuum again to remove the fine particulate lead that is unavoidably generated by any deleading process. The deleaded areas should be repainted. Encapsulant paints have recently become available for this purpose.

Most children detected in current screening programs are asymptomatic and fall into groups I, IIA, IIB, and III (Table 63-2). For those in groups I and II, the previously described measures and improved diet should suffice. Neither chelation therapy nor extensive removal of intact lead paint in good condition is likely to be of any benefit in group II. Chelation therapy may be of benefit in selected cases in group III.

Chelation Therapy

Chelation therapy is advised for all children in groups IV and V including the asymptomatic cases. Intramuscular therapy with CaEDTA is limited to 5 days at a daily dose of 1,000 mg/m^2/day, given in two divided portions when venous blood lead levels are greater than 40 μg/dL but less than 90 to 100 μg/dL of whole blood. Chelation therapy before the onset of symptoms may simplify treatment and lessen the risk of cerebral injury. Repeat courses of CaEDTA with intervals of at least 4 days between courses may be indicated for children with higher body lead burdens. Treatment with oral CaEDTA is contraindicated. The use of CaEDTA is regularly accompanied by transitory increases in serum transaminases and decreases in serum alkaline phosphatase.

CaEDTA has now been almost completely replaced by meso-2,3-dimercaptosuccinic acid (DMSA, succimer) for the treatment of asymptomatic children; this was approved by the Food and Drug Administration (FDA) in 1991. Whether the drug will be effective in symptomatic cases with blood lead levels greater than 100 μg/dL of whole blood has not been determined. The drug is given orally and has not been associated with serious adverse side affects. It does not induce acute zinc depletion as CaEDTA does. Nineteen-day courses are approved, with the priming dose of 1,050 mg/m^2/day given in three divided doses for the first 5 days, followed by a sustaining dose of 700 mg/m^2/day given in two divided doses for the next 2 weeks. In animals, DMSA is more effective than CaEDTA in reducing temporarily the lead content of the brain, kidney, and blood. For those with higher body lead burdens, multiple courses will likely be required. Under no circumstance should the drug be given on an outpatient basis to children concurrently overexposed to lead; increase in blood lead during DMSA therapy has been observed under these circumstances.

Patients with symptomatic plumbism (e.g., colic, seizures, acute encephalopathy) should be treated promptly with chelating agents on the basis of positive presumptive laboratory test results. Because the onset and clinical course of encephalopathy are unpredictable, the risk of delay far outweighs the risk of a few days of chelation therapy. If subsequent tests do not support the diagnosis of lead poisoning, treatment should be discontinued and the diagnosis reconsidered.

For acute encephalopathy or lead levels exceeding 90 to 100 μg/dL of whole blood, a regimen of 2,3-dimercaptopropanol (BAL) and CaEDTA is recommended. The dose for BAL is 500 mg/m^2 per 24 hours, and the dose for CaEDTA is 1,500 mg/m^2 per 24 hours. The drugs are injected simultaneously at separate deep intramuscular sites in six divided doses each day for 5 days after an initial priming dose of BAL only.

PROGNOSIS

The adverse effects of lead are not reversible. Sequelae are related to the degree and duration of excessive tissue levels as indexed by serial blood lead measurements or the lead content of shed deciduous teeth. Recurrence of clinical manifestations increases the chance of permanent injury. Residual brain damage or dysfunction may not be evident until the early elementary school years. Sequelae of encephalopathy include seizure disorders, impaired mentation and, rarely, blindness and hemiparesis. Some survivors may require residential care. Seizures tend to abate before adolescence, but intellectual deficits persist.

General agreement exists that blood lead levels, if sustained during early childhood at levels greater than 10 to 15 μg/L of whole blood (0.50 to 0.72 μmol/L), carry an unacceptable risk for long-lasting but subtle injury to the nervous system, even if no clinical symptoms are detected. Follow-up of a cohort of children at 18 to 20 years of age has revealed that those with the higher dentin lead content at 6 to 8 years of age were seven times more likely to have dropped out of school and six times more likely to have a reading disability than those with the lower dentin lead content during the elementary school years. Some of these children had blood lead values during the preschool years averaging 35 $\mu g/dL$ of whole blood. Attention deficits and reading disabilities have been identified in other cohorts of younger children.

CHAPTER 64
Apparent Life-Threatening Events

Adapted from Gerald M. Loughlin and John L. Carroll

An apparent life-threatening event (ALTE) describes a complex of observations and events that are perceived by the child's caretaker to be life-threatening. ALTE merely describes a manner of presentation for many different disorders (Table 64-1). In most studies of ALTE, a possible cause of the event is discovered in approximately 50% of cases. The occurrence of an ALTE most likely reflects a developmental immaturity in the regulation of cardiorespiratory responses. These infants appear to experience an exaggerated response to commonly occurring stressors in an infant's life.

APPROACH TO THE INFANT AFTER AN APPARENT LIFE-THREATENING EVENT

The first steps in evaluating these patient should focus both on ruling out treatable causes of life-threatening events and on determining if a life-threatening or dangerous event actually occurred. In many instances, parents have witnessed a normal physiologic variation that appears to be life-threatening to the inexperienced layperson. Normal infants can experience respiratory pauses lasting for up to 20 seconds during sleep. Many of these pauses are not associated with color change or desaturation, and they are frequently preceded by a sigh. To a parent waiting for a baby to start breathing again, however, even 10 seconds can seem like an eternity. Thus, this infant may be brought to medical attention in an urgent fashion and labeled as abnormal. The physician is confronted by an anxious parent or caretaker who believes that she or he has witnessed an event that has endangered the child's life. Somehow, the physician caring for this child must identify the infant at true risk.

TABLE 64-1. Some Causes of Apparent Life-Threatening Events

Cardiac
Congestive heart failure
Arrhythmia
Respiratory
Infection, pneumonia, respiratory syncytial virus
Respiratory failure
Sepsis
Gastrointestinal
Gastroesophageal reflux
Dysfunctional swallowing
Central nervous system
Seizures
Brainstem neoplasm or compression
Infection
Central hypoventilation syndromes
Metabolic disorders
Hypoglycemia
Medium-chain acyl-CoA dehydrogenase deficiency
Prematurity
Apnea of prematurity
Anemia
Child abuse
Poisoning

A detailed history of the event is essential. A description of the circumstances preceding the event is key. Was the patient awake or asleep? Events that occur when the child is awake are often found to be secondary to gastroesophageal reflux or a seizure. Was the event associated with body movements or unusual posturing? Again, this suggests a seizure disorder or gastroesophageal reflux. Was the child struggling to breathe (suggestive of airway obstruction), or were respiratory efforts absent?

An accurate description of the intervention required to reestablish normal respiration is important, because Oren and colleagues have demonstrated a strong association between the need for vigorous resuscitation and increased risk of recurrent severe spells and even death. Recovery spontaneously or with minimal intervention (i.e., touching the infant) is reassuring and may suggest that what was witnessed was most likely a normal physiologic event. Information about the time required to reverse the event and the infant's mental and physical status after the event is also important in planning subsequent therapy.

Was the infant premature? Was the delivery difficult? Was respiration initiated in normal fashion at birth? Was there evidence of prior respiratory difficulties? Has the child's growth and development been appropriate? These questions help to establish a predisposition to abnormalities in control of respiration and also help to identify a chronic condition.

A history of how the infant handles feeding is important. Dysfunctional swallowing is more common in preterm infants and can trigger reflex apnea and bradycardia by direct aspiration, stimulation of laryngeal chemoreceptors, or by reflux of formula into the nasopharynx. Apnea may be central or obstructive and often occurs during feeding in preterm infants. However, if reflux occurs, apnea may occur at varying intervals after feeding.

Is there a family history of sudden unexplained death in other siblings or relatives? Multiple deaths in a family should make one suspicious about the potential for child abuse or an inherited metabolic disorder. Is there a family history of snoring or obstructive sleep apnea? This information suggests a possible familial predisposition to respiratory control disorders.

Assessment of growth and development, along with a focus on cardiac, neurologic, and respiratory systems, is necessary to identify subtle signs of chronic conditions that may predispose to life-threatening events. Similarly, evidence of an acute infection (sepsis, central nervous system, respiratory) should be sought so that appropriate therapy can be initiated.

Overview of Laboratory Studies

A comprehensive laboratory evaluation should be reserved for infants whose history and physical examination suggest that a significant event took place. This can be a challenge, because the observer's report often does not help the physician to make these decisions. When the infant is brought to medical attention,

TABLE 64-2. Other Studies Possibly Indicated in Children with Apparent Life-Threatening Events

Study	Possible diagnosis
Chest radiography	Pneumonia, bronchiolitis, screen for cardiac disease
Barium swallow	Dysfunctional swallowing, gastroesophageal reflux, upper airway obstruction
Electroencephalography	Seizure disorder
Electrocardiography and echocardiography	Rule out cardiac disease or cor pulmonale
pH probe	Suspicion of gastroesophageal reflux
Documented cardiorespiratory monitoring	Unusual apnea, recurrent events or alarms, concerns about compliance, suspected child abuse
Polysomnography	Unusual apnea, need to assess oxygenation and ventilation, rule out obstructive apnea

a measure of acid–base status, either an arterial blood gas or a measurement of serum bicarbonate and a measurement of blood glucose (if the child has not eaten in several hours), should be obtained as soon as possible. Obviously, the longer the interval between the event and obtaining the sample lessens the value of the data, but it is still worth doing. A serum bicarbonate level is a particularly useful test. A low value suggests that the event may have been severe enough to result in a metabolic acidosis or may suggest the presence of an underlying metabolic disorder. On the other hand, elevation of serum bicarbonate is consistent with chronic compensation for respiratory acidosis. Hypoglycemia may indicate an underlying metabolic disorder such as medium-chain acyl-CoA dehydrogenase deficiency as the cause of the ALTE. A complete blood count with differential, looking for anemia, polycythemia, and signs of acute infection, should also be a part of this initial screening approach. A hematocrit in the high 30s or 40s in an infant aged 2 to 3 months whose hematocrit should be at physiologic nadir suggests underlying chronic hypoxemia. On the other hand, hematocrit values in the 20s have been associated with apnea and bradycardia in the preterm infant. The white blood cell count is a window on infection. Based on the report of Schwartz et al. on a relationship between prolonged QT interval and sudden infant death syndrome (SIDS) (12 of 24 infants who died from SIDS over a 20-year period were found to have a prolonged rate-corrected QT interval on an EKG that had been obtained at 3 days of age), including an EKG in the initial screening evaluation of a child with an ALTE is justified. Based on results of the initial screening tests, the history and physical examination, or subsequent observations, other studies may be indicated (Table 64-2).

MANAGEMENT

For infants who required minimal intervention or stimulation and have no evidence of infection or abnormality on physical examination, discharge from the emergency department or clinic may be possible without an extensive workup. However, sufficient time must be spent with the family to answer questions, explain the normal variations in respiratory patterns, and reassure them that their baby does not demonstrate evidence of underlying disease. Follow-up must be provided for the family if questions arise or the child has another event. If concern exists about the family's ability to handle even this minor event and the low risk of a recurrence, the child should be admitted to the hospital for observation, parental education, and reassurance.

An infant who experiences a severe ALTE should be monitored in a hospital for at least 48 hours after the event. Hospitalization allows for a period of close observation and parental education. All infants should be placed on both cardiac and respiratory monitors and should be easily observable by the medical and nursing staff. This initial monitoring must be done carefully because undocumented false alarms lead to increased anxiety for the family and may lead to additional and unnecessary studies. Hospitalization also allows the nursing staff to obtain important information on parent-child interactions and on feeding skills of the infant and parents and to observe the development of clinical symptoms of an underlying disease. Hospitalization permits time for the initial laboratory data to be analyzed and, if necessary, for secondary tests to be ordered.

Finally, many parents are frightened by these events and are quite concerned about the future. A brief hospital stay gives the appropriate medical and other support personnel time to talk with the family and to establish relationships that will form the basis for continuity of outpatient support. Furthermore, if a decision is made to initiate cardiorespiratory monitoring, there will be enough time to train the family in the use of the monitor and in infant CPR.

Home Monitoring

Although technically not a treatment, home cardiorespiratory monitoring has emerged as the most widely used approach to the problem of ALTEs. The use of monitoring has increased out of frustration about the unknown and unpredictable nature of these spells, coupled with an effort to alleviate parental fears and stress. Current indications for home monitoring are listed in Table 64-3.

No clear-cut guidelines exist on which to base the decision to initiate home monitoring for an infant with an ALTE. As discussed in the section on pneumograms, no tests clearly define the subgroup of infants with ALTE who are truly at risk of sudden death. Approximately 60% of infants who required vigorous resuscitation have been noted to have a second severe spell; consequently, this group should be monitored. For most infants reported to have an ALTE, however, the circumstances are unclear and the severity of the episode is difficult to assess.

Monitoring is also a mixed blessing for the family. The frequent false alarms are a particular problem, because there is no way to know that the alarm is false until an adult checks the infant. Monitors change the family's lifestyle. The mother often bears the major burden of responsibility for the child. Routine daily procedures like vacuuming and showering must be scheduled around times when someone is available to monitor the infant. Locating baby-sitters is a problem because the

TABLE 64-3. Current Indications for Home Monitoring

- Infants with severe apparent life-threatening events requiring vigorous resuscitation and for whom no treatable cause can be identified (monitoring for infants with milder spells and siblings of sudden infant death syndrome victims is somewhat controversial)
- Infants with tracheostomy younger than 1 year
- Infants with bronchopulmonary dysplasia on supplemental oxygen
- Infants with potential treatable causes of apparent life-threatening events to assess response to therapy
- Premature infants discharged on methylxanthine therapy for persistent apnea

idea of caring for a child who is at risk for a life-threatening event generally frightens away caretakers. Many baby-sitters are not CPR-certified. Thus, families often find themselves isolated.

The decision to discontinue monitoring is influenced by a variety of factors. If monitoring was initiated for an ALTE, it should be continued for at least 2 months beyond the last event or real alarm. Bradycardia caused by inappropriate alarm setting or shallow breathing interpreted as apnea by the monitor should not be counted. The infant should be at least 6 months old (the incidence of SIDS decreases rapidly after 6 months) and have had at least one diphtheria, pertussis, and tetanus immunization and one upper respiratory infection before discontinuing the monitor; these are considered by some to be stress tests. Although the diphtheria, pertussis, and tetanus vaccine has not been shown to increase the risk of SIDS, an apparent association exists between viral upper respiratory tract infections and SIDS.

Cessation of monitoring for other conditions is based on the natural course of the disease and the response to therapy. If drug therapy (methylxanthine, antireflux, or seizure medication) has been used, monitoring should usually be continued for at least 1 month after the drug therapy has been stopped. This guideline is somewhat arbitrary, and decisions must be individualized. Monitoring for a sibling of a SIDS victim generally continues until several weeks beyond the age at which the other child died.

Discontinuing the monitor may be difficult for some parents. Many families become dependent on it, so the physician and support team must frequently increase their involvement with the family to support them through the weaning process. Families anxious about stopping the monitor should start by not monitoring the infant during naps to facilitate the transition to no monitoring.

APPARENT LIFE-THREATENING EVENTS WITH NO DEFINABLE CAUSE

Infants who have ALTE with no definable cause are a major management dilemma for the practitioner. The data on the risks of subsequent spells and possible death are limited and somewhat biased by interventions. The physician has, at best, three therapeutic options: no intervention, the use of respiratory stimulants, or home monitoring. Doing nothing is not often a choice because of parental anxiety surrounding the risk of subsequent events. Because monitoring has not been demonstrated to reduce the incidence of SIDS, some have recommended a nonintervention approach once treatable or diagnosable conditions are eliminated. This choice is not popular with many families, but it is an option, assuming the family can be reassured and the physician is comfortable that the event is not severe or likely to recur. Unfortunately, many families and physicians are extremely uncomfortable with doing nothing. Stimulants have a limited role other than the use of theophylline in infants with persistent apnea of prematurity (AOP). In general, an ALTE of unknown cause is best handled with judicious use of home monitoring.

CHAPTER 65
Sudden Infant Death Syndrome

Adapted from John L. Carroll
and Gerald M. Loughlin

Sudden Infant Death Syndrome (SIDS) is what remains after a thorough postmortem investigation fails to reveal a cause of an infant's death; in other words, it is a diagnosis by exclusion. Currently, SIDS is defined as the sudden death of an infant younger than 1 year that remains unexplained after a thorough investigation including a performance of complete autopsy, examination of the death scene, and review of the clinical history. This definition restricts the age to infants younger than 1 year and requires a thorough investigation; it explicitly states that if no death-scene investigation is performed, a diagnosis of SIDS cannot be made. Noteworthy is that, although rare, sudden unexpected deaths do occur in infants older than 1 year. Unexplained death in older infants should prompt additional investigation for unusual disorders such as metabolic defects. The causes of SIDS are unknown. The search for the causes of SIDS has been complicated by the study of so-called infants at risk or high-risk infants, because identification of groups that are at risk is a matter of dispute. Much of the scientific data that have been proposed or assumed to describe infants at risk may or may not apply to most SIDS victims.

RISK FACTORS

Table 65-1 lists the environmental and infant risk factors associated with SIDS. The most substantial recent advance in the prevention of SIDS has been the recommendation to not allow infants to sleep in the prone position. The American Academy of Pediatrics (AAP) issued a policy statement in 1992 recommending that healthy infants be positioned on their sides or backs when placed down for sleep. In 1996, in response to new evidence that the side position conferred an increased risk for SIDS, the AAP issued a new policy statement recommending that healthy infants should sleep on their backs. In the 4 years after the 1992 AAP statement, the proportion of infants sleeping prone in the United States declined from approximately 75% to 20%, and the SIDS rate dropped approximately 40%.

TABLE 65-1. Risk Factors for SIDS

Environmental
Prone sleep position
Prenatal and postnatal smoke exposure
Unsafe sleeping environments
Soft mattresses and porous bedding material
Infection
Lack of breast-feeding
Poor nutrition
Illicit drugs
Over-the-counter medications
Antihistamines and phenothiazines
Infant Characteristics
Prematurity and low birth weight

GROUPS PROPOSED TO BE AT INCREASED RISK FOR SUDDEN INFANT DEATH SYNDROME

Traditional groups said to be at increased risk include premature infants, subsequent siblings of SIDS victims, survivors of an apparent life-threatening event (ALTE), and infants of substance-abusing mothers. Prematurity and low birth weight are potent risk factors for SIDS and are not in dispute.

PREDICTION

At present, SIDS risk cannot be predicted for individual infants. No test, including a pneumogram or polysomnography (sleep study), is useful for determining SIDS risk. Neither can any test predict SIDS risk for a family or a subsequent sibling. No test can determine which infants should receive home apnea monitoring or when a home monitor can be discontinued appropriately. However, we can predict increased risk for premature infants, low-birth-weight infants, infants placed to sleep prone or on their side, infants exposed to prenatal or postnatal tobacco smoke, and so on, opening the door for a variety of risk-reduction approaches.

HOME MONITORING

The question of home monitoring is unsettled. As currently used in the United States, home cardiorespiratory monitoring is intended to improve the outcome of any infant perceived to be at increased risk of sudden death. However, after decades, home monitoring has not decreased the incidence of SIDS. In 1986, the Consensus Development Conference on Infantile Apnea and Home Monitoring found no reports of scientifically designed studies of the effectiveness of home monitoring as regards ALTE, subsequent siblings of SIDS victims, premature infants, or other pathologic conditions; in 1998, this situation remains true.

Often, pediatricians are in doubt about the correct time at which to discontinue home monitoring. No tests, including pneumograms or polysomnography, will resolve this issue. Discontinuing monitoring is a clinical decision based on the overall clinical picture. In general, monitoring can be discontinued when no significant abnormal cardiorespiratory events have occurred for 2 or 3 consecutive months.

Memory monitors, which provide a hard-copy printout of all alarm events, are in common use today. Although the monthly cost is higher than that for conventional cardiorespiratory monitoring, often the overall cost is lower because most alarm events are false (artifact). Much of the guesswork is taken out of monitor decision making because physicians and parents can review the hard copy, can be reassured that serious cardiorespiratory events did not occur, and can discontinue use of the monitor sooner than they might have if conventional monitoring were being used.

CHAPTER 66

Child Maltreatment

Adapted from Lawrence S. Wissow

TYPES OF ABUSE

Neglect is thought to be the most common and probably the most lethal form of child maltreatment. Neglect is found in approximately 60% of confirmed reports of maltreatment. Neglect may take many forms, but the common feature is the failure of a parent or other caretaker to provide a child with basic shelter, supervision, or support. This failure can be passive such as not obtaining needed health care, or it can be active such as knowingly exposing a child to some hazardous situation.

Physical abuse is found in approximately 23% of confirmed abuse reports. It is defined as inflicting of physical injury through malicious, cruel, or inhumane treatment. Vigorous debate still rages over the boundary between acceptable forms of corporal punishment and physical abuse. In practice, punishments that result in injury (i.e., leave marks, break the skin or bones, involve real or perceived threats to life or health) are regarded as abusive.

Emotional abuse is found in approximately 4% of confirmed abuse cases. It is one of the more difficult types of maltreatment to define or detect and has had relatively little recognition in child abuse reporting laws. Garbarino offered one working definition that may be useful to the clinician: "The willful destruction or significant impairment of a child's feeling of competence or security" by a parent or other caretaker.

Sexual abuse is found in approximately 9% of confirmed reports of maltreatment, although its actual prevalence may be much greater. The definition of sexual abuse includes inappropriate exposure to sexual acts or materials, passive use of children as sexual stimuli for adults (i.e., child pornography), and actual sexual contact of children with older persons. A child's apparent "consent" to participate in sexual activity does not reduce the older person's responsibility or alter the diagnosis of abuse.

CAUSES OF ABUSE

Abuser's Childhood

Many abusive parents report having experienced what could be labeled emotional abuse during their own childhoods. This includes a consistent lack of empathy from their parents, a lack of support for their own development, and a chronic feeling of never having had their own needs met. Physical and sexual abuse appear to be more common in the childhoods of abusers than of nonabusers. Most abuse, however, is committed by persons who do not give a history of having been abused, and most persons abused as children do not grow up to become abusers.

Family Stresses and Supports

Another theory of abuse causation is that excessive stress on the parent or family causes a breakdown of inhibitions and a release of frustration on a child. Several factors were associated with families in which abuse did take place. Dissatisfaction with marriage and a frustrated expectation that the husband should be the dominant family decision maker were associated with a twofold increase in the rate of abuse. Abuse was also more likely to occur in families that approved of one spouse slapping another. Participation in social, business, or religious activity outside the family was associated with lower rates of abuse. These data support the theory that stresses alone do not cause abuse. Other forces such as poverty or poor self-esteem, may make a person more susceptible to stress and more prone to abuse, and better social support or a more positive history of dealing with crises makes maladaptive responses to stress less likely.

Socioeconomic Status

In the Family Violence Survey, job status classification and educational level had little to do with the occurrence of violence toward children. Low income, however, was associated with a marked increase in violence, and in other studies, it was associated with increased rates of child neglect and sexual abuse.

Maternal Age

Maternal age at the time of a child's birth appears to influence the likelihood of physical abuse but not of neglect. Mothers of abused children usually begin childbearing earlier than do nonabusing mothers, but the explanation for this association is uncertain. Younger parents may have less knowledge of normal child behavior, and they may be more likely to be frustrated or disappointed by their child's activities. Pregnancy at a younger age may be a sign of other dysfunction within the parent's family and an indication that the parent has had less of a chance to experience appropriate care.

Characteristics of Children at Risk for Abuse

Infants perceived by their parents as being fussier or as being slow to develop or to be in poor health appear to be at a higher risk of abuse, as do children labeled by their parents as having undesirable characteristics reminiscent of disliked family members. Increased rates of abuse have been reported among handicapped children. The families of handicapped children may need more emotional and logistical support to achieve feelings of satisfaction and competency in parenting. Particular points of stress may arise, as during school vacations when a sudden increase occurs in the family's need to provide care for the handicapped child. Work schedules may be disrupted, siblings may be conscripted against their wills into supervisory roles, and the handicapped child's behavior may change outside of a structured school environment.

Children who are socially, emotionally, and geographically isolated also appear to be at a higher risk for sexual abuse. These children may be more open to an abuser's advances, even if they perceive them to be wrong, as a substitute for other relationships. It may be harder for these children to reveal the abuse to others, or they may be less likely to get a supportive response to disclosure.

Medical History

The goals of the basic history are to establish immediate treatment needs and to begin formulating a level of suspicion of abuse. In many abuse cases, the history given is misleading or false. Improbable or inconsistent stories are important elements of diagnosing abuse, but they do not help diagnose a child's immediate medical problems. A careful and complete physical examination is needed, especially if the clinician suspects that the history is unreliable.

When interviewing adults, carefully establish the source of the information provided. Is the informant a regular caretaker for the child? What is his or her relationship? If the evaluation involves a question of trauma, was the informant actually a witness, or is the information given second hand? Be especially careful to ask for details of events, and do not volunteer or suggest answers. When inquiring about previous illnesses or treatments, try to obtain enough information so that the history can be verified if necessary. Include the name and location of hospitals, clinics, physicians, and schools and approximate dates when the services were used.

Be alert for aspects of the history that do not make sense when compared with clinical experience. Does the story fit the child's developmental age and abilities? Is the proposed mechanism of injury plausible? Have you seen other children with similar histories who had the same degree of injury to the same part of the body? Do the symptoms fit with any fairly common condition, or do you find yourself having to imagine combinations of unlikely conditions to explain the child's illness?

When considering potential abuse cases, a social worker is an invaluable resource for obtaining a detailed family and social history. However, the physician must often obtain this information to make a decision about referral or reporting.

Establishing the Plausibility of Injury

It is often difficult to assess a parent's story of how a child was injured. As has been described, one must be alert for a lack of detail or consistency in the story or for aspects that do not match the child's developmental abilities. Often, a visit to the alleged accident scene is required. Knowledge of patterns of injury in known accidents can also help. Injuries of any kind to children younger than 2 or 3 months are unusual, mostly because these children have such limited mobility. Few children can roll over before 2 months of age, and some still cannot at 4 months. Falls from the height of most household furniture rarely result in serious injury. In general, the presence of intracranial injury (subdural bleeding, anything other than very transient concussive symptoms) suggests greater force than generally occurs in household injuries. Falls to concrete floors or onto hard, pointed objects may be exceptions, but physical findings (e.g., abrasions, bruises corresponding to the shape of the object) may also be seen that corroborate the history.

BRUISES, BITES, AND LACERATIONS

Signs

Bruises and other skin lesions are the most common manifestations of physical abuse. Normal, active children may have many bruises and abrasions at any given time. These injuries are usually over bony areas such as the shins, knees, elbows, and forehead. Injuries in other areas, especially to soft tissues such as the abdomen, genitalia, buttocks, thighs, or mouth are more worrisome, because they are unusual in unintentional household trauma. Particularly worrisome are injuries to the inner aspects of the upper or lower arm. These surfaces may be injured when the arms are raised to protect the face from a blow. Bilateral injuries to the face raise the question of abuse. Because the prominence of the nose makes it difficult to accidentally strike both sides of the face at the same time, bilateral bruising may be a sign of multiple impacts, possibly of battering.

The shape of an injury may also be a clue to its cause. Some of the few lesions that are virtually diagnostic of abuse fall into this category. A looped cord leaves a characteristic mark in the shape of an oversized hairpin. The loop may have a double railroad track appearance if it was inflicted with an electrical cord or an abraded texture if it was made with a rope. Belt buckles leave characteristic marks, usually an erythematous band from the belt itself, terminating in a horseshoe-shaped mark from the buckle. A flat palm with spread fingers leaves a mark that the examiner can test by superimposing his own hand. Petechial lesions from the neck up, with or without bruising, or cordlike lesions on the neck may be a sign of strangulation.

Bites usually appear as a semicircular or crescent-shaped red area with or without breaking of the skin. The diameter and circumference of a bite may suggest that an adult or a child inflicted it. It is important to measure the bite or take a photograph with a ruler visible in the frame. If it seems that the bite will be important in trying to identify the abuser, a forensic dentist may be able to match the wound with a suspect's dentition. Serial photographs should be taken over several days because most bite wounds are crush injuries that darken and become more visible with time.

Differential Diagnosis

Trauma, intentional or accidental, is not the only cause of skin lesions. Alternative diagnoses must be carefully considered, because the skin findings may be signs of life-threatening illness, and because the accusation of abuse, once made, is not retracted easily. Perhaps the most commonly occurring similar lesions are mongolian spots, areas of purplish or dark brown discoloration frequently seen on the buttocks and lower back of black or Asian infants. They may also appear on the trunk, upper extremities, or face. These spots are entirely benign, unrelated to trauma, and usually have been observed since birth. The easiest way to differentiate them from bruises is to notice that they fail to change color over a period of days.

Thrombocytopenia from any cause, meningococcal disease, and Schönlein-Henoch purpura can cause bruise-like lesions. Especially if a child presents with altered mental status or seems to be acutely ill, these causes must be considered first or, at least, simultaneously with the diagnosis of trauma. A vasculitis associated with hypersensitivity can also produce streaky ecchymotic lesions on the extremities that look like welts. These patients often develop urticaria and other signs of systemic illness. Even if abuse is strongly suspected, it is usually reasonable to obtain a platelet count if bruising is the major sign pointing to the diagnosis. Although the clinician may not think that thrombocytopenia is likely, the platelet count may be useful in proving to a court that alternative diagnoses were carefully considered.

Hemophilia usually presents as joint or deep soft tissue bleeding, often after minor trauma. Coagulation study results are usually abnormal, although patients who are only carriers of the condition may require determinations of individual clotting factor levels to make the diagnosis. Even if abuse is strongly suspected as the cause of a soft tissue bleed, documenting normal coagulation studies may strengthen a case if it is brought to court.

Folk medicine practices from many cultures may leave cutaneous signs falsely suggestive of abuse. Cupping, the application of a heated cup to the skin to draw out an ailment, is practiced in some Middle Eastern, Latin American, Chinese, and Eastern European cultures. The procedure may leave circular red lesions, sometimes with petechiae, on the abdomen or other soft tissue areas. The skin within the circle may have been abraded before the cupping. Cao gio, coin rubbing, is a Southeast Asian practice that may leave linear red marks on the back resembling whip or stick welts.

BURNS

Burns are among the most serious forms of intentional injury. They may be inflicted by hot liquids or heated objects. In both cases, the shape of the injury and its depth (i.e., first, second, or third degree) may offer a clue that the cause was not accidental. Tap water or hot drinks cause most hot liquid burns. Many homes have hot water heaters set higher than 130°F to 140°F; water at this temperature can cause a third-degree burn in less than 10 seconds. Immersion in hot liquids as a punishment for messiness or lack of bowel control results in a typical pattern of injury. The burn, which is usually second or third degree, is uniform in depth and has a smooth border corresponding to the liquid's surface. The burn may have a glove or stocking distribution when the child's extremities are immersed. If the child is forcibly seated in a tub of hot water, there may be sparing of thicker skin and skin that protruded from the water or was pressed against the cooler surface of the tub. The soles, knees, and buttocks may be spared, whereas the rest of the legs, perineum, and lower back are burned. Clothing worn during immersion can prolong contact of the skin with hot water and result in unusual burn patterns; outlines of elastic waistbands or folds of cloth may be visible as deeper burns.

Spill or splash burns often show a pattern of flow of the hot liquid over the skin. Some areas may be burned more than others as the liquid cools on its way to and over the body. Splash burns often have satellite lesions from drops of liquid, unlike the large, smooth-bordered lesions of immersion burns.

Burns in the shape of hot solid objects often indicate abuse. Cigarettes, hair curlers, and heating devices are among the more common objects causing questionable burns. The physician is often asked to decide if these burns occurred by accident or if they were inflicted. Inflicted burns are rarely first degree (i.e., only redness and pain). People seeking to harm children with hot objects usually hold the object in place long enough for it to cause a deeper injury. Children are no less sensitive to pain than adults and withdraw from hot objects if given the chance. Some household appliances such as electric curling irons, attain surface temperatures in excess of 280°F, hot enough to cause a second- or third-degree burn in a matter of seconds, and they may remain hot for many minutes after they are unplugged. It may be difficult to differentiate intentional from unintentional injuries attributed to such devices.

The child's size and developmental abilities must be consistent with the history. Immersion burns of the lower extremities are frequently explained by saying that the child fell into the bathtub, often after turning on the water himself. Most children cannot climb until 14 to 16 months of age, and at that stage, they would most likely go face first over a high tub side, if they could get over it at all. It is only later that they learn to swing their legs up and have a chance to enter feet first. Ideally, a visit to the home can be made to see the bathtub and measure its height in relation to the child's height.

Cigarette burns may be difficult to differentiate from impetigo. The location may be helpful; both impetigo and accidental burns are rare on the palms or soles, although these may be prime places for punitively inflicted burns. Accidental brushing of a cigarette (and impetigo) produce injury only to the superficial layers of the skin. A deeper wound is more likely to represent an inflicted burn.

HEAD INJURIES

The child's head is especially vulnerable to intentional injury. During infancy, the head is large and heavy in relation to the rest of the body. The neck muscles are weak and cannot control the head's movements. The infant skull is pliable and more readily transmits force to the brain itself. Head injury must be considered any time a child presents with a change in level of consciousness or with a focal neurologic finding. Care must be taken to keep an open mind about diagnosis until conditions such as meningitis, encephalitis, seizure disorders, diabetic ketoacidosis, and other acute toxic or metabolic conditions have been considered. Patients waiting for computed tomography (CT), usually the definitive procedure to detect head injury, should be closely monitored and sometimes receive treatment for other disorders that cannot yet be ruled out.

Battle's sign (i.e., bruising over the mastoid process behind the ears), raccoon eyes, and blood behind the tympanic membranes may be signs of basilar skull fracture. Some depressed skull fractures can be palpated, although they are difficult to feel if the suspected fracture site is under an area of the scalp that is tender and swollen. Large, boggy areas of the scalp may be associated with blood escaping through a fracture line. However, serious intracranial injuries, even those caused by direct blows, may have few or no external signs of bruising or swelling.

An ophthalmologic examination is essential if head injury is suspected. Shaking of the head or violent compression of the chest may cause retinal hemorrhages. Their presence in the setting of minor head trauma suggests that the history given may be false. They are sometimes the only clue that a child suspected of having meningitis or metabolic disease may have suffered some trauma.

ABDOMINAL INJURIES

Blunt trauma to the abdomen can cause serious injury that is difficult to detect with a physical examination alone. Duodenal hematoma is the lesion most associated with child abuse. Blunt force compresses the small bowel against the vertebral column producing bleeding into the duodenal wall. In the absence of rupture and subsequent peritonitis, patients usually have a history of increasing abdominal pain and anorexia spanning a period of a few days. They are often thought to have a benign gastroenteritis until the hematoma becomes large enough to cause obstruction and bilious vomiting begins. Sometimes an upper abdominal mass is palpable, but the diagnosis is usually made radiographically. A flat plate of the abdomen may or may not show a mass effect, and the obstruction is high enough in the gastrointestinal tract that, with the stomach decompressed, none of the usual signs of obstruction may be present such as air–fluid levels in dilated loops of bowel. Oral contrast studies are most often used to demonstrate the lesion, although ultrasound, abdominal CT scans, and MRI may also be used.

SEXUAL ABUSE

Injuries to the Genitalia

Any injury to the genitalia raises the question of abuse, although this area of the body is also susceptible to unintentional injury. Most children who have been sexually abused have no detectable genital injury. A negative physical examination never rules out sexual abuse.

Female Genitalia

The examination of the prepubertal girl is usually restricted to an inspection of the external genitalia. Patients and parents should be reassured at the outset that an internal examination is not required and that the procedures used are basically the same as those involved in routine well-child care. Girls may be comfortable in the lithotomy position (without stirrups) or they may prefer the prone, knee-to-chest position. The first step in the examination is to inspect the external genitalia, with the labia majora slightly spread, and to document the location of any bruises, lacerations, irritation, or bleeding. Venereal warts, erythematous papules suggesting herpes infection, or chancres may be found.

The next step is to examine the anterior vagina and hymen. The labia minora are retracted until the hymen is visible. The normal hymenal opening may be round, U-shaped, slit-like, pinpoint, or irregular. Important observations include whether the hymen is irregular; the size of the opening; and whether there seems to be any bruising, bleeding, or scarring. Old scars may be visible to the naked eye as areas with a different coloration, as retracted areas or clefts in the hymen, or as adhesions of the hymen to the vaginal wall. Clefts in the lower quadrants of the hymen (from 3–9 o'clock) may be more significant for trauma than clefts in other locations, which are more likely to be normal anatomic variants. Friability or scars of the vaginal mucosa, especially in the posterior fourchette, should be observed. Increased vascularity of the mucosa may also be a sign of old trauma.

Male Genitalia

Penile bruising, erythema, or discharge may suggest abuse. Papules or ulcers may be signs of sexually transmitted diseases (STDs). Phimosis, or a swelling of the foreskin, may be caused by trauma or infection. Small infants may develop phimosis from a piece of hair that accidentally becomes wrapped around the penis. Subsequent swelling and tenderness may make it difficult to find or remove the hair.

Rectal Lesions

Visible injury to the rectum is rare in sexual abuse. Most pedophiles go to great lengths not to inflict trauma so that abuse remains undetected. The anus is expansive, and stools larger than the adult penis can be accommodated without injury. However, some signs may be present, especially after rape. The perirectal area should be examined for scars, warts, petechiae, bruising, and small skin tags. These tags develop as tears or hemorrhoidal bleeding resolve. Children who have been chronically sodomized may have thickening of the perianal skin. Rectal tone may be a clue to the presence of abuse. After forced penetration, the injured sphincter may remain lax for 2 to 4 hours and then go into spasm. Some children who have been chronically abused may develop reflex relaxation of the sphincter in response to a soft stroke on the adjacent buttocks, but this may also develop in children who have been examined repeatedly. Normal children may have an anal "wink," a reflex tightening of the sphincter, with the same stimulation. Few children, even those who have been repeatedly sodomized, have a patulous or lax rectum. An important exception is the child with a spinal cord lesion such as meningomyelocele. Interruptions of the cord in the area of the third sacral vertebra may result in flaccid paralysis of the internal sphincter. A digital examination is not required unless a rectal foreign body or impaction is suspected.

Laboratory Evidence in Cases of Sexual Abuse

Of all the types of child maltreatment, sexual abuse requires the most meticulous collection of laboratory and forensic evidence. Most of this collection is aimed at detecting STDs and other body fluids or tissues that may be transferred from the abuser to the victim during intimate sexual contact. Although this kind of evidence is found only in a minority of cases, it must be looked for carefully if sexual abuse is suspected because it is compelling evidence that abuse has taken place and may help to identify a specific person as being the abuser. A minority of sexually abused children is infected with an STD. Three organisms appear to be almost exclusively associated with sexual activity: *Chlamydia trachomatis*, *Neisseria gonorrhoeae*, and *Trichomonas vaginalis*.

It is important to have a fairly fixed protocol for diagnosis of STDs in sexual abuse cases. Cultures for gonorrheal and chlamydial infection should be obtained from the pharynx, anus, and genitals (i.e., vagina in prepubertal girls, cervix in postpubertal girls if a speculum examination is indicated, urethra from boys). If no symptoms exist and the child is anxious, cultures may be deferred until a follow-up visit a few days later. DNA probes for gonorrhea and chlamydia should be performed in possible cases of sexual abuse.

WET PREPS AND GRAM STAINS

Any obvious discharge should be put on a microscope slide, fixed, and Gram stained using standard procedures. If gonorrhea is found, the microscope slide should be labeled and kept as part of the permanent case records.

A drop of the secretions, diluted with more saline if necessary, should be immediately examined under the microscope for the presence of motile organisms (e.g., *Trichomonas* species) and for sperm. Another drop should be mixed with potassium hydroxide and examined for yeasts and hyphae. If any positive findings are made, another slide should be made and immediately placed in or sprayed with the fixative used for Papanicolaou (Pap) smears. This specimen should be sent to a cytopathology laboratory for official confirmation of the diagnosis. These tests should be coordinated with the other necessary examinations for cases of recent (i.e., within 72 hours) sexual assault.

URINALYSIS

A urinalysis is always indicated in the evaluation of child abuse. It may reveal evidence of retroperitoneal trauma (e.g., blood or heme) or urinary tract infection, or it may be contaminated with a vaginal discharge and help to diagnose a genital infection. Urine that shows signs of infection should be Gram stained and sent for culture.

SEROLOGY

A RPR test or some other screening test for syphilis should be performed, although it may be deferred for a few days if it would be traumatic to perform a venipuncture at the initial examination. If the suspected abuse is recent (i.e., within the last few weeks), a follow-up titer should be drawn 1 to 2 months later.

FORENSIC PROCEDURES

If abuse or assault has occurred within the past 48 to 72 hours, it may be possible to detect secretions or tissues from the abuser on the victim's body. This may provide important evidence to demonstrate that abuse has taken place and may even help to identify the abuser. The procedures must be carefully followed to collect and preserve available evidence. Many communities have referral centers that specialize in the collection and interpretation of forensic evidence in cases of possible sexual abuse. Children can be referred to these centers if the suspected abuse has occurred within 72 hours.

SKELETAL TRAUMA

Bone Lesions Highly Suggestive of Abuse

METAPHYSEAL INJURIES

Injuries to the metaphyses of the long bones are among the lesions thought to be most diagnostic of intentional injury. They occur when the limbs are subjected to pulling and torsional forces as a child is shaken or pulled violently causing fractures through newly forming bone just under (on the diaphysis side of) the growth plate. A thin disc of bone is formed just under the radiolucent growth plate and epiphysis. Projected onto radiographic film, the disk appears as tufts, arcs, or irregularities at the ends of the bone. The most common place to see these injuries is in the distal humerus and femur or the proximal tibia. The metaphysis appears irregular and may have spurs or displaced chips.

RIB FRACTURES

Rib fractures in young children are usually nondisplaced and visible only after healing has begun. They may occur posteriorly near the attachment to the spine, possibly as a result of a direct blow on the back or from squeezing the sides of the chest, or occur laterally in the midaxillary line, possibly from anteroposterior forces. Lateral fractures are difficult to see on standard chest radiographic films because they are hidden by the overlapping shadows of the curving ribs. Oblique views of the chest should be obtained if any question of irregularity exists.

COMPLEX SKULL FRACTURES

Simple, nondisplaced linear fractures of the parietal bone seem to occur from relatively minor trauma, although they can occur from abuse as well. Fractures that are wide (greater than 3 mm), complex (e.g., branching fracture lines, multiple fractures, involvement of skull suture lines), or occur outside the parietal bone suggest significant force. These findings are consistent with an automobile accident, a fall from a considerable height, or a forceful blow to the head. A history of minor trauma or no known trauma at all, combined with the finding of a complex fracture, strongly suggests abuse.

Bone Lesions Less Suggestive of Abuse

Spiral or oblique fractures of the long bones are frequently cited as signs of abuse. However, they may occur in any setting in which rotational force occurs on a bone. These forces frequently occur when the leg or arm is trapped under the rest of the body during a fall. Transverse fractures may actually be more common in abuse, because they imply a direct blow to the bone or the snapping of the bone over a fulcrum-like object. All of these fractures require careful attention to the details of the injury itself and an assessment of what other factors in the family may be grounds for suspecting abuse.

Bone Lesions Rarely Suggestive of Abuse

Two common injuries rarely indicate abuse. The "nursemaid's elbow" (i.e., subluxation of the head of the radius) occurs when force is applied to the already extended elbow joint. These injuries typically occur when toddlers are walking along with an adult and are being held by the hand. The toddler's arm is extended above his or her head. If the toddler trips and the adult holds on, pulling and twisting on the elbow can cause a dislocation. Some children appear to be congenitally susceptible to this injury and repeatedly dislocate the same elbow in the same fashion.

WHIPLASH OR SHAKEN BABY SYNDROME

Signs

The syndrome's major injuries are believed to occur when the infant is held by the chest and violently shaken. Flailing of the limbs causes metaphyseal lesions, and shaking of the head causes tears to bridging vessels and subdural bleeding. Variants of the syndrome may occur if the head strikes a solid object or if compression of the chest occurs. Skull and rib fractures, and retinal and intracranial hemorrhages, may then result.

Symptoms of brain injury are what usually cause parents to bring the child for medical care. Seizures or respiratory arrest may occur immediately or may develop over a period of days as a subdural fluid collection increases in size. Alternatively, the child may present with developmental abnormalities, irritability, and an enlarged head or bulging fontanelle (again, secondary to subdural fluid or hydrocephalus). It is important for the clinician to keep trauma in mind as a possibility while considering other diagnoses.

Parents usually relate no history of trauma, or only that of a minor fall. There may be a history of colic or other infant temperament, feeding, or sleeping problem that stresses caretakers. Usually no external findings of trauma are found. Often retinal hemorrhage is the only sign visible without radiologic studies.

Vital signs and laboratory studies may also be misleading. There may be instability of blood pressure and an elevation of the peripheral white blood cell count suggestive of infection. Bloody spinal taps may be ascribed to traumatic procedures, but the fluid should be centrifuged and the supernatant examined. A supernatant that is colored by broken-down red blood cells (i.e., xanthochromic) suggests that the blood is actually coming from within the central nervous system. Chest films obtained in the course of evaluation for sepsis should be carefully examined for rib fractures.

Differential Diagnosis

The most frequently raised alternative diagnosis to the shaken baby syndrome is that of birth trauma. Intracranial bleeding and the development of subdural hematomas or hydrocephalus are associated with precipitous vaginal deliveries of large babies, often to primiparous mothers. These injuries appear to be rare given current obstetric practices, but when they do occur, they usually present at 4 to 8 weeks of life with an enlarged head circumference and sometimes (especially if hydrocephalus is present) with neurologic findings. In contrast, the median age for presentation of the shaken baby syndrome is 6 months, and many of these children are acutely ill. Retinal hemorrhages may also occur during delivery, but they do not persist after the first weeks of life. The hemorrhages associated with trauma persist for long periods. Therefore, the most difficult cases are children in the first few months of life who have subdural effusions, normal development, and no history of precipitous or traumatic birth. At present, there seems to be no way to say whether these children have suffered intentional injury.

MUNCHAUSEN SYNDROME BY PROXY

Signs

Many presentations of the syndrome can occur. In some cases, long but vague histories of difficult-to-document medical complaints (e.g., hyperactivity, somnolence, seizures, or abdominal, chest, or head pains) are accompanied by doctor shopping, erratic compliance with suggested treatment, and lack of satisfaction with negative findings on evaluation. Bleeding, hematuria, and hematemesis are also common signs. Parents have been known to put their own blood in the child's urine or stool samples during the course of a workup. Cases have been reported of blood removal from indwelling central venous catheters. Presenting central nervous system problems, including drowsiness, coma, seizures, and apnea, may be symptoms of ingestion, head trauma (including the shaken baby syndrome), or suffocation. In some cases, laboratory test results may be returned with values that do not have ready physiologic explanations or that suggest too many simultaneously occurring illnesses to be likely. If real, the findings may be the result of salt or fluid poisoning; if factitious, they may be the result of "doctored" laboratory specimens.

Children hospitalized for mysterious conditions often get better in the hospital only to suddenly worsen when discharge is planned. In many cases of intentional poisonings, parents have continued administration of the toxic substance during the child's hospitalization.

Common Family Findings

The child's mother is often the perpetrator in cases of Munchausen syndrome by proxy. She is often perceived by the hospital staff as a model mother during the child's hospitalization; she is always helpful on the ward and solicitous of the staff. It is not clear if this represents a conscious effort to deceive the staff or is a reflection of the mother's abnormally great need for affection and belonging. She may have a history of medical illness or complaints similar to that of the child and may have been prescribed drugs that are used to poison the child. She may have a history of medical training or extensive contact with medical care settings giving her knowledge of symptoms that elicit attention from the staff and allowing her to give convincing descriptions of these symptoms.

In some cases, the syndrome seems to have its origins in an abnormally symbiotic mother-child relationship in which the mother creates a special sick-role bond between herself and her child. The child may adopt the sick role as a means of staying close to the mother. In this way, the Munchausen syndrome by proxy has much in common with school avoidance and other parent-child separation problems. The father may take a distant or passive role in all of the child's illnesses. He may leave medical decisions about the child to the mother and may seem to have little regard for the apparently serious illness being experienced by the child.

Diagnosis

Detection of the Munchausen syndrome by proxy requires a high index of suspicion. It should be considered if confronted with a medical history or constellation of symptoms that does not make sense or cannot be verified from previous records. Children with such problems are often hospitalized as a chance for further consultation and controlled observation of the symptoms. Hidden cameras are sometimes used to document the offense. During the hospitalization, the physician should inquire about illnesses in other family members, especially siblings. The occurrence of similar problems or the death of a sibling should be closely investigated. Independent confirmation of these facts and records from any previous source of medical care must be obtained.

Inquiries should be made about medications that may be in the home or illnesses of family members that may require toxic medications. Complete toxicology screens should be considered for patients with altered mental status, especially delirium. If the sensitivity of hospital testing is unknown, extra urine and serum samples should be obtained for freezing and further testing if required. If toxic drugs are known to be in the home, they should be mentioned specifically on the test requisition. This may help the laboratory to screen the samples more efficiently.

Ultimately, the diagnosis of Munchausen syndrome by proxy is usually made in one of two ways. The clinical team is able to confront the parent with incontrovertible evidence of induced or factitious illness (e.g., adult blood in the child's urine, a toxic substance discovered in the child's blood), or the parent is actually observed tampering with a specimen or injuring the child. Many such abusers still deny having caused the child's illness, even if they acknowledge that somehow the child was poisoned. Unless the evidence specifically links the parent to the injury, observation and entrapment may be the only way to prove the identity of the perpetrator or to convince social service authorities to take action to protect the child.

CHILD NEGLECT

Physical Neglect

Physical neglect includes the failure to provide basic food, shelter, and clothing. These requirements may be taken to mean food with calories and nutrients sufficient for normal growth; shelter that is safe, sanitary, and adequately ventilated or heated; and clothing that is in good repair and appropriate for the weather.

Children require adequate supervision for their safety and emotional well-being. Parents are given the responsibility of ensuring that this supervision is provided by themselves or by someone they designate. Substitute caretakers should have sufficient information to care for the child and to contact the parent in the case of an emergency. Preadolescent children are usually not suitable caretakers for their younger siblings, even on a short-term basis.

Medical Neglect

Failure to obtain recommended preventive care, lack of compliance with prescribed treatment, or delays in seeking care for acute illnesses may constitute medical neglect. The failure to obtain prenatal care or the use of harmful drugs or alcohol during pregnancy may also be considered medically abusive or neglectful. Making the determination of neglect in these situations may not be easy. The decision may be clouded by conflicts between the clinician and the parents or by judgments about the parents' lifestyle. By law, parents are not permitted to neglect their children's education, and in many jurisdictions, immunizations are also compulsory aspects of medical care that parents must provide.

Safe Placement of the Victim

A critical question is whether it is safe for an abuse victim to return home. If medical problems require hospitalization, an admission is indicated, and sometimes conditions that are otherwise treatable on an outpatient basis require admission for psychological support or because reliable care at home cannot be guaranteed. The hospital staff must be informed of the medical indications for such admissions. Patients who are labeled as social admissions may not receive appropriate medical and emotional support.

When it is medically appropriate for the victim to be discharged, several factors can be considered. Has the perpetrator been identified and, if so, can he or she be kept from contact with the victim? Can the victim receive sufficient support and protection in the home? The home environment must be physically safe, but it must also be emotionally supportive.

How did the abusive crisis occur? Is it a general symptom of the family's level of stress or lack of resources? If abusing parents, for example, continue to show extreme anxiety and inability to cope and if the stresses that contributed to abuse continue to exist, the risk of repeat abuse may be high. Families that have a long history of dysfunction or that have no immediately available outside contacts may prove to be at risk for repeat abuse.

Is there evidence of serious mental illness in the abuser? This includes abuse without any apparent stressors or risk factors, injuries that seem premeditated or are characterized by torture or sadism, evidence of sociopathic behavior (e.g., violent outbursts, frequent previous involvement with legal difficulties), and distorted views of reality (e.g., seeing the child as evil or inherently sick). Injuries justified by unusual or rigid moral or religious beliefs also present a high risk of recurrence.

Safety issues involving pedophiles and incest offenders may be especially difficult to evaluate. These persons typically go through cycles of offense, remorse, and repeat offense. In their remorseful state, they may convincingly seem to be under control and fully motivated to not offend again. A suppression effect often exists at the time of disclosure, and in the short-term, the offenders appear to lose interest in offending. However, pedophile or incest behavior can be seen as a habituated behavior such as alcohol or drug abuse, over which the abuser initially has little control. For this reason, regardless of the abuser's initial appearance, many therapists consider separation of the sex offender and victim mandatory, at least until the victim is psychologically prepared and adequate safety can be guaranteed.

Child Protective Services (CPS) agencies are given the authority and responsibility to protect children suspected of being abused or neglected. Their initial approach is often to make a contract, sometimes written, with a family, and voluntary arrangements are made for the child's safety and the abuser's conduct. The abuser may agree to stay out of the home, and the nonabusing parent may promise to call the police if the abuser returns. The parents may agree to have the child live with a close relative or family friend with whom his or her safety will be assured. If the family is unwilling, the CPS agency may go before a family or juvenile court and get an order, enforceable by the police, granting authority over the child's whereabouts to CPS. The child may still be placed at home, with relatives, or in a foster home, but the agency is given formal legal authority, and the parents' consent is not required.

Whenever possible, the offender, not the victim, should be removed from the home. However, placement of the victim is sometimes unavoidable. In this case, several steps can be taken to ease the difficulty of separation. To the extent possible, parents and children should be involved in the decision to place the victim outside of the home. Everyone should understand the rationale for placement, why other alternatives are not appropriate, and that the separation is temporary. Care must be taken that removal is not seen by the parents or children as a punitive step, but rather viewed as a move that is therapeutic for the victim and the abuser. The best placements are with close family members or with a member of the extended family who can come and live with the child in his or her own home. The person caring for the child must be prepared to help overcome the guilt feelings that the child may have about causing the separation and must be careful not to vilify the offending parent. If possible, siblings should remain together, and familiar objects and toys should accompany the children. Preliminary plans for visitation should be discussed before the actual separation takes place.

CHAPTER 67

Acute Head Trauma

Adapted from N. Paul Rosman

Pediatric head injuries are a very important cause of childhood morbidity and mortality in the United States, where 2 to 5 million children sustain some degree of head trauma each year. The frequency is greater in children from birth to 5 years than in those who are older. Such injuries—twice as frequent in boys as in girls—have many different causes including falls, bicycling and other recreational activities, competitive sports (e.g., football, ice hockey, and boxing), motor vehicle accidents, and assaults including child abuse. Every year in the United States, approximately 200,000 children are hospitalized with head injuries, and approximately 5,000 children die as a result of such trauma. Thus, mortality from pediatric head injuries has been estimated to be as high as 10 per 100,000 per year. Of these 5,000 deaths, approximately 1,500 occur from child abuse. For each fatality in the United States each year, five persons are hospitalized and 27 are examined but not hospitalized for brain injury. The worldwide incidence of brain injury may be as high as 500 million cases per year.

CLINICAL SYNDROMES IN ACUTELY HEAD-INJURED CHILDREN

Scalp Injuries and Swellings

Contusion and laceration are probably the most frequent complications of head injury. Lacerations should be cleaned thoroughly and sutured, if necessary. An underlying (depressed) skull fracture should be sought.

In older children, most scalp swellings after head trauma are the result of subgaleal hematomas, but other possibilities must be considered, particularly in newborns. In neonates, diffuse scalp swelling with decreased transillumination suggests a subgaleal hematoma, whereas diffuse scalp swelling with increased transillumination indicates a caput succedaneum. When the scalp swelling is focal, an affected newborn very likely has a cephalhematoma (subperiosteal hemorrhage), particularly when the swelling is parietal in location and transillumination is decreased. In approximately 5% to 25% of patients, an accompanying skull fracture is present. When the swelling is focal and transillumination is increased, a porencephalic or leptomeningeal cyst with an associated "growing" skull fracture is suggested.

No treatment is required for subgaleal hematoma, caput succedaneum, or cephalhematoma; in fact, aspiration of fluid from the scalp is contraindicated because of possible complicating infection. Cephalhematomas commonly calcify and are reabsorbed into the underlying bony calvarium. A leptomeningeal cyst must be treated surgically, however, with removal or replacement of protruding arachnoid and repair of the dural tear.

Skull Fractures

Six major varieties of skull fractures can occur in childhood: linear, depressed, compound, basal, diastatic, and growing. Linear skull fractures constitute approximately 75% of pediatric skull fractures; they are especially frequent in children younger than 2 years, and most are temporoparietal in location. Although they need not be treated themselves, such fractures may overlie serious intracranial pathologic conditions such as an epidural hemorrhage, for which treatment is urgently required. Thus, if a linear fracture involves the temporal bone or the sagittal suture, a CT scan should be performed promptly. Linear fractures heal within 1 to 2 months. When found in infants or young children, the possibility of neglect or inflicted injury must always be considered.

In depressed skull fractures, either continuity of the bony calvaria is disrupted or the skull may simply be indented, resulting in a ping-pong or pond fracture unaccompanied by a break in the cranial vault. Compound, or open-skull, fractures have a direct communication between a scalp laceration and the fracture site. These fractures are called penetrating if a tear in the dura is also present. These fractures are of urgent concern because of the danger of complicating infection.

Two main varieties of basal fractures are frontobasal and petrous. Because of the anatomic complexity of the base of the skull, only approximately 20% of basal skull fractures can be recognized on standard skull radiography. Although the addition of multiplanar tomography and thin-section CT substantially increases the frequency with which such fractures can be demonstrated radiographically, usually the firm diagnosis of basal skull fracture depends on the recognition of coexisting signs. This diagnosis can often be inferred, if not confirmed, by coexisting signs that include hemorrhage in the nose, nasopharynx, or middle ear; overlying the mastoid bone (Battle sign); or around the eyes ("raccoon eyes").

Diastatic skull fractures are traumatic separations of cranial bones at one or more suture sites. Most frequently, they affect the lambdoid suture and occur in the first 4 years of life. Such fractures should be followed closely in children younger than 3 years because they can become sites of so-called growing fractures. Growing skull fractures are caused by herniation of tissue through torn dura and an accompanying fracture (linear or diastatic) into the overlying scalp. Such fractures occur most often in the parietal region. The herniating tissue is either solid brain parenchyma or cystic in nature, usually a porencephalic cyst (communicating with a lateral ventricle) or (less often) a leptomeningeal cyst.

ACUTE INJURY TO BRAIN

Cerebral Concussion

Concussion is an alteration in mental state, with or without loss of consciousness, that occurs immediately after a head injury. Usually, the causative trauma is direct and blunt. Generally, the force of injury needed to produce a concussion is somewhat less than that required to produce a skull fracture. Concussion is much more likely to occur when the head moves freely after impact (acceleration-deceleration) than when the head is firmly in place (compression). Concussion can also occur in the absence of direct head trauma if sufficient force of whiplash type is applied to the brain. Concussive injuries cause an increase in intracranial pressure (ICP), followed by a temporary shear strain on the upper brainstem, resulting in an altered mental state. The brain that has received a concussive injury does not show any consistent morphologic abnormality, underscoring the probable subcellular basis of the disorder. Apparently, clinical state is caused by suddenly increased and unmet energy demands of the brain.

Confusion and amnesia are the hallmarks of concussion. Early symptoms of concussion (minutes to hours) include headache, dizziness, lack of awareness of surroundings, nausea, and vomiting. Concussion, when accompanied by loss of consciousness, is commonly associated with three types of amnesia: (a) temporary retrograde that antedates the head injury, sometimes by 2 years; (b) permanent retrograde that encompasses the few seconds to minutes immediately before the injury; and (c) temporary posttraumatic (anterograde) characterized by impaired ability to form new memories usually lasting for some hours after the accident. Late symptoms of concussion (days to weeks) include headache, lightheadedness, inattention, memory disturbance, fatigability, irritability, low frustration threshold, photophobia, impaired visual focus, sonophobia, tinnitus, anxiety, depression, and sleep disturbance.

CONCUSSION AND CONTACT SPORTS

The severity of concussion must be considered in deciding whether an injured player can return to athletic competition. Grade 1 concussion is characterized by transient confusion, no loss of consciousness, and clearing of mental status in less than 15 minutes. The characteristics of grade 2 concussion are the same as those for grade 1 except that mental status changes last longer than 15 minutes. In grade 3 concussion, a period of unconsciousness exists. On the basis of the severity of the concussion and the sideline evaluation of the athlete with a concussive injury (mental status testing, neurologic tests, provocative exercise tests), recommendations have been put forth by the Quality Standards Subcommittee of the American Academy of Neurology outlining the additional evaluations that can help in deciding when such players might be permitted to return to competitive play.

Among contact sports, concussion is particularly frequent in ice hockey and football. Most collected data have focused on football, for in the United States, 20% of high school football players and 10% of college football players sustain a cerebral concussion. The risk of sustaining a concussion in football is four to six times greater for a player with a previous concussion than for players who have no such history. Repeated concussions have been shown to cause cumulative neuropsychological and neuroanatomic damage, even when the incidents are separated by months or years. The so-called second-impact syndrome is the result of a second concussion while an affected individual is still symptomatic from an earlier event. One postulation is that the first insult disturbs the brain's autoregulatory mechanisms with consequent vascular congestion and poor brain compliance. Because of this presumed poor compliance, malignant brain swelling after a relatively minor second impact can result in a marked increase in ICP and in rapid deterioration. Such swelling is seen more commonly in children than in adults. The results of such second-impact injuries can be catastrophic with permanent disability or death.

POSTCONCUSSIVE SYNDROME

Although children with concussions should be followed closely for at least 24 hours, with particular attention given to alertness, responsiveness, and vital signs, most children who suffer an uncomplicated cerebral concussion recover uneventfully. Some children, however, can be fairly disabled if they develop postconcussion syndrome. Actually, two pediatric postconcussion syndromes can be seen: one in adolescents, the other in younger children. Symptoms in adolescents, which include headache, dizziness, irritability, and impaired concentration, are usually relatively mild and self-limited. By contrast, younger children show behavioral changes that can include aggression, disobedience, behavioral regression, inattention, and anxiety. The duration of such symptoms can vary from several days to several months and, on occasion, can persist.

The pathogenesis of the postconcussion syndrome is unsettled. Organic, environmental, and emotional factors have variously been cited. Evidence for an organic basis for this disorder is mounting, however, with minor physiologic and anatomic alterations of axons, primarily in brainstem, believed to be important in causation. The occurrence of attention deficits as a prominent manifestation of the postconcussion syndrome suggests persisting dysfunction of deep subcortical structures including the medial temporal lobes and upper brainstem. Because temporal lobe or partial complex seizures may follow head trauma, their presence must always be considered in a child with a posttraumatic behavioral change. Also, anticonvulsants, particularly phenobarbital, may affect a child's personality and behavior adversely.

A common triad of symptoms that often follows minor head injuries in young children includes lethargy, irritability, and vomiting, unaccompanied by loss of consciousness. These symptoms, attributed to torsion of the brainstem, usually subside within 48 to 72 hours.

Acute Epidural and Subdural Hematomas

The clinical points that aid in the diagnosis of and differentiation between acute epidural and subdural intracranial hematomas are outlined in Table 67-1. The relatively large volumes of extravasated blood in epidural and subdural hematomas typically produce symptoms and signs of increased ICP. These include irritability or lethargy, vomiting, fullness of the anterior fontanelle, headache and papilledema, and elevation of systolic blood pressure, with a decreased or increased pulse rate, and slowed, irregular respirations. With sufficient elevation of pressure in the supratentorial compartment, unilateral transtentorial herniation may occur. The signs and symptoms of such herniation were discussed.

TABLE 67-1. Clinical Features of Acute Epidural and Subdural Hematomas

Clinical feature	Epidural hematoma	Subdural hematoma
Supratentorial		
Frequency	Less than subdural	5–10 times greater than epidural
Skull fracture	70%	30%
Source of hemorrhage	Arterial or venous	Almost always venous
Age	Usually >2 yr	Usually <1 yr
Location	Usually temporoparietal	Usually frontoparietal
Laterality	Usually unilateral	75% bilateral
Seizures	<25%	75%
Preretinal and retinal hemorrhages	Uncommon	Very frequent
Increased intracranial pressure	Present	Present
Cranial computed tomographic configuration	Usually lenticular	Curvilinear or crescentic
Mortality	Relatively high	Usually lower than epidural
Morbidity	Low	High
Infratentorial		
Frequency	2–3 times greater than subdural	Less than epidural
Skull fracture	Almost always	Frequent
Source of hemorrhage	Venous	Venous
Impaired consciousness	Frequent	Frequent
Acute hydrocephalus/medullary compression	Variable	Variable
Other posterior fossa signs	Variable	Variable

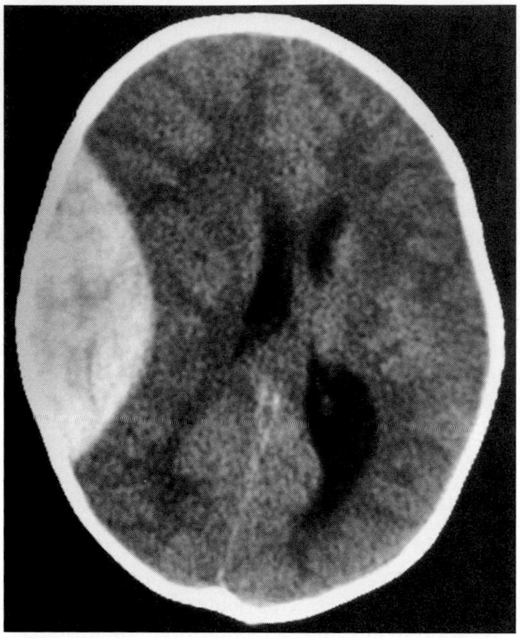

Figure 67-1. Cranial computed tomographic scan shows a large right-sided epidural hematoma with a characteristic biconvex appearance in a 10-month-old girl after a fall onto the back of her head. The midline structures are displaced to the left, causing effacement of much of the right lateral ventricle, with dilation of the frontal horns of both lateral ventricles and of the posterior portion of the left lateral ventricle.

Cranial CT is particularly valuable in differentiating between acute epidural and subdural hematomas. The former usually assumes a lens-like (biconvex) configuration (Fig. 67-1), contrasting with the curvilinear or crescentic shape of the latter; however, exceptions are common. Both types of hematomas may coexist in the same patient. The mortality in children with acute epidural hematoma has varied from 9% to 17%, but survivors tend to be relatively free of neurologic residua. Although mortality from acute subdural hematoma has occurred less frequently compared to acute epidural hematoma, in some series, it has been as high as 17% to 20%. Further, morbidity (i.e., motor deficits, seizures, cognitive impairment) is greater with the acute subdural hematoma because of the frequency of accompanying injury to the underlying brain.

When epidural hemorrhage is suspected clinically, usually the diagnosis should be confirmed by cranial CT; however, such hematomas may progress so rapidly with signs of acutely elevated ICP and progressive hemiparesis that immediate neurosurgical treatment is required [i.e., craniotomy, surgical removal of blood clot, and identification (if possible) of the bleeding source].

When subdural hemorrhage is suspected clinically, neurosurgical intervention is rarely needed before confirmation of the diagnosis by cranial CT. Occasionally, however, with acutely elevated ICP in infants in whom a subdural hematoma is suspected, the subdural space should be tapped as a combined diagnostic and therapeutic measure.

Subacute and Chronic Subdural Hematomas

In addition to acute subdural hematomas, in which symptoms appear during the first 48 hours, such hematomas can be subacute (symptoms appearing between 3 and 21 days) or chronic (symptoms appearing after 21 days). Unlike acute subdural hematomas, which are most frequent in infants, most chronic subdural hematomas occur in older children and adolescents. In these less acute hematomas, as in the acute, recurrent vomiting from intracranial hypertension can occur. Macrocrania, reflecting a longer-standing increase in ICP, is often present; additionally, the head may have a box-like appearance.

MRI is the ideal imaging modality to demonstrate these lesions. MRI findings depend on the predominant type of hemoglobin found in the hematoma, which varies with age. Initially, the hematoma is composed primarily of oxyhemoglobin and has a signal intensity that is isointense with brain on T1-weighted images and either isointense or hyperintense with brain on T2-weighted images. Over the first few hours, oxyhemoglobin is converted to deoxyhemoglobin with signal intensity that continues to be isointense on T1-weighted images but hypointense on T2-weighted images. Starting 2 to 4 days after the trauma, deoxyhemoglobin is then converted to methemoglobin, which shows increased signal intensity on T1-weighted images and low or increased signal intensity on T2-weighted images. Eventually, the red blood cells in the hematoma break down, and the clot becomes composed of extracellular methemoglobin, which is hyperintense on T1- and T2-weighted images. As subdural hematomas become chronic, a thick outer membrane and a thin inner membrane begin to develop at 1 and 3 weeks, respectively.

The methods of treatment used in the management of these hematomas include (a) subdural taps with aspiration of subdural fluid; (b) external drainage with shunting of fluid from the subdural space to the peritoneum or to a pleural cavity; and (c) burr holes (or occasionally craniotomy) with aspiration or surgical removal of subdural clots.

PROGNOSIS IN ACUTE BRAIN INJURIES

Most children hospitalized after a head injury with an accompanying concussion, skull fracture, or cerebral contusion will recover completely, usually within 1 to several days; a small number of such children, however, develop a postconcussion syndrome or posttraumatic seizures. An even smaller number will have sustained a severe head injury with prolonged coma followed by persisting cognitive, behavioral, or motor deficits.

Severe head injuries in children younger than 4 years and in adolescents produce a higher mortality than those in school-aged children. Similarly, morbidity is greater in preschool children than in children who are older. These differences can be explained, at least in large measure, by differences in the types of traumas sustained most often by children of different ages. In infants, toddlers, and young children, diffuse injuries and multiple insults are common (e.g., falls, child abuse). In school-aged children, injuries are often focal and less severe (e.g., bicycle accidents, sports injuries). Older children and adolescents, on the other hand, tend to suffer more impact injuries (e.g., motor vehicle accidents).

Duration of Posttraumatic Coma and Neurologic Outcome

Posttraumatic coma of less than 24 hours is rarely associated with permanent neurologic or neuropsychological sequelae in the head-injured child. In severely head-injured children age 10 or younger, the average length of coma for those returning to normal intelligence was 1.7 weeks; for borderline intelligence, 3 weeks; for mild retardation, 8 weeks; and for severe retardation, 11 weeks. Usually, children older than age 10 had longer durations of coma and a similar relationship between duration of coma and cognitive outcome. Such benchmarks notwithstanding, children and adolescents have a greater capacity than that of adults for recovering from severe head injuries and can show improvement in cognitive and social skills for more than 3 years.

The Glasgow Coma Scale (GCS) score obtained 12 months after a head injury is the outcome statistic compared most frequently in different series. Of those children who, by 12 months, had made a good recovery or who by then were moderately disabled, almost two-thirds had already reached this level within 3 months of the injury, and 90% had done so by 6 months. Only 10% of those children who were severely or moderately disabled at 6 months were in the next better category by 1 year. Only 5% improved sufficiently after 12 months to reach a better category.

Neurologic Outcome in Mild Head Injuries

Mild head injuries are caused by blunt trauma or sudden acceleration-deceleration with periods of unconsciousness for 20 minutes or less, a GCS score of 13 to 15, no intracranial complications, and cranial CT findings limited to skull fracture. Most children with these types of injuries appear to recover quickly and completely, although later neurologic deficits, often quite subtle, are sometimes found. These deficits include symptoms of postconcussion syndrome, temporary cognitive difficulties, behavioral changes, and occasional posttraumatic seizures.

CHAPTER 68
Status Epilepticus

Adapted from Daniel G. Glaze

Status epilepticus (SE) may be defined as seizure activity that lasts longer than 15 to 30 minutes or repeated seizures between which the child does not return to the baseline level of consciousness. In convulsive SE, the child has a prolonged, generalized tonic-clonic seizure or the repetition of such seizures without a return to full consciousness between episodes. In nonconvulsive SE such as absence status and complex partial status, the clinical presentation is a prolonged twilight or semicoma state. In epilepsia partialis continua, consciousness is preserved in the face of continuous, focal motor activity. Most SE episodes in children appear to be generalized convulsive in character. Of those SE episodes beginning with partial seizures, most secondarily generalize. Careful history taking and observation suggest that the majority (64% of adults and children) of all SE episodes begin as partial seizures that generalize so that the final character is generalized.

EPIDEMIOLOGY

The burden of SE is significant. One epidemiologic study estimated the overall (adults and children) incidence of SE to be 61 per 100,000 and that SE results in an estimated 42,000 deaths (children and adults) per year in the United States. The age distribution of SE suggests two age peaks: during the first year of life (the time of the highest frequency of SE) and in individuals 60 years or older. In children, 21% of all cases of SE occur in the first year of life and 64% in the first 5 years. Approximately 12% of patients with newly diagnosed epilepsy have a seizure lasting 30 minutes or longer. The greatest proportion of cases of SE occur in children, and less than 25% occur as idiopathic events. The occurrence of SE should prompt a full diagnostic workup.

MORBIDITY AND MORTALITY

Previously, overall mortality figures as high as 30% were reported but, more recently, investigators have reported a mortality of 3% to 6% in children. This decrease in mortality is the result of more rapid diagnosis and support combined with better medical treatment and improved intensive care. Death is usually attributable to the underlying cause of SE rather than to a prolonged seizure. When this information is considered, mortality related to prolonged seizures per se has been reported to be as low as 1% to 2%. SE can be associated with significant mortality and morbidity that can include epileptic brain damage, neurologic cognitive defects, and continuing recurrent seizures.

Three factors appear to be related to mortality and morbidity: duration of SE, age, and etiology. Greater mortality is observed if SE lasts longer than 1 hour. Prolonged seizures can lead to a series of metabolic derangements that can potentially cause neuronal damage. Tonic-clonic SE that progresses beyond 60 minutes may be associated with severe, permanent brain damage or death. The significance of prolonged SE, frequently defined as seizures of greater than 1 hour's duration, has been observed in humans and experimental animals. In animals with experimentally induced seizures of less than 1 hour's duration, reversible neuronal injuries are produced. However, if seizure duration is greater than 1 hour, neuronal death involving the hippocampus, amygdala, thalamus, and middle cerebral cortical layers is observed, even though reversible changes also occur in the cerebellum as a result of ventilation and metabolic support. Initial increases in cerebral blood flow and glucose consumption are followed after 60 to 120 minutes of seizure activity by decreased cerebral blood flow but continuing glucose consumption. Excessive enhancement of local metabolic rates may result in selective cell death. The initial systemic effects of SE include an increase in plasma catecholamines, an increase in blood pressure, tachycardia, and hyperpyrexia. These effects are self-correcting with the cessation of SE. Late effects that may be less amenable to correction include hypotension, hypoglycemia, acidosis, pulmonary edema, hyperpyrexia, and rhabdomyolysis. They may contribute to significant mortality and morbidity. These findings in humans and animal models emphasize the importance of prompt cessation of SE and the management and correction of the systemic effects of SE.

In most series, mortality is significantly lower in children. One study found that mortality was less than 5% in children versus 26% in adults and more than 50% in adults older than 80 years. Differences in etiology in children versus adults contribute to this observation. SE may occur in the setting of an acute illness, in patients with established epilepsy, or as a first unprovoked seizure. Etiologies can be classified as idiopathic, remote symptomatic, febrile, acute symptomatic, or associated with a progressive encephalopathy. Although 6% to 12% of SE episodes in children represent a first unprovoked seizure, a cause should be investigated. Infectious processes, toxic or metabolic disorders, and chronic forms of encephalopathy, as well as the sudden withdrawal of antiepileptic drugs, may underlie or precipitate this condition in children. In known epileptics, antiepileptic drug noncompliance or low levels should be considered. If a child has a known preexistent neurologic or other medical abnormality, complications (e.g., shunt malfunction, central nervous system hemorrhage or infection) should be considered. In adults, anoxic/hypoxic-ischemic insults account for significant mortality; these etiologies are observed in children infrequently. More frequent etiologic factors in children include central nervous system infections (meningoencephalitis), metabolic aberrations, febrile seizures, and "idiopathic" epilepsy. These factors have a lower incidence of associated mortality and morbidity. In children, most fatalities are associated with acute central nervous system insult or progressive neurologic disorders.

SEQUELAE

Neurologic sequelae in children with idiopathic or febrile SE are rare (1.5% versus 9.1% for all etiologies). In addition, incidence of recurrent seizures after SE in children is low. Risk of recurrent episodes of convulsive SE approaches 50% in neurologically abnormal children but is very low in neurologically normal children. After SE as the first unprovoked seizure in a neurologically normal child, no increased risk of seizure recurrence is observed. Some authors suggest that initiating long-term therapy for a normal child whose first seizure is an episode of SE is not necessary. Factors influencing a favorable outcome of SE in children may be related to advances in therapy, prompt and aggressive management of seizure and systemic abnormalities, and the resistance of the immature brain to damage from seizures.

TREATMENT

Tonic-clonic SE is a life-threatening situation and represents a neurologic emergency. The longer the seizure lasts, the more difficult it will be to stop. The therapeutic measures outlined here are appropriate in cases in which a seizure or repeated seizures continue unabated for 15 to 30 minutes. Some clinicians consider almost any tonic-clonic seizure to be an episode of SE and intervene with both supportive and drug therapy.

Therapy must address the immediate problem of stopping the seizure, providing supportive measures (supplemental oxygen, a clear airway, an intravenous glucose source, etc.), detecting and correcting any predisposing or precipitating factors, and incorporating a drug with a long half-life to prevent the recurrence of seizures once they have been arrested.

SUPPORTIVE MEASURES

The preservation of vital functions takes precedence:

- Blood pressure, respiration, and cardiac function are maintained to avoid hypoxic-ischemic damage to the brain. Resuscitation equipment should be available.
- Blood samples are obtained for electrolyte, glucose, blood urea nitrogen, calcium, and magnesium measurements and, if the patient has been treated previously for seizures, for antiepileptic drug level determinations.
- An intravenous line is inserted for the infusion of a glucose solution to maintain the blood sugar level at approximately 150 mg/dL. Fluids should be limited initially to 1,000 to 1,200 mL/m^2.
- Increased intracranial pressure is treated if evident.

DRUG THERAPY

Excluding infants who are younger than 2 to 3 months, diazepam in an intravenous dose of 0.25 to 0.30 mg/kg may be given (maximum dose 5 mg in children younger than 5 years and 10 mg in children 5 to 10 years old). In children who are 5 to 10 years old, an alternative method of calculating the dose is 1 mg per year of age to a maximum of 10 mg. Clinical experience suggests that intramuscular midazolam may be as effective as intravenous diazepam. A suggested dose of midazolam is 0.2 mg/kg. The intramuscular route may be particularly useful in the physician's office, in the prehospital setting, and for children with difficult intravenous access.

Because of its short half-life and characteristic distribution within body tissues, the effect of diazepam is short. The duration of action of intravenous diazepam is less than 1 hour. Seizures may recur within 20 to 30 minutes. Therefore, if seizures are arrested, an antiepileptic drug with a longer duration of action must be given. Fosphenytoin has replaced phenytoin as a drug of choice in the treatment of SE. Fosphenytoin is a prodrug of phenytoin with equal efficacy. It has a more neutral pH than phenytoin, is water soluble and rapidly converted to phenytoin, and has a low rate of injection site reactions. Fosphenytoin is given as phenytoin equivalents (PE), and the dose is 10 to 20 mg PE per kilogram given intravenously for the treatment of SE. Fosphenytoin can be given in normal saline or dextrose at a rate of 3 mg/kg/minute. A maximum dose of 150 mg/minute has been suggested, although levels are rapidly available after slower (50–100 mg/minute) administration. Side effects may include vomiting, somnolence, ataxia, nystagmus, and pruritus (typically perineal) and paresthesias. Although fosphenytoin is not reported to have significant cardiovascular side effects in children and infants, monitoring cardiac rhythm and vital signs is suggested. Intramuscular administration of fosphenytoin can give rapid, adequate levels of phenytoin, but it is not recommended for the treatment of SE. In children younger than 1 year, close monitoring of phenytoin levels is suggested based on reports of difficulties achieving and maintaining adequate serum levels with fosphenytoin in this age group. An advantage associated with the use of fosphenytoin is the general absence of sedation and respiratory depression. If seizures persist after the initial doses of diazepam and fosphenytoin are given, this combination may be repeated. If seizures continue after approximately 20 to 30 minutes, phenobarbital at a dose of 10 mg/kg at a rate of 50 to 100 mg/minute may be used. If this regimen is unsuccessful, neurologic consultation is appropriate.

In neonates and very young infants, intravenous phenobarbital at a dose of approximately 20 mg/kg is advised. The dose may be repeated up to a maximum of 40 mg/kg. If necessary, it may be followed by fosphenytoin given intravenously in doses starting at 10 mg PE per kilogram at rates of 1 mg/kg/minute. A dose of 10 mg PE per kilogram may be repeated if seizures continue.

The use of lorazepam, a long-acting benzodiazepine, as the initial drug in the treatment of SE is now widely accepted. Lorazepam has a rapid onset and a more prolonged duration of anticonvulsant action than does diazepam. Although its half-life of 10 to 15 hours is less than that of diazepam, lorazepam continues to achieve effective brain levels for 8 to 24 hours. The suggested dose is 0.05 to 0.10 mg/kg (maximum dose, 4 mg) given intravenously and repeated one or two times as needed. For many physicians, lorazepam has replaced diazepam as the drug of choice for patients with SE.

CHAPTER 69
Diabetic Ketoacidosis (DKA)

Adapted from Leslie Plotnick, MD

DKA can be defined as a blood glucose level usually greater than 250 mg/dL, pH less than 7.2 or 7.3, and plasma bicarbonate level of 15 or less. Severe DKA is defined as a pH of 7.1 or less and a bicarbonate level of 10 or less. Milder forms may be seen. Careful monitoring of blood glucose and urinary ketones, and appropriate treatment responses to early metabolic abnormalities can prevent a significant number of DKA episodes in patients with established type 1 diabetes. In new-onset type 1 diabetes, attention to early signs and symptoms of diabetes by the primary health care providers and families may help lower the number of newly diagnosed patients presenting with severe DKA.

The basic cause of DKA is absolute or relative insulin deficiency. Elevated levels of counter regulatory or stress hormones (e.g., glucagon, cortisol, growth hormone, catecholamines) are present. These hormonal abnormalities produce hyperglycemia (by increased glucose production and decreased use), which leads to an osmotic diuresis and dehydration, lipolysis and hyperlipidemia, acidosis caused by the production of ketones (i.e. acetoacetate, beta-hydroxybutyrate) from fatty acids, and electrolyte abnormalities caused by intracellular-extracellular shifts and urinary losses. Table 69-1 lists the common errors in DKA diagnosis and management.

CLINICAL CHARACTERISTICS

The usual manifestations of DKA include a history of classic signs and symptoms of polyuria, polydipsia, and weight loss. After patients are sufficiently ketotic and acidotic, they have the fruity breath odor of ketosis. Many also exhibit nausea, vomiting, and lethargy. State of consciousness may vary from awake and alert (with mild DKA) to drowsiness or coma. Hyperventilation and dehydration also occur. Abdominal pain and an elevation in leukocytes may be caused solely by DKA and may be confused with an acute abdomen. These clinical findings usually resolve with therapy of DKA, but if not, an underlying cause (e.g., appendicitis) must be sought. DKA must be considered in children who are vomiting and appear dehydrated but continue to urinate excessively.

In a known diabetic patient, DKA may be precipitated by an acute infection, but it is usually caused by omission of insulin that may be deliberate or based on a misconception that insulin doses should be eliminated or significantly decreased because of anorexia or vomiting. Careful monitoring of blood glucose levels and urinary ketones, and appropriate therapeutic response can help avoid many DKA episodes.

The degree of hyperglycemia does not necessarily correlate with the degree of acidosis, and patients may be severely acidotic but only minimally hyperglycemic. The diagnosis of DKA can be established rapidly at the bedside with a meter glucose reading and a urinary or serum ketone determination using strips or tablets.

TREATMENT

The basic components of DKA treatment are fluid and electrolyte replacement (with careful attention to potassium) and insulin, which must be performed with frequent monitoring of clinical and laboratory factors using a flow sheet (Table 69-2) and paying careful attention to details and trends.

Fluid Replacement

Dehydration affects virtually all patients with DKA. Water and electrolyte losses occur because of polyuria caused by the osmotic diuresis produced by glycosuria, hyperventilation, vomiting, and diarrhea. The best measure of dehydration is the patient's current weight compared with a recent, healthy weight. Dry mucous membranes, poor skin turgor, and orthostatic

TABLE 69-1. Common Errors in Diabetic Ketoacidosis Diagnosis and Management

Taking good urine output to mean the patient is not significantly dehydrated (usually occurs with new-onset type 1 diabetes)
Delay in starting insulin: waiting for all laboratory values to be done or waiting for infusion pump
Letting the blood glucose drop too low by not adding enough glucose to the intravenous fluids
Too-aggressive fluid intake (too rapid or too much)
Feeding patient too early, causing nausea and vomiting before gastric peristalsis normalizes
Decreasing the intravenous insulin rate or discontinuing intravenous insulin when the blood glucose has decreased but the patient is still acidotic
Not anticipating cerebral edema
Not heeding and treating symptoms of cerebral edema (e.g., worsened sensorium, severe headache)
Not carefully reviewing clinical and laboratory data and adjusting the treatment plan as needed (i.e., rigidly adhering to a predetermined treatment regimen)
Stopping the intravenous insulin before starting subcutaneous insulin
Not giving subcutaneous insulin before a meal or snack

TABLE 69-2. Diabetic Ketoacidosis Flow Sheet

Feature	Monitoring schedule
Clinical data	
Weight	Onset of treatment
Vital signs	Onset of treatment and every 1–2 hr initially
State of consciousness	Onset of treatment and every 1–2 hr initially
Laboratory data	
Electrolytes (Na, K, Cl, HCO_3), venous pH	Every 1–2 hr for the first 4–8 hr and then every 2–4 hr until diabetic ketoacidosis is cleared
Glucose	Hourly
Blood urea nitrogen, creatinine, calcium, phosphate levels	Every 4–8 hr depending on initial levels and type of fluids used
Urinary ketone level	Every void
Fluids	Type and rate; record hourly input
Urine output	Record every void
Potassium, phosphate, bicarbonate	Record amounts added to fluid
Insulin	Dose, rate, and route

hypotension are clinical indications of dehydration. Most patients with DKA are 5% to 10% dehydrated. Patients in shock may have greater degrees of dehydration.

Adequate intravenous fluid replacement is extremely important and should begin as soon as the diagnosis of DKA is established. Normal saline (NS) or Ringer lactate, an isotonic solution, is recommended initially because they help to restore the intravascular volume and, thereby, maintain blood pressure and kidney perfusion, which enhances glucose loss through the kidney resulting in a lower blood glucose level.

A variety of published recommendations exists for the amount and rate of fluid replacement. The recommendations discussed in this section are the ones most generally accepted. For initial rehydration or resuscitation, 10 to 20 mL/kg of NS is given in the first hour. Some clinicians prefer Ringer lactate. Rarely, colloid (i.e., albumin) may be needed for patients in shock. After the first hour, the patient's state of hydration should be reassessed. If evidence of poor perfusion is still present (e.g., hypotension, delayed capillary refill), another infusion of NS (10 to 20 mL/kg) may be needed in the second hour.

After this initial reexpansion, half isotonic saline (0.45 NS = 50% NS) should be used unless the patient is significantly hyperosmolar, then NS should continue. This phase of replacement and rehydration takes into account maintenance requirements, replacement of the fluid deficit, and if excessive, ongoing losses. Maintenance requirements of 1,500 to 2,000 mL/m^2/day plus the deficit can be given evenly over 24 to 36 hours. Slower replacement (over 48 hours) may be needed when marked hyperosmolality or high-calculated serum sodium levels are present. Recommendations for a maximum of 4 L/m^2/day of fluid have also been made (see paragraph on cerebral edema in Complications, later). Urinary catheters are rarely needed. Nasogastric tubes may be needed in obtunded, vomiting patients. For patients in shock, monitoring central venous pressure may be needed.

Insulin

Continuous low-dose insulin infusion is the method of choice. Short-acting (regular) insulin is used. The advantages of a continuous intravenous insulin infusion are the elimination of the problem of poor absorption from subcutaneous and intramuscular sites in a dehydrated patient and rapid clearance, allowing easy dose adjustment, which makes management more controllable. The usual recommended dose is 0.1 U/kg/hour. Sometimes a bolus of the same dose is given before starting the insulin infusion. Running the infusate (30–50 mL) through the tubing to saturate binding sites on the tubing is recommended. The insulin infusion is best given separately from the replacement fluids so the rates can be independently adjusted, and it is best to use an infusion pump. If no improvement in acidosis is seen within approximately 2 hours, the intravenous insulin rate should be increased to 0.15 or 0.20 U/kg/hour.

Glucose

A decrease in glucose should occur at a rate of approximately 75 to 100 mg/dL/hour. In the first hour or two of treatment, a decrease in glucose level from the initial rehydration fluids occurs as intravascular volume expands. The blood glucose level corrects to normal levels more quickly than does the acidosis, and intravenous insulin must be continued until the acidosis is cleared. Continuing the intravenous insulin infusion until urinary ketones are cleared may enable easier management after the infusion is discontinued and subcutaneous insulin is started. If the blood glucose level decreases to 250 mg/dL and acidosis is still present, glucose should be added to intravenous fluids starting with 5% dextrose and increasing as needed to 7.5% or 10.0% dextrose to keep the blood glucose at approximately 250 mg/dL. If the blood glucose level is less than 300 at the onset of treatment, adding 5% dextrose at the onset of therapy is useful. In some patients, despite the use of 10% dextrose, the blood glucose may fall too low (perhaps less than 100 mg/dL), and decreasing (not discontinuing) the intravenous insulin infusion rate becomes necessary.

Potassium

Patients with DKA have total-body potassium depletion, but the measured serum potassium may be high, normal, or low. An exchange of intracellular potassium ions for extracellular hydrogen ions occurs. Treatment with insulin causes potassium to move intracellularly causing a decrease in serum potassium. Both hypokalemia and hyperkalemia are potential causes of death, and, therefore, the serum potassium must be monitored every 1 to 2 hours; potassium should not be added to the intravenous fluids until the serum potassium level is known and the patient is voiding. Electrocardiography performed while awaiting the potassium level can help assess whether hypokalemia or hyperkalemia is present.

If serum potassium is elevated at the onset of treatment, adding potassium to the intravenous fluids should not be done until the serum potassium has fallen into the normal range. If the potassium is normal or low, potassium should be added to the intravenous fluids unless renal failure exists. Generally, 40 mEq/L is used. If the serum potassium is low, more than 40 mEq/L may be needed and careful monitoring (e.g., electrocardiography, frequent blood determinations) is, therefore, required. Potassium chloride, potassium phosphate, or potassium acetate may be used.

Sodium

Patients with DKA have lost sodium through the urine and have a total-body sodium loss. Most have low serum sodium levels, probably caused by hyperglycemia, which has osmotic pressure and causes dilution of the extracellular sodium. Lipemic serum falsely lowers the sodium level. During DKA treatment, serum sodium levels should be monitored closely to ensure the sodium concentration is not decreasing. A failure of serum sodium to increase as glucose levels decrease may be a marker for excess free water (see paragraph on cerebral edema in Complications, later). An increase in serum sodium as the glucose level falls helps prevent rapid osmolality changes. The osmolality should be calculated (2 [Na] + [glucose]/18) to ensure it remains in the normal (not low) range. Sodium replacement involves intravenous NS, 20 mL/kg during the first hour and 10 to 20 mL/kg during the second hour, if indicated. After this initial volume reexpansion, 50% NS is recommended· If serum osmolality drops, NS (instead of 50% NS) is needed.

Phosphate

Phosphate depletion occurs in DKA because of poor food intake, the catabolic state, and urinary losses. Insulin treatment causes phosphate to move intracellularly lowering serum phosphate levels. In clinical studies, routine phosphate administration has not been demonstrated to have any advantage in DKA treatment. Potential theoretical benefits for phosphate use exist; phosphate depletion can impair the central nervous system and myocardial function, cause insulin resistance, and shift the hemoglobin-oxygen dissociation curve to impair oxygen delivery to the tissues.

Phosphate replacement is indicated when the serum phosphate is very low, less than 2 mEq/L. Many clinicians recommend some phosphate replacement (not more than 1.5 mEq/kg/day) for approximately 8 to 12 hours after the initial fluid reexpansion with potassium added as half potassium chloride and half potassium phosphate. One advantage of using part potassium phosphate instead of all potassium chloride is that less chloride is given. When phosphate is given, a risk of hypocalcemia exists, and calcium levels must be monitored.

Bicarbonate

Treatment of DKA with bicarbonate to help correct acidosis has been controversial. The treatment of DKA with insulin generates bicarbonate as ketones are metabolized, and bicarbonate is not needed in mild or moderate DKA. These patients gradually correct their acidosis as insulin and fluid treatment proceed. Potential risks of bicarbonate include over treatment producing a metabolic alkalosis, greater risks of hypokalemia, and paradoxic cerebrospinal fluid acidosis. Clinical trials of bicarbonate in severe DKA have not shown improvement in DKA outcome whether or not bicarbonate was used. Bicarbonate use should be reserved for patients who are severely acidotic if the acidosis may threaten respiratory or cardiac function (e.g., pH less than 7.0 to 7.1 and bicarbonate less than 5) and only for a small partial correction (e.g., to raise the pH to 7.2, maximum). Generally, 1 to 2 mEq/kg of bicarbonate given over approximately 2 hours and added to the first bottle of 50% NS (not NS) can be given. The pH should be rechecked approximately 30 minutes after the infusion. Bicarbonate should not be given to hypokalemic patients until treatment with potassium is ongoing.

Converting to Subcutaneous Insulin

Patients should be continued on intravenous fluids and an intravenous insulin infusion until they are clinically stable with normal sensorium and normal vital signs until the acidosis is cleared (i.e., normal venous pH and bicarbonate), and until they can take fluids and food orally without vomiting. Any identified precipitating factor (e.g., infection) should have been treated. Subcutaneous insulin requires time to take effect, and the intravenous insulin infusion must be continued for 30 to 60 minutes after the first subcutaneous dose of insulin is given to prevent insulin levels from becoming too low, which would allow recurrence of lipolysis and ketogenesis. A dose of short-acting insulin between 0.10 and 0.25 U/kg is given before a meal.

The switch from intravenous to subcutaneous insulin is best done during the daytime. The subcutaneous insulin doses should all be followed within approximately 0.5 hour by a meal or snack, and doses of regular insulin are needed approximately every 4 to 6 hours. During this period of dose adjustment, frequent blood glucose measurements and urinary ketone checks are important. Dose adjustment depends on the patient's blood glucose responses to previous subcutaneous doses. When the patient's usual insulin requirement is known and the precipitating factor of the DKA is cleared, the patient may be able to resume his or her usual dose of insulin as soon as normal caloric intake is reestablished. For example, a well-controlled child who had an episode of moderate DKA because of a skipped insulin dose with a viral gastroenteritis could probably resume the usual insulin schedule fairly soon after the DKA has cleared, and he or she can eat normally. The usual morning dose may be satisfactory before breakfast. Some patients may need lower insulin doses after a DKA episode because of decreased caloric intake, but some may need more. Frequent monitoring of blood glucose and urinary ketones is imperative. Newly diagnosed patients need to have their current insulin requirements established.

Two common errors occur during this transition period. First, the intravenous insulin infusion is discontinued without giving subcutaneous insulin, and the patient becomes hyperglycemic, ketotic, and even acidotic within several hours. This decision is made because the blood glucose is normal or low and the acidosis is cleared. If this condition occurs during the night, 4 to 8 hours may transpire before the deterioration of the patient's metabolic control is appreciated. The second common error is to withhold regular insulin before a meal because the blood glucose is normal or low. When this is done, the blood glucose increases to high levels after eating, and the general response is then to give regular insulin to lower the blood glucose level, which may fluctuate over a wide range during the remainder of the day. The best approach is to give regular insulin before eating to prevent a postprandial glucose rise.

Prevention

Vigilance and careful monitoring of blood glucose and urinary ketones can prevent many episodes of DKA. Urinary ketones should be checked whenever blood glucose is elevated to approximately 250 mg/dL or higher and if the patient is feeling ill. This requirement cannot be overemphasized. When ketone test results become positive (moderate to large), extra regular insulin can be given until the ketones are clear. Failure to monitor, failure to recognize or pay attention to symptoms of illness, and failure to contact the health care team early may lead to episodes of DKA that could have been prevented. Proper sick day management can prevent DKA. Recurrent DKA is uniformly caused by deliberate insulin omission, often in dysfunctional families, but it may also be caused by putting too much responsibility for diabetes management on a child or adolescent without adequate parental supervision.

Other Management Topics

Ketones (e.g., acetoacetate) interfere with creatinine measurements. A child with DKA may have an elevated cretinine suggesting he or she is in renal failure when this is a spurious measurement. Creatinine should be rechecked as the ketoacidosis clears. Use of Acetest tablets to determine the presence of serum ketones is useful to rapidly establish a diagnosis of DKA. However, serum dilutions (titers) on Acetest tablets are not useful in establishing the severity of the acidosis. Acetest tablets (i.e., nitroprusside reaction) do not measure beta-hydroxybutyrate, which is the major ketone in DKA. Because DKA treatment causes a shift toward acetoacetate from beta-hydroxybutyrate, using this qualitative ketone method may suggest the patient's condition is worsening, although total ketones and acidosis are improving, and this method is not useful in following the course of DKA treatment. It is not necessary to wait for an infusion pump to arrive to start insulin. One hour's worth of insulin can be put in an intravenous solution and infused over 1 hour. If the timing is not exact, no harm occurs. Delay in starting fluids and insulin leads to worsening of the patient's clinical status.

The diagnosis of DKA can be established rapidly at the bedside by a meter blood glucose reading and a rapid assessment of serum ketones (i.e., Acetest method). Usually, a venous pH measure will be rapidly available. The initial fluid reexpansion can then be started. Insulin can be started immediately or delayed by 1 to 2 hours. Treatment should be started if the diagnosis of DKA is evident, without waiting for all the laboratory results. However, potassium should not be added to the intravenous fluids until the serum potassium level is known. Electrocardiography can help to rapidly establish whether the serum potassium level is low, normal, or high.

Complications

Cerebral edema is an unpredictable, often fatal, and uniformly feared complication of treating DKA. It usually occurs when biochemical abnormalities are improving. Cerebral edema probably accounts for one-half or more of DKA-associated deaths. Subclinical brain swelling often occurs during DKA treatment. Factors implicated, but not pinpointed as possible causes of cerebral edema, are too rapid a decrease in blood glucose decreasing the blood glucose to an excessively low level, excessive fluid administration, tonicity of intravenous fluids, failure of the serum sodium to increase during treatment, and the use of bicarbonate.

Rosenbloom's comprehensive review of 69 cases of intracerebral complications in DKA found that infants and children younger than 5 years and patients with new-onset diabetes made up an excessive proportion of cases. In this review, rate or tonicity of hydration fluids, rate of blood glucose decrease, amount of sodium given, degree of decrease in serum sodium concentration, or the use of bicarbonate could not be implicated as causes of cerebral edema. One-half of the patients had histories suggesting dramatic changes in neurologic status before respiratory arrest occurred, and treatment before respiratory arrest had a better outcome. This review indicated that close neurologic monitoring and treatment to decrease raised intracranial pressure, when definite signs of neurologic deterioration occur, could improve outcome.

Other studies have shown that fluid intakes above 4.0 L/m^2/day are associated with more cases of cerebral edema. Failure of serum sodium to increase in the face of decreasing glucose levels, which may indicate excess free water administration, occurs more frequently in patients with complications attributable to brain edema. Until the causes of cerebral edema are better defined, paying attention to all of these factors in DKA treatment seems prudent, but anticipating cerebral edema, knowing it occurs more commonly in infants and young children and with new-onset diabetes, is important. The physician should be prepared to recognize its signs and symptoms of increased intracranial pressure such as severe headache, arousal and sensorium or behavior changes, changes in blood pressure, dilated pupils, problems with temperature regulation, slow pulse, and onset of incontinence. Careful clinical monitoring is essential. Treatment involves intubation and hyperventilation to lower increased intracranial pressure and restriction of mannitol (probably 1 g/kg by intravenous bolus) and fluid. Mannitol should be located by the bedside or nearby for the first 24 hours of treatment. However, even early treatment did not prevent severe or fatal central nervous system damage in almost one-half of the patients in one study.

CHAPTER 70
Sepsis and Septic Shock

Adapted from Kenneth M. Boyer
and William R. Hayden

ETIOLOGY

Typically, sepsis and the various septic syndromes are caused by bacterial infections of an advanced or rapidly progressive nature. Contrary to popular belief, the majority of patients with sepsis do not have documented bacteremia, which accounts for some of the recent changes in definitions. However, the probability of positive blood cultures increases as one progresses down the classification list to septic shock and multiple organ dysfunction syndrome (MODS). Even with negative blood cultures, however, bacterial etiology can generally be established by positive Gram stains and cultures of purulent exudates, characteristic alterations in hematologic parameters, tests for the presence of capsular polysaccharide antigens, or clinical responses to empiric antimicrobial therapy.

The encapsulated organisms—*Streptococcus pneumoniae, Neisseria meningitidis,* and *Haemophilus influenzae* type b—are the most common causes of sepsis (and bacteremia) of occult origin. These organisms occur most frequently in children aged 3 months to 5 years and correspond to the nadir in transplacentally acquired maternal IgG antibodies. Commonly, such infections are preceded by a viral upper respiratory illness that results in a mucosal portal of entry for the organism (e.g., meningococcemia preceded by influenza).

A focus of infection should always be sought in patients with occult bacteremia. Often, the identity of a bloodstream isolate can be a clue to the origin. *Staphylococcus aureus* bacteremia, for example, should always suggest the possibility of osteomyelitis, endocarditis, or pericarditis.

In sepsis of focal origin, likely bacterial etiologies are suggested by the site of the infection and are often determined by the normal flora of a contiguous surface. For example, urinary tract infections are often caused by enteric flora. Generally, first episodes are caused by antibiotic-susceptible *Escherichia coli.* Recurrent episodes separated by periods of prophylactic antibiotics (to the extent that prophylaxis has altered enteric flora) will be caused by *Klebsiella* species, *Enterococcus* species, *Enterobacter* species, or *Pseudomonas aeruginosa* with multiple drug resistance.

Generally, sepsis associated with bacterial enteritis is caused by *Salmonella, Shigella,* or *Yersinia enterocolitica.* Often, *Salmonella* enteric fever is associated with bacteremia. *Shigellosis,* on the other hand, is rarely bacteremic but may be associated with sepsis and septic shock, especially if *Shigella dysenteriae* is involved.

Disruption of skin or mucosal barriers may be accidental or surgical. Bite wounds can be associated with unusual oral pathogens depending on the source. For example, dog bites are generally inoculated with *Staphylococcus* and oral anaerobes, but they may also be contaminated with *Pasteurella multocida* or *Capnocytophaga canimorsus.* Often, the latter two species are associated with bacteremia and sepsis. Generally, infections affecting surgical sites involve normal flora that contaminate surgically damaged tissue at the site of operation. For example, sepsis complicating craniofacial surgery is caused by the normal flora of the skin, scalp, and upper respiratory mucosal surfaces including staphylococci, *Haemophilus* species, *S. pneumoniae*, and oral anaerobes.

Sepsis has a broad differential diagnosis. Included are nonbacterial infections such as viral, rickettsial, and spirochetal infections, and responses to bacterial products such as vaccines. Although it is not a final diagnosis, sepsis is an appropriate problem statement for such conditions. Shock states that may be confused with septic shock include supraventricular tachycardia with cardiogenic shock (often triggered by an acute febrile illness) and gastroenteritis with hypovolemic shock (also commonly associated with fever). Recognizing the former is particularly important because aggressive fluid resuscitation can lead to deterioration, rather than improvement, in cardiovascular status.

Clinical Manifestations

Recognition of the septic child is difficult. The pediatrician's fundamental dilemma is differentiating the child with a potentially life-threatening infection from among the many children with self-limited or readily treated infections that are not life-threatening. An awareness of the presence of predisposing conditions to infection in individual children is probably the most helpful guide. However, not all seriously ill children have identified defects in their host defenses, particularly in infancy.

Most children with sepsis have obvious and significantly elevated temperatures. However, in the very young and those with advanced disease, temperatures actually may register in the hypothermic range. Rigors and hyperthermia (temperature greater than 41°C [105.8°F]) imply bacteremia.

Behavioral changes can be helpful indicators of serious illness. Four of the six items on the Yale Observational Scale—quality of cry, reaction to parent stimulation, state variation, and response to social overtures—are behavioral. Children with febrile illness, a weak cry, poor responsiveness, no smile, and lack of facial expression are likely to be septic. In most cases, these changes reflect compromised cerebral circulation; occasionally, they indicate complicating meningitis.

Although changes in respiratory pattern generally point to pulmonary disease, tachypnea and acrocyanosis may also reflect metabolic acidosis and poor peripheral perfusion—both characteristic of sepsis.

A careful evaluation of circulatory adequacy is important. Measurement of blood pressure is basic, but one should recognize that children often compensate well for early shock states, so that blood pressure may be in the normal range. Difficulty in measuring a child's blood pressure is more likely to be a reflection of marginal circulation than of a technical problem with the blood pressure apparatus. Even if measured blood pressure registers in the normal range, circulatory inadequacy is usually manifested by cool extremities, acrocyanosis, absent or diminished peripheral pulses, and capillary refill times of more than 3 seconds. Although "warm shock" is said to be seen early in sepsis, it is relatively unusual in children.

Cutaneous manifestations of sepsis may be extremely helpful as warning flags. Between 8% and 20% of patients with fever and petechiae have a serious bacterial infection, and 7% to 10% have meningococcemia or meningococcal meningitis. Purpuric lesions or ecchymoses of the distal extremities (purpura fulminans) raise these probabilities even higher. Diffuse erythroderma in the presence of fever and shock should suggest toxic shock syndrome.

Laboratory Abnormalities

Laboratory manifestations of sepsis include positive blood cultures and positive cultures from other sites such as urine, cerebrospinal fluid, stool, joint or bone aspirates, exudates, abscesses, and cutaneous lesions. Continuing efforts should be made to identify the site of origin of a septic process using multiple cultures of multiple sites if necessary. Blood cultures that are persistently positive in spite of adequate treatment imply resistant organisms or an endovascular origin of infection.

Hematologic parameters are useful in initial and continuing evaluations. Leukocytosis is the norm; leukopenia is more prognostically ominous. Often, leukopenia is the initial response, with remarkable leukocytosis the later response to successful therapy. Elevated band counts, toxic granulation, and Döhle bodies imply bacterial sepsis. Thrombocytopenia implies the presence of disseminated intravascular coagulation, which should be confirmed with documentation of prothrombin time, partial thromboplastin time, fibrinogen levels, and the presence of fibrin split products. Band counts (decreasing) and platelet counts (increasing) are useful serial studies implying successful treatment.

Metabolic acidosis, manifested by decreased serum bicarbonate, pH, and increased serum lactate, is a frequent biochemical manifestation of diminished end-organ perfusion. Persisting metabolic acidosis during therapy is an ominous indicator of inadequate tissue oxygen delivery. Compensatory respiratory alkalosis is a common early abnormality. Prerenal azotemia or uremia is the usual manifestation of diminished renal perfusion and acute tubular necrosis, respectively. Often, hypoalbuminemia develops during management of severe sepsis, the consequence of both a catabolic state and capillary leak of colloid into the interstitium.

THERAPY

The cornerstones of treatment for sepsis and septic shock are maintenance of adequate oxygen and nutrient delivery to vital organs and eradication of the infecting organisms. After recognition of the situation, an orderly but rapid sequence of initial interventions to achieve these goals is mandatory.

Patients with severe sepsis should be monitored for all five vital signs: respiration, heart rate, blood pressure, temperature, and oxygen saturation (by pulse oximetry). An adequate airway and peripheral oxygen saturation are top priorities. If abnormal, they should be supported immediately by oxygen administration and, if necessary, by an endotracheal tube and mechanical ventilation.

Circulation should also be assessed rapidly and, if it is marginal or inadequate, vascular access must be achieved by peripheral or central venous catheter or by the intraosseous route. Initial blood cultures should be obtained when access is achieved. If cardiogenic shock can be excluded reasonably, normal saline, 20 to 40 mL/kg, should be administered as bolus infusions.

Then, initial empiric antibiotic therapy by the parenteral route is indicated. An assessment of probable etiology should be made with consideration of the likely infecting organisms. The other key element in antibiotic choice is the likelihood of encountering resistance, the two major determinants of which are whether the infection was acquired in the hospital and whether the patient has received recent antimicrobial therapy. In the former instance, knowledge of previous bacterial isolates from a hospitalized child may be very helpful. In the latter, one can suspect an overgrowth phenomenon requiring an alternative drug or combination. Occult, community-acquired sepsis is treated appropriately with cefuroxime, cefotaxime, or ceftriaxone. Cefuroxime has superior activity against staphylococci, but it should not be used if the physician has not excluded the presence of meningitis. Nosocomial sepsis is best treated empirically with multiple agents. Vancomycin, a third-generation cephalosporin, and an aminoglycoside are the combinations commonly used.

The goals of initial empiric antimicrobial therapy are clearing of the bloodstream, penetration to infected sites, and control of the progress of the infectious process. With more definitive microbiological data, regimens should be changed to the specific drugs of choice for the organisms isolated—as single agents or synergistic combinations, depending on identity. Often, gram-positive organisms are treated effectively with single agents; gram-negative rods are managed best with synergistic combinations.

The elements of supportive care after intensive care unit admission include continued monitoring of vital signs and oxygen saturation. In addition, invasive monitoring of central venous pressure and arterial pressure is generally indicated. They enable rational management of intravascular volume status, ventilator settings, and pressor infusions.

Maintaining adequate nutrition is extremely important. Sepsis mediators create a hypermetabolic state that rapidly depletes body stores and exceeds the caloric content of conventional intravenous fluids. Early and aggressive parenteral nutrition is necessary to keep up with these demands and to provide sufficient calories to promote tissue regeneration and healing.

The most tantalizing advances in therapy for sepsis and septic shock involve the use of monoclonal antibodies directed against gram-negative endotoxin or receptor antagonists of the mediators of the sepsis inflammatory cascade. Monoclonal antibodies against lipopolysaccharides have shown some promise in clinical trials but only in population subgroups that have proven gram-negative infection. In one trial, mortality was actually higher in the treatment group. The benefit of such antibodies may be limited by the fact that they are likely to be administered at a time when pathogenic pathways are already far advanced. The possibility of using recombinant proteins that closely resemble the naturally occurring antagonists of TNF and IL-1 or of using monoclonal antibodies directed against these mediators has also generated enthusiasm. Although extensive clinical trials of these biologics have, to date, been disappointing, several new products (e.g., Fab antibody fragments directed against TNF) show promise.

SECTION

C

Diseases of Childhood

1

Infectious Diseases

A

General Topics

CHAPTER 71

Using the Bacteriology Lab

Adapted from Edward O. Mason, Jr.

RESPIRATORY CULTURES

Throat and Nasopharyngeal Cultures

Cultures of material from the throat and nasopharynx are processed for the detection of group A streptococci unless the laboratory is notified differently. Many laboratories use rapid screening procedures to detect group A streptococcal antigen in throat swabs. Positive results obtained with these kits have been shown to correlate with the isolation of *Streptococcus pyogenes* from the nasopharynx. If it is not routine laboratory policy, the physician may be advised to request a standard culture after a negative result is obtained from a screening test. These tests should be used only to detect group A streptococci in throat specimens unless otherwise stated by your laboratory. The validity of the test obtained from other sites has not been determined.

If infection with *Bordetella pertussis*, *Corynebacterium diphtheriae*, or *Neisseria gonorrhoeae* is suspected, the lab should be notified in advance. Fluorescent antisera are available to identify both *B. pertussis* and *C. diphtheriae* directly from culture swabs, but there is a high incidence of false-positive reactions and formal cultures should always be obtained.

Ear Cultures

The most reliable method for the diagnosis of the causative agent of otitis media is the culture of middle-ear fluid obtained directly by tympanocentesis. The next most reliable source of culture material is fluid obtained at myringotomy. Fluid obtained from the middle ear after myringotomy, however, may become contaminated inadvertently with flora from the external ear during collection. Gram stain of this material, followed by prompt processing, is crucial in the subsequent interpretation of culture results.

Cultures of nasopharyngeal isolates are poor predictors of the causative agent of otitis media and are, thus, not indicated.

STOOL CULTURES

Historically, the microbiology laboratory processed stool specimens exclusively for the detection of *Salmonella* or *Shigella* species. Failure to isolate either of these two species led to a report of "no enteric pathogens isolated." Because numerous organisms are now described as causing gastroenteritis, the physician should provide as much clinical information and guidance as possible to the lab. Identification of *Salmonella* and *Shigella,* as well as *Campylobacter fetus* subspecies *jejuni,* should be standard practice in every laboratory.

Other bacterial causes of acute gastroenteritis include the following. In general, the physician should notify the laboratory in advance if any of these organisms is particularly suspected. Local labs may require the aid of reference laboratories for identification of some of the following organisms.

- Enterotoxigenic *Escherichia coli,* causing a watery diarrhea as a result of a cholera-like enterotoxin
- Enterohemorrhagic *E. coli,* a shiga-like toxin causing hemorrhagic colitis and hemolytic uremic syndrome; O157:H7 serotype is well described.
- Enteroinvasive *E. coli,* causing a dysentery similar to that caused by *Shigella*
- Enteropathogenic *E. coli,* causing infantile diarrhea or disease in younger children
- Enteroaggregative *E. coli* associated with chronic diarrhea
- *Clostridium difficile*
- *Aeromonas hydrophila*
- *Bacillus cereus*
- *Staphylococcus aureus*
- *Vibrio cholerae*
- *Vibrio parahaemolyticus*
- *Yersinia enterocolitica*

BLOOD CULTURES

In children, the quantity of blood available for culture depends on the size of the child; in the neonate, that quantity is often limited to 1 mL. This quantity can be diluted in any amount of culture broth as long as the ratio exceeds 1:5 to 1:10. The quantity of blood cultured *does* influence the ability to detect bacteremia. The level of bacteremia is usually higher in children than in adults, however. Thus, bacteremia in children may be detected even when only small amounts of blood are available for culture.

At present, most laboratories use automated blood culture systems, which periodically measure metabolites of specific substrates contained in the broth medium. Detection of bacterial growth is monitored continuously allowing more rapid detection of positive culture results. Aerobic and anaerobic media are available, although studies have demonstrated that routine anaerobic culture of blood is probably not useful except for special circumstances. The evidence of efficacy for those culture bottles that contain "antimicrobial removal substances" is not overwhelming.

CEREBROSPINAL FLUID CULTURES

Cerebrospinal fluid (CSF) submitted for any purpose should always be cultured for bacteria, regardless of the clarity of the fluid or the results of the Gram stain or cell count. The specimen should be plated to blood and chocolate agar and to a broth medium. The preparation of two smears of a centrifuged pellet is advisable. One smear is stained immediately for bacteria, and the other is reserved for staining of mycobacteria, if indicated. Any bacteria found in CSF cultures should be identified and reported.

URINE CULTURES

The proper collection of urine from children is difficult and must be performed with utmost care to ensure meaningful bacteriologic results. Urine collected by any method must be transported to the laboratory and processed within 30 minutes. Refrigeration for as long as 2 hours is permitted if immediate transport is not possible. Depending on the age of the patient, the method of urine collection and specific clinical circumstances, quantitative culture results of 10^3 to 10^5 colony-forming units (CFU) per microliter are indicative of infection. For example, any quantity of bacteria recovered in a bladder aspirate is significant.

Culture kits for outpatient use exist and generally consist of dipsticks, paddles, or tubes containing a differential agar medium that is inoculated immediately on obtaining the urine sample. The results are semiquantitative and, depending on the individual test, may indicate the bacterial identity by differential growth or color changes in the agar medium. The specimen can be later transported to a laboratory for identification. Chemical urinalysis strips designed to detect bacterial nitrite, glucose oxidase, catalase, or leukocyte esterase are also available but have differential sensitivity and specificity depending on the age of the patient. Because the first three tests detect products or enzymes of the infecting bacteria, they require a specimen that has been in the bladder at least 4 hours (or overnight). This may be difficult to achieve in a very young child. Leukocyte esterase is an enzyme produced by the polymorphonuclear leukocytes that are usually present in response to infection. The leukocyte esterase test is the most reliable of the chemical tests, but it can generate a positive result in the absence of infection. Similarly, it can generate a negative result if no white blood cells are present in the urine, as may occur in patients with asymptomatic bacteriuria.

ANAEROBIC CULTURES

Proper collection and transportation of specimens is crucial to the successful diagnosis of anaerobic infection. Although some anaerobic species can survive prolonged exposure to oxygen, others are killed rapidly by even brief exposure to oxygen. Generally, containers in which all the oxygen has been replaced with nitrogen ensure optimal conditions for the recovery. The laboratory should be advised before the collection procedure to minimize the time between collection and culture. For example, notifying the laboratory from the operating room where the specimen is obtained is a common practice.

STAINS FOR MICROSCOPIC EXAMINATION

Gram Stain

Performed properly, the Gram stain quickly demonstrates the morphology and probable identity of many of the pathogenic bacteria. Interpretation of the Gram stain by an experienced observer is crucial.

In sputum and tracheal aspirates, the presence of many polymorphonuclear leukocytes indicates adequacy of the specimen and confirms the source as the lower respiratory tract. The presence of epithelial cells in sputum indicates buccal or salivary contamination and also indicates that the culture results may be misleading in distinguishing the true pathogen.

One bacterium per oil immersion field (magnified 1,000×) seen on the stained smear of uncentrifuged urine corresponds to a colony count of 10^5 CFU per milliliter.

Fluorescent Antibody Stains

The use of fluorescein-tagged antibodies directed at specific bacterial antigens can identify specific pathogens rapidly in clinical specimens or confirm the identity of bacteria from cultures. The technique requires a microscope with a UV light source and conjugated antisera.

Wet Mount Preparations

Wet mount preparations for the diagnosis of bacterial infection are performed most often on uncentrifuged urine. The presence of more than 20 bacteria per high-power microscopical field (magnified 400×) corresponds to a colony count of 10^5 CFU per milliliter and is a reliable indication of bacterial infection of the urinary tract.

AIDS TO DETERMINING ANTIBIOTIC THERAPY

Antibiotic Susceptibility Testing

QUALITATIVE METHODS

The disk diffusion susceptibility procedure described by Bauer and Kirby is a standardized, reliable method of assessing the susceptibility of rapidly growing bacteria to numerous antibiotics. Pure cultures of the bacteria are placed on an agar surface, and filter paper disks containing a known and precisely determined amount of antibiotic are applied. Antibiotic diffuses into the agar, and the bacteria grow to an area surrounding the disk to form a "zone of inhibition" correlated to the minimal inhibitory concentration (MIC) of that particular strain. The inhibitory zone is inversely proportional to the MIC. Knowledge of the pharmacokinetics of a particular antibiotic can then be used to define zones corresponding to susceptible, intermediate, and resistant classifications. In practice, the zone sizes are measured and reported as S (susceptible), I (intermediate), or R (resistant) in the laboratory report. These assessments of susceptibility are based on the level of antibiotic that can be achieved in the serum. Because antibiotic levels that can be achieved in the meninges, bone, and abscesses are less than those that can be achieved in serum, caution should be exercised in using disk susceptibility data to predict the efficacy of an antibiotic at other body sites.

A 1-μg oxacillin disk should be used to determine strains of *Streptococcus pneumoniae* that are resistant to penicillin. These strains are not detected readily with penicillin disks, and decreased susceptibility to penicillin is confirmed by quantitative methods that reveal the MIC to be greater than 0.1 μg/mL.

Beta-Lactamase Testing

Testing for the presence of penicillin-destroying enzyme (beta-lactamase) is useful for rapid determination of resistance to the beta-lactam antibiotics. The basis of the test is a colorimetric change in an indicator in response to an acid substrate resulting from cleavage of the beta-lactam ring. With any such test, proper controls consisting of known beta-lactamase-positive and -negative strains should be tested simultaneously. Bacterial species for which this testing is useful include *Haemophilus influenzae*, *N. gonorrhoeae*, *S. aureus*, and certain anaerobes.

QUANTITATIVE METHODS

Bacterial susceptibility can be measured quantitatively by adding a standard inoculum of the bacterial strain to serial twofold dilutions of antibiotic in test tubes. Inhibition is determined by the absence of growth in the broth, and this amount of antibiotic is defined as the MIC. The minimal bactericidal concentration (MBC) is determined by subculture of tubes where inhibition occurred and is defined as the lowest concentration of antibiotic that was bactericidal for the strain. Knowledge of the antibiotic concentration that can be achieved at different sites of infection and of the MIC and MBC of the infecting strain can then be used to guide the choice of antibiotic.

AUTOMATED METHODS

Automated methods such as microtiter trays with prediluted antibiotics, are now used for susceptibility testing. Results obtained with these systems have been found to be reproducible and reliable. The disadvantage of these systems becomes evident when fastidious strains are tested or the antibiotics requested for testing are not included in standard panels. These disadvantages are compounded when the laboratory has no alternative procedure that can be implemented rapidly and reliably. Examples of the most common problems encountered with automated systems include bacterial strains that require altered growth times, nutritionally fastidious strains, strains with heteroresistant populations, failure to detect the MBC, and failure to detect tolerance. Other difficulties arise when the antibiotics to be tested are selected by the manufacturer and cannot be altered easily, or the susceptibility ranges are predetermined and are not adequate for all bacterial species.

An alternative useful method for assessing antimicrobial susceptibility is the Elipsometric test or E-test (AB Biodisk, Solna, Sweden). It can be performed with the flexibility and ease of the disk diffusion method, yet it produces MIC results that have been shown to correlate well with results obtained by conventional methods.

Antibiotic Levels

Measurement of antibiotic levels in serum is indicated routinely when potentially toxic agents such as the aminoglycosides are used in therapy. The procedure can be used to monitor the effects of inadvertent overdoses, antibiotic absorption from the gastrointestinal tract, and compliance with therapy.

Modern testing methods based on radioimmunoassay, enzyme-multiplied immunoassay, fluorescence polarization, and high-pressure liquid chromatography are highly specific and are not affected by the presence of other drugs or antibiotics. The physician must be cognizant of any reported drug interference, however, and of the procedure used in a particular laboratory.

The timing of the collection is of utmost importance. Trough levels (the lowest level) are determined on specimens collected just before the antibiotic is administered. The time of specimen collection for peak level determination depends on the antibiotic and the route of administration. In general, peak levels of antibiotics administered intravenously are determined on samples collected immediately after completion of the infusion. Peak levels for intramuscular antibiotics are reached 1 hour after injection. Peak serum levels for oral antibiotics are determined on samples collected 1.5 to 2.0 hours after ingestion and can be affected by the timing and content of meals.

CHAPTER 72
Fever and Its Treatment

Adapted from Martin I. Lorin

Fever is an elevation of body temperature as part of a specific biological response mediated and controlled by the central nervous system (CNS). This definition distinguishes fever from other types of elevated body temperature such as heat stress and heat illness.

PATHOPHYSIOLOGY

Fever is only one of a large array of responses elicited by chemical mediators of the inflammatory process. Of these *endogenous pyrogenic cytokines*, the best-known are interleukin-1alpha and interleukin-1beta (collectively are known as *interleukin-1*, IL-1). IL-1 is synthesized by blood and tissue macrophages. In addition to inducing fever, IL-1 and other pyrogenic cytokines increase the synthesis of acute-phase proteins by the liver, decrease serum iron and zinc levels, provoke leukocytosis, and accelerate skeletal muscle proteolysis. IL-1 also induces slow-wave sleep, perhaps explaining the somnolence frequently associated with febrile illnesses.

IL-1 and other mediators are synthesized by phagocytic cells in the blood or tissues. Molecules of IL-1 enter the blood and are carried to the CNS, where they induce an abrupt increase in the synthesis of prostaglandins, especially prostaglandin E_2, in the region of the anterior hypothalamus. This increase results in elevation of the set-point (or reference point) of the thermostat mechanism in this area of the brain. The temperature control region of the anterior hypothalamus then reads current body temperature as too low in comparison to the new set-point and initiates a series of events to elevate body temperature to a height equal to the new set-point. In response, increased metabolic rate and increased muscle tone and activity occur to increase heat production. Decreased heat loss also occurs, primarily through diminished perfusion of the skin. Body temperature rises until a new equilibrium is achieved at the elevated set-point.

FEVER: FRIEND OR FOE?

The question often posed is: Is fever a friend or a foe? A more appropriate question would be: Under what conditions is fever beneficial and under what conditions is it harmful?

The growth or survival of some pathogenic bacteria or viruses is impaired at temperatures in the range of 40°C (104°F). Many pathogenic bacteria require iron for their growth, and fever has been shown to be associated with a decrease in serum iron and simultaneous increase in serum ferritin resulting in minimal levels of free iron in the blood. *In vitro* studies have demonstrated enhancement of several human immunologic functions at moderately elevated ambient temperatures. These functions include increased lymphocyte transformation response to mitogen, increased bactericidal activity of polymorphonuclear leukocytes, and increased production of interferon. However, as temperatures approached 40°C (104°F) in these experiments, most of the functions decreased to below baseline levels. In one study of rabbits infected with *Pasteurella multocida*, survival increased with moderate fever, but with fevers greater than 2.25°C above baseline, survival rates were lower than in the euthermic state. Thus, fever of moderate degree appears to enhance several aspects of the immunologic response. At high body temperatures, however, these effects may be diminished or even reversed.

Fever often makes patients uncomfortable. It is associated with an increased metabolic rate, increased oxygen consumption and carbon dioxide production, and increased demands on the cardiovascular and pulmonary systems. However, for the child with an underlying disorder, especially of the heart or lungs, these increased demands may be significantly detrimental. Fever can precipitate febrile convulsions in susceptible children. These are typically benign but may cause great anxiety in families.

TREATMENT OF FEVER

Clearly, fever need not always be treated, and body temperature need not always be restored completely to normal. Wisdom dictates that one treat high fever [40°C (104°F) or greater] in children at risk for febrile convulsions, with underlying neurologic or cardiopulmonary disease, with septic shock, and in any situation in which a component of heat illness is a consideration. It is common practice to treat milder fevers that make patients uncomfortable. While this practice likely creates no advantages in the management of the illness, patient comfort is important to caretakers of children. Furthermore, the practice should not be condemned until data suggests that, when done properly, it is unsafe.

Once a decision is made to treat a patient's fever symptomatically, the choice of a specific therapeutic modality should be based on several considerations. Because fever is the result of an elevation of the set-point in the hypothalamic thermoregulatory center, the most rational way to treat fever is to restore this set-point to normal. Although agents such as aspirin, acetaminophen, and ibuprofen all work on this basis, aspirin will not be discussed as it should not be used in children to decrease fevers except for clinical situations (due to association with Reye syndrome). Studies have shown a somewhat greater and more prolonged reduction in fever with ibuprofen as compared to acetaminophen, but this difference has not been shown to be clinically important. Acetaminophen should be prescribed on a weight-based dosage, the dose being 10 to 15 mg/kg PO or PR every 4 to 6 hours. Some sources suggest limiting the total dosage to no more than five times per day. Many over-the-counter preparations exist and care should be taken to note the concentration or dosage strength. In large overdoses, acetaminophen can lead to hepatic toxicity and necrosis. Some reports have raised concern of acute liver injury secondary to excessive *therapeutic* dosage of acetaminophen over the course of several days. The half-life of many drugs is significantly prolonged in the newborn and very young infant; therefore, antipyretics should be used with caution and at a reduced dosage in these age groups.

TABLE 72-1. Use of External Cooling in Treating Elevated Temperature

Cooling method	Indications
Tepid sponging *instead of* antipyretic drugs	Very young infants Severe liver disease History of hypersensitivity to antipyretic drugs
Tepid sponging *plus* antipyretic drugs	High fever [>40°C (104°F)] History of febrile seizures, neurologic disorders, or brain damage Infection plus suspicion of overheating or overwrapping Septic shock*
Cold sponging alone	Heat illness

*May require cold sponging.

Recommended antipyretic doses of ibuprofen are also based on body weight at 5–10 mg/kg/dose PO every 6 to 8 hours. Many over-the-counter preparations exist and care should be taken to note the concentration or dosage strength.

Under certain circumstances, the use of external cooling, generally by sponging, to reduce body temperature is advisable, either in addition to or instead of antipyretic drugs (Table 72-1). External cooling is the treatment of choice for heatstroke and other forms of heat illness. However, for fever, external cooling is indicated only in specific situations. External sponging is advisable in any situation in which suspicion exists that the cause of the elevated temperature may be a form of heat illness. Some patients with infections may also have a component of heat illness from over wrapping, dehydration, or drugs.

For the previously well child with a nonlife-threatening febrile illness, sponging may cause discomfort. Sponging with ice water is particularly discomforting and is not necessary for fever. The antipyretic effect of oral acetaminophen plus sponging with tepid water is only slightly more rapid than the effect of oral acetaminophen alone. In very young infants, sponging may be preferable to using any antipyretics. Sponging should be done with tepid water [generally at approximately 30°C (85°F)]. Alcohol should not be used because its fumes are absorbed across the alveolar membrane and possibly across the skin too, resulting in CNS toxicity.

CHAPTER 73
Fever without Source

Adapted from Mark W. Kline and Martin I. Lorin

Fever is one of the most common pediatric complaints. Between 5% and 20% of febrile children have no localizing signs on physical examination and nothing in the history to explain the fever. Fever without source (FWS), like febrile illness in general, is most common in children younger than age 5, with a peak prevalence occurring between 6 and 24 months of age.

Fever without a source is best defined as fever of relatively brief duration, arbitrarily 7 or fewer days, without an apparent source on history or physical examination. If the unexplained fever persists for longer than 7 days, it is commonly termed *fever of undetermined origin* (FUO). Although overlap exists between FWS and FUO, the differential diagnosis and the clinical approach are somewhat different.

In most cases, FWS resolves spontaneously without a specific diagnosis being established and is presumably caused by a viral infection. In some cases, a relatively minor infectious process, either focal (e.g., otitis media, pharyngitis) or nonfocal (e.g., roseola), becomes apparent as the cause of the fever. Because the duration of FWS is, by definition, relatively brief and because so many children with self-limited viral infections present with FWS, the percentage of children who have FWS and serious persistent infections (e.g., osteomyelitis) or noninfectious chronic inflammatory conditions (e.g., juvenile rheumatoid arthritis) is much lower than the percentage of children who have FUO. A young child presenting with FWS should be examined for the clinical criteria of Kawasaki syndrome, an important vasculitis syndrome of unknown etiology (Chapter 116).

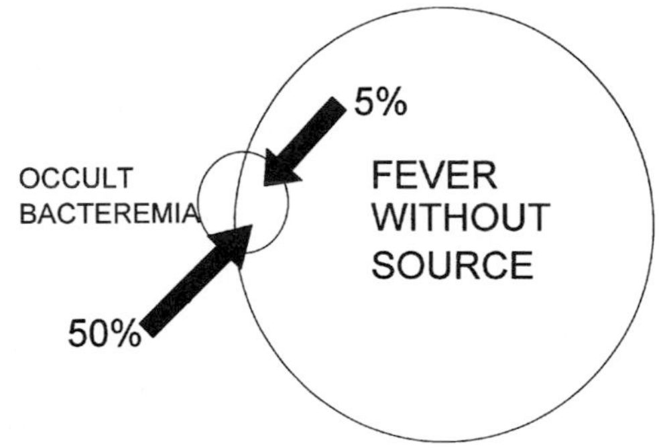

Figure 73-1. Relation of fever without source (FWS) and occult bacteremia. Many more cases of FWS than of occult bacteremia occur. Only 5% of cases of FWS are associated with occult bacteremia, but more than 50% of patients with occult bacteremia have FWS.

There is a trend for higher fevers to be associated with a greater risk of bacteremia, but one must remember that most children with fevers (even high fevers) do not have a serious bacterial illness. Viral illness is much more common. A careful diagnostic approach is, therefore, always warranted.

The concern over making the diagnosis of occult bacteremia is the potential for a child to suffer sequelae including meningitis, septic arthritis, osteomyelitis or possibly endocarditis. In studies done before the practice of routine immunization against *H. influenzae*, up to 5% of children with occult bacteremia developed purulent meningitis, and another 5% developed other significant soft tissue infections such as periorbital cellulitis or osteomyelitis. Approximately 15% were found to have persistent bacteremia at the time of reexamination. The relative risk, however, of subsequent meningitis was greater with *H. influenzae* bacteremia than it currently is with *S. pneumoniae* bacteremia.

OCCULT BACTEREMIA

A small but clinically significant percentage of children with bacteremia cannot be identified by ordinary clinical examination alone. These children have *occult bacteremia*, which should be defined as the presence of a positive blood culture in children who look well enough to be treated as outpatients and in whom the positive blood culture results are not anticipated. Specifically, the child does not have any focal findings that would ordinarily be associated with bacteremia but the child may have a minor infection such as otitis media. Although only approximately 5% of children with FWS have occult bacteremia, somewhat more than 50% of the children with occult bacteremia come from the pool of children with FWS (Fig. 73-1).

Streptococcus pneumoniae is responsible for the majority of occult bacteremia. *Neisseria meningitidis*, salmonellae, and *H. influenzae* account for most of the remaining cases, but due to wide-spread vaccination, *H. influenzae* type is very uncommon. Not surprisingly, therefore, many of the characteristics of occult bacteremia associated with *S. pneumoniae* are statistically true for occult bacteremia in general: peak prevalence between 6 and 24 months, association with high fever, and a high leukocyte count. No racial, geographic, or socioeconomic predilection for occult bacteremia is apparent. The exact prevalence of occult bacteremia in different series of outpatients varies depending on the selection criteria for the study. Figures have generally been in the range of 3% to 6% of highly febrile young children.

In one series, 3% of febrile children with evidence of upper respiratory tract infections had occult bacteremia, in contrast to those with FWS, for whom the prevalence was 9%.

DIAGNOSIS

Many of the diagnostic studies used to evaluate children with FWS are directed at excluding the presence of bacteremia. However, the indiscriminate use of diagnostic tests causes unnecessary effort, expense, and discomfort for the patient.

Several investigators have suggested that the use of clinical scoring systems (e.g., the Yale Observation Score) for children with FWS may permit the selection of a subgroup of patients who appear well and have only a small or negligible risk of bacteremia or other serious bacterial illnesses. These clinical features include the child's appearance (e.g., normal hydration, lack of apparent toxicity, and lack of distress) and behavior (e.g., alert, playful, and eating and drinking well). A study dealing only with children with "nonfocal, nontoxic-appearing illness (or uncomplicated otitis media)" treated as outpatients found that the Yale Observation Score was not clinically useful in detecting occult bacteremia. Therefore, many children with FWS undergo some level of laboratory evaluation. (A full discussion on the management of children with FWS can be found at the following reference: Baraff LJ, Bass JW, Fleisher GR, et al. Practice guidelines for the management of infants and children 0 to 36 months of age with fever without source. *Pediatrics* 1993; 92:1.)

Two types of laboratory tests are used in evaluating children for bacteremia: *indirect tests* such as the white blood cell (WBC) count and *direct tests* such as blood culture, the gold standard for detection of bacteremia. Indirect laboratory tests serve only as screening tests to identify a subgroup of children at high risk of bacteremia. In a population with a low prevalence of a disease—as is the case with febrile children and bacteremia—even a sensitive and specific screening test will have a low positive predictive value. For children with FWS, a WBC count of 15,000 cells per microliter or greater has sensitivity and specificity of approximately 85% and 75%, respectively, for the detection of bacteremia. The positive predictive value, however, is only approximately 15%. Nevertheless, the WBC count is the most widely used and probably the most practical screening test available.

Other laboratory tests may be indicated in certain situations. Neonates and young infants, in particular, may fail to manifest signs of meningeal irritation even in the presence of confirmed bacterial meningitis; hence, a high index of suspicion for that disease must be maintained, and a lumbar puncture should be performed if any concern for meningitis exists, regardless of the *absolute* age of the young patient. Urinalysis is indicated in the neonate and the all female infants with unexplained fever to exclude urinary tract infection. Beyond approximately 6 months of age, boys with unexplained fever have a lower risk of urinary tract infection. Chest roentgenogram is not indicated routinely for infants and children with FWS, but it may be considered for very young infants and for patients with very high fever, tachypnea out of proportion to fever, or markedly increased WBC count (suggestive of pneumococcal disease).

ANTIBIOTIC TREATMENT

Expectant antibiotic therapy may be justified for the child with FWS and high fever, WBC count greater than 15,000 per microliter, or other risk factors for occult bacteremia (*Pediatrics* 1993; 92:1). Empiric antibiotic therapy should be directed against the most common bacterial pathogens. Given concerns over penicillin-resistant pneumococcal strains, the most widely used empiric coverage is a single injection of ceftriaxone (50–75 mg/kg). This provides 24 hours of coverage against *S. pneumoniae, H. influenzae,* and *N. meningitidis* without concern over compliance or vomiting. Regardless of therapy, careful follow-up care is essential, and affected children should be reevaluated immediately if the clinical condition deteriorates, if signs or symptoms of serious focal infection develop, or if the blood culture yields any potential pathogen.

CHAPTER 74

Fever of Unknown Origin

Adapted from Martin I. Lorin and Ralph D. Feigin

The definition of fever of unknown origin (FUO) in children has evolved over the past few decades. The term FUO best describes the condition of children who are febrile for 8 or more days and in whom a careful history, physical examination, and preliminary laboratory evaluation fail to reveal a probable cause for the fever. Children who have been febrile without explanation for fewer than 8 days should be considered as having fever without a source (FWS), which carries a different set of diagnostic probabilities and requires a different clinical diagnostic approach (see Chapter 73).

GENERAL PRINCIPLES

Most children with FUO *do not* have rare or exotic diseases. This finding has been true even in series from major pediatric referral centers. Although the relative frequencies are somewhat different, the three most commonly identified causes of FUO in children are the same as those in adults: infectious diseases, rheumatologic disorders, and malignancies. Whereas the prognosis in children is somewhat better than in adults, FUO may represent a serious condition. Mortality was 9% in the series of Pizzo and colleagues and 17% in that of Lohr and Hendley. McClung reported that 40% of the children in his study had "serious or lethal diseases." In many cases of FUO in children, a specific diagnosis is never established and the condition eventually resolves spontaneously.

INITIAL APPROACH TO CLINICAL EVALUATION

The approach to the child with FUO should be individualized for each patient. For most patients, the diagnostic evaluation may be initiated in the office or the clinic. However, young infants, children who appear toxic or chronically ill, and children who have been febrile for a prolonged period should be hospitalized for evaluation. Hospitalization is useful not only for expediting laboratory tests, but also for providing an opportunity to document fever, exploring the history further, repeating the physical examination at different intervals, and maintaining constant observation.

The patient's history should be searched carefully for any possible clues, however trivial or remote. Animal contact is always important. Dogs can harbor brucellosis or leptospirosis, and cats are vectors for cat-scratch disease (Bartonella) and toxoplasmosis. Rodents carry tularemia and leptospirosis. A history of travel, even in the distant past, is notable. Endemic diseases in Africa, India, and Asia include malaria, amebiasis, and schistosomiasis, which may manifest months to years after returning from an endemic area. Coccidioidomycosis is endemic in the southwestern portion of the United States.

EVALUATION

After a careful and thorough history and physical examination have been conducted, evaluation of the child with FUO can be performed simultaneously as three processes: follow-up of all diagnostic clues, performing screening tests, and observation with reexamination.

Follow-Up of Diagnostic Clues

The most important aspect of the evaluation of a youngster with FUO is meticulous and complete follow-up of all potential clues, however insignificant they may appear. The results of the history and physical examination and all available laboratory data must be scrutinized closely for any abnormalities or positive features. Pizzo and colleagues found that in one-half of their cases, failure to use existing laboratory data correctly was a major reason for failure to establish the proper diagnosis before hospitalization. As an example, even a mild peripheral eosinophilia may be a clue to parasitic infection, immunodeficiency, or occult malignancy.

Screening Tests

When no clues exist to guide the workup, the physician must rely on an initial battery of screening tests. Basic screening tests include a complete blood count with examination of the blood smear, erythrocyte sedimentation rate and/or C-reactive protein, chest roentgenography, urinalysis and culture, tuberculin skin test, blood culture (done in triplicate if endocarditis is a consideration), analysis of levels of hepatic enzymes and alkaline phosphatase, and analysis of blood urea nitrogen and creatinine. Further tests could include, as warranted, those for serum antibody titers against brucellosis, tularemia, rickettsia, Epstein-Barr virus, and HIV. Screening for rheumatic disease is often associated with false positives and poor predictive value. One must remember that tests such as serum rheumatoid factor results are usually negative in patients with the acute systemic form of juvenile rheumatoid arthritis (JRA). If these tests fail to yield a diagnosis, a gallium scan should be considered to look for a focus of inflammation. Other imaging studies such as bone scan, radiographic skeletal survey, roentgenography of the sinuses and mastoids, and abdominal ultrasound or computed tomographic (CT) examination, should generally be performed only when specific clues or indications are present or fever persists for an inordinate period of time. Bone marrow aspiration is generally most useful in diagnosing or ruling out hematologic disorders such as leukemia and hemophagocytic syndrome, but it rarely yields an unexpected organism on culture.

Hospitalization, Observation, and Reexamination

Hospitalization for the child who requires it, whether for clinical indications or because of persistent fever with an unrevealing outpatient workup, affords an opportunity not only to facilitate diagnostic testing, but also to obtain additional historical data from the patient, parents, and even other family members who may visit. The patient must have a complete physical examination on admission and a relatively complete follow-up examination at least daily. Often, pulmonary rales, cardiac murmurs, skin rashes, areas of tenderness, pain on motion of a joint, and even abdominal masses appear during the hospitalization. All available data should be reviewed continually for clues that were not initially apparent. The pattern of fever should be observed. A high, spiking fever that spikes once or twice a day may be an indication of an occult abscess or the systemic form of JRA.

The response to antipyretic agents should be noted. Lack of response may indicate factitious fever or a neurologic basis for the fever. Temperature elevations secondary to neurologic dysfunction are often unresponsive to antipyretic drugs (central fever).

ETIOLOGY

In up to one-fourth of all the cases of FUO in children, no definite diagnosis is ever established. Most of these cases resolve spontaneously. In the remainder, the following causes should be considered. This list is not inclusive of all diagnoses. More detailed information on these diagnoses may be found in other chapters of this text.

- Infectious Causes
  - Localized Infections
    - Sinusitis
    - Otitis Media
    - Tonsillitis
    - Urinary Tract Infection
    - Osteomyelitis
    - Occult abscess (subdiaphragmatic, periappendiceal)
  - Systemic Infections
    - Epstein-Barr virus
    - CMV
    - Hepatitis
    - HIV infection
    - Spirochetes (leptospirosis, rat-bite fever, syphilis)
    - Rickettsial infections
    - Tuberculosis
    - Salmonellosis
    - Brucellosis
    - Tularemia
    - Parasitic infections

Connective Tissue Diseases

Connective tissue disorders and vasculitis are the second leading cause of FUO in children, and JRA accounts for most pediatric cases of rheumatologic diseases presenting as FUO. Although all three clinical forms of this disorder (acute systemic, pauciarticular, and polyarticular) may be associated with fever, the acute systemic form is most likely to present as FUO. The classic fever pattern in this disorder is one or two temperature spikes daily. Most serologic test results for rheumatoid factor are negative in children with the acute systemic form of JRA rendering the disease difficult to diagnose. The diagnosis is often made clinically by observation over a prolonged period.

Malignancy

Malignancies are the third most frequent cause of FUO in children. Most cases are caused by leukemia or lymphoma. Rarely, neuroblastoma or other cancers such as hepatoma, rhabdomyosarcoma, and atrial myxoma may present as unexplained fever.

Factitious Fever

A child who looks well, has no tachycardia, and does not feel warm at the time of alleged fever may have factitious fever. In the age of the electronic thermometer, the attendant routinely remains at the bedside while measuring the temperature making it difficult for the patient or parent to factitiously elevate the temperature reading. However, the oral reading can still be influenced by ingesting hot liquids before the temperature measurement is taken. The ingenuity of some patients or parents in falsifying temperature readings and feigning illness is extraordinary, and, undoubtedly, such individuals will find ways to circumvent modern technology. In bizarre cases, the parent may actually induce fever by injecting the child with infectious or noxious materials.

Periodic Disorders

Familial Mediterranean fever is an exceedingly rare autosomal recessive disorder seen mostly in Arabs, Armenians, and Sephardic Jews. Familial Mediterranean fever is characterized by acute episodes of fever and inflammation of serosal tissue such as the peritoneum, pleura, or joint synovia. Episodes occur at irregular intervals. In contrast, most other periodic disorders are characterized by recurrent episodes of fever at fairly regular intervals. In many cases, the febrile attacks initially tend to occur 3 or 4 weeks apart, but as the illness persists, the interval between episodes often lengthens to 5 or 6 weeks. Between episodes, the patient is normal and asymptomatic. Some patients have neutropenia at the time of fever suggesting a variant of cyclic neutropenia. Others may have arthralgias, pharyngitis, aphthous stomatitis, or cervical lymphadenopathy with each episode of fever. The nature of most of these periodic disorders remains unknown, but some cases of periodic fever in children, with or without stomatitis and adenopathy, are now recognized as being associated with the hyperimmunoglobulinemia D syndrome.

Other Causes

Other causes of FUO include serum sickness, drug reactions, inflammatory bowel disease, thyrotoxicosis, Behçet syndrome, histiocytosis, sarcoidosis, ectodermal dysplasia, diabetes insipidus, and subdural hematoma. Several cases of infants receiving furosemide who have had otherwise unexplained fever lasting for many months have been reported.

Mucocutaneous lymph node syndrome (Kawasaki syndrome) should be considered in the differential diagnosis of any young child with FUO, but it can usually be diagnosed or ruled out by the presence or absence of clinical features.

Infrequently, an apparent FUO is only an exaggerated normal circadian temperature pattern; a misinterpretation of normal temperature readings, which may be as high as 38°C (100.48°F) in infants or young children, or an unfortunate (but not remarkable) series of self-limited viral infections.

CHAPTER 75
Mycoplasma pneumoniae

Adapted from W. Paul Glezen

Mycoplasmas are classified as bacteria, but they are unique because they lack a rigid cell wall. For this reason, their morphology depends on the environment in which they grow, they do not take usual bacterial stains, and they are not susceptible to antibiotics that act on the cell wall such as the penicillins.

Only three mycoplasmas have been associated with disease in humans. *Mycoplasma pneumoniae* causes primary atypical pneumonia and is the only pathogen of this group that is an important cause of disease in children. *Mycoplasma hominis* and *Ureaplasma urealyticum* are genital mycoplasmas.

MYCOPLASMA PNEUMONIAE

Epidemiology

M. pneumoniae is the most common cause of pneumonia and tracheobronchitis in older children and young adults treated in the outpatient setting. The average annual rate is approximately 5 in 1,000 school-aged children. *M. pneumoniae* is an uncommon cause of lower respiratory tract disease in infants.

Sporadic infections can occur throughout the year but epidemics of *M. pneumoniae* disease may begin in the summer with peak activity reached in autumn. In experimentally inoculated volunteers, the incubation period from the day of infection to the onset of pneumonia was approximately 14 days, but the average interval between the onset of an index case and the onset of a secondary case in the same household is closer to 3 weeks and may be as long as 3 months.

Pathogenesis

Infection of a susceptible person probably occurs through contact with *M. pneumoniae*-containing droplet nuclei that are coughed into the environment. Infection of humans by aerosol may be accomplished by as little as one colony-forming unit (CFU). The concentration of organisms in sputum specimens from patients with pneumonia has ranged from 10^2 to 10^6 CFU per milliliter.

The organism attaches to ciliated respiratory epithelial cells by a specialized tip. The attachment protein has been isolated, and specific antibodies have been demonstrated in serum and respiratory secretions of immune subjects. These antibodies apparently block attachment and, thereby, prevent infection. Uninhibited attachment of *M. pneumoniae* to ciliated cells leads to ciliostasis, then loss of cilia and, eventually, the desquamation of epithelial cells. Mononuclear cells infiltrate the submucosa of affected bronchi and bronchioles. An exudate consisting of debris from the desquamated cells, polymorphonuclear leukocytes, macrophages, and mucus develops as the disease progresses and may lead to a productive cough. Bacterial superinfection may occur.

Clinical Features

The main clinical features of *M. pneumoniae* disease are fever, malaise, sore throat, and a dry, hacking cough. The onset is usually gradual over several days. The affected school-aged child may not appear particularly ill, and the examiner may be surprised when chest auscultation reveals rales and rhonchi. The chest roentgenogram may show peribronchial thickening and infiltration of one or both lower lobes with some subsegmental atelectasis. Pleural effusion is not a prominent finding but may be present. The peripheral white blood cell count is usually in the normal range.

Some children not known to wheeze previously may have expiratory wheezing on examination. Children with existing asthma may have a severe exacerbation of wheezing requiring aggressive therapy. A nondescript rash may accompany the infection. A few children present with acute otitis media or bullous myringitis. The total course of the illness with or without treatment may encompass 2 weeks with a bothersome night cough persisting even longer.

Complications

A wide variety of extrapulmonary complications has been attributed to *M. pneumoniae* infection. The complication best documented in children is Stevens-Johnson syndrome; the organism has been isolated from skin lesions on occasion. Hemolytic anemia with or without renal failure has been reported in adults. A plethora of neurologic syndromes, including meningoencephalitis, Guillain-Barré syndrome, transverse myelitis, and cerebral infarction, have been attributed to the infection; in most cases, however, the only evidence of infection is either an increase in the level of complement-fixing (CF) antibodies or a single high titer. Some cases have been reported in the absence of evidence of significant respiratory tract infection. The neurologic diseases that occur in the presence of cold agglutinin-positive pneumonia, at least, are more acceptable as putative neurologic complications. Isolation of the agent from respiratory secretions should be required to establish the association between *M. pneumoniae* infection and a neurologic condition.

Diagnosis

The diagnosis of *M. pneumoniae* infection can be suspected in a child who has the typical clinical picture described previously. The clinical impression can be reinforced by the presence of cold agglutinins in the serum at a titer of 1:64 or greater. Cold agglutinins are immunoglobulin M antibodies that may appear early in the course of the infection, probably because the organism has an antigen similar to the I antigen on the red blood cell membrane. Cold agglutinins are not specific for *M. pneumoniae* infection and are present in only approximately 50% of affected persons.

A specific diagnosis can be made by isolating the organism. *M. pneumoniae* can be grown and identified on enriched agar containing antibiotics to inhibit normal pharyngeal bacterial flora. Approximately 1-2 weeks is required for the growth of colonies.

Serologic diagnosis had traditionally been accomplished by documenting a fourfold increase in the level of CF antibodies between acute and convalescent serum. Newer assays for IgM and IgG specific to *M. pneumoniae* are widely available. Caution should be used in interpretation as the *M. pneumoniae* IgM response may last several months and, thus, not be related to the acute illness. Furthermore, antibodies to *M. pneumoniae* may cross react with other antigens leading to false-positive results.

A specific and sensitive polymerase chain reaction (PCR) is available for *M. pneumoniae* in certain labs.

Treatment

The treatment of choice for children with *M. pneumoniae* infection is a macrolide antibiotic. Therapy should be started early for optimal response, which may not be dramatic even under the best of circumstances. Controlled clinical trials have shown that use of either erythromycin or tetracycline shortens the clinical course and hastens improvement of the chest roentgenographic findings. Treatment may not eradicate the organism; it is often possible to recover *M. pneumoniae* from respiratory secretions after therapy is discontinued. The prognosis is generally good, and few sequelae of infection have been reported.

CHAPTER 76
Chlamydial Infections

Adapted from Margaret R. Hammerschlag

Chlamydiae are obligate intracellular bacteria. Members of the genus possess both DNA and RNA, divide by binary fission, contain their own ribosomes, have a cell wall (but no detectable peptidoglycan or muramic acid), and are susceptible to antimicrobial agents.

The genus now contains four species: *Chlamydia psittaci, Chlamydia trachomatis, Chlamydia pneumoniae* (TWAR strain), and *Chlamydia pecorum.* The first three species are capable of causing infection in humans. The routes of transmission, susceptible populations, and clinical presentations differ markedly for the three species that cause infection in humans (Table 76-1).

INFECTIONS CAUSED BY *CHLAMYDIA PSITTACI*

C. psittaci is widespread in the animal kingdom, where it is a major cause of both respiratory and genital disease. Humans usually contract the disease from infected birds. The birds may be ill, but unapparent infection can also occur. Psittacosis is likely to occur in poultry workers, veterinarians, and bird fanciers. Person-to-person spread is unusual. The clinical course of psittacosis varies with incubation periods of 7 to 15 days or longer. Often, it starts suddenly with chills and high fever (38°C–40.5°C). Headache, often diffuse and severe, is a common chief complaint, as are malaise and nausea. A persistent dry, hacking cough is usually present. The physical findings may belie the extent of the pulmonary involvement as seen on chest radiography. Rales may be heard, but changes indicative of consolidation are not usually seen. Chest radiography reveals soft, patchy infiltrates radiating from the hilum or, less frequently, a reticulonodular pattern.

Once psittacosis is suspected (usually as an atypical pneumonia or epidemiologically because of contact with birds), the best and most available method of diagnosis is serologic. A fourfold rise in the complement-fixing antibody titer is diagnostic. A single titer of 1:32 or greater in patients with a compatible illness is very suggestive. Early treatment may delay antibody response for several weeks. The treatment of choice is tetracycline given for 21 days. Erythromycin may be an alternative but may also be less effective.

INFECTIONS CAUSED BY *CHLAMYDIA TRACHOMATIS*

Trachoma

Trachoma is probably the greatest single preventable cause of blindness in the world. It is endemic in the Middle East and Southeast Asia. The disease is spread from eye to eye; flies are a frequent vector. Trachoma starts as a follicular conjunctivitis, usually in early childhood. The follicles heal leading to

TABLE 76-1. Characteristics of Three Chlamydial Species that Cause Disease in Humans

Characteristic	*C. trachomatis*	*C. psittaci*	*C. pneumoniae*
Number of serovars	15	At least 4 avian serovars	1
Percent DNA homology to *C. pneumoniae*	<5	<10	94–100
Plasmid	Yes	Yes	No
Contains glycogen	Yes	No	No
Resistant to sulfonamides	Yes	No	No
Morphology of elementary body	Round	Round	Round or pear shaped
Natural host	Humans	Birds, mammals	Humans
Population	Sexually active adults, infants	Poultry workers, veterinarians, bird fanciers	All ages
Mode of transmission	Sexual, mother to infant	Aerosol: animal to person	Aerosol: person to person
Diseases	Nongonococcal urethritis, cervicitis, salpingitis, epididymitis, neonatal conjunctivitis, infantile pneumonia, lymphogranuloma venereum	Pneumonia: "psittacosis"	Pneumonia, bronchitis, pharyngitis, otitis media

conjunctival scarring, which may result in turning of the eyelid so that the lashes abrade the cornea (entropion and trichiasis). Eventually, corneal ulceration secondary to the constant trauma leads to scarring and blindness.

Trachoma can be diagnosed clinically. The World Health Organization suggests that at least two of the following four criteria be met for diagnosis: lymphoid follicles on the upper tarsal conjunctivae, typical conjunctival scarring, vascular pannus, and limbal follicles. The diagnosis is confirmed by culture or staining methods during the active stage of the disease. As socioeconomic conditions improve, the incidence of the disease decreases substantially.

Lymphogranuloma Venereum

Lymphogranuloma venereum (LGV) is a systemic, sexually transmitted disease caused by the LGV biovar of *C. trachomatis*. Fewer than 1,000 cases of LGV are reported in adults in the United States each year. LGV strains have a predilection for lymph node involvement.

The first stage of LGV is characterized by the appearance of the primary lesion, a painless, usually transient papule on the genitals. The second stage is characterized by lymphadenitis or lymphadenopathy. Most patients are seen at this time with enlarging, painful buboes, usually in the groin. The nodes may break down and drain. Men are more likely to have this symptom. In women, the lymphatic drainage of the vulva is to the retroperitoneal nodes. Fever, myalgia, and headache are also common. In the tertiary stage, a full-blown genitoanorectal syndrome is seen with rectovaginal fistulas, rectal strictures, and urethral destruction.

LGV can be diagnosed either through culture of *C. trachomatis* from a bubo aspirate or serologically. The recommended therapy is 2 to 3 weeks of tetracycline or sulfisoxazole. Tetracycline should not be given to children younger than 9 years.

Oculogenital Infections in Adults

The trachoma biovar of *C. trachomatis* is also responsible for a large spectrum of diseases that occur in sexually active adults. In men, it is the cause of 30% to 50% of all cases of nongonococcal urethritis. The symptoms are less acute than those of gonorrhea, and the discharge is usually mucoid rather than purulent. Asymptomatic urethral infection is frequent in sexually active men. As many as 50% of men with gonorrhea are coinfected with *C. trachomatis*, however. Autoinoculation from the genitals to the eyes can lead to inclusion conjunctivitis in both men and women.

In women, *C. trachomatis* infects the endocervix; women may have mucopurulent cervicitis but are frequently asymptomatic. The prevalence of cervical chlamydial infection among sexually active women has been reported to range from 2% to 35% depending on the population studied. Some of the highest prevalence rates have been found in adolescent girls. *C. trachomatis* can also infect the urethra leading to the urethral syndrome of dysuria with "sterile" pyuria. Complications of genital chlamydial infections in women include perihepatitis (Fitz-Hugh-Curtis syndrome) and salpingitis. The latter may cause significant morbidity leading to infertility and ectopic pregnancy.

The definitive diagnosis of genital chlamydial infection in adults is by isolation of the organism in tissue culture from the urethra in men and the endocervix in women. Several nonculture methods are available for the diagnosis of chlamydial conjunctivitis. They include enzyme immunoassays (EIA) and direct fluorescent antibody tests. Most of these tests are approved only for testing with urethral and cervical specimens from adults. A DNA probe is also widely available and its performance has been similar to most of the approved EIAs. Also, three nucleic acid amplification tests are approved for only genital sites and urine in adults. Polymerase chain reaction (PCR) assays, ligase chain reaction assays, and transcription-mediated amplification exist.

A single 1-g dose of azithromycin or a 7-day course of doxycycline (100 mg twice daily) is now recommended by the Centers for Disease Control and Prevention (CDC) as a first-line regimen for the treatment of uncomplicated genital infection in men and nonpregnant women. Amoxicillin or erythromycin is recommended as the first-line regimens for treatment of pregnant women. Sexual partners should be treated as well.

Perinatally Transmitted Infections

An infant may acquire infection during passage through an infected birth canal. The overall risk of transmission is near 50%. The organism can be inoculated into the conjunctivae, nasopharynx, rectum, and vagina. Clinically, the infant may have conjunctivitis or pneumonia.

Inclusion Conjunctivitis

C. trachomatis is the most frequent identifiable infectious cause of neonatal conjunctivitis. The incubation period is 5 to 14 days after delivery. The presentation varies extremely, ranging from mild conjunctival infection with scant mucoid discharge to severe conjunctivitis with copious purulent discharge. The conjunctivitis must be differentiated from gonococcal ophthalmia. At least 50% of infants with chlamydial conjunctivitis also have nasopharyngeal infection. The best diagnosis is made by culture of a conjunctival scraping or by one of the antigen detection methods. Oral erythromycin, 50 mg/kg/day for 14 days, is the therapy of choice. It permits better and faster resolution of the conjunctivitis and also treats any concurrent nasopharyngeal infection, which will prevent the potential development of pneumonia. Additional topical therapy is not needed.

Ocular prophylaxis with silver nitrate, erythromycin, or tetracycline ointments or drops is not effective for the prevention of neonatal chlamydial conjunctivitis or pneumonia. Identification and treatment of pregnant women before delivery appear to be the best methods of preventing chlamydial infection in infants.

Pneumonia

Pneumonia develops in approximately 10% to 20% of all infants born to women with active chlamydial infection. *C. trachomatis* is one of the most common causes of pneumonia in infants younger than 6 months. The onset of chlamydial pneumonia is usually between 1 and 3 months of age and is characterized by persistent cough, tachypnea, and lack of fever. Auscultation reveals bilateral rales. The finding of peripheral eosinophilia (greater than 400 cells per microliter) is common. The most consistent finding on chest radiography is hyperinflation accompanied by interstitial or alveolar infiltrates. Erythromycin given for 14 days is the treatment of choice and results in clinical improvement and elimination of the organism from the respiratory tract.

Culture of chlamydia from the conjunctiva or nasopharynx is diagnostic. Nasopharyngeal specimens can be obtained with a posterior nasopharyngeal swab or by aspiration of the nasopharynx. Direct fluorescent antibody and EIA techniques can also be used for conjunctival and nasopharyngeal specimens. These tests appear to perform well at these sites with sensitivities and specificities of not less than 90%.

Infections in Older Children

Children who have been sexually abused may acquire anogenital infection. These infections are usually asymptomatic. Accumulating evidence, however, suggests that perinatally acquired rectal and vaginal infections may persist for at least 3 years; thus, the presence of *C. trachomatis* in the vagina or rectum of a prepubertal child cannot be used as absolute evidence of sexual abuse. Cultures should be obtained from these sites only when a prepubertal child is being evaluated. The direct fluorescent antibody and EIA tests have both been associated with many false-positive results when used on specimens from these anatomic sites.

INFECTIONS CAUSED BY *CHLAMYDIA PNEUMONIAE*

DNA studies have found less than 5% relatedness between *C. pneumoniae* and *C. trachomatis* and *C. psittaci*. *C. pneumoniae* appears to be a primary human respiratory pathogen; no zoonotic reservoir has been identified. Transmission is thought to occur person-to-person through respiratory droplets. *C. pneumoniae* may be responsible for up to 20% of community-acquired "atypical" pneumonia (including acute chest syndrome in children with sickle cell disease), 10% of bronchitis, and 5% to 10% of pharyngitis. Clinically, infections caused by *C. pneumoniae* cannot be differentiated readily from those caused by other agents, especially *Mycoplasma pneumoniae*. Coinfections may be present. Asymptomatic respiratory infection occurs in 2% to 5% of adults and children. Serologic surveys have documented a rising prevalence of *C. pneumoniae* antibody beginning in school-aged children and reaching 30% to 45% by adolescence suggesting that clinically unapparent infection may be fairly common. However, infection as documented by culture is as frequent in young children as in adults. Respiratory infection with *C. pneumoniae* has been associated with reactive airway disease in patients with no history of asthma and causing acute exacerbations in individuals with asthma.

The specific diagnosis of *C. pneumoniae* infection is based on isolation of the organism in tissue culture. The optimum site for culture appears to be the posterior nasopharynx, and the specimen should be collected with wire-shafted swabs in a manner similar to that for *C. trachomatis*.

C. pneumoniae is sensitive *in vitro* to macrolides, tetracycline, and quinolones. Currently macrolides (erythromycin, clarithromycin and azithromycin) and tetracyclines (in children age 8 years and older) are recommended as first-line therapy. Quinolones are not approved for use in children younger than age 18 years.

CHAPTER 77
Rickettsial Infections

Adapted from Ralph D. Feigin and Marc L. Boom

The rickettsial diseases described in this chapter are Rocky Mountain spotted fever and Ehrlichiosis. Rickettsiae are microorganisms that have characteristics of both bacteria and viruses. Like viruses, they rely on the intracellular milieu for growth and reproduction. Like bacteria, they contain both DNA and RNA; they multiply by transverse binary fission; possess enzymes of protein synthesis and electron transport, and their growth can be inhibited by a variety of antibacterial agents.

ROCKY MOUNTAIN SPOTTED FEVER

Rocky Mountain spotted fever (RMSF) is a disease caused by *Rickettsia rickettsii*. It was recognized in areas of Idaho and Montana but its occurrence is not limited to the Rocky Mountain area. In fact, the disease is most prevalent in the southeastern United States, where the majority of cases is now seen. The annual incidence of RMSF per 1 million U.S. population is estimated to be between 2 to 5 cases. Nearly two-thirds of all patients with Rocky Mountain spotted fever are 15 years old or younger. Rocky Mountain spotted fever is the most common fatal tick-borne disease in the United States. Despite the use of antibiotics for treatment, Rocky Mountain spotted fever has an overall case fatality rate of 4.0%. A considerable number of the deaths can be attributed to failure to consider and establish the diagnosis early enough for appropriate therapy to be beneficial.

Etiology, Epidemiology, and Transmission

R. rickettsii is a small coccobacillary microorganism measuring 0.3 to 0.4 μm in length and 0.3 to 0.5 μm in diameter. Because Rocky Mountain spotted fever rickettsiae are primarily parasites of ticks, human disease is generally associated with the biology of the ticks that transmit it. However, disease can be transmitted by the aerosol route in the laboratory or by blood transfusion.

The dog tick (*Dermacentor variabilis*) is the primary vector in the East. The wood tick (*Dermacentor andersoni*) is the primary vector in the West. Rocky Mountain spotted fever rickettsiae do not kill the arthropod host, but they can be passed from generation to generation of ticks transovarially. Most cases occur during the period of greatest tick activity between April and September.

Pathogenesis

Rickettsiae multiply within the endothelial cells lining small blood vessels and are disseminated widely by the bloodstream causing a vasculitis. Vascular lesions account for the more prominent clinical features noted including rash, mental confusion, headache, heart failure, and shock. Pneumonia can be acquired by laboratory inhalation.

The vascular lesions are found everywhere, but they are appreciated most readily in the skin, adrenal glands, and gonads. Inflammation can also cause vasculitis of the heart (causing interstitial myocarditis) and nervous system.

Hyponatremia may be profound. Etiologies include a loss of sodium by the urine, a shift in water from the intracellular to the extracellular space, and an exchange of sodium for potassium at the cellular level.

Clinical Manifestations

Fever, headache, and rash are the hallmarks of Rocky Mountain spotted fever, although the complete triad may be present in only half of cases. Mental confusion and myalgia are also notable. The onset of disease in children may be gradual or abrupt and usually occurs 2 to 8 days after a bite from an infected tick. Persistent body temperature elevations to 40°C are often noted.

The characteristic rash generally appears by the second or third day of illness, although it may be delayed for a week. Initially, the lesions are erythematous macules that can blanch on pressure. The lesions rapidly become petechial and, in untreated patients, even hemorrhagic. The rash appears peripherally on the wrists and ankles (and may involve the palms and soles), spreading quickly to the extremities and trunk. The absence of rash, however, does not exclude a diagnosis.

Muscle tenderness (myalgia) is a common feature of Rocky Mountain spotted fever. Characteristically, the patient complains when the calf or thigh muscles are squeezed.

Persistent, intractable headache in older children and adults is a characteristic finding. Young children may not complain of this symptom. Signs of meningoencephalitis include irritability, restlessness, signs of mental confusion or delirium. Meningismus may be present, but is not generally accompanied by abnormalities in the cerebrospinal fluid. Cardiac involvement is frequent including congestive heart failure and arrhythmias are common.

Pulmonary involvement occurs in 10% to 40% of reported cases and may be associated with abnormal chest radiographic results and abnormal arterial blood gas measurements.

Enlargement of the liver and spleen are unusual. Gastrointestinal symptoms and signs, including nausea, vomiting, abdominal pain, and diarrhea, arise frequently.

Diagnosis

Laboratory evaluations do not permit a specific cause to be identified before therapy must be instituted. *R. rickettsii* can be identified by immunofluorescent techniques in skin specimens obtained by biopsy on days 4 through 8 of the illness. Practically, and due to false, negative testing, a positive immunofluorescent test is a means to confirm the illness before a specific serologic diagnosis can be made. Since specific serologic results are not usually positive before day 10 or 12 of the illness, and the majority of the 20% of patients who die will do so before this time, it is emphasized again that the provision of appropriate therapy can never await a definitive diagnosis.

Nonspecific serologic testing includes the Weil-Felix test, which will exhibit positive results as early as, or earlier than, any other specific tests in a high proportion of patients with untreated Rocky Mountain spotted fever. This test depends on the fact that rickettsiae possess antigens in common with certain strains of Proteus bacteria.

Specific diagnosis can be obtained by using a complement fixation test, indirect hemagglutination reaction, microimmunofluorescence tests, and latex agglutination and microagglutination tests. Each of these tests has limitations with regard to sensitivity or specificity.

A microtiter enzyme-linked immunosorbent assay (ELISA) has been developed to characterize the IgG and IgM response in Rocky Mountain spotted fever. The ELISA is both sensitive and accurate. The value of this test is limited, however, because IgG and IgM seroconversions cannot be demonstrated until 6 days after the onset of illness. A polymerase chain reaction (PCR) assay that enables the detection of specific sequences of DNA has been developed and is available through selected labs.

Selected laboratory clues may be helpful. During the first 4 or 5 days after the onset of disease, the white blood cell (WBC) count is normal or may reveal a leukopenia. As the disease progresses, secondary bacterial infections may occur, and leukocyte counts may increase to as high as 30,000 cells per microliter. Thrombocytopenia of varying severity develops in most cases. Hyponatremia, as mentioned above, may be seen.

Differential Diagnosis

Meningococcemia is the disorder most frequently confused with Rocky Mountain spotted fever. Differentiation from meningococcemia can be difficult because WBC counts may be low or normal and signs of meningeal irritation and moderate pleocytosis may be seen in both diseases. The inability to differentiate meningococcemia from Rocky Mountain spotted fever does not justify delaying antimicrobial therapy because both diseases are potentially fatal. Treatment should be initiated promptly with antimicrobials to treat both infections.

Measles may also be considered in the differential of Rocky Mountain spotted fever.

Therapy

Tetracyclines are highly effective when they are given early in the course of the disease and in an appropriate dosage. Of the tetracyclines, doxycycline is the drug of choice. The 2003 Report of the Committee on Infectious Diseases of the American Academy of Pediatrics (AAP) allows for the use of doxycycline in RMSF in children who are younger than 8 years. The duration of therapy is usually 7 to 10 days. Doxycycline has the additional advantage of also being the treatment of choice for ehrlichiosis, which can be confused clinically with Rocky Mountain spotted fever. Chloramphenicol is effective for RMSF, but it has become difficult to obtain in the United States and is associated with a risk of idiosyncratic aplastic anemia while requiring monitoring of serum levels.

The need for supportive care cannot be overemphasized. Careful evaluation of serum and urine electrolyte levels, body weight, and renal function is important to guide fluid therapy. Hyponatremia is treated best by providing maintenance fluids or, in the case of severe hyponatremia, by instituting modest fluid restriction. The administration of sodium-rich fluids may cause cardiac decompensation and pulmonary edema. Hypoalbuminemia may need to be addressed with albumin infusions. Disseminated intravascular coagulation may require the administration of vitamin K, fresh frozen plasma, and platelet transfusions.

Prevention

Avoidance of contact with ticks is the most effective means of prevention. Ticks must be attached and feeding for 4 to 6 hours or more before they can transmit the disease, so early tick removal after activity is useful.

Killed vaccines have been valuable in preventing death, but they do not reliably protect against the acquisition of disease. No vaccine is currently commercially available. A prior infection of Rocky Mountain spotted fever is followed by solid immunity.

Prognosis

The mortality from Rocky Mountain spotted fever is approximately 25% if untreated. If appropriate antibiotics are provided before the end of the first week of illness, recovery is generally the rule. The overall mortality remains 4% to 7%, however, principally because diagnosis and therapy are delayed in many patients until the second week of illness. When death occurs, it is usually the result of heart failure, vascular collapse, renal failure, or thrombocytopenia, either alone or in combination. Central nervous system involvement and disseminated intravascular coagulation are common.

EHRLICHIOSIS

Two human tick-borne diseases caused by *Ehrlichia* species have been recognized in the United States since 1986. The two diseases, human monocytic ehrlichiosis (HME) and human granulocytic ehrlichiosis (HGE), have similar presentations including fever, headache, myalgias, and anorexia with associated leukopenia or pancytopenia.

Organism

Currently, as many as three tick-borne bacteria are responsible for human ehrlichiosis. Human monocytic ehrlichiosis is caused by *E. chaffeenisis* while human granulocytic ehrlichiosis is caused by *Anaplasma phagocytophila* and *E. ewingii*. These are gram-negative cocci that are obligate intracellular microorganisms.

Epidemiology and Transmission

Illness occurs in the months when ticks are prevalent, from March to October. The Lone Star tick (*Amblyomma americanum*), whose distribution is the Southeast and South central United States, is the likely principal vector of *E. chaffeenisis* and *E. ewingii*. Deer and livestock are the preferred hosts of *A. americanum*, and proximity to a wildlife reserve is a risk factor for HME in some case clusters. HGE infections have been reported most commonly in Wisconsin, Minnesota, and Connecticut among other states. The deer tick (*Ixodes scapularis*), also the vector for the causative agent for Lyme disease (*Borrelia burgdorferi*), is the primary vector for HGE.

Pathogenesis and Pathology

Granulocytes are the primary target cells for HGE, and macrophages are the primary target cells for HME.

Ehrlichia enter the cytoplasm of host cells and multiply in phagosomes into elementary bodies. These individual *Ehrlichia* organisms multiply by binary fission into immature inclusions called *initial bodies*. Mature groups of elementary bodies form morulae that are released by rupture of the cell to reinitiate the infecting process.

Intraleukocytic inclusions have been observed in lymphocytes, monocytes, and neutrophils in some cases of human infection.

Clinical Manifestations

HUMAN MONOCYTIC EHRLICHIOSIS

The estimated incubation period for HME is 12 to 14 days. HME is an acute febrile illness that causes fever, headache, anorexia with or without vomiting, and myalgias (Table 77-1). Rash in children is common and may be macular, maculopapular, or petechial involving both the trunk and the extremities.

Meningitis may occur with cerebrospinal fluid pleocytosis ranging from approximately 50 to 1,000 WBCs, with a predominance of either neutrophils or lymphocytes, mildly elevated protein levels (85–120 mg/dL); and a normal to slightly low glucose value.

Affected adults and children often have mild leukopenia and thrombocytopenia. Usually, thrombocytopenia is not associated with clinical bleeding; however, disseminated intravascular coagulopathy has been reported. Elevations of liver function and renal function tests may occur in addition to hyponatremia, and hypoalbuminemia. These manifestations are a consequence of the generalized vasculitis that accompanies the infection.

TABLE 77-1. Clinical and Laboratory Features of Adult and Pediatric Monocytic Ehrlichiosis

Feature[a]	Percentage of cases	
	Adult (N = 46)	Pediatric (N = 20)
Fever	96	100
Anorexia	76	78
Headache	80	100
Myalgia	74	67
Rash	20	65
Leukopenia[b]	61	72
Thrombocytopenia[c]	52	78
Elevated aspartate amino-transferase levels[d]	76	83

[a]Some features were not specified for all patients.
[b]White blood cell count less than 4,000 per microliter.
[c]Platelets less than 150,000 per microliter.
[d]More than 55 U/L.
Reprinted with permission from Edwards MS, Feigin RD. Rickettsial disease. In: Feigin RD, Cherry JD, eds. *Textbook of pediatric infectious diseases*, 4th ed. Philadelphia: Saunders, 1998:2239.

HUMAN GRANULOCYTIC EHRLICHIOSIS

The clinical features of HGE include fever, malaise, myalgia, and headache. However, rash occurs in only 10% of cases, and hepatosplenomegaly and cardiac murmurs are uncommon. Thrombocytopenia occurs in the majority of patients, mild leukopenia occurs in approximately 50%, and elevated serum aspartate aminotransferase levels occur in 90% of patients. The mortality for HGE ranges from 5% to 10%.

DIAGNOSIS AND DIFFERENTIAL DIAGNOSIS

The diagnosis of ehrlichiosis can be established by the isolation of an *Ehrlichia* organism from blood or CSF. Polymerase chain reaction may also be used for both *E. chaffeenisis* and *A. phagocytophila*. Alternatively, documenting a fourfold increase in *Ehrlichia* antibody titer between acute and convalescent serum is confirmatory. A single titer of at least 1:64 in a patient with intracytoplasmic bacterial inclusions (morulae) is also diagnostic.

Clinically, ehrlichiosis is less likely than RMSF to be manifest by rash and more likely to have leukopenia or pancytopenia as a laboratory feature. The similarity of ehrlichiosis and Rocky Mountain spotted fever is emphasized by two retrospective serosurveys in which approximately 10% of the specimens taken from patients lacking the serologic criteria for the diagnosis of Rocky Mountain spotted fever fulfilled the criteria for the diagnosis of ehrlichiosis. Other tick-borne illnesses such as Lyme disease, babesiosis, Colorado tick fever, relapsing fever, and tularemia, should be included in the differential diagnosis.

TREATMENT

The treatment of choice for human ehrlichiosis is a tetracycline, preferably doxycycline. The dosage is the same as that for spotted fevers. The 2003 Report of the Committee on Infectious Diseases of the American Academy of Pediatrics allows for the use of doxycycline in RMSF in children who are younger than 8 years. The duration of therapy is usually 7 to 10 days.

B
Bacterial Infections

CHAPTER 78
Bacterial Meningitis Beyond the Newborn Period

Adapted from Ralph D. Feigin
and Joseph H. Schneider

Meningitis is an inflammation of the meninges. Between 1986 and 1995, the United States incidence of bacterial meningitis in children aged 1 month to 5 years decreased 87%, primarily because of the introduction of conjugate vaccine for *Haemophilus influenzae* type b (Hib). Meningitis is still, however, a feared childhood infection.

ETIOLOGY AND EPIDEMIOLOGY

Common causes of bacterial meningitis in children older than 1 month of age are *Neisseria meningitidis, Streptococcus pneumoniae* and, until recently, Hib. The highest risk of infection is in infants aged 6 to 12 months. Before the introduction of conjugate Hib vaccine, approximately 65% of U.S. bacterial meningitis was caused by Hib with the remainder caused primarily by *N. meningitidis* and *S. pneumoniae*. Nonspecific risk factors for meningitis from these organisms include young age, close contact with carriers or those with invasive disease, and host factors such as asplenia or immunodeficiency.

Approximately 90% of meningococcal disease is caused by groups A, B, and C. The incidence in U.S. children aged 1 to 23 months is 4.5 per 100,000 per year; with mortality estimated at 8%. There is a secondary peak in incidence in the later teens. The disease is generally acquired from carriers who can harbor the organism for months. The U.S. carriage rate is 15% but, during outbreaks, it can increase to more than 30%. The disease generally occurs in newly infected individuals rather than by breakthrough in chronic carriers. The risk of severe meningococcal disease is 1% in family contacts, approximately 1,000 times greater than the community risk. The incubation period is from 1 to 10 days. Host factors such as terminal complement deficiency (C5–C9), complement-depleting diseases, or properdin deficiency increase susceptibility to disease.

S. pneumoniae is a gram-positive diplococcus with approximately 90 capsular polysaccharide serotypes. Sepsis and meningitis occur most frequently with serotypes 4, 6B, 9V, 14, 18C, 19F, and 23F. Before the universal vaccination with conjugated pneumococcal vaccine, meningitis rate in U.S. children aged 1 to 23 months was 6.6 per 100,000. The U.S. childhood mortality has been estimated at 15%. The risk of meningitis in the U.S. black population is increased five to 36 times. Carriage of pneumococcus is transient and is a risk factor for infection. Host factors such as sickle cell disease, may increase susceptibility to infection.

Hib is a gram-negative coccobacillus. Historically, it was the leading cause of bacterial meningitis in many developed countries. The incidence in children younger than 5 years ranged from 20 to 30 per 100,000 in certain countries to 409 per 100,000 in Alaskan Eskimos. In the United States, the current incidence is approximately 0.7 per 100,000 in children between 1 and 23 months. The previous carriage rate of 2% to 5% has also declined because the vaccine also protects against nasopharyngeal colonization.

Other bacteria such as group B streptococcus, *Listeria monocytogenes,* and *Salmonella,* can cause meningitis in normal children. Host factors, both congenital and acquired, can be important in meningitis caused by these bacteria. For example, skin flora should be suspected in children with a dermoid sinus, meningomyelocele, or hydrocephalus and a cerebrospinal fluid (CSF) shunt. Children with sickle cell disease, or congenital asplenia are especially susceptible to *S. pneumoniae* and *Salmonella* infection.

PATHOLOGY AND PATHOPHYSIOLOGY

Initially, upper respiratory tract infection occurs. Bacteremia follows, with opsonization and phagocytosis inhibited by bacterial capsules. Meningeal seeding occurs most likely in the cerebral capillaries and choroid plexus. Invasion from a contiguous infection (e.g., mastoiditis) can also occur. Meningitis after otitis media is usually from bacteremia rather than direct invasion. Meningitis can also develop subsequent to skull or vertebral column osteomyelitis.

Organisms are initially found in the lateral and dorsal longitudinal (sagittal) sinuses. A meningeal exudate eventually occurs over the brain. The spinal cord may be encased in pus. Purulent material may develop in the ventricles (ventriculitis).

Cerebral cortex damage produces the neurologic sequelae of meningitis such as impaired consciousness, seizures, retardation, and nerve deficits. Deafness, vestibular disturbances and optic nerve involvement may also occur. Transtentorial herniation may cause nerve compression.

Cerebral edema results from vasogenic, interstitial, and cytotoxic processes. Vasogenic edema results from increased blood–brain barrier permeability. Interstitial edema occurs with decreased CSF resorption as proteins, leukocytes, and debris interfere with the function of the arachnoid villi. Cytotoxic edema results from host and bacterial toxic factors, which increase intracellular water and sodium and loss of intracellular potassium.

Increased ICP often exceeds 300 mm H_2O. Hypoxemia and ischemia from decreased perfusion may result. In some cases, meningitis is associated with the syndrome of inappropriate antidiuretic hormone release (SIADH) causing water retention and electrolyte abnormalities.

Hypoglycorrhachia (low CSF glucose) and acidosis result, in part, from increased glucose use and decreased glucose transport across the inflamed choroid plexus. Acidosis may contribute to loss of cerebral autoregulation and tissue damage. Increased CSF protein is partly caused by flow of albumin-rich fluid into the subdural space secondary to inflammation and increased vascular permeability.

Host inflammatory responses in the CSF seem to rely on two mechanisms to clear bacteria. One requires a type-specific antibody, a functional classic complement system for opsonization and competent neutrophils for phagocytosis. The second system is dependent on the interaction of nonspecific antibody and the alternative complement system for opsonization of the organism. Clearance by this system occurs without neutrophils. The host inflammatory response remains only partially understood and appears to be somewhat different for each type of organism. It includes a complex interaction of leukocytes, cytokines, complement, arachidonic acid products, platelet-activating factor (PAF), nitric oxide (NO), toxic oxygen products, and excitatory amino acids.

Antibiotic therapy results in a large release of bacterial fragments, which promotes production of the cytokines interleukin-1beta (IL-1beta) and tumor necrosis factor-alpha (TNF-alpha). These cytokines trigger a cascade of mediators, Interleukin-1beta (IL-1beta) and tumor necrosis factor-alpha (TNF-alpha) also stimulate endothelial cells to activate receptors that promote leukocyte attachment leading to leukocyte migration into the CSF. Complement is involved early in the host response. The complement cascade product C5a is a potent early chemoattractant for leukocytes.

CLINICAL MANIFESTATIONS

Meningitis can develop slowly over several days or it can be fulminant with onset within hours.

Fever and meningeal inflammation symptoms occur in 85% of patients. These include headache, irritability, confusion, hyperesthesia, photophobia, nuchal rigidity, and seizures. Nuchal rigidity may appear late, especially in a young child. Seizures occur in 20% to 30%. Infants may have only restlessness, irritability, poor feeding, or unstable temperature. They may also exhibit a bulging fontanelle. Older children frequently have headaches, and symptoms may proceed to altered mental status. Adolescents may present with behavioral abnormalities that may be confused with drug abuse or psychiatric disorders. Papilledema is rare; if present, a search for other processes (e.g., brain abscess, venous sinus occlusion, subdural empyema) should be performed.

Kernig sign (while supine with the leg flexed at the hip to 90 degrees and the knee flexed, pain occurs on leg extension beyond 135 degrees) and Brudzinski sign (while supine, leg flexion occurs when the neck is flexed) may be absent in 50% of cases, especially if antibiotics have been given.

Other symptoms and signs may be present. Subdural effusions may occur in 50% of cases. Although usually asymptomatic, they may cause increasing head circumference, vomiting, seizures, full fontanelle, focal neurologic signs, or persistent fever. Facial cellulitis, pneumonia, epiglottitis, and endophthalmitis can also be presenting signs of meningitis. In one study of buccal cellulitis, 8% of patients had bacterial meningitis, most without meningeal signs.

In one-half or more cases of meningococcal disease, the patient may have purpura or petechiae (a nonblanching rash) during the course, but it may occur in any vasculitic process. Shock with profound hypotension may occur in 5% of meningococcal and Hib meningitis cases, but it can be associated with any overwhelming bacteremia. Disseminated intravascular coagulation may occur.

DIAGNOSIS

No single symptom or sign is pathognomonic for meningitis because any, none, or all of the clinical manifestations described previously may be present. Definitive diagnosis is established by positive identification of the organism in the CSF by culture or by other diagnostic techniques.

Lumbar Puncture

A lumbar puncture (LP) must be performed if meningitis is suspected. Increased numbers of neutrophils and increased protein and decreased glucose concentrations suggest bacterial infection. Usual initial CSF findings in CNS suppurative diseases are shown in Table 78-1.

Contraindications to an LP are cardiopulmonary compromise, signs of possible increased ICP (e.g., papilledema, altered respiratory efforts, focal neurologic signs), and skin infection over the LP site. Herniation may occur with increased ICP. In children with suspected increased ICP or altered mental status, antibiotics should be given immediately after taking blood cultures and an emergency computed tomographic (CT) scan should be done before the LP. If an LP cannot be performed, meningitic doses of antibiotics should be administered until the procedure can be performed.

When an LP is performed, CSF pressure should be measured. In one study, the mean pressure was 180 $\pm$ 70 mm H_2O, twice the upper normal limit. When ICP is elevated significantly, the minimum amount of fluid necessary for studies should be removed.

Microscopy should include a total leukocyte count and differential. In children older than 12 months, a normal CSF leukocyte count is less than seven cells per milliliter. If the LP is traumatic, a safe approach is to wait for culture results. A Gram stain should be performed. Most Gram stains, if done properly, will be positive in a child with bacterial meningitis not yet pretreated with antibiotics.

Normal CSF may be found in up to 10% of cases of meningococcal meningitis; hence, a strong index of suspicion is necessary. Cultures should be performed regardless of fluid appearance or cell count. If an organism cannot be identified from an LP, alternative identification methods can be used.

CSF glucose values of less than two-thirds of the blood glucose level are frequently found. Several studies of meningococcal meningitis have reported normal glucose values in approximately 50% of patients. CSF protein is usually elevated. Normal protein levels in children older than 2 months are less than 40 mg/dL.

Rapid detection tests exist but are not necessary for all patients. They may be helpful in situations such as a traumatic LP or in a patient who has been pretreated with antibiotics. Latex particle agglutination tests of the CSF are widely available, but reported sensitivities and specificities vary substantially. A negative latex particle agglutination result rarely affects the decision to give antibiotics.

TREATMENT

Because of increasing penicillin resistance by *S. pneumoniae*, most centers now use cefotaxime (225–300 mg/kg/day in three to four divided doses) or ceftriaxone (100 mg/kg/day in two divided doses) for children older than 3 months. In children aged 1 to 3 months, ampicillin (400 mg/kg/day in four divided doses) should be added because of possible *L. monocytogenes* or enterococcal infection. Vancomycin (60 mg/kg/day in four divided doses) is often given with cefotaxime or ceftriaxone to address the possibility of cephalosporin resistant pneumococci until sensitivities are known.

In the United States, approximately 46% of *S. pneumoniae* strains are now relatively resistant to penicillin. Resistance is not beta-lactamase mediated. In some U.S. locations, up to 25% resistance to third-generation cephalosporins has been found. Although cefotaxime and ceftriaxone are effective against most penicillin-resistant pneumococci, caution is urged. Ceftriaxone and cefotaxime are third-generation cephalosporins with broad antimicrobial activity against gram-positive and gram-negative organisms. They penetrate the blood–brain barrier well and have excellent CSF bactericidal activity. Because of its long serum half-life, ceftriaxone may be given every 12 to 24 hours. In meningitis, every 12 hours is recommended.

TABLE 78-1. Initial Usual Cerebrospinal Fluid Findings in Suppurative Diseases of the Central Nervous System and Meninges

Condition	Pressure (mm H_2O)	Leukocytes per microliter; predominant type	Protein (mg/dL)	Glucose (mg/dL)	Specific findings
Acute bacterial meningitis	Elevated; average, 300	0–60,000; average, a few thousand; PMNs	100–500; occasionally >1,000	<40 in more than one-half of cases	Organism seen on smear or culture in 90% of cases
Subdural empyema	Elevated; average, 300	<100 to a few thousand; PMNs	100–500	Normal	No organisms seen
Brain abscess	Elevated	10–200; lymphocytes	75–400	Normal	Fluid is rarely acellular
Ventricular empyema (rupture of brain abscess)	Considerably elevated	Several thousand to 100,000; >90% PMNs	Several hundred	<40	Organism may be seen on smear or culture
Cerebral epidural abscess	Slightly elevated	Few to several hundred; lymphocytes	50–200	Normal	No organisms seen
Spinal epidural abscess	Reduced with spinal block	10–100; lymphocytes	Several hundred	Normal	No organisms seen
Thrombophlebitis (associated with subdural empyema)	Often elevated	Few to several hundred; PMNs and lymphocytes	Slightly elevated	Normal	No organisms seen
Bacterial endocarditis (with embolism)	Normal to slightly elevated	Few to <100; PMNs and lymphocytes	Slightly elevated	Normal	No organisms seen
Acute hemorrhagic encephalitis	Elevated	Few to >1,000; PMNs	Moderately elevated	Normal	No organisms seen
Tuberculous infection	Elevated; may be low with dynamic block in advanced stages	25–100; rarely, >500; 80% PMNs in early stages, then lymphocytes	100–200; may be higher if dynamic block	Reduced; <50 in 75% of cases	Acid-fast organisms may be seen on smear of protein coagulum or culture
Cryptococcal infection	Elevated; average, 225	0–800; average, 50; lymphocytes	20–500; average, 100	Reduced in >50% cases; average, 30	Organisms seen in India ink preparation and Sabouraud culture medium
Syphilis (acute)	Elevated	Average, 500; lymphocytes with rare PMNs	Average, 100; gamma-globulin often high	Normal (rarely reduced)	Positive reagin test result; no organisms seen by usual techniques
Sarcoidosis	Normal to considerably elevated	0 to <100; monocytes	Slight-to-moderate elevation	Normal	No specific findings

PMNs, polymorphonuclear neutrophils.
Adapted with permission from Feigin RD, Cherry JD, eds. *Textbook of pediatric infectious diseases,* 4th ed. Philadelphia: Saunders, 1997.

Vancomycin combined with ceftriaxone or cefotaxime appears to be synergistic. It should not be used as monotherapy. Meropenem, a carbapenem, either alone (120 mg/kg/day every 8 hours) or in combination with other drugs, may be effective for patients who cannot tolerate vancomycin.

Duration of antibiotic therapy depends on the causative agent and clinical response. Minimal duration for Hib and S. pneumoniae is 10 days. A minimum of 7 days is required for meningococcal meningitis. The patient should be afebrile for 5 days before halting therapy. Most other forms of Gram-negative meningitis should be treated for a minimum of 3 weeks.

ADJUNCTIVE THERAPY

In experimental meningitis, corticosteroids reduce meningeal inflammation, thereby reducing ICP and significantly increasing cerebral perfusion.

Sensorineural hearing loss is an important sequela of bacterial meningitis. In children with Hib meningitis, numerous studies have shown that dexamethasone (0.15 mg/kg per dose every 6 hours for 2 days) given rapidly just before or with administration of antibiotics significantly reduces hearing loss. Corticosteroids are not universally recommended for pneumococcal or meningococcal meningitis to reduce sensorineural hearing loss or other neurologic sequelae. The Committee on Infectious Diseases of the American Academy of Pediatrics states that dexamethasone may be beneficial for Hib meningitis and should be considered in pneumococcal meningitis after the risks and benefits have been assessed.

SUPPORTIVE CARE

In addition to critically following vital signs, the patient's body weight, urine specific gravity, serum electrolytes (sodium, potassium, chloride, and bicarbonate), and osmolality of serum and urine should be measured on admission and every 6 to 12 hours for the first 24 to 36 hours. A complete blood count with differential and platelets should be performed on admission and repeated as indicated. Coagulation factors should be checked if petechiae, purpura, or abnormal bleeding is present.

A complete neurologic evaluation should be performed on admission, followed by brief neurologic checks every 2 to 4 hours for the first several days. Complete neurologic evaluation should be performed daily. In children younger than 18 months, daily head circumference measurements should be done to detect hydrocephalus.

A careful intake and output record is required. All patients should be assessed carefully for hydration status and development of SIADH. The best indicators of SIADH are absence of signs of dehydration, increased body weight, decreased serum osmolality, and continued sodium excretion despite hyponatremia. Fluid restriction is the preferred therapy for SIADH, but routine fluid restriction should not occur in all patients with bacterial meningitis. Antidiuretic hormone secretion in bacterial meningitis may be secondary to dehydration. If dehydration is present, maintenance fluids plus sodium and water deficit replacement over 24 to 48 hours can be given. In patients with septic shock, fluid must be provided to maintain circulation and blood pressure.

When increased ICP signs such as a bulging anterior fontanelle or progressive lethargy occur, head elevation to 30 degrees may help. Increased ICP with mental status deterioration or cerebral herniation signs may be treated with intravenous mannitol (0.5 g/kg over 30 minutes repeated as necessary) and, if necessary, placement of an ICP monitoring device. ICP should be kept at less than 20 mm Hg.

Subdural effusions are part of the normal pathophysiology of the disease. Subdural empyema should be drained and treated with antibiotics. Indications for CT scan include focal neurologic signs, prolonged obtundation, focal seizures, rapidly increasing head circumference, persistently increased CSF protein, persistent CSF granulocytosis, or chronically recurring meningitis.

PROGNOSIS AND SEQUELAE

Death rates vary widely. Rates up to 55% have been reported in developing countries. In the United States, a metaanalysis found the death rate to be approximately 4% for Hib, 8% for N. meningitidis, and 15% for S. pneumoniae. Similar results from other developed countries have been reported.

Meningitis sequelae include hearing loss, mental retardation, seizures, spasticity and paresis, hydrocephalus, blindness, behavior disorders, and neuropsychological or auditory dysfunctions that adversely affect academic performance. In one U.S. metaanalysis, sequelae were present in only 16% of cases. In a large prospective study, 33% of cases had detectable neurologic abnormalities, including paralysis, seizure, ataxia, hydrocephalus, and vision or auditory problems at discharge. Five years later, only 11% of cases had a detectable neurologic deficit, although this rate increased to 14% at 15 years because of the occurrence of late seizures. Even major neurologic deficits may resolve with time. The incidence of sequelae varies by organism. In one study, discharge morbidity was 21% for Hib, 9% for N. meningitidis, and 38% for S. pneumoniae. Hearing loss is the most common neurologic sequela with deafness present in approximately 10% of survivors.

PROPHYLAXIS

Prophylaxis can prevent spread of *N. meningitis* and *H. influenzae*. Pneumococcal prophylaxis is not recommended because contacts are not at significantly increased risk of infection. Anyone who develops fever after exposure to patients with any form of bacterial meningitis should get prompt medical attention.

N. meningitis prophylaxis with rifampin (10 mg/kg, with a 600 mg maximum, every 12 hours for 2 days) should be given within 24 hours of case recognition. Household, day care, and close contacts of the patient in the previous 7 days should receive rifampin, but casual school or work contacts should not. Often, deciding who had close contact is difficult because infections have occurred after exposure on school buses and school trips. Medical personnel exposed to the patient's secretions in the first 24 hours after the start of antibiotics should receive prophylaxis. Rifampin may turn urine, sweat, and tears orange. Contact lenses may stain permanently, and serum levels of oral contraceptives and other drugs may be reduced. Ciprofloxacin (500 mg orally in one dose) can be used for contacts older than 18 years. Ceftriaxone (125 mg intramuscularly in those younger than 15 years and 250 mg for those older than 15 years) is an effective alternative to rifampin and can be used during pregnancy. The index patient should receive prophylaxis on discharge unless treated with ceftriaxone or cefotaxime.

Hib prophylaxis with rifampin (20 mg/kg, with a 600 mg maximum, once daily for 4 days) eliminates most nasopharyngeal carriage of Hib. Rifampin is recommended for all nonpregnant household contacts, including adults, if a vaccinated child of any age or unvaccinated child younger than 48 months lives in the home. Rifampin should be given to day care or nursery school contacts if two or more cases occur within 60 days. Children who have received Hib vaccine should receive prophylaxis.

For the latest information and details regarding chemoprophylaxis, see the 2003 Report of the Committee in Infectious Diseases (Red Book®) from the American Academy of Pediatrics.

VACCINES

Conjugated (protein-capsular polysaccharide) vaccine for Hib and *S. pneumoniae* exist as part of the universal immunization schedule in the United States. Information on these vaccines can be obtained in chapters dealing with these specific organisms.

N. meningitidis vaccine is recommended for individuals at high risk for disease (e.g., people traveling to hyperendemic areas, those with terminal complement or properdin deficiency, or in an epidemic of known type). The American College Health Association has recommended that college students should consider vaccination against meningococcal disease. The vaccine is given to members of the U.S. armed services.

A quadrivalent vaccine is available and consists of 50 μg of capsular polysaccharides A, C, Y, and W135 in each 0.5-mL dose. It is also available in monovalent A, monovalent C, and bivalent A and C forms. The vaccines are highly protective in the short term, but revaccination should occur at 1 year for children younger than 4 years and at 5 years for children older than 4 years.

CHAPTER 79

Campylobacter and *Helicobacter*

Adapted from Guillermo M. Ruiz-Palacios and Larry K. Pickering

Campylobacter and *Helicobacter* are among the most common bacterial pathogens that infect humans. Their spiral shape and motility of these organisms are adaptations that permit them to penetrate and colonize mucus.

CAMPYLOBACTER

Originally regarded as a rare, opportunistic pathogen, *Campylobacter* has been shown to be one of the leading causes of bacterial enteritis in the world. The incidence of diarrhea caused by

TABLE 79-1. Species of *Campylobacter* and *Helicobacter* that Infect Humans

Species	Affected human hosts	Common disease produced in humans
C. fetus	Extremes of age; immunocompromised	Bacteremia, meningitis, vascular infections; less commonly diarrhea
C. jejuni/C. coli	All ages; cases tend to cluster	Diarrhea, fever, abdominal pain; less commonly bacteremia
C. jejuni subspecies *doylei*	Predominantly in children	Diarrhea, fever, abdominal pain; less commonly bacteremia
C. upsaliensis	All ages	Diarrhea, abdominal pain; less commonly bacteremia, abscesses
C. lari	All ages	Diarrhea, abdominal pain; less commonly colitis, appendicitis
C. hyointestinalis	All ages	Diarrhea, vomiting, abdominal pain; less commonly bacteremia
C. concisus	All ages	Diarrhea, fever, vomiting; less commonly bacteremia
C. sputorum	All ages	Abscesses
H. pylori	All ages	Gastritis, peptic ulcer disease
H. fennelliae	All ages	Diarrhea, abdominal cramps, proctitis; less commonly bacteremia
H. cinaedi	All ages	Diarrhea, abdominal cramps, proctitis; less commonly bacteremia

C. jejuni in the United States is similar to or greater than that of *Salmonella* and surpasses that of *Shigella*.

Etiology

Campylobacter are slender, spirally curved, microaerophilic, motile, gram-negative bacilli with a flagellum on one or both ends. The family Campylobacteraceae comprises two genera, *Campylobacter* species and *Arcobacter* species. Twenty-one species have been identified in the family Campylobacteraceae, but only 12 cause disease in humans. *C. jejuni*, *C. coli*, *C. upsaliensis*, and *C. jejuni* subspecies *doylei* are the most common species isolated from children (Table 79-1).

Epidemiology

Animals serve as the reservoir for *C. jejuni* and *C. coli*, which have been isolated from the gastrointestinal tracts of cattle, sheep, pigs, and numerous commercially raised fowl. Contamination of meat during slaughter may be the way bacteria enter the human food chain. The main source of *C. jejuni* and *C. coli* infection in humans is poultry, although pet dogs, cats, and hamsters are potential sources. Transmission occurs by the fecal-oral route through contaminated food and water or by direct contact with fecal material from infected animals or people.

Outbreaks of diarrhea caused by *C. jejuni* and *C. coli* have been associated with consumption of undercooked poultry or red meat, unpasteurized milk, and contaminated water. In the United States, *C. jejuni* is the most common species of *Campylobacter* isolated in those patients with disease. Rates of asymptomatic carriage are low in developed countries.

Pathogenesis

After ingestion, *C. jejuni* are killed rapidly by hydrochloric acid indicating that gastric acid is an effective barrier against infection. Controlled studies have shown a wide variation in the number of *C. jejuni* organisms needed to produce an infection. Organisms must then attach to the intestinal mucosa for infection to persist; this can occur because of the ability of *C. jejuni* to penetrate the mucous layer and to adhere to epithelial cells.

After *C. jejuni* adhere to epithelial cells, the organisms are capable of causing illness by three postulated mechanisms. The first involves cell attachment and production of an enterotoxin, similar to cholera toxin, with subsequent secretory diarrhea. Second, like *Shigella*, bacteria can penetrate and proliferate within the intestinal epithelium and produce at least two cytotoxins causing cell damage and death, which can be manifested as bloody diarrhea. In the third mechanism, referred to as *translocation*, bacteria may penetrate the epithelial lining without causing cellular damage and proliferate in the lamina propria and mesenteric lymph nodes, reaching the bloodstream to cause extraintestinal infection such as mesenteric adenitis, arthritis, meningitis, and cholecystitis.

Clinical Manifestations

Acute diarrhea is the most common clinical presentation, and more than 90% of cases are caused by *C. jejuni*. After an incubation period of 1 to 7 days, patients typically experience prodromal symptoms of fever, headache, and myalgia. Diarrhea, accompanied by nausea, vomiting, and abdominal cramps, usually occurs within 24 hours with stools that vary from loose and watery to grossly bloody. The frequency of stools varies, but can be more than ten stools per day. Acute resolution is the rule, but diarrhea lasts longer than 2 weeks in 20% of cases, and chronic diarrhea accompanied by failure to thrive has occurred. Abdominal pain can be severe enough to mimic appendicitis. Occasionally, the illness can be confused with inflammatory bowel disease.

Immunoreactive complications have been described that include Guillain-Barré syndrome; the Miller-Fisher syndrome, a variant characterized by ophthalmoplegia, areflexia, and ataxia; reactive arthritis; Reiter syndrome; and erythema nodosum.

Bloodstream and extraintestinal infections are uncommon occurring more frequently in malnourished children or patients with chronic debilitating illnesses or immunosuppression. If bactermeia does occur, focal infections such as meningitis, pneumonia, endocarditis, or thrombophlebitis, can result.

Diagnosis

Clinical diagnosis of *Campylobacter* diarrhea is difficult because of variation in the clinical presentation from watery to grossly bloody diarrhea. However, when inflammatory diarrhea with bloody stools, fever, and abdominal pain occurs, *Campylobacter* should always be considered in the differential diagnosis. Direct examination of stool with Wright stain often shows the presence of fecal leukocytes. A Gram stain of stool may show spiral and curved organisms, which may lead to a tentative diagnosis.

Ideally, for isolation of *Campylobacter* from feces, two systems are used: a selective enrichment medium containing antibiotics to specifically suppress the colonic microflora and a filtration method using cellulose membranes. Although all *Campylobacter* species grow at 37°C, the optimal temperature for growth of a thermophilic group of *Campylobacter* composed of *C. jejuni*,

C. coli, and *C. lari* is 42°C. Because *C. jejuni* is the species that usually causes intestinal illness, many laboratories place stool specimens on one of the selective media and incubate stool cultures at 42°C to help select for this organism.

Several methods using polymerase chain reaction (PCR) for detection of *Campylobacter* in feces have been developed; PCR has been shown to be more sensitive than culture, and it can also be used to differentiate species.

Isolation of *Campylobacter* from blood and other sterile body sites does not present the same problem as does isolation from feces. Growth occurs in standard blood culture media, but slow growth requires that bottles be kept for at least 2 weeks.

Treatment

Rehydration and correction of electrolyte abnormalities are the mainstay of treatment for patients with *C. jejuni* enteritis. Debate continues over the use of antimicrobial agents in uncomplicated infections. Treatment can shorten the course of the illness and limit spread, therefore, it may be indicated if patients are acutely ill at the time of bacteriologic diagnosis or if they have complications, systemic infection, or immunosuppression. Treatment of toddlers in child-care centers may also be reasonable to prevent secondary spread of the organism. When antimicrobial therapy is indicated, erythromycin or azithromycin are the recommended agents. Several placebo-controlled studies have shown erythromycin therapy to be of no clinical benefit if given late in the course of disease, except for decreasing fecal shedding. Excretion of the organism can persist for 2 weeks to 3 months in immunocompetent hosts not treated with antibiotics.

HELICOBACTER

Helicobacter pylori infection is often acquired during childhood and persists for decades. In children, the infection is usually asymptomatic, but it may be associated with nausea, vomiting or chronic persistent abdominal pain. *H. pylori* has been further implicated as a cause of gastritis and as an important contributing factor in the pathogenesis of peptic ulcer disease, gastric carcinoma, and gastric lymphoma.

Etiology

H. pylori is a gram-negative, microaerophilic bacteria. The Helicobacteriaceae family has several other recognized species, in addition to *H. pylori*. *H. acinonyx* has been identified in cheetahs with gastritis and *H. felis* from cats and dogs.

Epidemiology

H. pylori infects humans and occasionally domestic animals such as kittens, puppies, and pigs, which may become infected through human feces. *H. pylori* is a ubiquitous pathogen with prevalence rates that differ among populations and ethnic groups. There is an age-related increase in prevalence of antibodies to *H. pylori*, and antibody response is more common in developing countries with as many as 65% positives among children younger than 10 years.

Transmission of *H. pylori* to humans is not completely understood. Evidence of iatrogenic (e.g., fiber optic endoscopes), fecal–oral, and oral–oral transmission exists. If a parent is infected, children have a 40% chance of becoming infected, as compared with only 3% among children from uninfected parents. During the first 18 months of life, however, when greater intimate contact occurs between mother and child, children of infected mothers seldom become infected. Prevalence of infection rapidly increases after this age, especially in developing countries, suggesting that other factors in the household influence transmission to children. The chance of *H. pylori* infection is greater in crowded conditions.

H. pylori may also be transmitted by animals, as suggested by the higher prevalence of infection among slaughterhouse workers who have direct contact with freshly cut animal parts, among persons exposed to cattle, or persons who consume internal organs.

Pathogenesis

Gastritis associated with *H. pylori* primarily affects the mucus-secreting antral-type gastric epithelium and eventually involves the stomach fundus. These lesions are known as type B or nonspecific gastritis. The histologic changes of gastritis associated with detection and isolation of *H. pylori* revert with specific antimicrobial treatment and, if reinfection occurs, the changes return.

The presence of gastric-like tissue in the duodenum also provides a supportive milieu for *H. pylori* colonization. The active inflammation results in development of a duodenal ulcer. In patients with recurrent duodenal ulcers, *H. pylori* is always found in the margins of the ulcer and in the inflamed antral mucosa.

Sufficient epidemiologic evidence shows a high risk of gastric carcinoma in adults infected with *H. pylori*. A significant association has been observed between gastric cancer incidence and mortality and *H. pylori* seropositivity. A low-grade mucosa-associated lymphoid tissue (MALT) lymphoma, is a neoplasia that occurs less frequently than gastric carcinoma, but it has an even stronger association with *H. pylori* infection. Early stages of MALT lymphoma are cured by eradication of *H. pylori* with antibiotics.

Clinical Manifestations

Little information exists on the natural history of *H. pylori* infection in its early stages during childhood when the infection is often acquired. Most descriptions of patient symptoms are based on adult infection. In children, primary infection appears to be mainly asymptomatic. Furthermore, infection with *H. pylori* in childhood apparently does not last a lifetime but is often spontaneously cleared, although children can become reinfected.

In symptomatic *H. pylori* infection in children, one of the most frequent clinical symptoms is chronic, recurrent abdominal pain; however, most recurrent abdominal pain in children is not associated with *H. pylori* infection. The infection in young infants can present as an acute illness characterized by protracted vomiting that can be confused with upper gastrointestinal tract obstructive disorders. Clinical entities that have been associated with *H. pylori* infection include asymptomatic gastritis; acute active gastritis; and chronic gastritis, duodenitis, and peptic ulcer.

Diagnosis

Invasive tests for *H. pylori* infection are based on direct assessment of gastric biopsies, and noninvasive tests are based on immunologic response (antibodies), on detection of metabolic products (urease activity), or on detection of a stool antigen.

For isolation of *Helicobacter* species from clinical specimens, at least two homogenized biopsies from the gastric antrum should be placed in a selective and enriched medium at 37°C under microaerobic conditions for 2 to 5 days. PCR can also be used to amplify *H. pylori* DNA in gastric mucosa, as well as other specimens such as saliva, stools, and gastric juice.

Organisms can usually be visualized easily on histologic sections using Gram, hematoxylin-eosin, silver, Giemsa, or acridine orange staining. For a presumptive diagnosis, several commercial tests are available for detection of urease production in biopsy specimens, although their sensitivity and specificity are lower than those of silver stains of histologic preparations.

Noninvasive, commercially available tests include serum antibody (IgG) detection by enzyme immunoassay and the carbon 13 and carbon 14 urea breath tests. The basis of the breath test is as follows. *H. pylori* hydrolyze urea, which is metabolized to ammonia and bicarbonate. The bicarbonate is absorbed and excreted as CO_2 by the lungs. If urea is labeled with ^{13}C or ^{14}C and the labeled urea is metabolized, it can be detected in the breath as labeled CO_2, which can be measured and used as a marker for *H. pylori* infection.

Treatment

Multiple therapeutic regimens have been shown to be effective in curing patients infected with *H. pylori*. Use of single agents has been found to be ineffective for curing infection in the majority of patients. Two or three drugs for 14 to 21 days are recommended for treatment.

Treatment is indicated only in symptomatic children in whom *H. pylori* infection has been confirmed by culture, serology, or breath test. Treatment is not recommended in asymptomatic children or in children with nonspecific gastrointestinal tract symptoms. Success in treatment of *H. pylori* infection depends on several factors. The susceptibility of the isolate must be determined or at least the resistance pattern in the specific geographic area where the patient lives should be known.

The goal of treatment is eradication of *H. pylori*. Eradication can be achieved only with a multidrug therapy consisting of a proton-pump inhibitor and two of the following drugs in various combinations: clarithromycin, metronidazole, or amoxicillin or, in adults or older children, tetracycline. Controlled studies of treatment in children are limited, and because most recommendations are based on the large clinical studies in adults, treatment in children should be closely followed. Of the triple regimens available for adults, the one containing tetracyclines should be avoided in children.

CHAPTER 80

Cat-Scratch Disease

Adapted from Kenneth M. Boyer

Cat-scratch disease is a subacute, regional lymphadenitis syndrome that occurs after cutaneous inoculation with a fastidious proteobacterium, *Bartonella henselae*. Contact with cats, in the form of a scratch by claws or teeth, is strongly associated with the illness, although cases without known cat contact have been reported. The disease usually undergoes spontaneous resolution after a 2 to 3 month course. Complications may occur.

ETIOLOGY

B. henselae was first identified in 1990 in patients with acquired immunodeficiency syndrome (AIDS) who had unique opportunistic infections such as bacillary angiomatosis. Studies suggested that the organism was most closely related to *Bartonella quintana* (the cause of trench fever) and *Bartonella bacilliformis* (the cause of bartonellosis). After successful cultivation, the organism was named *B. henselae*.

EPIDEMIOLOGY AND TRANSMISSION

Cat-scratch disease is transmitted by cutaneous inoculation, a cat scratch or bite often by a kitten younger than 6 months. Cat-scratch disease is more common in children than in adults. Cats are the zoonotic reservoir of B. henselae. In one study, 81% of cat sera were positive for antibodies. In another, 41% of apparently healthy cats were bacteremic. Fleas are the major vector for transmission among cats. Human to human transmission is not reported.

PATHOLOGY

Both the primary inoculation site and the draining regional lymph node show central avascular necrosis surrounded by lymphocytes and histiocytes. Generalized node enlargement and granuloma formation eventually lead to central necrosis and formation of large, pus-filled sinus cavities. The capsule of the node may ultimately rupture resulting in a fibrotic inflammatory reaction.

CLINICAL MANIFESTATIONS

After an incubation period ranging from 3 to 30 days (usually between 7 and 12 days), one or more 2 to 5 mm red papules develop at the site of cutaneous inoculation. Although often overlooked, such primary lesions were uncovered in more than 90% of affected patients after a careful search in one series. They persist until the development of lymphadenopathy, which generally occurs in 1 to 4 weeks.

Chronic lymphadenitis is the hallmark of cat-scratch disease, most frequently affecting the first or second sets of nodes draining the site of inoculation. The sites affected most frequently, in decreasing order of incidence, are the axillary, cervical, submandibular, preauricular, epitrochlear, femoral, and inguinal lymph node groups. At a given site, approximately one-half of all cases will involve a single node, and the other half will involve multiple nodes.

Usually, affected nodes are tender, and the overlying skin becomes warm, red, and indurated. Between 10% and 40% of the nodes eventually suppurate. The duration of lymph node enlargement is 4 to 6 weeks with persistence of up to 12 months in exceptional cases. The majority of patients lack constitutional symptoms. Elevated temperatures are documented in approximately 30% of patients. Other nonspecific symptoms may include malaise, anorexia, fatigue, and headache.

A distinctive manifestation of cat-scratch disease is Parinaud oculoglandular syndrome. The site of primary inoculation is the conjunctiva of one eye or the eyelid. Mild to moderate conjunctivitis accompanies the primary lesion. Preauricular lymph nodes are the corresponding unilateral site of adenopathy. Although the oculoglandular syndrome may be induced by other agents, notably Francisella tularensis, the most common cause appears to be cat-scratch disease.

The most serious complication of cat-scratch disease is involvement of the central nervous system in the form of encephalopathy or encephalitis. High fever and convulsions develop within 6 weeks of the onset of lymphadenopathy, followed by alteration in the level of consciousness, headache, and muscle weakness. The cerebrospinal fluid is normal or shows minimal pleocytosis or elevated protein content. Recovery has occurred without residua in nearly all the well-documented cases in the literature. A few patients have had a prolonged convalescence and required anticonvulsant therapy for persistent seizure foci. The incidence of encephalopathy is low, but it can be the presenting manifestation of cat-scratch disease.

Osteolytic bone lesions have been noted at sites anatomically remote from the site of primary inoculation, suggesting hematogenous spread.

Granulomatous hepatitis may present as fever of unknown origin with or without lymphadenopathy. The reported cases have shown characteristic multiple hypodense lesions in the liver on computed tomographic scanning.

DIFFERENTIAL DIAGNOSIS

Eliciting a history of cat exposure and a careful clinical evaluation for a site of inoculation may be all that is needed to make a strong clinical case for a diagnosis of cat-scratch disease. The differential diagnosis of cat-scratch disease can include all known causes of lymphadenopathy. As a general rule, the diagnosis is favored by chronicity, unilateral occurrence, tenderness, and characteristic sites of involvement such as axillary, epitrochlear, and preauricular nodes.

Serologic tests are available to aid in clinical diagnosis but are best done at reference labs or the Centers for Disease Control and Prevention (CDC). *B. henselae* can be detected by polymerase chain reaction (PCR). If tissue is available from a biopsy, *B. henselae* may be seen by using the Warthin-Starry stain, but this test is nonspecific. The cat-scratch skin test (a skin antigen test prepared by using pus from aspirated nodes of patients) should be considered obsolete and no longer be used.

TREATMENT AND PROGNOSIS

Cat-scratch disease is often considered when acute lymphadenitis fails to respond to treatment with an antibiotic that covers Gram-positive organisms. *In vitro*, *B. henselae* has been demonstrated susceptible to penicillin G, amoxicillin, gentamicin, rifampin, erythromycin, clarithromycin, and azithromycin. One controlled trial demonstrated more rapid resolution of enlarged lymph nodes in children treated with azithromycin.

Suppurative nodes are treated best by needle aspiration, which should be repeated when necessary. Generally, surgical excision of affected nodes is unnecessary. Incision and drainage should not be performed, as this procedure leads to prolonged drainage and scar formation. In most patients, cat-scratch disease follows a benign course. Usually, systemic symptoms last less than 2 weeks. Affected nodes may be painful for several weeks and may remain enlarged for a number of months. Generally, patients with complications such as encephalopathy or bone lesions, run a more prolonged course but also have a good long-term prognosis.

PREVENTION

The only preventive approach might be to avoid contact with cats, particularly play with young kittens where scratching is common.

CHAPTER 81
Diphtheria

Adapted from Julia A. McMillan
and Ralph D. Feigin

In susceptible human hosts, *Corynebacterium diphtheriae* can infect the skin or the respiratory tract via an extracellular protein toxin.

C. diphtheriae is a gram-positive pleomorphic bacillus. During infection, local invasion occurs. However, widespread complications such as neuropathy, carditis with arrhythmias, and adrenal hemorrhage, are due to the protein exotoxin. The toxin is produced only in *C. diphtheriae* that are lysogenic for a phage carrying the gene for toxin production.

EPIDEMIOLOGY

Humans are the only known reservoir, although other "diphtheroids" are ubiquitous in nature. In the United States, approximately 125,000 cases were reported per year during the 1920s with approximately 10,000 deaths annually. Frequency of disease fell sharply after widespread use of diphtheria toxoid vaccine so that, during the 1980s, five or fewer cases of respiratory disease were reported per year (27 total cases) with three fatalities.

C. diphtheriae is acquired through contact with respiratory secretions or skin of an infected or colonized individual. Asymptomatic carriage occurs but is infrequent in countries where vaccine use is prevalent. Immunization of 70% to 80% of a population is postulated to prevent endemic spread of disease.

Historically, diphtheria was a disease of children, but in highly immunized populations, more adults and elderly individuals are susceptible because of waning vaccine-related immunity.

The incubation period after exposure is approximately 2 to 5 days. Communicability among untreated infected persons continues for up to 2 weeks and is reduced to fewer than 4 days with treatment.

PATHOGENESIS

C. diphtheriae can enter the mucosal surfaces of the nose, mouth, eye, skin or genitalia. Toxin is elaborated and released after an incubation period of approximately 2 to 5 days. Diphtheria toxin is a protein made up of two fragments. The B fragment attaches to host cell receptors and brings about entry of the toxin into the cell. The A fragment interrupts cellular protein synthesis by preventing elongation of amino acid chains.

Toxin acts locally to produce necrosis and edema. In the mouth or throat, a patchy exudate appears, followed by deeper tissue involvement and the development of a gray-black, adherent membrane composed of epithelial cells, fibrin, inflammatory cells, erythrocytes, and organisms. The membrane may become so extensive that it causes upper airway obstruction and even suffocation. At the site of a cutaneous infection, an ulcer with sharp borders develops and becomes covered with a gray membrane.

Toxin is disseminated by the hematogenous route and through the lymphatics to reach distant organs. Effects of toxin on cardiac and nervous tissue can be life-threatening. In the heart, cellular infiltrate develops, particularly involving the conducting system. Clinically apparent cardiac involvement may be present during the first few days of illness, although it often is delayed until the second week or later. Fatty degeneration of the myelin sheaths of nerves can cause paralysis both locally (in the muscles of the palate and hypopharynx) and at distant sites (including the muscles of respiration). Neurologic consequences of toxin are not generally seen until 2 to 3 weeks after onset of infection and may appear as late as 10 weeks.

Antitoxin neutralizes circulating diphtheria toxin, but it has no effect once toxin has entered cells. To be effective, it should be given as early as possible.

CLINICAL MANIFESTATIONS

Tonsillar and pharyngeal diphtheria are most common; symptoms begin with a sore throat, usually in the relative absence of other systemic complaints, but low-grade fever, malaise, dysphagia, and headache can occur. In nonimmune, infected individuals, membrane formation begins after the 2- to 5-day incubation period and grows to involve the pharyngeal walls, tonsils, uvula, and soft palate. It may even extend to the larynx and trachea causing airway obstruction and eventual suffocation. Marked edema of the neck may lead to a bull-neck appearance with a distinct collar of swelling. Swallowing may be made difficult by unilateral or bilateral paralysis of the muscles of the palate. If toxin production is unopposed by antitoxin, early localized signs and symptoms give way to circulatory collapse, respiratory failure, stupor, coma, and death. If antitoxin is given promptly, less severe disease resolves with the sloughing of the membrane within 7 to 10 days (or earlier). Disseminated effects of toxin, including myocarditis and nervous system complications, may occur late in the illness, even if the initial respiratory disease was mild.

The larynx and the nares are other less likely sites of infection.

Cutaneous diphtheria may occur at one or more sites, usually localized to areas of previous mild trauma or bruising. It is more common in tropical climates. Pain, tenderness, and erythema at the site of infection progress to ulceration with sharply defined borders and formation of a brownish gray membrane. Local disease may persist for weeks to months. Antitoxin prevents systemic complications but has little effect on skin lesions.

COMPLICATIONS

Airway obstruction by the diphtheritic membrane and peripharyngeal edema combine to pose a risk of death for patients with diphtheria. Toxin-related complications can occur despite the use of appropriate antibiotics, especially if antitoxin administration is delayed.

In historical series, cardiac involvement has been thought to be responsible for 50% to 60% of the deaths associated with diphtheria. The first sign of toxin-induced cardiomyopathy is tachycardia disproportionate to the degree of fever. A variety of dysrhythmias and congestive heart failure may be a consequence of myocardial inflammation. In patients who survive, cardiac muscle regeneration and interstitial fibrosis lead to recovery of normal cardiac function, unless toxic damage has led to a permanent arrhythmia.

Demyelination of nervous tissue is seen in all fatal cases of diphtheria. Frank paralysis, typically of the palate and hypopharyx, occurs in 10% to 20% of patients. Difficulty swallowing and nasal speech are often the first indication of neurologic impairment. Involvement of other cranial nerves can result in oculomotor paralysis and blurred vision. Motor deficits due to involvement of the anterior horn cells of the spinal cord may be seen as late as 3 months after initial disease. Involvement of the phrenic nerve may cause diaphragmatic paralysis at any time between the first and seventh weeks of illness. Recovery from neurologic damage is usually complete in patients who survive.

DIAGNOSIS

In patients whose clinical presentation suggests diphtheria, a portion of the membrane or a swab specimen of material beneath the membrane should be sent for culture. In addition to media selective for *C. diphtheriae*, a blood agar plate should be inoculated so that concomitant infection with group A streptococcus can be identified. If suspicious diphtheria organisms are isolated, a test should be performed to determine whether the isolate is a toxigenic strain. The gel diffusion test (Elek test) is commonly used, or toxin may be demonstrated by intradermal guinea pig inoculation. Coryneform bacteria are frequent contaminants, but if such organisms are isolated from patients with suggestive disease, they should be identified to the species level.

If neuropathy is present, the CSF protein may be slightly elevated and a mild CSF pleocytosis may exist.

Pharyngeal diphtheria may be distinguished from streptococcal pharyngitis, adenovirus, and mononucleosis by the presence of a firmly attached membrane and by the initial relative paucity of fever and other systemic complaints in patients with diphtheria. Clinical findings usually prevent confusion with other pharyngeal infections and their complications including mucositis in patients treated with chemotherapy, oropharyngeal candidiasis, Vincent angina, retropharyngeal or peritonsillar abscess, and jugular vein thrombophlebitis. Conditions involving the trachea and larynx, including severe laryngotracheobronchitis, bacterial tracheitis due to staphylococci or streptococci, epiglottitis, foreign-body aspiration, and masses (e.g., laryngeal papillomas, hemangiomas, and lymphangiomas), are best distinguished from diphtheria by the presence or absence of an adherent membrane seen at laryngoscopy.

TREATMENT

Both neutralization of toxin using equine antitoxin and eradication of the organism with antibiotics are important in achieving effective therapy. The dose of antitoxin recommended depends on the location and size of the diphtheritic membrane, the degree of toxicity, and the duration of illness. For patients who have been ill for at least 48 hours, 20,000 to 40,000 units should be administered for pharyngeal or laryngeal diphtheria and 40,000 to 60,000 units for nasopharyngeal lesions. Patients with extensive involvement, including extensive swelling of the neck, or illness of at least 3 days' duration, should receive 80,000 to 120,000 units. Some experts recommend that 20,000 to 40,000 units be used in patients with cutaneous diphtheria, as toxic sequelae have been reported, but antitoxin is probably of no value in isolated skin disease. Antitoxin should be administered intravenously.

Approximately 10% of individuals have preexisting hypersensitivity to horse serum, the only preparation available in the United States. Immediate hypersensitivity and serum sickness can occur. Before antitoxin administration, a test for sensitivity should be performed using a scratch test, which, if negative, is followed by intradermal administration of 0.02 mL of a 1:1,000 dilution of antitoxin in saline. Sensitivity is indicated by a wheal surrounded by an area of erythema at least 3 mm larger than a negative physiologic saline control injection in either the scratch test or the intradermal test.

If the patient's history or the sensitivity tests suggest a risk for reaction, desensitization protocols are available such as one recommended in 2003 by the Committee on Infectious Diseases of the American Academy of Pediatrics (Red Book®).

Antibiotic therapy should be used concomitantly to eradicate the organism. Both erythromycin (40–50 mg/kg/day orally or parenterally, to a maximum of 2 g/day for 14 days) and penicillin (penicillin G, 100,000–150,000 U/kg/day intravenously in four divided doses, or procaine penicillin, 25,000–50,000 U/kg/day intramuscularly, to a maximum of 1.2 million units in two divided doses for 14 days) are acceptable therapies for respiratory or cutaneous diphtheria. Because patients may not develop effective immunity after infection, diphtheria toxoid should be administered once patients have recovered to complete the recommended series of immunizations.

Patients with respiratory diphtheria should be placed in isolation, and droplet precautions should be followed. Contact precautions are recommended for patients with cutaneous diphtheria.

Public health officials should be notified when diphtheria is suspected. Nasal and pharyngeal swab cultures should be obtained from all close contacts, regardless of immunization status, to identify asymptomatic carriers. Public heath officials will then typically outline treatment of carriers and future schedules for repeat cultures.

PROGNOSIS

Death due to mechanical airway obstruction or cardiac involvement with circulatory collapse occurs in at least 10% of patients with respiratory tract diphtheria. For patients in whom disease is recognized on day 1 and therapy is initiated promptly, the mortality is approximately 1%. If appropriate treatment is withheld until day 4, the mortality rises to 20%.

PREVENTION

Diphtheria toxoid is prepared by formaldehyde treatment of toxin followed by adsorption to aluminum salts to enhance potency. The toxoid used for immunization of children younger than 7 years should be administered at 2, 4, and 6 months of age with booster doses given at 15 to 18 months and again before school entry at 4 to 6 years of age. Because of a higher likelihood of adverse reactions, children aged 7 years and older and adults should receive only the reduced dose. For those who have completed the initial immunization series, diphtheria toxoid should be administered every 10 years along with tetanus toxoid (dT). Multiple studies performed in countries in which universal childhood immunization is recommended, or provided without cost to patients, have demonstrated inadequate antitoxin antibody concentrations in adults, presumably because of waning immunity and inadequate adult immunization.

CHAPTER 82
E. coli Diarrhea

Adapted from James P. Nataro and Larry K. Pickering

Escherichia coli is the predominant aerobic gram-negative organism of the human intestine. Whereas most *E. coli* isolates are harmless intestinal commensals, several have evolved the ability to cause a spectrum of human diseases. The diarrheagenic *E. coli* can be subdivided into six distinct categories, each with a characteristic mode of pathogenesis (Fig. 82-1), epidemiology, and clinical presentation (Table 82-1).

Diagnosing any of the diarrheagenic *E. coli* pathotypes can be challenging as all stool flora *E. coli* can be recovered easily from clinical specimens. Specialized tests exist to identify specific virulent strains or toxins.

ENTEROTOXIGENIC *ESCHERICHIA COLI*

Enterotoxigenic *E. coli* (ETEC) causes mild to severe watery diarrhea and is the major cause of diarrhea in travelers to developing countries.

Epidemiology

ETEC is a ubiquitous contaminant of food and water sources in some places, particularly the developing world. Fortunately, short-lived immunity develops to ETEC surface antigens, thereby confining most symptomatic disease to immunologically naive travelers and weaning infants in developing countries.

Pathogenesis

ETEC colonizes the surface of the small bowel mucosa and elaborates enterotoxins, giving rise to a secretory state. The enterotoxins belong to one of two groups: so-called heat-labile enterotoxins (LTs) and heat-stable enterotoxins (STs). Strains may express an LT only, an ST only, or both enterotoxins. LTs are closely related to the cholera enterotoxin expressed by Vibrio cholerae. Two unrelated classes of STs (STa and STb) differ in structure and mechanism of action. Only STa has been associated with human disease.

ETEC adheres to the intestinal mucosa via one or more proteinaceous fimbrial colonization factors, or CFAs. These organelles may have the appearance of rigid rods (of approximately 7 nm in diameter), thinner wiry structures, or wavy bundles of filaments.

Clinical Manifestations

The incubation period of ETEC diarrhea is 1 to 3 days in adult volunteers. Diarrhea usually begins abruptly and is watery in nature without blood, mucus, or fecal leukocytes. Patients may experience vomiting, but they generally do not have fever. ETEC infection is usually self-limited to less than 5 days.

Diagnosis

If necessary, ETEC is best diagnosed by detection of the enterotoxins ST or LT. Several phenotypic and immunologic tests exist to identify the toxins. Enzyme immunoassays are available commercially. Genetic detection techniques are available in research and reference laboratories and include DNA probes and polymerase chain reaction (PCR).

Treatment

Maintaining adequate hydration is the cornerstone of management of ETEC diarrhea. Antibiotics to which ETEC is susceptible will hasten resolution of symptoms. Trimethoprim-sulfamethoxazole has been traditionally recommended; however, increasing resistance to this agent has been documented, and alternative agents such as fluoroquinolones, ampicillin, and cefixime may be considered.

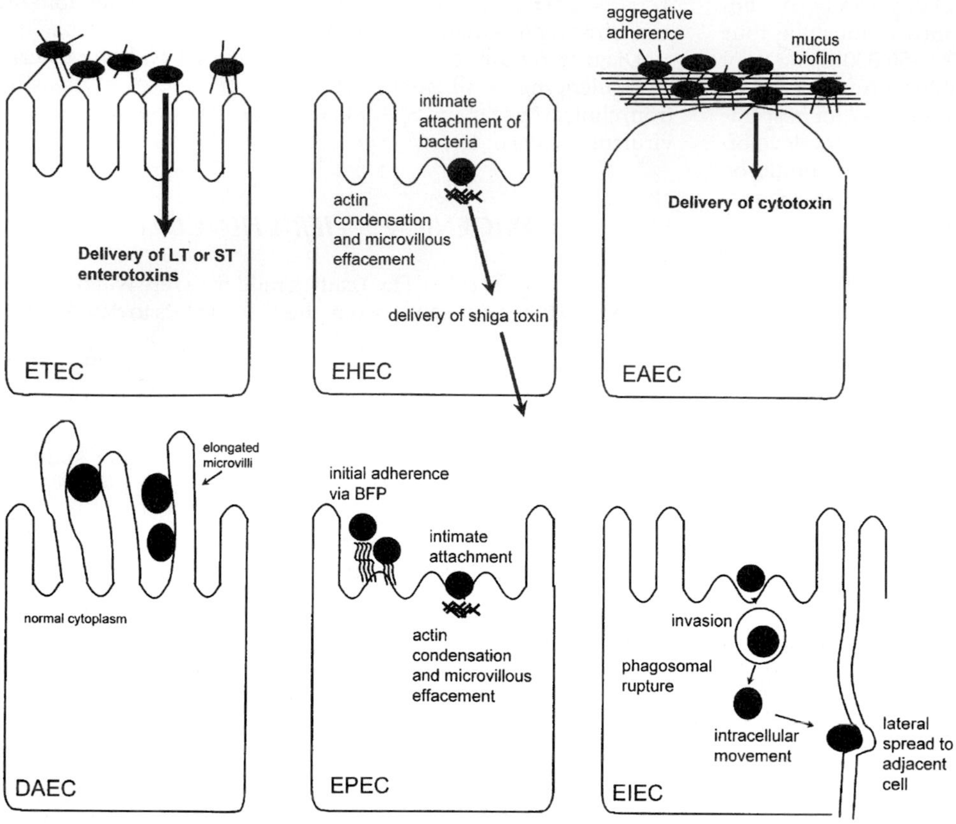

Figure 82-1. Pathogenic mechanisms of diarrheagenic *E. coli*. The six pathotypes of diarrheagenic *E. coli* have distinct pathogenic strategies, illustrated here as their respective interactions with an intestinal epithelial cell. Enterotoxigenic *E. coli* (ETEC) adheres to the small bowel mucosa and delivers secretory enterotoxins. Enterohemorrhagic *E. coli* (EHEC) adheres intimately to the colonic mucosa ("attaching and effacing") and transduces a signal resulting in secretory diarrhea: Concurrently, the organism releases shiga toxin resulting in local and systemic effects. Enteroaggregative *E. coli* (EAEC) adheres in a thick mucous gel and causes intestinal secretion and damage. Diffusely adherent *E. coli* (DAEC) has been shown to elicit elongation of microvilli *in vitro*, although this effect has not been demonstrated *in vivo*. Enteropathogenic *E. coli* (EPEC) elicits the attaching and effacing lesion in the small bowel resulting in intestinal secretion. Enteroinvasive *E. coli* (EIEC) invades the colonic mucosa giving rise to an inflammatory enteritis. BFP, bundle-forming pilus. (Reprinted with permission from Nataro JP, Kaper JB. Diarrheagenic *Escherichia coli*. *Clin Microbiol Rev* 1988;11:1.)

ENTEROPATHOGENIC *ESCHERICHIA COLI*

Enteropathogenic *E. coli* (EPEC) is a common cause of watery diarrhea among infants in the developing world and is defined as *E. coli* that causes a characteristic "attaching and effacing" (AE) lesion in the small bowel. EPEC does not secrete the enterotoxins or shiga toxin.

Epidemiology

EPEC is primarily an infection of infants younger than 2 years. In the 1940s and 1950s, EPEC caused outbreaks of severe, watery diarrhea in nurseries in the developed world, but since the 1970s, most EPEC disease has been shown to occur as sporadic endemic diarrhea in developing areas. The vehicle for EPEC transmission is not known with certainty.

Pathogenesis

The full mechanism of pathogenesis of EPEC is not understood, but the AE histopathology is thought to be central to the pathogenic process. This striking phenotype is characterized by effacement of the microvillous brush border and intimate adherence between the bacterium and the epithelial plasma membrane. How the development of the AE lesion leads to diarrhea remains unclear.

Clinical Manifestations

EPEC causes vomiting, low-grade fever, and watery diarrhea without fecal leukocytes. The incubation period is 1 to 5 days. Some studies suggest that EPEC may elicit a chronic diarrhea with malabsorption and sustained AE histopathology throughout the small intestine.

TABLE 82-1. Categories of Diarrheagenic *Escherichia coli*

Category	Clinical syndrome	Epidemiology	Diagnosis
Enterotoxigenic *E. coli*	Watery diarrhea	Weaning infants and travelers to developing countries	Detection of heat-stable or heat-labile toxins by enzyme immunoassay or genotype
Enteropathogenic *E. coli*	Watery diarrhea	Infants younger than 2 years, mostly in developing countries	Adherence to HEp-2 cells; gene probe, PCR
Enterohemorrhagic *E. coli*	Watery diarrhea, hemorrhagic colitis, hemolytic uremic syndrome	Epidemic and sporadic diarrhea, mostly in developed countries	Detection of characteristic serotypes (i.e., O157:H7, O111:H8, O26:H11); detection of shiga toxin; gene probe, PCR
Enteroaggregative *E. coli*	Watery, persistent diarrhea	All ages but predominantly infants	Adherence to HEp-2 cells; gene probe, PCR
Enteroinvasive *E. coli*	Watery diarrhea, dysentery	All ages; occurs in developing and developed countries	Invasion of cells in culture or guinea pig eye; gene probe, PCR
Diffusely adherent *E. coli*	Watery diarrhea	Older children	Adherence to HEp-2 cells; gene probe, PCR

PCR, polymerase chain reaction.

Diagnosis

EPEC can be identified using genotypic or phenotypic methods. The most common genetic assay is detection of the plasmid-borne adhesin genes with a DNA probe or PCR.

Treatment

Antibiotic therapy lessens the severity of symptoms and decreases the duration of shedding, but proper hydration and supportive care are the most important aspects of management. Nonabsorbable aminoglycosides (especially colistin sulfate) have been the mainstay of therapy.

ENTEROHEMORRHAGIC *ESCHERICHIA COLI*

Enterohemorrhagic *E. coli* (EHEC, also known as verotoxigenic or shiga toxin-producing *E. coli*) are defined as organisms that form an AE lesion and elaborate shiga toxin. EHEC causes two distinctive syndromes: hemorrhagic colitis and hemolytic uremic syndrome (HUS), which may be preceded by hemorrhagic colitis or watery diarrhea. Like EPEC, EHEC elicits an AE lesion of the intestinal mucosa (but in the colon). All EHEC strains produce shiga toxin, which induces hemorrhagic colitis and is responsible for the systemic sequelae of this infection.

Epidemiology

Large outbreaks of EHEC accompanied by deaths from HUS have focused public attention on issues of food safety. EHEC can be isolated from bovine species and, as such, the pathogen may contaminate beef products or other foods in contact with bovine-exposed soil. Beef products (particularly ground beef), other meats, vegetables, and apple cider have been implicated in outbreaks. EHEC outbreaks have also been linked to fecally contaminated drinking and recreational water (water parks). The infectious dose required to initiate EHEC infection is extremely low (less than 100 organisms), enabling large point-source outbreaks and person-to-person transmission. EHEC infects patients of all ages, but HUS is most common in children and elderly adults.

EHEC infection has a geographic distribution with high rates occurring in Canada and the northern tier of the United States. EHEC appears to be unusual in most of the developing world. Most outbreaks of EHEC infection have been linked to O157:H7 strains, suggesting that this serotype is in some way more virulent or more transmissible than are other serotypes, but other serotypes have been implicated in both sporadic disease and outbreaks.

Pathogenesis

The prominent features of EHEC pathogenesis include development of the AE lesion (see Enteropathogenic *Escherichia coli*, Pathogenesis) on the colonic mucosa, followed by elaboration of shiga toxin. The latter accounts, at least in part, for the severe mucosal damage that distinguishes EHEC enteritis from the less severe EPEC disease. EHEC also imparts epithelial cell signal transduction events that are similar to those elicited by EPEC.

The shiga toxin family contains two related but immunologically non-cross-reactive groups called Stx1 and Stx2. A single EHEC strain may express Stx1 only, Stx2 only, or both toxins. Stx1 from EHEC is identical to shiga toxin from Shigella dysenteriae 1.

The shiga holotoxin is composed of one A subunit, conferring the enzymatic activity, and five B subunits, conferring binding to the glycolipid receptor, Gb3. The A1 peptide is an N-glycosidase that removes a single adenine residue from the 28S rRNA of eukaryotic ribosomes, thereby inhibiting protein synthesis and causing cell death. The presence of the Gb3 receptor on enterocytes and renal endothelial cells is thought to account for the clinical manifestations of EHEC infection and its sequelae. Shiga toxin is believed to damage the glomerular endothelial cells leading to narrowing of capillary lumina and occlusion of the glomerular microvasculature with platelets and fibrin.

Clinical Manifestations

EHEC enteritis comprises a clinical spectrum ranging from mild watery diarrhea to severe hemorrhagic colitis. EHEC infection typically begins with the development of watery diarrhea, vomiting and abdominal cramps after an incubation period of 1 to 5 days. The diarrhea then becomes bloody (defining hemorrhagic colitis) in the majority of patients, and typically the illness lasts 4 to 10 days. Intestinal hemorrhage may be profuse, and colonic necrosis and perforation may occur.

HUS consists of the triad of microangiopathic hemolytic anemia, thrombocytopenia, and renal failure, but partial forms have been described. Two percent to 13% of pediatric patients with O157:H7 infection develop HUS, typically in the second week of illness and after diarrhea has resolved. The typical human renal histopathology includes swollen glomerular endothelial cells and deposition of platelets and fibrin within the glomeruli. Of the patients who develop HUS, chronic renal failure persists in 4% to 10%; other forms of chronic renal disease or hypertension persist in 12% to 39%.

Other complications of EHEC infection include cholecystitis, pancreatitis, posthemolytic biliary lithiasis, rectal prolapse, and appendicitis.

Diagnosis

Most O157:H7 isolates do not ferment sorbitol, therefore, cultivation of *E. coli* on sorbitol MacConkey medium is a convenient method for detection of this serotype, but confirmation of presumptive isolates with O157:H7 antiserum is required. Several other assays are available to detect O157 or its products in stool; these tests include enzyme immunoassays for O157 and shiga toxin, latex agglutination tests for the O157 antigen, and rapid strip-mounted monoclonal antibodies to detect the O157 antigen in stools. All of these tests have been shown to have good sensitivity and specificity in EHEC detection, with the caveat that analysis of stool for the presence of the pathogen should be performed as early as possible in the diarrheal illness. Studies suggest that by 1 week after the onset of EHEC diarrhea (and before most cases of HUS are manifest), most stools no longer yield the pathogen. All patients with bloody diarrhea should have their stools cultured for EHEC. The clinician should notify the laboratory personnel of this possibility.

Treatment

The approach to a patient with O157:H7 infection is somewhat controversial. Some studies have suggested that treatment with antibiotics increases the risk of HUS. A recent metaanalysis, however, failed to support this conclusion. It is likely that treatment with antibiotics offers little benefit to the patient. Because of the potential for doing more harm than good, most pediatricians withhold antibiotics for all but the sickest patients with bloody diarrhea, during which time, supportive care is administered. If a stool pathogen is identified as 0157:H7 and the patient is improving, treatment with antibiotics should be withheld. The administration of antimotility agents during the diarrhea should be avoided. When HUS supervenes, aggressive support can be lifesaving, and early dialysis is associated with improved outcome.

ENTEROAGGREGATIVE *ESCHERICHIA COLI*

Enteroaggregative *E. coli* (EAEC) is an established cause of watery diarrhea in infants. EAEC are defined as *E. coli* that do not secrete enterotoxins LT or ST and that adhere to HEp-2 cells in an aggregative pattern.

Epidemiology

EAEC is associated with acute and, especially, persistent diarrhea (longer than 14 days) among children in the developing world. The vehicle for sporadic EAEC disease is not known, but several foodborne outbreaks of EAEC diarrhea have been described in developed countries.

Pathogenesis

EAEC pathogenesis is not thoroughly understood, but EAEC characteristically enhances mucus secretion from the small and large bowel mucosa with trapping of the bacteria in a mucus-containing biofilm.

Certain EAEC strains can cause shortening of villi, hemorrhagic necrosis of the villous tips, and a mild inflammatory response. A high-molecular-weight (greater than 100 kd) enterotoxin/cytotoxin has been described. An ST-like toxin (EAST1) may also be involved in intestinal secretion by EAEC.

Diagnosis

EAEC diagnosis can be difficult for several reasons. First, asymptomatic shedding of EAEC is common. It is also likely that not all organisms that exhibit the typical aggregative adherence pattern are, in fact, pathogenic. Thus, an EAEC strain should not be presumed to be the cause of a patient's diarrhea unless the organism is isolated repeatedly in the absence of another pathogen. Molecular methods have been developed for diagnosis of EAEC infection, yet none of these tests is as sensitive as the adherence assay.

Clinical Considerations

The diarrhea (mucoid, watery or occasionally bloody) often persists for 2 weeks or more and may even continue for several days after the administration of appropriate antibiotic therapy.

Treatment

Fluid and nutritional support are the mainstays of therapy. The effectiveness of antibiotic therapy for EAEC infection is unclear. EAEC is frequently resistant to antimicrobial agents, but nonabsorbable aminoglycosides and fluoroquinolones are likely to be effective agents.

ENTEROINVASIVE *ESCHERICHIA COLI*

Enteroinvasive *E. coli* (EIEC) is closely related to Shigella species and is defined by its ability to invade epithelial cells. EIEC may cause watery diarrhea but also an invasive inflammatory colitis and, occasionally, dysentery.

Epidemiology

Foodborne or waterborne outbreaks have been described. The infectious dose for EIEC in volunteers is higher than that for Shigella and, thus, the potential for person-to-person transmission is lessened.

Pathogenesis

The current model of EIEC pathogenesis comprises (a) epithelial cell penetration, followed by (b) lysis of the endocytic vacuole, (c) intracellular multiplication, (d) directional movement through the cytoplasm, and (e) extension into adjacent epithelial cells. Although EIEC is invasive, dissemination of the organism past the submucosa is rare.

Clinical Manifestations

EIEC can occasionally cause dysentery syndrome with fecal blood, mucus, and polymorphonuclear cells, but, more commonly, the infection manifests as secretory or mild inflammatory diarrhea. The infection is usually self-limiting. Antibiotic therapy is effective in ameliorating symptoms and decreasing the duration of shedding. Trimethoprim-sulfamethoxazole is the preferred agent when the strain is susceptible; ampicillin, cefixime, and quinolones are alternatives.

Diagnosis

EIEC can be detected by phenotypic or genotypic analyses of lactose-negative *E. coli* isolated from stool. Gene probes and PCR assays are available.

DIFFUSELY ADHERENT *ESCHERICHIA COLI*

Diffusely adherent *E. coli* (DAEC) is defined by its characteristic diffuse pattern of adherence to HEp-2 cells in culture. Whether DAEC strains are true diarrheal pathogens is unclear because adult volunteers fed these strains have not developed diarrhea and no outbreaks have been documented.

CHAPTER 83
Gonococcal Infections

Adapted from Lori E. R. Patterson

MICROBIOLOGY

Neisseria gonorrhoeae is a gram-negative, aerobic, nonmotile, oxidase-positive bacterium that appears as a small diplococcus with flattened adjacent surfaces. The outer lipid membrane contains pili, lipooligosaccharide, and several distinct proteins. The most prevalent of these, porin (previously called outer membrane protein I), acts as an anion channel through the hydrophobic cell membrane. Other outer-membrane proteins facilitate adherence and block host humoral immunity to the gonococcus. Pili also contribute to adherence; nonpiliated strains are avirulent. There are more than 100 distinct strains of *N. gonorrhoeae*. Resistance to antibiotics may be conferred either by chromosomal alterations or by plasmid-mediated mechanisms.

PATHOPHYSIOLOGY

Once exposed to mucosal surfaces, the gonococcus adheres to the host cell aided by outer membrane pili. The bacteria penetrate by endocytosis through or between epithelial cells disrupting the mucosal integrity. Lipooligosaccharide exerts a toxic effect on the ciliated epithelial cells. An intense inflammatory response with influx of neutrophils produces the characteristic profuse exudate. As gonococci invade the subepithelial space, deeper tissue destruction occurs through the action of extracellular enzymes and the cytotoxic and endotoxin-like effects of lipooligosaccharide. Invasion of local blood vessels and lymphatics may lead to dissemination. Eventually, scarring and fibrosis develop in the untreated patient.

Specific host defenses against gonococcal infection are not fully understood. Humoral and secretory immunoglobulins against *N. gonorrhoeae* appear in response to infection, but they are not fully protective against subsequent episodes. Complement activation may play a role in protecting against disseminated disease, as complement-deficient patients are at increased risk for developing gonococcemia. The role of cellular immunity in defense against the gonococcus is undetermined.

EPIDEMIOLOGY

More than 500,000 cases of gonorrhea are tallied annually by the Centers for Disease Control and Prevention (CDC) making it the infectious disease reported most commonly in the United States. Because of asymptomatic infection, authorities estimate that 1 to 2 million cases actually occur each year. Young adults account for the most cases, followed closely in incidence by older adolescents. Young women aged 15 to 19 years have the highest incidence of any group. Demographic risk factors for gonococcal disease include young age, unmarried status, nonwhite race, urban residence, low socioeconomic status, and male homosexuality. Gonorrhea incidence rates have been falling or remained stable since the late 1970s.

Gonorrhea is transmitted through direct physical contact with infected mucosa. In adolescents and young adults, this spread occurs via sexual contact. Usually, neonates and young children are infected intrapartum or by sexual abuse, respectively. Conjunctivitis in older children occurs by autoinoculation. Rectal gonorrhea may be acquired by receptive anal intercourse or by perineal contamination by genitourinary secretions. Pharyngeal infection presumably follows orogenital contact. Transmission by fomites has been implicated in nursery outbreaks. The incubation period is generally 2 to 7 days.

Since the late 1970s, the prevalence of antibiotic-resistant strains of *N. gonorrhoeae* has risen markedly. In 1992, gonococci with plasmid-mediated resistance to penicillin or tetracycline, plus those with chromosomally mediated resistance to these drugs, accounted for roughly one-third of all isolates, an increase of approximately 70% in just 4 years.

CLINICAL PRESENTATION AND COMPLICATIONS

Ophthalmia Neonatorum and Other Neonatal Disease

Ophthalmia neonatorum, the most common form of neonatal gonorrhea, usually occurs after intrapartum contact with the mother's infected genital secretions, but cesarean delivery does not preclude its development. Usually, onset of the conjunctivitis occurs at age 2 to 5 days. The ocular discharge is classically bilateral, mucopurulent, and profuse; marked eyelid edema and chemosis are present. Without prompt treatment, corneal ulceration and invasion of deeper ocular structures occur with subsequent loss of vision. Invasive infection (sepsis, meningitis) also occurs in neonates, albeit rarely. A form of neonatal septic arthritis usually appears 1 to 4 weeks after delivery and after several days of prodromal symptoms, involves one to four distal joints, and is not associated with skin lesions.

Vaginitis and Cervicitis

Uncomplicated gonococcal infection of the female genital tract presents with mild to profuse vaginal discharge, local pruritus, and dysuria. Many infections produce no symptoms. Pelvic examination may or may not reveal a purulent endocervical discharge in postpubertal girls. Edema, erythema, and tenderness of the vulva are common in young children. Localized labial swelling and tenderness may reflect infection of the Bartholin's gland. Systemic symptoms and signs are rare.

The most serious complication of genital gonorrhea, seen in 10% to 20% of infected female patients, is pelvic inflammatory disease (PID). Ascent of the gonococcus from the vagina or cervix leads to endometritis, salpingitis and, occasionally, pelvic or abdominal abscesses. The resultant fallopian tube fibrosis leads to obstruction and sterility in 12% of first-time infections, increasing to 50% to 75% after three episodes. Other women later have an increased incidence of ectopic pregnancy or chronic pelvic pain. PID is suggested clinically by lower abdominal pain, discomfort on motion of the cervix, and tenderness of the adnexal structures, which may show a mass-like enlargement. Fever and genital bleeding or discharge may also be present. More extensive spread of the gonococcus, with or without other organisms, leads to perihepatitis (i.e., Fitz-Hugh–Curtis syndrome) with fever and right upper quadrant tenderness.

Urethritis

Purulent urethral discharge and dysuria are hallmarks of urethral infection and are seen in either gender, though the infection is rarely confined here in female patients. Urinary frequency and urgency are not seen. A significant percentage of infected men are asymptomatic. Epididymitis and prostatitis are unusual complications, but scarring may result in urethral strictures.

Disseminated Gonococcal Infection (DGI)

Hematogenous spread of gonococci to joints and other sites occurs more frequently in children and adolescents than in adults. DGI usually occurs after asymptomatic infection. Unlike the arthritis in neonates, joint symptoms in older children mimic the adult presentation and take one of two forms. The first, "arthritis-dermatitis syndrome," consists of migratory polyarthralgia, tenosynovitis, skin lesions, and systemic symptoms. Knees, ankles, and wrists are most commonly involved. The skin lesions are usually distributed sparsely on the dorsal extremities and appear as painful papules or petechiae that rapidly become hemorrhagic, pustular, necrotic, or ulcerated. Usually, blood and skin biopsy cultures are positive, but no growth is obtained from synovial fluid. The second syndrome is characterized by a monoarticular purulent arthritis with minimal systemic signs. A joint aspirate is likely to show gonococci on smear or culture, but bacteremia is not demonstrable. This is the most common form of septic arthritis in young adults.

DIAGNOSIS

The patient history should make note of risk factors for gonorrhea and details of alleged abuse. In adolescents, information must be obtained about sexual activity and symptoms in partners. The patient should be examined gently but thoroughly for urogenital discharge and signs of trauma. Isolation of *N. gonorrhoeae* from the infected site confirms the diagnosis. Samples should be collected from the urethra in male patients, the vagina in prepubertal female patients, the endocervix in older female patients, and other sources (e.g., rectum, pharynx, joint fluid, blood, skin biopsy) as appropriate. Use of gel lubricants or cotton swabs may interfere with isolation of the gonococcus and should be avoided; warm water and synthetic swabs are suitable alternatives. A first-void urine may also be centrifuged, then the sediment can be cultured.

Gonococci do not tolerate drying. Success in isolation requires immediate plating of clinical specimens onto room-temperature media. Generally, modified Thayer-Martin medium (i.e., chocolate agar plus vancomycin, colistin, trimethoprim, and nystatin) is used for isolation. The added antibiotics suppress growth of accompanying normal flora, but they also may impair isolation of vancomycin-sensitive strains of *N. gonorrhoeae*. If the specimen is taken from a normally sterile site (e.g., synovial fluid), chocolate agar alone is sufficient. Optimal growth occurs at 35°C to 37°C in an atmosphere enriched with 5% carbon dioxide, which may be obtained with use of an incubator and a candle jar.

A Gram stain of purulent secretions that shows gram-negative diplococci within neutrophils is helpful in diagnosing gonococcal urethritis and conjunctivitis but is less so in other clinical conditions. *N. gonorrhoeae* cannot be distinguished from the nonpathogenic *Neisseria* by appearance alone. After isolation, specific species of oxidase-positive, gram-negative diplococci should be determined by their pattern of acid production from carbohydrates (i.e., gonococcus metabolizes glucose but not maltose, lactose, or sucrose). Other tests for definitive identification of clinical isolates include chromogenic enzyme substrate systems, rapid coagglutination techniques using monoclonal antibodies against the gonococcus, and fluorescence-tagged monoclonal antibodies. Because of the medicolegal ramifications in the diagnosis of pediatric gonorrhea, at least two of these culture-based identification methods should be performed. Enzyme immunoassay or nucleic acid probes can detect the gonococcus directly in clinical specimens. DNA amplification testing of clinical specimens is also available.

TREATMENT

Historically, penicillin has been the drug of choice for most gonococcal infections, but trends in antibiotic resistance have forced the abandonment of this approach. Treatment strategies now focus on using drugs that have an efficacy approaching 100% for all strains after a single dose. Treatment options generally consist of third generation cephalosporins or quinolones for older patients; other regimens may be effective. The reader is directed to the most recent CDC Guidelines for the treatment of sexually transmitted diseases at http://www.cdc.gov/std/treatment/default.htm (Accessed 4/30/03). "Test of cure" cultures are unnecessary after standard therapy, but performing follow-up cultures several weeks after treatment is advisable in patients who remain sexually active, as reinfection is common.

Regardless of disease form, a medical and legal imperative is finding and treating the source of pediatric gonorrhea. The possibility of sexual abuse must always be considered, and all household members should be evaluated for gonorrheal infection. The partners of sexually active adolescents must be notified and treated. Concurrent empiric therapy for this chlamydia is also recommended.

PROGNOSIS

When treated promptly with appropriate antibiotics, most gonococcal infections can be cured. Usually, permanent sequelae (e.g., blindness from ophthalmia neonatorum, sterility from PID) are the result of delay in seeking medical attention.

PREVENTION

Interrupting the spread of gonorrhea from mother to neonate may be accomplished best by identifying women who harbor infection at the first prenatal visit. High-risk persons should be cultured again in the third trimester and should be retreated if reinfection has occurred. Partners should be treated as well. Extensive experience has proved the efficacy of the Credé procedure (instillation of 1% silver nitrate solution into the conjunctival sac within 60 minutes of birth) in preventing gonococcal ophthalmia neonatorum. The use of topical 0.5% erythromycin ophthalmic ointment has been advocated as alternative prophylaxis because this agent does not cause chemical conjunctivitis and appears to be as effective. Neither agent reliably protects against nonocular infection or chlamydial conjunctivitis.

Among sexually active adolescents, use of condoms and spermicide should be encouraged as a means of preventing gonorrhea and other sexually transmitted diseases. Every effort should be made to identify and treat the sexual contacts of known gonorrhea patients. However, asymptomatic persons rarely seek treatment, thus, serving as an ongoing source of infection and increasing their own risk of complications.

CHAPTER 84
Haemophilus influenzae

Adapted from Sheldon L. Kaplan

Haemophilus influenzae is a fastidious, gram-negative, pleomorphic coccobacillus that is responsible for serious systemic and local infections in children.

MICROBIOLOGY

Encapsulated strains of *H. influenzae* are classified by capsular polysaccharides types a through f. The polysaccharides are high-molecular-weight polymers that comprise repeating subunits of a disaccharide. In the prevaccine era, approximately 95% of invasive diseases were caused by the type b strain, for which the repeating subunit is polyribosyl ribitol phosphate (PRP). Unencapsulated strains (i.e., nontypable strains) are primarily etiologic agents in upper respiratory tract infections such as otitis media and sinusitis, but they also cause systemic disease, especially in the neonate or immunocompromised host.

H. influenzae organisms have several outer membrane proteins (OMP) and based on the OMP pattern, 21 subtypes of *H. influenzae* type b (Hib) can be described. OMP patterns have proven useful for epidemiologic investigations. *H. influenzae* contain a lipopolysaccharide. This lipopolysaccharide is an additional virulence factor for Hib.

H. influenzae appears to have several adherence factors that promote colonization. Approximately one-third are capable of expressing pili that bind to receptors on the host's respiratory cells.

EPIDEMIOLOGY

In the United States, approximately 20,000 cases of systemic Hib infection occurred yearly before the introduction of the Hib protein conjugate vaccines. Most cases were bacterial meningitis in children aged 6 to 11 months.

During 1987 to 1995, the incidence of invasive *H. influenzae* disease decreased 96% (Fig. 84-1). As a result, nontypable strains and other non-b serotypes (especially type f) now cause a higher proportion of invasive *H. influenzae* infections. Serotype f has been associated with meningitis and pneumonia in children younger than 5 years; almost 25% of them have an underlying illness.

African-American, Hispanic, and Native American children have higher rates of infection with Hib than do white, nonHispanic children. The highest endemic incidence of disease occurs among native Alaskan Eskimos. Children younger than 4 years who are household contacts of a patient with Hib disease have a much higher risk for this disease than does the general population. Children with underlying immune deficiencies and anatomic or functional asplenia (e.g., hemoglobinopathies) are more likely to develop systemic *H. influenzae* infections. Other risk factors for invasive Hib infections are day care attendance, crowded households, frequent infections, and socioeconomic status. Additional risk factors for developing local infections due to nontypable *H. influenzae* include viral respiratory infections, allergies, exposure to smoke, and anatomic abnormalities such as cleft palate.

Breast-feeding for infants between 2 and 5 months of age appears to be a relatively protective factor.

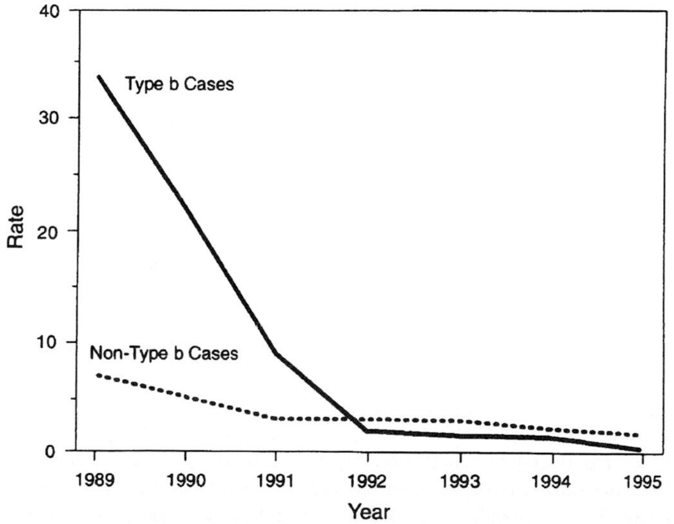

Figure 84-1. Race-adjusted incidence of rate (per 100,000 children younger than 5 years old) for invasive *Haemophilus influenzae* type b and nontype b disease detected through active laboratory-based surveillance in the United States, 1989 to 1995.

PATHOGENESIS AND IMMUNITY

Invasive disease caused by Hib frequently followed a viral upper respiratory infection, which may disrupt mucosal barriers and interrupt the normal activity of respiratory cilia. After it passes the mucosal barrier, the organism can directly invade the bloodstream. In a susceptible host, bacteria multiply readily, and after a critical bacterial density is reached, dissemination occurs.

For local infections caused by unencapsulated strains, a preceding viral upper respiratory infection frequently disrupts the normal physiologic clearance mechanisms and permits invasion of the sinuses or middle ear by normal respiratory flora such as nontypable *H. influenzae*. However, certain nontypable strains may possess one or more virulence factors.

Antibody to the capsular polysaccharide (PRP) is a major component of the host defense against Hib. Antibody to PRP is an important opsonin, is bactericidal in combination with complement, and promotes neutrophil chemotaxis. Antibodies to other noncapsular polysaccharide antigens such as OMPs and lipooligosaccharides, may play some role in immunity against *H. influenzae*.

INFECTIONS CAUSED BY *HAEMOPHILUS INFLUENZAE* TYPE B

After Hib bacteremia developed, invasion of most sites in the body could occur, but certain sites of infection predominated.

Hib was the leading cause of bacterial meningitis and a common cause of pneumonia in children between the age 4 years and younger in the United States. Neither of these two focal Hib infections could be clinically differentiated from infection with other organisms such as *S. pneumoniae*.

Septic or Pyogenic Arthritis

Hib caused septic arthritis, primarily of large joints such as the knee, hip, ankle, and elbow, in children younger than 2 years. Hib was an uncommon cause of osteomyelitis.

Cellulitis

Many children displayed a pattern of upper respiratory infection, followed by the acute onset of cellulitis. Usually, no history of trauma existed. The cheek or buccal region and the periorbital area were the most common sites of infection. Why Hib was related to buccal cellulitis is unknown. The area of cellulitis typically has indistinct margins and is tender and indurated. A violaceous or blue-purple color is common. Concomitant infections, especially meningitis, may complicate the diagnosis. Blood culture results are positive in as many as 80% of the patients, and Hib can often be recovered from an aspirate of the cellulitis.

Pericarditis

Hib can cause bacterial pericarditis. These patients are usually between 2 and 4 years of age and often have had an antecedent upper respiratory tract infection. Fever, respiratory distress, and tachycardia are consistent findings. Associated infections are also common. The etiologic diagnosis may be established by blood culture or by culture of pericardial fluid. Optimal management includes pericardiectomy.

Other Infections

Acute epiglottitis was frequently associated with Hib. Occult bacteremia, urinary tract infections, bacterial tracheitis, endocarditis, soft tissue abscess, and brain abscesses can all be caused by Hib.

INFECTIONS CAUSED BY NONTYPABLE *HAEMOPHILUS INFLUENZAE*

Upper Respiratory Tract Infections

Unencapsulated *H. influenzae* remains a common cause of acute otitis media and acute sinusitis in children. In older children and adults, nontypable *H. influenzae* is associated with bronchitis. Nontypable strains are also common causes of conjunctivitis in children.

In the neonate, nontypable *H. influenzae* sepsis, pneumonia, respiratory distress syndrome, meningitis, and conjunctivitis have been reported.

Bacteremia, meningitis, lung cyst, rectal abscess, septic arthritis, and cerebrospinal fluid shunt infections may be caused by nontypable *H. influenzae*. Systemic infections caused by unencapsulated *H. influenzae* occur predominantly in immunocompromised hosts, although pneumonia caused by nontypable strains is common in children living in developing countries. Invasive infections caused by nontype b *H. influenzae* should prompt an investigation for an underlying anatomic or immune defect.

DIAGNOSIS

Cultures of sterile body sites yield *H. influenzae* in most children with invasive infections. Gram stain may demonstrate the characteristic pleomorphic coccobacilli of *H. influenzae*. Polysaccharide for Hib antigen can be detected by latex agglutination in a variety of body fluids, but these tests suffer from poor sensitivity and specificity.

TREATMENT

Approximately 30% to 40% of *H. influenzae* strains are resistant to ampicillin. The typical mechanism of resistance is beta-lactamase production and is more common among isolates recovered from children younger than 5 years. A small but growing percentage of ampicillin-resistant strains has a mechanism of resistance related to altered penicillin-binding proteins. These strains test negative for beta-lactamase but are resistant to ampicillin.

Cefuroxime, cefotaxime, and ceftriaxone are parenteral cephalosporins with proven efficacy in the treatment of systemic *H. influenzae* infections. Trimethoprim-sulfamethoxazole, cefpodoxime, cefuroxime axetil, the combination of amoxicillin and clavulanic acid (a beta-lactamase inhibitor), and newer macrolides such as azithromycin are oral agents useful for treating infections caused by ampicillin-resistant *H. influenzae*. Several treatment options are available for the initial management of the child with suspected invasive infection caused by Hib. Cefotaxime or ceftriaxone should be used for bacterial meningitis. Cefuroxime should be avoided due to inadequate penetration into the CSF.

The initial treatment of upper respiratory infections possibly caused by *H. influenzae* is usually with high dose amoxicillin. If the physician suspects that ampicillin-resistant strains are involved, any one of the oral agents previously mentioned can be administered.

PREVENTION

The development of the Hib protein conjugate vaccines has been one of the most important advances in preventive pediatrics. Children younger than 2 years do not develop protective antibodies to polysaccharide vaccines. However, conjugating the PRP capsular polysaccharide to a protein enhances the immunogenicity in infants by converting a T-cell-independent antigen to a T-cell-dependent one. Currently, multiple Hib protein conjugate vaccines, which differ in composition, are available. A combination vaccine of Hib (PRP-OMP) and hepatitis B is available (COMVAX®, Merck, West Point, Pa.).

The American Academy of Pediatrics (AAP) and the Centers for Disease Control and Prevention (CDC) recommend routine immunization beginning at 2 months of age. The vaccine administration schedules are different because of differences in the kinetics of antibody response. For a full discussion of immunization details, the reader is referred to the 2003 Report of the Committee on Infectious Diseases (Red Book®) from the AAP.

To prevent secondary infection, rifampin prophylaxis is indicated for all family contacts of persons with Hib disease if another family member younger than 4 years who has not completed the Hib immunization series is residing in the same household. Rifampin is administered to children at a dose of 20 mg/kg (not to exceed 600 mg) once daily for 4 consecutive days. Parents are given 600 mg/day for 4 days. The index patient should receive rifampin because systemic antibiotics do not reliably eradicate nasopharyngeal colonization of Hib. Parents should be told that an increased risk of secondary infection exists in the household and that they should seek prompt medical attention for any suspicious signs or symptoms in their child. Parents of children exposed to a single case of systemic Hib infection in a child-care center or nursery school should be similarly warned. Although not perfect, rifampin prophylaxis is effective in preventing secondary infections.

CHAPTER 85
Legionella

Adapted from Morven S. Edwards

A constellation of illnesses caused by *Legionella* has been defined since the late 1970s. When epidemic pneumonia was diagnosed among delegates attending the 1976 American Legion convention in Philadelphia, the descriptive term *legionnaires' disease* was coined. An estimated 182 people developed pneumonia, and 29 died. A 3-year-old child was among those with documented seroconversion. Within months, a "new" bacterium was discovered: *Legionella pneumophila*. Serologic testing revealed that the bacillus had existed for decades and accounted for a number of previously unexplained outbreaks of pneumonia. Many of the members of the genus *Legionella* are recognized agents of human infection. Legionnaires' disease and Pontiac fever are caused by *L. pneumophila*.

MICROBIOLOGY

Legionella are small, pleomorphic, gram-negative bacilli. Of the 40 species of *Legionella*, *L. pneumophila* is the most pathogenic and accounts for 90% of legionellosis cases. *L. pneumophila* has 14 serogroups, each of which has been associated with human infection. Serogroup 1 accounts for 80% of reported infections. Legionella from clinical specimens are not visible by Gram stain. Special stains such as the Gimenez and Dieterle silver impregnation, are necessary for visualization.

EPIDEMIOLOGY AND TRANSMISSION

Legionella spreads by the airborne route, and legionnaires' disease is transmitted by inhalation, particularly of water vapor containing aerosolized bacteria. Outbreaks have been linked to the evaporative condensers of air-cooling systems, which amplify spread of the bacteria.

The incidence of legionnaires' disease peaks in the late summer and early fall and has a male population predominance. Person-to-person spread has not been documented. Infection is uncommon in the first two decades of life. Risk factors for infection in adults include smoking and alcoholism. Major predisposing features for all ages include organ transplantation, immunosuppression, malignancy, and renal disease. Underlying respiratory disease may be a risk factor in childhood.

Seroconversion to *L. pneumophila* or a closely related or cross-reacting organism in association with mild or unapparent clinical infection appears to be common among young children. In one longitudinal 5-year study, more than one-half of the participants younger than age 4 years at enrollment developed a fourfold or greater rise in titer that was not associated with acute illness. The infrequency with which *L. pneumophila* can be implicated as a cause of acute pneumonia in normal children was illustrated by a study of 110 children who ranged in age from 1 week to 17 years and were hospitalized with pneumonia. Only two cases of legionnaires' disease—one confirmed and one possible—were identified.

PATHOPHYSIOLOGY

Legionnaires' disease is initiated by inhalation of *L. pneumophila*. The bacillus gains entry into the cytoplasm of macrophages through phagocytosis and has the capacity to resist monocytic microbicidal mechanisms and to replicate intracellularly. The resultant cellular infiltrate in the alveolar spaces consists of macrophages and neutrophils. On radiography, this mode of invasion causes a patchy lobular consolidation, which may progress to severe multilobular involvement and bilateral consolidation. A nodular infiltrate occurs in some 20% of patients.

Bacteremic spread is the proposed route for dissemination of infection in immunocompromised patients. The reticuloendothelial system is often involved in fatal infections. Focal involvement of other organs such as the heart (e.g., myocardium, pericardium, endocardium), kidneys, brain, and peritoneum has been observed. Cellular immunity has a major role in host defense.

CLINICAL MANIFESTATIONS

The incubation period for legionnaires' disease is 2 to 10 days. Prodromal symptoms include malaise, myalgias, and headache. The illness is characterized by sudden onset of high fever and shaking chills with systemic toxicity. A dry, nonproductive cough is usually apparent by the second day of illness. Without intervention, pulmonary signs become more prominent and may progress to consolidation. In the normal host, spontaneous resolution of symptoms begins on days 7 to 10 of the illness.

Most symptomatic pediatric infections have been diagnosed in children with identifiable risk factors for legionnaires' disease, but cavitary pneumonia can occur in immunocompetent hosts. In immunocompromised children, symptoms may progress rapidly to respiratory failure with fatal outcome, often accompanied by renal failure and neurologic manifestations.

The usual laboratory features include leukocytosis (i.e., 15,000–20,000 leukocytes per cubic millimeter) with a neutrophil predominance, hyponatremia due to inappropriate secretion of antidiuretic hormone, hypophosphatemia, and abnormal liver function tests. Chest radiography reveals distal air space disease, usually in a segmental or lobar distribution. Small pleural effusions may be evident, particularly early in the course of infection.

Pontiac fever is a self-limited disease and has been diagnosed only in epidemic situations. The onset of influenza-like symptoms occurs so rapidly after exposure (i.e., 6 hours–2 days) that symptoms may represent a toxic or allergic response to the bacillus rather than a response to replication of the bacteria in pulmonary macrophages.

DIAGNOSIS

Legionellosis can be diagnosed by isolation of the organism, direct staining techniques, detection of antigen, or demonstration of a rise in specific antibody titer in paired sera. Blood, lower respiratory tract secretions, and lung tissue are the best sources.

Direct fluorescent antibody techniques use fluorescein-labeled antibodies to *L. pneumophila* to detect the organism in sputum, pleural fluid, and fresh or formalin-fixed lung specimens. Sensitivity ranging from 25% to 75% and specificity exceeding 90% is reported. A monoclonal-antibody direct fluorescent antibody reagent is available commercially (Genetic Systems, Sanofi Diagnostics Pasteur, Chaska, MN).

Tests to detect *L. pneumophila* serogroup 1 antigen in urine also permit a rapid diagnosis. Commercially manufactured legionella urinary antigen tests are available as a radioimmunoassay and an enzyme immunoassay (Binax, Portland, ME). They have high sensitivity (=70%) and specificity (99%). Antigen remains detectable in urine for days or weeks, even during the administration of antibiotics.

Assays based on the polymerase chain reaction (PCR) have been used to detect legionella in clinical samples such as bronchoalveolar lavage fluid. The PCR-based tests are highly specific, but they are not more sensitive than a culture.

Legionellosis may be diagnosed during convalescence by indirect fluorescent antibody techniques. The reagents for measuring IgG and IgM were developed and standardized by the Centers for Disease Control and Prevention (CDC). A fourfold rise between acute and convalescent antibody titers obtained at least 3 weeks after the onset of illness to a titer of 1:128 or more is diagnostic. Among some patients, seroconversion may not occur until the sixth week of illness.

TREATMENT

Erythromycin has been the drug of choice for the treatment of *legionella* infections. Initially and for the first week of therapy, it should be administered intravenously at a dosage of 40 mg/kg/day (maximum, 2–4 g/day) in divided doses every 6 hours. The 2- to 3-week course of treatment may be completed using the same regimen orally. The newer macrolides, especially azithromycin, have *in vitro* activity and lung-tissue penetration that is superior to that of erythromycin. Rifampin (15 mg/kg/day; maximum, 600 mg/day) should be used with erythromycin as adjunctive therapy for patients with severe infection, but it should not be given as a single agent because resistant strains may emerge. Penicillins, cephalosporins, and aminoglycoside antibiotics are ineffective for legionella infections.

Appropriate supportive care should be provided for lower respiratory tract infection, respiratory failure, or inappropriate secretion of antidiuretic hormone.

OUTCOME

Clinical response is usually evident within 2 to 5 days after initiation of therapy. Fever may persist for as long as 1 week. The resolution of pneumonia proceeds slowly and may require 1 month. The overall fatality rate for patients managed appropriately is 15% to 25%, but rates as high as 80% have been reported for immunocompromised patients. Apparent relapses have been encountered with a 2-week treatment course and are an indication for retreatment with erythromycin.

CHAPTER 86

Listeriosis

Adapted from Morven S. Edwards

The first perinatal infection due to *Listeria monocytogenes* was described in 1936. The organism was called *Listerella* at that time; the current designation was adopted in 1939 in honor of Lord Lister.

MICROBIOLOGY

L. monocytogenes is a short, non-spore-forming, gram-positive bacillus, which grows well on most laboratory media. Somatic and flagellar antigens have been used to classify *L. monocytogenes* into serovars, designated numerically. Currently, at least 17 have been identified, with types 1a, 1b, and 4b accounting for 90% of listeriosis.

EPIDEMIOLOGY AND TRANSMISSION

L. monocytogenes is found in dust, soil, water, sewage, and vegetation. It has caused naturally acquired infection in more than 50 species of animals and has been isolated from insects, but insects are not considered an important vector of infection. Between 1% and 5% of asymptomatic adults harbor this organism in the gastrointestinal tract.

The incidence of human infection is highest in spring and summer months. Infection in humans is sporadic and cannot usually be traced to animal contacts. Most cases probably result from soil-borne infection. The acquisition of *L. monocytogenes* beyond the neonatal period likely results in asymptomatic colonization or infection of the mucous membranes of the throat or gastrointestinal tract. Among neonates, infection may be acquired transplacentally or perinatally after delivery through the birth canal of a colonized parturient. *Listeria* may be transmitted genitally from person to person, but transmission by the respiratory route has not been documented. Epidemic neonatal listeriosis may be transmitted between infants by contact with the hands of hospital personnel.

Numerous food-borne outbreaks have been documented. In one of these, cabbage used in coleslaw was contaminated, presumably from the manure of a flock of sheep, one of which had died from listeriosis. Pasteurized milk was the source in another outbreak. The milk came from dairy cows that had suffered from *Listeria* encephalitis.

PATHOPHYSIOLOGY

Many people are exposed to *L. monocytogenes*, although few develop invasive infection. Most infections are observed in neonates and older persons, suggesting a host-associated immune defect. Persons with reticuloendothelial dysfunction caused by diabetes, malignancy or other immunosuppressive states are also predisposed. The propensity for listeriosis in persons with T-cell dysfunction demonstrates the critical role of thymus-derived lymphocytes and mononuclear phagocytes in host response to this intracellular pathogen. Listeria replicates within the cytoplasm of host cells and usurps their actin-based contractile mechanism to form filopods ingested by adjacent cells. This cell-to-cell spread avoids direct spread with the extracellular environment. Thus, cell-mediated immunity is highly important in listeriosis. Immune globulins and complement also function in host defense, but only limited protection is conferred by these T-cell-independent mechanisms.

Invasion of the bloodstream from a gastrointestinal tract source is the most likely route. The organism has tropism for the central nervous system (CNS), particularly the meninges. Among neonates, hematogenous maternal infection is presumed to seed the placenta and to cause fetal infection through the umbilical vein with dissemination to multiple organs. In neonates, the liver is usually involved diffusely, and granulomas are also observed in the lungs, spleen, adrenal glands, and lymph nodes. The organisms cause necrosis followed by proliferative activity of cells of the reticuloendothelial system. The granulomas undergo central necrosis. At the periphery of the necrotic focus, chronic inflammatory cells and organisms may be seen.

CLINICAL MANIFESTATIONS

Listeria infections affecting children can be divided into three broad categories: maternal infections, neonatal infections, and infections beyond the neonatal period in children with or without predisposing conditions.

Maternal Infections

Maternal infection is manifested as an influenza-like illness with chills, fever, vomiting, myalgia, and headache that occurs in the days or weeks before abortion or delivery. Intrauterine infection can cause amnionitis, premature labor, spontaneous abortion, stillbirth, or early-onset neonatal infection.

Neonatal Infections

Three syndromes of listeriosis occur in neonates: granulomatosis infantisepticum, early-onset sepsis with or without pneumonia, and late-onset meningitis.

Granulomatosis infantisepticum is the designation for classic disseminated listeriosis, with generalized septicemia, extensive pustular or petechial rash, and marked hepatomegaly. This overwhelming form of listeriosis frequently results in death *in utero.* Live-born infants are often depressed at birth and usually die in the first hours of life due to respiratory distress, meningitis with seizures, or shock. In one report, 15 of 21 infants born alive had fatal outcomes.

Early-onset listeriosis is defined by the onset of symptoms within the first 7 days of life. Most infants are symptomatic at or within hours after delivery. Respiratory distress and shock with cardiac dysfunction are the predominant symptoms. Meningitis can occur. Serovars 1a and 1b predominate in early-onset disease, although outbreaks due to type 4b have also been described. The mortality, even in series reported since the late 1980s, ranges from 20% to 40%.

Late-onset listeriosis occurs 2 to 4 weeks after delivery (mean, 2 weeks). The mode of acquisition of the organism is through a birth canal with colonized disease. Also called the *meningitic* form of disease, late-onset listeriosis generally occurs in full-term infants whose mothers have had a benign obstetric course. It is manifested almost always as meningitis or meningoencephalitis with symptoms typical of purulent meningitis including fever, irritability, and poor feeding. Serovar 4b predominates in late-onset disease. With proper treatment, the fatality rate is less than 10%, but some infants sustain neurologic damage from meningitis.

INFECTION AFTER THE NEONATAL PERIOD

Listeriosis in childhood or adolescence is uncommon. Series suggest that approximately one-half of all infections occur in normal hosts. Infection may present as bacteremia with no focus; as focal infection such as endocarditis, osteomyelitis, peritonitis, or ocular infection; or as CNS infection.

Several CNS manifestations of listeriosis have been described. With its propensity to affect the brain or brainstem, *Listeria* may cause a diffuse encephalitis or rhombencephalitis characterized by dizziness, vomiting, and cranial nerve palsies. Primary involvement of the brainstem follows a biphasic pattern in which a nonspecific prodrome of headache, vomiting, and fever is followed by cranial nerve palsies most commonly involving the sixth, seventh, ninth, and tenth nerves. Food-borne transmission is now recognized as a major source of human listeriosis manifesting as gastroenteritis. Outbreaks have been associated with unwashed raw vegetables; with ready-to-eat foods including soft cheese, deli foods, and pâté; and with unpasteurized milk. After an incubation period of approximately 24 hours, the common symptoms are fever, chills, nonbloody diarrhea, and abdominal cramps.

DIAGNOSIS

L. monocytogenes infection can be diagnosed reliably by isolating the organism from clinical specimens. For suspected early-onset neonatal infection, the placenta, amniotic fluid, and maternal vagina may provide evidence of infection. Neonatal surface cultures from the throat, conjunctivae, or feces are indicative only of colonization, which may or may not be associated with invasive infection and are not clinically useful. A Gram stain of CSF or purulent collections that reveals short, gram-positive coccobacillary organisms supports the diagnosis. Cultures usually yield the organism within 24 to 48 hours of incubation, but a longer interval may be required. Serologic tests have not been useful for establishing a diagnosis of *Listeria* infection in individual patients.

Although other *in utero* infections such as disseminated cytomegalovirus infection, should be considered in the differential diagnosis, the features of granuloma infantisepticum are usually so distinctive as to be pathognomonic. The septicemic form of early-onset listeriosis, with or without respiratory distress, cannot be differentiated clinically from septicemia associated with other bacteria that cause early-onset infection, particularly group B streptococci and the Enterobacteriaceae. Similarly, *Listeria* meningitis cannot be differentiated from other bacterial infections of the meninges.

TREATMENT

Successful treatment of *L. monocytogenes* infection with ampicillin or penicillin alone has been reported. However, because of reported *in vitro* tolerance or resistance to penicillin alone and studies showing *in vitro* synergy and increased clinical efficacy, combination therapy with ampicillin and gentamicin is the initial regimen of choice. In neonates, an ampicillin dose of 150 to 200 mg/kg/day for nonmeningeal infections or 300 to 400 mg/kg/day for *Listeria* meningitis is indicated. The higher dose is appropriate for treating infection in immunocompromised hosts. After clinical response occurs or for less severe infections in normal hosts, ampicillin or penicillin alone may be given. The optimal therapeutic regimen, however, has not been determined. Treatment should be continued for 10 days for bacteremia without a focus, for 14 to 21 days for meningitis or meningoencephalitis, and for 4 to 6 weeks for such serious focal infections as brain abscess or endocarditis. Untreated, listeriosis is usually fatal within 4 days. With treatment, the usual duration of illness is 10 days for septicemia, 2 to 3 weeks for meningitis or meningoencephalitis, and 4 to 6 weeks for more severe illness such as brain abscess or endocarditis.

Among patients with underlying immunosuppression and those with granuloma infantisepticum, the fatality rates are 60% to 70%. Proportionately lower rates are found among neonates and otherwise healthy older children.

CHAPTER 87
Lyme Disease

Adapted from Barbara W. Stechenberg

Lyme disease, recognized in 1975, was first brought to medical attention by the inquiries of two women from Lyme, Connecticut, who were concerned about an illness spreading in their community. An infectious cause that was probably bacterial and associated with a vector was sought due to the epidemiologic characteristics of the disease. In 1982, Burgdorfer and colleagues isolated a spirochete from the midgut of the tick Ixodes scapularis. Its etiologic role was soon confirmed by isolation of the spirochete from blood, skin, and cerebrospinal fluid of patients with Lyme disease. The organism was designated *Borrelia burgdorferi.*

EPIDEMIOLOGY

The major areas where this organism is found are the eastern seaboard, the upper Midwest, and the West. The deer tick, I.

scapularis, is the vector in the eastern and midwestern United States. In the West, the tick associated with this disease is *Ixodes pacificus*. In Europe, cases of EM, with or without neurologic findings, have occurred primarily in the geographic range of the Ixodes ricinus tick.

The occurrence of Lyme disease peaks during summer and early fall. Cases cluster in sparsely settled and wooded areas. As many as 67% of the patients in many studies do not report a history of tick bite, probably because of the small size (i.e., no larger than a pinhead) of the unengorged tick.

PATHOGENESIS

Lyme disease results from direct infection by *B. burgdorferi* and the host's response to infection. In order to progress to the next life stage, various forms of the tick need to take a blood meal. During this blood meal, *B. burgdorferi* in infected ticks migrates to the salivary glands. As the tick is excreting excess water into the host, the B. burgdorferi in the salivary glands is passed into the host resulting in infection. Transmission of *B. burgdorferi* occurs 36 hours or more after tick attachment making prolonged attachment necessary to infect the host.

After an incubation period of 3 to 32 days, the spirochete may invade or migrate to the skin causing erythma migrans (EM, see below), or it may enter the bloodstream and migrate to distant sites.

CLINICAL MANIFESTATIONS

The clinical findings in Lyme disease can be divided into three stages; early localized, early disseminated, and late disease.

In early localized disease, the most common clinical finding is the skin rash (EM) (Fig. 87-1), which usually begins 4 to 20 days after the tick bite. An erythematous macule or papule forms at the site of the bite and gradually enlarges to form a large, plaque-like erythematous annular lesion with a median diameter of 16 cm. The middle of the lesion is often clear, but it can be indurated. EM may be associated with systemic symptoms such as malaise, fatigue, headache, stiff neck, and arthralgia. Fever is usually low grade, but it may be as high as 40°C. Symptoms usually resolve over several days, but they may occur intermittently for several weeks. Fewer than 50% of individuals with EM recall a tick bite.

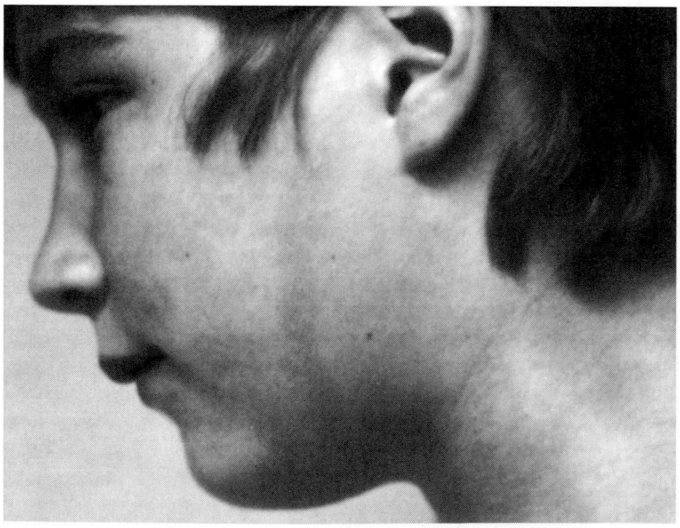

Figure 87-1. An enlarging lesion and multiple smaller annular lesions on the face of an 11-year-old boy diagnosed with Lyme disease who had been hiking in Westchester, NY.

Early disseminated disease can occur 3 to 5 weeks after the tick bite and is most often seen as multiple EM lesions reflective of the blood borne stage of the spirochete. Aseptic meningitis with headache and meningismus, and cranial nerve palsies (typically VII nerve) may occur. Cardiac abnormalities occur in a small percentage of patients. These abnormalities range from fluctuating degrees of atrioventricular block to myocarditis and left ventricular dysfunction. Systemic symptoms such as low-grade fever, arthralgia and myalgia can also be seen.

Late disease is usually seen as arthritis of the large joints, particularly the knee. Attacks may be recurrent and, although unlikely, can occur even after successful treatment in the earlier stages. Neurologic abnormalities such as neurocognitive dysfunction and peripheral neuropathy have been described in late Lyme disease.

Maternal-to-fetal transmission has been documented but currently no conclusive evidence exists for a congenital Lyme disease.

DIFFERENTIAL DIAGNOSIS

If the characteristic EM rash is not identified, it may be confused with cellulitis, erythema multiforme, or erythema marginatum.

Forms of arthritis that may be confused with Lyme disease are pauciarticular juvenile rheumatoid arthritis; reactive arthritis associated with Salmonella, Shigella, or Yersinia; Reiter syndrome; or postinfectious arthritis associated with several viral illnesses. From the standpoint of a systemic illness, Lyme disease is usually easily differentiated from rheumatic fever.

The major neurologic manifestation of aseptic meningitis may be confused with enteroviral, leptospiral, or early tuberculous meningitis. Facial palsy has been associated with EBV infection.

DIAGNOSIS

The diagnosis of Lyme disease is best made on clinical and epidemiological (history of tick bite or exposure) grounds, particularly in a patient with a characteristic skin rash or facial palsy. Decisions to treat may be made on this basis. Routine screening laboratory test are generally normal. In a patient with suspected meningitis, examination of cerebrospinal fluid may reveal a pleocytosis with a predominance of mononuclear cells, elevated protein, and an elevated opening pressure.

Specific serologic diagnosis may be used for patients. Many laboratories offer an ELISA test with high sensitivity that screens for "total Lyme antibody," not specific to IgM or IgG. If this test is positive, than a specific Western blot analysis is performed to detect IgM and IgG response to Borrelia. IgM is typically detected early but may not yet be present in early localized (EM) disease. Peak IgM response is typically 4 to 6 weeks after infection. IgG response occurs more slowly and is generally positive for many years even after Borrelia are eradicated.

Polymerase chain reaction (PCR) also exists and may be useful in certain clinical settings.

TREATMENT

For children older than 8 years with early localized disease, the treatment is oral doxycycline, 100 mg twice a day for 14 to

21 days. Amoxicillin in a dosage of 30 to 50 mg/kg/day in two divided doses for 14 to 21 days is also recommended with cefuroxime axetil, 30 to 40 mg/kg/day in two divided doses, as an alternative.

For patients with isolated facial palsy (without CSF pleocytosis) or other manifestation of early disseminated disease (such as multiple EM), a similar regimen can be used for the longer duration, typically 21 to 28 days.

Children with acute arthritis should be treated with amoxicillin or doxycycline in doses above for 28 days.

As recommended by the 2003 Report of the Committee on Infectious Diseases of the American Academy of Pediatrics (Red Book®), children with persistent or recurrent arthritis, cardiac disease or other neurologic sequelae such as meningitis or encephalitis should be treated with ceftriaxone (75–100 mg/kg IV or IM once per day) for 14 to 21 days or penicillin, 300,000 Units/kg/day, IV to be divided every 4 hours (maximum 20 million Units/day) for 14 to 28 days.

PREVENTION

Avoiding contact with the tick vectors prevents Lyme disease, as well as many other tick-borne illnesses. After exposure occurs, however, detachment is particularly important, because at least 36 hours of attachment are required to allow transmission of the organism. Judicious use of insect repellents such as N, N-diethyl-meta-toluamide (DEET, in concentrations of 10% or less for children) for skin and clothing may be helpful. Routine prophylactic antimicrobial therapy after a tick bite is currently not routinely recommended. For those individuals who have had prolonged tick attachment from hyperendemic areas, one 200 mg dose of doxycycline has been shown to prevent early localized disease.

In 1998, a novel Lyme disease vaccine was FDA approved. Because of low demand from physicians and their patients, the vaccine was removed from the market by the manufacturer in 2002.

CHAPTER 88

Meningococcal Infections

Adapted from Morven S. Edwards and Carol J. Baker

Great strides have been made in our understanding of the meningococcus since the initial descriptions of "epidemic cerebrospinal meningitis" by Vieusseux in 1805 and of "petechial or spotted fever" the following year by Elisha North. However, *Neisseria meningitidis* still causes fulminant infections that are fatal within hours after the onset of symptoms, and many problems must be resolved before meningococcal disease can be successfully eradicated.

MICROBIOLOGY

Neisseria is a member of the family Neisseriaceae. *N. meningitidis* is differentiated from Neisseria gonorrhoeae and the less pathogenic Neisseria species on the ability to ferment glucose and maltose. N. gonorrhoeae ferments only glucose.

N. meningitidis is a gram-negative, biscuit-shaped or coffee bean-shaped diplococcus with rounded outer and flattened inner margins. Specific capsular polysaccharide antigens allow the classification of meningococci into at least 13 serogroups, of which three—designated A, B, and C—are responsible for 90% of human disease. The other ten groups are designated D, X, Y, Z, W135, 29-E, H, I, K, and L. The principal noncapsular cell wall antigens include lipooligosaccharide (LOS), which is analogous to the lipopolysaccharide of enteric gram-negative bacilli, and the outer membrane protein (OMP). The OMPs are part of a lipoprotein-lipopolysaccharide complex that is responsible for the endotoxin-like effect observed in invasive infection. Meningococci also contain pili or fimbriae that enhance attachment to nasopharyngeal epithelial cells.

EPIDEMIOLOGY

In general, an inverse relation exists between age and attack rate with the exception of an increased incidence among 15- to 19-year-old adolescents. More than 50% of the patients are younger than 4 years, and the highest age-specific attack rate is found among infants 6 to 12 months of age. Infection is unusual during the first 2 months of life. Approximately two-thirds of the cases occur during the winter and spring months, and increased disease activity may follow an outbreak of influenza A.

Meningococcal disease has a worldwide distribution. The incidence of disease varies from year to year because of the superimposition of 3- to 5-year epidemic cycles on the base of endemic disease activity. Epidemic disease activity has been reported with group A, B, and C strains.

Sporadic cases are usually caused by serogroup B or C. Since the mid-1980s, serogroup C strains have predominated in endemic disease.

Infections that develop within 24 hours of onset in the index case are designated as coprimary, whereas onset at least 24 hours after exposure to the index case is referred to as a secondary case. Sporadic cases are to be distinguished from a cluster of cases, in which two or more cases of the same serogroup occur more closely than expected in a population, and from an outbreak, in which increased transmission of infection in a population occurs.

PATHOGENESIS AND PATHOLOGY

Humans are the only natural host for meningococcal infection, and the oropharynx is its reservoir. Acquisition of nasopharyngeal infection by inhalation or direct contact results in transient, intermittent, or chronic carriage. The prevalence of asymptomatic carriage during nonepidemic periods ranges from 2% to 38%, and the median duration of carriage is 10 months. In most hosts, infection of the upper respiratory tract elicits formation of serum bactericidal antibody 7 to 10 days later. This immune response does not eliminate carriage, but it does protect the host from symptomatic infection. Susceptibility to invasive disease exists in the interval between acquisition of the organism in the nasopharynx and development of bactericidal antibody in the serum. Pili mediate the attachment of meningococci, and parasite-directed endocytosis promotes their entry into nonciliated cells of the nasopharyngeal mucosa. Dissemination occurs when the organism penetrates the nasopharyngeal mucosa of the nonimmune host and enters the bloodstream, where it replicates. From there, it may disseminate to the meninges, joints, myocardium, or elsewhere. Injury to the nasopharyngeal mucosa by preceding respiratory viral infection may promote invasiveness, but this hypothesis is contested.

Maternally derived antibody provides protection for most infants during the first few months of life. Passively acquired antibody concentrations reach a nadir between the ages of 6 and

24 months, when the incidence of invasive infection is greatest. Nasopharyngeal carriage of meningococci from serogroups with low pathogenicity may elicit cross-reactive antibodies that protect against invasiveness of pathogenic serogroups A, B, and C. Similarly, gastrointestinal colonization with bacteria containing antigens that cross-react with meningococci may contribute to the development of naturally acquired immunity.

Specific antibody and complement are important for immunity. Specific bactericidal IgG antibodies bind to meningococci and may activate the classic or alternative complement pathways. Bacterial killing can be mediated by serum bactericidal activity, which requires the membrane attack complex, or by phagocytes. Patients who are deficient in specific antibody must rely more heavily on the integrity of complement-dependent bactericidal activity. Fatal meningococcemia has been associated with congenital deficiencies of properdin or of terminal complement pathway components C5 through C9. These hosts must kill the organism by phagocytic rather than complement-mediated mechanisms.

The predominant pathologic feature of fulminant meningococcemia is diffuse vascular damage and disseminated intravascular coagulation (DIC). Histopathologically, the vascular changes consist of endothelial damage, vessel wall inflammation, necrosis, and thrombosis. These changes are presumably mediated by the effects of endotoxin. Endotoxic shock resulting in circulatory collapse and myocardial dysfunction is the major cause of death.

CLINICAL MANIFESTATIONS

The clinical expression of meningococcal disease in children may be categorized as bacteremia without sepsis, meningococcemia without meningitis, meningitis, and other manifestations. The initial replication of meningococci in the bloodstream usually causes the nonspecific symptoms of fever, malaise, myalgia, and headache. Bacteremia without a focus may be considered as a possible diagnosis and, depending on the degree of toxicity, these patients may be sent home with or without antimicrobial therapy. The bloodstream may clear without antimicrobial therapy.

Acute meningococcemia without meningitis begins with influenza-like symptoms but, within hours, affected children are septic. Most of them have cutaneous manifestations, which may initially take the form of a nonspecific maculopapular, morbilliform, or urticarial rash. Evolution to a petechial or purpuric rash within hours or days is the rule. Purpura, usually most extensive on the buttocks and lower extremities, is a feature of fulminant disease. In fulminant disease, hypotension, oliguria, DIC, myocardial dysfunction, and vascular collapse (often irreversible) lead to death in approximately 20% of the patients. When the course is less fulminant and shock is responsive to therapy, the occasional fatal infection is usually due to the consequences of direct invasion of the myocardium, manifested by congestive failure, poor contractility, and pulmonary edema.

Only one-third to one-half of the children with meningococcal meningitis have petechiae or purpura at the time of initial evaluation. Among the remainder, the clinical presentation is that of bacterial meningitis characterized (except in very young infants) by nuchal rigidity, altered level of consciousness, and signs or symptoms of increased intracranial pressure. Most children (95%) with meningococcal meningitis survive. The most common cause of death is cerebral edema with herniation.

Children with meningitis or meningococcemia have quantitatively higher-grade bacteremia than do those with occult bacteremia or other manifestations of infection. However, at the time of hematogenous dissemination, other sites may be seeded. The primary presentation reflects the particular focus in which a nidus for infection was established. Primary meningococcal pneumonia, periorbital cellulitis, pericarditis, peritonitis, cervical adenitis, endocarditis, purulent conjunctivitis, and endophthalmitis are rare, but they have been reported in children. Occasionally, manifestations of disease usually attributed to *N. gonorrhoeae* such as vulvovaginitis or pelvic inflammatory disease, prove to be caused by *N. meningitidis*. A syndrome of chronic meningococcemia exists, in which persistent meningococcal bacteremia is associated with fever, skin lesions resembling gonococcemia, and arthritis.

DIAGNOSIS

The diagnosis of a confirmed case of infection with N. meningitidis is established by growth of the organism from blood, cerebrospinal fluid (CSF), synovial fluid, petechial or purpuric lesion, or other usually sterile sites. The presence of gram-negative diplococci in stained smears of CSF, petechiae, buffy coat of blood, and other usually sterile fluid defines a presumptive case. The diagnosis of a probable case is established by a positive antigen test (unfortunately, these tests have very poor sensitivity and specificity) in blood or CSF in the setting of a clinical illness consistent with meningococcal disease.

Meningococcemia should be considered in any child with fever and a petechial rash. Rocky Mountain spotted fever, ehrlichiosis, staphylococcal sepsis, viral infections, Kawasaki disease, idiopathic thrombocytopenic purpura, Henoch–Schonlein purpura, vasculitis and drug reactions are other diagnostic considerations.

Early in the course of infection, meningococcal skin lesions may be exclusively macular or maculopapular. Meningococcemia should be considered in any child with signs of toxicity, even if the rash appears benign.

TREATMENT

Penicillin G at a dose of 300,000 U/kg/day I.V. is the treatment of choice for meningococcal infections. Cefotaxime (200 mg/kg/day) or ceftriaxone (100–150 μg/kg/day) is also effective. For the penicillin-allergic child, in whom a cephalosporin may pose some risk for cross-allergenicity, chloramphenicol (75–100 mg/kg/day) is an alternative antimicrobial. Strains of N. meningitidis with reduced sensitivity or resistance to penicillin (minimal inhibitory concentration, 0.1–1.0 μg/mL) have been recovered with increasing frequency; these strains are sensitive to cefotaxime. Routine penicillin susceptibility testing, however, is not recommended in the United States.

Meningococcemia constitutes a medical emergency. Antibiotics should be administered immediately. Supportive care should be directed toward anticipating or treating shock as many patients develop shock shortly after the initiation of antimicrobial therapy. The advisability of administering steroids to patients with possible adrenal hemorrhage is debated, but this probably does not favorably affect the outcome in critically ill patients. For meningococcemia or meningococcal meningitis, generally 5 to 7 days of parenteral drug therapy are required.

OUTCOME AND COMPLICATIONS

Approximately 20% of children with meningococcemia die. The usual cause of death is irreversible shock, and most deaths occur within 48 hours of hospital admission. Fatality rates for children with meningococcemia plus meningococcal meningitis are lower (approximately 5%), presumably because these patients constitute a subset who have survived meningococcemia long enough to develop meningeal seeding.

The complications of meningococcal infections may be classified as early and late. Early complications include myocarditis, pericarditis, pneumonia, hemorrhage, and arthritis. Meningococcal meningitis may be complicated acutely by seizures, cranial nerve palsies (particularly of the third, fourth, and sixth cranial nerves), ataxia, or cerebral herniation. Subdural effusion, almost universally sterile, may be seen during convalescence. The most common neurologic residual of meningococcal meningitis is deafness, which is usually bilateral, sensorineural, and permanent. Residual cranial nerve palsy or retardation occurs occasionally.

Late, allergic, hypersensitivity, immune complex-mediated, and reactive all are terms that have been used to describe the complications of meningococcal disease that occur during recovery from infection. Late complications, manifested as cutaneous vasculitis, arthritis, pericarditis or, rarely, as episcleritis, occur in 10% of the survivors. The treatment consists of drainage (only if needed for symptomatic relief) and administration of nonsteroidal antiinflammatory agents. Occasionally, prednisone may be required to reduce inflammation in patients with pericarditis.

PREVENTION

Antimicrobial Prophylaxis

Chemoprophylaxis to eradicate the nasopharyngeal carriage interrupts the spread of meningococcal infections. Among household contacts, the secondary attack rate varies from 3 per 1,000 for sporadic disease to 3 per 100 exposed persons in epidemic situations. High-risk contacts of index cases of invasive meningococcal disease for whom chemoprophylaxis is recommended include household contacts (especially young children and those who have slept or eaten in the same dwelling as the index patient or had secretion contact with the patient), child-care or nursery-school contacts (within the 7 days before the index patient's admission), and those who have had unprotected contact during mouth-to-mouth or intubation resuscitation efforts. Chemoprophylaxis is not recommended for school contacts, indirect contacts, or medical personnel who have not been directly exposed to secretions. However, a few outbreaks among school classmates have been reported and, in this setting, chemoprophylaxis should be undertaken only after consultation with local public health authorities. Because high-dose penicillin suppresses colonization of the nasopharynx only transiently, the index patient should receive treatment for nasopharyngeal carriage eradication at the conclusion of parenteral therapy, unless the infection was treated with ceftriaxone or cefotaxime.

Rifampin is the antimicrobial often used for chemoprophylaxis in children (Table 88-1). Rifampin eradicates the carrier state rapidly, but resistant strains have emerged. The drug is usually well tolerated, but recipients should be alerted that it stains urine and tears red-orange. Ceftriaxone administered as a single dose intramuscularly is an alternative to rifampin that is also highly effective in eradicating carriage. It is not recommended for routine use because efficacy has been documented only for serogroup A. Sulfisoxazole has proved efficacious for eradicating colonization and preventing secondary disease, but widespread sulfa resistance has resulted in the restriction of its use to situations in which the disease-producing strain has documented susceptibility. A single 500-mg dose of ciprofloxacin orally is effective in eliminating carriage, but currently it is approved for use only in patients who are 18 years or older.

TABLE 88-1. Chemoprophylaxis Regimens for High-Risk Contacts and Index Cases

Age of patient	Dose	Duration
Rifampin		
≤1 mo	5 mg/kg orally every 12 hr	2 d
>1 mo	10 mg/kg (maximum, 600 mg) orally every 12 hr	2 d
	or	
	20 mg/kg (maximum, 600 mg) orally every 24 hr	4 d
Ceftriaxone		
≤2 yr	125 mg intramuscularly	Single dose
>12 yr	250 mg intramuscularly	Single dose
Sulfisoxazole*		
<1 yr	500 mg orally daily	2 d
1–12 yr	500 mg orally every 12 hr	2 d
>12 yr	1 g orally every 12 hr	2 d

*May be used if the organism is known to be susceptible.

Monthly injections of benzathine penicillin G have prevented recurrence of invasive disease in patients with a terminal complement protein deficiency.

Immunoprophylaxis

The only vaccine currently available in North America for immunoprophylaxis against invasive meningococcal infection is a quadrivalent preparation containing polysaccharides of groups A, C, Y, and W135 *N. meningitidis* (trade name: Menomune). As of the writing of this manuscript, there have been interruptions in the availability of this vaccine. Administration of vaccine may be considered an adjunct to chemoprophylaxis among household and intimate contacts. Immunization is recommended for persons older than 2 years who have anatomic or functional asplenia and deficiencies of properdin or terminal complement components. It is also recommended for those traveling to areas with hyperendemic or epidemic meningococcal disease.

College freshmen are at slightly increased risk for meningococcal disease. This is particularly true of those living in dormitories or residence halls. Physicians should educate their patients and families about meningococcal disease and offer the family the opportunity to make an individualized decision about receiving the vaccine.

A meningococcal Group C conjugated vaccine was introduced into the immunization schedule in the United Kingdom in November 1999. It is known to be immunogenic in children as young as two months of age. This vaccine may be available for use in the United States in the future.

CHAPTER 89

Pasteurella multocida

Adapted from Morven S. Edwards

Pasteurella multocida, first isolated by Kitt in 1878 and subsequently by Pasteur, are common commensals in the respiratory tract of animals. Human infection can usually be linked to contact with animals.

MICROBIOLOGY

P. multocida includes three subspecies: *multocida, septica,* and *gallicida*. *P. multocida* is the most virulent species in animals. Most human *Pasteurella* infections are caused by organisms identified as *P. multocida* subspecies *multocida* and subspecies *septica*. *Pasteurella* grows well on a variety of routine media. *P. multocida* is a small, nonmotile, gram-negative rod that occurs singly, in pairs, or in short chains, and may exhibit bipolar staining. These organisms may be confused microscopically with *Haemophilus influenzae*, *Neisseria* species, and *Acinetobacter* species.

EPIDEMIOLOGY AND TRANSMISSION

The incidence of asymptomatic respiratory tract or oral cavity colonization with *P. multocida* approximates 90% in cats, 70% in dogs, 50% in pigs, and 15% in wild rats. Carriage has been documented in larger and a variety of other animals including horses and cattle.

Most *P. multocida* infections in humans are the result of direct inoculation by animal bites or scratches, and this pathogen has been implicated in 80% of infected cat bites and 50% of infected dog bites. Occasionally, asymptomatic upper respiratory tract colonization may precede dissemination of infection in humans, and *P. multocida* has been isolated from asymptomatic persons who have frequent contact with animals. Close contact with the family cat during breast-feeding was the source for transmission through oropharyngeal colonization to an infant who developed meningitis and bacteremia due to *P. multocida*. In rare cases, no animal contact can be established for diagnosed *Pasteurella* infection. Although exquisitely susceptible to direct sunlight, the organism can survive in water or soil for approximately 3 weeks. Human-to-human transmission has not been documented, but an animal-soil-human route could account for some cases that cannot be linked directly to animals.

PATHOGENESIS AND PATHOLOGY

Inoculation of organisms beneath the skin is likely to be deeper and perhaps penetrate the periosteum or a joint space if the source is a cat bite (i.e., puncture wound injury) than if it is a dog bite (i.e., laceration wound). The rapidly established and intensely painful local cellulitis that results may be attributed, in part, to the production by *P. multocida* of neuraminidase and endotoxin.

Nasopharyngeal colonization with *P. multocida* may precede respiratory tract infection. Invasive infection occurs almost exclusively in the setting of underlying respiratory tract disease such as chronic bronchitis or bronchiectasis.

CLINICAL MANIFESTATIONS

The three major clinical manifestations of *P. multocida* infections are focal soft tissue, respiratory tract, and disseminated infections. Cellulitis due to *P. multocida* characteristically has a rapid onset, often within a few hours after an animal bite or scratch. The average time of onset is 12 to 24 hours with a range of 3 hours to 3 days. Erythema, exquisite pain, edema, and discharge described as watery and gray, odorous, or serosanguineous. Abscess formation, tenosynovitis, arthritis, osteomyelitis, and regional adenopathy may occur. The extremities are usually affected, but osteomyelitis and brain abscess have complicated a bite wound to the head of children. Joint stiffness with cellulitis of the hand is a sign of tendon sheath involvement, and surgical exploration should be undertaken. Even with appropriate drainage, wound infections due to *P. multocida* heal slowly, particularly if poorly vascularized tissues such as the tendon, are involved.

Respiratory tract infections occur in the setting of chronic pulmonary disease such as bronchitis or bronchiectasis, and are rare in children.

Meningitis with or without bacteremia is the most common manifestation of disseminated infection in children. Most of the reported cases have occurred in infants younger than 1 year. A history of nontraumatic animal contact such as facial licking by household pets, is commonly elicited.

DIAGNOSIS

The diagnosis of *P. multocida* infection is established by culture of the organism, a wound, abscess, or sterile body site. Laboratory personnel should be alerted to the possibility of *Pasteurella*. Clinically, the features of rapid onset and grayish drainage aid in differentiating between cellulitis due to *P. multocida* and staphylococcal or streptococcal wound infections. Tularemia, plague, and cat-scratch disease are differential considerations, each of which has a longer incubation period than do *Pasteurella* infections.

TREATMENT

Penicillin is the drug of choice for *P. multocida* infections. Some wounds may be managed as an outpatient, but if wound severity warrants hospitalization, aqueous penicillin G should be administered. Parenteral therapy is always indicated if bite wounds are associated with signs of systemic toxicity; if involvement of tendon, bone, or joint is a consideration; if wound cellulitis has progressed despite oral therapy; and in children with impaired immune function, particularly splenic dysfunction.

Although *Pasteurella* is almost uniformly sensitive to penicillin, susceptibility testing should be confirmed in serious infections or in those patients who fail to show the expected response to therapy because rare isolates may be penicillin-resistant. Other antimicrobials to which isolates of *P. multocida* are susceptible include the penicillin derivatives ampicillin, ticarcillin, piperacillin, and mezlocillin; the second- and third-generation parenteral cephalosporins; and trimethoprim-sulfamethoxazole. Semisynthetic penicillin, erythromycin, clindamycin, vancomycin, and the aminoglycosides are inadequate. Consider that *P. multocida* may be part of a polymicrobial infection and antibiotic coverage for Staphylococcal and Streptococcal species may be warranted. Clinically, amoxicillin-clavulanate and ampicillin-sulbactam fulfill these requirements.

OUTCOME

Recovery is the rule, but bone and joint infections due to *P. multocida* may have residua consisting of decreased joint mobility or ankylosis and chronic osteomyelitis depending on the extent of the initial injury. Most survivors of meningitis have had a normal outcome, but hemiparesis has been reported.

CHAPTER 90
Pertussis

Adapted from James D. Cherry

Pertussis (i.e., whooping cough) is an acute, communicable, respiratory illness that affects susceptible persons of all ages but is particularly serious in infants.

ETIOLOGY AND EPIDEMIOLOGY

Pertussis is caused by *Bordetella pertussis* and, less frequently, by *Bordetella parapertussis*. Both are fastidious gram-negative aerobic coccobacilli that require special media for growth.

Humans are the only known hosts of *B. pertussis*. Transmission occurs from person to person by respiratory secretion droplets, and contagion is extremely high in nonimmunized populations. Spread occurs from patients with disease to susceptible contacts; asymptomatic carriers are not important in transmission. Adults with protracted cough illnesses (i.e., atypical pertussis) are an important source of *B. pertussis* infection among nonimmunized or partially immunized children.

In nonvaccinated populations, approximately 10% of reported cases occur in children younger than 1 year, 40% in children 1 to 4 years old, 45% in children 5 to 9 years old, and 5% in persons at least 10 years of age. Reported pertussis in persons older than 15 years is rare. In highly immunized populations such as in the United States, nearly 40% of the reported cases occur in the first year of life, another 20% occur before age 5, and 25% occur in children 10 years of age or older and in adults.

Pertussis is an endemic disease with epidemic cycles occurring at intervals of 2 to 5 years. In the prevaccine era in the United States, the average yearly reported attack rate was 157 per 100,000 persons. If an allowance was made for underreporting, the actual rate can be estimated to have been approximately 900 cases per 100,000. During the vaccine era, the reported rate of illness has ranged from 0.5 to 2.3 per 100,000 persons. The major mortality from pertussis occurs among infants. Of reported pertussis cases in the United States, nearly 0.6% of the patients younger than 1 year die. The clinical attack and mortality rates of pertussis are higher for females than for males.

PATHOPHYSIOLOGY

Pertussis is predominantly a disease of the ciliated epithelium of the respiratory tract. In the pathogenesis of pertussis, four steps are important: attachment, evasion of host defenses, local damage, and systemic disease.

After the airborne transmission of respiratory secretions containing *B. pertussis*, the organisms attach to the cilia of the respiratory epithelial cells of the new host. Filamentous hemagglutinin (FHA), pertussis toxin (PT), pertactin (i.e., 69-kd outer membrane protein), and fimbriae (types 2 and 3) are *B. pertussis* antigens that are important in the attachment process. After attachment, the infection proceeds because of the profound adverse effect on host immune effector cell function by organism adenylate cyclase and PT. Another *B. pertussis* toxin, tracheal cytotoxin, disrupts normal clearance mechanisms allowing infection to persist.

Three *B. pertussis* toxins contribute to local tissue damage of the ciliated respiratory epithelium: tracheal cytotoxin, dermonecrotic toxin, and adenylate cyclase. Pertussis is a unique disease in that systemic manifestations are rare. The characteristic lymphocytosis is caused by PT.

CLINICAL MANIFESTATIONS

Classic pertussis is a lengthy illness, commonly lasting 6 to 8 weeks and characterized by three stages: catarrhal, paroxysmal, and convalescent. The catarrhal stage has its onset after an incubation period of 7 to 10 days. The onset of illness is subtle and resembles a mild upper respiratory tract infection with coryza, mild conjunctival injection, and mild cough.

The paroxysmal stage is manifested by increasingly forceful coughing in the form of episodic paroxysms, which are particularly frequent at night. In classic pertussis, episodes of repetitive severe coughing are followed by a single sudden massive inspiration. The characteristic whoop sound results from the forceful inhalation and a narrowed glottis. Each coughing paroxysm consists of ten to 30 forceful coughs in a staccato series. The patient's face becomes increasingly cyanotic, the tongue protrudes to the maximum, and mucus, saliva, and tears stream from nose, mouth, and eyes, respectively. Episodes of paroxysmal cough may be singular or several may occur in rapid succession. Twenty or more sessions of paroxysmal cough may occur each day. The paroxysmal episodes are exhausting, and young children appear apathetic and dazed after attacks. Between attacks, patients usually show few signs of illness, and fever is not characteristic of uncomplicated cases. In young infants, a whoop is less likely to occur after a paroxysm.

After the paroxysmal stage, which lasts from 1 to 4 weeks or more, the convalescent stage is heralded by a lessening in the severity and frequency of paroxysms. The duration of the convalescent stage varies. Paroxysmal-type coughing often occurs for 6 months or more after the occurrence of pertussis in association with other respiratory infections. Weight loss or failure to gain weight is a conspicuous feature of severe pertussis, especially in infants. Studies indicate that only 50% to 60% of pertussis cases in children have the classic picture and that the other cases are mild with cough durations of less than 4 weeks.

COMPLICATIONS

Complications of pertussis are common and can be grouped into three categories: respiratory, central nervous system, and secondary pressure effects. The rate of complications is inversely related to age. Bronchopneumonia, the most common complication, is caused by secondary infection with common respiratory pathogens or it can be caused by a more extensive *B. pertussis* infection. Carefully performed follow-up studies provide little evidence that permanent pulmonary sequelae occur.

Central nervous system complications are relatively common during the paroxysmal stage of pertussis. Data indicate that 1.9% of infants experience seizures with pertussis, and approximately 0.2% suffer encephalopathy. After encephalitis-like illness, permanent sequelae are common. Approximately one-third of patients die, one-third survive with residua, and one-third survive and appear normal. Sequelae include mental retardation, seizure disorders, and changes in personality and behavior.

Secondary pressure effects during the paroxysmal stage of severe pertussis may cause epistaxis, melena, petechiae, subdural hematoma, umbilical or inguinal hernias, and rectal prolapse.

DIAGNOSIS

Typical pertussis can be reliably diagnosed clinically on the basis of characteristic history and physical findings. A careful history will usually reveal contact with a person or persons (often a young adult) having a prolonged illness with cough.

The absence of or only minimal fever suggests that pertussis rather than an illness caused by a respiratory virus. In classic pertussis, the leukocyte count is elevated because of lymphocytosis. Leukocytosis develops at the end of the catarrhal and during the paroxysmal stages of the disease and, although characteristic, this is not a sensitive nor specific diagnostic feature. Absolute lymphocyte counts are usually greater than 10,000 and are often more than 30,000 cells per deciliter.

The specific diagnosis of pertussis depends on isolation of the organism or its demonstration by a rapid identification method. *B. pertussis* can be isolated from nasopharyngeal secretions during the catarrhal and early paroxysmal stages of disease. Specimens for culture should be obtained from the nasopharynx with the use of Dacron or calcium alginate swabs or by nasal aspiration. These specimens should be inoculated directly onto or into selective media. Alternatively, appropriate transport medium should be inoculated and the specimen transported to a diagnostic laboratory. Prior antibiotic treatment may markedly reduce the isolation rate.

Direct fluorescent antibody identification of *B. pertussis* in nasopharyngeal specimens is particularly useful if antimicrobial therapy has been given, decreasing the likelihood of obtaining a positive culture. In some studies, the polymerase chain reaction (PCR) has been shown to be more sensitive than is culture.

Pertussis can also be diagnosed serologically, but because all standard tests usually depend on the demonstration of an increase in antibody titer, these techniques are not usually useful for early diagnosis. The demonstration of a fourfold rise in agglutinin titer is firm evidence that the illness was pertussis.

TREATMENT

B. pertussis is susceptible to erythromycin and other macrolides, and the administration of these antibiotics to children during the incubation period or the catarrhal stage may prevent or modify clinical disease. Erythromycin therapy may also alter the clinical course of pertussis if treatment is initiated early in the paroxysmal stage. Treatment initiated later in the paroxysmal stage does not lessen the duration or severity of clinical illness, although patients should be treated to reduce the risk of spread to other susceptible contacts. The dosage of erythromycin is 40 to 50 mg/kg/day (adults, 1 g/day), given in four doses for a total of 14 days. This regimen should be used for treatment and prophylaxis.

Because pertussis is a highly contagious infectious disease, patients should be placed in respiratory isolation, which should be maintained for 5 days after the initiation of erythromycin therapy. If erythromycin therapy is not given because of a contraindication, the patient should remain in isolation until 3 weeks after the onset of paroxysms.

Most infants should receive oxygen, and gentle suction should be used to remove secretions. Supportive care includes avoidance of situations that provoke attacks of coughing and maintenance of hydration and nutrition. Although corticosteroids and salbutamol (albuterol) have been used as adjuncts to therapy and, in uncontrolled studies, have reduced coughing paroxysms, no controlled data have indicated the usefulness of either type of medication.

PREVENTION

Universal immunization with pertussis vaccine in children has been extraordinarily successful in controlling epidemic pertussis in the United States. Older vaccines of inactivated *B. pertussis* cells (i.e., whole-cell vaccines) are no longer used. Acellular pertussis vaccines (DTaP) are now licensed for the primary immunization of infants in the United States. DTaP vaccines are less reactogenic than DTP vaccines. Pertussis vaccines are available routinely in the United States only in combination with diphtheria and tetanus toxoids. A successful immunization program for children consists of five doses of DTaP. The primary immunization series consists of an initial three doses given at approximately 2, 4, and 6 months of age with a fourth dose at 15 to 18 months. The fifth dose (i.e., booster) is given at the time of school entry, at 4 to 6 years of age. The duration of vaccine-produced immunity is relatively short, although illness is usually less severe in previously vaccinated persons than in nonvaccinated individuals. DTaP vaccines are given intramuscularly in a volume of 0.5 mL per dose.

Currently, pertussis immunization is not performed routinely in persons 7 years of age or older because severe pertussis is a disease of young children. In the future, the successful control of pertussis will probably necessitate booster immunizations in adolescents and adults, as is recommended for diphtheria and tetanus toxoids.

Reactions associated with DTP immunization were common and included pain at the injection site, possible high fever, and febrile seizures (1/1,750). The most significant concern to parents and physicians were the so-called pertussis vaccine encephalopathy and sudden infant death syndrome (SIDS) occurring after immunization. After rigorous epidemiologic investigation, instances of alleged pertussis vaccine encephalopathy have actually proved to be neurologic diseases attributable to other causes and are only temporally related to immunization. No evidence supports the concept of pertussis vaccine encephalopathy. SIDS is a catastrophic event that occurs at a rate of 1.4 to 1.9 per 1,000 live births. Because DTP immunizations are carried out at the age of peak occurrence of SIDS, by chance alone, many cases occur after DTP immunization. Studies have shown no correlation between DTP immunization and SIDS.

In general, reactions after DTaP administration are markedly less frequent and less severe than after DTP administration and occur at a rate and magnitude similar to that after DT immunization. DTaP can cause local reactions, which are more frequent after the fourth and/or fifth doses. Mild systemic reactions such as fever and drowsiness, can occur but are much less common than with DTP. For example, fever of less than 101°F is reported in 3% to 5% of DTaP recipients versus 16% of DTP recipients. Moderate to severe systemic events such as fever greater than 105°F, febrile seizures, persistent crying lasting more than 3 hours, and hypotonic hyporesponsive episodes are rarely reported after DTaP, and are much less frequent than with DTP.

CONTRAINDICATIONS TO VACCINE

Although an area of much confusion and distress among practitioners, recent CDC guidelines clearly outline contraindications to further vaccination with DTaP. An absolute contraindication is anaphylaxis to a prior dose of vaccine or vaccine component and encephalopathy not due to another identifiable cause within 7 days of vaccination.

A moderate to severe acute illness is considered a precaution to vaccination at that visit (but children should be quickly rescheduled). Often this is over interpreted and children go unimmunized. It is important to note that children with mild illness such as otitis media or upper respiratory infection, should be vaccinated.

There remain infrequent adverse events following pertussis vaccination that will generally contraindicate subsequent doses of pertussis vaccine. The CDC defines these events as:

- Temperature greater than 40.5°C (105°F) within 48 hours not due to another identifiable cause.
- Collapse or shock-like state (hypotonic-hyporesponsive episode) within 48 hours.
- Persistent, inconsolable crying (lasting more than 3 hours, occurring within 48 hours).
- Convulsions with or without fever occurring within 3 days.

DTaP should never be substituted in children who have a valid contraindication to DTP. If any valid contraindication exists to DTaP, DT should be used for the remaining doses in the schedule.

CHAPTER 91
Pneumococcal Infections

Adapted from Ralph D. Feigin
and Warren K. Brasher

Streptococcus pneumoniae is the leading cause of otitis media and a frequent cause of pneumonia, bacteremia, and meningitis in children. The emergence of pneumococcal strains resistant to multiple antibiotics has complicated the therapy of suspected and proved *S. pneumoniae* infections.

MICROBIOLOGY

S. pneumoniae is a gram-positive, lancet-shaped diplococcus that usually occurs in pairs and possibly chains. *S. pneumoniae* is encapsulated and exhibit alpha-hemolysis on blood agar. Pneumococci may be grown aerobically or anaerobically. The Quellung reaction permits rapid identification of pneumococci. This reaction is carried out by mixing equal volumes of the suspension of bacteria, antiserum, and methylene blue on a slide and examining the bacteria by light microscopy. Capsular swelling identifies genus, species, and serotype.

EPIDEMIOLOGY

S. pneumoniae, which are present in the pharynx of normal people, are spread from person to person in droplets from respiratory secretions. The prevalence of colonization has typically been found to be between 25% and 50% with some studies finding rates as high as 97%. Most children develop colonization at some point during their first few years of life. Rates of colonization gradually increase with age over the first 1 or 2 years of life, the highest rates being associated with children receiving institutional care. Factors implicated in the colonization with resistant pneumococci include residence in a chronic-care facility, attendance in a child-care facility, recent hospitalization, recent therapy with antimicrobial agents, and age younger than 2 years.

More than 80 serotypes of *S. pneumoniae* have been identified. There is a difference between serotypes causing infections in adults versus those in children. Serotypes 6, 9, 14, 18, 19, and 23 are associated most commonly with infections in the pediatric age group. These same serotypes have also been found to account for the majority of organisms with antibiotic resistance. In one study, these six serotypes accounted for greater than 85% of the drug-resistant pneumococci.

Immunity to *S. pneumoniae* depends on the presence of type-specific antibody to the capsular antigen of the organism. Immunity during the first few months of life is derived from maternal antibody. Children younger than age 2 respond poorly to the capsular polysaccharide antigen. This finding may explain the frequency of pneumococcal bacteremia in children between ages 6 months and 2 years.

PATHOGENESIS

Pneumococci may invade from a site of colonization by hematogenous spread or direct extension. Pneumococcal meningitis usually follows pneumococcal bacteremia, but it can also result from direct spread to the meninges as a result of a temporal or basilar skull fracture. Pneumococcal otitis media usually results from the spread of pneumococci colonizing the nasopharynx by the eustachian tube into the middle ear. Pneumococcal pneumonia is caused by aspiration of pneumococci that reside in the pharynx. Several studies document that a viral infection may compromise pulmonary defense mechanisms and predispose the individual to invasion by pneumococci.

The capsule of *S. pneumoniae* is known to aid the pneumococci by resisting phagocytosis. Specific serotypes associated with large capsules appear to be more virulent and to cause greater morbidity and mortality than serotypes characterized by smaller capsules. Rough strains of pneumococci lacking a capsule are avirulent.

Most researchers concur that the cell wall elements are responsible for the initiation of the inflammatory response seen with pneumococcal infection. Specifically, peptidoglycan and teichoic acid have been found to be the two most potent inflammatory components of the cell wall and appear to initiate an inflammatory response by activating complement factor C3 via the alternative pathway.

Numerous pneumococcal proteins that may serve as virulence factors have been identified. Pneumolysin, an intracellular protein, is the best characterized of these. Although it is not secreted by pneumococci, it is released on cell lysis as the infection progresses or on initiation of antimicrobial therapy. *In vitro*, pneumolysin can form transmembrane pores and results in lysis of most of the cell types found in the lung. It has also been shown to inhibit ciliary motion, to disrupt epithelial membranes, to interfere with neutrophil and lymphocyte function, and to stimulate the production of inflammatory cytokines.

Pneumococcal disease is much more prevalent among persons with anatomic or functional asplenia and is particularly prevalent in patients with sickle cell disease and other hemoglobinopathies. These patients appear to be unable to activate C3 by the alternative pathway or to fix opsonin to the pneumococcal cell wall. Ineffective clearance of blood-borne bacteria in the absence of type-specific antibodies and abnormal activation of the alternate pathway for complement metabolism place the asplenic patient at risk for overwhelming infection. The efficacy of phagocytosis for *S. pneumoniae* is diminished in patients with B-cell and T-cell deficiency syndromes that lack opsonic anticapsular antibody and fail to produce agglutination and lysis of bacteria.

Within body tissues, particularly the lung, the spread of infection is enhanced by the antiphagocytic properties of the capsular-specific soluble substance. Edema-promoting factors also play important roles in the pathogenesis of infection within the lung. After infection is established, the alveoli fill with serous fluid. Subsequently, polymorphonuclear leukocytes accumulate in the infected alveoli causing consolidation. Ultimately, macrophages replace the leukocytes, and the exudate resolves. This sequence of events evolves over 7 to 10 days, but it can be modified by the use of appropriate antimicrobial therapy.

CLINICAL MANIFESTATIONS

Otitis media, sinusitis, pharyngitis, abscesses, pericarditis, bacteremia, empyema, peritonitis, mastoiditis, epidural abscess, and meningitis have been reported as results of infections with *S. pneumoniae*. Pneumococcal bacteremia may occur in children who are between ages 6 months and 2 years and have unexplained fever and no localizing signs or symptoms Bacteremia may be followed by septic arthritis, osteomyelitis, endocarditis, or brain abscess. Epiglottitis due to *S. pneumoniae* has been observed in immunocompromised children. Rarely, pneumococcal infection is an uncommon but well-described etiologic agent in hemolytic uremic syndrome.

DIAGNOSIS

The isolation of pneumococci from the nasopharynx does not permit a diagnosis of pneumococcal disease because pneumococcal carriage is so prevalent. Pneumococci can be identified in selected body fluids by Gram stain as gram-positive, lancet-shaped diplococci. Cultures of selected fluids confirm the diagnosis. A direct Quellung test using pneumococcal omniserum helps to establish a definitive diagnosis rapidly. Latex particle agglutination test can also establish a diagnosis rapidly, but these tests lack sensitivity and specificity. As a result, their clinical utility is limited to special circumstances such as patients who have been pre-treated with antibiotics before cultures.

TREATMENT AND PROGNOSIS

Penicillin remains the drug of choice for patients with pneumococcal disease caused by penicillin-sensitive strains. In the past decade, a rapid increase in the prevalence of both penicillin-nonsusceptible (minimal inhibitory concentration, 0.1–1.0 μg/mL) and penicillin-resistant (minimal inhibitory concentration, greater than 2 μg/mL) strains has occurred throughout the world. Penicillin kills *S. pneumoniae* by binding cell wall penicillin binding proteins (peptidoglycans). This process eventually leads to disintegration of the organism. Resistant strains of pneumococcus have altered peptidoglycans, and the binding of penicillin is reduced. Thus, inhibiting cell wall production requires higher penicillin concentration. In addition, many of these strains have also displayed resistance to other antibiotics including cephalosporins, erythromycin, trimethoprim-sulfamethoxazole, tetracycline, chloramphenicol, and rifampin. The prevalence of antibiotic-resistant strains continues to increase with more than 50% of isolates found either nonsusceptible or resistant to penicillin in some areas of the United States and the world. Because of the high rates of resistance, all pneumococci isolated from normally sterile body fluids should have antibiotic sensitivity patterns evaluated.

Except for central nervous system infections, pneumococcal infection by both penicillin-susceptible and penicillin-nonsusceptible strains may usually be treated successfully with penicillin. The recommended dosages of penicillin G are as follows: for such infections as otitis media, 100,000 U/kg/day; for bacteremia or other serious nonCNS infections, 200,000 to 300,000 U/kg/day Macrolide antibiotics may be used for mild pneumococcal disease in children who are allergic to penicillin. Treatment of pneumococcal infections by resistant organisms, with the exception of meningitis, should be guided by susceptibility testing of the organism isolated and based on clinical response.

For children with presumed bacterial meningitis or with positive CSF Gram stains for gram-positive cocci, empiric antibiotic coverage should be directed at the treatment of a possible penicillin- or cephalosporin-resistant organism. Initial antibiotics should include a third-generation cephalosporin (e.g., cefotaxime or ceftriaxone) and vancomycin. This combination can be continued until antibiotic sensitivities are available. Recommended dosages for intravenous administration are as follows: cefotaxime, 300 mg/kg/day given in three to four divided doses; ceftriaxone, 100 mg/kg/day given in one to two divided doses; and vancomycin, 60 mg/kg/day given in four divided doses. Once sensitivities are available, treatment should be based on those results. Penicillin-sensitive organisms can be treated with penicillin alone. Penicillin-nonsusceptible and -resistant organisms should be treated with cefotaxime or ceftriaxone alone, and vancomycin should be discontinued when sensitivity to cephalosporins is established. *S. pneumoniae* isolates resistant to third-generation cephalosporins should be treated with the combination of vancomycin and cefotaxime or ceftriaxone. Vancomycin should not be used alone for therapy of meningitis.

The prognosis of pneumococcal disease depends on the age of the host, integrity of the immune system, virulence of the infecting organism, site of infection, and adequacy of therapy.

PREVENTION

Since 1983, a 23-valent pneumococcal polysaccharide vaccine is available commercially. Current recommendations are to provide pneumococcal vaccine to children aged 2 years and older with functional or anatomic asplenia, including patients with sickle cell disease and other hemoglobinopathies, and to children with nephrotic syndrome or chronic renal failure, conditions associated with immunosuppression, human immunodeficiency virus infection, and CSF leaks.

Other patients for whom pneumococcal vaccine should be considered are children with chronic cardiovascular, pulmonary, or hepatic disease. The currently available polysaccharide vaccines for *S. pneumoniae* are poorly immunogenic in young children, especially those younger than aged 2 years.

Pneumococcal conjugate vaccine (PCV7) has been available in the United States since 2000. It contains the capsular polysaccharide of 7 serotypes of *S. pneumoniae* (4, 6B, 9V, 14, 18C, 19F, 23F) conjugated to a protein (a nonvirulent variant of diphtheria toxin, CRM197).

A pneumococcal polysaccharide conjugate vaccine containing 11 serotypes is currently under investigation. The vaccine is recommended as part of the universal immunization series in all children less than 24 months old. Recommendations for other uses of this vaccine can be found at the Centers for Disease Control and Prevention (CDC) National Immunization Program: www.cdc.gov/nip

CHAPTER 92
Salmonella Infections

Adapted from Enrique Chacon-Cruz and Larry K. Pickering

The genus *Salmonella* contains more than 2,000 serotypes. Non-*typhi Salmonella* organisms cause disease of the gastrointestinal tract and are distributed widely in nature in the gastrointestinal tracts of wild and domestic mammals, birds, reptiles, and insects. These organisms are important public health problems in industrialized countries, where ingestion of contaminated foods often results in large outbreaks of disease. Other *Salmonella* serotypes, *S. typhi* and *S. paratyphi*, are adapted to humans and have no other known natural hosts. These organisms, which are associated with prolonged enteric fever, are endemic in undeveloped countries that lack safe drinking water and food.

ETIOLOGY

Salmonellae are gram-negative, nonspore-forming, facultatively anaerobic bacilli that belong to the Enterobacteriaceae family. The single species *S. enterica* is subclassified into seven subgroups. Almost all serotypes pathogenic for humans are classified into subgroup I. *Salmonella* can be subdivided into serotypes on the basis of three types of surface antigens: cell-wall somatic or O antigens, flagellar or H antigens, and polysaccharide or Vi antigens. Generally, *Salmonella* serotypes were named for the city in which they were defined. Most hospital laboratories perform agglutination reactions that define specific O antigens into serogroups designated as *Salmonella* A, B, C_1, C_2, D, and E. This grouping confirms genus identification and may be useful epidemiologically, but it is not helpful in clarifying whether an organism is associated with enteric fever. For instance, *S. enteritidis*, a cause of diarrhea, and *S. typhi*, a cause of enteric fever, are both in group D; both *S. typhimurium*, a cause of diarrhea, and *S. paratyphi*, another cause of enteric fever, are in group B. *S. typhimurium* and *S. enteritidis* (group D) are common causes of human *Salmonella* infections in the United States. Other common serotypes include *S. newport* (group C_2), *S. heidelberg* (group B), *S. infantis* (group C_1), *S. hadar* (group C_2), and *S. agona* (group B).

EPIDEMIOLOGY

Animals, including poultry, livestock, and pets, are the major reservoirs for nontyphoidal *Salmonella*. Other sources include contaminated animal products, meat-processing plants, contaminated water, and infected humans. Methods of transmission include ingestion of contaminated food, milk, water, medications, or dyes; contact with an infected animal; fecal-oral transmission resulting in person-to-person spread; and, more rarely, contact with contaminated medical instruments or even blood transfusions. Volunteer studies using adults have shown that between 10^5 and 10^6 viable organisms must be ingested for clinical disease to occur.

Approximately 45,500 infections with nontyphoidal *Salmonella* were reported in 1996 to the Centers for Disease Control and Prevention (CDC). Before 1996, a passive surveillance system in the United States estimated that 800,000 to 3.7 million infections occurred annually. In 1996, an active surveillance system for food-borne illness, referred to as the Foodborne Diseases Active Surveillance Network (FoodNet), was established by the CDC. In 1997, *Salmonella* was second to *Campylobacter* in the incidence of laboratory-confirmed cases of enteric pathogens.

Age-specific attack rates peak in the first year of life and are higher for children younger than aged 5 years and for persons from ages 25 to 64 years. Most reported cases of *Salmonella* infection are sporadic, but transmission by contaminated food and water frequently results in outbreaks of disease. Many outbreaks of S. enteritidis have been associated with ingestion of contaminated eggs. *S. enteritidis* infects the upper oviduct and contaminates the contents of clean, intact shell eggs. Morbidity and mortality after infection are more common at the extremes of age and in those patients who are immunosuppressed or have chronic gastrointestinal disorders.

S. typhi and *S. paratyphi* colonize only humans; therefore, disease can be acquired only through close contact with a person with typhoid fever or with a carrier of one of these organisms or through ingestion of food or water contaminated with human feces from a carrier. In the United States today, disease with *S. typhi* is uncommon compared to nontyphoidal salmonellosis. The majority of U.S. cases of typhoid fever are associated with foreign travel; most domestically acquired cases result from contact with food contaminated by a chronic carrier. Worldwide typhoid fever is a major health problem with an estimated 12.5 million cases occurring per year.

The incubation period for *Salmonella* gastroenteritis is 6 to 72 hours (usually less than 24 hours). The incubation period for enteric fever is 3 to 60 days (usually 7–14 days).

PATHOGENESIS

Exposure to normal gastric acidity (pH less than 3.5) is lethal to *Salmonella*. In some situations such as achlorhydria, gastric surgery, or antacid therapy, sufficient bacteria may enter the small intestine.

Symptoms of *Salmonella* infection are associated with mucosal invasion with inflammation or production of toxins. Some *Salmonella* strains elaborate a heat-labile toxin that may function as an enterotoxin or cytotoxins that inhibit protein synthesis. Once attached, *Salmonella* are internalized by epithelial cells, which is an important mechanism for transcytosis across the intestinal mucosal barrier. After several weeks of infection, Peyer patches enlarge and become necrotic and are most likely responsible for the abdominal pain that occurs during the course of typhoid fever. As *Salmonella* organisms invade through Peyer patches, they are transported in phagocytic cells to mesenteric lymph nodes and through the thoracic duct to the bloodstream; circulating bacteria are removed by reticuloendothelial cells in liver, spleen, and bone marrow. Some organisms can reach distant target organs or tissues such as the gallbladder, where they can multiply and secondarily seed the intestine bile. Symptoms of typhoid fever occur when a critical number of organisms have replicated. Serotypes vary in their potential to invade the bloodstream. Many *Salmonella* contain a wide variety of plasmids and genes that encode virulence factors and antimicrobial resistance.

CLINICAL MANIFESTATIONS

The clinical syndromes caused by various *Salmonella* serotypes are: the chronic carrier state; acute gastroenteritis; bacteremia; enteric fever including typhoid and paratyphoid fevers; and dissemination with localized suppuration, which manifests as intravascular infection, abscesses, osteomyelitis, arthritis, or meningitis. These clinical syndromes may overlap.

Every serotype can produce any of the clinical patterns. The transient asymptomatic carrier may be more common than gastroenteritis. By the third month after infection, more than 90% of infected persons have stopped excreting the organism. A higher proportion of neonates have prolonged carriage. Persons who excrete the organism for longer than 1 year are considered to be chronic carriers.

Salmonella most commonly causes gastroenteritis. Diarrheal stools can range from a few stools to profuse bloody diarrhea to a cholera-like syndrome. Usually, diarrhea is self-limited and lasts 3 to 7 days. In uncomplicated gastroenteritis, bacteremia occurs in 5% to 10% of cases with higher rates in groups at high risk.

The term typhoid fever refers to illness caused by *S. typhi*. Enteric fever is most often produced by *S. typhi*, *S. paratyphi* A, or *S. paratyphi*, but it may be caused by any serotype. Typically, the onset of enteric fever is gradual with elevated fever, headache, malaise, anorexia including constipation, and (less frequently) diarrhea. The presence of an erythematous pharynx, hepatosplenomegaly, and lymphadenopathy with or without the presence of rose spots (faint salmon-colored maculopapular rash on the trunk) are common signs. Without antimicrobial therapy, most infections resolve without development of complications after 4 weeks of infection.

With *Salmonella* bacteremia, the primary concern is development of a focal infection. Focal infections occur in approximately 10% of patients with *Salmonella* bacteremia. Osteomyelitis and meningitis are the most common focal infections, followed in descending order by pyelonephritis, endocarditis, vascular infections, pneumonia, both septic and reactive arthritis, and abscesses in other organs.

DIAGNOSIS

Gastroenteritis caused by *Salmonella* can be made by stool culture. The diagnosis of *Salmonella* bacteremia is made by obtaining cultures of blood and bone marrow aspirate and, in enteric fever, cultures from any foci of infection, including rose spots, urine, and stools, are also useful. Approximately 90% of patients with typhoid or paratyphoid fever have positive blood or bone marrow cultures during the first week of illness. This condition slowly diminishes over time with a concomitant increase in positive stool and urine cultures. Bone marrow culture is the most sensitive procedure for recovery of *S. typhi*.

Often, serologic tests for *Salmonella* agglutinins are part of the febrile agglutinin panel, which includes the Widal test. This procedure, which measures the antibody response to somatic and flagellar antigens of *S. typhi*, is unreliable because of frequent false-positive and false-negative results.

TREATMENT

The use of antimicrobial agents should be considered in patients with gastroenteritis if the disease appears to be evolving into enterocolitis or into one of the systemic syndromes. Antimicrobial agents are also recommended in severely malnourished children; in neonates; in patients with hemoglobinopathies; and in immunosuppressed patients who have uncomplicated gastroenteritis, in whom the risk of developing bacteremia or metastatic infection is high. Antimicrobial agents should not be used in most patients with gastroenteritis and in persons who are nontyphoid *Salmonella* carriers.

Despite *in vitro* activity, first- and second generation cephalosporins and aminoglycosides have been ineffective in the therapy of patients with *Salmonella* infection and should not be used. The selection of antimicrobial agents for therapy is complicated by the emergence of *Salmonella* strains that are resistant to multiple antibiotics. Agents such as trimethoprim-sulfamethoxazole, cefotaxime, ceftriaxone, and fluoroquinolones are often used.

Candidates for antibiotic treatment of *Salmonella* infection include patients with typhoid fever, bacteremia by nontyphoid strains, dissemination with localized suppuration, selected patients with acute gastroenteritis (as above), and persons who are chronic carriers of *S. typhi*. Ciprofloxacin is the drug of choice for chronic adult carriers of *S. typhi*, whereas in children with normally functioning gallbladders without cholelithiasis, ampicillin or amoxicillin combined with probenecid is the treatment of choice.

PREVENTION

The most important aspects of prevention of *Salmonella* infection are education and avoidance. Proper food handling and storage techniques should be used, especially for raw eggs. All dairy products should be pasteurized before ingestion. *Salmonella* usually grow at 35°C to 37°C, but they can grow at much lower temperatures. To minimize problems, foods should be held at or below 2°C to 5°C at all times.

Three typhoid vaccines are available for use in the United States: (a) an oral live-attenuated vaccine manufactured from the Ty21a strain of *S. typhi* by the Swiss Serum and Vaccine Institute; (b) a capsular polysaccharide vaccine for intramuscular use; and (c) a heat-phenol-inactivated vaccine for subcutaneous use that has been widely used for many years. A fourth vaccine, an acetone-inactivated parenteral vaccine, is currently available only to the armed forces. Typhoid fever vaccination is indicated for administration to travelers who go to typhoid-endemic regions and may be exposed to contaminated food and drink, household contacts of known *S. typhi* carriers, and microbiology laboratory technicians who work with *S. typhi*.

TABLE 92-1. Typhoid Vaccines

Vaccine	Type	Route	Age at receipt (yr)	Number of doses	Interval between doses	Boosting interval (yr)
Ty21a	Live-attenuated	Oral	≥6	4	2 d	Every 5
ViCPS	Polysaccharide	IM	≥2	1	—	Every 2

CPS, capsular polysaccharide; IM, intramuscular.

Several field trials have demonstrated the efficacy of each vaccine. Table 92-1 shows a comparison of the main characteristics of live oral vaccine Ty21a and parenteral Vi polysaccharide vaccine. The parenteral heat-phenol-inactivated vaccine causes frequent adverse reactions such as fever, headache, pain, and swelling, limiting its usefulness.

New strains of *S. typhi* with precise attenuating mutations are being engineered. They may immunize successfully after administration of a single oral dose, but trials are ongoing.

CHAPTER 93
Shigellosis

Adapted from Thomas G. Cleary and Henry F. Gomez

Although *Shigella* had been described in the late 1880s, the genus was eventually named after Kiyoshi Shiga because of his 1898 description of the organism and epidemiology of bacillary dysentery.

MICROBIOLOGY

All shigellae are gram-negative, aerobic, nonmotile bacteria. The *Shigella* genus consists of four species. Group A, *Shigella dysenteriae*, has 13 serotypes. Group B includes *Shigella flexneri* serotypes. Group C, *Shigella boydii*, has 18 serotypes, and group D, *Shigella sonnei*, has one serotype. These organisms are traditionally discussed together because of their microbiological and clinical similarities.

EPIDEMIOLOGY

Shigellae can survive in water for up to 6 months and are spread by the fecal-oral route. The inoculum size required to cause illness is very low, perhaps as few as 10 organisms. Shigellae are passed easily from person to person.

The peak incidence of symptomatic *Shigella* infection occurs during the first 4 years of life. Infants in the first few months of life are rarely infected symptomatically with shigellae. In the United States, an incidence of 463 cases per 1 million children younger than 4 years was reported for 1995.

American Indians have a risk of shigellosis that is approximately four times that of the remainder of the population. Day care centers are an important focus for outbreaks of shigellosis in the United States. The peak occurrence of *Shigella* infection occurs between July and October in the United States.

In the United States, most shigellosis is caused by *S. sonnei* with *S. flexneri* the second most important cause. In most of the developing world, *S. flexneri* is more common than *S. sonnei*.

PATHOGENESIS

All shigellae have the ability to invade mammalian cells. A small number of polypeptides are coded for by a virulence plasmid but the exact function of each of these proteins is not known. Shigellae also have chromosomally encoded traits that enhance pathogenicity (e.g., Lipopolysaccharide). *Shigella* species also produce multiple toxins. Shigatoxin, produced by *S. dysenteriae* serotype 1, may account for the severity of infection caused by this serotype compared with other shigellae. This toxin is involved in the pathogenesis of the hemolytic uremic syndrome (HUS), a major complication of *S. dysenteriae* serotype 1 infection.

Immune responses to shigellae are both humoral and cellular. Antibodies to lipopolysaccharides and the invasion plasmid antigens are produced during natural infection.

PATHOLOGY

The rectosigmoid and distal colon have the most obvious pathologic changes, typically more than the proximal areas. Erythema, mucosal edema, friability, focal hemorrhages, and adherent mucopurulent pseudomembranes may all be found. The microscopical findings include edema, capillary congestion, capillary thromboses, focal hemorrhages, crypt hyperplasia, crypt abscesses, mononuclear and polymorphonuclear infiltrates, shedding of epithelial cells, and ulcerations. The cellular infiltrate persists for a month or more.

CLINICAL MANIFESTATIONS

The usual incubation period is 12 to 48 hours. *Shigella* enteric infection has several typical clinical presentations. Some children have a biphasic illness presenting with abdominal cramps, fever and watery diarrhea, followed in 24 to 48 hours by colitis with abdominal pain, and small-volume, bloody stools whose passage is associated with tenesmus (an ineffectual urge to defecate). Other children present with a picture of colitis. In still others, watery diarrhea never progresses to the colitic phase. Why some children have predominantly watery diarrhea and others have dysentery is not known. In adult volunteer studies, the dose of organisms that causes watery diarrhea in some patients causes dysentery in others. Overall, only approximately 40% of children with *Shigella* infection have blood in their stools; approximately one-half have emesis.

Physical findings include fever, evidence of toxicity, dehydration, and lower quadrant abdominal tenderness. Rectal examination may demonstrate an unusual degree of tenderness. Without therapy, fever and diarrhea may persist for a week or more. Mild dehydration and electrolyte disturbances are common. Hyponatremia (most common with *S. dysenteriae*) and hypoglycemia are the two major metabolic abnormalities that occur with shigellosis. Shigellosis causes protein-losing enteropathy, which can aggravate or provoke malnutrition and lead to death.

In various series, 10% to 35% of the affected children have seizures or other neurologic symptoms. Encephalopathy can occur during an enteroinvasive *E. coli* infection or a *Shigella* infection. Seizures have been considered the most frequent extraintestinal manifestation of shigellosis. Their frequency is disproportionate to the expected incidence of febrile convulsions, which suggests that shigellae produce a neurotoxin. In the past, Shigatoxin was considered to cause seizures; however, it is now clear that *Shigella* species isolated from patients with seizures do not produce Shigatoxin. Lethargy and seizures often precede development of diarrhea.

The development of HUS is associated with *S. dysenteriae* serotype 1. Hemolysis and thrombocytopenia are triggered by vascular damage caused by inhibition of protein synthesis caused by Shigatoxin. Some *E. coli* (e.g., *E. coli* O157:H7, *E. coli* O26:H11) are like *S. dysenteriae* serotype 1 in that they produce Shigatoxin. These *E. coli* are associated with an afebrile hemorrhagic colitis and HUS.

Bacteremia is uncommon in watery diarrhea caused by *Shigella* species. However, sepsis complicates enteritis in 1% to 10% of severe dysentery cases. Bacteremia during shigellosis may be caused by either the *Shigella* or other enteric organisms. Children infected with *S. dysenteriae* serotype 1 are at least twice as likely to develop bacteremia as those infected with other serotypes. Bacteremia-associated mortality ranges from 50% to 85%.

The mortality of isolated enteric infection is well below 1% in industrialized societies. In developing countries, however, 10% to 30% of the children with severe dysentery die. Complications that can lead to death include intestinal perforation, dehydration, sepsis, hyponatremia, hypoglycemia, encephalopathy, HUS, pneumonia, and malnutrition. These are more common with *S. dysenteriae* type 1.

DIAGNOSIS

Many *Shigella* infections are not detected with current methods of stool culture. Stool cultures may be unrevealing in 20% of ill patients who have ingested shigellae. Optimal recovery of shigellae from stool or rectal swab specimens is achieved by promptly inoculating selective and nonselective media. Complete identification of shigellae depends on biochemical and serologic criteria.

The fecal leukocyte exam is positive in many children with *Shigella*. Blood counts often show leukocytosis with a left shift; approximately one-third of the children have more than 25% band forms. Leukemoid reactions with leukocyte counts greater than 50,000 occur in as many as 10%. Cerebrospinal fluid examinations of children who have seizures are usually normal, although a few have a mild lymphocytic pleocytosis.

TREATMENT

Shigellosis should be treated routinely with antibiotics. Treatment clears the organism from the feces, diminishing the chances of secondary cases, and allows recovery more rapidly. Whether treatment prevents complications such as hemolysis or HUS is not known. The major disadvantages associated with treatment are cost, drug toxicity, and possible selection of resistant organisms.

The emergence of resistant shigellae has been a recurring theme since the late 1950s. The usual choice of therapy has been trimethoprim-sulfamethoxazole (TMP-SMX), but the incidence of isolates resistant to TMP-SMX has been increasing worldwide and in the United States. TMP-SMX is no longer an appropriate empiric choice.

A third-generation cephalosporin may currently be the best empiric choice for suspected shigellosis of unknown susceptibility. Both oral and parenteral third-generation cephalosporins are efficacious. The newer quinolones have been used successfully in the treatment of shigellosis in adults and children. They are not approved for use in children and these drugs should be reserved for very ill children who have a *Shigella* known to be resistant to all other agents.

The timing of therapy can be problematic. Patients with suspected *Shigella* may be started empirically on antibiotics before cultures are available. This is particularly true if local epidemiology suggests an outbreak of cases. There is some evidence, however, that empiric treatment of children with *E. coli* 0157:H7 infection may increase the risk of HUS. In these cases, it would be prudent to wait for stool culture results while providing supportive care to the patient. If *Shigella* was not suspected initially because of a watery diarrhea syndrome without colitis, therapy should be started after cultures suggest that *Shigella* is the likely cause.

Single-dose regimens are almost as effective as multiple-dose regimens in relieving symptoms in older children, but single doses are less effective in clearing the feces of the organism. For this reason, multiple doses are typically used. Regardless of the antibiotic chosen, a 5-day course of therapy is recommended.

As a general rule, antimotility agents such as loperamide (Imodium) should be avoided in children, although some data in adults suggest it is useful. Agents such as diphenoxylate hydrochloride with atropine (Lomotil), appear to prolong fever and excretion of the organism.

PREVENTION

Because day care centers represent a source of *Shigella* infection in young children, attention to infection control measures is mandatory. An emphasis on hand washing, exclusion of sick children, and exclusion of food preparers from diaper changing duty is recommended. Parents should also be instructed about the importance of hand washing. In developing nations, the best means of preventing infection of the young child appears to be prolonged breast-feeding. Whether breast-feeding decreases shigellosis by preventing the consumption of contaminated food, by providing secretory IgA and lactoferrin and, thus, impairing bacterial virulence, by loading the gut with receptor glycolipids that bind Shigatoxin, or by nonspecific gut flora-modifying factors remains uncertain.

CHAPTER 94
Staphylococcal Infections

Adapted from Christian C. Patrick

Staphylococci may colonize and may be pathogenic for humans and animals. *Staphylococcus aureus* is the predominant pathogen causing a variety of infections. Coagulase-negative staphylococci (CoNS) are pathogens in neonates, the compromised host, and patients with foreign bodies.

MICROBIOLOGY

Staphylococci are gram-positive, nonmotile, aerobic, or facultative anaerobic bacteria. They grow well on ordinary media. All members are catalase positive. Staphylococci are categorized by their ability to produce coagulase; *S. aureus* is coagulase positive. Currently, 29 species are CoNS.

EPIDEMIOLOGY

Staphylococci are widely distributed in nature and are common inhabitants of the normal human flora. *S. aureus* is found in the nares, fingernails and, occasionally, skin. *S. aureus* is carried by 20% to 40% of adults; 30% are long-term carriers.

Staphylococci are usually tolerated by the human body but may cause localized disease or systemic infections. Viral respiratory infection may alter the natural host defense and allow the development of staphylococcal pneumonia. Recurrent staphylococcal infections can be caused by autoinfection from an asymptomatic carrier state.

Staphylococcal infections can occur as an epidemic or as a sporadic event. Person-to-person spread appears to be the most common form of transmission, although airborne transmission can occur.

PATHOGENESIS

The pathologic effects of *S. aureus* can be attributed to direct tissue invasion or toxin production and liberation. Colonization factors allow *S. aureus* to adhere to host surface-binding proteins such as fibrinogen. This allows *S. aureus* to bind to indwelling foreign bodies (catheters) as well.

Some enzymes (catalase, hyaluronidase, beta-lactamase, lipase) produced by *S. aureus* are virulence factors. Hyaluronidase or spreading factor facilitates spread of infection in the early stages. Beta-Lactamase inactivates a class of antibiotics. Catalase converts H_2O_2 to H_2O and O_2, reducing H_2O_2 as a host defense mediator in phagocytosis. Lipase facilitates invasion.

S. aureus produces five membrane-damaging toxins (alpha, beta, delta, and the leukocidins). Other toxins include the enterotoxins A through E, epidermolytic toxins A and B, and toxic syndrome toxin 1. The enterotoxins cause food-borne diseases; however, enterotoxins B and C are associated with toxic shock syndrome (TSS). The epidermolytic toxins cause scalded skin syndrome.

CLINICAL MANIFESTATIONS

The clinical manifestations vary with the portal of entry of the organism and the immune status and general health of the patients.

S. aureus infections of the skin include impetigo, bullous impetigo, folliculitis, furuncles (i.e., boils), carbuncles, paronychia, and cellulitis. Toxin mediated diseases of the skin include staphylococcal scalded skin syndrome, staphylococcal scarlatiniform eruption, and TSS.

S. aureus is the most frequent cause of acute osteomyelitis and diskitis. In most cases, the bacteria reach the bone by hematogenous spread but can occur from a contiguous focus of infection. The organism usually localizes in the metaphyseal end of a long bone.

Staphylococcal bacteremia usually occurs with a source of infection such as the skin, respiratory tract, or intravenous access. Septic arthritis is also frequently caused by *S. aureus* and most commonly involves the hip, knee, ankle, and elbow. Muscle abscesses (pyomyositis) usually present with a subacute onset of moderate muscle pain followed by fever. An associated increase in serum muscle enzymes without evidence of septicemia occurs.

Staphylococcal pneumonia occurs as a primary infection or secondary to a viral infection. Radiographic findings are perhaps unique in staphylococcal pneumonia and include pneumatocele, pneumothorax, and abscesses.

Staphylococcal enterocolitis is a food poisoning that is caused by ingestion of contaminated food. When left at room temperature, certain foods (e.g., dairy products, bakery products, meats) are fertile soil for the production of enterotoxins. The illness has a sudden onset, occurring 1 to 6 hours after ingestion of preformed toxin in contaminated food. The illness is manifested by profuse diarrhea, abdominal cramps, and nausea. Symptoms improve within 8 to 24 hours.

Central nervous system (CNS) infections that may be caused by *S. aureus* include meningitis, brain-subdural-epidural abscesses, and cerebral venous thrombosis. Meningitis caused by *S. aureus* is rare and generally results from hematogenous spread after surgery in patients with a foreign body, but it can occur by contiguous extension of otitis media, sinusitis, mastoiditis, or osteomyelitis of the skull and vertebrae.

Cardiovascular infections include endocarditis, pericarditis, and septic thromboses.

S. aureus is the second most frequent cause of infections in foreign body infections after *S. epidermidis*, caused by items such as central venous catheters, CNS shunts, and peritoneal dialysis catheters.

Infection by *S. aureus* in neonates includes omphalitis, breast abscess, parotitis, and cervical adenitis.

DIAGNOSIS

Gram stain of clinical material (e.g., aspirate of pus, sputum, and blood) should reveal gram-positive cocci. A definitive diagnosis depends on isolation of the organism from an otherwise sterile site or aspiration from a wound or lesion.

The diagnosis of staphylococcal food poisoning is usually made on a clinical basis. Suspicion of the disease can be substantiated by Gram stain and culture of the presumed food source and by demonstration of toxin-producing staphylococci.

TREATMENT

The therapy for staphylococcal infections depends on the general health and immune status of the patient, the site of infection, and the results of antimicrobial susceptibility testing. Focal infections with collections of purulent material require adequate drainage. Serious staphylococcal infections require systemic bactericidal antibiotics. Staphylococcal infections can persist and recur; then prolonged antibiotic therapy may be required.

Penicillin G is active against penicillin-susceptible, staphylococci and is the treatment of choice. However, approximately 90% of community- and hospital-acquired staphylococci are resistant to penicillin.

For organisms resistant to penicillin, the semisynthetic penicillins such as methicillin, nafcillin or oxacillin, and for oral use, cloxacillin or dicloxacillin, are administered.

Methicillin-resistant *S. aureus* necessitates the use of vancomycin, which is the drug of choice for treating organisms resistant to penicillin or to penicillin derivations. For severe infections, vancomycin should be used in areas of high levels of methicillin-resistant *S. aureus* before antimicrobial susceptibility test results are known.

Clindamycin may be used in penicillin allergic patients without CNS disease.

PREVENTION

The possibility of a vaccine against *S. aureus* appears realistic. Capsular polysaccharide conjugate vaccines can promote antibody production in humans.

Good personal hygiene and hand washing with an effective detergent containing hexachlorophene is effective in reducing recurrent soft tissue infection. Mupirocin antibiotic ointment has been used to eradicate the nasal carriage state.

INFECTIONS CAUSED BY COAGULASE-NEGATIVE STAPHYLOCOCCI

Historically, CoNS have been regarded as harmless commensals, but certain species are now considered pathogens and are implicated in a wide range of infections. *S. epidermidis* is the prominent species in infections.

CoNS are a primary cause of nosocomial bacteremia in neonates and immunocompromised patients with cancer or after a bone marrow transplant. CoNS are also the major pathogens in patients with an infected central venous catheters, CNS shunts, or peritoneal dialysis catheters. Two nonnosocomial infections caused by CoNS are recognized: *S. epidermidis* can cause native valve endocarditis and *S. saprophyticus* causes urinary tract infections in young, sexually active women.

Certain species of CoNS adhere to catheters and secrete a slime substance or glycocalyx that coats the staphylococci allowing them to evade their host's defenses.

With regard to therapy, methicillin resistance of CoNS can be interpreted as resistance to all beta-lactam antibiotics. Vancomycin is the drug of choice for organisms resistant to penicillinase-resistant penicillin and is also recommended for empiric treatment of severe infections.

TOXIC SHOCK SYNDROME

TSS is an acute febrile illness with an erythroderma rash, multisystem involvement, and a high complication rate.

Etiology

TSS toxin-1 and other mediators produced by *S. aureus* including enterotoxins B and C act as superantigens that stimulate the host response.

Epidemiology

TSS was first described in 1978. In 1980, it was recognized with increasing frequency in young, menstruating women using a particular brand of tampons. TSS can occur at any age but has been recognized more frequently in teenage and young adult women. Any individual with focal infection caused by *S. aureus* can be at risk.

Clinical Manifestations

Patients with TSS describe a prodrome of nausea and vomiting, sore throat, profuse watery diarrhea, and myalgia. Prominent fever ($\geq$38.8°C), conjunctivitis, pharyngeal hyperemia and a diffuse sunburn-like rash are common. Eventually, hypotension leads to multiple organ system dysfunction. Desquamation of the palms, soles, fingers, and toes occurs 2 to 4 weeks after the onset of the illness.

Diagnosis

The major criteria for diagnosis are: (a) fever of 38.8°C or higher, (b) rash or erythroderma with subsequent desquamation, and (c) hypotension. Minor criteria require any three of the following: (a) mucous membrane inflammation (vaginal, oropharyngeal, or conjunctival hyperemia), (b) gastrointestinal abnormalities (vomiting or diarrhea), (c) muscle abnormalities (elevated creatine kinase, severe myalgia), (d) CNS abnormalities (obtundation, coma, no focal findings), (e) hepatic abnormalities (elevated bilirubin or transaminases twice the upper limit for age), (f) renal abnormalities (urinalysis with =5 white blood cells per high-power field or blood urea nitrogen or serum creatinine greater than twice the upper limit for age), and (g) hematologic (platelet count of less than 100,000 per microliter). Additionally, culture results must be negative for other etiologies except for *S. aureus* and negative serologic test results for Rocky Mountain spotted fever, leptospirosis, and measles, as indicated. A focus of *S. aureus* infection should be aggressively sought.

The 1997 Centers for Disease Control and Prevention (CDC) case definition for TSS is available at http://www.cdc.gov/epo/dphsi/casedef/toxicsscurrent.htm (accessed 05/05/03).

Treatment

Appropriate antibiotics such as nafcillin should be administered in addition to intervention for shock. Drainage of the infected sites or removal of a potentially infectious device is imperative. Clindamycin may also be given to inhibit staphylococcal protein synthesis and, thus, toxin production. In severe cases, intravenous immunoglobulin (to provide potential antitoxin antibodies) and methyl prednisolone (to suppress cytokine production) may be used.

CHAPTER 95
Group A Streptococcal Infection and Rheumatic Fever

Adapted from Julia A. McMillan and Ralph D. Feigin

MICROBIOLOGY

Streptococcus pyogenes (group A streptococcus) is a gram-positive coccus that produces clear (beta) hemolysis on blood agar.

Group A hemolytic streptococci differ from other hemolytic streptococci by their group-specific cell wall carbohydrate. More than 60 types of group A streptococci (GAS) have been identified based on distinct surface proteins (i.e., M proteins). The M protein plays a role in the pathogenesis of infection rendering the organism resistant to phagocytosis.

The carbohydrate substance that is responsible for group specificity is found in the cell wall. The group A carbohydrate is a polymer of rhamnose units with side chains of N-acetylglucosamine.

The GAS release many biologically active extracellular products into surrounding media. Streptolysin O (i.e., oxygen-labile hemolysin) and streptolysin S (i.e., oxygen-stable hemolysin) can injure cell membranes. Three erythrogenic or pyrogenic toxins (A, B, and C) with similarities to endotoxin may be elaborated.

Other extracellular products of GAS include DNAases, the streptokinases, a hyaluronidase, an amylase, and proteinase. Several of these are antigenic and measuring antibodies to these antigens has proven useful in documenting clinical infection.

TRANSMISSION

Close contact is required for the spread of streptococcal pharyngitis; direct projection of large droplets or physical transfer of respiratory secretions containing the bacteria is necessary. Airborne route plays little or no role.

Children with streptococcal pharyngitis are most contagious during the acute stage of illness. If penicillin is begun, the patient can be considered much less contagious after 24 to 48 hours of therapy. Children can return to school at that time with little risk of spreading of the organism.

Prolonged pharyngeal carriage (weeks to months) of GAS has been reported in approximately 10% to 20% of school-aged children. Anal carriers of GAS have also been identified.

Group A streptococci are often found on normal skin, but they do not produce disease unless some means of access exists. Skin infections with GAS require disruption of the epithelium by trauma, insect bites, etc.

EPIDEMIOLOGY

Streptococcal impetigo is most common in preschool children, but streptococcal pharyngitis is predominantly a disorder of school-aged children.

Tonsillitis and pharyngitis caused by streptococci are particularly common in cold and temperate climates. Streptococcal impetigo and pyoderma occur with greater frequency in tropical climates.

PATHOGENESIS

The development of pharyngitis appears to depend on the attachment of GAS to epithelial cells. The streptococci must compete with the other pharyngeal flora.

Skin lipids are lethal for GAS *in vitro* and may provide a barrier against the establishment of streptococcal infection of the skin under normal conditions.

The rash of scarlet fever has been attributed to the elaboration of erythrogenic toxin. Streptococcal toxic shock syndrome may result from a direct influence of the pyrogenic exotoxins or the M protein acting as a "super antigen" to cause polyclonal stimulation of T-cells that mediate the production of a variety of lymphokines (e.g., tumor necrosis factor-beta, interleukin-2, and gamma interferon).

CLINICAL MANIFESTATIONS

Streptococcal pharyngotonsillitis is a relatively brief illness with incubation periods of several hours to 3 or 4 days. The infection varies in severity from subclinical (i.e., no symptoms) to severe symptoms of nausea, vomiting, high fever, and hypotension. The onset is often abrupt and, in addition to sore pharyngitis, may include headache, fever, and abdominal pain, particularly in children. The tonsils and pharynx generally appear inflamed. Halitosis is often present but nonspecific. Exudate, appearing by the second day of the disease, is present in 50% to 80% of patients. Swollen and tender anterior cervical lymphadenopathy affects 30% to 60% of the patients. Clinical manifestations of the disease usually subside in 3 to 5 days. Nonsuppurative complications such as acute nephritis may be seen in 10 days and rheumatic fever, an average of 18 days after the onset of group A streptococcal pharyngitis.

A form of streptococcal infection known as streptococcal fever or streptococcosis may occur in infants. This illness is characterized by a chronic low-grade fever, generalized lymphadenopathy, persistent mucoserous nasal discharge, and little evidence of localized pharyngeal inflammation.

Scarlet fever is unusual in infancy, possibly because of the transplacental transfer of maternal antibody to erythrogenic toxins. It usually presents with fever, nausea, vomiting, and the appearance of the typical rash. Abdominal pain and vomiting may precede the development of the rash by 12 to 48 hours. Sore throat is usually present, but it may not be as troublesome as in patients with pharyngitis alone. The erythematous maculopapular rash usually begins on the trunk and spreads to cover the entire body within hours to days. The rash has the texture of sandpaper. The forehead and cheeks are flushed, and the area around the mouth is pallid (i.e., circumoral pallor). The rash generally fades on pressure and may ultimately desquamate. Deep red, nonblanching, or petechial lesions may be seen in the folds of the joints (i.e., Pastia's lines) or in other parts of the extremities. Early in the course of illness, the dorsum of the tongue has a white coat, through which edematous and red papillae project (i.e., white strawberry tongue). Several days later, the white covering subsides, and the tongue becomes swollen, red, and mottled (i.e., red strawberry tongue). A scarlatiniform rash may also appear in patients with streptococcal wound infections or impetigo. The rash may desquamate over 7 to 21 days. Eosinophilia is common during the recovery phases from scarlet fever; the number of eosinophils may reach 30% of the differential leukocyte count in this disorder.

Streptococcal impetigo may develop up to several weeks after a strain of GAS is detected on normal skin. The patient is usually afebrile and the lesion is painless. The lesion appears initially as a superficial vesicle with little surrounding erythema and progresses to a pustule that becomes thick and yellow. A secondary staphylococcal infection is possible.

Erysipelas is a streptococcal infection of the skin. Erysipelas is characterized by an elevated red lesion often associated with bullae filled with yellowish fluid that may crust over after rupture. A well-demarcated advancing border, which appears redder and more edematous at the edge than centrally, is seen. Erysipelas usually involves the face and or neck; the extremities and the rest of the body are affected less often. The acute onset of erysipelas is often accompanied by systemic toxicity. The lesion may persist for several days to several weeks.

Acute poststreptococcal nephritis can follow impetigo or other forms of streptococcal skin infection, or streptococcal pharyngitis. This disorder is produced by specific nephritogenic strains of streptococci. Rheumatic fever has not been associated with streptococcal skin infections. The latent period for acute nephritis is longer after skin infection (average, 3 weeks) than after throat infection (average, 10 days).

Toxic shock syndrome can be caused by GAS and cases of this have increased recently. This syndrome is characterized by high fever (greater than 38.9°C), diffuse macular erythroderma, hypotension, and involvement of at least three of the following organ systems: gastrointestinal, muscular, renal, mucous membranes, hepatic, hematologic, and central nervous system.

Other infections that may be caused by GAS include otitis media, sinusitis, mastoiditis, pneumonia, empyema, necrotizing fasciitis, septicemia without localized infection, and meningitis. The currently accepted case definition of streptococcal toxic shock syndrome appears in Table 95-1.

TABLE 95-1. Case Definition for the Streptococcal Toxic Shock Syndrome*

I. Isolation of group A streptococci (*Streptococcus pyogenes*)
- A. From a normally sterile site (e.g., blood, cerebrospinal, pleural, or peritoneal fluid, tissue biopsy, surgical wound)
- B. From a nonsterile site (e.g., throat, sputum, vagina, superficial skin lesion)

II. Clinical signs of severity
- A. Hypotension: systolic blood pressure $\leq$90 mm Hg in adults or <fifth percentile for age in children

and
- B. Two or more of the following signs:
  - Renal impairment
  - Coagulopathy
  - Liver involvement
  - Adult respiratory distress syndrome
  - Generalized erythematous macular rash that may desquamate
  - Soft tissue necrosis, including necrotizing fasciitis or myositis, or gangrene

*An illness fulfilling criteria IA and II (A and B) can be defined as a *definite* case. An illness fulfilling criteria IB and II (A and B) can be defined as a *probable* case if no other etiology for the illness is identified.

STREPTOCOCCAL RESPIRATORY CARRIER STATE

Many normal persons harbor GAS in the upper respiratory tract for prolonged periods without evidence of disease or an immunologic response. Approximately 10% of school-aged children are carriers, and that rate may increase to as high as 30% during periods of peak streptococcal activity in the community. Carriers only rarely spread the organism to close contacts. The risk of a carrier developing rheumatic fever appears to be significantly less than that of a person with active streptococcal pharyngeal infection. Streptococcal pharyngitis is often diagnosed mistakenly in patients who are colonized by group A streptococcus but whose symptoms are caused by a viral infection. The carrier state may be recognized by culturing the throat after symptoms have resolved.

DIAGNOSIS

For patients with acute pharyngitis or tonsillitis, the physician must rely on the clinical appearance of the patient, culture results, and epidemiologic findings to confirm the probability of streptococcal infection. The physician's problem in identifying group A streptococcal pharyngitis is difficult because these organisms are found in the throats of normal children (i.e., carriers) and those whose clinical findings are caused by many other agents including gonococci, Epstein-Barr virus, and *Mycoplasma pneumoniae*. As an example, in young adults, pharyngitis caused by *Arcanobacterium haemolyticum* may mimic streptococcal pharyngitis, and the rash often associated with this infection may be indistinguishable from scarlet fever.

Most streptococcal infections are short-term illnesses. Antibody responses appear relatively late, and streptococcal antibody titers are useful only retrospectively in supporting the diagnosis of nonsuppurative complications of GAS disease such as acute nephritis and rheumatic fever. The measurement of antibody titers may be useful if obtaining a culture of the primary site of infection (e.g., osteomyelitis) is difficult or if the patient has been treated with antibiotics to which the group A streptococcus is susceptible.

Clinical manifestations that suggest streptococcal disease include high fever, exudative pharyngitis, tender anterior cervical nodes, a history of contact with a documented case of streptococcal infection, and a scarlatiniform rash. The concurrent findings of hoarseness, cough, rhinorrhea, or conjunctivitis render the diagnosis of streptococcal pharyngitis less likely.

The diagnosis of streptococcal pharyngitis can be confirmed by culture, but recovery of GAS from the pharynx does not in itself differentiate the streptococcal carrier state from streptococcal disease. A number of rapid techniques (i.e., 5–60 minutes) for identifying group A streptococci in the upper respiratory tract are available commercially. These techniques involve extraction of the group-specific carbohydrate from the cell wall of the organism and subsequent identification of the organism by agglutination or immunologic reaction detected by a color change. Currently available data suggest that the specificity for these tests exceeds 90% and that the sensitivity ranges from 85% to 95%. These tests have the advantage of rapid identification of GAS and are particularly appealing because more rapid treatment is clearly associated with an earlier clinical response. Because the sensitivity of these rapid tests is not 100%, however, a negative result in a patient whose symptoms suggest group A streptococcal pharyngitis should be followed by a confirmatory throat culture. Rapid antigen detection tests can also be useful in the detection of GAS from streptococcal pyoderma-like lesions.

In impetigo, GAS is the only pathogen isolated in 5% of cases, whereas *S. aureus* is the sole isolate in 50% to 60% of cases. Occasionally, the vesicles of chickenpox resemble those of a bullous impetigo, but the former are usually less transient and tend to involve the trunk more than the extremities. The lesions of chickenpox tend to itch, and the crusts are not as thick as those of streptococcal impetigo. However, the lesions of varicella can be infected secondarily with streptococci.

Elaboration of antibody to the M protein is important because it is the basis of immunity to or protection against reinfection from the same serologic type. Type-specific antibody may also be transferred from the mother to the fetus. The development of type-specific antibody can be inhibited by prompt treatment with penicillin.

In the process of supporting the possibility of a preceding GAS infection in patients with rheumatic fever or glomerulonephritis, the antistreptolysin O titer is the streptococcal antibody test used most frequently. The test is not specific for group A infection. The antistreptolysin O response is weak in patients with streptococcal impetigo and pyoderma, but anti-DNAase B and antihyaluronidase responses are measurable after both skin and throat infections.

The Streptozyme (Carter-Wallace, Inc., Cranbury, NJ) agglutination test is based on the antibody agglutination of erythrocytes coated with a mixture of streptococcal extracellular antigens. This test has the appeal of speed, simplicity, and reaction with a variety of streptococcal antigens. Antibody responses measurable by this assay have been demonstrated within the first 7 to 10 days after the onset of infection. This contrasts with the development of neutralizing antibody titers to streptolysin O, which appear after 3 to 6 weeks, and to anti-DNAase B, which appear after 6 to 8 weeks. Because of problems with standardization of this reagent, producing variable results with different lots, this test should be interpreted with caution.

TREATMENT

Penicillin remains the drug of choice for the treatment of group A beta-hemolytic streptococcal infections unless the patient is allergic. No strains of group A streptococcus resistant to penicillin have been isolated. Although penicillin tolerance has been described, its clinical significance has not been defined. Eradication of GAS from the nasopharynx or the upper respiratory tract may be difficult because of noncompliance with prescribed antibiotics, reinfection from family or classroom contacts, or persistence of colonizing group A streptococcus. Also, beta-lactamase-producing organisms in the nasopharynx or the production of inhibitory substances by other organisms may allow the persistence of the group A streptococcus.

Erythromycin is the drug of choice in patients who are allergic to penicillin. Group A beta-hemolytic streptococci resistant to erythromycin have been reported, and in countries where the use of erythromycin is higher than that in the United States (Japan, Spain, Finland), resistance rates as high as 20% have been found. In the United States, less than 5% of group A streptococcal strains are resistant to erythromycin and the other macrolides.

The rationale for the use of penicillin in the treatment of streptococcal pharyngitis is to relieve symptoms and prevent the development of acute rheumatic fever, which can be accomplished with low-dose therapy maintained over a rather long period. A 10-day course of oral penicillin is the treatment of choice. Alternatively, administration of a single intramuscular injection of benzathine penicillin G is another method of accomplishing this objective.

In patients who are allergic, a 10-day course of macrolide therapy is recommended. If azithromycin is used, 5 days of therapy is recommended by the manufacturer.

Patients with streptococcal bacteremia, deep soft tissue infections, erysipelas, pneumonia, or meningitis should be treated with penicillin parenterally, preferably intravenously. The dosage and duration of therapy must be based on the nature of the disease process, and daily dosages as high as 400,000 U/kg/day may be required in the most severe infections. Intravenous clindamycin, in addition to intravenous penicillin, has been recommended by some experts to treat streptococcal toxic shock syndrome and necrotizing fasciitis.

In patients with streptococcal impetigo, oral or parenteral penicillin or oral erythromycin should be used. Local skin care such as removal of crusts and use of special bacteriostatic soaps, should be performed but its efficacy probably depends on thoroughness. These measures, with use of local antibiotic ointments, may be sufficient for the management mild cases but are not recommended for those with more widespread impetigo. A topical antibiotic ointment [e.g., mupirocin (Bactroban)] is effective therapy for some patients with localized impetigo, even when parenteral therapy has not been initiated.

Patients with skin infection caused by a nephritogenic streptococcal strain may develop nephritis despite penicillin therapy.

PREVENTION

Streptococcal disease cannot yet be prevented by immunization. The spread of GAS is decreased by limiting the density of persons living within the home environment, isolating the contagious patient and, especially, treating with antibiotics patients known to have this infection. For populations with streptococcal infection occurring at an epidemic level over an extended period (e.g., selected military populations), institution of mass prophylaxis, usually with injections of benzathine penicillin, may be necessary.

INFECTIONS CAUSED BY STREPTOCOCCI OTHER THAN GROUPS A AND B

The classification of streptococci can be confusing because of their separation on the basis of hemolysis and their separate identification by Lancefield typing. These two methods of identification are not mutually exclusive; Table 95-2 shows classification of streptococci by Lancefield type and by the hemolytic reactions on blood agar, and their correlation with human colonization and disease.

RHEUMATIC FEVER

Rheumatic fever (RF) is a delayed, nonsuppurative sequela to upper respiratory infection with GAS. It is a diffuse inflammatory disease of the connective tissue that involves principally the heart, blood vessels, joints, central nervous system, and subcutaneous tissues.

Several factors predispose to RF: age, family history, season, recurrent streptococcal infections, and host factors affecting susceptibility. The first attack usually occurs in patients between 5 and 15 years of age. RF is rare in children younger than 4 years. No gender preference exists unless chorea is included, in which case, the incidence is slightly greater among girls.

RF may affect more than one member in the same family. It is possible that the same housing conditions predispose several persons to recurrent streptococcal infections. Constitutional susceptibility may be a factor but, currently, no evidence for genetic markers in rheumatic patients exists. Similar to streptococcal pharyngitis, RF occurs more commonly in the winter and spring.

Recurrent streptococcal infections are the most important predisposing factor in the occurrence and recurrence of RF. Approximately 1% to 5% of streptococcal throat infections are followed by RF. Skin infections are unlikely to produce the disease.

Because RF develops after streptococcal pharyngitis in a relatively small percentage of patients, host predisposition is probably a factor. After RF is acquired, its reactivation after subsequent streptococcal infections is much more likely. The recurrence rate per infection is approximately 50% during the first year after the initial attack; it decreases sharply after that. The rate levels off after several years to approximately 10%. This persistently high attack rate after RF suggests acquired hyperreactivity.

MECHANISM PRODUCING RHEUMATIC FEVER

RF is thought to be an autoimmune disease. The requirements for its development include group A beta-hemolytic streptococcal infection in the throat with antibody response indicative of recent infection and persistence of the organism in the pharynx for a period sufficient to produce an immunologic response. The magnitude of the antibody response is a major factor determining the attack rate of RF after streptococcal infection. The predisposing organism has antigens immunologically similar to proteins in the human heart, and the antibodies produced against the streptococci react with the heart (i.e., cross-reactive immunity). A plethora of streptococcal cellular components cross-reacting with various mammalian tissues has been described. The hyaluronate capsule is identical to human hyaluronate. Antibodies to the cell wall polysaccharide cross-react with glycoproteins of heart valves. Membrane antigens cross-react with the sarcolemma and smooth muscles of endocardial and myocardial arteries. Antibody to the streptococcal group A polysaccharide persists in the serum of patients with rheumatic valvular disease in contrast to its more rapid decline in patients with RF without cardiac involvement.

TABLE 95-2. Correlation of Streptococci Identified by Lancefield Grouping and Hemolytic Reactions with Sites of Human Colonization and Disease

Lancefield group	Species	Usual reaction on sheep blood agar	Usual human habitat	Most common human disease
A	*S. pyogenes*	Beta-hemolysis	Pharynx, skin, rectum	Pharyngitis, erysipelas, impetigo, septicemia, wound infections, rheumatic fever, acute glomerulonephritis, necrotizing fasciitis, cellulitis, otitis media, meningitis, pneumonia, conjunctivitis, acute endocarditis
B	*S. agalactiae*	Beta-hemolysis	Pharynx, vagina	Puerperal sepsis, endocarditis, neonatal sepsis, meningitis, otitis media, osteomyelitis, pneumonia
C	*S. equi, S. equisimilis, S. dysgalactiae, S. zooepidemicus*	Beta-hemolysis	Pharynx, vagina, skin	Wound infection, puerperal sepsis, cellulitis, endocarditis
D	*Enterococcus faecalis, E. faecium; S. bovis*	Gamma	Colon contents	Endocarditis, urinary tract infection, biliary tract infection, intestinal infection, peritonitis
E	*S. infrequens*	?	?	?
F	*S. minutus anginosus*	Beta-hemolysis	Mouth, pharynx	Sinusitis, meningitis, brain abscess, pneumonia
G	*S. canis*	Beta-hemolysis	Pharynx, vagina, skin	Puerperal infection, skin or wound infection, endocarditis
H	*S. sanguis**	Alpha-hemolysis	Mouth	Endocarditis, brain abscess
K	*S. salivarius**	Alpha-hemolysis	Mouth	Endocarditis, sinusitis, meningitis, brain abscess
L		Beta- or alpha-hemolysis	Mouth	Endocarditis, abscess, parotitis, neonatal sepsis
M		Beta- or alpha-hemolysis	Mouth, pharynx, vagina	Endocarditis, septicemia
N	*S. lactis-cremoris*	Alpha-or gamma-hemolysis	Pharynx	Meningitis, septicemia?
O		Alpha- or beta-hemolysis	Pharynx, conjuctiva, vagina	Pneumonia, endocarditis, septicemia
Nontypable	*S. viridans*	Alpha-hemolysis	Pharynx	Endocarditis, intravascular catheter-related infections
Nontypable	*S. mutans*	Alpha-hemolysis	Pharynx	Endocarditis, intravascular catheter-related infections
Nontypable	*S. pneumoniae*	Alpha-hemolysis	Nasopharynx	Sepsis, meningitis, otitis media, pneumonia, sinusitis

*These organism are isolated frequently from the bloodstream as alpha-hemolytic streptococci. Along with many nongroupable alpha streptococci, they are often called *S. viridans,* a term that incorrectly implies a specific species. Nevertheless, as a group, they cause most episodes of endocarditis and are usually exquisitely sensitive to penicillin.
Adapted from Keusch GT, Weinstein L. *Streptococcal disease.* Kalamazoo, MI: Upjohn Company, 1973.

CLINICAL CHARACTERISTICS

Antecedent Streptococcal Infection

The interval between the onset of pharyngitis and the symptoms of RF is 1 to 5 weeks (average, 3 weeks). However, clinical evidence for a preceding streptococcal infection may be lacking. Approximately one-third of patients have had no apparent illness during the preceding month.

Polyarthritis

Inflammation affects the large joints and moves from one to another. The affected joint is hot, red, tender, and swollen. The arthritis characteristically leaves the joints without any sequelae and responds almost immediately to salicylates. The severity of joint involvement is inversely proportional to the severity of cardiac involvement.

Carditis

In contrast to the seriousness of its prognosis, rheumatic carditis, unless it causes heart failure or pericarditis, produces no symptoms of its own and is usually diagnosed during examination of a patient with arthritis or chorea.

Chorea

Rheumatic or Sydenham chorea, a late manifestation of RF, is more common among female than male patients. Chorea may last from 1 week to more than 2 years. Chorea is never seen simultaneously with arthritis, but it may coexist with carditis. If there is no carditis, the sedimentation rate is not elevated. In such cases, the ASO and other streptococcal antibody titers may not be increased, probably because chorea appears only after a latent period as long as 6 months after the streptococcal infection and, by that time, the acute-phase reactants and the streptococcal antibody titer may have returned to normal.

Involuntary, uncoordinated, jerky movements are present and are accompanied by hypotonia and emotional disturbances with abrupt alterations between laughter and tears. Flexion at the wrist and dorsiflexion of the fingers occur in the outstretched hands. Objects often fall from the hands. The patient, after protruding the tongue for inspection, may withdraw it rapidly, snapping the jaws over it.

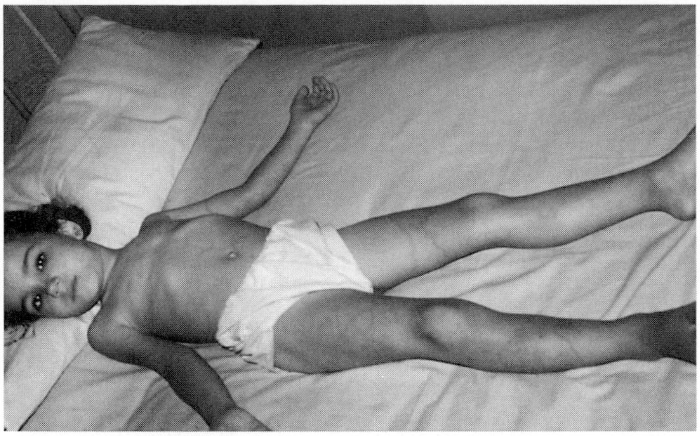

Figure 95-1. A 6-year-old girl with erythema marginatum has acute rheumatic fever with severe carditis. (Courtesy of Dr. Samir Kassem, Alexandria Medical School.)

TABLE 95-3. Duckett Jones Criteria for the Diagnosis of Rheumatic Fever

Requirements for diagnosis
Two major criteria
or
One major plus two minor criteria
plus
Evidence of previous streptococcal infection (e.g., elevated antistreptolysin O titer)

Major criteria	Minor criteria
Carditis	Previous rheumatic fever
Arthritis	Arthralgia
Chorea	Fever
Erythema marginatum	Elevated erythrocyte sedimentation rate
Subcutaneous nodules	Elevated leukocyte count
	Prolonged PR interval
	C-reactive protein

Subcutaneous Nodules

Now rarely seen, subcutaneous nodules usually indicate severe carditis. The nodules are attached to the tendon sheaths and occur on the extensor surfaces and bony prominences of the arms and legs and on the scapula and the mastoid processes. Histologically, they consist of collections of Aschoff's bodies.

Erythema Marginatum

The rash of erythema marginatum generally appears as an area of erythema. The margins progress as the center clears. The rash occurs chiefly over the trunk and the proximal parts of the limbs (Fig. 95-1).

DIAGNOSIS

Laboratory tests typically show a high erythrocyte sedimentation rate, anemia, leukocytosis, and C-reactive protein. The ASO antibody is elevated abnormally in 70% to 85% of patients with RF. A single value of 500 units indicates recent streptococcal infection, and a value of 333 units is of borderline significance. If the ASO titer is 333 units or less, additional antistreptococcal antibody assays such as antiDNase and antihyaluronidase should be obtained.

The diagnosis of RF is important because serious cardiac disease can be prevented or minimized by long-term antistreptococcal therapy. No single diagnostic test for RF exists. The laboratory tests indicate recent streptococcal infection, but diagnosis of RF rests on the ability to satisfy the Duckett Jones criteria (Table 95-3). It is mandatory to demonstrate recent streptococcal infection (usually by elevation of ASO titer) and to find one major and two minor criteria or to identify two major criteria. The minor manifestations are less specific for the illness.

Diagnosis of recurrent attack of RF has been suggested if there is evidence of recent group A streptococcal infection and the presence of one major or two minor Duckett Jones criteria in a patient with rheumatic heart disease. A presumptive diagnosis of recurrent attacks of RF may be made when a patient presents with one minor criterion and several other manifestations such as anemia, abdominal pain, rapid sleeping pulse rate, tachycardia out of proportion to fever, malaise, epistaxes, precordial pain, and an elevated level of IgG, IgA, C3, and circulating immune complexes.

COURSE AND PROGNOSIS

RF usually follows a characteristic clinical course. The latent period is short for disease complicated with arthritis and erythema marginatum, longest for RF with chorea, and midlength for RF with carditis and subcutaneous nodules. The duration of active disease is usually less than 3 months. Fewer than 5% of patients with RF have disease that remains active for more than 6 months, a condition known as chronic active carditis. The prognosis is excellent for the patient who does not develop carditis during the initial attack. The prognosis becomes poorer with increasing severity of initial carditis.

Over the years, changes have occurred in the epidemiology of RF and in its severity, presentation, and clinical manifestations. RF is less common in developed countries and, when it occurs, it tends to be mild. In tropical and subtropical countries, RF and rheumatic heart disease are common and assume more malignant forms.

TREATMENT

Prophylactic Therapy

Prevention of RF is achieved by improving socioeconomic circumstances and sanitation. The aim of primary prophylaxis is to prevent initial attacks of RF by prompt and accurate recognition and treatment of streptococcal pharyngitis or by antibiotic prophylaxis using benzathine penicillin intramuscularly for members of a susceptible population. Modern outbreaks in the United States were blamed, in part, on diminished adherence to conventional recommendations for penicillin, which is highly effective in preventing RF caused by pharyngeal infections.

Secondary prophylaxis is the prevention of recurrences of RF by continuous chemoprophylaxis. The most effective method is a single monthly intramuscular injection of 600,000 to 1,200,000 units of benzathine penicillin. RF recurs in approximately 0.45% of individuals who use benzathine penicillin prophylaxis, compared with 11.5% of those who do not comply with treatment. In areas where RF is endemic, twice monthly (or once every 3 weeks as advised by the World Health Organization) benzathine penicillin prophylaxis was found to significantly decrease the recurrence rate of RF, compared with monthly injections. The incidence of allergic reactions is approximately 3%, but anaphylaxis occurs after only 1 in 10,000 injections. Oral penicillin prophylaxis can be provided by 500 to 1,000 mg of penicillin G administered twice daily. If the patient is allergic to penicillin, prophylaxis can be achieved by 250 mg of erythromycin given twice daily. The injectable form of prophylaxis is more effective than the oral forms because patient compliance is superior and the medication is not affected by variations in intestinal absorption. The duration of secondary prophylaxis depends on the variables that influence the recurrence rate and the degree to which the heart has been affected. The risk of recurrence declines with age.

Curative Therapy

Bed rest is required until the signs and symptoms of acute inflammation disappear. Salt is restricted if signs of heart failure are observed.

A course of antibiotics should be initiated after a throat culture has been obtained. Antibiotics should be administered even in the absence of positive throat culture results. One intramuscular injection of benzathine penicillin (600,000–1,200,000 units) or a 10-day course of oral penicillin G (500–1,000 mg, four times daily) is recommended. Patients who are allergic to penicillin should receive erythromycin (250–500 mg, four times daily) for 10 days.

The selection of an antirheumatic drug is not critical to the outcome of RF. Salicylates and corticosteroids are valuable symptomatic drugs, but they are not curative and may actually prolong the course of the disease.

Acetylsalicylic acid (aspirin) is analgesic and antipyretic and reduces malaise. It causes such dramatic improvement of the arthritis that it can be given as a therapeutic test, but it has no effect on carditis. Aspirin is given to patients with or without mild carditis, if side effects or contraindications to corticosteroids are present, and during and after withdrawal from corticosteroids. The dosage is 60 to 120 mg/kg/day given in six divided doses and administered until a satisfactory clinical response is obtained. The dosage is then reduced by one-third and continued until all laboratory findings return to normal, which usually requires 6 to 9 weeks. The dosage is decreased gradually to avoid the rebound that occurs if the drug is stopped abruptly.

Corticosteroids do not markedly shorten the course of illness or diminish the likelihood of cardiac damage. Corticosteroids do produce prompt control of the subcutaneous nodules, erythema marginatum, fever, and arthritis. Corticosteroids are indicated for patients with severe carditis. The dosage of prednisone or prednisolone is 2 mg/kg/day (not to exceed 60 mg/day) for 3 to 4 weeks. Shortly before or at the time corticosteroid therapy is discontinued, aspirin (90–120 mg/kg/day) should be given, and it should be continued for 1.5 to 6 months, probably until active inflammation subsides.

Chorea

The patient with chorea should be maintained in a quiet atmosphere, protected from self-injury. Haloperidol (butyrophenone), a centrally acting drug, is the most effective in controlling chorea, but severe, adverse extrapyramidal reactions have been reported. Patients with concomitant rheumatic activity should be given salicylates.

Heart Failure

Heart failure may be an indication for the use of corticosteroids or diuretic agents. Operative repair or replacement of a severely compromised cardiac valve may be necessary during acute RF if signs and symptoms of severe congestive heart failure are unresponsive to medical therapy.

CHAPTER 96
Syphilis

Adapted from Christian C. Patrick and Jonathan A. McCullers

Syphilis, a venereal disease of adolescence and adulthood, is of major importance in pediatrics as an acquired and a congenital infection. *Treponema pallidum*, the etiologic agent of syphilis, was described in 1905; symptoms specific to syphilis were not determined until 1938 because of frequent dual infection with gonorrhea. Humans are the sole natural host of *T. pallidum*.

MICROBIOLOGY

T. pallidum is a member of the genus *Treponema* (order *Spirochaetales*). Treponemes are microaerophilic gram-negative bacteria that exhibit a characteristic corkscrew motility. They reproduce by transverse fission. Treponemes cannot be grown *in vitro*.

EPIDEMIOLOGY

Syphilis may be transmitted via sexual contact. Acquisition by direct contact with an infected lesion is rare. Congenital syphilis occurs by transplacental passage of *T. pallidum* from an infected mother to a fetus or by contact with an infectious lesion in the birth canal.

Epidemics of crack cocaine use and HIV infection caused high syphilis infection rates in the late 1980s; these decreased in the first half of the 1990s. During this epidemic, the number of cases of congenital syphilis increased due to the rising incidence of acquired syphilis in women of childbearing years.

PATHOGENESIS

T. pallidum penetrates the skin or mucous membrane at a site of exposure. The organism multiplies locally and spreads through the perivascular lymphatic system to the systemic circulation, which disseminates the infection widely even before a primary lesion is evident. Within 3 to 4 weeks, a local inflammatory response is initiated as a result of an invasion by mononuclear and plasma cells. This response produces a red, ulcerated lesion with surrounding induration: the chancre. A concomitant cellular proliferation in the regional lymph nodes produces adenopathy.

Secondary lesions of syphilis, a consequence of dissemination, are caused by an inflammatory response in ectodermal tissue of skin, mucous membranes, and the central nervous system (CNS). The host response to these lesions is similar to that which occurs to primary lesions.

Tertiary syphilis is caused by slowly developing immune-mediated host responses to the infection. This stage is characterized by a diffuse, chronic inflammation in affected tissues, generally skin, CNS, and cardiovascular tissues. Organisms are not found within the tertiary syphilis lesions.

Congenital syphilis occurs mainly by transplacental passage of treponemes during maternal spirochetemia, although transmission by contact with an infected lesion at birth is possible. Transmission can occur as early as 9 to 10 weeks of gestation, and pathologic changes can be observed as early as 15 weeks. Spontaneous abortion of syphilitic fetuses generally occurs some time after 18 weeks of gestation. The organs affected most severely include bone, brain, liver, lung, and the skeletal system.

CLINICAL MANIFESTATIONS

In primary syphilis, after a mean incubation period of 21 days (range, 3–90 days), the chancre appears, usually single and nontender. This occurs most often on the genitalia and is associated with nontender lymphadenopathy. Regional lymphadenopathy is particularly important when present in women with a cervical chancre, as it may be the only sign or symptom of syphilis. Primary syphilis heals spontaneously in 3 to 12 weeks.

Symptoms of secondary syphilis appear 6 to 12 weeks after the onset of primary syphilis and are caused by the dissemination of treponemes. Symptoms include low-grade fever, malaise, and diffuse lymphadenopathy, and a polymorphous rash that inevitably harbors organisms. The classic rash is maculopapular, begins on the trunk and eventually involves the palms and soles. Neurologic manifestations of meningeal and cranial or spinal nerve involvement appear during secondary syphilis but are reversible with proper therapy.

Tertiary infection occurs after a latent period of at least 1 year (termed the early latent period) or, more frequently, 3 to 10 years (the late latent period). The classic lesion of tertiary syphilis, called the gumma, comprises a necrotic center surrounded by plasma cells, lymphocytes, and monocytes. Involvement of nonvital structures such as skin, soft tissue, and bone, which is called benign late syphilis, occurs in 15% of the cases of late syphilis. Cardiovascular syphilis, including syphilitic aortitis with medial necrosis, occurs in 10% of patients with late syphilis. Neurosyphilis with multiple presentations that may include tabes dorsalis, paresis, meningitis, or transverse myelitis develops in perhaps 7% of patients with late syphilis.

Although as many as two-thirds of newborns with congenital syphilis are asymptomatic at birth, early congenital syphilis can affect many organ systems by widespread dissemination of the organisms from maternal spirochetemia. Hepatosplenomegaly occurs in more than 90% of affected infants, although liver function usually remains normal. Generalized nonsuppurative lymphadenopathy, including epitrochlear adenopathy, is evident in as many as 50% of infants. Mucocutaneous lesions produce snuffles (i.e., a rhinitis loaded with spirochetes) after the first week of life. Nasal cartilage destruction can lead to a saddle-nose deformity. Dermatologic lesions include pemphigus syphiliticus, condylomata lata, or the classic copper-brown maculopapular rash on the palms and soles. Ocular involvement presents most commonly as chorioretinitis, but congenital glaucoma and uveitis are also seen. CNS disease may occur after the neonatal period.

The organ system involved most frequently is the skeletal system. Involvement is usually multiple and symmetric and affects the metaphyses and diaphyses of long bones. Pain associated with bony involvement can be striking and can lead to pseudoparalysis, termed pseudoparalysis of Parrot.

Late congenital syphilis has several manifestations. Dental anomalies include Hutchinson teeth (peg-shaped, notched central incisors) and mulberry molars (multicuspid first molars). Eye involvement leads to interstitial keratitis between ages 4 and 30, secondary glaucoma, or corneal scarring. Eighth nerve deafness can develop, usually between ages 8 and 10. These three disorders—Hutchinson teeth, interstitial keratitis, and eighth nerve deafness—comprise the Hutchinson triad. The scars that remain after the occurrence of snuffles in early congenital syphilis are called rhagades. Clutton joints are symmetric synovial effusions, usually localized to the knees. Another lesion of bone and joints, saber shins, is secondary to persistent periostitis. A classic sign of late congenital syphilis is perforation of the hard palate. CNS involvement can include meningovascular involvement and paresis.

DIAGNOSIS

The definitive laboratory diagnosis is made by direct visualization of treponemes by dark-field microscopy of exudate from a primary chancre or by an active secondary lesion or by direct fluorescent antibody of clinical specimens. The probable diagnosis, however, is often made by clinical findings and/or positive findings on treponemal-specific or nonspecific serology (Table 96-1).

Specific tests for antibody to *T. pallidum* include the fluorescent treponemal antibody absorption (FTA-ABS) test and the treponemal-specific microhemagglutination test. They are positive in 75% to 85% of patients with primary syphilis and in 100% of patients with secondary syphilis. The nontreponemal tests for syphilis involve detection of antibodies to cardiolipin, a component of membranes and mammalian tissue. The two nontreponemal tests currently in use are the rapid plasma reagin (RPR) test and the VDRL test. The RPR is positive in approximately 85% of cases of primary syphilis and in 98% of cases of secondary syphilis, whereas the VDRL test is positive in approximately 80% of primary cases and in 95% of secondary cases. Titers can be followed (not available with FTA-ABS), and they decrease with treatment allowing monitoring of therapy during latent or tertiary syphilis. In rare cases, a serofast state in which a positive VDRL test exists despite adequate therapy occurs. The RPR is used more often in screening, but the VDRL test is the only one approved for testing reactivity of spinal fluid. Both acute and chronic false-positive reactions are seen. False-negative results can also occur when a high concentration of antibody inhibits agglutination (the prozone phenomenon), which can be avoided with serial dilutions of the serum. Because of the high false-positive rate of nontreponemal tests, specific treponemal tests are used to confirm the clinical diagnosis in the absence of definitive laboratory confirmation.

The diagnosis of congenital syphilis relies on history, clinical findings, and laboratory data and is achieved best through direct identification of *T. pallidum* from a lesion on the mother or infant by either dark-field microscopy or direct fluorescent

TABLE 96-1. Diagnostic Tests for Syphilis

Diagnostic identification of *Treponema pallidum*
Dark-field examination of exudate
Direct fluorescent antibody to *T. pallidum* (exudate)
Specific treponemal serologic tests
Fluorescent treponemal antibody absorption test (FTA-ABS)
Microhemagglutination test for *T. pallidum* (MHA-TP)
Nontreponemal serologic tests
VDRL test
Rapid plasma reagin card test

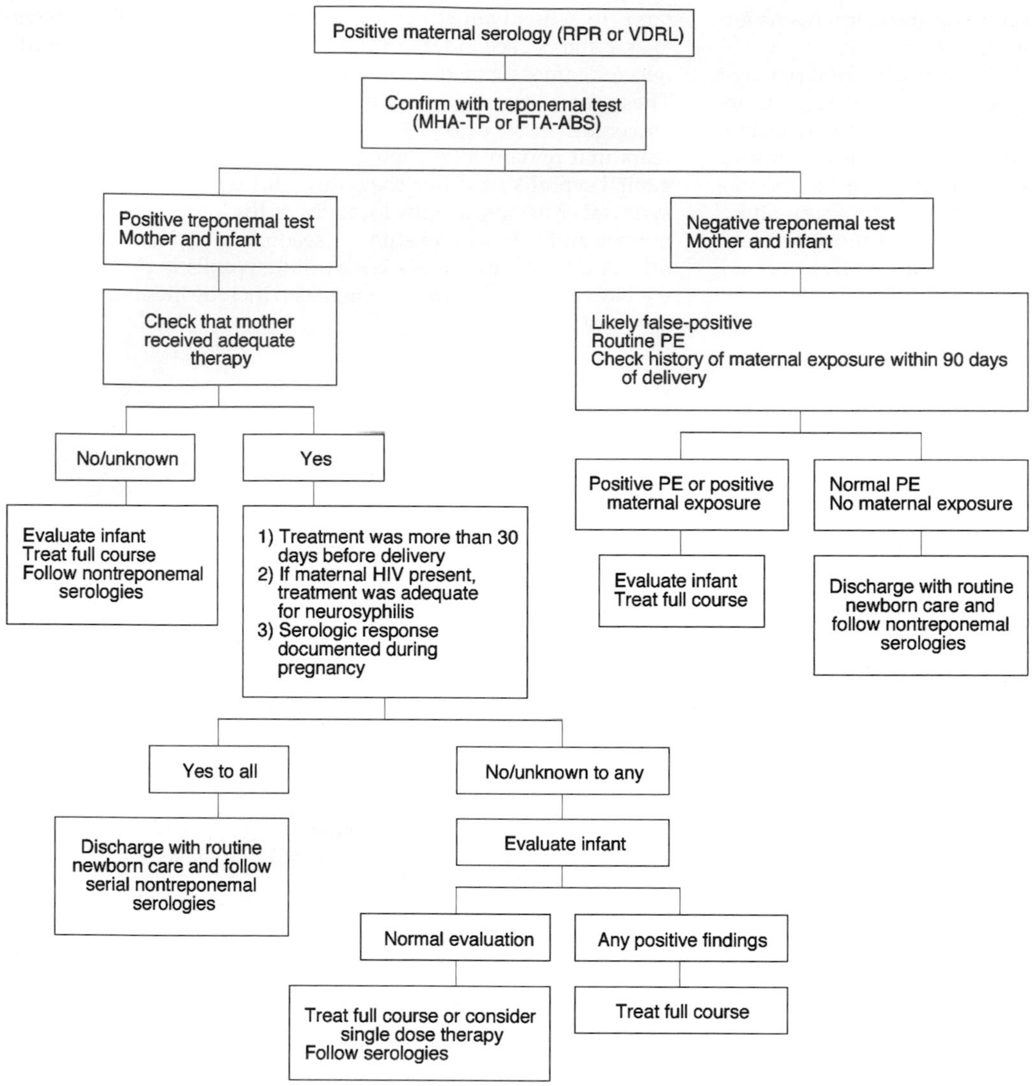

Figure 96-1. Algorithm for serologic diagnosis and treatment of congenital syphilis. FTA-ABS, fluorescent treponemal antibody absorption test; HIV, human immunodeficiency virus; MHA-TP, microhemagglutination test for *T. pallidum*; PE, physical examination; RPR, rapid plasma reagin test.

antibody techniques. Making serologic diagnosis is difficult in infants because transplacentally acquired maternal immunoglobulin G may lead to false-positive results. If the titer of the infant's RPR or VDRL test is four times that of the mother, the presence of active infection is assumed, although a titer lower than the mother's does not exclude infection. The maternal titer should fall at least fourfold with adequate treatment. If positive serologies in the infant are derived maternally, the test will usually become negative within 3 months. The FTA-ABS or treponemal-specific microhemagglutination test may be persistently positive but may remain maternally derived for up to 6 months; a positive test at 15 months indicates a probable active infection. The decision whether to treat the infant when maternal serologies are positive depends on numerous factors including any therapy the mother may have received, the timing of the therapy, and the mother's response to the therapy; the infant's physical examination and laboratory work; and social factors such as a stable home environment ensuring good follow-up care. Fig. 96-1 may be used as a guide for treatment decisions and workup for congenital syphilis.

The infant with suspected congenital syphilis should receive a thorough physical examination looking for clinical signs and symptoms, as discussed. Laboratory work aside from the serologies includes a complete blood cell count, platelet count, liver function tests, urinalysis, and lumbar puncture. In cases of neurosyphilis, the cerebrospinal fluid (CSF) shows increased leukocytes and increased total protein. A positive VDRL test can be seen, but this test on the CSF is relatively insensitive and may be negative in as many as one-half of the cases of neurosyphilis. A chest radiograph should be obtained if pneumonia is a possibility. Radiography of the long bones should be obtained and has been reported to be the most sensitive screening assay for congenital syphilis. Additional tests such as cranial ultrasonography, ophthalmologic examination, or auditory brainstem responses, should be considered when indicated. Infants with signs of disease on physical examination, radiographic evidence of disease, a reactive CSF VDRL test, an elevated CSF white blood cell count or elevated CSF protein, a quantitative nontreponemal serologic titer at least fourfold higher than the mother's titer, or infection of the placenta should be considered symptomatic and should receive a full course of treatment.

TREATMENT

Acquired primary, secondary, or early latent syphilis of less than 1 year's duration can be treated with 50,000 U/kg of benzathine penicillin G intramuscularly in a single dose (not to exceed 2.4 million units). Pregnancy mandates treatment with penicillin because insufficient erythromycin may pass through the placenta to the fetus. Tetracycline or doxycycline are alternative therapies for nonpregnant patients who are older than 9 years and allergic to penicillin. Erythromycin may also be used. The Jarisch-Herxheimer reaction of fever, headache, and malaise can occur 2 to 12 hours after therapy for active syphilis. The reaction is thought to be produced by the release of treponemal endotoxin by the action of penicillin.

Latent or tertiary syphilis existing for more than 1 year with no evidence of neurosyphilis can be treated with benzathine penicillin G at a dosage of 50,000 U/kg/week (not to exceed 2.4 million units), administered intramuscularly for 3 successive weeks. In patients who are allergic to penicillin, either tetracycline or doxycycline should be given for 4 weeks only in cases in which neurosyphilis has been excluded by lumbar puncture.

The recommended regimen for treatment of neurosyphilis in adults is aqueous crystalline penicillin G, 12 to 24 million U/day (2–4 million units every 4 hours) intravenously for 10 to 14 days. If compliance can be assured, patients may be treated with an alternative regimen of 2.4 million units of procaine penicillin intramuscularly as a single daily dose combined with probenecid, 2.0 g/day orally in four divided doses, both for 10 to 14 days.

Treatment programs for congenital syphilis are tailored to the clinical and laboratory data (Fig. 96-1). The maternal serology should be confirmed by a specific treponemal test. Infant serology should be used to confirm the results. If a baby has positive specific treponemal serologies, the treatment strategy is based on the adequacy of maternal therapy, the timing of the maternal treatment, any further maternal exposure to primary syphilis, the infant's appearance, and the results of laboratory studies, especially the lumbar puncture. If the mother has inadequate or undetermined therapy, has received therapy during the last 4 weeks of pregnancy, was treated with an antibiotic other than penicillin, or had serologic titers that either were not documented or did not show a fourfold decrease in titers, the infant should be treated. If the mother was exposed to a person with primary or secondary syphilis within 90 days of delivery, the infant should be treated.

The treatment of congenital syphilis is aqueous crystalline penicillin G at a dose of 200,000 to 300,000 U/kg/day intravenously (divided into every-6-hour doses) for 10 to 14 days. This regimen should also be used to treat children who are older than 1 year and have late and previously untreated congenital syphilis. Some experts suggest giving such patients benzathine penicillin G, 50,000 U/kg intramuscularly, in three weekly doses following the 10- to 14-day treatment course of intravenous penicillin. These dosage recommendations also apply to the infant with neurosyphilis.

Follow-up examinations for early congenital syphilis should be at 1, 2, 4, 6, and 12 months after treatment. If titers of nontreponemal serologies do not decrease or if symptoms and signs persist, the infant should be retreated. Treated infants with congenital neurosyphilis and initially positive CSF VDRL tests or abnormal or noninterpretable CSF cell counts or protein concentrations should undergo repeat clinical evaluation and CSF examination at 6-month intervals until their CSF examinations are normal. A reactive CSF VDRL test at 6 months is an indication for retreatment. If cell counts are still abnormal at 2 years or are not decreasing at each examination, retreatment is again indicated.

PREVENTION

Case reporting and thorough investigation of contacts in association with local health care authorities are important preventive measures. All pregnant women should undergo serologic screening early in pregnancy and again at delivery. Women at high risk for syphilis should undergo testing again at 28 weeks' gestation. Acquired syphilis in children warrants an investigation for sexual abuse.

CHAPTER 97
Tuberculosis

Adapted from Jeffrey R. Starke

Tuberculosis remains the most important chronic infectious disease in the world in terms of morbidity, mortality, and cost. An estimated 1 to 2 billion people worldwide are infected with the tubercle bacillus and 1 to 3 million deaths from tuberculosis occur annually. Children in developing countries account for 1.3 million cases and 450,000 deaths annually from tuberculosis. In the United States, 20,000 people develop tuberculosis each year, and 2,000 die from the disease.

After *Mycobacterium tuberculosis* enters the lung and begins to multiply, the person has tuberculosis infection. The hallmark of tuberculosis infection is a positive tuberculin skin test result, but chest radiography is normal or reveals only a healed granuloma and the child is free of signs and symptoms. Tuberculosis disease occurs when clinical manifestations of pulmonary or extrapulmonary tuberculosis become apparent by chest radiography or clinical findings. The word tuberculosis usually refers to disease. Most untreated infected persons never develop disease. The time between the onset of tuberculosis infection and the beginning of disease may be several weeks or many years. In adults, usually a clear distinction between infection and disease exists. However, among children in whom disease usually develops as an immediate complication of the primary infection, the two stages are less distinct. An infected child with radiographic or clinical manifestations consistent with tuberculosis is considered to have disease, even if no symptoms are present.

ETIOLOGY

Tubercle bacilli are nonmotile, nonspore-forming, pleomorphic, weakly gram-positive, curved rods approximately 2 to 4 μm long. The cell wall of mycobacteria contains 20% to 60% lipids bound to proteins and carbohydrates. This lipid-rich cell wall accounts for hydrophobic properties and resistance to the bactericidal actions of antibody and complement.

Identification of mycobacteria is based on their growth characteristics, staining properties, and biochemical or metabolic characteristics. In most modern mycobacteriology laboratories, the identification of *M. tuberculosis* is established by a DNA probe of colonies on a plate or organisms in broth.

EPIDEMIOLOGY

The incidence of tuberculosis in the United States declined 5% to 6% each year for several decades until 1985, when it leveled off. From 1986 to 1992, the reported number of cases increased to 26,000 per year. From 1992 to 1997, case numbers again declined to approximately 19,000 in 1997. From 1985 through 1997, more than 80,000 additional cases of tuberculosis were reported in the United States than would have been expected if the previous decline had continued. Three major factors are often cited to explain the increase during this period. One cause is the human immunodeficiency virus (HIV) epidemic because coinfection with HIV infection is the greatest risk factor known for the development of tuberculosis disease in an adult infected with the tubercle bacillus. An increasingly important factor is the increase in the number of immigrants to the United States from countries with a high prevalence of tuberculosis. Finally, the general decline in public health services and access to medical care in parts of the United States has hindered rapid diagnosis, treatment, and completion of contact investigations.

In the early twentieth century, the risk of being exposed to an adult with infectious tuberculosis was higher and more uniform across the entire population than it is currently. Tuberculosis has retreated into fairly well-defined groups of high-risk persons. This group includes homeless persons, residents of correctional institutions, and users of IV drugs. Although tuberculosis case rates in the United States have generally increased with patient age, a trend toward an increased case rate in young adults, especially among urban minority populations, has occurred. Case rates are always lowest among children 5 to 14 years of age; most childhood tuberculosis occurs among children younger than 5 years.

Children with tuberculosis represent 5% to 6% of the total annual number of cases. Since 1976, the decline in incidence of childhood tuberculosis had been slower than that for older populations. The pediatric tuberculosis case rate reflects the effect of the disease on childhood health and serves as a public health marker of ongoing tuberculosis transmission within a community. As long as the disease persists in adults, susceptible children will become infected. The epidemiology of childhood tuberculosis in the United States has remained fairly constant. Approximately 60% of childhood cases occur in children younger than 5 years.

M. tuberculosis is transmitted from person to person, usually by droplets of mucus that become airborne when an infected person coughs, sneezes, laughs, or sings. Occasionally, transmission occurs by direct contact with infected discharges (e.g., urine or purulent sinus tract drainage) or with a contaminated fomite. Adults with cavitary disease harbor the greatest number of tubercle bacilli for the longest time. Most adults are no longer infectious after several days to 2 weeks of therapy, but this period may increase for patients with advanced cavitary disease who continue to cough. Children with pulmonary tuberculosis rarely infect other children. Tubercle bacilli are sparse in the endobronchial secretions of children who usually do not cough with sufficient force to transmit infection.

PATHOGENESIS

The primary (Ghon) complex of tuberculosis consists of disease at the portal of entry and the regional lymph nodes that drain the area of the primary focus. The primary site of infection is the lung in more than 95% of cases. In the alveoli or alveolar ducts, bacilli multiply and an inflammatory exudate is present. While the primary complex is developing, tubercle bacilli spread by the bloodstream and lymphatics to many parts of the body. This dissemination can involve large numbers of bacilli leading to miliary tuberculosis or, more commonly, small numbers of bacilli that leave tuberculous foci scattered in various tissues. After 4 to 8 weeks, cell-mediated immunity usually develops. At this time, the primary complex usually heals to the extent that it is not visible on chest radiography, and further dissemination is arrested. These events usually produce no signs or symptoms.

The parenchymal portion of the primary complex often heals completely after undergoing caseating necrosis and encapsulation. The nodal component has a decreased tendency to heal completely. Even after calcification, viable tubercle bacilli may persist for many years in the node or in distant sites. Although children usually develop tuberculosis disease during the primary infection, most cases in adults are caused by endogenous regrowth of latent bacilli (i.e., adult or postprimary tuberculosis). The most common form of postprimary tuberculosis affects the apical region of the lung.

Without specific therapy, tuberculosis disease develops in 5% to 10% of immunologically normal adults with tuberculosis infection at some time during their lives. The risk for children is greater; as many as 40% of children younger than 1 year with untreated tuberculosis infection develop radiographic evidence of disease, compared with 24% of children between the ages of 1 and 5 years, and 15% of children between the ages of 11 and 15 years.

A predictable timetable of tuberculosis infection and its possible complications exists. Massive lymphohematogenous spread leading to miliary or acute meningeal tuberculosis occurs approximately 3 to 6 months after the initial infection. Endobronchial tuberculosis, with segmental pulmonary changes, occurs within 9 months. Clinically important lesions of bones or joints do not appear until at least 1 year after infection, and renal lesions develop 5 to 25 years after initial infection. In general, complications in children occur within the first 5 years (especially the first year) after initial infection.

DIAGNOSIS

The diagnosis of tuberculosis disease in adults is mainly bacteriologic, but in children, it is usually epidemiologic and indirect. In the absence of a positive culture result, the strongest evidence for tuberculosis in a child is history of exposure to an adult with contagious disease. The importance of an adequate history and exposure tracings cannot be overemphasized. Less direct methods such as the tuberculin skin test and other laboratory tests, offer supportive information.

Tuberculin Skin Test

A positive tuberculin skin test result is the hallmark of tuberculosis infection. Two major techniques for tuberculin skin testing exist. The first is the multiple-puncture test, which involves the intradermal delivery of tuberculin antigen by metal prongs coated with the antigen. Most commercially available tests use PPD (purified protein derivative) as the antigen (e.g., Aplitest, Tine Test). There is great variability in amount of antigen left in the skin and reaction size. Results should be read as positive, negative, or questionable. The false-positive rates may be as high as 10% to 20%, and false-negative rates are 1% to 10%. Because of the lack of standardization in dose administration, sometimes low sensitivity and specificity, and their potential to create larger subsequent reactions after repetitive testing (i.e., booster phenomenon), the use of multiple puncture skin tests should be eliminated.

The gold standard tuberculin test is the Mantoux, an intradermal injection of 5 tuberculin units (TU) of PPD in 0.1 mL of diluent containing the stabilizing agent polysorbate 80. This test is standardized and quantitative; results are interpreted as the transverse diameter of induration at 48 to 72 hours. The Mantoux test is subject to a variety of influences related to the test procedure (Table 97-1). Approximately 10% of adults and children with culture-documented tuberculosis do not react initially

TABLE 97-1. Factors that Can Influence Mantoux Test Results

Factors related to the host
Presence of other infections (viral, bacterial, fungal)
Recent inoculation with live virus vaccine
Metabolic derangements
Malnutrition
Immunuosuppression by disease or drug treatment
Age (very old young)
Overwhelming tuberculosis disease
History of bacille Calmette-Guérin vaccination
Factors related to the environment
Prevalence of nontuberculous mycobacteria
Factors related to the testing procedure
Improper administration or interpretation
Antigen overload with simultaneous tests
Boosting exerted by previous skin tests
Loss of strength of purified protein derivative because of improper storage
Variations in commercial products

to PPD; delayed hypersensitivity often appears after appropriate treatment is started. In adults, initial anergy to tuberculin is related to a poor prognosis, but this does not appear to be true for children. A negative skin test result never rules out tuberculosis.

Recent exposure to environmental nontuberculous mycobacteria (NTM) can result in cross-sensitization and a false-positive reaction to PPD. This problem is especially common in the southeastern United States, where NTM occur in the environment, especially the soil. Cross-sensitization with NTM usually causes a reaction of less than 10 mm to a 5-TU Mantoux test, although reactions up to 15 mm can occur. This cross-sensitization tends to wane over a period of months. Prior immunization with bacille Calmette-Guérin (BCG) may also cause a significant Mantoux reaction, which is often smaller than 10 to 12 mm and usually wanes within 3 to 5 years. Because the effect of BCG on the skin test is variable and a reaction of 10 mm or more in a previously BCG-vaccinated child usually indicates infection with M. tuberculosis, the interpretation of the skin test result should be the same for a BCG-vaccinated child as it would be for a comparable, nonvaccinated child. Prior receipt of a BCG vaccine is not a contraindication to receiving a tuberculin skin test.

The important issue in interpreting the Mantoux test result is the amount of induration that should be considered as likely to indicate tuberculosis infection. The critical information is epidemiologic. Has exposure occurred? The only way to answer this question is by vigorous contact tracing in the child's environment looking for the infectious case.

False-positive and false-negative Mantoux results will always occur, no matter what amount of induration is selected. Because of the critical contribution of epidemiology to the interpretation of the skin test, the size of induration considered positive varies for different risk groups. For adults and children at the highest risk of having tuberculosis infection progress to disease—induration of 5 mm or more is classified as positive, indicating likely infection with M. tuberculosis. For other high-risk groups including all infants, and for children living with high-risk adults, induration of 10 mm or more is a positive result. The American Academy of Pediatrics (AAP) and Centers for Disease Control and Prevention (CDC) recommend that children from low-prevalence populations with no specific risk factors should not be tested routinely, but if they are tested, 15-mm or larger indurations should be considered positive.

Laboratory Tests

Routine laboratory tests rarely aid in the diagnosis of tuberculosis. Abnormalities on serum liver enzyme tests may help diagnose miliary tuberculosis. Analyses of infected body fluids demonstrating lymphocytes, elevated protein, and decreased glucose suggest tuberculosis. These fluids and sputum should be examined microscopically with acid-fast stain to detect mycobacteria.

The most important laboratory test for the diagnosis and management of tuberculosis is the mycobacteria culture. Isolation of M. tuberculosis is not essential to the diagnosis of tuberculosis in children if epidemiologic, skin test, clinical, and radiographic findings are compatible with the disease. If culture and susceptibility tests are available from the adult source case, cultures from the child add little to management. However, when the source case is unknown, especially in areas with high drug resistance, attempts should be made to isolate the organism from the child. Cultures should be obtained in any child with suspected extrapulmonary tuberculosis to confirm the diagnosis. Sputum produced by an older child or adolescent with pulmonary tuberculosis often yields M. tuberculosis. Younger children rarely produce sputum. Gastric aspirates yield the organism in 30% to 40% of patients; the yield is even greater in infants. When obtained correctly, gastric aspirates have a greater yield than do bronchial samples. Aspiration should be done early in the morning, as the child awakens, before the overnight accumulation of secretions swallowed from the respiratory tract is emptied from the stomach. The aspirates should be collected using saline-free fluid, and the pH should be neutralized if processing will be delayed for more than several hours.

Traditional culture methods require 4 to 6 weeks for isolation of the organism and another 2 to 4 weeks for susceptibility testing. Many laboratories now use DNA probes to identify and speciate mycobacteria after they have been isolated in media. The sensitivity and specificity of these probes when used on isolated organisms approaches 100%. Unfortunately, the sensitivity decreases precipitously when these probes are used directly on patient samples. The technique of nucleic acid amplification (NAA) markedly increases the sensitivity of DNA testing on patient samples.

Diagnostic Criteria

The diagnosis of tuberculosis disease in children is often based on epidemiologic, clinical, radiographic, and skin test information, rather than mycobacteriologic data. The diagnosis of tuberculosis disease is confirmed if *M. tuberculosis* is isolated from any body site or if the clinical, radiographic, or histologic findings are consistent with tuberculosis and at least two of the following criteria are met: (a) a 5-TU Mantoux test yields more than 5 mm of induration, (b) other disease entities are ruled out and the subsequent clinical course and response to therapy are consistent with tuberculosis, and (c) an adult source case with contagious tuberculosis is discovered.

CLINICAL FORMS OF TUBERCULOSIS

Endothoracic Disease

ASYMPTOMATIC PRIMARY TUBERCULOSIS

Asymptomatic, primary tuberculosis is an infection associated with tuberculin skin reactivity in the absence of clinical or significant radiographic findings. In infected older children, 80% to 95% of have clinically silent tuberculosis, but only 50% to 60%

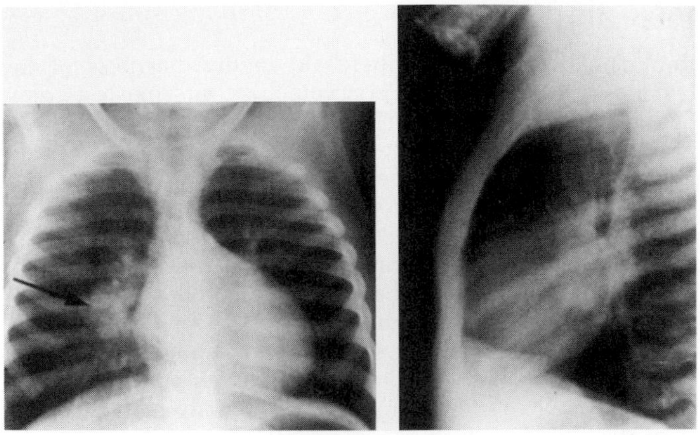

Figure 97-1. Chest radiographs of hilar adenopathy (*arrow*) caused by a primary tuberculous infection in an infant. Notice the mass lesion at the hilum, seen best in the lateral view. (Courtesy of Dr. Katharine H. K. Hsu.)

of infected infants are asymptomatic. These children are usually treated with a single antituberculosis drug. Contact tracing to determine the etiology of the infection is important.

PRIMARY PULMONARY TUBERCULOSIS

The initial pulmonary complex includes the parenchymal focus and regional lymphadenitis. Approximately 70% of primary foci are subpleural. All segments of the lung are at equal risk of being seeded. In 25% of cases, multiple primary foci are present in the lungs. The infection spreads early to regional (usually hilar or mediastinal) lymph nodes. The hallmark of primary tuberculosis in the lung is the relatively large size and importance of the adenitis compared with the relatively small size of the initial parenchymal focus.

In most cases, the parenchymal infiltrate and adenitis resolve early. In some children, especially infants, the hilar lymph nodes continue to enlarge (Fig. 97-1). Bronchial obstruction may occur as the nodes enlarge. The nodes may erode through the bronchial wall. The radiographic findings may be similar to those seen with foreign body aspiration.

Occasionally, the beginning of infection is marked by low-grade fever and mild cough. As the primary complex progresses, nonspecific symptoms such as fever, cough, weight loss, and night sweats may occur. Pulmonary signs are usually absent. Some children have localized wheezing or diminished breath sounds, which may be accompanied by tachypnea or rarely by frank respiratory distress. Most cases of tuberculous bronchial obstruction in children resolve fully. Occasionally, residual calcification of the primary focus or regional lymph nodes are present. Calcification implies that the lesion has been present for at least 6 months. Progressive primary pulmonary tuberculosis is a rare but serious complication when the primary focus enlarges steadily and develops a large caseous center. Liquefaction may result in the formation of a thin-walled primary cavity associated with large numbers of tubercle bacilli. A tension cavity may develop as a result of a valve-like mechanism allowing air to enter but not escape the cavity. The enlarging focus may slough necrotic debris into an adjacent bronchus leading to further intrapulmonary dissemination. Rupture into the pleural cavity leads to bronchopleural fistula or pyopneumothorax; rupture into the pericardium or mediastinum can also occur.

PLEURAL EFFUSION

Localized pleural effusion occurs so frequently in primary tuberculosis that it is almost a component of the primary complex. Clinically significant pleurisy with effusion occurs in 5% to 30% of young adults with tuberculosis but is infrequent in children younger than 6 years and very rare in those younger than 2 years. Pleurisy is caused by extension of a subpleural focus.

CHRONIC PULMONARY DISEASE

Chronic pulmonary tuberculosis (i.e., adult or reactivation tuberculosis) represents endogenous reinfection from a site of tuberculosis infection established previously in the body. This form of tuberculosis has always been rare in childhood, but it may occur in adolescence. Children with a healed tuberculosis infection acquired before 2 years of age rarely develop chronic pulmonary disease, which is more common in those who acquire their initial infection after 7 years of age.

CARDIAC AND PERICARDIAL TUBERCULOSIS

Although rare, the most common form of cardiac tuberculosis is pericarditis. Involvement of the myocardium may occur in miliary disease. Direct extension of tuberculosis to the myocardium from mediastinal nodes or lung parenchyma is exceedingly rare. Tuberculous endocarditis has been described only in several case reports.

LYMPHOHEMATOGENOUS SPREAD

Tubercle bacilli are disseminated to distant sites from the lymphadenitis or primary focus of the primary complex in all cases of tuberculosis infection. The clinical picture produced by the lymphohematogenous dissemination depends on the host immune response and the quantity of organisms released.

OCCULT LYMPHOHEMATOGENOUS SPREAD

Occult lymphohematogenous spread is the most common form, and it occurs in all cases of asymptomatic tuberculosis infection. This event may lead to the development of extrapulmonary tuberculosis months or years after the initial infection.

MILIARY TUBERCULOSIS

Miliary tuberculosis arises when massive numbers of tubercle bacilli are released into the bloodstream resulting in simultaneous disease in two or more organs. It is usually an early complication of primary infection occurring within 2 to 6 months after the initial infection. This disease is most common in infants and young children.

The pathologic picture of miliary tuberculosis is caused by tubercle bacilli entering the bloodstream from a caseous focus that erodes through a blood vessel. The organisms lodge in small capillaries in various sites and form tubercles of relatively uniform size ranging from 2 mm to several centimeters. Different tissues have different susceptibilities to infection. Lesions are larger and more numerous in the lungs, spleen, liver, and bone marrow than in other tissues. Most often, the clinical onset is insidious with weight loss, anorexia, malaise, and low-grade fever. Early in the course, few abnormal physical signs are present. Hepatosplenomegaly and generalized lymphadenopathy then develop in approximately one-half of patients. Within 3 to 4 weeks after symptom onset, the lung fields usually become filled with tubercles. The child may develop respiratory distress and diffuse rales or wheezing. Pneumothorax, pneumomediastinum, and pleural effusion can also complicate miliary tuberculosis. Signs or symptoms of meningitis or peritonitis are found in 20% to 30% of these patients. These patients may present with a fever of unknown origin. As many as 30% of these patients have a negative tuberculin skin test result, especially late in the course of disease. Early sputum cultures have a low sensitivity; the yield from gastric aspirates or bronchial washings is greater. Biopsy of the liver or bone marrow may facilitate a more rapid diagnosis. As always, the most important clue may be a history of a recent exposure to an adult with contagious tuberculosis.

Extrathoracic Disease

CENTRAL NERVOUS SYSTEM TUBERCULOSIS

Several different forms of CNS tuberculosis, including meningitis, tuberculoma, and brain abscess, exist.

Tuberculous meningitis complicates 1 in 300 untreated tuberculosis infections in children. This disease is almost unheard of in infants younger than 4 months because it takes at least that long for the inciting pathologic events to develop. It is most common in children younger than 4 years and usually occurs within 3 to 6 months of the initial infection.

The pathogenesis of CNS tuberculosis results from formation of a metastatic caseous lesion in the cerebral cortex or meninges during the occult lymphohematogenous dissemination of the initial infection. This lesion (Rich focus) may increase in size and discharge tubercle bacilli into the subarachnoid space. A thick, gelatinous exudate infiltrates the cortical or meningeal blood vessels producing inflammation, obstruction, or infarction. The brainstem is usually the site of greatest involvement. Cranial nerve findings may be seen. The basal cisterns usually become obstructed leading to hydrocephalus.

The most important aid to the correct diagnosis is a history of recent contact with an adult who has active tuberculosis. The tuberculin skin test result is negative in as many as 50% of patients, especially infants and young children. The CSF leukocyte count ranges from 10 to 500 cells per microliter, lymphocytes often predominate. The glucose level is typically less than 40 mg/dL and the protein level is elevated. The lumbar CSF protein is not indicative of the ventricular CSF protein, which is often normal or only slightly elevated. Acid-fast stains of spun CSF are more likely positive if 5 to 10 ml of CSF is sampled. Culture of other sites such as gastric aspirates or urine, may help confirm the diagnosis.

SKELETAL TUBERCULOSIS

Skeletal tuberculosis results from lymphohematogenous dissemination of tubercle bacilli early in the course of the initial infection. Occasionally, bone infection is initiated by direct extension from a contiguous lymph node or by extension from a neighboring infected bone. Involvement of bone complicates 1% to 2% of untreated infections in childhood, usually occurring within 12 to 24 months of formation of the primary complex.

The most commonly affected bones are the vertebrae, causing tuberculosis of the spine (i.e., Pott disease). Usually, the body of the vertebra is affected, causing destruction and collapse. Paraspinal abscess, psoas abscess, or retropharyngeal abscess may develop from the bone lesion.

RENAL TUBERCULOSIS

Renal tuberculosis does not develop for several years after the initial infection. Tubercle bacilli reach the kidney during lymphohematogenous dissemination. Small caseous tubercles develop in the renal parenchyma and discharge tubercle bacilli into the tubules. Usually no symptoms are present early in the course of renal tuberculosis. The development of "sterile" pyuria, hematuria, dysuria, or vague flank pain first suggests the infection. Superinfection with other bacteria may cause delay in diagnosing the underlying tuberculosis. The urine culture result is almost always positive for M. tuberculosis, although cultures may be positive intermittently. Microscopical examination of sediment from an adequately large early morning urine specimen frequently reveals acid-fast bacilli. The tuberculin skin test result should be positive. Surgical intervention is rarely required for diagnosis or treatment if adequate chemotherapy is given.

SUPERFICIAL LYMPH NODE TUBERCULOSIS

Tuberculosis of the superficial lymph nodes (i.e., scrofula) complicates 3% to 6% of infections. In most cases, it is an early manifestation of lymphohematogenous dissemination occurring within 6 to 9 months of the primary infection.

In the early stage of infection, the lymph nodes are firm, discrete, and nontender. Scrofula in the neck is usually unilateral, but because of the drainage patterns of lymphatics from the chest, it may be bilateral. Other than low-grade fever, systemic signs and symptoms are usually absent. The lymph nodes may enlarge gradually but, occasionally, rapid enlargement associated with high fever, tenderness, and fluctuation occurs. The initial presentation of a fluctuant mass with overlying cellulitis or discoloration of the skin is usually more suggestive of bacterial adenitis.

Many other conditions, including infection caused by NTM, cat-scratch disease, tularemia, brucellosis, malignant tumor, and pyogenic infection, can be confused with tuberculous adenitis. The most frequent problem in diagnosis is differentiating infection caused by M. tuberculosis from NTM adenitis in geographic areas where NTM are common. Evidence of thoracic lymph node or pulmonary involvement on chest radiography is more common in tuberculosis but can occur with NTM disease. The induration caused by a 5-TU PPD Mantoux test is usually greater than 15 mm with M. tuberculosis infection and less than 10 mm with NTM disease; reactions of 10 to 15 mm can be caused by either infection. The most important part of an evaluation is determining whether exposure to a tuberculous adult has occurred. In many cases, the correct diagnosis can be established only by biopsy and culture of tissue from the involved lymph node.

If left untreated, tuberculous adenitis causes caseation and necrosis of the lymph node. The capsule breaks down leading to the spread of infection to adjacent lymph nodes. The skin overlying this mass of lymph nodes becomes thin, shiny, and erythematous. Rupture through the skin may result in formation of a sinus tract. Lymphadenitis caused by M. tuberculosis responds well to antituberculosis chemotherapy, although the lymph nodes may not return to normal size for months or years. Surgical removal is not adequate therapy because the lymph node disease is but one part of a systemic infection.

PERINATAL TUBERCULOSIS

True congenital tuberculosis caused by the spread of infection through the placenta or amniotic fluid can occur but is rare. This hematogenous "inoculation" of the fetus leads to miliary tuberculosis. The major site of disease is the liver. Pulmonary disease, generalized lymphadenopathy, and meningitis occur in approximately 50% of these patients. The exact clinical manifestations depend on the infecting "dose" of bacilli and the time of transmission. Symptoms most commonly begin around the second week of life and include lethargy, decreased feeding, nasal discharge, jaundice, respiratory distress, and abdominal distention from hepatosplenomegaly. Congenital tuberculosis can also be caused by aspiration of amniotic fluid infected with M. tuberculosis from a mother with tuberculous endometritis.

Perinatal tuberculosis caused by inhalation of tubercle bacilli expelled by an adult who handles the infant is much more common than true congenital tuberculosis. The newborn infant should be separated from any adult known or thought to have pulmonary tuberculosis until the disease is no longer contagious. If significant exposure has occurred or is likely to occur, the infant should have baseline chest radiography and then be started on isoniazid for 3 months after the last possible exposure. A Mantoux tuberculin test is then performed. If the test result is positive, isoniazid is continued as in standard therapy of tuberculosis infection; if the test result is negative, the drug is discontinued.

TREATMENT

Most cases of tuberculosis can be cured. The limiting factor is often human behavior: poor adherence to treatment leading to relapse and the emergence of drug resistance.

Chemotherapeutic Agents

A variety of chemotherapeutic agents are available for treating patients with tuberculosis (Table 97-2). The first-line drugs, which include isoniazid, rifampin, pyrazinamide, ethambutol, and streptomycin, are most often used for initial treatment. The second-line drugs, including paraaminosalicylic acid, ethionamide, capreomycin, kanamycin, fluoroquinolones (ciprofloxacin and ofloxacin), and cycloserine, are used when drug resistance or intolerance is encountered. First-line drugs are described below. Doses are found in Table 97-2.

Isoniazid

Treatment with isoniazid provides a high degree of antituberculous activity that persists in the plasma and sputum for many hours. Concentrations in the CSF, even in the absence of inflammation, are 50% to 100% of plasma concentrations.

Most children tolerate isoniazid so well that only clinical monitoring is necessary. Transient elevation of hepatic enzymes has been documented in 10% of adult patients with overt clinical hepatitis occurring in only 1%. Both problems are rare in children, but they are slightly more common in adolescents. Routine serum liver enzyme testing is unnecessary for children taking isoniazid unless they have a history of liver disease, are taking other hepatotoxic drugs (especially anticonvulsants), or develop clinical signs and symptoms of toxicity.

Peripheral neuritis, caused by the competitive inhibition of pyridoxine metabolism, can occur when isoniazid is given to patients with poor nutrition. Although this problem is fairly common in adults, children's pyridoxine levels are depressed, but clinical manifestations are rare. Children with balanced diets do not need pyridoxine supplementation. However, breast-fed infants receiving isoniazid should always receive supplementation because of the low pyridoxine concentrations in breast milk.

Rifampin

Rifampin is absorbed readily from the gastrointestinal tract. Rifampin diffuses readily into all body tissues and fluids achieving CSF concentrations of 60% to 90% of plasma levels. Its metabolism and excretion occur in the liver and kidneys, respectively.

Rifampin is usually well tolerated. Hepatic toxicity is rare (less than 1%) unless rifampin is used in conjunction with isoniazid. Gastrointestinal irritation, leukopenia, thrombocytopenia, and a peculiar influenza-like syndrome that is immunologically mediated may occur. Rifampin can render oral contraceptives inactive and may interact adversely with several other drugs including quinidine, sodium warfarin, and corticosteroids. The preparation is an orange-red dye that stains all body fluids including urine, tears, sweat, and feces. It may permanently stain contact lenses.

Pyrazinamide

First developed in 1949, pyrazinamide has been rediscovered as an important antituberculosis drug. Pyrazinamide is an unusual drug that is not bactericidal *in vitro* but does contribute to killing M. tuberculosis *in vivo*. It is active only at a pH of approximately 5.5, which is the pH inside macrophages. It is metabolized by the liver, and hepatotoxicity may occur.

TABLE 97-2. Antituberculosis Drugs Used in Children

Drug	Dose (kg/d)	Route of administration	Drug toxicity	Available preparations
Isoniazid	5–15 mg	Oral, intravenous, intramuscular	Hepatotoxicity; peripheral neuritis; rash	100- and 300-mg scored tablets; 10 mg/mL suspension
Rifampin	10–20 mg	Oral	Hepatotoxicity; staining of contact lenses; flulike syndrome	150- and 300-mg capsules
Pyrazinamide	20–40 mg	Oral	Hepatotoxicity; arthritis or arthralgias; gout	500-mg scored tablets
Streptomycin	20 mg up to 1 g total	Intramuscular	Eighth nerve damage (vestibular loss more common than hearing loss)	1-g vials
Ethambutol	15–25 mg	Oral	Optic neuritis; red-green color blindness	100- and 400-mg scored tablets
Ethionamide	10–20 mg	Oral	Gastric irritation; teratogenic	250-mg tablets
Capreomycin	10–15 mg	Intramuscular	Nephrotoxicity; eighth nerve damage (hearing loss more common than vestibular loss)	1-g vials
Kanamycin	15–30 mg	Intramuscular	Nephrotoxicity; eighth nerve damage (hearing loss more common than vestibular loss)	100-mg, 500-mg, and 1-g vials
Cycloserine	10–20 mg up to 1 g total	Oral	Neurologic and psychiatric	250-mg capsules
Paraamino-salicylic acid	250–300 mg	Oral	Severe gastric irritation	Packets (three per day is the adult dose)

Streptomycin

Streptomycin (given only intramuscularly) penetrates inflamed meninges well, but CSF levels are low in the absence of inflammation. The principal adverse effect is eighth nerve toxicity. Auditory acuity should be monitored if streptomycin is used for more than a few weeks.

Ethambutol

Ethambutol can cause optic neuritis or red-green color blindness, but these toxicities are extremely rare in children. Ethambutol is not used routinely in small children, because it is difficult to monitor their visual activity and color perception, but it should be used in cases of drug-resistant tuberculosis or when the risk of resistance is high.

Rationale for Multidrug Therapy

The traditional approach to antituberculosis chemotherapy is combined use of a potent bactericidal drug, usually isoniazid, with a second drug given to prevent the emergence of resistance to isoniazid. Some drugs such as pyrazinamide and streptomycin, can kill *M. tuberculosis* but are not as effective in preventing emergence of resistance to other drugs. Rifampin, isoniazid, ethambutol, and paraaminosalicylic acid effectively prevent the development of resistance to other agents. This approach required 12 to 24 months of treatment to produce a bacteriologic cure.

Short-Course Therapy

Treating patients for the shortest possible period is important for several reasons. Expense and resource utilization is decreased markedly compared with longer therapy, and patients are exposed to potentially toxic drugs for less time. Numerous short-course therapy trials have been conducted on adults with drug-susceptible pulmonary tuberculosis. Nine months of treatment with isoniazid and rifampin cures 98% of cases. Therapy with isoniazid and rifampin lasting less than 9 months has led to unacceptably high relapse rates (10%) in adults. Shorter durations can be successful if more than two drugs are used initially. For some patients, it is important that intermittent therapy (such as twice weekly dosing) be under direct observation (directly observed therapy).

Other intensive, short-course antituberculosis therapy has proven to be highly effective for children with drug-susceptible pulmonary tuberculosis. The reader is directed to the latest edition of the Report of the Committee of Infectious Diseases (Red Book®) from the AAP.

Drug Resistance

Primary resistance occurs when a person is infected with an organism that is already resistant to a drug. Secondary resistance occurs when drug-resistant organisms emerge as a dominant population during therapy. Poor patient adherence or improper administration of medications by the physician lead to secondary resistance.

Patterns of drug resistance among children mirror those found in adults in a given population. Certain epidemiologic factors such as immigration from a country with a high resistance rate or history of prior treatment for tuberculosis, correlate with drug resistance in adult patients and their contacts. When drug resistance is suspected, initial therapy must include at least three or four drugs. Subsequent therapy must be tailored to the resistance pattern.

Corticosteroids

Although data on their efficacy are relatively sparse, corticosteroids have found a place in the treatment of some forms of tuberculosis. However, they should never be used unless effective antituberculosis drugs are given simultaneously. Corticosteroids may be of benefit if the host inflammatory reaction is contributing to tissue damage or impairment of function. Convincing evidence suggests that corticosteroids aid patients with tuberculous meningitis and increased intracranial pressure caused by brainstem inflammation and resultant hydrocephalus.

PREVENTION

Bacille Calmette-Guérin Vaccination

BCG was derived from a strain of M. bovis that was attenuated through years of serial passage in culture. BCG vaccine activates host cell-mediated immunity to mycobacterial antigens in an attempt to prevent infection or progression to disease if a subsequent infection with M. tuberculosis occurs.

The efficacy of the BCG vaccines in preventing subsequent tuberculosis disease in children has ranged from 0% to 80% in various studies. BCG is given to newborns in some countries, to 1-year-old children in others, and to adolescents in still others. The most important and consistent effect of the BCG vaccines is to limit significantly the development of serious disseminated tuberculosis (e.g., miliary disease, meningitis) in young children. Vaccinated children who subsequently develop tuberculosis tend to have localized thoracic disease.

Adverse reactions to BCG are uncommon in immunocompetent children. Localized ulceration, adenitis, and osteomyelitis have been reported. Disseminated infection and death have been reported only in children with severe immunodeficiencies.

The BCG vaccine is rarely used in the United States. BCG can produce transient hypersensitivity to tuberculin and a positive Mantoux reaction (usually less than 12 mm) that may persist for as long as 5 years. Because a skin test reaction caused by BCG cannot be differentiated from one caused by infection with M. tuberculosis, the safest course is to attribute any significant reaction to tuberculosis infection, regardless of the BCG status of the patient.

Treatment of Latent Tuberculosis Infection (LTBI)

The treatment of asymptomatic, tuberculin-positive patients to prevent development of tuberculosis disease is an established practice in the United States. The widespread use of the term chemoprophylaxis is unfortunate, because it is actually treatment of a subclinical infection. Therapy with isoniazid does not alter the tuberculin reaction in most children infected with M. tuberculosis, but extensive clinical trials have demonstrated that 1 year of daily isoniazid therapy prevents the development of active tuberculosis for at least 30 years.

Isoniazid is indicated for children with a positive tuberculin test result but no clinical or radiographic evidence of disease, children with a negative tuberculin test result who have had known recent exposure to an adult with contagious tuberculosis, and persons of any age who show recent conversion (from negative to positive) of the tuberculin skin test after exposure to a contagious case. For established infection in children, isoniazid is given for 9 months. Daily or twice-weekly directly observed therapy is acceptable.

C
Viral Infections

CHAPTER 98
Adenoviruses

Adapted from James D. Cherry

Adenoviruses cause a diverse array of diseases in children, most commonly respiratory and gastrointestinal illnesses. Certain clinical manifestations of adenovirus infections are distinctive, although most illnesses are difficult to differentiate from those caused by other viral and bacterial pathogens.

ETIOLOGY

Adenoviruses are DNA viruses; 49 types are known to infect humans. Six subgroups have been defined. Clinical specimens from infected tissues produce a characteristic cytopathic effect in 1 day to 4 weeks.

EPIDEMIOLOGY

Adenoviral infections occur throughout the world. In temperate climates, sporadic disease occurs year round; epidemic disease commonly occurs in winter, spring, and early summer. Seasonal variation with adenoviral gastroenteritis has not been described.

Transplacental antibody appears to be protective in early infancy. However, when adenoviral infection occurs in the neonate, severe and rarely fatal pulmonary or multiorgan system diseases may occur. Adenoviral infections in children are commonly caused by types 1, 2, 3, and 5. Types 6 and 7 occur slightly less frequently. Incidence of adenoviral infection peaks between ages 6 months and 5 years. An increased susceptibility to adenoviruses is reported in neonates and small infants, in immunocompromised patients, and occasionally in male subjects.

Transmission of adenoviruses occurs by small droplets or the fecal-oral route and is facilitated by closed environments. Contaminated swimming pool water has been implicated in the spread of pharyngoconjunctival fever. The incubation period of adenoviruses is between 3 and 7 days. Virus may be shed from the respiratory tract up to 2 days before and 5 days after clinical symptoms develop. Virus may be found in the stool for several months. Adenoviruses are commonly isolated from the throat, conjunctiva, and stool.

PATHOPHYSIOLOGY

Characteristics of adenoviral infections vary with infecting serotype and immune status of the host. Infection usually involves the upper respiratory tract and the conjunctivae. Spread to the lower respiratory tract may occur by progression or viremia. Rashes and multiorgan infections may also result from viremia. Swallowed virus is thought to cause gastrointestinal infection. Autopsy material from lethal infections has revealed necrotizing bronchitis, bronchiolitis and pneumonia, focal hepatic necrosis, and cerebral edema with perivascular lymphocytic infiltrates.

CLINICAL MANIFESTATIONS

Respiratory Infections

Serologic surveys indicate that 10% of respiratory infections in children are caused by adenoviruses. Rarely, adenoviruses cause common colds. Usually, respiratory infections with adenoviruses are characterized by fever and pharyngitis. Symptoms that occur with acute adenoviral pharyngitis include malaise, headache, sore throat, cough, cervical adenopathy, abdominal pain, and coryza, especially in the young. Pharyngeal exudates may be thin and spotty or thick and membranous. Laryngotracheitis, bronchitis, pneumonia and, rarely, bronchiolitis may occur concomitantly with pharyngeal disease. Illness of 5 to 7 days is common, although symptoms may persist for 2 weeks.

Pulmonary infection with adenoviruses can be severe, especially in infants, toddlers, and immunocompromised patients. Manifestations of extrapulmonary involvement including meningitis, encephalitis, hepatitis, myocarditis, nephritis, and exanthems may be present.

Pertussis-Like Syndrome

Adenoviral infections are occasionally associated with illness characterized by paroxysmal cough with associated posttussive whoop, vomiting, apnea or hypoxemia, and lymphocytosis. The illness often begins with mild coryza without fever. Convalescence occurs in usually 1 to 3 months. Studies suggest that most and probably all of these pertussis-like illnesses are Bordetella infections in which the adenovirus is a coinfecting agent.

Pharyngoconjunctival Fever

The constellation of acute fever, conjunctivitis, coryza, pharyngitis, and cervical adenitis occurring historically in summer epidemics, usually associated with inadequately chlorinated swimming pools, can be ascribed with some certainty to adenoviral infection. Both the bulbar and palpebral conjunctivae are involved. Bacterial superinfection of the conjunctiva is rare, and resolution is complete.

Epidemic Keratoconjunctivitis

Numerous adenoviruses can cause epidemics of keratoconjunctivitis (KC), commonly type 8, although type 37, Adenoviral KC, is nonseasonal, primarily affects adults (but infants and young children can be affected), and is transmitted by fomites, ophthalmic instruments and solutions, and bodies of fresh water. After 4 days to 2 weeks of incubation, a follicular conjunctivitis develops with symptoms of lacrimation, photophobia, and foreign-body sensation. Hyperemia and edema of the conjunctiva are present, and preauricular adenopathy is common. Keratitis with punctate epithelial and sometimes subepithelial lesions develops as the conjunctivitis resolves. Visual disturbances may occur and persist for several years.

Skin Manifestations

Several types of adenoviruses cause exanthematous disease, usually an erythematous maculopapular rash. Exanthems of confluent morbilliform, petechial, and Stevens-Johnson syndrome have been reported.

Genitourinary Manifestations

Hemorrhagic cystitis caused by adenovirus begins acutely with dysuria and frequency; hematuria develops within 24 hours. Suprapubic pain, fever, and upper respiratory tract symptoms may be present. Resolution occurs in several days to 2 weeks and appears to be complete. This illness is not seasonal. Boys are affected more frequently than girls.

Nephritis has been reported in cases of disseminated adenoviral infections and in rare instances with respiratory infections.

Adenoviruses have reportedly been isolated from genital lesions that clinically resemble herpes genitalis and from cervicitis occurring with pharyngoconjunctival fever. Hemolytic-uremic syndrome has been associated with adenoviral infection.

Gastrointestinal Manifestations

The adenoviral types commonly associated with respiratory illnesses may also cause vomiting and diarrhea. Adenovirus types 40 and 41, along with rotavirus, are thought to cause most gastroenteritis in infants and young children. These enteric adenoviruses are most easily identified by electron microscopy or enzyme-linked immunosorbent assay because they do not grow in commonly used tissue cultures. Watery diarrhea usually lasts 1 to 2 weeks and, in the initial days, may be associated with vomiting.

Mesenteric lymphadenitis with abdominal pain, fever, and other symptoms suggestive of appendicitis can be seen with adenoviral infections. Adenoviruses have been isolated from intraoperative specimens of mesenteric lymph nodes and the appendix. Acute and chronic adenoviral appendicitis occurs. Hepatitis has been reported with adenoviral infection in infants, young children, and immunocompromised patients.

Neurologic Manifestations

Although uncommon, both meningitis and encephalitis may be the major manifestations of adenoviral infections. Alternatively, neurologic illness may be associated with marked disease at other body sites.

Immunocompromised Host

Severe disseminated disease occurs and includes fulminant disease with multiorgan involvement, notably severe necrotizing pneumonia and hepatitis with disseminated intravascular coagulation.

Congenital and Neonatal Infections

Congenital and neonatal adenoviral infections may be severe with multiple organ involvement. Illnesses suggest early-onset sepsis with hepatomegaly, progressive pneumonia, hepatitis, and thrombocytopenia.

DIAGNOSIS

Differential diagnosis for adenoviral illnesses differs with various clinical manifestations. Pharyngoconjunctival fever and keratoconjunctivitis are often recognized as adenoviral infections based on clinical findings because of their characteristic symptom complex and epidemic nature. The features of Adenoviral pharyngitis are less specific. Adenoviral pneumonia may be clinically difficult to distinguish from illness caused by other viral and bacterial pathogens. Because of the occurrence of fever, lymphadenopathy, and exanthem and enanthem, adenoviral infections are frequently confused with Kawasaki disease.

Specific diagnosis is commonly achieved by tissue culture methods, specific antigen detection, or seroconversion. Respiratory adenoviruses can be isolated in most clinical laboratories. Specimens for culture should be obtained from the affected conjunctiva or throat by vigorous swabbing with cotton or Dacron, or respiratory secretions, urine, or tissue may be submitted. Rapid diagnostic tests (indirect fluorescent antibody test, enzyme-linked immunosorbent assay, DNA probes, radioimmunoassay) are available. In general, their sensitivity is relatively low compared with culture, but specificity is high.

The serologic diagnosis of adenoviral infection is achieved by demonstrating an increase in complement-fixing antibody to the adenovirus-type–common hexon antigen or the demonstration of specific IgM serum antibody in a single serum by enzyme-linked immunosorbent assay.

TREATMENT

No treatment beyond supportive care exists for adenoviral infections. Corticosteroids should be avoided, and immunosuppressive regimens should be reduced or suspended. Depending on clinical findings, some ophthalmologists treat keratoconjunctivitis with topical steroids. Experimental treatment of severe adenoviral infections has included administration of immunoglobulins with high titers against the specific adenovirus and intravenously administered ribavirin.

PREVENTION

Although there is no universal immunization directed against adenovirus infections, live attenuated viruses in enteric-coated capsules are effective and are used to immunize military recruits against adenovirus types 4 and 7. Subsequent asymptomatic intestinal infection protects against respiratory disease in military subjects. Trials of these vaccines in children show similar efficacy.

CHAPTER 99

Acquired Cytomegaloviral Infections

Adapted from Stuart P. Adler

CMV, a member of the herpes family of viruses is ubiquitous in the human population. CMV usually causes little or no disease, but it may induce illness as a primary infection, reactivation infection in a immunocompromised host, or a secondary infection after reinfection with a second viral strain. CMV is excreted in nearly all body fluids including urine, saliva, and semen. Disease associated with CMV infection occurs most often when the immune system is compromised because of immaturity, immunocompromised host (HIV) or because of iatrogenic causes (as occurs in transplant patients).

Only a single serotype of CMV is known (i.e., antibodies directed against one viral isolate cross-react with almost all other isolates). Genetically, however, thousands of different strains probably exist. Each unrelated isolate of CMV differs genotypically from all other epidemiologically unrelated isolates. These genotypic differences have been important epidemiologic tools in tracking the virus as it is transmitted from one individual to another.

EPIDEMIOLOGY AND TRANSMISSION

In the United States, approximately 1% to 2% of the population acquires a CMV infection each year and, thus, by age 70 years, nearly all individuals become infected with CMV. In many areas of the world, nearly 100% of the population is infected with CMV by age 2 years. Between 1% and 2% of all newborns worldwide are infected with CMV at birth, a minority of total CMV infections. Newborns can be infected due to primary maternal infection or reactivation infection of latent CMV in mothers. If a woman's first CMV infection occurs during pregnancy, the CMV transmission rate from mother to fetus is approximately 50%; but for women initially infected with CMV before pregnancy, the transmission rate to the fetus is only 1% to 3%. Congenital CMV infection is covered in Chapter 29.

Postnatal Transmission

CMV is acquired postnatally from two major sources. One source is cervical and vaginal secretions of a mother who is excreting CMV. Perinatal acquisition of CMV via this mode by full-term healthy newborns causes no apparent disease. CMV transmission from mother to infant also occurs via breast milk. Between 25% and 50% of seropositive women who breast-feed transmit CMV to their infants. Infants acquiring CMV via breast milk also exhibit no apparent disease.

Peer-to-Peer Transmission

Child-to-child transmission and intrafamilial transmission of CMV occurs. Of preschool children who attend large group day care, between 10% and 70% acquire a CMV infection from other children in the same group. These children, especially those younger than 2 years, in turn transmit the virus to their caretakers including parents and day-care workers. Infection rates for previously uninfected day-care workers are between 10% and 20% per year, compared with an annual infection rate of approximately 2% for the general population.

CMV transmission by young children is facilitated by the prolonged duration of viral excretion in both saliva and urine. For children younger than 2 years who acquire a CMV infection postnatally, CMV is excreted for an average of 18 months (range, 6–40 months). In contrast, for older children and adults who acquire a primary CMV infection, viral excretion in urine and saliva usually occurs for only a few days to several weeks.

Due to viral shedding in semen and vaginal secretions, CMV transmission occurs via sexual activity. CMV infections are associated with increased sexual activity among adolescents and those attending clinics for sexually transmitted diseases.

Nosocomial Transmission

Nosocomial transmission of CMV within the hospital occurs infrequently and CMV transmission from infected patients to hospital personnel has not been observed. Patient-to-patient transmission is rare. Thus, CMV-seronegative women caring for young children who may be excreting CMV can be reassured that little or no risk exists of acquiring CMV from patients.

Transfusion Transmission

CMV may be transmitted by transfusion of whole blood. CMV is located in the white cell fraction. For immunocompromised patients requiring transfusion, the risk of CMV acquisition from a blood donor is eliminated either by selecting donors who are seronegative for CMV or using blood products with the white cells removed.

CYTOMEGALOVIRUS INFECTIONS IN THE IMMUNOCOMPETENT HOST

Although most CMV infections are totally inapparent, disease manifestations, when present, may be associated with an infectious mononucleosis-like syndrome. Mild flu-like symptoms with low-grade fever and malaise, or lymphadenopathy, hepatosplenomegaly, atypical lymphocytosis, pharyngitis and, occasionally, a rash may occur.

Symptomatic adults or children with acquired CMV infections experience resolution of symptoms over several weeks or days without sequelae. Adults with acquired CMV infections are more likely to have disease manifestations and especially infectious mononucleosis-like syndrome. Both this syndrome and a variety of unusual manifestations associated with CMV infections are relatively rare occurring in less than 1% of infected individuals.

DISEASE IN THE IMMUNOCOMPROMISED HOST

CMV infections are a frequent cause of morbidity and mortality in immunocompromised patients. A compromised immune system may produce CMV disease in any organ or tissue system.

Patients who have had organ transplants, malignancy, or those patients with immunodeficiency are at risk. Symptoms include fever, lymphadenopathy, hepatitis, pneumonia, or gastrointestinal infections with either gastritis or colitis. Arthritis, encephalopathy and retinitis may be present.

Immunosuppression leads to the reactivation of latent virus. Among solid organ transplant recipients, latent CMV reactivates from the seropositive donor organ more than 90% of the time. CMV-seronegative patients who have received an organ from a CMV-seropositive donor are at highest risk for CMV disease. Depending on the immunosuppressive therapy used to prevent graft rejection, seropositive recipients of seronegative organs may also reactivate latent CMV after transplantation and develop CMV disease. Among bone marrow transplant recipients, CMV always reactivates posttransplantation if either the donor or recipient was seropositive, and reactivation is often accompanied by severe CMV disease, especially pneumonitis. HIV-infected patients have particular difficulties with CMV pneumonia, retinitis, gastrointestinal disease and, occasionally, neuropathy and encephalitis.

Among transplant recipients, CMV infections may enhance organ rejection and graft-versus-host disease. CMV enhances both cytoplasmic and surface expression of HLA class 1 antigens *in vitro* and also induces many classes of autoantibodies. However, whether CMV infection is central in triggering rejection or is simply activated after immune suppression or treatment for rejection is unknown.

DIAGNOSIS

After a primary CMV infection, immunocompetent individuals make IgG antibodies to CMV. These antibodies are usually detected 2 to 4 weeks after a primary CMV infection and increase to levels that are generally sustained for life. A primary infection can also be identified among immunocompetent individuals by detecting IgM in the serum. IgM antibodies are not specific for primary infection because the antibodies may also occur after reactivation of CMV. However, when this reactivation occurs, patients rarely have disease.

Culture Methods

The diagnosis of CMV can be supported but not confirmed by detecting the virus in secretions, particularly in urine or saliva. Viral culture in human fibroblasts in tissue culture is the traditional method, and it is easy to perform, but often time consuming, requiring 2 to 4 weeks to detect traditional cytopathic effects in tissue culture. A more rapid culture method, called the shell vial assay, is based on the detection of a protein made in the early stages of CMV infection. This test allows the detection of CMV in body fluids as rapidly as 48 hours after obtaining specimens. Hence, in an immunocompetent patient with a suspected CMV infection, one should use serologic techniques for detecting both IgG and IgM antibodies, as well as virologic techniques for detecting CMV in urine, saliva, or other fluids. IgG should be absent or at low levels early in the course of illness because of primary infection and should increase during the ensuing 2 to 4 weeks.

Among immunocompromised patients, the diagnosis of CMV disease, as opposed to CMV infection, is much more difficult to establish. Seropositive immunocompromised patients often reactivate CMV after immunosuppression. Thus, the detection of antibodies of CMV in serum or the detection of virus in urine, saliva, or even in blood is sufficient to diagnose a CMV infection but not to diagnose *disease* caused by CMV. The detection of CMV antigenemia in the plasma of patients, particularly those who have received organ transplants, has a good association with CMV disease.

The diagnosis of CMV disease in immunocompromised patients requires two factors. First, all other possible causes of inflammation or disease must be eliminated. Second, CMV must be detected in a biopsy specimen. The presence of CMV in inflamed tissues is suggested by classic intranuclear inclusions. These cells are called owl-eye cells and indicate high levels of virus in the infected tissue. CMV can also be detected by in situ nucleic acid hybridization or by the polymerase chain reaction (PCR), both targeted to CMV DNA. These nucleic acid techniques are very sensitive and detect low levels of virus that, although clearly establishing tissue infection, may not always establish disease. Thus, the presence of owl-eye cells in a diseased tissue such as lung, liver, and brain without the presence of another microorganism that may be producing the patient's symptoms is usually sufficient for a diagnosis of CMV disease.

PROGNOSIS AND THERAPY

No specific therapy is required for immunocompetent persons with a resulting good prognosis. For immunocompromised patients, the outcome depends on the level and duration of immune suppression. Hence, antiviral therapy against CMV is important for immunocompromised patients. Two forms of therapy are available. One is chemotherapy using drugs that inhibit CMV DNA replication. Ganciclovir is the most commonly used drug and is structurally similar to acyclovir but with greater inhibitory activity against CMV. Ganciclovir has been used to successfully treat CMV infections in immunocompromised patients and is licensed in the United States for the treatment of severe CMV infections. Cellular enzymes phosphorylate ganciclovir to a triphosphate, and the triphosphate acts as a competitive and reversible inhibitor of viral DNA synthesis with little, if any, effect on cellular DNA replication. Ganciclovir reduces or eliminates the amount of virus excreted in urine and saliva and generally clears CMV from the blood. After ganciclovir therapy is stopped, viral excretion, viremia, or both rapidly reappear. In patients with AIDS, CMV relapses are common after ganciclovir therapy, and long-term administration of ganciclovir is often required. Oral ganciclovir is available and is used primarily to treat CMV retinitis. The common adverse effects associated with ganciclovir include mild leukopenia and neutropenia. Another drug for treating CMV retinitis in HIV-infected patients is foscarnet, which also inhibits CMV DNA synthesis, although by a different mechanism.

Another treatment for CMV infections among immunocompromised patients is immunoglobulin with high levels of IgG antibodies to CMV. Immunoglobulin is usually administered concurrently with ganciclovir and is especially important for patients who have had bone marrow or solid organ transplants.

No specific therapy is available for the treatment of congenital CMV disease, and studies investigating the use of ganciclovir in these infants are under way.

PREVENTION

A live attenuated CMV vaccine, called the Towne strain, is effective prophylactically in preventing or significantly reducing the incidence of CMV disease among seronegative patients who have received a kidney from a seropositive donor. Unfortunately, this vaccine is not commercially available. Thus, many transplant centers use a combination of passive immunization with immunoglobulin and prophylactic administration of ganciclovir to preemptively prevent CMV after organ transplantation. Work is in progress to develop other vaccines against CMV.

CHAPTER 100
Epstein–Barr Virus

Adapted from John L. Sullivan

In 1964, Anthony Epstein and Yvonne Barr isolated a new herpesvirus from Burkitt lymphoma tumor cells. This herpesvirus (the fifth to be described) was named *Epstein–Barr virus* (EBV) and, in 1968, Werner and Henle demonstrated that seroconversion to EBV occurred during the course of infectious mononucleosis (IM).

VIRUS

EBV is a double-stranded DNA virus. Infection of human B lymphocytes with EBV results in a latent infection characterized by the persistence of the viral genome. EBV is also known to infect T lymphocytes, smooth-muscle cells, and Reed-Sternberg cells in Hodgkin's disease. EBV infection of cells may result in a lytic virus-producing infection or a latent nonvirus-producing infection. In the majority of circumstances in which EBV infection is associated with malignant transformation of cells, the infection is primarily a latent infection.

EPIDEMIOLOGY

EBV is spread primarily by contact with oropharyngeal secretions. EBV has also been recovered from the genital tract suggesting a sexual mode of transmission. EBV infection may be transmitted through blood transfusions in which latently infected B lymphocytes serve as the source of infecting virus.

Seroepidemiologic studies have demonstrated a wide variation in the age at which EBV infection is established. In many areas of the developing world, EBV infection occurs in early infancy, and by 2 years of age, more than 80% of children have experienced primary EBV infection. The majority of these infections are asymptomatic. Passively acquired maternal antibody is apparently protective with the majority of primary infections occurring after 4 to 6 months of age. In some areas of the developed world, primary infection does not occur until adolescence. In the United States, approximately 10% to 15% of susceptible college students become infected each year, and the majority of these infections are associated with a mononucleosis syndrome.

PATHOGENESIS

EBV is an acute infection characterized by the immunologic control of viral replication and the induction of viral latency in the lymphoreticular system (Fig. 100-1). EBV-infected B lymphocytes disseminate throughout the lymphoid system. Persistence of EBV infection in epithelial cells and B lymphocytes has been demonstrated for the lifetime of an infected individual.

In acute EBV-induced IM, the onset of clinical symptoms (fever, sore throat, etc.) is associated with the presence of atypical lymphocytes in the peripheral blood. EBV infects and replicates primarily in the B-lymphocyte fraction of blood mononuclear cells. EBV-infected B lymphocytes account for only a minority of the atypical lymphocytes found in the peripheral blood during acute EBV-induced IM, yet nearly 20% of all B cells in the circulation may be infected with the virus.

During the acute phase of EBV-induced IM, a marked depression of cell-mediated immunity exists that can be clinically demonstrated by anergy to delayed cutaneous hypersensitivity skin tests. *In vitro*, T-lymphocyte responses to mitogens, the mixed leukocyte reaction, and responses to soluble antigens are markedly depressed. In acute EBV-induced IM, atypical lymphocytosis is the result of intense *in vivo* T-cell stimulation by EBV-infected and transformed B cells.

LABORATORY DIAGNOSIS

In the majority of young adults with IM, atypical lymphocytosis and heterophil antibodies are present. However, in young infants and children with primary EBV infection (whether or not associated with IM), heterophil antibody responses are frequently absent. Primary infection in childhood frequently requires EBV-specific serologic tests. A common approach to a patient suspected of having a primary EBV infection is to first perform a rapid slide test for heterophil antibodies; if the test result is positive, EBV-specific serology is unnecessary, but if the rapid slide test result is negative, the serum sample should be tested for EBV-specific antibodies.

Antibodies

Antibodies to three specific EBV antigens have been thoroughly studied and found to be of diagnostic importance: (a) viral capsid antigen (VCA), (b) early antigens (EAs), and (c) EBNAs. Individuals experiencing acute EBV-induced IM and the EBV-associated malignancies (Burkitt lymphoma and nasopharyngeal carcinoma) have been thoroughly studied, as well as normal controls, and certain characteristic antibody patterns have been described.

Figure 100-2 shows the characteristic antibody patterns observed in young adults experiencing EBV-induced IM. Before EBV infection, all three antibodies are absent, but during the

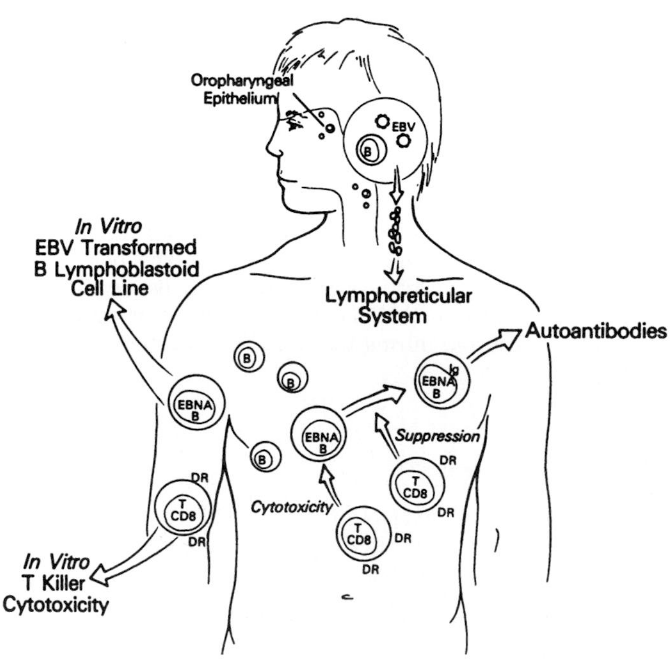

Figure 100-1. Immunopathogenesis of acute Epstein–Barr virus (*EBV*)-induced infectious mononucleosis. DR, HLA-DR antigen; EBNA, Epstein–Barr nuclear antigens.

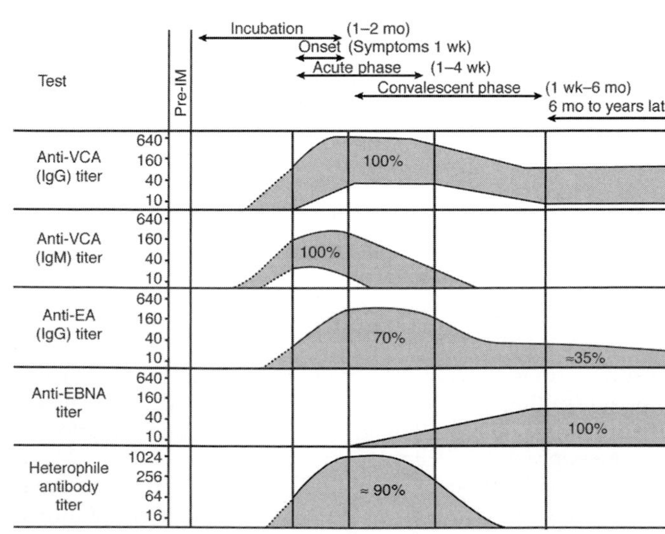

Figure 100-2. Characteristic Epstein–Barr virus-specific antibody responses observed in young adults with acute infectious mononucleosis (*IM*). EA, early antigens; EBNA, Epstein–Barr nuclear antigens; VCA, viral capsid antigen. (Adapted from Henle G, Henle L, Horowitz CA. Epstein–Barr virus-specific diagnostic tests in infectious mononucleosis. *Hum Pathol* 1974;5:551.)

acute phase of infection, high titers of IgM and IgG antibodies to VCA are seen. IgM antibodies are transient and disappear after a few months. The majority of persons develop transient IgG antibodies against EAs, and many normal persons maintain moderate (1:20–1:40) antibody titers to EAs for years after primary infection. Antibodies directed against the EBNA proteins are produced early in infection; however, detectable titers by indirect immunofluorescence are not usually found until 1 to 2 months after acute infection. Healthy persons who have had past infection with EBV show VCA-IgG antibodies. VCA-IgM responses may be seen in only 60% and EA responses in approximately 50% of young infants during acute EBV infection.

In general, acute or recent primary infection is indicated by the following: (a) the presence of VCA-specific IgM antibodies; (b) high titers of VCA-specific IgG antibodies (1:320 or greater); (c) detection of anti-EA antibodies (1:10 or greater); and (d) the absence of anti-EBNA. Convalescent serum samples should be obtained to demonstrate the disappearance of VCA-IgM and the appearance of EBNA antibodies. EBV antibody titers should not be used to make a diagnosis of chronic IM or other EBV-associated syndromes on the basis of mild to moderate elevation of VCA (1:160–1:320) or EA (1:20–1:40) antibodies because normal persons may show such titers years after uncomplicated infection. Elevated EBV titers are also seen in patients with EBV-associated malignancies and those patients with virtually any condition associated with suppression of cellular immune function [i.e., allograft recipients, patients receiving chemotherapy, patients with human immunodeficiency virus (HIV) infection]. Past infection is indicated by the presence of VCA-IgG and EBNA-IgG antibodies.

PRIMARY EPSTEIN–BARR VIRUS INFECTION IN INFANTS AND CHILDREN

Primary EBV infections in young infants and children are frequently asymptomatic. When symptoms do occur, a variety of syndromes have been observed including otitis media, diarrhea, abdominal complaints, upper respiratory infection, and IM (Fig. 100-3). These syndromes may occur without the production of heterophil antibodies. Most of the children had clinical evidence compatible with IM (significant cervical adenopathy and tonsillar pharyngitis). Complications of EBV IM occur in approximately 20% of children. Table 100-1 lists the frequency of complications noted in one series of patients.

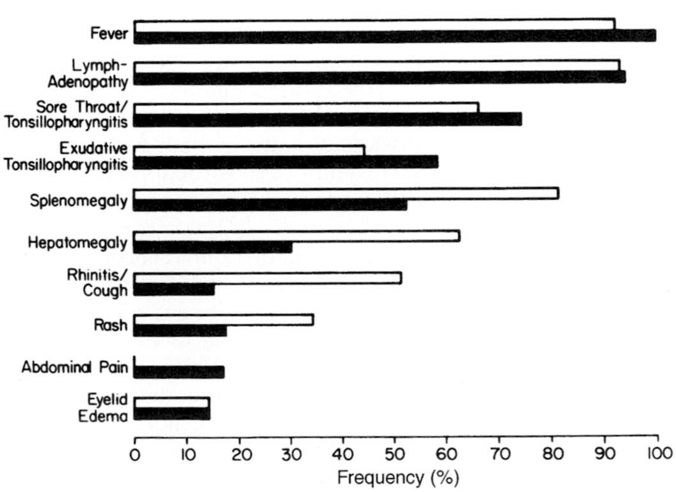

Figure 100-3. Frequency of clinical findings in two age groups: less than 4 years old (*open bars*) and 4 to 6 years old (*solid bars*). (Reprinted with permission from Sumaya CV, Ench Y. Epstein–Barr virus infectious mononucleosis in children: I. clinical and general laboratory findings. *Pediatrics* 1985;75:1003.)

TABLE 100-1. Complications Present in Childhood Epstein–Barr Virus Infectious Mononucleosis

Complication	Number of children (%)
Respiratory tract	
Pneumonia	6 (5.3)
Severe airway obstruction[a]	4 (3.5)
Neurologic	
Seizures	4 (3.5)
Meningitis/encephalitis	2 (1.8)
Peripheral facial nerve paralysis	1 (0.9)
Guillain-Barré syndrome	1 (0.9)
Hematologic	
Thrombocytopenia with hemorrhages	4 (3.5)
Hemolytic anemia	1 (0.9)
Infectious	
Bacteremia	1 (0.9)
Recurrent tonsillopharyngitis	3 (2.7)
Liver: jaundice	2 (1.8)
Renal: glomerulonephritis	1 (0.9)
Genital: orchitis	1 (0.9)
Total	31[b]

[a]Criteria consisted of nasal alar flaring suprasternal retractions, or stridor.
[b]Because four children had more than one of these complications, this total is composed of 24-different children, or 21.2% of the study group.
Reprinted with permission from Sumaya CV, Ench Y. Epstein-Barr virus infectious mononucleosis in children: I. Clinical and general laboratory findings. *Pediatrics* 1985;75:1003.

INFECTIOUS MONONUCLEOSIS IN THE ADOLESCENT

The IM syndrome appearing in adolescents is characterized by fever, anterior and posterior cervical lymphadenopathy, exudative pharyngitis, and fatigue. The syndrome is self-limited lasting an average of 2 to 3 weeks. An estimated 30% to 50% of students entering college in the United States are susceptible (seronegative) to EBV. Approximately 10% to 15% of seronegative persons become infected each year, and the majority of those infected show signs and symptoms of classic IM. Studies conducted on West Point cadets have demonstrated an association of clinically apparent IM with the likelihood of being under stress.

Individuals experiencing acute IM may develop morbilliform rashes when treated with ampicillin or penicillin during the acute phase of the disease. Hepatosplenomegaly is commonly present and may be severe but only rarely results in splenic rupture, after trauma and fulminate hepatitis secondary to periportal necrosis. One of the most common causes of hospitalization during acute IM is severe pharyngitis with concern for airway obstruction. This complication, which usually resolves in 24 to 72 hours, may be severe enough to warrant empiric treatment with intravenous corticosteroids.

X-LINKED LYMPHOPROLIFERATIVE SYNDROME

The XLP syndrome is characterized by a selective immunodeficiency to EBV manifested by severe or fatal IM and acquired immunodeficiency. Prospective studies in male subjects before

EBV infection have demonstrated normal cellular and humoral immunity. During acute EBV infection, male subjects with XLP syndrome demonstrate vigorous cytotoxic cellular responses, which predominantly involve activated cytotoxic CD8 T cells. Fatal EBV infections in male subjects with XLP syndrome usually result from extensive liver necrosis, and those who survive acute EBV infection demonstrate global cellular immune defects with deficient T-cell, B-cell, and NK-cell responses. Genetic studies have localized the XLP gene to the Xq25 region of the X chromosome. The protein encoded by the XLP gene has been identified in T lymphocytes and has been named signaling lymphocyte activation molecule-associated protein (SAP). This protein appears to play an important role in T-lymphocyte signal transduction events.

BURKITT LYMPHOMA

Burkitt lymphoma is the most common childhood malignancy in equatorial Africa and was first described in 1958 by the British surgeon Denis Burkitt. This unmistakable tumor typically presents in the jaws of young patients, and the majority of endemic cases occur in discrete geographic climates located along the malaria belt in Africa. Malaria is hypothesized to provide a chronic stimulator for proliferation of B lymphocytes, some of which carry latent EBV. In the rare instance during B-cell division that a specific reciprocal chromosomal translocation involving the c-myc locus on the long arm of chromosome 8 and one of the immunoglobulin loci on chromosome 14, 2, or 22 occurs, a Burkitt lymphoma may result. The ability of EBV to "growth transform" human B cells, along with the potential to induce malignant lymphomas in New World monkeys, makes EBV a strong candidate for contributing the remaining transforming factors in the multistep process of Burkitt lymphoma development.

More than 95% of endemic Burkitt lymphoma tumor cells contain copies of the EBV genome, whereas only 15% to 20% of sporadic (outside high-incidence areas) cases of Burkitt lymphoma contain EBV genomes. Analysis of the EBV genome terminal repeat frequency in endemic Burkitt lymphomas has demonstrated that the tumors originate in the lineage of a single EBV-infected B cell.

MALIGNANCIES AND HUMAN IMMUNODEFICIENCY VIRUS INFECTION

NonHodgkin's Lymphomas

In the setting of immunodeficiency associated with HIV-1 infections, nonHodgkin's lymphomas have been shown to occur approximately 60- to 100-fold more frequently than expected. A study conducted in Los Angeles County from 1984 to 1992 showed that EBV was associated with 39 of 59 (66%) HIV-related systemic lymphomas.

Given the profound immune defects in HIV-infected patients, along with the known role of cytotoxic T lymphocytes in controlling EBV-induced proliferation, it is not surprising that the number of EBV-infected B cells in the peripheral blood of those patients with HIV infection is higher than in the general population. HIV-associated nonHodgkin's lymphoma, usually of B-cell origin, is a relatively late manifestation of HIV infection. For unknown reasons, the majority of EBV-associated nonHodgkin's lymphomas in HIV-infected patients have presented as primary central nervous system lymphomas.

Oral Hairy Leukoplakia

Another EBV-induced disease in HIV-infected individuals is oral hairy leukoplakia, an unusual wart-like disease of the lingual squamous epithelium. Virus replication is evident only in the upper layers of the epithelium and is effectively inhibited by acyclovir. Interestingly, the lesions of oral hairy leukoplakia appear to be relatively specific to HIV-related immunodeficiency; the disease is only rarely observed in patients with other immunodeficiencies.

HODGKIN'S DISEASE

EBV genomic DNA was first reported in Hodgkin's disease in 1987. More recent evidence supports a role for EBV in the pathogenesis of Hodgkin's disease in which the malignant cells, including Reed-Sternberg cells, contain the EBV genome in up to 50% of Western cases. As with Burkitt lymphoma, the association of EBV with Hodgkin's disease appears to vary geographically, as 94% of cases of classic Hodgkin's disease occurring in Peru contain EBV transcripts within Reed-Sternberg cells. Healthy Western populations are infected with predominantly type 1 EBV and, not surprisingly, the majority of EBV detected in Hodgkin's disease is type 1. However, current information suggests that the link between EBV and Hodgkin's disease may apply only to certain histologic subtypes because the frequent presence of EBV in Hodgkin's disease is usually associated with only the mixed cellularity and nodular sclerosing subtypes.

T-CELL LYMPHOMA

Until the mid-1990s, there was little evidence that normal T-cell lymphocytes were susceptible to EBV infection. Studies have demonstrated EBV-infected tonsillar T lymphocytes in individuals with acute IM. This observation is consistent with the description of T-cell lymphomas in individuals with chronic EBV infection.

TREATMENT

Symptomatic and Antiinflammatory

Supportive care is the mainstay of treatment. Acetaminophen or nonsteroidal antiinflammatory agents are recommended for the treatment of fever, throat discomfort, and malaise. The use of corticosteroids in the treatment of EBV-induced IM has been controversial. A trial of corticosteroids in individuals with impending airway obstruction due to lymphoid obstruction (manifested clinically by difficulty breathing or dyspnea in the recumbent position) is generally warranted.

Some experienced clinicians recommend that corticosteroids should be administered in routine cases of IM, but these recommendations are based on anecdotal experience. The clinical illness of IM reflects the immune response to EBV, an agent that establishes lifelong latency and has oncogenic potential. For this reason, the administration of immunomodulating agents such as corticosteroids during primary infection, is theoretically contraindicated because of the possibility of altering the immune response and predisposing the patient to a long-term lymphoproliferative complication. Indeed, studies in individuals with IM who received corticosteroids many weeks earlier have demonstrated diminished numbers of B cells and T cells including diminished numbers of CD4 helper T and CD8 cytotoxic/suppressor T cells. Because no long-term data obtained on individuals who receive corticosteroids during primary EBV infection are available, it would seem prudent, despite the potential of short-term improvement, to withhold such treatment from most individuals given the self-limited nature of this infection in the vast majority of cases.

Antiviral Treatment

Acyclovir is a nucleoside analogue that inhibits permissive EBV infection through inhibition of EBV DNA polymerase but has no effect on latent infection.

Specific therapy of acute EBV infections with intravenous and oral formulations of acyclovir has been studied. Although short-term suppression of viral shedding can be demonstrated, significant clinical benefit has been lacking.

CHAPTER 101
Herpes Simplex Virus

Adapted from Steve Kohl

THE VIRUS

Herpes simplex virus (HSV) is a moderately large virus consisting of an icosahedral capsid enclosing a core of double-stranded DNA and protein surrounded by a lipid-containing envelope. Two subtypes are distinguishable—types 1 and 2—with approximately 50% DNA homology. Although type 1 is regarded as the oral type and type 2 as the genital type, changing sexual habits and possibly other factors blur this distinction. Thus, the virus type is not a reliable indicator of the anatomic site of isolation. The large HSV genome (approximately 100×10^6 kd) encodes for more than 90 polypeptides. Replication occurs after viral penetration and uncoating by an orderly cascade of gene products. The virus is assembled in the nucleus and buds through the nuclear membrane acquiring its envelope and is released at the cell surface. Like all the herpesviruses, HSV assumes a state of persistent latency in neural tissue (ganglion) after primary infection of the host.

EPIDEMIOLOGY

Although highly infectious, HSV is not transmitted casually from person-to-person. The virus is relatively unstable at atmospheric conditions, and close interpersonal contact is usually required for transmission. HSV can be transmitted via body fluids such as saliva and can certainly be acquired by direct apposition of infected with uninfected integument or mucous membranes. For example, the virus has been transferred directly between wrestlers (herpes gladiatorum) and rugby players (herpes rugbeiorum or "scrum pox"). Nurses and respiratory therapists may acquire HSV infections of the paronychial region (herpetic whitlow), presumably from ungloved hand contact with oropharyngeal secretions. Children with gingivostomatitis may acquire HSV whitlow by nail biting or thumb sucking. Newborns may acquire HSV infection during passage through a virus-infected birth canal. Genital and anal HSV infections are acquired and transmitted through direct contact with infected genitalia or in connection with oral-genital, genital, or oral-anal contacts. In all such cases, transmission may occur when the infected parties are asymptomatic and unaware of their own HSV infections. The presence of active lesions is associated with high titers of virus, which probably increases the likelihood of transmission. Few data, however, implicate inanimate sources as important reservoirs of virus persistence and spread.

If the uninfected exposed skin or mucous membranes are abraded, damaged, or otherwise altered, the risk of transmission and spread is enhanced. For example, burned or abraded skin is more susceptible to HSV infection than intact skin. Infants may acquire HSV infections in the area of a diaper rash; infants and children with eczema are at risk for serious disseminated HSV infections (Kaposi varicelliform eruption) (Fig. 101-1).

The epidemiology of HSV is dominated by symptomatic and asymptomatic infection in a huge pool of latently infected individuals. Symptomatic recurrences and asymptomatic shedding ensure continued spread of HSV. Approximately 1% of individuals shed HSV orally, and 0.2% to 0.5% of women shed HSV genitally at any time. The numbers are higher for individuals who are high risk or immunocompromised. Seroepidemiologic studies reveal that HSV infections are found in all populations.

Most neonatal HSV infections are acquired from maternal genital strains and, thus, are usually caused by HSV-2. After the neonatal period, HSV-1 infections predominate and, depending on social and economic factors, 40% to 60% of young children of lower socioeconomic status are seropositive by age 5 years. Most of such individuals exhibit HSV-1 antibodies by adulthood.

The incidence of HSV genital infection has increased markedly since the late 1970s. Approximately 300,000 to 500,000 new cases occur annually in the United States. In studies of

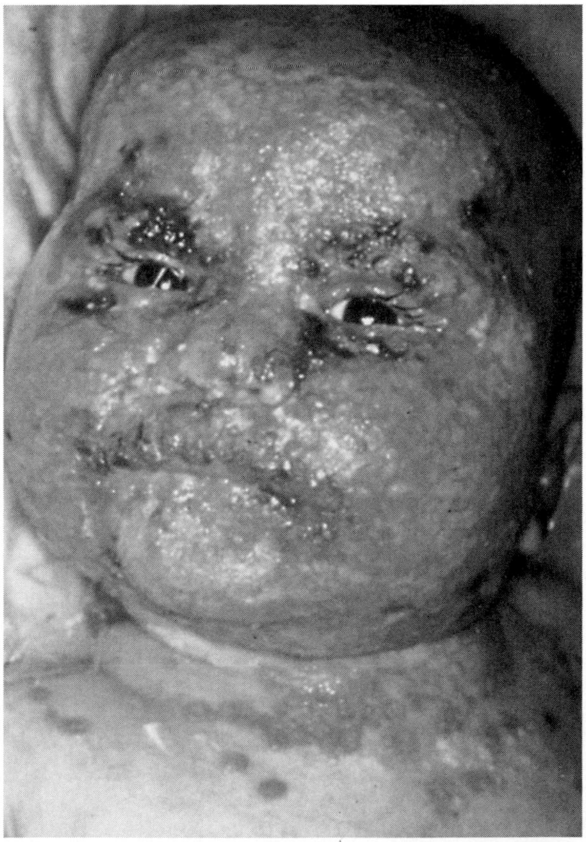

Figure 101-1. Extensive herpes simplex virus infection in an infant with atopic eczema (Kaposi's varicelliform eruption). (Reproduced with permission from Kohl S. Postnatal herpes simplex virus infection. In: Feigin RD, Cherry JD, eds. *Textbook of pediatric infectious diseases*, 4th ed. Philadelphia: Saunders, 1998:1709.)

sexually active university students, 4 to 8 per 1,000 acquire genital HSV infection annually.

Risk factors for HSV-2 acquisition in North America include gender (female subjects greater than male subjects), race (higher in blacks), lower socioeconomic status, multiple sex partners, and failure to use condoms. Transmission of HSV-2 from an infected individual to an HSV-2-seronegative individual occurs annually in approximately 10% of stable heterosexual couples.

Reactivation of latent HSV infection is associated with a variety of influences including exposure to sunlight (ultraviolet), certain febrile illnesses, local trauma, menstruation, and immunosuppression. These influences, therefore, define additional epidemiologic factors pertinent to HSV infections.

PATHOGENESIS AND PATHOLOGY

In most cases, initial viral replication occurs at the entry site, usually in skin or mucous membranes. Because HSV has a predilection for cells that originate in embryonic ectoderm, these viruses may involve the central nervous system (CNS). Encephalitis may accompany or follow primary HSV infection, but it can be seen with reactivation of latent virus.

The incubation period for primary infection varies from 2 to 20 days in most HSV infections. After primary HSV infection, the virus remains latent in sensory neural ganglia that innervate portions of the skin or mucous membranes originally involved. Thus, an individual with recurrent HSV almost always experiences reactivation of the HSV lesions in the identical region. In immunologically intact individuals, the recurrence is generally less severe than the primary infection. In individuals previously infected with one type of virus (e.g., HSV-1, orally), infection with a second type (e.g., HSV-2, genitally) is less severe than in a host who has never been infected with either. Similarly, an individual can acquire a reinfection with the same type (e.g., a second infection with a new strain of HSV-2 genitally in a patient with preexisting genital HSV-2 infection). Generally, the reinfection is mild and is often dismissed as an endogenous recurrence. These strains can be differentiated by DNA endonuclease restriction analysis of viral isolates.

After primary HSV infection, immunocompetent individuals have an early nonspecific response followed by a specific immunologic response. The former consists of mobilization of polymorphonuclear and mononuclear leukocytes to the site of infection. The latter consists of specific antiviral antibodies being produced after several days.

The immune response to recurrent infection is not well characterized. It does not appear to be associated with marked alterations in antibody production, although fourfold titer rises and reemergence of IgA and IgM antiviral antibody may occur. Natural killer cell activity and lymphokine production increase. In the host with cellular immune defects, recurrences are common and result in long duration and increased severity but often do not cause widespread dissemination.

CLINICAL MANIFESTATIONS

Gingivostomatitis

Gingivostomatitis is the most common form of HSV-induced primary illness seen in children. Usually, it is seen in young children between ages 6 months and 3 years, a time at which the child is no longer protected with maternal antibody. The infection is often acquired from a family member with active primary or recurrent oral HSV infection. The incubation period covers a few days, and the illness is ushered in by fretful behavior and fever. Usually, affected infants refuse to eat and may even refuse fluids. Vesicular lesions appear on and around the lips, along the gingiva, on the anterior tongue, and on the anterior (hard) palate (Fig. 101-2). Often, cervical and submental nodes are swollen and tender. Vesicles eventually lead to 1- to 3-mm shallow gray ulcers on an erythematous base. Generally, the gums are mildly hypertrophic, ulcerated, and often bleed. Often, the breath emits a foul smell (fetor oris). If fluids are refused, such children may require hospitalization to maintain adequate hydration (dehydration is often complicated by fever). The process evolves for 4 to 5 days, and resolution requires at least an additional week. Autoinoculation may cause lesions on the hands (whitlow) and, less commonly, on the trunk or genital area.

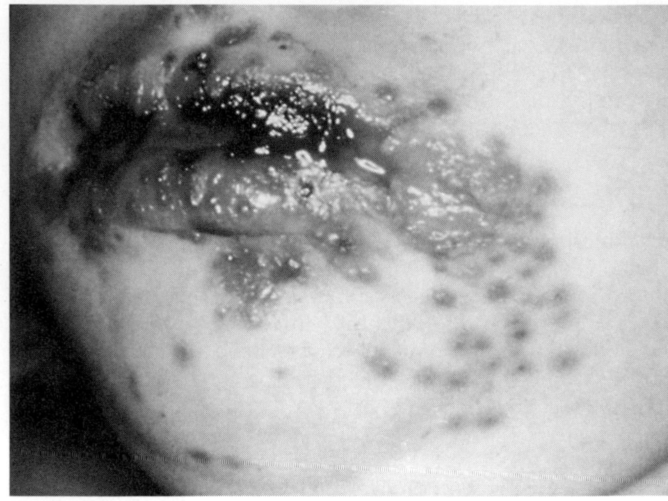

Figure 101-2. Primary herpes gingivostomatitis in a normal toddler at the ulcerative vesicular stage. (Reproduced with permission from Kohl S. Postnatal herpes simplex virus infection. In: Feigin RD, Cherry JD, eds. *Textbook of pediatric infectious diseases,* 4th ed. Philadelphia: Saunders, 1998:1706.)

HSV gingivostomatitis is differentiated from herpangina, a manifestation of enteroviral infection, by the predominance of ulcers in the anterior and posterior portion of the oropharynx; usually, herpangina is a posterior pharyngeal ulcerative condition. In addition, unlike HSV infection, herpangina often has a more acute onset, shorter duration, and seasonal occurrence. Although enterovirus-mediated hand-foot-and-mouth disease can present with oral ulcers and a vesicular eruption on the distal portion of extremities, the bilaterally symmetric distribution should differentiate it from HSV gingivostomatitis and concurrent HSV autoinoculation of a digit.

In adolescents and especially in college-aged patients, primary HSV infection often manifests as a posterior, occasionally exudative pharyngitis. The characteristic findings are shallow tonsillar ulcers with a gray exudate. In this setting, it must be differentiated from streptococcal infection, Epstein-Barr virus, adenovirus, Arcanobacterium and, rarely, diphtheria or tularemia-induced pharyngitis.

Vulvovaginitis

Herpetic vulvovaginitis rarely occurs in infants and children. HSV may be introduced inadvertently in handling the genital area with contaminated hands. Genital herpes, however, may reflect sexual abuse of young children. The occurrence of genital HSV in young children warrants investigation.

The incidence of genital infection in adolescents and young adults has increased markedly since the late 1970s. HSV-1 accounts for approximately 25% of primary genital HSV infections with HSV-2 the majority. The incubation period is 2 to 14 days. Primary illness is accompanied by fever, headache, malaise, and myalgias. Local genital symptoms include severe pain, itching, dysuria, vaginal or urethral discharge, and tender inguinal adenopathy. In primary illness, lesions begin as painful vesicles or pustules and progress to wet ulcers and then to healing ulcers with or without crusts. Usually, crusts occur only on squamous epithelium. Lesions tend to last for 2 to 3 weeks before complete healing. Virus shedding occurs for a mean of 11.5 days.

Systemic symptoms may also include an aseptic meningitis syndrome (11%–35%) that is mild, self-limited, and not associated with neurologic residua unlike herpes encephalitis. Other complications of primary HSV genital infection include sacral autonomic nervous dysfunction (manifested as poor rectal sphincter tone, constipation, sacral anesthesia, urinary retention, impotence), extragenital lesions, secondary yeast infections in women, and pharyngitis.

Many other complications exist. Perhaps the most important is the possibility that maternal HSV may be transmitted to newborns (Chapter 30). HSV genital ulcer lesions can increase the risk for human immunodeficiency virus infection. Finally, the emotional aspects of HSV infection should not be underestimated. Although some individuals cope easily with the illness and the likelihood of recurrent disease, a sizable number exhibit profound depression, poor self-esteem, complete abstention from sexual activity, and general withdrawal.

Other Primary Herpes Simplex Virus Skin Infections

Herpes may infect virtually any part of the skin or mucous membranes, particularly areas that are damaged by abrasions or thermal or chemical burns. Vesicular lesions spread throughout the affected skin, usually crusting and resolving in approximately 1 week. In normal wrestlers, herpes gladiatorum usually involves the head (73%), extremities (42%), and trunk (28%). The illness accompanying eczema herpeticum can be severe and even fatal, although in most cases, the infection resolves without specific therapy and leaves no sequelae (Fig. 101-1).

Herpetic whitlow is a painful, erythematous, swollen lesion occurring on the terminal phalanx of fingers (69%) and thumb (21%). The painful white swellings appear to be filled with pus but, when opened for drainage, they are found to contain little fluid and no purulent material. Occasionally, the whitlow, which may persist for 7 to 10 days, is initially accompanied by a few vesicles that may give a clue to the etiology of the infection. Whitlows are seen in four typical situations. First, infants with herpetic gingivostomatitis may autoinoculate their fingers (Fig. 101-3). Second, whitlows are encountered in infants without obvious oral disease, sometimes caused by infected adults kissing their children's fingers. Third, in sexually active patients, more often the whitlow is a manifestation of concurrent genital disease. Fourth, dentists, respiratory therapists, nurses, and pediatricians who sometimes examine oral cavities without wearing gloves are at risk for herpetic whitlow. Because of the epidemiology of HSV, whitlow in children is usually caused by HSV-1. Appropriate diagnosis is important (clinical diagnosis or culture) because whitlows should not be incised and drained.

Herpes Simplex Virus of the Eye

Primary HSV infection of the eye may manifest as a blepharitis or a follicular conjunctivitis, often accompanied by preauricular lymphadenopathy. If restricted to the conjunctiva, the infection, which can be accompanied by vesicular herpetic lesions elsewhere on the face or in the nose or mouth, usually resolves without sequelae. Herpetic infection of the eye may, however, progress to involve the cornea with more serious potential consequences. For this reason, ophthalmologists should always examine and evaluate such cases.

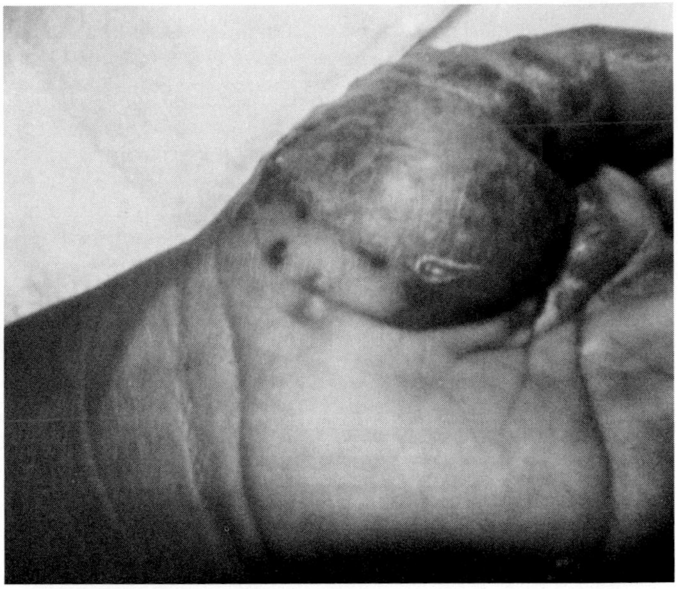

Figure 101-3. Herpetic whitlow in a toddler with oral herpes simplex virus infection. (Reproduced with permission from Kohl S. Postnatal herpes simplex virus infection. In: Feigin RD, Cherry JD, eds. *Textbook of pediatric infectious diseases*, 4th ed. Philadelphia: Saunders, 1998:1710.)

Herpes Simplex Virus Infections of the Central Nervous System

HSV accounts for 2% to 5% of all cases of encephalitis in the United States but up to 20% of all etiologic diagnoses (60%–70% of cases of encephalitis remaining without a diagnosis). The case-fatality rate associated with untreated HSV encephalitis is approximately 70%, and survivors generally exhibit considerable permanent neurologic disability. The spread of HSV-1 to the CNS seems to proceed via neurogenic pathways. Although HSV encephalitis may involve virtually any area of the brain, it shows a striking tendency to involve the frontal and temporal lobes after the neonatal period.

An important step is to differentiate the HSV-induced aseptic meningitis syndrome—usually caused by HSV-2 and usually a complication of primary genital infection—from HSV encephalitis. In the former, signs of meningitis, including headache, photophobia, and stiff neck, appear shortly after genital lesions are noted. Usually, seizures and focal CNS findings are absent. The cerebrospinal fluid (CSF) examination reveals a lymphocytosis with 300 to 2,600 white blood cells (WBCs) per cubic millimeter and sometimes a low glucose level. This syndrome may recur with genital recurrences. Usually, complete recovery occurs without specific therapy. HSV may occasionally be grown from the CSF.

In contrast to meningitis, HSV encephalitis is a highly lethal disease. In 96% of cases, it is caused by HSV-1. It may be a result of primary (30%) or recurrent (70%) infection. One-third of cases occur in the pediatric age range. HSV encephalitis has no seasonality. It is an acute illness with fever, malaise, irritability, and nonspecific symptoms lasting 1 to 7 days, progressing to signs and symptoms of focal CNS involvement in 3 to 7 days, and finally to coma and death. Fever and altered behavior in any child should evoke suspicion of encephalitis. Meningeal signs are uncommon. The presence of oral or genital lesions is not helpful in the diagnosis or exclusion of HSV encephalitis.

A mild CSF pleocytosis (50-2000 WBC/mm^3) with lymphocyte predominance often exists. Early in the infection, neutrophils may predominate. In 75% to 85% of cases, red blood cells reflecting the hemorrhagic necrosis are seen in the CSF. Between 5% and 25% of patients have hypoglycorrhachia, and 80% have elevated CSF protein levels (median, 80 mg/dL), which rise to striking levels with disease progression. The CSF is normal in 2% to 3% of patients with early HSV encephalitis. HSV may not grow from lumbar CSF specimens. HSV polymerase chain reaction (PCR) should be requested in addition to culture.

Other neurodiagnostic tests may aid in the diagnosis. A "typical" pattern of unilateral or bilateral focal spikes against a background of slow activity is associated with HSV encephalitis. In 80% to 90% of patients, the EEG finding is not only abnormal but localizing. Early in the course of illness, CT scan of the brain may be normal. Magnetic resonance imaging (MRI) (Fig. 101-4), is the radiologic technique of choice for early diagnosis of HSV encephalitis. The finding of focal abnormality on EEG, and magnetic resonance imaging is very suggestive of HSV encephalitis. Although brain biopsy is considered the gold standard for diagnosis, HSV DNA PCR diagnosis of spinal fluid samples performed in reliable laboratories has been shown to be more than 98% sensitive and 94% specific.

Recurrent Herpes Simplex Virus Infections

All the sites discussed in connection with primary HSV disease may also be involved in recurrent infections. The most common manifestation of recurrent HSV infection is herpes labialis ("cold sores," "fever blisters"). Most individuals experience a prodrome burning or tingling at the site lasting 6 hours to several days. Then a progression from papules (lasting 12–36 hours) to vesicles (usually gone by 48 hours) to ulcers and crust (lasting 2–4 days) follows. Most outbreaks are healed by 5 to 10 days. Recurrences generally occur on the lips or mucocutaneous junction. A differential diagnosis of the condition also includes aphthous ulcers, ulcers caused by cyclic neutropenia, and ulcers associated with celiac disease, inflammatory bowel disease, and Behçet syndrome.

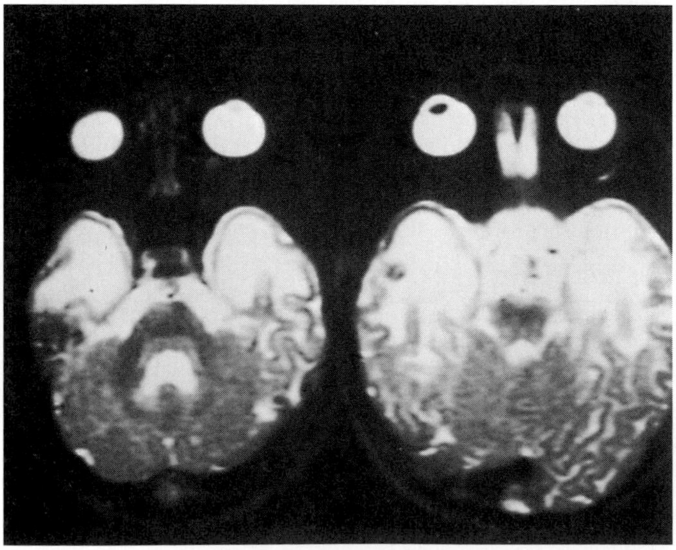

Figure 101-4. Magnetic resonance image of patient with early herpes simplex virus encephalitis. Note the bilateral temporal lobe enhancement. (Reproduced with permission from Kohl S. Herpes simplex encephalitis. *Pediatr Clin North Am* 1988;35:465.)

Recurrent genital HSV is more common after primary HSV-2 (90%) than after HSV-1 (55%) infection. The mean rate of recurrence is 0.1 episodes per month after primary genital HSV-1 and 0.3 episodes per month after primary HSV-2 genital infection. Subclinical recurrences are very common and account for one-third of total days of viral reactivation.

Only 5% to 12% of individuals with recurrent genital HSV have constitutional symptoms. Local symptoms include pain (averaging 4–6 days), itching, dysuria, adenopathy, and lesions lasting 4 to 5 days and progressing to crusting and healing by 9 to 11 days. Virus is shed for an average of 3 to 4 days. In dry areas, vesicles are seen but, in wet areas, the vesicles rapidly break down into ulcers. Generally, symptoms are milder and their duration is shorter than in primary genital disease.

Erythema Multiforme and Herpes Simplex Virus Infection

Erythema multiforme is known to be precipitated by recurrent HSV infection, perhaps due to an allergic response. Several studies document HSV antigen-antibody immune complexes present in the serum and skin of patients with erythema multiforme after HSV infection. HSV DNA has been detected in the biopsy samples of skin lesions of patients with erythema multiforme. Skin manifestations may last for 14 to 21 days.

Herpes Simplex Virus Infection in the Immunocompromised Host

Patients with skin abnormalities (eczema, burns) or immunologic defects, primarily in the cell-mediated aspects of the immune system, are a risk for severe HSV infections. Immunodeficiencies known to be associated with significant HSV infection are severe combined immunodeficiency syndrome (SCID), agammaglobulinemia, and Wiskott-Aldrich syndrome. Other conditions associated with unusually severe HSV infections are transplantation, malignancy, and immunosuppressive therapy. Many of these patients are candidates for prophylactic antiviral therapy.

Several major syndromes are attributable to HSV in immunocompromised patients, with some overlap, and occasional progression from one to another. The first is a local, chronic, often extensive cutaneous or mucocutaneous infection. The second is infection of one organ, usually contiguous to an orifice (e.g., esophagitis or pneumonitis). The most serious is widespread dissemination involving distant areas of skin or visceral organs (lungs, liver, adrenals) and the CNS. Except in the most immunosuppressed patients, disseminated disease probably (most often) represents primary infection, whereas the local syndromes may represent primary or (more often) recurrent illness.

Esophagitis caused by HSV has been reported in normal children, but it is relatively common in immunocompromised patients. HSV pneumonia is a rare premortal diagnosis and occurs almost exclusively in immunosuppressed patients. In immunocompromised patients, meningoencephalitis caused by HSV may occur as part of widely disseminated disease or may be a localized condition. The most severe form of HSV infection in the immunocompromised host is widely disseminated disease involving the liver, adrenals, lungs, spleen, kidney, marrow, and (often) the brain. Usually, the clinical presentation is one of initial fever and mucocutaneous involvement that, instead of healing as expected, disseminates. In approximately 20% of cases of disseminated disease, skin lesions are absent. The major target organs involved give rise to syndromes of hepatitis, pneumonia, shock, bleeding, disseminated intravascular coagulopathy, seizures, coma, renal failure, hypothermia, and death in days to weeks.

DIAGNOSIS

The finding of HSV in certain secretions does not mean that the clinical condition is caused by HSV. In general, the virus must be isolated from the tissue in question to confirm the diagnosis, especially in immunosuppressed hosts.

Rapid, Nonspecific Methods

Electron microscopy and cytologic examination are rapid and very suggestive diagnostic modalities, but they are not entirely specific. Electron microscopy of vesicular fluid or tissue preparations may reveal the characteristic virus of the herpes family, but it cannot differentiate HSV from other herpesviruses.

In most series, 40% to 60% of culture-positive specimens are cytologically positive if examined by an experienced observer. False-positive examination results are unusual but do occur.

Nonspecific methods include electron microscopy and cytologic exam. Cytology can reveal typical multinucleated giant cells, but these findings may also be seen with cytomegalovirus and varicella-zoster virus. Electron microscopic exam of vesicular fluid may demonstrate a herpesvirus but cannot fully differentiate HSV from others in the family.

Several specific tests (based on antigen detection) include fluorescent antibody methods, enzyme-linked immunosorbent assays (ELISAs). Generally, these tests use specific hyperimmune serum to HSV or monoclonal antibodies to specific HSV glycoproteins.

Polymerase chain reaction (PCR) allows for sensitive detection of viral DNA. Since mucocutaneous HSV is often a clinical diagnosis, perhaps the most useful role for PCR is detection of HSV DNA in spinal fluid of patients with possible HSV encephalitis (since viral cultures of CSF in patients with HSV encephalitis are generally negative). If a reliable laboratory reports a positive PCR result, the need for a brain biopsy test is obviated. The major problem with PCR is false-positive responses, primarily caused by poor laboratory technique.

The reference standard for HSV diagnosis outside of the CNS remains tissue culture. Mucocutaneous sites can be cultured and specimens transported in specific viral transport media. HSV grows rapidly (mean, 2–3 days) in viral culture producing a typical cytopathic effect. Definitive viral characterization is then accomplished by antisera reaction. Typing can be accomplished using specific monoclonal antibodies or endonuclease restriction patterns.

A variety of antibody tests can be used to document *primary* HSV infection. Several precautions must be observed in analyzing the serologic response. Patients with documented prior HSV infections may have fourfold titer rises with recurrences, and they may have IgM or IgA responses with recurrences. Rarely, severely immunosuppressed patients do not produce antibody. Thus, only when a patient's serum converts from negative to positive can a primary infection be diagnosed with confidence. Generally, patients with prior HSV infection (symptomatic or asymptomatic) remain seropositive for life (probably reflecting existing latency) with minor fluctuations. However, in some of the most important conditions—HSV encephalitis or early disseminated HSV in immunosuppressed hosts—serology is relatively useless because of a slow titer rise or late conversion. In addition, a significant percentage of these conditions represents recurrent and not primary disease.

Endonuclease Restriction Analysis takes advantage of HSV DNA having a specific cleavage pattern or "fingerprint" when digested by endonuclease restriction enzymes. These cleavage patterns can be used to type the virus and to demonstrate relatedness or differences (strains) among isolates from different persons for epidemiologic purposes ("outbreaks," nosocomial transmission), among isolates obtained from different sites in the same individual during one illness, or among isolates obtained from the same site over time.

PROGNOSIS, COMPLICATIONS, AND SEQUELAE

Outside of the fetal and neonatal period, HSV infections are an annoyance but usually not life-threatening. On the other hand, HSV encephalitis outcome can be grave ranging from extensive and permanent neurologic disability to death. In immunocompromised patients, it is a major cause of morbidity and mortality.

THERAPY

Acyclovir (Zovirax and generic) is the standard for antiviral therapy of HSV infections (Table 101.1). This is an inactive drug that requires phosphorylation to inhibit DNA synthesis. HSV thymidine kinase is much more active than its mammalian counterpart. Thus, acyclovir becomes a specific antiviral agent in the presence of thymidine kinase-positive viruses. It is important to note that mutant, thymidine kinase-negative acyclovir-resistant isolates of HSV have been recovered from patients in the course of acyclovir therapy for genital HSV infections.

Newer agents such as valacyclovir and famciclovir are being used increasingly, primarily due to their improved bioavailability over traditional acyclovir. As of this manuscript, neither of these drugs is FDA approved for use in children, but these drugs may be used in adolescents (Genital Herpes Simplex Virus Infection below).

Oral Herpes Simplex Virus

Oral acyclovir for infants and children with primary HSV gingivostomatitis results in decreased duration of oral lesions, and a more rapid disappearance of fever, extraoral lesions, and eating and drinking problems. It can also reduce the number of days of viral shedding. Intravenous acyclovir has been used in patients with severe primary gingivostomatitis when hospital admission was required to maintain hydration.

Oral acyclovir has minimal effects on the course of recurrent oral HSV infection in normal hosts and is probably not warranted.

Symptomatic therapy for gingivostomatitis includes antipyretics and oral hydration with bland liquids and ice slurries. Oral anesthetics (lidocaine) are often used but must be done so with caution.

Herpes Simplex Virus Keratitis

Trifluridine (a pyrimidine nucleoside) in a 1% ophthalmic solution inhibits HSV DNA synthesis and is the drug of choice for the local treatment of primary and recurrent HSV eye disease such

TABLE 101-1. Therapy of Herpes Simplex Virus Infection in Children

Genital disease
Primary
Oral acyclovir, 200 mg five times daily for 7–10 days (1 capsule = 200 mg)[a] or 400 mg three times daily for 10 days
Valacyclovir, 1 g twice daily for 10 days[a]
Famciclovir, 250 mg three times daily for 7–10 days[a]
Intravenous acyclovir, 15 mg/kg/d in three divided doses for 5–7 days
Recurrent
Oral acyclovir, 200 mg five times daily for 5 days or 400 mg three times daily for 5 days[a]
Oral valacyclovir, 500 mg twice daily for 5 days[a]
Oral famciclovir, 125 mg twice daily for 5 days[a]
Suppressive
Oral acyclovir, 200 mg three to five times daily or 400 mg two to three times daily for up to 5 years[a]
Oral valacyclovir, 500 mg/d[a] or 1,000 mg/d or 250 mg twice daily[a]
Oral famciclovir, 250 mg twice daily[a]
Oral disease
Primary: same as for primary genital infection. Oral dose for children should not exceed 80 mg/kg/d of acyclovir (15 mg/kg five times daily). (No pediatric dosing guidelines are available for valacy-clovir or famciclovir).
Recurrent: penciclovir, topical, every 2 hours while awake for 4 days
Encephalitis
Intravenous acyclovir, 30 mg/kg/d in three divided doses for 14–21 days[b]
Neonatal disease
Intravenous acyclovir, 45–60 mg/kg/d in three divided doses for 14–21 days[b]
Immunocompromised patients
Intravenous acyclovir, 15–30 mg/kg/d in three divided doses; duration as warranted clinically
Oral acyclovir, 200 mg three to five times daily, not to exceed 80 mg/kg/d; duration as warranted clinically
Acyclovir-resistant isolates
Intravenous foscarnet, 120 mg/kg/d in three divided doses until infection resolution[c]
Ocular infection
Trifluorothymidine (Viroptic), 1% ophthalmic solution, one drop every 2 hours to a maximum of nine drops, then one drop every 4 hours (five drops daily), not to exceed 21 days
Vidarabine (Vira-A), 3% ophthalmic ointment, five times daily; change to different agent if no healing in 7–9 days
Iododeoxyuridine (Stoxil), 0.1% ophthalmic solution or 0.5% ophthalmic ointment. Solution: one drop each hour during the day and every 2 hours during the night. Ointment: five times daily, every 4 hours and before bedtime; change to different agent if no healing in 7–9 days

[a]These are adult doses. No licensed guidelines exist for pediatric doses in this condition. Oral acyclovir dose for children should not exceed 80 mg/kg/d. No pediatric dosing guidelines are available for valacyclovir or famciclovir.
[b]The large dose has been found effective and nontoxic in these particular clinical conditions and patients.
[c]This is an unlicensed use, and controlled trials in children have not been performed.
Adapted with permission from Kohl S. Postnatal herpes simplex virus infection. In: Feigin RD, Cherry JD, eds. *Textbook of pediatric infectious diseases*, 2nd ed. Philadelphia: Saunders, 1987:1577.

as keratitis, keratoconjunctivitis, and eyelid lesions. Caring for HSV eye disease should involve the care of a qualified ophthalmologist. Other topical antiviral agents exist. Furthermore, some ophthalmologists will carefully use corticosteroids for keratitis.

Herpes Simplex Virus Encephalitis

Intravenous acyclovir is the drug of choice in the treatment of children with HSV encephalitis. In addition to antiviral therapy, multidisciplinary intensive care optimizes the outcome of these patients. Often, direct intracranial pressure measurement by ventricular catheter or epidural bolt is necessary to monitor and treat increased intracranial pressure effectively. The use of steroids remains controversial. The care of children with HSV encephalitis most often requires a team of pediatric intensivists, neurologists, neurosurgeons, and infectious-disease experts in a tertiary-care setting.

Genital Herpes Simplex Virus Infection

Intravenous acyclovir or oral acyclovir can significantly reduce viral shedding, lesion formation, duration of lesions, and duration and severity of symptoms in primary infection (Table 101-1). Dosing guidelines also exist for valacyclovir and famciclovir, and these agents may be preferable because of improved bioavailability and less frequent dosing. All three drugs are approved for recurrent HSV treatment, as well as suppressive dosing.

Symptomatic therapy of HSV lesions should be directed at reducing local discomfort, preventing autoinoculation, and superinfection. Keeping lesions clean and dry is an important local measure. Urination can be made less painful by urinating in a bathtub or sitz bath.

Herpes Simplex Virus Infection in Immunocompromised Hosts

Both oral and intravenous acyclovir are efficacious in HSV infections in immunocompromised hosts. Intravenous acyclovir is the drug of choice for treating moderate or severe HSV infections in this setting. In very serious disease (e.g., dissemination to visceral organs or the CNS), the typical dose should be doubled. The major toxicity has been renal with a reversible obstructive nephropathy and transient rises in serum creatinine levels (5%–10% of patients). Usually, adequate hydration prevents this problem.

Acyclovir Resistance

Three HSV mutations give rise to acyclovir resistance. These include altered viral DNA polymerase, altered thymidine kinase, and absent thymidine kinase. The overwhelming majority of significant clinical isolates of acyclovir-resistant viruses is due to absence of thymidine kinase. These isolates have occurred and resulted in acyclovir-unresponsive illness in immunocompromised children who have usually been treated with chronic or recurrent courses of acyclovir. Usually, this outcome manifests as lesions that fail to heal and will worsen during the course of adequate acyclovir therapy. Resistance should be assumed in a patient who fails to improve and alternate therapy must be considered. Currently, foscarnet is the agent of choice for treating acyclovir-resistant HSV infection in immunocompromised hosts.

PREVENTION

Environmental Control or Barrier Prevention

Use of antiseptics, soap and hot water, or chlorine decreases the risk of transferring the virus in settings such as the home, spas, pools, and hospitals. Patients with skin lesions (such as wrestlers) should be excluded from participation until herpes infection is cleared or ruled out. Medical and dental personnel who handle respiratory or oral secretions should wear gloves and wash hands. Other hospital personnel with active cold sores or herpetic whitlow should not care for immunosuppressed patients. Care should be taken to avoid exposure to HSV in those patients with extensive dermatitis (eczema) or burns.

Immunoprophylaxis

Currently there are no products available for passive prophylaxis or active (vaccine) immunoprophylaxis for HSV.

Chemoprophylaxis

Daily oral acyclovir can suppresses recurrences of HSV in immunodeficient patients. Oral or intravenous acyclovir used at times of maximum immunosuppression, for example, in the first months after organ transplantation or during periods of neutropenia in individuals receiving antineoplastic chemotherapy, nearly completely prevents the predictable rate of HSV recurrence in seropositive individuals.

Daily oral acyclovir, famciclovir, or valacyclovir can decrease recurrence of genital HSV. Breakthrough recurrences are typically mild. When therapy is discontinued, HSV recurrences revert to pretreatment frequency.

CHAPTER 102
HIV Infection

Adapted from Gwendolyn B. Scott
and Wade P. Parks

Perinatal HIV infection in the United States has declined because of the use of zidovudine in pregnant women infected with HIV-1. An explosive increase in pediatric HIV-1 infection worldwide, particularly in Asia and Africa, continues to occur.

TRANSMISSION

HIV-1 can be transmitted perinatally by blood (possibly free virus) and by lymphoid cells from infected pregnant women; similarly, blood or blood products may transmit infection to a transfusion recipient or to a health care worker. HIV-1 is also a sexually transmitted disease (STD) spread by either homosexual or heterosexual contact.

Mother-to-Child Transmission

The placenta serves as a barrier to HIV-1 infection of the fetus, but transmission can occur. A considerable range of perinatal transmission rates has been reported from studies around the world, but, without treatment, the average is 25% to 30%. Increased transmission rates occur with prolonged rupture of the membranes (greater than 4 hours) and breast-feeding. The use of antiretroviral agents such as zidovudine, that inhibit the HIV-1 reverse transcriptase (RT), are thought to be effective because they protect the fetal cells from infection rather than because they significantly lower maternal virus levels.

Adolescent Sexual Transmission

Although kissing is not a significant route of transmission, probably receptive oral sex can transmit infection by contact with the virus or cellular contents of seminal fluid. The oral route of sex cannot be considered "safer sex." The highest rate of sexual transmission is associated with receptive anal intercourse in which the likelihood of exposure to virus or cells is greatly increased because of the relative thinness of the rectal mucosa.

Vaginal intercourse also carries a significant risk of HIV-1 transmission, which is estimated to be at least 20-fold greater for young women than for their male partners. A latex condom, preferably with an anti-HIV spermicide, is strongly recommended for vaginal intercourse.

EPIDEMIOLOGY

HIV-1 infection in pregnant women and perinatal transmission are the major sources of infant infection with HIV-1. The number of infected infants is rapidly declining in the United States due to antiretroviral chemoprophylaxis used in the mother before and during delivery and in the infant after birth (Prevention of Perinatal Transmission). As opposed to the worldwide pattern of epidemic spread, HIV-1 infection in the United States has moved from an epidemic to an endemic STD infecting the same populations (minority populations and from the lowest socioeconomic groups) as do other STDs such as syphilis.

Sources of adolescent HIV-1 infection include young women who have sex with older men or with intravenous drug users. Another population is young men who have sex with men. Often, other STDs are found in these populations.

ETIOLOGIC AGENT AND PATHOGENESIS

HIV-1 is a member of the Lentivirus subfamily of retroviruses. Lentiviruses replicate in macrophages, and HIV-1 can also replicate in $CD4^+$ lymphocytes. Two HIV-1 proteins RT and protease are the targets of current antiretroviral therapy. RT transcribes the viral RNA into double-stranded DNA in an error-prone manner. RT is important only in cells that are being infected because RT enables the infecting RNA to become DNA. After making the DNA copy, RT is not essential to the subsequent production of virus. In contrast, the protease is important only in cells that are already infected and making virus. Without the protease, the virus cannot be assembled and released from infected cells.

The infidelity of reverse transcription by RT results in highly variable populations of viruses with very complex genetic patterns. Individuals can have dual infections suggesting that any future HIV-1 vaccine will have to be polyvalent and continuously updated, as is the case for influenza vaccines. With modern technology, the detection of molecular genetic differences is possible.

Both macrophages and $CD4^+$ lymphocyte cell types have CD4 molecules that are the primary receptors for virus attachment. After the initial cellular infection and replication, a rapid spread or dissemination of the virus in lymphoid tissues occurs. Replication continues unchecked until the host immune system responds and begins to control viral replication.

Due to, among other factors, a less mature immune system, children have higher levels of viral RNA than adults. This increased viral replication poses a treatment challenge in children. With increased replication, the potential for mutation and selection of antiretroviral-resistant HIV-1 increases.

The assessment of HIV-1 replication can be measured sensitively by levels of viral RNA in plasma or serum. As with the measurement of CD4+ counts, RNA are relative and are of most value when repeated over time.

Specific immune responses to HIV-1 are both humoral and cellular. The cellular responses control or eliminate infected cells but are not sufficient to completely eliminate viral replication.

The humoral response is also vigorous, and antibody synthesis can be detected in infected infants within a few weeks after birth. The transplacental immunoglobulin G (IgG) from the mother predominates the infant's early antibody response. Most children with HIV-1 infection develop hypergammaglobulinemia. Much of this response is specific for HIV-1 viral antigens, but infants with hypogammaglobulinemia have a poor prognosis.

DIAGNOSIS OF HUMAN IMMUNODEFICIENCY VIRUS 1 INFECTION

The laboratory test used for diagnosing pediatric HIV infection depends on the age of the child. Serologic tests for HIV-1 remain positive through 18 months of age because of passively transferred maternal IgG. Thus, in this age group, antibody tests for HIV only indicate exposure and not necessarily infection. The diagnosis of infection should be made by detecting the virus or viral products. HIV DNA polymerase chain reaction (PCR) is available commercially and is used commonly for diagnosing HIV-1 in infants. A positive test result should always be confirmed on a different blood specimen. Approximately 40% of infected infants have a positive HIV DNA PCR result at birth, whereas the remainder have positive results after 2 to 6 weeks of age. Repeated negative PCR results after 2 months of age suggest the absence of HIV-1 infection.

After the child reaches 2 years of age, an HIV enzyme-linked immunosorbent assay antibody test with a confirmatory immunoblot test is the standard method for diagnosing HIV-1 infection in children.

CLINICAL MANIFESTATIONS

HIV-1 infection is a chronic, multisystem infection, and the presentation of clinical disease is extremely varied. The Centers for Disease Control and Prevention (CDC) have published a pediatric classification system that outlines the spectrum of clinical disease (Tables 102-1 to 102-3). Numerous nonspecific findings that may herald the onset of clinical disease include failure to thrive, generalized lymphadenopathy, hepatosplenomegaly, persistent oral candidiasis, recurrent or chronic diarrhea and, rarely, parotitis.

Pneumocystis carinii pneumonia (PCP) is the most serious opportunistic infection in children with HIV-1 infection. If HIV-1 infection is acquired by the perinatal route, PCP can occur in the first year of life with associated high morbidity and mortality. Fever and tachypnea are often the presenting signs. Bilateral interstitial perihilar infiltrates are seen on chest x-ray. Diagnosis is made by demonstrating the organism in endotracheal aspirates, bronchial washings, or lung tissue. PCP can be prevented by using chemoprophylaxis.

Candida esophagitis may present with poor oral intake, dysphagia, vomiting, and fever. A barium swallow suggests the diagnosis, which can be confirmed by endoscopy with biopsy and appropriate culture. Other common opportunistic infections are listed in Table 102-1.

Lymphocytic interstitial pneumonitis (LIP) is characterized by the presence of bilateral reticulonodular infiltrates with or without hilar lymphadenopathy. Diagnosis is confirmed by lung biopsy, although in most instances, the diagnosis is made presumptively on the basis of persistent typical radiographic findings and failure to demonstrate infectious agents. The onset is usually insidious and the disease may be static or progressive resulting in chronic lung disease with the development of hypoxemia and pulmonary hypertension.

Children infected with HIV-1 are at risk for severe or recurrent infections with common childhood pathogens, particularly Streptococcus pneumoniae. Infections can include bacteremia, meningitis, septic arthritis, osteomyelitis, pneumonia, otitis media, and deep and superficial abscesses. Gram-negative enteric infections may also occur.

Central nervous system abnormalities have been described in as many as 50% to 90% of children infected with HIV-1. Neurodevelopmental abnormalities range from mild developmental delay to progressive encephalopathy. The encephalopathy may be static or progressive and is characterized by loss of developmental milestones, motor weakness, seizures, ataxia, myoclonus, and extrapyramidal rigidity. HIV-1 encephalopathy likely results from direct invasion of HIV-1 into the brain.

Nephrotic syndrome with renal failure can occur early in children with HIV. Cardiomyopathy also occurs as either an acute or subacute process. Other associated clinical manifestations include anemia, leukopenia, and thrombocytopenia. Numerous cutaneous viral infections such as herpes simplex stomatitis, herpes zoster, molluscum contagiosum, and condylomata may be presenting, persistent, or recurrent problems.

MANAGEMENT OF THE CHILD AT RISK FOR HUMAN IMMUNODEFICIENCY VIRUS INFECTION

Medical monitoring is important to provide routine care, diagnostic testing for HIV-1, early recognition of complications of HIV-1, and prophylaxis against PCP. After maternal treatment with AZT in the antepartum and peripartum periods, parents should be instructed about the importance of giving the infant zidovudine for 6 weeks. Varicella vaccine should not be given to children with HIV-1 infection. Measles vaccine should not be administered to children with severe immunosuppression (CDC immune category 3; Tables 102-2 and 102-3).

Diagnostic testing using DNA PCR for HIV-1 detection should be done at birth, between 1 and 2 months of age, and between 4 and 6 months. Trimethoprim-sulfa prophylaxis should be started at 4 to 6 weeks of age for prevention of PCP in all infants at risk for HIV-1. In infants who have negative PCR test results through the first 6 months of life and who are clinically and immunologically normal, PCP prophylaxis can be discontinued at that time. These children are presumptively HIV-1-negative, and they should be followed until two negative HIV-1 antibody test results are documented. Maternal antibody to HIV-1 disappears in uninfected infants by a median age of 10 months and disappears in virtually all uninfected infants by 18 months of age. Infants infected with HIV-1 who are documented by two positive DNA PCR test results should be treated with antiretroviral therapy, while viral load, CD4 counts and percentage, and clinical status are monitored.

TREATMENT

Prophylactic medications are available for preventing opportunistic infections, and children should receive prophylaxis against PCP, M. avium-intracellulare complex, Candida infection, varicella, herpes simplex, recurrent bacterial infections, and cytomegalovirus, according to the published guidelines: (2001

TABLE 102-1. Clinical Categories for Children with Human Immunodeficiency Virus Infection

Category N: not symptomatic
Children who have no signs or symptoms considered to be the result of HIV infection or who have only one of the conditions listed in category A

Category A: mildly symptomatic
Children with two or more of the conditions listed below but none of the conditions listed in categories B and C
- Lymphadenopathy (≥0.5 cm at more than two sites; bilateral = one site)
- Hepatomegaly
- Splenomegaly
- Dermatitis
- Parotitis
- Recurrent or persistent upper respiratory infection, sinusitis, or otitis media

Category B: moderately symptomatic
Children who have symptomatic conditions other than those listed for category A or C that are attributed to HIV infection. Examples of conditions in clinical category B include but are not limited to
- Anemia (<8 g/dL), neutropenia (<1,000 per microliter), or thrombocytopenia (<100,000 per microliter) persisting ≥30 days
- Bacterial meningitis, pneumonia, or sepsis (single episode)
- Candidiasis, oropharyngeal (thrush), persisting (>2 months) in children >6 months of age
- Cardiomyopathy
- Cytomegalovirus infection, with onset at <1 month of age
- Diarrhea, recurrent or chronic
- Hepatitis
- Herpes simplex virus stomatitis, recurrent (more than two episodes within 1 year)
- Herpes simplex virus bronchitis, pneumonitis, or esophagitis with onset at <1 month of age
- Herpes zoster (shingles) involving at least two distinct episodes or more than one dermatome
- Lymphoid interstitial pneumonia or pulmonary lymphoid hyperplasia complex
- Nephropathy
- Persistent fever (lasting >1 month)
- Toxoplasmosis, onset at <1 month of age
- Varicella, disseminated (complicated chickenpox)

Category C: severely symptomatic
Children who have any condition listed in the 1987 surveillance case definition for acquired immunodeficiency syndrome, with the exception of lymphoid interstitial pneumonia
- Serious bacterial infections, multiple or recurrent (i.e., any combination of at least two culture-confirmed infections within a 2-year period), of the following types: septicemia, pneumonia, meningitis, bone or joint infection, or abscess of an internal organ or body cavity (including otitis media, superficial skin or mucosal abscesses, and indwelling catheter–related infections)
- Candidiasis, esophageal or pulmonary (bronchi, trachea, lungs)
- Coccidioidomycosis, disseminated (at a site other than or in addition to lungs or cervical or hilar lymph nodes)
- Cryptococcosis, extrapulmonary
- Cryptosporidiosis or isosporiasis with diarrhea persisting >1 month
- Cytomegalovirus infection with onset of symptoms at age >1 month (at a site other than liver, spleen, or lymph nodes)
- Encephalopathy (at least one of the following progressive findings present for at least 2 months in the absence of a concurrent illness other than HIV infection that could explain the findings): (a) failure to attain or loss of developmental milestones or loss of intellectual ability, verified by standard developmental scale or neuropsychological tests; (b) impaired brain growth or acquired microcephaly demonstrated by head circumference measurements or brain atrophy demonstrated by computerized tomography or magnetic resonance imaging (serial imaging is required for children <2 years of age); (c) acquired symmetric motor deficit manifested by two or more of the following: paresis, pathologic reflexes, ataxia, or gait disturbance
- Herpes simplex virus infection causing a mucocutaneous ulcer that persists for >1 month; or bronchitis, pneumonia, or esophagitis for any duration affecting a child >1 month of age
- Histoplasmosis, disseminated (at a site other than or in addition to lungs or cervical or hilar lymph nodes)
- Kaposi sarcoma
- Lymphoma, primary, in brain
- Lymphoma, small, noncleaved cell (Burkitt), or immunoblastic or large cell lymphoma of B cell or unknown immunologic pheno-type
- *Mycobacterium tuberculosis,* disseminated or extrapulmonary
- *Mycobacterium,* other species or unidentified species, disseminated (at a site other than or in addition to lungs, skin, or cervical or hilar lymph nodes)
- *Mycobacterium avium-intracellulare* complex or *Mycobacterium kansasii,* disseminated (at site other than or in addition to lungs, skin, or cervical or hilar lymph nodes)
- *Pneumocystis carinii* pneumonia
- Progressive multifocal leukoencephalopathy
- Salmonella (nontyphoid) septicemia, recurrent
- Toxoplasmosis of the brain with onset at >1 month of age
- Wasting syndrome in the absence of a concurrent illness other than HIV infection that could explain the following findings: (a) persistent weight loss >10% of baseline, *or* (b) downward crossing of at least two of the following percentile lines on the weight-for-age chart (e.g., 95th, 75th, 50th, 25th, fifth) in a child ≥1 year of age, *or* (c) <fifth percentile on weight-for-height chart on two consecutive measurements, ≥30 days apart, *plus* (a) chronic diarrhea (i.e., at least two loose stools per day for ≥30 days) *or* (b) documented fever (for ≥30 days, intermittent or constant)

HIV, human immunodeficiency virus.
From Centers for Disease Control and Prevention. 1994 Revised classification system for human immunodeficiency virus infection in children less than 13 years of age. *MMWR Morb Mortal Wkly Rep* 1994;43(Rr-12):1.

TABLE 102-2. Immunologic Categories Based on Age-Specific CD4+ T-Lymphocyte Counts and Percentage

	Age of child					
	<12 mo		*1–5 yr*		*6–12 yr*	
Immunologic category	*Number*	*Percentage*	*Number*	*Percentage*	*Number*	*Percentage*
1: No evidence of suppression	≥1,500	≥25	≥1,000	≥25	≥500	≥25
2: Evidence of moderate suppression	750–1,499	15–24	500–999	15–24	200–499	15–24
3: Severe suppression	<750	<15	<500	<15	<200	<15

From Centers for Disease Control and Prevention. 1994 Revised classification system for human immunodeficiency virus infection in children less than 13 years of age. *MMWR Morb Mortal Wkly Rep* 1994;43(Rr-12):1.

TABLE 102-3. Pediatric Human Immunodeficiency Virus Clinical Classification

Immunologic category	N: No signs or symptoms	A: Mild signs or symtoms	B: Moderate signs or symptoms	C: Severe signs or symptoms
1: No evidence of suppression	N1	A1	B1	C1
2: Evidence of moderate suppression	N2	A2	B2	C2
3: Severe suppression	N3	A3	B3	C3

From Centers for Disease Control and Prevention. 1994 Revised classification system for human immunodeficiency virus infection in children less than 13 years of age. *MMWR Morb Mortal Wkly Rep* 1994;43(Rr-12):1.

USPHS/IDSA Guidelines for the Prevention of Opportunistic Infections in Persons Infected with Human Immunodeficiency Virus).

Combination antiretroviral therapy should be used to prevent the emergence of drug resistance. Furthermore, when using combination therapy, drugs with different mechanisms of action and different toxicities should be used whenever possible. Several drugs are approved for use in children younger than 13 years. Medications can be divided into the following groups (drugs shown have received approval for pediatric use); nucleoside analogue reverse transcriptase inhibitors NRTIs including zidovudine, didanosine, stavudine, lamivudine, and abacavir; nonnucleoside analogue reverse transcriptase inhibitors NNRTIs such as nevirapine and efavirenz; protease inhibitors PIs such as ritonavir, nelfinavir, and amprenavir; and the fusion inhibitor enfuvirtide.

The treatment of adolescents with HIV-1 infection is similar to that recommended for adults. A detailed discussion of recommended antiretroviral drugs and treatment regimens is beyond the scope of this text. Guidelines for selection and information on medications for pediatric use can be found at http://aidsinfo.nih.gov/

In the case of drug toxicity, an effort should be made to continue the drug if the toxicity is not life-threatening. As an example, in the case of anemia or neutropenia, erythropoietin or granulocyte colony-stimulating factor, respectively, can be used to maintain blood counts. With "appropriate" therapy, the expectation is that the clinical status will remain stable, the CD4 counts will increase or remain stable, and the viral load will become undetectable (less than 400 RNA copies per milliliter of plasma) or have at least a 1 log decrease from baseline.

In children, other issues need to be considered for optimal treatment. Compliance may be difficult for families, particularly when basic needs are not met and the child is on a complex regimen with multiple medications.

PROGNOSIS AND OUTCOME

Pediatric HIV-1 infection is a chronic disease. Markers of disease progression include the clinical, immunologic, and virologic statuses. As HIV-1 disease progression occurs, the CD4 count and percentage decline, and patients with severe immune suppression have the poorest prognosis. The CD4 lymphocyte count should be monitored at least every 3 months, because this value will guide decisions regarding antiretroviral therapy, primary prophylaxis of PCP in a child older than 1 year, and initiation of prophylaxis against atypical M. avium-intracellulare complex. Viral load is used to make decisions regarding the efficacy of treatment and changing drug regimens. Thus, an important consideration is the biological variation when interpreting HIV RNA assay results, and any change in the values over baseline should be confirmed by a second determination.

The prognosis of HIV-1-infected children continues to change with the advent of new antiretroviral therapies.

PREVENTION OF PERINATAL TRANSMISSION

The ability to reduce perinatal transmission of HIV-1 to approximately 8% by administering zidovudine during pregnancy and delivery, and to the newborn for the first 6 weeks of life, has been a major breakthrough. The success of this regimen depends on recognizing women with HIV-1 before or during pregnancy, so they can be counseled regarding therapy for their own disease and using zidovudine for reducing perinatal transmission.

This regimen has become the standard of care for pregnant women in many industrialized countries. However, this regimen is too complex for many developing countries. Studies have shown that shorter courses of zidovudine can reduce perinatal transmission.

Delivery of HIV-1-infected women by elective cesarean section (before rupture of membranes) may reduce perinatal transmission of HIV-1 by as much as 50%. This intervention might be particularly beneficial in a woman who is identified with HIV-1 infection late in pregnancy, does not have the benefit of zidovudine prophylaxis, or both.

Studies have also determined that a single oral dose of nevirapine given to the mother at the onset of labor, with subsequent dosing in her infant with nevirapine within hours of birth, can reduce perinatal transmission rates.

As a better understanding of the mechanisms of perinatal HIV-1 transmission is gained, simpler, more effective and less expensive interventions will likely be developed. This is particularly critical for developing countries where perinatal HIV-1 transmission remains a serious problem.

CHAPTER 103

Influenza Viruses

Adapted from James D. Cherry

Influenza viruses cause acute respiratory infections that usually occur in outbreaks or epidemics. Influenza viral infections in children are associated with considerable morbidity and mortality, and the spectrum of clinical illness is broad.

Influenza viruses are orthomyxoviruses. Three major antigenic types (A, B, and C) and multiple antigenic subtypes have been identified. The surface of the virus is composed of numerous hemagglutinin and neuraminidase "spikes." Inside the virus is a lipid bilayer, a matrix protein, and an RNA nucleocapsid. The nuclear protein is the antigenic basis for typing strains as A, B, or C. Hemagglutinin and neuraminidase antigens are subtype-specific and variable.

Fifteen different hemagglutinin subtypes (H1–H15) and nine neuraminidase subtypes (N1–N9) occur in nature. Each of these subtypes has the potential to combine through genetic reassortment to yield a different viral strain. However, since 1874, only three separate hemagglutinins, H1, H2, and H3, and two separate neuraminidases, N1 and N2, have been recognized in influenza A viruses causing epidemics in humans. Variation in these two antigens (hemagglutinin and neuraminidase) is the basis for antigenic drift and shift in the prevalent viruses. *Drift* implies a minor change in an antigen without a change in subtype; *shift* implies a major change in either hemagglutinin or neuraminidase or both antigens resulting in a change in subtype. Antigenic drift occurs in influenza A and B viruses, but shift occurs only in influenza A.

Nomenclature for the classification of influenza virus strains specifies type, host (for strains of animal origin), geographic source, strain number, and year of isolation. To this, the code designations of hemagglutinin and neuraminidase subtypes are appended. In 1998, prevalent human influenza viral types were represented by A/Wuhan/359/95 (H2N2), A/Bayern/07/95 (H1N1), and B/Beijing/184/93 (H3N2).

EPIDEMIOLOGY

Pandemics of influenza A (such as the one on 1918) result from irregular antigenic shift, the last occurring in 1977. After pandemic influenza of a new subtype, epidemics of generally lesser intensity occur approximately every 2 to 3 years in association with antigenic drift. Outbreaks of influenza B are more variable, occur at roughly 4- to 7-year intervals, and are the result of antigenic drift. Infection with influenza C virus is common in children, but the epidemiologic pattern of this virus is not determined.

Populated areas generally experience some influenza viral activity each year. Epidemics and outbreaks usually occur at times of cooler weather; in the tropics, epidemic disease usually occurs during the rainy season. The highest attack rate of influenza usually occurs in children, followed by secondary peaks of illness in adult populations. Case-fatality rates are greatest in infants and the elderly. Influenza is more likely to be fatal in persons with preexisting heart disease, chronic pulmonary disorders, diabetes mellitus, chronic renal disease, neuromuscular disorders, and neoplasms.

Influenza is spread from person-to-person via the respiratory route. The most common mechanism is inhalation of large airborne particles produced by coughing and sneezing. Spread may also occur by direct or indirect contact with fine-particle aerosols.

PATHOPHYSIOLOGY

The major site of infection is the ciliated epithelium of the respiratory tract. There is early necrosis of nasal and tracheal ciliated cells followed by edema and infiltration with inflammatory cells. Secondary bacterial infection is common.

Pneumonia may result from primary influenza viral infection, bacterial superinfection, or combined bacterial-viral infection. The heart, brain, and lymphoid tissues are sometimes involved in fatal cases of influenza. Specifically, focal and diffuse myocarditis and diffuse cerebral edema have been observed. In addition, Reye syndrome (diffuse encephalopathy and fatty degeneration of the liver) is a complication of influenza, particularly that caused by type B virus in children.

Humoral, secretory, and cell-mediated mechanisms all are involved in influenza infection. In general, natural immunity against influenza A strains lasts approximately 4 years. As increasing antigenic drift occurs, previously infected persons are likely to have symptomatic reinfections; when antigenic shift occurs, antibody from the previous infection offers no protection.

CLINICAL MANIFESTATIONS

Clinical manifestations of influenza follow a 2- to 3-day incubation period. In general, the manifestations of influenza in children fall into two categories based on age. In school-aged children and adolescents, the illness is similar to that which occurs in adults (classic influenza). Illness onset is abrupt with fever, chills, headache, myalgia, and malaise. Temperature varies between 39°C and 41°C and is generally lower in older patients. Systemic complaints, on the other hand, are generally more severe in the older patient. Initially, dry cough and coryza occur, but these symptoms are of lesser concern to the patient than the severe systemic manifestations. Approximately one-half of patients complain of sore throat, which is associated with a nonexudative pharyngitis. Ocular symptoms are common and include tearing, photophobia, burning, and pain with eye movement. In uncomplicated illness, the fever lasts from 2 to 5 days. Occasionally, the temperature shows a biphasic pattern that may or may not be caused by secondary bacterial complications.

The course of illness changes by day 2 to 4 of illness, when the respiratory symptoms become more prominent and the systemic complaints begin to subside. Major coughing—dry and hacking—usually persists for up to a week.

The leukocyte count in uncomplicated influenza is usually normal, but frequently leukopenia (less than 4,500 cells per microliter) occurs. Approximately one-third of patients have a relative lymphopenia, and one-third have a relative neutropenia. In general, approximately 10% of older children have clinical signs and radiographic evidence of pulmonary involvement.

In younger children and infants, the manifestations of influenza viral infections are frequently similar to those of other common respiratory viral infections. Laryngotracheitis, bronchiolitis, and pneumonia all occur. Frequently, primary infection is an undifferentiated febrile upper respiratory illness. Temperature usually exceeds 39.5°C. Affected children appear mildly toxic and have cough, coryza, and irritability. On examination, pharyngitis is usually noted and pulmonary involvement is common. Other findings include vomiting, diarrhea, otitis media, and fleeting erythematous or erythematous maculopapular discrete rashes.

In neonates, influenza infection cannot be distinguished clinically from bacterial sepsis. Lethargy, poor feeding, petechiae, poor peripheral circulation with mottling of skin, and apneic spells all occur.

COMPLICATIONS

Bacterial infections of the respiratory tract (pneumonia, otitis media, and sinusitis) are the most common complications. Acute myositis (influenza B) may occur and is characterized by severe pain and tenderness in the calves and thighs of both legs. Serum creatinine phosphokinase and aspartate immunotransferase levels may be increased.

Although the pathogenesis is obscure, Reye syndrome is a complication of both influenza A and B infections. Other rare complications of influenza viral infections include neurologic manifestations (encephalitis, Guillain-Barré syndrome, and transverse myelitis), pericarditis and myocarditis, and sudden death.

DIAGNOSIS

A clinical diagnosis of influenza can often be made in the community epidemic. The definitive diagnosis of influenza depends on either isolation of virus from respiratory secretions or a significant increase in serum antibody titer during convalescence. Rapid detection techniques (fluorescent antibody and enzyme immunoassay) for influenza antigens in nasopharyngeal epithelial cells are increasingly available.

TREATMENT

Rest, adequate hydration with oral fluids, control of fever and myalgia with acetaminophen, and maintenance of comfortable breathing by means of humidified air and, occasionally, nasal decongestants are the mainstays of treatment. With knowledge of side effects, the physician may prescribe cough suppressants.

Bacterial superinfections are suggested by a prolonged febrile course or recrudescence of fever during early convalescence. Before antibiotic therapy is begun, the site of infection should be identified and appropriate cultures obtained. Most infections are caused by *Streptococcus pneumoniae*, *Streptococcus pyogenes* or, less commonly, *Staphylococcus aureus*.

Antiviral therapy for both prophylaxis and treatment is available for children. These drugs should be strongly considered in children with underlying medical problems (as mentioned above), as this population is at greater risk of complications from influenza. Their use in normal children is increasing but remains more a matter of practice. All drugs show their greatest effectiveness if used within 48 hours form the start of symptoms. Therefore, rapid diagnostic tests should be available.

Amantadine was the first agent approved for children, and it is available for both treatment and prophylaxis in children 1 year old or greater. Amantadine has activity only against influenza A and has CNS side effects (anxiety, lightheadedness) in some patients. Rimantidine is also effective against only influenza A but has fewer side effects than Amantadine. It is approved for prophylaxis for children 1 year old or greater and for treatment of children age 14 or greater. Two newer agents [oseltamivir (Tamiflu) and zanamivir (Relenza)] are neuraminidase inhibitors. Both of these agents are effective against influenza A and B. Oseltamivir is approved for the treatment of influenza A and B in children aged 1 year or greater and for prophylaxis in children age 13 or greater. Zanamivir is approved for the treatment of influenza in patients age 12 or greater. Zanamivir is available only as an oral powder Diskhaler and is not generally recommended in patients with underlying airway diseases.

PREVENTION

Inactivated (split-virus) influenza viral vaccines are safe and effective in preventing influenza if the antigens in the vaccine correlate with circulating influenza viruses. Historically, routine immunization of normal children or adults was not recommended, but this is changing rapidly. In the 2002 to 2003 influenza season, the CDC Advisory Committee on Immunization Practices encouraged influenza vaccine for all children aged 6 to 24 months "whenever feasible." This statement is based on the data suggesting a high rate of hospitalization and complications in this age group. A full policy statement is expected in the near future. Influenza vaccine continues to be recommended for those children with chronic illness, especially cardiovascular disease, chronic pulmonary disease, metabolic diseases such as diabetes, renal insufficiency and neurologic disorders in which weakness or paralysis of respiratory muscles occurs. A live attenuated, cold-adapted nasal influenza vaccine is scheduled to be released in 2003. An extensive discussion on prevention and control of influenza was published in 2002 and is available at http://www.cdc.gov/mmwr/preview/mmwrhtml/rr5103a1.htm

Antiviral agents may be used for chemoprophylaxis in those patients too young for immunization or for those in whom the vaccine is contraindicated, generally those with severe hypersensitivity reactions to vaccine component or eggs. These agents should also be considered when the need for protection against influenza is immediate, as it takes up to 14 days for a vaccine recipient to develop an immune response.

CHAPTER 104
Mumps

Adapted from Larry H. Taber
and Gail J. Demmler

Mumps is a contagious viral illness characterized by swelling of the salivary glands, particularly the parotid glands. In 1934, experiments by Johnson and Goodpasture discovered mumps virus. A vaccine was prepared and licensed in 1968. Mumps is a single-stranded RNA virus, a member of the family Paramyxoviridae, as is measles.

EPIDEMIOLOGY

Mumps is transmitted by direct contact or by infected droplets from the oropharynx. Patients are typically contagious 1 to 2 days (as long as 7 days) prior to parotid swelling and 7 to 9 days after onset of parotid swelling. The incubation period of mumps is approximately 18 days. When endemic in the prevaccine era, mumps had its highest attack rate in 5- to 9-year-old children. Inapparent infection may occur in 40% of infected individuals.

PATHOGENESIS AND PATHOLOGY

After entry into the oropharynx, viral replication takes place with subsequent viremia and involvement of glands or nervous tissue. Affected glands show edema and lymphocyte infiltration.

CLINICAL MANIFESTATIONS

Parotitis

The classic illness of mumps is swelling of the parotid gland (i.e., parotitis). Low-grade fever, headache, malaise, anorexia, and abdominal pain are often present. Unilateral swelling usually occurs first, followed by bilateral parotid involvement. The angle of the jaw is usually not palpable on exam due to parotid swelling. Occasionally, simultaneous involvement of both parotid glands occurs. Unilateral parotid disease occurs in less than 25% of patients. Fever subsides within 1 week and disappears before swelling of the parotid gland resolves, which may require as long as 10 days. Other salivary glands may be involved including both submaxillary and sublingual, and orifices of the ducts may be erythematous and edematous.

Orchitis

Approximately one-third of postpubertal male subjects develop unilateral orchitis, generally following parotitis. Bilateral orchitis occurs much less frequently and, although gonadal atrophy may follow orchitis, sterility is rare even with bilateral involvement. Prepubertal boys may develop orchitis, but it is uncommon in those younger than 10 years.

Orchitis is accompanied by high fever, severe pain, and swelling. Nausea, vomiting, and abdominal pain are not uncommon. Fever and gonadal swelling usually resolve in 1 week, but tenderness may persist.

Meningoencephalitis

Central nervous system infection with mumps is more often characterized by aseptic meningitis rather than a true encephalitis. It usually occurs in the first week after parotitis. Headache, fever, nausea, vomiting, and meningismus are common. Marked changes in sensorium and convulsions are present in encephalitis. In clinically diagnosed meningoencephalitis, a CSF mononuclear pleocytosis occurs. CSF glucose is usually normal. Mumps virus may be isolated from CSF early in the illness. Mumps meningoencephalitis carries a good prognosis and is usually associated with an uneventful recovery.

Other uncommon clinical manifestations of mumps include pancreatitis, thyroiditis, oophoritis, and mastitis.

DIFFERENTIAL DIAGNOSIS

Parotitis caused by other viruses—coxsackieviruses, influenza viruses, and parainfluenza viruses—cannot be differentiated clinically from mumps parotitis. In suppurative parotitis commonly caused by bacteria, involvement is more often unilateral, the parotid gland is very tender, and the overlying skin is erythematous.

Calculus of Stensen's duct, tumors of the parotid gland, and Mikulicz syndrome (a rare benign illness characterized by enlargement of the head and neck glands) should be considered in the differential diagnosis. Mumps meningoencephalitis is indistinguishable from that caused by many other viruses, unless parotitis is present.

DIAGNOSIS

In the past, the diagnosis of mumps was typically made clinically. Today, as mumps is rarely seen in the United States, the lab is often called upon to aid in the diagnosis. Elevations in salivary or pancreatic amylase are usually seen with involvement of these sites. Serum assays for mumps IgM and IgG are readily available through reference labs using enzyme immunoassay technique. Mumps virus can also be grown readily from saliva or swabs of material expressed directly from Stensen's duct and from urine and CSF. Positive viral cultures confirm the diagnosis.

TREATMENT

Treatment of mumps parotitis and other glandular involvement is supportive with analgesica and antipyretics as necessary. Antibiotics are not recommended for parotitis, orchitis, or aseptic meningitis. Respiratory isolation of the hospitalized patient is advised. Patients are considered no longer contagious 9 days after onset of parotid swelling.

PREVENTION

Mumps vaccine, as a component of measles-mumps-rubella vaccine (MMR), is part of the universal immunization schedule in the United States. All children should receive MMR at 12 to 15 months of age. More than 95% of persons receiving a mumps vaccine develop antibody. A second dose of MMR vaccine should be administered at age 4 to 6 years.

Children who have recently received immunoglobulin (IG) should have mumps vaccine delayed at least 3 months, as IG interferes with the immune response to the vaccine.

Allergic reactions to mumps vaccine are not common and few are associated with anaphylaxis. Previous contraindications included egg allergy (as mumps vaccine is produced in chick embryo cell culture) and neomycin allergy. Current recommendations suggest that egg allergy is no longer an absolute contraindication to mumps vaccine (as MMR). It may be prudent to discuss specific cases with an allergist, with the additional consideration of giving MMR vaccine in a controlled setting capable of responding to allergic emergencies.

Adverse reactions with mumps vaccine administration are uncommon, but encephalitis and meningitis have been reported.

For detailed recommendations or contraindications for vaccine administration, the reader is referred to the American Academy of Pediatrics' 2003 report of the Committee on Infectious Diseases (Red Book®).

CHAPTER 105
Parainfluenza Viruses

Adapted from Sarah S. Long

Parainfluenza viruses most often cause simple upper respiratory tract infections but can cause significant morbidity. It is estimated that parainfluenza viruses may be responsible for two-thirds of all cases of croup and up to one-half of upper respiratory tract illnesses

CHARACTERISTICS/IMMUNE RESPONSE

Parainfluenza viruses are single-stranded RNA viruses of the paramyxovirus family. Four types (1, 2, 3, and 4) exist. Surface glycoproteins are important for attachment to host cells and are used for type-specific identification of the viruses. Unlike influenza viruses, parainfluenza viruses have primarily stable antigenic determinants. Primary infection with parainfluenza virus elicits type-specific serum antibody. Infections with parainfluenza viruses do not confer lifetime immunity. Reinfections are common, but involvement of the lower respiratory tract in children is less likely with reinfection.

EPIDEMIOLOGY

Seasonal Occurrence

Parainfluenza virus infections occur year round. Type 1 parainfluenza virus produces epidemics of laryngotracheitis (croup) in young children and laryngitis in older individuals in the late summer to fall. Parainfluenza virus type 2 appears more sporadically and only occasionally rises to epidemic proportions. Parainfluenza virus type 3 predominates in spring and summer in temperate climates and is a major cause of lower respiratory tract disease in infants in the first year of life, second only to respiratory syncytial virus as a cause of bronchiolitis and pneumonia.

Age Incidence

Type 3 parainfluenza virus is one of the most common respiratory tract pathogens of infancy. One-half to two-thirds of infants experience primary infection by 12 months of age. Young infants appear to be protected against types 1 and 2 parainfluenza viruses in the first 6 months of life. Primary infection with types 1 and 2 occurs more gradually infecting one-third of children by age 4 and three-fourths of school-aged children. Primary infections with parainfluenza viruses and reinfections can occur throughout childhood; almost all adults having been infected with types 1 and 3, and the majority having contracted type 2.

TRANSMISSION AND PATHOGENESIS

Transmission occurs readily with close person-to-person contact through direct or indirect contact with large droplets or infected secretions. If protected from drying, parainfluenza virus can remain infectious for up to 10 hours on nonporous surfaces and for much shorter periods on porous surfaces and skin.

The virus attaches to nasal and pharyngeal epithelium and then spreads locally to the larynx and trachea by cell-to-cell transfer. The incubation period is 2 to 6 days. In limited pathologic reports in children, marked necrosis of respiratory tract epithelium, inflammatory edema, and fibrinous exudate are predominant findings. Early mononuclear cell-inflammatory response can be followed by neutrophilic predominance if necrosis or secondary bacterial infection ensues.

Viral shedding is of the highest density and longest duration in young children during primary infection and severe disease. Average duration of shedding for parainfluenza type 1 is 4 to 7 days and for type 3 is 8 to 9 days; however, virus shedding can persist for 2 and 3 weeks, respectively, in previously healthy children and longer in immunodeficient individuals.

CLINICAL MANIFESTATIONS

Upper Respiratory Tract Disease

The common cold is the most frequent clinical manifestation of parainfluenza viruses. Although fever is slightly more common, rhinorrhea, sneezing, sore throat, and cough are indistinguishable from symptoms of rhinovirus. Laryngitis with loss of voice is highly associated with parainfluenza. Acute otitis media and sinusitis are complications of parainfluenza virus infections, sometimes caused directly by the virus but more often by secondary bacterial infection.

Laryngotracheitis and Laryngotracheobronchitis

CLINICAL MANIFESTATIONS

Acute laryngotracheitis and laryngotracheobronchitis are caused most commonly by parainfluenza viruses resulting in the croup syndrome. Initial symptoms are nasal stuffiness and sore throat. Fever ranging from 37.8°C to 40.0°C follows within 24 hours; then hoarseness and a harsh cough become the predominant symptoms. For most patients, the illness progresses no further, and symptoms abate over 3 to 5 days. On examination, affected children have a barking cough, hoarseness, and coryza and, possibly, stridor. In severe disease, progressive obstruction can lead to hypoxia, restlessness, and cyanosis, or prolonged incomplete obstruction can lead to eventual fatigue and respiratory failure.

DIAGNOSIS

The CBC is generally normal. Lateral neck radiography may show distention of the hypopharynx and narrowing and haziness of the subglottic trachea. The epiglottis should be normal.

Virus can be isolated from nasopharyngeal secretions in tissue culture usually within 4 to 7 days. Rapid identification of viral

TABLE 105-1. Clinical Characteristics of Infectious Causes of Upper Airway Obstruction

	Epiglottitis	Laryngotracheitis	Bacteria tracheitis	Retropharyngeal abscess
Peak age	2–7 yr	7–36 mo	7–36 mo	3–24 mo
Prodrome	None to nonspecific URI	Coryza, cough	Coryza, cough	Nonspecific URI
Onset of fever	Sudden, high	Gradual, variable	Variable, frequently with sudden high rise	Sudden, high
Striking feature	Stridor	Stridor or cough	Stridor	Drooling, respiratory distress ± stridor
Other major symptoms				
Hoarseness	–	+++	++	–
Cough	–	+++	++	–
Drooling	+++	–	–	+++
Dysphagia	+++	±	±	+++
Major signs	Severe obstruction, toxicity	Obstruction, mild to no toxicity	Obstruction, toxicity	Toxicity, obstruction
Associated findings	Visibly swollen epiglottis, sniffing	Rhinorrhea, mild pharyngitis	Rhinorrhea, mild pharyngitis	Rhinorrhea, bulging posterior pharynx
Preferred position	Sitting	None	None	Hyperextension of neck

–, not present; ±, sometimes present; ++, frequently present; +++, ballmark of disease; URI, upper respiratory tract infection.

antigen in nasopharyngeal secretions is possible by immunofluorescent and enzyme immunoassays. Serologic diagnosis requiring acute and convalescent specimens is not practical and results may be difficult to interpret due to heterotypic antibodies.

DIFFERENTIAL DIAGNOSIS

Viral laryngotracheitis must be differentiated from the more fulminant infectious disease that can also present with stridor (e.g., epiglottitis, bacterial tracheitis, diphtheria, and retropharyngeal abscess), from life-threatening obstruction by a foreign body, and from spasmodic croup. These distinctions are made on clinical grounds with skillful, unobtrusive examinations and with selective roentgenographic and laboratory tests (Table 105-1). Bacterial tracheitis usually occurs as a secondary infection following viral laryngotracheobronchitis.

TREATMENT

Depending on the patient population considered, a very small percentage of children with acute viral laryngotracheitis require hospitalization. In studies examining those who are hospitalized, less than 10% of these children require tracheal intubation, and less than 1% of these hospitalized children die. In the hospital, therapy is primarily supportive with the following considerations:

- Examinations should be performed rapidly with as few disturbances as possible. The comforting parent should not be separated from the child.
- Although unproven, mist therapy has the potential benefit to soothe the airway and loosen secretions. Oxygen is administered if hypoxemia is documented.
- Antibiotics are not indicated in croup. Their use should be reserved for concern over other infectious processes such as retropharyngeal abscess or bacterial tracheitis.
- Nebulized racemic epinephrine has a short-term beneficial effect to diminish airway mucosal edema. Patients requiring this therapy should be carefully observed after the drug's effect has decreased because of concerns for rebound edema or worsening of their clinical course.
- Steroids have been shown to reduce airway obstruction and the need for hospitalization. Children who are brought in for urgent care for croup should receive a glucocorticoid. A single dose (0.15–0.6 mg/kg) of dexamethasone given intramuscularly or orally or budesonide (2–4 mg) given by nebulization has been shown to be efficacious.

Lower Respiratory Tract Disease

Bronchiolitis caused by parainfluenza viruses (predominantly type 3) progresses from signs of the common cold to wheezing and respiratory distress. These children are clinically indistinguishable form those with respiratory syncytial virus. Parainfluenza virus pneumonia can occur in normal children but can be fatal in children with congenital immunodeficiencies.

Miscellaneous Infections

Parainfluenza viruses have been recovered from infants with acute apneic onset of respiratory tract illnesses and from infants who experience sudden infant death. Parotitis simulating disease caused by mumps virus is associated with parainfluenza virus infection.

PREVENTION

Strict adherence to infection control procedures (contact precautions, in addition to standard precautions) should control nosocomial transmission. Infections with parainfluenza are unavoidable, but parents, children, patients, and staffs of hospitals, schools, child-care centers, and other settings in which children congregate should be careful to wash their hands.

No current vaccine is available but investigation continues.

CHAPTER 106
Parvovirus

Adapted from James D. Cherry

Parvovirus B19 is the cause of erythema infectiosum (fifth disease) and transient red blood cell aplasia (aplastic crisis), as well as other less common clinical manifestations. The virus is a small (23 nm), single-stranded DNA, nonenveloped virus.

EPIDEMIOLOGY

Erythema infectiosum outbreaks are most prevalent in the winter and spring and last for 3 to 6 months. The mode of spread is by droplet via the respiratory tract. The case-to-case interval of erythema infectiosum is usually between 4 and 14 days, and the attack rate is high. Antibody studies indicate the following prevalence data: in children younger than 5 years old, 2% to 9%; in children and adolescents 5 to 18 years old, 15% to 35%; and in adults older than 18 years, 40% to 60%. The studies suggest that many infections are either asymptomatic or unrecognized as B19 viral infections.

PATHOPHYSIOLOGY

After infection via the respiratory tract, viremia occurs in which 10^{10} or 10^{11} viral particles per milliliter of blood may be found. Seven to 10 days after infection, a reticulocytopenia occurs associated with viremia. Early erythrocyte precursor cells are susceptible to B19 virus infection. Neutropenia, lymphopenia, and thrombocytopenia may occur in conjunction with the reticulocytopenia. During the second week of infection, hemoglobin values decrease slightly.

In erythema infectiosum, the exanthem occurs approximately 17 to 18 days after infection. At this time, virus can no longer be detected in throat swabs or blood specimens. At the time of rash, virus-specific 1gM antibody is present. Parvovirus B19 infection is unique, in that no cell-mediated immune response has been demonstrated. In immunocompromised patients who fail to produce effective neutralizing antibodies, persistent infections occur.

CLINICAL MANIFESTATIONS

Erythema Infectiosum

Studies in volunteers suggest that erythema infectiosum is a biphasic illness. Approximately 1 week after infection, a nonspecific febrile illness with headache, chills, malaise, and myalgia occurs. These symptoms last 2 to 3 days, followed by an asymptomatic interlude of approximately 7 days, and then the exanthematous phase of the illness begins.

The exanthem occurs in three stages. The first stage is the appearance of a fiery red rash on the cheeks ("slapped-cheek" appearance) and a relative circumoral pallor. The second stage follows the onset of facial involvement by 1 to 4 days as an erythematous maculopapular rash on the trunk and extremities. Initially, this rash is discrete, but soon it takes on a characteristic lacy or reticular pattern. The third stage of the exanthem is characterized by changes in the intensity of the rash with periodic evanescence and recrudescence. The rash is often pruritic, especially in adults, and is generally more prominent on the extensor surfaces. Occasionally, slight desquamation is noted in some patients. As for other symptoms, joint pain and swelling and myalgia are particularly troublesome in adults.

Arthritis

The most common complication of erythema infectiosum is arthropathy. It is much more common in adults (80%) than children (10%). The illness ranges in severity from mild arthralgia to frank arthritis. Symptoms are usually transient, but some adults may persist for weeks to months. Arthritis is more common in women than in men and most often involves the knees, ankles, and proximal interpharyngeal joints; involvement is usually bilateral. The onset of arthritis usually occurs 1 to 6 days after the onset of the rash, but it has occasionally been noted before the exanthem. Many adults have arthritis without skin manifestations of infection.

Aplastic Crisis

In individuals with hemolytic anemias, acute B19 infection may result in critical depression of hemoglobin concentrations. This transitory arrest of erythrocyte production is termed aplastic crisis and can occur in any individual whose erythrocytes have a short lifespan such as sickle cell anemia, hereditary spherocytosis, and acquired hemolytic anemias. Most patients have fever, malaise, and gastrointestinal symptoms; some also have respiratory symptoms. Typical erythema infectiosum is rare.

Laboratory studies in afflicted patients reveal reticulocyte counts between 0% and 1% and hemoglobin values 10% to 30% less than baseline values.

Intrauterine Infection

Infection in pregnancy may result in fetal hydrops, fetal death, and miscarriage. Studies indicate that maternal B19 virus infections result in a transpiacental transmission rate of 33% and a fetal death rate of 9%.

DIAGNOSIS

Although sometimes confused with scarlet fever or enteroviral infections, erythema infectiosum is a clinical diagnosis. In patients with chronic hemolytic anemia, occurrence of an aplastic crisis is generally assumed to be caused by B19 virus infection. Other causes should be considered such as systemic bacterial infections and marrow-suppressive drugs.

The specific diagnosis of a B19 viral infection can be made by demonstrating B19-specific 1gM antibody in the serum. Polymerase chain reaction (PCR) is becoming readily available. Past infection and immunity is determined by presence of specific B19 serum IgG antibody.

TREATMENT AND PREVENTION

No specific treatment is available for B19 viral infections. Patients with aplastic crisis may require transfusion; otherwise, B19 viral infections rarely require therapy. Arthritis or arthralgia can be treated with nonsteroidal antiinflammatory agents.

In erythema infectiosum outbreaks, pregnant women should, when possible, avoid contact with susceptible school-aged children. If B19 virus infection occurs during pregnancy, the pregnancy should be carefully monitored. At delivery, examination of cord blood or blood from the neonate for virus and IgM antibody reveals whether *in utero* infection occurred. Babies infected *in utero* should be examined periodically for delayed sequelae. Because congenital malformation has not been found to be causally related to B19 virus infection, therapeutic abortion is not indicated for infection during pregnancy.

During erythema infectiosum outbreaks, isolation of exanthematous patients is not useful because the patient is no longer contagious by the time the exanthem occurs. On the other hand, patients with aplastic crisis or immunodeficiency may still be excreting virus and should be isolated from other patients when hospitalized.

CHAPTER 107

Polioviruses

Adapted from James D. Cherry

Polioviruses are a subgroup of the enteroviruses. When a susceptible person is infected with a poliovirus, one of the following responses may occur: inapparent infection, minor illness (abortive poliomyelitis), nonparalytic poliomyelitis (aseptic meningitis), or paralytic poliomyelitis. Infection with and disease caused by polioviruses can be controlled completely by universal immunization. Polioviruses are single-stranded RNA viruses. They are 20 to 30 nm in size and consist of a naked protein capsid and a dense central core of RNA. The three distinct antigenic types of polioviruses are types 1, 2, and 3. Infection with a poliovirus results in lifelong immunity to the homologous virus type, but it confers no immunity to the other two viral types.

EPIDEMIOLOGY

The general epidemiology of polioviruses is similar to that of other enteroviruses and is discussed more fully in Chapter 108, Nonpolio Enteroviruses. Historically, unrecognized infections were the main source of the spread of the virus. In populations with poor sanitation and hygiene, epidemics of poliomyelitis did not occur, but widespread dissemination of polioviruses occurred continually. In such populations, immunizing infections with all three poliovirus types occurred in infants who were usually protected from significant clinical disease by transplacentally acquired antibodies. In populations with improved standards of hygiene, immunizing infections of infants no longer regularly occur, so pools of susceptible children build up in the population. When poliovirus is introduced into such a population, infection occurs in these older children, and poliomyelitis may occur.

The universal use of oral polio vaccines since the early 1960s has resulted in the elimination of infection with wild polioviruses in the Western Hemisphere and much of the developed world. In areas of the world where polio vaccine control measures are not sufficient such as developing countries, endemic and epidemic poliomyelitis continues to occur.

PATHOPHYSIOLOGY

The general pathophysiology of enteroviral infections is presented in Chapter 108, Nonpolio Enteroviruses.

The virus can be recovered from the blood, throat, and feces of the infected person 3 to 5 days after exposure. At this time, minor illness may occur, or the infection may be unrecognized. Major illness with central nervous system (CNS) involvement has its onset approximately 10 days after infection. The neuropathology of poliomyelitis is usually pathopneumonic. Neuronal lesions, caused by multiplication of the virus in the cells, are most common in the anterior horn cells of the spinal cord.

CLINICAL FINDINGS

In susceptible persons, 90% to 95% of infections are inapparent, approximately 4% to 8% are classified as minor illness (abortive poliomyelitis), and rarely does nonparalytic poliomyelitis (aseptic meningitis) or paralytic poliomyelitis develop.

Abortive poliomyelitis (minor illness) is similar to many other enteroviral infections. The illness is mild and nonspecific with low-grade fever, malaise, anorexia, and sore throat. On physical examination, no significant abnormalities are noted.

Nonparalytic Poliomyelitis (Aseptic Meningitis)

Nonparalytic poliomyelitis is similar to aseptic meningitis caused by many other enteroviruses. After a brief flu-like prodrome, the neck, back, and hamstrings become stiff, and sometimes hyperesthesia and paresthesia occur. On physical examination, nuchal rigidity can be observed. The reflexes are usually normal, but observing these over time is important as changes may indicate impending paralysis. The CSF cell count range usually varies from 20 to 300 cells per microliter with a possible predominance of neutrophils early in the illness. In the usual case, recovery occurs in 3 to 10 days.

Paralytic Poliomyelitis

The initial findings in paralytic poliomyelitis are similar to those in nonparalytic poliomyelitis except, occasionally, findings are more pronounced. Fever is likely to be higher, and muscle pain is more conspicuous. Before the onset of actual muscle weakness, superficial and deep tendon reflexes diminish or disappear. Patients destined to develop paralytic poliomyelitis often appear acutely ill, are restless and flushed, and have an anxious expression. Biphasic illness with a symptom-free interlude of several days between the initial illness phase and the occurrence of paralysis is common in paralytic poliomyelitis. The onset of paralysis may be sudden with complete loss of function within a few hours, or it may progress gradually over 3 to 5 days. In general, lower limbs are affected more commonly than upper limbs. Sensory abnormalities usually do not occur.

In bulbar disease, the tenth cranial nerve nuclei are involved most commonly resulting in paralysis of the pharynx, soft palate, and vocal cord. Facial paralysis is less common, and ocular palsies are unusual.

COMPLICATIONS

The most feared complication of paralytic poliomyelitis is respiratory insufficiency. Myocardial failure may occur, but is less common. Patients who have had paralytic poliomyelitis may develop what appear to be new neuromuscular symptoms (weakness) later in life. These symptoms are a result of routine attrition of remaining anterior horn cells associated with aging rather than persistent neural infection with polioviruses.

DIAGNOSIS

If poliovirus infection is ever suspected, specimens for viral studies should be obtained from the throat, stool, and CSF. Since requests to laboratories to isolate poliviruses are unusual, one should check with a hospital or reference lab to verify the lab's capabilities. Poliovirus grows readily in appropriate tissue culture systems, and the presence of an enterovirus is usually noted in 3 to 4 days. Its identification as a poliovirus usually takes another week or so.

The cause of the illness can also be confirmed by examining acute and convalescent serum antibody titers to any or all of the three polioviral types. A fourfold increase in neutralizing antibody titer is indicative of infection. In acute illness, specific IgM neutralizing antibody for a specific poliovirus type is also diagnostic.

TREATMENT

The treatment of nonparalytic poliomyelitis is supportive. Patients with paralytic disease should be hospitalized and closely observed for impaired ventilation. Mechanical ventilation or tracheostomy may be needed. Patients with poliomyelitis are usually fully conscious and aware. All procedures relating to their care should be explained to them to reduce anxiety.

PREVENTION

Poliomyelitis is a vaccine-preventable disease. Its control has been achieved in many areas of the world. In 1988, the World Health Assembly set an objective of global polio eradication by the year 2000. Although this goal has not yet been achieved, progress is being made. The program is based on four components: (a) maintenance of high vaccine coverage, (b) development of effective disease surveillance, (c) supplementary vaccine doses to all children during national immunization days, and (d) "mopping-up" vaccination campaigns in high-risk areas.

Polio vaccines are available in two forms, trivalent live oral poliovirus vaccine (OPV) and trivalent formalin-inactivated parenterally administered poliovirus vaccine (IPV). OPV induces intestinal immunity, is simple to administer, is well accepted by patients, and results in immunization of some contacts of vaccinated persons. In rare instances, however, (approximately 1 case per 800,000 first doses of vaccine), administration of OPV causes paralysis in healthy recipients or their contacts. This phenomenon is referred to as vaccine-associated paralytic polio (VAPP). In contrast with OPV, IPV is less likely to result in herd immunity, is more difficult to administer, and produces a lesser degree of intestinal immunity; it lacks the ability to immunize contacts of some immunized persons and necessitates booster doses in older children and adults.

Because of concerns for VAPP, the 2003 universal immunization schedule approved by the American Academy of Pediatrics and the Centers for Disease Control and Prevention (CDC) Advisory committee on Immunization Practices includes only IPV to be given at 2 months, 4 months, 6 to 18 months and 4 to 6 years (4 total doses). More information on polio vaccine is available at http://www.cdc.gov/nip/publications/pink/polio.pdf

CHAPTER 108
Nonpolio Enteroviruses

Adapted from James D. Cherry

The nonpolio enteroviruses consist of coxsackieviruses, echoviruses, and enteroviruses. They are grouped together because their natural habitat is the alimentary tract; they share common features in their epidemiology, clinical spectrum, and pathogenesis. The enteroviruses belong to the Picornaviridae (pico, small; RNA, ribonucleic acid) family; they are single-stranded RNA viruses. Twenty-three coxsackieviruses compose group A, and six coxsackieviruses compose group B; 32 echoviruses and four more newly identified enteroviruses (designated enteroviruses 68–71) also exist.

EPIDEMIOLOGY

Human spread is from person to person (child to child) by fecal–oral and, possibly, oral–oral (respiratory spread) routes. The incidence of infection and disease is inversely related to age. Epidemics and outbreaks depend on new susceptible individuals in the population; type-specific immunity is thought to protect against symptomatic reinfection. In temperate climates, enteroviral infections occur primarily in the summer and fall; in the tropics, infections regularly occur throughout the year.

PATHOPHYSIOLOGY

After an individual is exposed, an enterovirus attaches in the pharynx and the lower alimentary tract. The infection quickly spreads to the regional lymph nodes, the virus multiplies, and a minor viremia occurs on approximately the third day. This viremia results in involvement in many secondary infection sites, and viral multiplication in these sites coincides with the onset of clinical symptoms 4 to 6 days after exposure. As the virus multiplies at the secondary infection sites, a major viremia begins during days 3 to 7 of infection. Central nervous system involvement may occur as a result of the initial minor viremia, or it may be delayed and be the result of major viremia. Major viremia usually lasts for 3 to 7 days. Cessation of viremia correlates with the appearance of antibody and the beginning of clinical recovery. Infection may continue, however, in the lower intestinal tract for prolonged periods.

Enteroviral illnesses vary from clinically unrecognized to severe fatal illnesses. The most striking findings in severe cases are in the heart (myocarditis), brain and spinal cord (meningitis and encephalitis), lungs (pneumonitis), adrenals (cortical necrosis), and liver (hepatic necrosis).

CLINICAL FINDINGS

Virtually all children have one or more enteroviral infections each summer and fall. Many illnesses and syndromes can be caused by different coxsackieviral, echoviral, and enteroviral types. In a few instances, clinical characteristics indicate one or two specific enteroviral types.

Enteroviruses may be excreted in stool for months after acute infection, and the finding of an enterovirus on a particular day is no indication of when the infection first occurred. Although most enterovirus infections appear to go unrecognized, likely most affected persons have some symptoms, but usually the illnesses are trivial. The available data suggest that, on average, 50% or less of all infections are asymptomatic.

Nonspecific Febrile Illness

Nonspecific febrile illness is the most common manifestation of nonpolio enteroviral infections. Fever usually lasts 2 to 4 days and ranges in between 38.3°C and 40.0°C. Headache, malaise, anorexia, nausea, vomiting, and diarrhea may occur.

Respiratory Manifestations

The most common respiratory manifestation of enterovirus infection (particularly in summer) is pharyngitis. Headache and myalgia are frequent in older children. Symptoms in younger children are not often referable to the throat, and the presentation may be nonspecific such as fever, malaise, etc.

Herpangina is an enteroviral pharyngitis with a characteristic enanthem. Vesicles and ulcers 1 to 2 mm in diameter appear on the anterior tonsillar pillars, soft palate, uvula, tonsils, pharyngeal wall and, occasionally, the posterior buccal surfaces. Group A coxsackieviruses, most group B coxsackieviruses, and many echoviruses also cause herpangina.

The common lower respiratory illnesses of children such as croup, bronchiolitis, and pneumonia may be caused by enteroviral infections. Infection with enterovirus may act as a trigger for asthma in the susceptible child.

Pleurodynia (Bornholm disease) is a another specific enteroviral syndrome. Although an epidemic disease in the past, today in the United States, most cases occur sporadically and outbreaks are rare. Furthermore, many adults and older children (the typical age group) are probably diagnosed incorrectly. The onset of illness is characterized by sudden occurrence of muscular, variable intensity pain, typically located in the chest or upper abdomen. The pain can be severe and may occur in spasms that last from a few minutes to several hours. During spasms, patients may have pallor, rapid, shallow, grunting respirations that suggest pneumonia or pleural inflammation. In older children and adults, the pain is often described as stabbing or knife-like; in adults, the illness can be confused with a heart attack. The symptoms usually last only 1 to 2 days but, frequently, the illness is biphasic, so a patient apparently recovers only to have a recurrence several days later.

Gastrointestinal Manifestations

Gastrointestinal manifestations are almost universal in nonpolio enteroviral infections. Some manifestations such as nausea, vomiting, and diarrhea are very common but not usually severe and are only a part of a more general overall illness.

Ocular Manifestations

Mild conjunctivitis occurs frequently in many enteroviral illnesses, but it is not usually troublesome. A specific acute hemorrhagic conjunctivitis, however, may occur in major epidemics, often in school-aged children. This illness is caused mainly by enterovirus 70 or coxsackievirus A24. The illness has a sudden onset with severe eye pain, photophobia, blurred vision, lacrimation, erythema and congestion of the eye. Subconjunctival hemorrhages occur, and transient punctate epithelial keratitis, conjunctival follicles, and preauricular lymphadenopathy are frequently noted. The illness lasts 7 to 12 days.

Cardiovascular Manifestations

Pericarditis and myocarditis are infrequent but important, severe manifestations of nonpolio enteroviruses. The group B coxsackieviruses have been implicated most frequently. Group B coxsackieviruses are also an etiologic factor in some cases of acute myocardial infarction in young adults.

Genitourinary Manifestations

Group B coxsackieviruses are second only to mumps as causative agents of orchitis. Orchitis frequently occurs as a second phase in a biphasic illness; the initial phase is usually nonspecific febrile illness, aseptic meningitis, or pleurodynia.

Skin Manifestations

The nonpolio enteroviruses cause a variety of skin manifestations. In summer and fall, enteroviruses are the leading cause of exanthem in children.

Echovirus 9 is the agent most commonly associated with exanthem in children. This exanthem is erythematous, maculopapular, and usually discrete. Often the exanthem is petechial and is noted in association with aseptic meningitis. The illness mimics meningococcemia.

The hand-foot-and-mouth syndrome, which is most commonly caused by coxsackievirus A16, is a clearly recognizable enteroviral illness. The exanthem is predominantly vesicular and located on the hands, feet, and buttocks. The enanthem usually involves the anterior mouth and consists of large ulcerative lesions (herpangina).

Neurologic Manifestations

Aseptic meningitis is the most common form of neurological illness from the nonpolio enteroviruses. Paralytic illness similar to that caused by the polioviruses is also an occasional manifestation of the nonpolio enteroviruses. Paralysis caused by the nonpolio enteroviruses is usually less severe and causes less residual damage.

Neonatal Infections

Although neonatal infections with enteroviruses may be mild, a significant number are particularly severe, and deaths are not uncommon. In particular, the infections may be generalized with both myocarditis and meningoencephalitis. Of particular importance is a sepsis-like illness characterized by fever, poor feeding, abdominal distention, irritability, rash, lethargy, and hypotonia. Patients may also have diarrhea, vomiting, seizures, and apnea. Severe fatal illness are most often caused by echovirus 11. In fatal cases, jaundice, hepatitis, disseminated intravascular coagulation, thrombocytopenia, and hypotension occur.

Chronic Enteroviral Infections in Patients with Agammaglobulinemia

Chronic unusual infections in children with agammaglobulinemia caused by a variety of enteroviruses have been reported. The most common illness is meningoencephalitis; arthritis and polymyositis also frequently occur. Echovirus 11 has been the most common cause of chronic infection.

DIAGNOSIS

Enteroviral diseases can often be suspected based on the season of the year, geographic location, exposure, incubation period, and clinical symptoms. Because some enteroviral infections mimic severe but treatable bacterial illnesses (meningitis and septicemia), situations frequently occur for which treatment with antimicrobial therapy should be administered until a bacterial etiology is ruled out.

Specimens for viral culture should be collected from multiple sites such as throat, stool and CSF or other fluid (if available). Isolation of an enterovirus as a cause of a specific illness frequently takes less than 1 week. Polymerase chain reaction (PCR) for the rapid diagnosis of enteroviral infections is becoming more available. This test may be helpful in avoiding unnecessary hospitalization and therapy for some illnesses that appear to be bacterial in origin. Many commercial laboratories offer serologic diagnostic panels for enteroviruses. These panels are expensive and lack sensitivity and specificity leading to erroneous diagnoses. Only in certain circumstances when specific etiologies are suspected, will an antibody titer increase be useful in confirming a clinical diagnosis.

Therapy

Therapy generally consists of supportive care for these infections. In severe enteroviral infections such as those that occur in neonates, one may consider giving intravenous immune globulin to the patient, but true efficacy is not proven. Immune globulin has a limited beneficial effect in the treatment of subacute and chronic enteroviral infections in patients with immune deficiencies.

Prevention

Because killed and live viral vaccines for the polioviruses have been extraordinarily effective, similar vaccines could be developed for other enteroviruses. If a specifically virulent enteroviral type were to emerge, a new vaccine could possibly be developed.

CHAPTER 109

Respiratory Syncytial Virus

Adapted from Sarah S. Long

RSV is the most important lower respiratory tract pathogen of early life. Three million children younger than 4 years are infected annually, approximately 100,000 require hospitalization, and 2% to 5% of those hospitalized develop respiratory failure.

CHARACTERISTICS OF THE VIRUS

RSV is an RNA virus closely related to measles. Two RSV groups (A and B) differ primarily in the largest surface glycoprotein, the G protein, whereas the fusion glycoprotein, the F protein, is conserved.

Infection with the virus stimulates both humoral and cellular immune responses. Cellular response appears to be important in halting viral replications, and humoral response is most important in preventing symptomatic reinfection. Antibody delivered passively by placenta gives protection against disease transiently. Immunity after infection is variable, incomplete, and not durable.

EPIDEMIOLOGY

Age Incidence

Studies detail that the RSV infection rate is 69% in the first year of life and 83% in the second year of life. Approximately one-half of the children have a recurrence of RSV infection by age 2 years. Rates of infection, severe disease manifestations, and mortality are highest at 2 to 6 months of age. Infants and adults can have recurrent RSV infection during the same season. Although lower respiratory tract symptoms and fever are less frequent with age and reinfection, adults usually display some symptomatology.

Seasonal Occurrence

In temperate regions, outbreaks of bronchiolitis peak annually in midwinter to spring (December through April, with local variations from late fall). There is a near absence of RSV activity from August through October. Group A and B viruses circulate in the same season, but infection with group A viruses appear to produce more severe disease. During epidemic periods, 80% or more of cases of bronchiolitis are caused by RSV; in nonepidemic periods, less than 50% are RSV related.

Transmission

Human transmission is usually by direct or close contact with contaminated nasal secretions. Large droplets play a more important role than small-droplet aerosols. A major mode of transmission is via hand contact with contaminated secretions or fomites to the eyes or nasal mucosa of one's self or another person. Virus can remain infectious on nonporous surfaces for more than 6 hours and at least 30 minutes on skin. The period of viral shedding is usually 3 to 8 days, but it can be longer, especially in young infants (and immunocompromised individuals) who may shed virus for up to 3 to 4 weeks. Hospital patients and staff are major vectors in the transmission of RSV.

PATHOPHYSIOLOGY

The virus has tropism for ciliated respiratory epithelium, eventually leading to varying degrees of pulmonary obstruction, due to peribronchial inflammation and mucosal plugging of lumens caused by edema. This can lead to the classic findings of bronchiolitis with areas of emphysematous overaeration and atelectatic underaeration. Interstitial pneumonia may be present.

Pathologic and clinical manifestations likely result from both direct viral infection and host immune response. Immunocompromised individuals may have fatal infection. Immunopathologic mechanisms are suggested by recovery of RSV-specific IgE antibody in nasal secretions in infants with bronchiolitis and the infrequent manifestation of bronchiolitis in RSV-infected immunocompromised individuals.

CLINICAL MANIFESTATIONS

RSV causes many forms of clinical illness including upper respiratory tract infection, acute otitis media, laryngotracheobronchitis, bronchiolitis, and pneumonia. Young infants are at risk for apnea or may manifest a sepsis-like syndrome with lethargy, fussiness, and poor feeding. Manifestations such as myocarditis and central nervous system disease are rare in RSV infection but have been reported.

Bronchiolitis

Bronchiolitis, the most commonly diagnosed illness caused by RSV, is a clinical manifestation of acute viral infection in which obstruction of small airways is the predominant feature.

CLINICAL PRESENTATION

A timeline of bronchiolitis caused by RSV is presented in Fig. 109-1. Rhinorrhea is the usual initial event, followed by fever in at least 50% of cases, fussiness, poor feeding, and cough. Cough progresses over 3 to 5 days, wheezing occurs, and dyspnea ensues. Respiratory distress is the reason for hospitalization of most infants. The chest may be barrel shaped and grunting and wheezing can be audible. Auscultation reveals bilateral diffuse high-pitched expiratory wheezes and changeable inspiratory rhonchi and rales. Otitis media, pharyngeal hyperemia, and conjunctivitis can be present. Hyperinflation of the lungs may push the liver and spleen into palpable positions in the abdomen.

Apnea appears to occur at an increased frequency with RSV bronchiolitis. Respiratory pauses of 15 seconds and longer have occurred during hospitalization in nearly 20% of patients in retrospective studies. Apnea is occasionally the reason for hospitalization; almost invariably it disappears within 48 hours of hospitalization. Premature or very young infants and those with a history of apnea are more prone to this event.

LABORATORY FINDINGS

Abnormalities in the peripheral white blood cell count are so variable as to be of little use. Chest radiography often shows overinflated lungs and flattened hemidiaphragms. Peribronchial thickening is common. Atelectasis is common, peripheral interstitial infiltrates are less frequent, and lobar consolidation is even less common.

Virus is present in nasal secretions for 24 hours before the onset of symptoms and persists for 4 to 21 days. Rapid confirmation of specific RSV etiology is useful clinically, aids cohorting of infected children, and reduces nosocomial spread. Both enzyme immunoassays and a direct immunofluorescent antibody technique identify at least 85% of cases subsequently confirmed by virus isolation; fluorescent antibody is slightly more sensitive and specific. The sensitivity of antigen detection tests and culture is only as good as the specimen; nasal wash by instillation of 5 mL of isotonic saline and aspiration (by aspirator bulb or suction catheter) is superior to nasal swab. Because RSV is associated with the cell, epithelial cells must be abundant in the specimen to ensure an adequate examination.

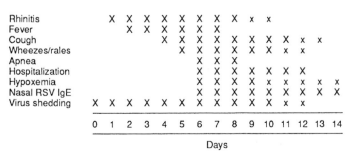

	0	1	2	3	4	5	6	7	8	9	10	11	12	13	14
Rhinitis		X	X	X	X	X	X	X	X	x	x				
Fever			X	X	X	X	X	X							
Cough					X	X	X	X	X	X	X	X	x	x	
Wheezes/rales						X	X	X	X	X	X	x	x		
Apnea							X	X	X						
Hospitalization							X	X	X	X	X	X	X		
Hypoxemia							X	X	X	X	x	x	x	x	x
Nasal RSV IgE							X	X	X	X	X	X	X	X	X
Virus shedding	X	X	X	X	X	X	X	X	X	X	X	x	x		

Days

Figure 109-1. Average duration of signs, symptoms, and laboratory findings for untreated respiratory syncytial virus (*RSV*) bronchiolitis. X, feature; x, diminished feature.

COURSE OF ILLNESS

Fever generally resolves over the first 2 days and respiratory symptoms may worsen for 3 days then show gradual improvement. Mild wheezing may be present for a week or more.

The course of RSV disease may be severe in those patients with congenital heart disease, especially when pulmonary hypertension exists. Mortality from RSV bronchiolitis in these patients is as high as 30%. Children with bronchopulmonary dysplasia, certain congenital anomalies, neuromuscular disorders, malnutrition, and congenital or acquired abnormalities of immunologic function also have excessive morbidity and mortality.

TREATMENT

Supportive care is the cornerstone of treatment for RSV bronchiolitis. Parenteral fluids, used judiciously, may be required for those infants unable to feed due to respiratory distress. Pulmonary fluid volume is increased by the disease process and excessive administration of fluid can interfere with gaseous exchange, especially in children with lung or congenital heart disease. Humidified oxygen is generally given to maintain the oxygen saturation greater than 94%. Frequent nasal suctioning often relieves upper airway obstruction and can help with respiratory distress.

The antiviral drug Ribavirin is approved for hospitalized children with RSV infection, but this drug suffers from high cost and a cumbersome delivery system. Its use has fallen out of favor recently, but it should still be considered for those children with severe disease or underlying conditions that put them at great risk for high morbidity and mortality with RSV.

The use of corticosteroids in the treatment of RSV bronchiolitis has been shown to be of no benefit in controlled studies. As secondary bacterial infections are unusual, antibiotic therapy is not warranted for most children with RSV bronchiolitis.

Bronchodilator Therapy

A subgroup of infants (difficult to identify prior to therapy) may respond to these agents. As a result, a carefully monitored trial of a bronchodilators (usually aerosolized) seems warranted for most patients. The physician should carefully monitor for any side effects and should discontinue the drug if it has no perceived benefit.

OUTCOME

The relationship of bronchiolitis in infancy to recurrence of wheezing in infancy and childhood (rate of greater than 50%) has been appreciated for some time; reasons appear to be multifactorial. Long-term studies have documented persistent abnormalities of pulmonary function and airway hyperreactivity for months to years after infection.

PREVENTION

Passive Prophylaxis

RSV intravenous immune globulin (RSV-IGIV), prepared from donors selected for high titers of RSV-neutralizing antibody, was approved by the Food and Drug Administration in 1996 for use in prevention of severe RSV in those children younger than 24 months with bronchopulmonary dysplasia or a history of premature birth ($\leq$35 weeks of gestation). Monthly infusions of RSV-IGIV (750 mg/kg) from November through March resulted in an approximate 50% reduction of significant RSV illness and

TABLE 109-1. Recommendations for Prophylactic Use of Palivizumab or Respiratory Syncytial Virus Intravenous Immune Globulin*

Should be considered for infants and children <2 years with chronic lung disease (CLD) who have required medical therapy within the 6 months before the anticipated respiratory syncytial virus season. Those with more severe CLD may benefit from prophylaxis for two respiratory syncytial virus seasons.
Infants born ≤32 weeks' gestation without CLD may benefit; risk factors to consider are gestational age and chronologic age at start of RSV season.
Infants born at ≤28 weeks' gestation may benefit from prophylaxis up to 12 months of age.
Infants born at 29 to 32 weeks' gestation may benefit from prophylaxis up to 6 months of age.
Children with severe immunodeficiencies may benefit.

*Prophylaxis is not approved by the Food and Drug Administration for patients with congenital heart disease. Prophylaxis may benefit children who have an indication for its use who have asymptomatic acyanotic congenital heart disease.
Summarized from the American Academy of Pediatrics, Committee on Infectious Diseases, Committee on Fetus and Newborn. Prevention of respiratory syncytial virus infections: indications for the use of palivizumab and update on the use of RSV-IGIV. *Pediatrics* 1998;102:1211.

associated hospitalization. Studies of infants with congenital heart disease suggested modest benefit for those with acyanotic disease and possible detriment for those with cyanotic disease; RSV-IGIV is currently contraindicated in the latter group. Monthly infusions of this drug are extraordinarily costly in dollars and resources. As a result, and because of the development of monoclonal antibody, use of RSV-IGIV is currently limited.

In mid-1998, a genetically engineered RSV monoclonal antibody (palivizumab) was approved for use similar to that of RSV-IGIV. Palivizumab is a mouse monoclonal antibody to the fusion glycoprotein of RSV that is grafted onto a human immunoglobulin backbone. In a multicenter trial involving 1,500 children, monthly intramuscular injections of palivizumab, 15 mg/kg per dose, compared with saline placebo, were associated with 55% overall reduction in RSV-related hospitalizations. For most circumstances, palivizumab is favored over RSV-IGIV by the American Academy of Pediatrics (AAP) because of the convenience of intramuscular injection, elimination of primary risks of IGIV (which is a blood product), and lack of interference with the immunization schedule. Indications for use are similar (Table 109-1); monthly injections from fall through spring (depending on RSV activity in the practice area) are still required.

Vaccine

There is currently no approved vaccine for RSV, but research is ongoing.

Control Measures

In hospitals, early identification and isolation or cohorting of patients with documented RSV infection is important to reduce risk for susceptible children. Contact precaution isolation procedures include care providers wearing gowns, gloves, and often masks. Meticulous hand washing and caregiver care to avoid self-inoculation is also necessary.

CHAPTER 110
Rhinoviruses

Adapted from Robert L. Atmar, Elliot C. Dick, and Rebecca L. Byers

Rhinoviruses (RVs) cause approximately 30% to 50% of all acute respiratory illness. RVs are associated primarily with the common cold, but they may also be involved in bronchitis, sinusitis, pneumonia, and acute exacerbations of asthma.

First isolated in 1954, at least 101 serotypes of RV have been identified. The genus name reflects the prominent nasal involvement. After attaching to a cell, the RV is likely endocytosed within a vesicle, then the RNA is released into the cytoplasm. Viral replication occurs in the cytoplasm, and viruses are released by cell lysis.

EPIDEMIOLOGY

RV infections are found in varying degrees year round, but they show the greatest incidence from spring through early fall. Several RV serotypes usually circulate simultaneously and frequently coincident with other respiratory viruses. Unlike some major respiratory viruses [e.g., parainfluenza types 1 and 3 and respiratory syncytial virus (RSV)], individual RV serotypes seldom recur within a population from year to year. The incidence of RV infections is highest in infants and lowest in older individuals. Prevalence studies show RV antibodies begin to appear early, increase throughout childhood and adolescence, peak in early adulthood, then stabilize for years.

TRANSMISSION

School children are the most important reservoir of RVs; home and school are locations of the highest rate of transmission. Long-term contact with individuals with RV infections may be required for transmission to occur. Even then, transmission rates approach only 50%. Thus, short contacts such as those that occur when shopping, attending movies, and visiting a physician's waiting room are reasonably risk free.

PATHOGENESIS AND COURSE OF INFECTION

Most infection is presumed to be by the respiratory route, although infection by the conjunctival route has been demonstrated. The incubation period is normally 2 to 3 days. RVs replicate well in the upper respiratory tract and generally cause rhinorrhea and nasal obstruction. Cough is usually present even in mild RV colds. RVs have been found in the lower bronchi, but no compelling evidence exists of viral replication in the lower respiratory tract.

RVs may be shed in large amounts (1,000–1 million infectious particles per milliliter of nasal washing) during the first 2 to 3 days of a cold and may continue to be produced for nearly a month. RVs seem to cause only mild pathologic changes in cells of the respiratory tract, even when producing a marked local response. Local secretion of kinins or other cytokines such as the interleukins can cause varied symptoms of inflammation. Approximately 24 hours after infection, a sharp increase in nasal IgA secretion occurs. After approximately 1 week, virus-specific antibody, predominantly IgA, appears in the nasal passages, tears, and parotid saliva. Serum antibody, usually IgG, appears at approximately 1 week and peaks at 1 month; however, specific serum antibody may not form in as many as 50% of cases. The presence of serum antibody correlates positively with immunity, and resistance to infection is related to amount.

CLINICAL MANIFESTATIONS

RV infections in any age group usually cause only mild respiratory tract illnesses (i.e., common colds with simple coryza). Complete recovery usually occurs in 1 or 2 weeks. However, since the discovery of the first RV serotypes, these viruses have been shown to cause serious lower respiratory illness, especially in young children. RVs are implicated in exacerbations of asthma and cases of bronchiolitis, pneumonia, sinusitis, and acute otitis media. In some studies, RV illnesses could not be differentiated clinically from severe lower tract illnesses attributable to RSV.

Acute otitis media (AOM) is primarily a bacterial disease, but it is often preceded or accompanied by a viral upper respiratory illness. Evidence for viral extension from the nasopharynx to the middle ear exists. From 1987 through 1988, pediatricians in Finland used traditional cell culture methodology to study the role of RVs in children with AOM. Viruses were detected in 42%; RV predominated over RSV by 24% to 13%.

DIAGNOSIS

RV infections cause such a wide spectrum of respiratory illness that diagnosing them clinically is not possible. Subclinical shedding from well children in the United States ranges from 0.8% to 11.0%. If an attempt to isolate the virus is clinically useful, nasal specimens are superior to throat swabs for RV. The virus can be isolated relatively easily if details of specimen collection and culture procedures are followed; however, because more than 100 serotypes exist and none is predictably predominant, clinical diagnosis by serologic methods is impractical because it is costly. Use of the polymerase chain reaction (PCR) has increased the identification of RV infections 50- to 200-fold compared with culture alone. No methods currently exist for rapid diagnosis of RV infection.

PREVENTION AND THERAPY

Because of the number of serotypes, development of a conventional vaccine is unlikely. Several potential antiviral drugs are in clinical trial. Interferon-alpha is a protein produced as part of the host's natural antiviral defense and is now produced by genetic recombinant methods. It can be administered by nasal spray to family members after symptoms appear in an index case; studies have shown this to be effective in preventing 80% of secondary RV colds. A combination of rapid diagnosis and family prophylaxis with interferon-alpha may be especially helpful for family members with asthma or a propensity to complications from rhinovirus infections.

CHAPTER 111
Roseola and Human Herpesviruses

Adapted from Julia A. McMillan and Charles F. Grose

GENERAL FEATURES OF ROSEOLA

Typically, roseola affects infants and young children between the ages of 6 months and 3 years with 80% of the cases occurring before age 18 months. Characteristically, roseola is manifested by an initial fever that may have an abrupt onset. The fever may reach 40.0°C to 40.5°C (104°F–105°F) and typically persists, either continuously or intermittently, for 3 to 4 days. During this febrile period, some infants will be described as intermittently irritable, while others maintain near-normal appetite and behavior.

There are few distinguishing findings during the febrile period. Sometimes, palpebral edema is described, and careful examination usually reveals suboccipital lymphadenopathy. Mild erythema of the pharynx may be seen in approximately one-third of affected patients. Sometimes, a bulging or tense fontanelle is noted in young infants with roseola. In this case, investigation and presumptive treatment for meningitis may be indicated. If laboratory studies are undertaken, a low to low-normal white blood cell count with a predominance of lymphocytes may be noted.

The rash of roseola coincides with the abrupt termination of the febrile period. The rash is pale pink (rose) with discrete macules or, less commonly, maculopapules, predominantly on the neck and trunk. It persists for 1 to 2 days, but it may last only a few hours. Pruritus and desquamation are not seen. The complication associated most frequently with roseola is simple febrile seizure.

EPIDEMIOLOGY

Most frequently, roseola occurs in the spring and fall. Historically, investigators demonstrated that blood or serum obtained during the febrile period from a child with roseola could produce a similar clinical illness when injected into another child with no history of roseola. These individuals and subsequent investigators have suggested that roseola is transmitted to infants and young children when a latent virus is shed intermittently by mother or other adult caregiver, probably in the saliva.

HUMAN HERPESVIRUS 6

Until 1986, the family of human herpesviruses included five members: herpes simplex viruses type 1 (oral) and type 2 (genital), varicella-zoster virus, cytomegalovirus, and Epstein-Barr virus. In 1986, a novel virus was isolated from the white blood cells of adult patients with various lymphomas associated with HIV. The virus had several characteristics in common with other herpesviruses, and DNA sequence analysis indicated some homology with the human CMV genome. The new virus was designated *human herpesvirus type 6* (HHV-6); HHV-6 has been divided into two subgroups called *strain A* and *strain B*. The primary cell tropism is the T lymphocyte ($CD4^+/CD8^-$).

In 1988, HHV-6 was isolated from the white blood cells of four otherwise healthy infants with clinical roseola syndrome and suggested that HHV-6 is the etiologic agent of the long-suspected viral disease. Subsequent serologic studies indicated that maternally derived antibody to HHV-6 is present in most infants at time of birth; after these titers decline, infection with HHV-6 commonly occurs during the first 18 months of life.

Primary HHV-6 infection has been associated with a variety of clinical illnesses in addition to roseola. Isolation of HHV-6 from peripheral blood mononuclear cells concomitant with a rise in antibody against HHV-6 has been reported for 14% of the children younger than 2 years and presenting with fever to a pediatric emergency center. Subsequently, rash was observed in only a minority of these children, but many of them had otitis media. HHV-6 infection has also been documented during illness associated with rash but no fever. Other findings described in infants with primary HHV-6 infection include diarrhea, pneumonia, hepatomegaly, hepatocellular dysfunction, intussusception and, most important, febrile seizures. Complete recovery from infection in these patients has been the rule. Once infected, immunity to HHV-6 is thought to be lifelong.

DIAGNOSIS AND ANTIVIRAL TREATMENT

Roseola is a clinical diagnosis that most often needs no virologic confirmation. If necessary, the most available approach for diagnosis of HHV-6 infection is measurement of specific serum IgM and IgG antibody. HHV-6 can be diagnosed by isolating the virus from white blood cells but this is cumbersome. Polymerase chain reaction (PCR) of HHV-6 DNA in lymphocytes is widely available.

Most cases of HHV-6 infection presenting as clinical roseola need no specific treatment but for supportive care. In a few instances such as severe HHV-6 hepatitis, antiviral treatment is a consideration with medications already approved for the treatment of other herpesviruses. Preliminary results show that HHV-6 behaves, as does CMV; that is, HHV-6 replication is inhibited readily by both ganciclovir and foscarnet but is not affected by acyclovir. However, it should be noted that ganciclovir and foscarnet are not approved for serious HHV-6 infection in humans (as of May 2003).

CHAPTER 112
Rubella

Adapted from Larry H. Taber
and Gail J. Demmler

Rubella is an acute infectious disease characterized by low-grade fever, erythematous maculopapular rash, and adenopathy. Attenuated rubella virus vaccine was developed in the late 1960s and licensed in the United States in 1969. Vaccine use in children and in women of childbearing age dramatically reduced the number of cases of postnatally acquired rubella and congenital rubella. Congenital rubella syndrome is discussed elsewhere in this book. Rubella refers to a single type of RNA virus.

POSTNATALLY ACQUIRED RUBELLA

Pathogenesis and Epidemiology

Natural infection with rubella virus occurs only in humans. Oral droplets are the primary means of transmission in acquired rubella. Congenital rubella is transmitted transplacentally. The virus replicates in nasopharyngeal mucosa, then involves regional lymphatics with a subsequent viremic phase. An infected person is most contagious 1 week prior to development of rash. This period of maximum communicability ends a week after the appearance of the rash.

Infected hosts develop both humoral and cell-mediated immunity. After infection, antibodies in both IgM and IgG classes develop rapidly after the appearance of the rash. Rubella-specific IgM antibody usually persists for approximately 12 weeks and may aid in the diagnosis of an acute infection. Antibodies of the IgG class persist for life.

After widespread immunization with rubella vaccine, incidence rates of reported rubella decreased steadily and reached an all-time low in 1988. In the 1990s, however, outbreaks of rubella have been described in Pennsylvania and California. Rubella incidence has increased in persons older than 15 years with Hispanics being a particular risk group. Data from outbreaks suggest that failure to vaccinate, not primary or secondary vaccine failure, was responsible for this increase in rubella.

Clinical Manifestations

Incubation periods for postnatal rubella range from 14 to 21 days. Inapparent infection may occur in 25% or more of infected individuals. Prodromal symptoms (1–5 days before rash) are seen more commonly in older children and adults. These symptoms consist of low-grade fever, coryza, conjunctivitis, cough, and lymphadenopathy. An enanthem of rubella (Forschheimer spots) consists of discrete, erythematous, pinpoint or larger lesions found on the soft palate in the prodromal period or on the first day of rash. These lesions are not pathognomonic for rubella.

The lymphadenopathy associated with rubella may appear as early as 7 days before the appearance of the rash. The suboccipital, posterior auricular, and cervical nodes are most commonly involved, but generalized lymphadenopathy may occur. The exanthem of rubella may be the first indication of this infection in young children. It begins on the face and moves rapidly downward to the trunk and lower extremities. The exanthem lasts approximately 3 days; it may persist for 5 days or disappear within the first day. The rash of rubella is erythematous, discrete, and maculopapular, and it generally does not coalesce or darken as in rubeola. It is occasionally pruritic. Fever in rubella is low grade and may be present for less than 24 hours.

Arthritis may occur and is more common in adults and adolescents. Female subjects tend to get arthritis more frequently. Joint involvement is usually multiple (large and small joints) and appears as the rash nears resolution with symptoms generally resolving in 2 weeks.

Other complications of rubella are encephalitis (1/6,000 infections) and Thrombocytopenic purpura.

Differential Diagnosis

No pathognomonic findings occur in rubella and, with the reduced incidence of rubella, physicians must have a high index of suspicion to make the diagnosis. Helpful epidemiologic factors include age of patient, history of contact cases, documented status of immunization, season of year, and period of incubation.

Included in the differential diagnosis are illnesses associated with enterovirus, mild rubeola, mild scarlet fever, mononucleosis, toxoplasmosis, *Mycoplasma pneumoniae* infection, and human parvovirus B19 infection.

Diagnosis

Rubella virus may be isolated (through viral culture) from nasopharyngeal secretions in postnatal rubella. The diagnosis of rubella is often determined by serologic testing of acute and convalescent sera obtained 10 to 14 days apart. Enzyme immunoassay (EIA), latex agglutination, and indirect immunofluorescence are all used. Tests to detect rubella-specific IgM antibody are also commercially available. Test results on paired sera with a fourfold rise in titer, or the determination of rubella-specific IgM antibody, indicates a recent infection with rubella virus.

Treatment

Treatment is largely supportive and includes use of antipyretics/analgesics for fever and arthralgia. Hospitalization is rarely required but may be necessary for complications.

RUBELLA PREVENTION

Control Measures

The primary method of control is immunization. In addition to universal childhood vaccination, emphasis should also be placed on determining immunity in women of childbearing age when they present for medical service, regardless of anticipated pregnancy.

Patients with rubella are generally considered infectious for 1 week after the onset of rash. Infants with congenital rubella should be considered contagious for 1 year, unless viral cultures show otherwise. Rubella is a reportable disease, and every effort should be made to diagnose and report all suspected cases.

Vaccine Recommendations

The live rubella virus vaccine [administered most commonly in combination with measles and mumps vaccines (MMR)] induces lifelong antibody in more than 98% of recipients. The Committee on Infectious Diseases of the American Academy of Pediatrics (AAP) recommends the first dose of MMR vaccine should be administered at 12 to 15 months of age, followed by administration of a second dose of MMR vaccine at age 4 to 6 or on entry into school. Rubella vaccine may also be administered alone when indicated. Susceptible children who reside in households with pregnant women may be immunized, as may children with minor illness. Adverse reactions to rubella vaccine include rash, fever, and adenopathy in a very small number of children 7 to 10 days after immunization. Postvaccine arthralgias may occur 2 to 3 weeks after vaccine, are transient, and are most likely to occur in postpubertal female subjects. Human immunodeficiency virus (HIV) patients (symptomatic or asymptomatic) should be immunized with MMR at the appropriate age. In general, other immunodeficiencies are a contraindication to this live virus vaccine. Pregnancy is a contraindication for rubella vaccine; if pregnant women are immunized inadvertently or if they become pregnant within 3 months after immunization, they should be advised of the theoretical risk to the fetus. Congenital rubella after rubella vaccination during pregnancy has yet to be documented, although it remains a theoretical consideration.

For detailed recommendations or contraindications for vaccine administration, the reader is referred to the 2003 *Report of the Committee on Infectious Diseases* (American Academy of Pediatrics, 2003).

CHAPTER 113
Rubeola

Adapted from Larry H. Taber
and Gail J. Demmler

Measles virus was isolated in 1954. Vaccine trials in the late 1950s led to vaccine licensure in 1963. Infection with measles virus produces an illness characterized by a prodrome of fever, coryza, cough, conjunctivitis, enanthem (Koplik spots), and development of a confluent, erythematous, maculopapular rash. Measles virus is an RNA paramyxovirus.

EPIDEMIOLOGY

Measles is highly contagious and transmission of the virus between individuals occurs by droplets of respiratory secretions. The highest period of infectivity is 3 to 5 days before the appearance of the exanthem.

With the widespread use of measles vaccine in the mid 1960s, the incidence of measles fell remarkably. In 1989 and 1990, however, the incidence of measles increased dramatically in all age groups and reached epidemic proportions in many areas of North America. This increase in measles was most striking among unvaccinated preschool-aged children, but outbreaks also occurred in large groups of vaccinated school-aged children, adolescents, and young adults.

PATHOGENESIS AND PATHOLOGY

Measles virus infection of the nasopharynx respiratory epithelium spreads to regional lymphatics, eventually resulting in viremia. The respiratory tract, skin, and conjunctivae are major sites of infection, but other organs may be involved. Viral replication peaks in all organs and the blood at approximately the same time that the rash appears, which coincides with development of immune responses and subsequent curtailment of the illness.

In natural infection, IgG antibody responses appear at approximately 14 days and peak several weeks later with a range of 4 to 6 weeks. Antibody in the IgM serum component appears early but is often not sensitive within the first 72 hours of rash. It rarely persists beyond 90 days. Infected hosts develop cell-mediated immunity and interferon response in the serum.

Immunocompromised hosts with T-lymphocyte dysfunction, in particular, may have a prolonged course with measles, prolonged excretion of virus, and high incidence of morbidity and mortality.

CLINICAL MANIFESTATIONS

Persons with measles virus infection fall into four distinct groups: typical measles in the normal host, modified measles in the host with antibody, atypical measles in the host who received killed vaccine, and measles in immunocompromised persons. The clinical illness may be the same in each group, but it is usually very different.

Typical Measles

The incubation period in typical measles is approximately 10 days, starting with 3- to 5-days of increasing symptoms of malaise, fever, cough, coryza, and conjunctivitis. Fever can range from 39.4°C to 40.6°C. Approximately 2 days before the rash appears, Koplik spots (white pinpoint lesions on a bright red buccal mucosa) appear opposite the lower molars and quickly spread to involve the entire buccal and lower labial mucosa. Koplik spots resolve by the third day of the exanthem. The exanthem of measles starts approximately 14 days after exposure and appears first behind the ears and at the hairline of the forehead. The rash progresses downward to the face, neck, upper extremities, and trunk and reaches the lower extremities by the third day. Initially, the rash is discrete, erythematous, and maculopapular, but it becomes confluent in the same progression as its spread. Eventually, the rash undergoes a brownish discoloration that does not blanch with pressure and may undergo desquamation. The exanthem lasts 6 to 7 days, and resolution of the rash begins on the third day in the same order as that of its appearance. In uncomplicated measles, the elevated temperature falls by either crisis or lysis; increased temperature beyond the third to fourth day of the exanthem suggests a complication.

Pharyngitis and generalized lymphadenopathy may be seen during the period of the exanthem. Splenomegaly is common. Diarrhea, vomiting, and abdominal pain may be prominent symptoms of measles, especially in young children. Leukopenia is often present.

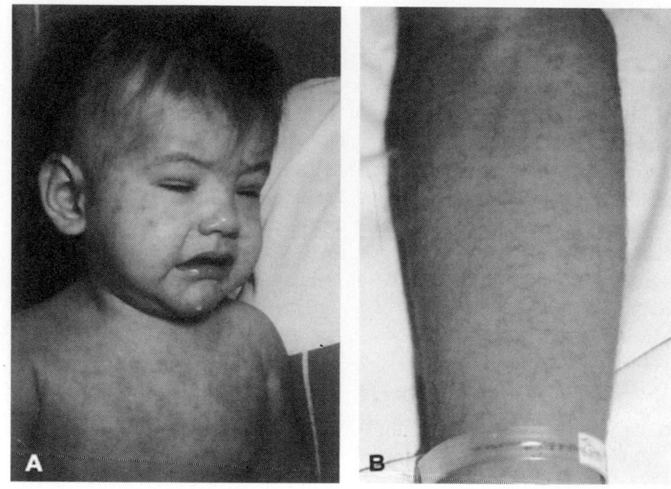

Figure 113-1. Maculopapular rash. **A:** Typical measles. (Courtesy of Dr. Gail J. Demmler.) **B:** Atypical measles.

Modified Measles

Modified measles occurs in children who have received serum immune globulin (IG) on exposure to measles or in young infants who still have transplacentally acquired maternal measles antibody. In addition, vaccine-modified mild measles, a form of secondary vaccine failure, can occur in individuals who were vaccinated appropriately with the live measles virus vaccine. In mild or modified measles, the prodrome period is shortened, symptoms are not as severe, and Koplik spots do not usually occur; if present, they fade rapidly. The exanthem follows the progression of regular measles, but it does not become confluent.

Atypical Measles

Atypical measles may occur in persons immunized with killed measles vaccine and exposed to natural measles. Killed measles virus vaccine was used from 1963 to 1967. Many of these individuals were never reimmunized with live virus vaccine.

The illness is characterized by sudden fever (39.4°C–40.6°C). Headache, myalgias, nonproductive cough, extreme weakness, and abdominal pain may be present. The rash of atypical measles appears first on the distal extremities and is pronounced on wrists and ankles. The rash may remain localized or may spread to involve the upper and lower extremities and the trunk. The palms and soles are also involved.

The rash of atypical measles may be erythematous and maculopapular (Fig. 113-1); it may be vesicular, petechial, or purpuric in nature. Urticaria has been described. Edema of the hands and feet and severe hyperesthesia have also been described. Koplik spots are rarely seen.

Pulmonary involvement may occur with a nodular pneumonia, hilar adenopathy, and pleural effusion.

Measles in Immunocompromised Hosts

Pneumonitis is a common complication of measles in immunocompromised hosts. It may occur in the absence of an exanthem, as has been described in children with symptomatic infection with human immunodeficiency virus (HIV). The pneumonia may have an insidious or a fulminant onset.

COMPLICATIONS OF MEASLES

Complications of measles include pneumonia (viral or superimposed bacterial), otitis media, laryngitis, laryngotracheobronchitis, and bronchiolitis. Myocarditis, pericarditis, appendicitis, corneal ulcerations, and thrombocytopenic purpura are also described.

Encephalitis occurs in approximately 1 in every 1,000 to 2,000 cases of measles. It usually becomes apparent during the period of the exanthem, but onset may occur in the prodromal period. High incidences of convulsions, cerebral edema, and other neurologic deficits occur in measles encephalitis. Usually, a mononuclear cell pleocytosis of the cerebrospinal fluid (CSF) and a slightly elevated protein occur.

Subacute sclerosing panencephalitis (SSPE) is an uncommon degenerative central nervous system (CNS) disease associated with persistent measles virus infection of the CNS. The risk of SSPE is approximately 1 per 100,000 infections with natural measles and 1 per 1 million immunizations in vaccine-associated SSPE. The incubation period is shorter with vaccine-associated SSPE than with natural measles. SSPE has an insidious onset with intellectual deterioration, myoclonic jerks, and progression to dementia and (finally) decorticate rigidity. The clinical picture, the typical electroencephalogram, and exceptionally high titers of measles antibody in serum and CSF are the basis for the diagnosis.

DIFFERENTIAL DIAGNOSIS

The differential diagnosis includes infections with viruses that may cause erythematous maculopapular rashes: the enteroviruses, adenoviruses, rubella, erythema infectiosum, and infectious mononucleosis. Also considered in the diagnosis are infections with Mycoplasma pneumoniae and drug eruptions accompanied by fever. More likely is that these illnesses would be confused with the clinical presentation of modified measles rather than typical measles. Atypical measles has also been confused with Rocky Mountain spotted fever. In atypical measles, the age of affected patients and a history of repeated measles immunizations (in which killed vaccine may have been administered several times) may help to confirm the diagnosis.

DIAGNOSIS

Measles virus may be isolated in tissue culture, but infections are generally documented serologically. To test antibody, a serum sample should be obtained immediately and a paired serum should be drawn in 2 to 3 weeks from patients with suspected measles. The presence of IgM antibody or a rising titer of IgG antibody (in the setting of a suggestive clinical illness) confirms a serologic diagnosis of measles. IgM antibody is typically detectable for 1 month from the onset of rash.

TREATMENT

Supportive care with antipyretics and careful attention to fluid intake is the rule. Antibiotics should not be given except when bacterial complications are present. Children with serious complications of measles (e.g., pneumonia, encephalitis, croup) should be hospitalized. In immunocompromised children, treatment with the antiviral agent ribavirin has been used on a compassionate basis to treat severe measles. Controlled trials have never been conducted.

Administration of Vitamin A is recommended by the World Health Organization (WHO) for those children with measles who reside in areas where Vitamin A deficiency is prevalent. This has been shown to decrease mortality from childhood measles in these populations. Although Vitamin A deficiency is not a public health problem in the United States, certain populations of children such as those with malabsorption syndromes may be at risk. Moreover, since severe measles in normal child hosts has been associated with low Vitamin A levels, the Committee on Infectious Diseases (COID) of the American Academy of Pediatrics (AAP) recommends that children less than age 2, hospitalized with a measles complication, be supplemented with Vitamin A. Guidelines also exist for supplementation of those children thought to be at risk for Vitamin A deficiency. Further information is available in the 2003 report of the Committee on Infectious Diseases (Red Book®).

Children with measles are still considered contagious for 5 days after the appearance of the rash, and measures should be taken to prevent their exposure to susceptible individuals. Immunocompromised persons with measles may be contagious longer.

MEASLES PREVENTION

General Considerations

Most physicians training today have not seen a patient with measles. Therefore, a high index of suspicion is necessary when confronted with patients with fever and a maculopapular exanthem, particularly if the patient may be unimmunized.

Prevention of measles is possible by maintaining a high level of immunization among children aged 15 months or older. Although some measles-susceptible persons of all age groups are found in the United States, the phenomenon of herd immunity plays a role in preventing the spread of measles through the population. Unimmunized individuals may be present because of parental or physician delay of immunization. Adults born after 1956 may never have been immunized or have had natural measles and, thus, are susceptible to infection. Persons immunized before 1977 may have been immunized at age 12 months or younger and may not be immune. Persons who were immunized with killed measles vaccine (1963–1967) may not have been reimmunized with attenuated vaccine. In addition, current attenuated vaccine causes an antibody response in 95% to 98% of individuals, meaning 2% to 5% primary vaccine failure rate. Protection increases to 99% after two doses, hence the recommendation for a second measles vaccine (see below).

Vaccine Recommendations

The combined measles-mumps-rubella (MMR) vaccine is part of the universal immunization schedule. The first dose of MMR vaccine should be administered at age 12 to 15 months. The second dose of MMR vaccine should be administered at age 4 to 6 years.

Vaccine Contraindications

Children who have recently received immunoglobulin (IG) should have measles vaccine delayed 8 to 11 months as IG interferes with the immune response to the vaccine.

Allergic reactions to measles vaccine are not common and few are associated with anaphylaxis. Previous contraindications included egg allergy (as measles vaccine is produced in chick embryo cell culture) and neomycin allergy. Current recommendations suggest that egg allergy is no longer an absolute contraindication to measles vaccine. The only absolute contraindication is an anaphylaxis event to a prior measles vaccine. This should preclude additional doses of MMR. It may be prudent to discuss specific cases with an allergist with the additional consideration of giving MMR vaccine in a controlled setting capable of responding to allergic emergencies.

As many as 15% of vaccinees may have fever 5 to 12 days after vaccination. Usually, fever lasts 1 to 5 days. A small number of vaccinees develop a transient rash. The frequency of CNS complications is 1 per 3 million doses of administered vaccine.

PREVENTION FOR EXPOSED INDIVIDUALS

If given in the first 72 hours after exposure, live measles virus vaccine may prevent infection. IG may be given to prevent or modify illness in exposed individuals if given within 6 days of exposure. The recommended dose is 0.25 mL/kg (maximum dose, 15 mL). Immunocompromised children should receive 0.5 mL/kg (maximum total dose, 15 mL). Special circumstances apply to children with HIV infection. For detailed recommendations or contraindications for vaccine administration, the reader is referred to the 2003 report of the Committee on Infectious Diseases (Red Book®).

CHAPTER 114

Varicella-Zoster Virus

Adapted from Charles F. Grose

Chickenpox is the common childhood exanthem caused by the human herpesvirus varicella-zoster virus (VZV). In the United States, varicella vaccine is recommended as part of the universal immunization schedule. When a person is exposed to varicella, either by infection or presumably immunization with live-virus vaccine, the virus remains in a latent state in the dorsal root ganglion cells for decades. As immunity wanes in late adulthood, occasionally the virus reactivates and causes the dermatomal exanthem known as *shingles* or *zoster*. Zoster can occur in children who are immunosuppressed.

THE VIRUS AND ITS PATHOGENESIS

VZV is a herpesvirus. The route by which primary VZV infection causes disease is illustrated in the schema for pathogenesis (Fig. 114-1). The interval between infection and appearance of the vesicular rash (incubation period) is usually 14 to 15 days with a range of 10 to 20 days. The initial site of infection is the conjunctivae or upper respiratory tract. Then the virus replicates at a local site in the head or neck for approximately 4 to 6 days. Thereafter, the virus is transmitted throughout the body during the primary viremia. After a second cycle of replication, the virus is released in larger amounts 1 week later (secondary viremia) and quickly invades the cutaneous tissues. As the virus exits the capillaries and enters the epidermis, characteristic vesicles of chickenpox appear on the skin.

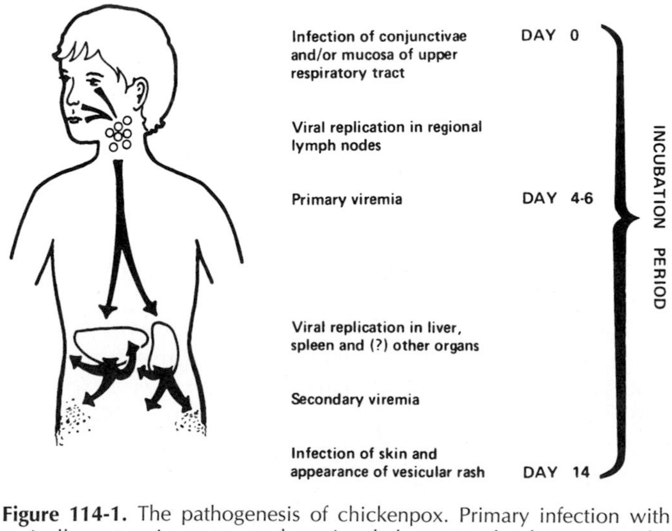

Figure 114-1. The pathogenesis of chickenpox. Primary infection with varicella-zoster virus occurs when virus-laden water droplets contact the respiratory mucosa or conjunctivae of a susceptible host. The pathogenesis most likely includes a biphasic course with a primary and secondary viremia followed by typical vesicular exanthem of chickenpox. Based on this schema, varicella-zoster immune globulin must be given before primary viremia to prevent chickenpox in the exposed host. (From Grose C. Varicella-zoster virus infections: chickenpox [varicella], shingles [zoster], and varicella vaccine. In: Glaser R, ed. *Human herpesvirus infections.* New York: Marcel Dekker, 1994:117.)

TRANSMISSION OF CHICKENPOX

Chickenpox is transmitted by virus droplets aerosol between individuals. In general, children are contagious two days before the eruption of the rash and remain infectious through day 6 of rash, a time at which all vesicles have generally crusted over. Susceptible individuals can contract varicella from patients with zoster. Before large-scale immunization, communities would typically have outbreaks of chickenpox annually from January to May.

CLINICAL FEATURES OF CHICKENPOX

The characteristic feature of chickenpox is the vesicle. In healthy children, the exanthem develops over 3 to 6 days, usually beginning along the hairline on the face. Each lesion begins as a macule that progresses to papule and vesicle, then to a crusted vesicle. Lesions in different stages of development are present throughout the first week. The rash is often more confluent wherever the skin has been abraded previously such as the diaper area.

Usually, the prodrome is mild with malaise and low-grade fever. When the rash erupts, the average number of skin lesions ranges between 200 and 300 in the index case within a family. Secondary cases may have a more severe course with up to 500 or more pox, presumably because such patients receive a larger inoculum of virus from infected siblings. By the end of the first week, children are usually afebrile, and the lesions are crusted. Infants, older teenagers, and adults may have more severe disease. More severe disease is also seen in children with immunosuppression, even those taking glucocorticoids for asthma. The mortality for chickenpox in otherwise healthy children (ages 1 through 14 years) is approximately 1 in 50,000, whereas that for infants younger than 1 year is 1 in 13,000.

The most frequent complication of chickenpox in a healthy child is skin and soft tissue infection. The most common infecting organism is group A streptococcus, although staphylococcal infections also occur. More serious, but less common, bacterial sequelae include septic arthritis and osteomyelitis, streptococcal necrotizing fasciitis, and staphylococcal pyomyositis. The onset of bacterial disease may be rapid, sometimes within 2 days of the appearance of the exanthem. Usually, this complication is heralded by a sudden rise in temperature and local signs of inflammation. Diagnosis of fasciitis and myositis, once a difficult procedure, is facilitated by magnetic resonance imaging.

Other systemic complications include pneumonitis, hepatitis, arthritis, pericarditis, glomerulonephritis, orchitis, and involvement of the nervous system. Usually, pneumonitis develops late in the first week of disease in those patients who have the most florid exanthem.

Neurologic manifestations include meningoencephalitis, myelitis, and polyneuritis. In particular, the acute cerebellar ataxia is the most common VZV-induced neurologic disease in children. Symptoms include unsteady gait, vomiting, speech changes, nystagmus, vertigo, and tremor. Usually, ataxia begins during the second week of the illness, but it can precede the exanthem. Chickenpox has also been temporally associated with Reye syndrome.

The variable outcome of chickenpox in children infected with human immunodeficiency virus (HIV) depends on the immunologic status of the patient. In HIV-seropositive children without symptoms of acquired immunodeficiency syndrome (AIDS), chickenpox usually follows its typical course. In children with very low CD4 lymphocyte counts and AIDS, chickenpox may be severe and progressive.

CONGENITAL VARICELLA INFECTION

Chickenpox in pregnant women can lead to intrauterine infection, especially during the first 20 weeks of gestation. The risk of fetal involvement in pregnant women with chickenpox is less than 3% by most surveys. The most common deformities are hypoplasia and paresis of one of the extremities, together with cicatricial scarring over the skin on the involved limb. Neurologic complications such as microcephaly or hydrocephalus may occur. Ophthalmic complications include cataracts and chorioretinitis. Documenting the diagnosis of congenital varicella syndrome is difficult because infants do not usually excrete virus and the VZV-specific IgM response is short-lived postnatally.

ZOSTER (SHINGLES)

Zoster is the dermatomal exanthem that occurs when VZV reactivates from its site of latency and travels down a sensory nerve to the skin. Zoster is unusual in children unless they are immunosuppressed (malignancy, medications, HIV). The younger the child at the time of chickenpox, the more likely that child will develop zoster later in childhood. Zoster in younger children often occurs in dermatomes supplied by the cervical and sacral dermatomes with the rash frequently seen on the arms and hands or in the groin and lower extremities.

DIAGNOSIS

Chickenpox is typically a clinical diagnosis. When necessary, the virus can be identified by obtaining samples of the vesicle fluid for inoculation in cell culture where cytopathic effect is usually observable 3 to 7 days later. Using VZV-specific monoclonal antibody infection can be diagnosed within 2 to 3 hours by a rapid antigen detection technique. The Tzanck smear is less valuable and is rarely required. Recent infection can be documented by obtaining acute and convalescent serum samples and demonstrating a fourfold or greater rise in VZV-specific antibody titer. Likewise, past infection can be demonstrated by persistence of antiVZV antibody.

TREATMENT

Modalities Including Varicella-Zoster Immune Globulin

Chickenpox in healthy children is most often not a serious disease. In the realm of supportive care, aspirin should be avoided because of its link with Reye syndrome. Most children never need to be seen by a physician. Topical and systemic medications to reduce pruritis are often recommended (Calamine lotion, Diphenhydramine).

The approach to exposed children receiving corticosteroids or chemotherapy for cancer or AIDS is much more emergent. Varicella-zoster immune globulin (VZIG) is the therapy of choice for passive immunization of these children at risk of developing progressive chickenpox. VZIG must be administered by intramuscular injection within 3 to 4 days after exposure to chickenpox. If VZV-susceptible patients are beyond the fourth day after exposure, no beneficial effect derives from passive immunization with VZIG. Therapy is then directed at chickenpox if it erupts. If given within the first 24 to 48 hours of illness, intravenous acyclovir blocks further viral replication within 24 to 48 hours, thereby preventing serious complications of progressive chickenpox.

Oral acyclovir is FDA approved for treatment of chickenpox in normal children. Treated children have been shown to have fewer total pox lesions, a shorter duration of new lesion formation, as well as 1 day less of fever. Chickenpox is less common today than it was when this drug was approved (1992). Despite practice controversies about whether a child with uncomplicated varicella should be treated, most agree that certain groups of children should be strong candidates for acyclovir: children during the first year of life, adolescents who are known to be at a higher risk, siblings of any age who sequentially contract chickenpox within the same household, children who have chronic conditions (e.g., eczema, asthma, diabetes), particularly if they need long-term aspirin therapy (rheumatoid arthritis), and children receiving inhaled corticosteroids.

VARICELLA VACCINATION

A live attenuated VZV vaccine called Varivax (Merck, West Point, PA) was approved in March 1995 for distribution in the United States. Before approval in the United States, studies in Japan (where it was licensed in 1988) observed that humoral immunity was maintained at least 7 to 10 years after vaccination, and that exposure of vaccine recipients to chickenpox in the community may provide a booster effect over time.

The current recommendation is that all healthy children between the ages of 12 and 18 months receive one dose of the live attenuated varicella vaccine (Varivax) by subcutaneous injection. Children who are older than 12 months and have not had chickenpox can also be given varicella vaccine. Children at age 13 or older require two doses of vaccine given 4 to 8 weeks apart. In most cases, varicella vaccine should not be administered to children receiving corticosteroids or other immunosuppressive therapies. There are many special circumstances for which varicella vaccine may be appropriate for children and adults. A full discussion of this can be found at http://www.cdc.gov/nip/publications/pink/Varicella-sm.pdf For example, an indication exists to give a nonimmune individual varicella vaccine within 3 to 5 days of exposure. This postexposure prophylaxis has been reported to be 70% to 100% effective.

Many experts feel immunity is permanent in persons who have received the vaccine. Approximately 1% of vaccinees per year will "breakthrough" with mild chickenpox infection, however. Side effects include a varicella like rash in 5% of those patients who receive the vaccine. In addition, a few cases of zoster have occurred in American vaccine recipients; some have been caused by the vaccine strain, whereas others are associated with community-acquired VZV strains. Overall, the rate of zoster is thought to be 5 times lower in vaccine recipients compared to those who have had wild-type varicella.

CHAPTER 115

Viral Gastroenteritis

Adapted from David O. Matson, Larry K. Pickering, and Douglas K. Mitchell

Acute viral gastroenteritis is a common illness that occurs in both endemic and epidemic forms worldwide. Four categories of viruses are recognized as medically important causes of human gastroenteritis: rotaviruses, enteric adenoviruses, caliciviruses, and astroviruses. These viruses exhibit important differences in epidemiology and pathogenesis.

ROTAVIRUS

Discovered in 1973, human rotavirus has been reported worldwide as a cause of acute diarrhea in humans. The name is derived from the Latin word *rota* ("wheel"), which describes the appearance of the virus on electron microscopy. Rotavirus is a double-stranded RNA virus. Differences in the antigenic properties of inner and outer capsid proteins allow rotaviruses to be classified into groups, subgroups, and serotypes. The most general category is the group of which there are six (A, B, C, D, E, and F).

Most human rotavirus infections are caused by group A rotavirus, the group detected by commercially available assays. Nongroup A rotaviruses, including groups B and C, also cause human disease, but their distribution is more limited worldwide, and few cases have been recognized in North America.

Epidemiology

Rotavirus diarrhea can occur in all age groups, but peak occurrence of symptomatic illness is in children 6 to 24 months of age. Rotavirus infection accounts for 15% to 50% of cases of acute diarrhea in children presenting to hospitals in tropical countries and for 35% to 60% of cases in temperate areas. The wide range of prevalence reflects differences in age groups studied, methods of detection, geographic locations, and time of year. Other community-based studies demonstrate that rotavirus causes 5% to 10% of diarrhea episodes during the first 2 years of life. In the United States, rotavirus causes some 70,000 hospitalizations each year of children younger than aged 5 years.

Rotavirus diarrhea shows seasonality in temperate climates and a lack of seasonality within ten degrees of the equator. In the United States, rotavirus season typically begins in October, or November in Mexico and the southwestern United States. It spreads as a wave of illness spreading across North America from the Southwest to the Northeast ending in May in the Maritime provinces of Canada.

Rotavirus has a mean incubation period of 2 days (range, 1–3 days) in children and in experimentally infected adults. Excretion of rotavirus in stool frequently precedes development of symptoms and continues after symptoms of illness resolve. Children can shed rotavirus in their stool and be asymptomatic. The titer of virus in stools is approximately 10^{11} infectious particles per gram shortly after the onset of illness, whereas only 10 to 200 particles are needed for infection. The usual duration of illness is 5 to 7 days; chronic infections with rotavirus can occur in immunodeficient children.

Rotaviruses are transmitted by the fecal-oral route, usually from person to person. Crowding is a risk factor and environments such as day care centers lead to spread infection. Asymptomatic individuals excrete fewer viral particles and are, therefore, less contagious than symptomatic infections.

Clinical Manifestations

Multiple infections in children in the first few years of life are expected but, in general, severity of symptoms decreases as the number of infections increases. Infections in the first few months of life tend to be asymptomatic because transplacental antibody and breast-feeding are protective for the newborn. After waning of transplacental antibody early (first or second) infections can be severe. Additional asymptomatic infections induce protective immunity for future infections. In infants and young children, clinical symptoms typically consist of fever and abrupt onset of explosive vomiting and watery diarrhea. Other common clinical features include dehydration (generally isotonic), compensated metabolic acidosis, and malabsorption, generally of carbohydrate and fat.

Stools infrequently contain blood or fecal leukocytes; mucus occurs occasionally. Fat malabsorption can lend a foul odor to stools. In immunocompromised hosts, rotaviruses may cause a chronic, protein-losing diarrhea, and infection of the liver and kidneys. Although reported for years, recent evidence is beginning to define a causal association of rotavirus with aseptic meningitis and encephalitis. The link of rotavirus to other disorders such as inflammatory bowel disease, hemolytic-uremic syndrome, Kawasaki syndrome, and neonatal necrotizing enterocolitis is less clear. Table 115-1 summarizes several characteristics of viruses, including rotavirus, that cause gastroenteritis.

Diagnosis

Stools collected early in the course of illness are most likely to contain virus, whereas stools collected 8 or more days after the onset of illness rarely contain detectable virus. Numerous, reliable, sensitive enzyme immunoassays and latex agglutination tests for detection of rotavirus in stool specimens are available commercially.

Human rotavirus can be isolated in tissue culture, but the technique is cumbersome. Electron microscopy can identify rotavirus, but the technique is not suitable for examination of a large number of specimens.

Treatment and Prevention

As in all children with acute diarrhea, prevention of dehydration with careful attention to oral fluid replacement (with glucose-electrolyte solutions) is necessary. For those children with clinically important dehydration (with or without acidosis), therapy for rotavirus is no different than for other forms of acute diarrhea. Parenteral fluids may be required in moderate to severe cases and should be administered if there is an inability to give enteral fluid replacement (oral rehydration therapy) and/or the child has evidence of significant intravascular volume depletion. Hospitalized patients should be on contact precautions to prevent spread. Breast-feeding is the most important preventive strategy available today. In 1998, the first rotavirus vaccine was licensed by the U.S. Food and Drug Administration (FDA). It was incorporated into the universal immunization series for 1999. Postmarketing surveillance studies suggested that administration of the vaccine (RotaShield®, Wyeth-Lederle) led to an increased incidence of intussusception in infants. Further case-control studies led credibility to this finding and in late 1999, the Advisory Committee for Immunization Practices (ACIP) from the Centers for Disease Control and Prevention (CDC) recommended against routine administration of rotavirus vaccine to children. The vaccine was subsequently removed from the market by the manufacturer but is currently still licensed by the FDA. Future vaccines are under study.

TABLE 115-1. Characteristics of Viruses that Cause Gastroenteritis

Enteric characteristic	Rotavirus	Adenoviruses	Caliciviruses	Astroviruses
Age group commonly involved (mo)	6–24	6–24	All ages	6–24
Incubation period (d)	1–3	1–3	1–2	1–3
Duration of illness	3–7 d	3–8 d	12 hr to 5 d	1–5 d
Method of transmission	Fecal-oral	Fecal-oral	Fecal-oral, food-borne	Fecal-oral, food-borne
Method of identification commercially available?	Yes	Yes	Special reference laboratories	Special reference laboratories
Immunization available?	Being tested	No	No	No

ENTERIC ADENOVIRUSES

Adenoviruses are double-stranded DNA viruses. There are 47 serotypes of human adenoviruses with enteric adenoviruses being members of group F, with designated serotypes 40 and 41. After rotavirus, enteric adenovirus is the next most common cause of viral gastroenteritis in infants and children.

Epidemiology and Clinical Features

Enteric adenoviruses are transmitted by the fecal-oral route. Symptoms are adenoviral diarrhea and are indistinguishable from symptoms of rotavirus infection but are perhaps less severe. Blood and mucus are generally not present in stools. Infections show no seasonal pattern and usually involve children less than age 2. Seasonality has not been recognized for enteric adenovirus diarrhea.

Diagnosis

Enteric adenoviruses are most often identified by immunoassays. Electron microscopy and viral culture may be used.

Treatment and Prevention

As with rotavirus, supportive care is the general rule. If necessary, fluid therapy (enteral or parenteral) should be used to replace volume and electrolyte abnormalities. Hospitalized patients should be isolated.

Measures that reduce spread of enteric adenovirus are similar to those recommended for all viral gastroenteritis pathogens. These measures include training care providers, routinely cleaning food preparation areas and diaper-changing tables, excluding ill care providers or food handlers, hand washing, and excluding or cohorting ill children.

CALICIVIRUSES

Caliciviruses are RNA viruses, the name of which is derived from the characteristic surface cups or chalice-like indentations observed by electron microscopy. The caliciviruses are divided into four genera. The Norwalk-like caliciviruses include strains known primarily for causing outbreaks of illness in adults and are associated with contaminated food (especially seafood) and water. The Sapporo-like caliciviruses primarily cause pediatric gastroenteritis. Rabbit-like and vesicular exanthem of swine-like caliciviruses are the other two genera and occur primarily in animals.

Numerous caliciviruses cause a wide spectrum of illness beyond diarrhea including vesicular exanthem, hemorrhagic pneumonia, a stunting syndrome, aphthous ulcers, and myositis. The most widely known, Norwalk virus, was first identified in 1972 in samples collected from an outbreak of gastroenteritis in a secondary school in Norwalk, Ohio.

Epidemiology and Clinical Manifestations

Caliciviruses have a worldwide distribution and are a common cause of water-borne and food-borne outbreaks of acute, nonbacterial gastroenteritis. Many calicivirus infections go undiagnosed.

Calicivirus outbreaks tend to occur in closed populations (child-care centers, cruise ships) and have a high attack rate. Outbreaks have occurred in association with contaminated water and food, particularly shellfish and salads. Secondary transmission may then occur from person to person via the fecal-oral route. Symptoms are generally mild and, especially in adults, can be of short duration and resemble staphylococcal food poisoning. In children, symptoms are indistinguishable from other causes of gastroenteritis. Characteristically, stools are not bloody and lack mucus. Leukocytes are not seen in fecal smears. The incubation period is 12 hours to 4 days. Excretion lasts 5 to 7 days after the onset of symptoms in one-half of the infected patients and can extend to 13 days. Virus excretion may continue for 4 days after symptoms cease.

Diagnosis and Treatment

Detection for calicivirus infections may require reference or research laboratories. Electron microscopy has been used in the past, but newer techniques include immunoassays and molecular modalities such as polymerase chain reaction (PCR).

Treatment is supportive. Hospitalized patients should be isolated, and infected individuals attending child-care centers or similar institutions should be cohorted. Virus may be inactivated with a 1-minute exposure to 0.1% sodium hypochlorite.

ASTROVIRUSES

Astroviruses are RNA viruses and are named for their star-like appearance when visualized by direct electron microscopy. Eight antigenic types of astroviruses have been identified. Antigenic types 1 and 2 are the most common types and are detected both in sporadic infections and astrovirus outbreaks.

Epidemiology and Clinical Manifestations

Human astroviruses have a worldwide distribution and have been known to cause outbreaks of gastroenteritis in all settings. Outbreaks in closed populations such as child-care centers have a high attack rate (as high as 90%). Most astrovirus infections have been detected in children younger than aged 4 years, and many infections can be asymptomatic. Transmission is via the person-to-person and fecal-oral routes. Outbreaks associated with water and food have been documented.

Symptoms are often mild but not distinguishable from other forms of diarrhea. The incubation period is 1 to 2 days. Excretion lasts for 5 days after onset of symptoms in one-half of the infected cases. The duration of asymptomatic excretion after onset of illness is uncertain.

Diagnosis and Treatment

In the United States, detection for astroviruses typically requires reference or research laboratories. Available techniques include reverse transcriptase PCR, enzyme immunoassays, and electron microscopy.

Treatment is supportive. Enteric precautions are recommended, and control measures are the same as those for rotavirus.

OTHER VIRAL AGENTS

Numerous other enteric viruses are associated with gastroenteritis. These include some picornaviruses, coronaviruses, toroviruses, parvoviruses and parvo-like viruses, and pestiviruses. Information supporting the causative role varies for each agent. For some, lack of diagnostic techniques, inability to cultivate the virus in cell culture, and a paucity of virus-containing samples have limited investigation of their relative importance and features.

D
Disorders of Unknown Etiology

CHAPTER 116
Kawasaki Syndrome

Adapted from Ralph D. Feigin and Frank Cecchin

Kawasaki syndrome (KS) is an acute, febrile, syndrome of unknown etiology that predominantly afflicts children younger than 9 years. The disease has also been termed the *mucocutaneous lymph node syndrome* (MCLNS). The diagnosis is based on clinical features because no specific laboratory findings are present.

The disease was first recognized by Tomisaku Kawasaki in 1967. Subsequently, KS has become the most common cause of acquired heart disease in children in North America.

EPIDEMIOLOGY

There is a racial predilection for KS. The incidence per 100,000 children 8 years or younger is three times higher in Asian-American than in black children and more than six times higher in Asian-American than in white children. The male-to-female ratio is 1.5:1. KS has not been detected in newborn infants, but the incidence increases steadily to peak at approximately ages 13 to 24 months, then falls off in almost linear fashion until age 12 years, after which occurrence of KS is most unusual. This incidence pattern suggests that transplacental antibody may offer some protection in young infants.

KS is seen in all seasons of the year. Clustering of cases of KS has been observed and has been reported in several cities in the United States, Australia, and Japan. One outbreak in Japan started in Tokyo and spread northward and southward to involve the entire country within 6 months. Secondary or co-primary cases are rare, and nosocomial infection has not been reported.

ETIOLOGY

The cause of KS is currently unknown. Most investigators have favored the possibility of an infectious agent or a dysregulated immune response to an infectious agent (superantigen theory). Laboratory features such as elevated white blood cell (WBC) count with a left shift, elevated levels of acute-phase reactants (CRP, ESR), and pyuria suggest an infectious etiology or immune system activation.

KS, however, does not respond to treatment with antibiotics. Many viruses have been implicated, among them, the herpesviruses. At present, no definitive data exist to implicate a specific bacterial or viral agent.

As mentioned above, the immunologic and clinical manifestations of KS bear similarity to diseases associated with superantigen production. The classic example is toxic shock syndrome, in which the staphylococcal enterotoxin functions as a superantigen that induces massive expansion of T cells. This event, in turn, leads to excess cytokine production causing clinical illness. Patients with acute KS have been shown to have selective expansion of T cells expressing T-cell-receptor variable regions $V\beta2$ and $V\beta8$.

KS has not been associated consistently with exposure to environmental pesticides, chemicals, heavy metals, toxins, or pollutants. Usually, poisoning with environmental agents does not simulate an acute infectious disease, although similarities between acrodynia (mercury poisoning) and KS have been noted. An outbreak of KS in Denver was considered to be associated with the use of rug shampoo. Eleven of 23 patients with the syndrome had been exposed to rug shampoo in the 30 days before the onset of illness. Some additional studies have demonstrated a significant association of KS with rug shampoo while others have not.

A similarity exists between infantile periarteritis nodosa and KS. Distinguishing infantile periarteritis nodosa with coronary artery involvement from fatal infantile KS is pathologically impossible. Clinically, however, most patients with infantile periarteritis nodosa associated with coronary artery involvement do not meet the other criteria established by the Centers for Disease Control and Prevention (CDC) for KS.

PATHOLOGY

Cardiac hypertrophy, multiple single bead-like or fusiform aneurysms of the coronary arteries, pericarditis, myocarditis, endocarditis, valvulitis, and conduction system inflammation are observed with polymorphonuclear infiltrates. If coronary inflammation is present, it resolves near day 30 with subsequent granulation formation. Coronary artery scarring, stenosis, and endocardial fibroelastosis are described after day 40. Aneurysms of other arteries such as the renal, iliac, and brachial arteries may be found.

CLINICAL MANIFESTATIONS

The clinical manifestations of KS in accordance with the CDC diagnostic criteria are given in Table 116-1. KS occurs in four discrete phases. In the first phase, previously healthy children become febrile and irritable. Fever is relentless, and the temperature exceeds 40.6°C (105.8°F) in 40% of such patients. Nonsuppurative cervical lymphadenopathy, usually in the anterior triangle and frequently bilateral, may be present but may disappear rapidly. Within several days, rash and bilateral conjunctival injection appears.

The second phase begins at approximately the fourth day of illness and is characterized by continuing high, spiking fever that is unresponsive to standard antipyretic regimens or to antibiotics. The mean duration of fever is 12 days if the patient is not treated with aspirin or gamma globulin. The child is febrile and irritable and may appear ill. Cervical lymphadenitis may be present and appears in at least 50% of patients. Bilateral injection of the conjunctivae, primarily bulbar, is impressive, and unilateral subconjunctival hemorrhage may occur. Anterior uveitis may be found in 80% of all such patients evaluated by slit-lamp examination. The patients' lips become bright red, dry, and cracked. A strawberry tongue may be apparent.

A rash particularly prominent over the trunk may be maculopapular, morbilliform, urticarial (erythema multiforme has been described). The rash is hardly ever vesicular or pustular and the presence of such rash should make the evaluator consider other diagnoses. Early in the illness, an erythematous, at times, desquamating rash may be seen in the diaper area, axillae or neck fold.

Diarrhea may occur in the early phases of the illness. Right upper quadrant or generalized abdominal pain may be seen, perhaps due to the well-described hydropic changes of the gall bladder. As the second phase progresses, erythema of the palms and soles may develop (Fig. 116-1). The hands and feet become edematous, and arthralgia and arthritis of large joints may be noted.

Laboratory evaluation reveals an elevated WBC with a left shift. A peripheral smear may reveal toxic neutrophils. The erythrocyte sedimentation rate, C-reactive protein is elevated, which may help to distinguish KS from viral infections. Transaminase levels may be elevated, but they are not usually more than three times the upper limit of normal. Urinalysis may reveal proteinuria and moderate pyuria, usually reflecting urethritis. In male patients, meatitis may be seen.

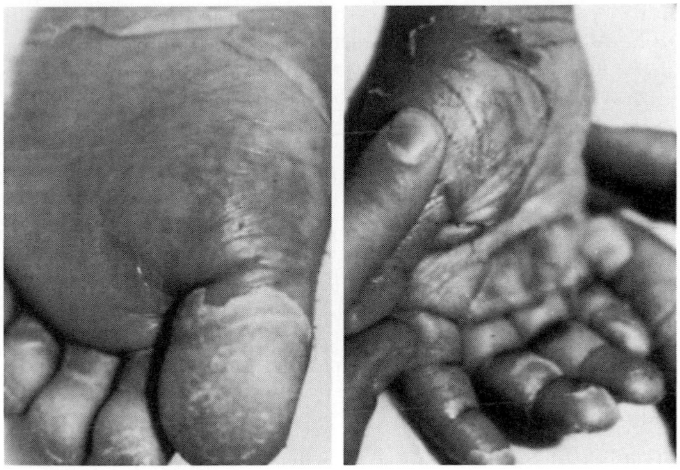

Figure 116-1. Erythema and edema of the feet and hands characteristic of the second phase of KS.

TABLE 116-1. Diagnostic Criteria for Kawasaki Disease

Fever of 5 or more days duration associated with at least four of the five following changes
- Bilateral conjunctival injection
- One or more changes of the mucous membranes of the upper respiratory tract, including pharyngeal injection, dry fissured lips, injected lips, and "strawberry tongue"
- One or more changes of the extremities, including peripheral erythema, peripheral edema, periungual desquamation, and generalized desquamation
- Rash, primarily truncal
- Cervical lymphadenopathy

Disease not explained by some other known disease process

*A diagnosis of Kawasaki disease can be made if fever and any of the changes listed are present in conjunction with coronary artery disease documented by two-dimensional echocardiography or coronary angiography.
Modified from previously published diagnostic criteria for Kawasaki disease from the Centers for Disease Control and Prevention and the American Heart Association Committee on Rheumatic Fever, Endocarditis, and Kawasaki Disease.

Nuchal rigidity and lethargy are occasionally present raising the possibility of infectious meningitis. In patients who have lumbar punctures, finding of aseptic meningitis can be seen with elevated CSF white blood cell count (predominantly mononuclear cells) and normal protein and glucose levels. As aseptic meningitis is a known complication of intravenous gammaglobulin (IVIG), at times it is impossible to know if abnormal CSF findings are related to KS or to IVIG in the previously treated patient.

Electrocardiograms are abnormal in many patients with KS, particularly those with pancarditis. Some common abnormalities are initially flattened T waves, followed by peaked T waves in convalescence; first-degree heart block; ST segment elevation or depression; and QT interval prolongation.

Disappearance of the rash and resolution of the adenopathy herald the end of the second phase of illness.

On approximately day 12 of the illness, the third phase occurs and is heralded by desquamation. Typically, this is seen in the periungual region, although other parts of the body may be involved. Thrombocytosis is another common feature of the third phase of illness with platelet counts ranging from 500,000 to 3 million per cubic millimeter. Thrombocytosis is rarely seen in the first week of illness. Usually, it appears in the second week, peaks in the third week, and returns gradually to normal approximately 1 month after onset in uncomplicated cases.

The fourth phase of illness is recognized in only a minority of cases. This phase is characterized by ongoing inflammation, subacute vasculitis, and an increased incidence of death from cardiac involvement.

COMPLICATIONS

The most serious complications of KS are cardiovascular and include aneurysms of the coronary arteries and other large arteries, aneurysmal rupture, hemopericardium, myocarditis, coronary thrombosis, pericardial effusions, cardiac tamponade, mitral valve disease, and arrhythmias. Aneurysm of other peripheral arteries have been described.

Acalculous cholecystitis has been noted and the diagnosis can be made by ultrasonography. Most cases resolve spontaneously.

DIFFERENTIAL DIAGNOSIS

Children who meet the CDC criteria should be strongly considered to have KS. Infants and older children are less likely to have a classic presentation than toddlers in the usual age group. These children who don't fully meet clinical criteria may be considered to have atypical Kawasaki syndrome and a high index of suspicion, for the diagnosis is, thus, needed to prevent serious sequelae.

The most common condition that mimics KS is group A beta-hemolytic streptococcal infection. Other disorders with which KS can be confused initially include rubeola, roseola, meningococcemia, Rocky Mountain spotted fever, leptospirosis, rubella, infectious mononucleosis, selected viral infections caused by the enteroviruses, rat-bite fever, toxoplasmosis, acrodynia, collagen vascular diseases (particularly infantile polyarteritis nodosa), Reiter syndrome, and Behçet syndrome. Toxic shock syndrome may need to be excluded. Drug reactions have also been confused with KS. Infantile papular acrodermatitis (Gianotti syndrome) can be confused with KS during the early stages of the disorder.

TREATMENT

The goals of therapy for KS are to decrease the inflammatory response and to reduce the severity of the cardiovascular complications. The combination of intravenous gamma globulin and aspirin effectively meets these goals.

Giving intravenous gamma globulin within the first 10 days of the onset of fever significantly decreases the incidence of aneurysm development. Current recommendations call for a single dose of gamma globulin at 2 g/kg given in a 10- to 12-hour infusion. The mechanism by which intravenous gamma globulin suppresses coronary artery lesions is not entirely clear. Possible mechanisms include Fc receptor blockade, neutralization of the etiologic agent, an antitoxic effect, alteration of the immune effect via antiidiotypic antibodies or induction of suppressor T cells, and decreased cytokine production by activated immune cells. Treatment with gamma globulin reduces the risk of coronary artery aneurysm to 2% to 3% compared to 20% of patients who are not treated.

Aspirin is also an important therapeutic modality. It can help to reduce the height and duration of fever and may serve as an important antithrombotic agent. The recommended aspirin dose in the United States is 80 to 100 mg/kg/day until defervescence. Some clinicians will keep a patient on this high dose aspirin for 7 to 14 days, at which point, the dose may be increased to 3 to 5 mg/kg/day to maintain an antiplatelet effect.

The use of steroids for treating KS is controversial, and the general consensus is that steroids should not be part of initial treatment. However, pulsed doses of methylprednisolone may be effective in reducing cardiac sequelae in children with persistent or recrudescent fever after treatment with intravenous gamma globulin.

Close follow-up after discharge from the hospital is essential to monitor for cardiac sequelae and persistent or recrudescent disease. The persistence or recrudescence of fever occurs in approximately 5% to 10% of children and should warrant retreatment with intravenous gamma globulin.

A complete blood count (to monitor WBC and platelet count) should be monitored once or twice per week in the recovery phases of the illness. Monitoring of C-reactive protein may also be useful as high C-reactive protein levels have been shown to correlate with an increased risk of cardiac sequelae, especially in infants younger than 12 months. Serial monitoring of the sedimentation rate immediately after IVIG may not be useful as it will often remain elevated. Later monitoring of the ESR is recommended by some.

Early cardiac involvement can be evaluated by obtaining a baseline echocardiogram at the time of diagnosis, as well as a follow-up approximately 2 weeks from the first. This schedule may need to be individualized for every patient. Angiography is indicated if significant coronary dilation or aneurysm formation occurs. The presence of coronary aneurysms predisposes an individual to platelet deposition, embolic phenomena, and progressive intimal fibrosis with luminal obstruction, which may lead to decreased coronary artery blood flow with resultant angina and myocardial infarction. Subtle coronary endothelium changes not visible on angiography may predispose to the development of coronary atherosclerosis during the second or third decade of life. Long-term evaluation of all patients with KS is recommended to detect the early onset of coronary artery disease or renovascular hypertension.

E
Fungal Infections

CHAPTER 117
Candidiasis

Adapted from Walter T. Hughes

The spectrum of candidiasis extends from benign superficial infections to life-threatening disseminated (systemic) mycosis. Most often candidiasis is seen as an opportunistic fugal infection in infants and young children.

ETIOLOGY

Candida albicans is the usual causative agent, but many other species of candida exist. Organisms such as *C. tropicalis*, *C. pseudotropicalis*, *C. paratropicalis*, *C. parapsilosis*, and *C. glabrata* have become more widely known due to their importance in immunocompromised patients.

EPIDEMIOLOGY

In addition to humans, *C. albicans* has been isolated from a variety of wild and domestic animals. Transmission of *Candida* involves direct contact with a colonized site. Oral thrush in neonates results from organisms that are acquired during passage through the birth canal or from colonized nipples of the mother or a nursing bottle. Colonization with *Candida* is not necessarily associated with discernible illness. Although mucosal surfaces are colonized easily, the normal skin is relatively resistant to colonization and infection with *Candida* species.

The immune system actively defends against *Candida* in healthy hosts. Secretory and humoral IgA antibodies are generated, as are specific anticandidal IgE, IgG, and IgM antibodies. The organism can activate an alternate complement pathway. Neutrophils, monocytes, and eosinophils can ingest and kill the yeast. The organism can induce the formation of suppressor and mitogen-stimulated lymphocytes and, thereby, produce a lymphokine that will kill it. Healthy individuals are at increased risk for candidiasis of the mucous membranes during infancy, pregnancy, and old age. Patients with congenital or acquired immunodeficiencies are a great risk for *Candida* infections. Disseminated candidiasis has been encountered in 7% of children infected with the human immunodeficiency virus and in 11% of recipients of bone marrow transplants.

PATHOLOGY

The initial step in infection is adherence of the yeast form of *Candida* to an epithelial cell surface. After the development of a filamentous or pseudohyphal form, the organism becomes invasive. Mucosal lesions may progress to well-demarcated ulcers, especially in the intestinal tract. Organisms may invade blood vessels and disseminate to any organ in the body in immunosuppressed patients. A multisystem disease may develop with the kidneys, lungs, liver, brain, and spleen affected most frequently.

CLINICAL MANIFESTATIONS

The clinical features of candidiasis are: mucous membrane involvement, skin infection, and systemic infection.

Mucous Membrane Candidiasis

Oropharyngeal candidiasis (thrush) is characterized by patches of pearly white pseudomembranes resembling curds of milk on the mucosal surfaces of the mouth. This pseudomembrane is composed of epithelial cells, leukocytes, keratin, food debris, and both yeast and pseudohyphal forms of *Candida*. Removal of the pseudomembrane leaves a denuded erythematous lesion. The buccal mucosa, dorsal and lateral areas of the tongue, gingiva, and pharynx are involved most frequently. *C. albicans* is the species that usually causes thrush. Any portion of the gastrointestinal tract may be affected, but extensive infection is usually seen in severely immunosuppressed patients.

Vaginal candidiasis causes pruritus and a whitish, watery vaginal discharge. Finally, the mucosal surface of the respiratory tract may be colonized with *Candida* at any site.

Cutaneous Candidiasis

Diaper dermatitis involving the groin, perineum, and lower abdominal areas is the most common form of cutaneous candidiasis. Often, the rash is a confluent papulovesicular reaction with well-demarcated borders. Other sites frequently involved include the intertriginous areas of the axilla and sites around the umbilicus.

Abnormal host immune status should be considered in cases of refractory candiasis. Chronic mucocutaneous candidiasis is an uncommon syndrome that reflects an underlying immunodeficiency or endocrinopathy.

Systemic Candidiasis

After becoming blood borne from a mucousal or skin entry site, *Candida* may involve any organ but most commonly involves the lungs, liver, spleen, kidney, and brain. Patients with this form of candidiasis are typically immunosuppressed, debilitated or premature infants.

DIAGNOSIS

Thrush is a clinical diagnosis. Other mucous membranes and skin lesions can be confirmed by direct examination of swabbed or scraped debris or by culture of the specimens. Ten percent potassium hydroxide (KOH prep) can be used to examine for budding yeast forms and pseudohyphae. The diagnosis of systemic candidiasis requires the isolation of *Candida* species from otherwise sterile body fluids; the demonstration of invasive yeasts or pseudohyphae in biopsy specimens; or both. Computed tomography (CT) is useful in demonstrating lesions in the liver, spleen, kidneys, and brain. Often, such lesions are sufficiently characteristic to permit that a presumptive diagnosis be made. The usefulness of methods to detect *Candida* antigenemia has been limited. Although molecular probes using polymerase chain reaction (PCR) methods offer promise, no generally accepted serologic method has evolved for the diagnosis of invasive disease. Determination of D-arabinitol/L-arabinitol ratios in urine have been reported as predictive of invasive disease.

TREATMENT

The type and location of candidiasis are important in determining the appropriate approach to treatment.

Mucous Membrane Candidiasis

Oropharyngeal candidiasis is treated with oral nystatin, 200,000 to 500,000 units every 4 to 6 hours for 1 week or longer. Clotrimazole troches are also effective. Nystatin troches, 200,000 units per tablet, are now available, although comparative studies of results in children are lacking. Vaginal candidiasis is treated with clotrimazole or nystatin suppositories. Esophageal, gastric, and intestinal candidiasis can be treated in the same manner as that used for treating oropharyngeal candidiasis, provided that the nystatin suspension is swallowed.

Fluconazole, given orally or intravenously, has been effective in oral and esophageal candidiasis and should be considered for use in severe cases and in patients who are not responsive to the nonabsorbable drugs. The efficacy of itraconazole has been found equal to that of fluconazole in the treatment of esophageal candidiasis.

Cutaneous Candidiasis

Cutaneous candidiasis can be treated with topical nystatin, amphotericin B, or clotrimazole preparations. Chronic mucocutaneous candidiasis in some cases may be treated effectively with oral ketoconazole.

Systemic Candidiasis

Candidiasis with deep organ involvement or hematogenous spread is treated systemically with amphotericin B. No drug has been shown to be more effective. The dosage of amphotericin B is 0.5 to 1.0 mg/kg/day as a daily infusion given over 4 to 6 hours.

Before this dose is initiated, a test infusion of 0.25 mg/kg/day is given over a period of 6 hours to assess the extent of possible adverse reactions to the preparation. Some physicians recommend the use of flucytosine in addition to amphotericin B in hepatosplenic candidiasis. Flucytosine is given orally at a dosage of 150 mg/kg/day in four divided doses. Both compounds should be administered over a period of 4 to 6 weeks or even longer in some cases. Especially important is the monitoring of patients who are receiving amphotericin B for adverse effects of the drug, which will be reflected in electrolyte imbalance and nephrotoxicity, and the observation of patients who are receiving flucytosine for effects on bone marrow suppression.

In randomized studies, fluconazole and amphotericin B were associated with similar clinical response rates and survival in the treatment of candidemia among nonneutropenic and neutropenic patients. However, drug-related adverse effects were more frequent with amphotericin B. Fluconazole may be used as an alternative to amphotericin B for systemic cases of candidiasis in patients other than those with *C. krusei* infections. The drug may be given orally or intravenously at a dosage of 3 to 6 mg/kg/day with the understanding that studies of its use in children are limited.

Lipid formulations of amphotericin B (lipid complex or colloidal dispersion) are now commercially available for patients with treatment-limiting toxicity and certain treatment failures from the standard amphotericin B preparation.

CHAPTER 118
Dermatophytoses

Adapted from Bernhard L. Wiedermann

Dermatophytosis refers to colonization of the skin with members of the dermatophytic fungi of the genera *Trichophyton*, *Microsporum*, and *Epidermophyton*. Clinical disease may appear as a consequence of the host's response to this colonization. The condition has been recognized since antiquity and was termed *herpes* by the Greeks, in reference to the tendency of lesions to creep in a circular fashion. Later, the Romans used the term *tinea*, meaning "worm" or "moth," to indicate a presumed association of the disease with insects. The modern term *ringworm* is a combination of these two historical names.

The affected body site is incorporated into commonly used clinical nomenclature. Thus, *tinea capitis* refers to dermatophytosis of the scalp, lesions of the trunk and extremities are termed *tinea corporis*, foot involvement is named *tinea pedis*, perineal disease is known as *tinea cruris*, and dermatophytosis of the nails is called *tinea unguium*.

ETIOLOGY

To date, approximately 40 different dermatophytes have been identified, but only 11 commonly cause disease in humans. The most common organisms causing disease in the United States are *Trichophyton tonsurans*, *Trichophyton rubrum*, *Trichophyton mentagrophytes*, *Microsporum canis*, and *Epidermophyton floccosum*.

EPIDEMIOLOGY

Age is a determinant for some dermatophyte infections. For example, tinea pedis is common in adults but rare in children. In contrast, tinea capitis is common in children but rarely occurs after puberty. Environmental issues such as using oils on the head, animal exposure, presence of trauma, or immunocompromising conditions (particularly those involving cell-mediated immunity) may predispose to dermatophytosis.

PATHOGENESIS AND PATHOLOGY

Infecting organisms are acquired from soil, animal, or human sources and colonize keratin-containing tissues. The dermatophytes possess the ability to use keratin for growth. During the initial incubation period, the organism grows in the stratum corneum of the skin. The site of disease enlarges and spreads locally. In circular lesions of the skin, active fungal growth and invasion occur at the rim of the lesion; the center of the lesion contains relatively few organisms. Histopathologic exam shows a mixed infiltrate of lymphocytes, histiocytes, eosinophils, and plasma cells in the stratum corneum. Fungal elements may be visualized using periodic acid–Schiff or methenamine silver staining.

CLINICAL MANIFESTATIONS

Tinea Capitis

Ringworm of the scalp in the United States is usually caused by *T. tonsurans*. In the noninflammatory variety, the lesion begins at the base of the hair shaft as an erythematous papule that then spreads peripherally as hairs break just above the level of the scalp leaving areas of alopecia, often appearing as black dots. Pruritus is common. The inflammatory type, more commonly associated with M. canis, may result in a pustular folliculitis and regional lymphadenopathy. Kerions are inflammatory, tender, purulent boggy masses that form as a result of the host's immune response (PMN infiltration) and generally do not represent secondary bacterial infection.

Tinea Corporis

Tinea corporis refers to dermatophytosis involving the skin of any part of the body with the exception of the palms, soles, and groin. The most frequent causes are *T. mentagrophytes*, *T. rubrum*, and *M. canis*. The typical ringworm lesion is pruritic and appears as an erythematous, annular lesion with an elevated, scaly, papular, and sometimes vesicular border spreading in a centrifugal manner while clearing centrally.

Tinea Cruris

Tinea cruris (jock itch) is similar to tinea corporis, except that tinea cruris appears almost exclusively in adolescent boys and adult men. The lesions are localized to the groin and are often associated with tight-fitting underclothing. The erythematous, slightly indurated patch spreads, forming tiny vesicles at the peripheral border. The lesions are intensely pruritic and may be painful. Secondary bacterial infection can occur.

Tinea Pedis

Tinea pedis (athlete's foot) is relatively uncommon in young children and occurs most frequently in adolescents. Use of communal baths, pools, and similar areas is a risk factor. *T. rubrum* and *T. tonsurans* are the most common etiologic agents. Fissuring, maceration, and scaling of the interdigital space of the toes is usually seen. These lesions are often intensely pruritic and may be painful. *T. rubrum* can cause a chronic hyperkeratotic rash of the sole of the foot in a so-called moccasin distribution, sometimes involving both feet and one hand. Secondary bacterial infection may complicate tinea pedis, and the condition may be confused with contact dermatitis or eczema.

Tinea Unguium

Tinea unguium is uncommon in children, but youngsters can be infected during household epidemics. The most common etiologic agent is *T. rubrum*. A yellow or brown discoloration of the nail is seen with thickening and friability beginning at the distal and lateral borders of the nail. Tinea unguium may be confused with candidal infection of the nail, psoriasis, or Reiter syndrome.

DIAGNOSIS

Diagnosis is typically on the basis of clinical features. Atypical features may require further study, however. For tinea capitis, Wood's light examination is no longer particularly useful because the major pathogen, *T. tonsurans*, does not fluoresce. (*M. canis* and *M. audouinii*, among others, fluoresce bright green but, since the late 1950s, they have been much less common causes of tinea capitis.) If necessary, specimens of hair or skin can be collected by gently scraping with a scalpel or by gently brushing (a toothbrush is often useful) a lesion. Nail clippings may also be examined. KOH examination of material might be useful if fungal hyphae are demonstrated, but a negative examination does not exclude the diagnosis. Dermatophyte test medium changes color from yellow to red within approximately 14 days of inoculation of clinical material containing dermatophytes.

TREATMENT

With the exception of tinea capitis and most cases of tinea unguium, dermatophyte infections are treated topically.

Tinea Capitis

Although it can resolve spontaneously, tinea capitis should be treated. Griseofulvin is the drug of choice given orally for 4 to 12 weeks. Other oral drugs such as ketoconazole, itraconazole, and terbinafine can also be effective.

Tinea Corporis

Tinea corporis can be treated with any of several topical antifungal preparations including miconazole and clotrimazole. Topical terbinafine may also be used. Severe cases of tinea corporis require griseofulvin orally for several weeks.

Tinea Cruris

The patient with tinea cruris should wear loose clothing that allows good aeration. The topical preparations listed for tinea corporis can also be used for tinea cruris.

Tinea Pedis

Tinea pedis can usually be treated with topical powders such as tolnaftate or undecylenic acid. Additionally, the affected child should wear clean, absorbent socks and should keep the feet as dry as possible. Severe or unresponsive cases may require treatment with griseofulvin or another systemic antifungal.

F
Parasitic Diseases

CHAPTER 119
Entamoeba histolytica

Adapted from Bradley Howard Kessler

Infection with *Entamoeba histolytica* (amebiasis) affects as much as 10% of the worldwide population with the highest prevalence seen in underdeveloped countries. Many individuals can be asymptomatic carriers of *E. histolytica*.

ETIOLOGY

Two forms of the protozoan parasite *E. histolytica*, cysts and trophozoites, are found in stool specimens. Trophozoites are motile, variably shaped organisms and may be found in patients with symptomatic or asymptomatic amebiasis. In individuals with symptomatic amebiasis, the pathogenic trophozoites may contain ingested red blood cells in vacuoles.

Infection occurs only with ingestion of cysts. On ingestion, after excystation in the small bowel, each single cyst results in eight trophozoites. Unlike the trophozoite, which is destroyed rapidly by external environmental conditions and gastric acid, the cysts are resistant to gastric acid and to the chlorine concentrations commonly used in domestic water purification, as well as to extreme temperature and drying. Cysts may survive outside the host for several weeks in a moist environment.

EPIDEMIOLOGY

E. histolytica is a leading parasitic cause of death in the world with as many as 50 million cases recorded annually. Humans are the natural host and reservoir for *E. histolytica*. Fecal-oral transmission occurs frequently through contaminated water or foods. Outbreaks have been associated with pollution of the water supply by sewage. Infected food handlers play a major role in transmitting the infection. Amebic infection is common in homosexuals infecting as much as 30% of this population with *E. dispar* (nonpathogenic) being the predominant species.

PATHOGENESIS AND PATHOLOGY

Pathogenesis of invasive amebiasis occurs through a number of steps: colonization of the colonic mucous blanket, penetration or depletion of the mucous layer with disruption of the epithelial barrier, and parasite lysis of responding host inflammatory cells, followed by deeper tissue penetration. The factors that determine whether ingestion of *E. histolytica* will produce no infection, a commensal state, symptomatic colitis, or hepatic abscess are not well defined.

Trophozoites may cause diarrhea by stimulating intestinal secretion. As the process continues, classic flask-shaped ulcers with undermined edges are formed. When amebae move into the bowel wall, some may be picked up in the portal circulation and become disseminated, first to the liver and then throughout the body.

The pathologic lesions described most frequently are ulcers that are scattered throughout the colon, which affect predominantly the cecum and ascending colon. As the disease progresses, the ulcer enlarges and extends into the submucosa and muscular coat. On rare occasions, this extension can lead to perforation.

An amebic liver abscess is usually solitary with the right lobe of the liver being involved most often. The material within an abscess has been described as resembling anchovy paste or chocolate syrup. The parasite is rarely found in aspirated abscess fluid.

CLINICAL FEATURES

Most infections are asymptomatic. Luminal colonization and elimination of the parasite from the gastrointestinal tract occurs within 12 months. For clinical illness, the incubation period is generally 2 to 4 weeks with varying degrees of severity. Most patients with invasive amebiasis describe a gradual onset of cramping, abdominal pain, malaise, tenesmus (with rectal involvement), and frequent stools. Stools are usually bloodstained and mucoid. Diarrhea may persist for weeks but can wax and wane with alternating periods of constipation. In some patients, the onset of symptoms may be acute with fever; profuse, bloody, mucoid diarrhea; dehydration; and electrolyte abnormalities. This fulminant picture may mimic that seen in toxic megacolon, acute inflammatory bowel disease, and bacillary dysentery. Possible complications include intestinal perforation, hemorrhage, stricture, inflammation, peritonitis, and a local inflammatory mass or ameboma. On physical examination, tenderness is usually present throughout the lower abdomen.

Hepatic amebiasis and abscess are characterized by fever, abdominal pain, pleuritic pain, respiratory distress, and hepatomegaly in a patient with a history of GI symptoms. The pain is usually localized to the right upper quadrant with radiation to the right shoulder and laterally to the chest. Chest radiographs may show elevation of the right hemidiaphragm. Laboratory evaluation may reveal anemia with an elevated leukocyte count and a left shift. The most common finding on physical examination is a large, tender liver. Complications involve the pleural cavity or intraabdominal extension of the abscess.

DIAGNOSIS

Microscopical examination of repeated stool specimens is the definitive diagnostic test. When the test is performed correctly, the results of more than 90% of stool examinations are positive in infected patients. Stool samples should be examined immediately after defecation or should be preserved in a fixative for later examination. An experienced examiner competent in the diagnosis of parasitic infections should be consulted to differentiate *E. histolytica* from other amebae that are rarely pathogenic. Many patients undergo sigmoidoscopy or colonoscopy to evaluate for ulcerative colitis. In this case, rectal mucosal scrapings can be examined as trophozoites can be seen on colonic biopsies in approximately 50% of cases. If stool examination results are negative and a high level of suspicion exists for intestinal amebiasis, serologic testing such as an indirect hemagglutination (IHA) test should be done. IHA test results are strongly positive (titer greater than 1:256) in 85% to 90% of patients with invasive colonic disease or liver abscess. A limitation of the IHA test is that the results can remain positive for more than 20 years and, therefore, may represent earlier illness. Colonization with nonpathogenic strains rarely provides a serologic response.

Infection Recognition

The key to recognizing an amebic liver abscess is suspecting the diagnosis in patients with fever and an enlarged, tender liver. Patients with a liver abscess do not usually have concurrent diarrhea. Laboratory test results are generally nonspecific with serum alkaline phosphatase, bilirubin, and transaminases being mildly elevated. Ultrasound or CT scan of the liver will make the diagnosis of abscess.

TREATMENT

The specific therapy for infection with *E. histolytica* depends on the site of involvement (luminal, intramural, or systemic). An asymptomatic carrier should be treated with iodoquinol (formerly diiodohydroxyquin), 30 to 40 mg/kg/day (maximum, 2 g/day) in divided doses given every 8 hours for 20 days. Invasive amebiasis of the intestine, liver, or other organs requires the additional use of a tissue amebicide such as metronidazole (Flagyl). This is administered at a dosage of 35 to 50 mg/kg/day in divided doses given every 8 hours for 10 days. Because metronidazole is a less effective luminal amebicide, patients should receive iodoquinol (as outlined earlier) for 20 days.

An uncomplicated, deep, unruptured liver abscess may be treated medically. Liver abscess or other forms of extraintestinal disease should be treated with metronidazole followed by iodoquinol (as outlined earlier). The patient's clinical condition will usually improve within 72 hours of the initiation of medical therapy. In all cases, positive contacts should be screened.

Prophylaxis for travelers to endemic areas is not recommended. The best prophylaxis is exercising caution in unsanitary conditions and endemic environments.

CHAPTER 120

Cryptosporidiosis

Adapted from Walter T. Hughes

Cryptosporidiosis is a common enteric infection caused by the coccidian protozoan *Cryptosporidium*. The infection came to prominence in the early 1980s because of its association with the acquired immunodeficiency syndrome (AIDS). *Cryptosporidium* is a frequent cause of diarrhea in otherwise normal children, especially those attending day-care centers.

ETIOLOGY

The oocyst form of *Cryptosporidium* resides in the feces and is the infective stage. Sporozoites within the oocyst mature, undergo sporulation, and are released into the intestine, where, as trophozoites, they attach to the microvillar surface of epithelial cells. Merogony, gametogony, and sporogony occur. Macrogametes and microgametes develop and, on fertilization, develop into an oocyst with four sporozoites. The oocyst is passed into the feces. At least six species of *Cryptosporidium* exist with *Cryptosporidium parvum* believed to cause the infection in humans.

EPIDEMIOLOGY

The organism appears to be highly transmissible from human to human, and some outbreaks have been traced to contaminated water supplies. Animal-to-human and human-to-animal transmission of *Cryptosporidium* has also been reported.

Sources

Carrier prevalence rates of *Cryptosporidium* range from 0.6% to 4.0% in North America and from 4% to 20% in developing countries. Because the oocyst is highly stable in the environment, contaminated drinking water, apple cider, and swimming pools are sources of outbreaks of infection. A contaminated public water supply resulted in an epidemic of nearly 400,000 cases of cryptosporidiosis in Milwaukee. Some studies indicate that *Cryptosporidium* oocysts are present in 65% to 95% of surface water (i.e., rivers, lakes, and streams) tested throughout the United States.

In the United States, 13% of children younger than 5 years, 38% of those 5 to 13 years of age, and 58% of adolescents 14 to 21 years of age are seropositive for antibodies to *C. parvum*. *Cryptosporidium* is frequently responsible for outbreaks of diarrhea in day-care centers.

Enteric isolation precautions for hospitalized patients with *Cryptosporidium* are necessary given possible person-to-person spread.

CLINICAL MANIFESTATIONS

Infection with *Cryptosporidium* may be asymptomatic or symptomatic. When the infection becomes clinically evident, the extent of the signs and symptoms is generally related to the degree of patient immunocompetence. Normal children and adults have either asymptomatic infection or a self-limited illness, which is similar to giardiasis with watery diarrhea, abdominal pain, malaise, myalgias, weight loss, and anorexia. In these illnesses, the incubation period is generally 1 week and the duration of the illness is approximately 12 days.

Patients with AIDS or other severe immunodeficiency states usually have chronic diarrhea, often with cholera-like features. Diarrhea is commonly profuse, watery, and without blood. Fluid losses may be extensive, as much as several liters per day in adults. These patients may also have abdominal pain, anorexia, nausea, and vomiting, but they are rarely febrile.

DIAGNOSIS

The differential diagnosis for cryptosporidiosis includes all causes of diarrhea. The diagnosis of cryptosporidiosis is established by the demonstration of *Cryptosporidium* oocysts in fecal specimens in the absence of other enteric pathogens. The clinician must bear in mind that *Cryptosporidium* can be found in asymptomatic individuals. If examination of the feces does not reveal the oocysts, specific concentration techniques should be used. The technique used most frequently is the Sheather sugar flotation method. An experienced microbiology lab is generally familiar with this procedure. Serologic tests for antibody to *Cryptosporidium* have been developed but are not in general use at this time and are not of diagnostic value.

A fluorescein-labeled antibody test that uses monoclonal antibody to *Cryptosporidium* (Meridian Laboratories, Cincinnati, OH) is available and is the most sensitive and specific test for the organism in stool specimens.

TREATMENT

No specific therapy is available for cryptosporidiosis. Oocyst excretion can persist for as long as 2 weeks after clinical recovery occurs. For this reason, hospitalized patients should be isolated. In most immunocompetent children, the course is self-limited, but immunosuppressed patients may require intensive and prolonged supportive management. Studies have yielded equivocal results from the use of drugs such as azithromycin, paromomycin, and nitrazoxanide. Experimental preparations of hyperimmune bovine colostrum and bovine transfer factor have undergone preliminary trials with some evidence of efficacy. Effective antiretroviral treatment of AIDS is associated with resolution of cryptosporidiosis symptoms.

Severely immunocompromised patients should avoid swimming in and drinking from lakes and rivers. Because chlorination does not kill the organism, the use of boiled tap water (1 minute) or the filtration of drinking water with submicron (1 micron) personal-use filters is suggested. Commercially available bottled water is not standardized for microbial purity.

CHAPTER 121
Giardia lamblia

Adapted from William J. Klish

DISTRIBUTION

Giardia lamblia has worldwide distribution and is an important cause of traveler's diarrhea. *Giardia* is the most common intestinal parasite found in the United States. Its prevalence may be increasing. The states in which it appears most frequently are located in the Midwest and Northwest. *Giardia* is also prevalent in the mountainous western United States where infection can be contracted by drinking water from mountain streams that have been contaminated by feces from humans, dogs, and other species susceptible to *G. lamblia*. The beaver acts as a reservoir for the organism during the summer months by becoming infected (presumably from humans) and then defecating directly into streams. Boiling water for 10 minutes kills all organisms.

Giardia can also be spread by close person-to-person contact in which fecal contamination may occur such as in day-care centers and residential institutions. In addition, contaminated food may act as a vector for this parasite. Human milk may contain secretory *anti-Giardia* antibodies that can prevent symptoms of diarrhea but not *Giardia* infection in breast-fed infants.

THE ORGANISM

Three species of *Giardia* have been described with *G. lamblia* being specific to humans. *G. lamblia* is the name used for the species infecting humans in North America. This same organism is called *G. intestinalis* in Europe and *Lamblia intestinalis* in Russia and Eastern Europe. It has also been called *G. duodenalis* and *G. enterica*.

G. lamblia is a motile flagellate protozoan with four pairs of flagella. Attachment to mucosa seems to be mediated through the cytoskeleton by contractile filaments and microtubules to lectin-binding sites. The organism also exists in a cyst form, which results when the trophozoite rounds up and elaborates a cyst wall. These cysts allow the organism to survive passage out of the host. *Giardia* cysts are resistant to destruction and can survive for more than 2 months in water at 8°C. When cysts are ingested, the excystation process is induced by gastric acid and is completed in the duodenum with the emergence of trophozoites. Infection is established if the trophozoite can survive, attach to the intestinal mucosa, and multiply. This process may require nutrients within the intestinal fluid.

CLINICAL FEATURES OF GIARDIASIS

Acute symptoms of giardiasis include watery diarrhea, nausea, bloating, belching (described as sulfurous), cramping, abdominal pain, and weight loss; these symptoms usually occur 1 to 2 weeks after the ingestion of cysts. The illness usually is self-limited, lasting 2 to 6 weeks, but may recur intermittently or become chronic. Chronic symptoms can include fatigue, weight loss, growth retardation, steatorrhea, lactose intolerance and, rarely, protein-losing enteropathy. Chronic giardiasis is frequently associated with immunodeficiency syndromes such as IgA and IgM deficiencies and the acquired immunodeficiency syndrome. Individuals who are carrying the disease may be chronically asymptomatic. The pathogenesis of diarrhea and steatorrhea in giardiasis is not understood completely.

DIAGNOSIS

Routine laboratory values are generally normal or nonspecific. Direct examination of feces in physiologic saline for the presence of *G. lamblia* cysts or trophozoites remains the hallmark for diagnosis. Because *Giardia* cysts and trophozoites are not excreted continuously, however, even the best laboratories report a significant number of stool specimens as negative in patients with disease. If the diagnosis is suspected strongly, at least three stools should be collected on different days. With examination of each stool, the chance of diagnosis is approximately 75% from one stool, 90% from two stools, and 97% from three stools.

The diagnosis is made readily by direct examination of the upper small intestine, either by mucosal biopsy or through the collection of jejunal contents. *Giardia* trophozoites can be seen in histologic sections of the small bowel. Jejunal aspirates obtained by intubation can also be examined microscopically for the presence of *Giardia* trophozoites.

An enzyme-linked immunosorbent assay on stool is available. These tests are proving to be more sensitive than the other tests being used routinely for diagnosis.

TREATMENT

Treatment is indicated whenever *Giardia* is found to cause acute diarrhea, chronic intermittent disease, subclinical symptoms, or infection in others. Generally, treatment of asymptomatic carriers is not recommended. Children with nondiarrheal giardiasis, however, who exhibit other gastrointestinal symptoms or who have evidence of malabsorption should be considered for therapy. Public health considerations might also require that asymptomatic carriers be treated.

The treatment of choice in both asymptomatic and symptomatic patients is metronidazole (Flagyl), administered for 1 week in adults and children. An alternative drug is quinacrine (Atabrine), administered for 7 days in adults and children. Another drug that can be used is furazolidone (Furoxone), administered for 7 to 10 days in both adults and children. Other therapies exist.

CHAPTER 122
Toxocara Infections

Adapted from B. Keith English

Human infection with the larval stage of the common dog roundworm, *Toxocara canis*, is the principal cause of two distinct clinical syndromes: visceral larva migrans (VLM) and ocular toxocariasis or ocular larva migrans.

EPIDEMIOLOGY AND TRANSMISSION

Toxocara canis, a nematode roundworm parasite, which infects dogs and is prevalent in all 50 states in the United States. Female worms produce up to 200,000 eggs per day and the eggs can become infective in 2 to 5 weeks. Adult worms live for approximately 4 months in the proximal small intestine of dogs.

Acquisition

Dogs may acquire *T. canis* infection by transplacental migration of larvae, transmammary passage (nursing pups drinking infected milk from their mother), ingestion of infected eggs, ingestion of infected larvae in animals such as pigs, mice, rats and lamb, and ingestion of late-stage larvae or immature adult worms.

Larvae

In adult dogs, eggs hatch into larvae in the stomach and small intestine. Then they penetrate the intestinal mucosa, travel via the portal circulation to the liver, and enter the systemic circulation reaching the heart and lungs 3 to 5 days after infection. Some larvae penetrate the bronchioles, travel to the trachea and pharynx, are swallowed, and develop into adult worms in the small intestine. Other larvae invade the pulmonary vein, travel back to the heart, and spread via the systemic circulation throughout the body. In puppies, the tracheal route predominates, accounting for their importance in the transmission of disease to other hosts.

In humans and paratenic hosts (including mice, rats, lambs, and pigs), the tracheal route of migration leading to the development of adult worms does not occur. Larvae do travel to the liver via the portal circulation and to the systemic circulation via the lungs, however, lodging in small blood vessels in somatic organs. The larvae then bore through the walls of the blood vessels and migrate through the tissues.

Nearly all human toxocaral infections occur by ingestion of infective eggs from soil that is contaminated with excreta from puppies or from contaminated hands or fomites. Ingestion of uncooked organ and muscle meat from paratenic hosts (pigs, lambs, rabbits, snails and, perhaps, chickens) is a documented (but uncommon) source for human infection. Pica for dirt (geophagia) is the principal risk factor for VLM in children and adults.

Seroprevalence rates (for antibodies to *T. canis*) increase with rural residence, crowding, and lower socioeconomic status. The epidemiologic features of VLM and ocular toxocariasis are strikingly different. Although both are associated with exposure to puppies, only VLM is associated clearly with pica. Patients with VLM are usually 1 to 4 years old, whereas patients with ocular toxocariasis have a mean age of 7 to 8 years. Most patients with ocular toxocariasis have no history of a syndrome similar to VLM, although ocular involvement may occur concomitantly with VLM, especially in very young children with severe disease or many years after VLM.

PATHOGENESIS

Dead or dying larvae provoke a particularly intense inflammatory response. Eosinophilic granulomas develop and surround larvae in various stages of disintegration. Most often in humans, the liver is the site of greatest involvement, but involvement of the lungs is also frequent. Eye involvement is an important complication of *T. canis* infection and occurs in many different forms.

Studies in paratenic hosts have confirmed the importance of the host immune response in the development of tissue injury in this disease.

CLINICAL FEATURES

Visceral Larva Migrans

Classic manifestations of VLM included fever, hepatomegaly, eosinophilic leukocytosis, pruritic rash, and hypergammaglobulinemia. Seizures were reported in more than 25% of patients in one early series. The majority of *T. canis* infections in children are now understood to be asymptomatic, and only a small number of symptomatic infections result in the full-blown VLM syndrome.

Toxocariasis can lead to granulomatous hepatitis. The most common symptoms of VLM are pulmonary and often mimic those of asthma or pneumonia. Chest radiographs demonstrate infiltrates in one-half of the patients with pulmonary symptoms and may reveal a nodular pattern. Ocular disease is unusual in association with VLM but may occur in severe cases.

Leukocyte counts of 30,000 to 100,000 per cubic millimeter with pronounced eosinophilia are common. The percentage of eosinophils is usually greater than 20% in acute cases of VLM and may reach 90%; eosinophilia can persist for months or years after symptoms resolve. Hypergammaglobulinemia is often present with elevations of IgE, IgM, and IgG. Isohemagglutinin titers (anti-A, anti-B) are often elevated because the T. canis larva expresses surface antigens that cross-react with epitopes of the blood group antigens.

The prognosis in most cases of VLM is excellent, complete recovery being the rule. Severe and even fatal cases have been reported, however. Myocardial involvement is rare but has been reported in several fatal cases and as an incidental finding at the time of open-heart surgery in two patients. Although seizures may occur as a complication of VLM, this complication appears to be much less frequent than early reports suggested.

Ocular Toxocariasis

Ocular toxocariasis usually occurs in young school-aged children (mean age, 7–8 years). A history of pica is not frequently present, and eosinophilia is uncommon. Usually, only one eye is involved, but bilateral disease has been reported. Patients commonly complain of decreased visual acuity

Toxocara endophthalmitis, which is characterized by a yellow-white mass, retinal detachment, and cells in the vitreous, is the most common pattern. A feared complication of this condition is the formation of a cyclitic membrane, which may lead to complete vision loss.

Two syndromes often recognized as consequences of *T. canis* ocular disease are posterior retinochoroiditis and peripheral retinochoroiditis. Other clinical patterns include optic papillitis, diffuse unilateral subacute neuroretinitis, the motile chorioretinal nematode syndrome (so-called ocular larva migrans), keratitis, conjunctivitis, and lens involvement.

DIFFERENTIAL DIAGNOSIS

Other animal roundworms such as *Toxocara cati* (cats) and *Toxascaris leonina* (dogs and cats) can cause both visceral and ocular larva migrans. Infection with other nematodes whose life cycle includes a tissue migratory phase (e.g., *Ascaris lumbricoides*, *Trichinella*, and hookworms) may cause marked eosinophilia and may mimic toxocaral VLM. Silent or preceding *T. canis* infection should be considered in the differential diagnosis of unexplained persistent eosinophilia.

The most difficult and important problem for the ophthalmologist is the distinction between *T. canis* endophthalmitis and retinoblastoma. Although retinoblastoma is more frequently bilateral and calcified than ocular toxocariasis, enough overlap exists to render these features unreliable. *Toxocara* endophthalmitis is not usually associated with much pain or photophobia.

Although a presumptive diagnosis of VLM can be supported by abnormalities on a variety of laboratory tests (eosinophilia, hypergammaglobulinemia, elevated isohemagglutinin levels), such tests are nonspecific and are usually normal in cases of ocular disease. The development of ELISA tests, which detects *Toxocara* antibodies in serum, has improved greatly the diagnosis of *T. canis* infections. The ELISA has reported sensitivity and specificity of 78% and 92%, respectively.

The serologic diagnosis of ocular toxocariasis remains problematic. The ELISA can be 90% sensitive and 91% specific if a titer greater than 1:8 is considered indicative of infection. Elevated titers in the absence of disease or false-positive results (representing asymptomatic *T. canis* infection in association with ocular disease of another etiology) can occur. Aspiration of aqueous humor or vitreous humor may confirm the diagnosis by ELISA testing of these fluids. Imaging techniques (such as ultrasonography and computed tomography) have been used to characterize *T. canis* ocular lesions but do not appear to distinguish these lesions clearly from other diagnoses including retinoblastoma.

THERAPY

The overall prognosis for VLM is excellent. Treatment with albendazole or mebendazole typically leads to satisfactory recovery. When severe symptoms occur (e.g., severe respiratory distress) or when involvement of critical organs (myocardium, brain) is noted, corticosteroids may be indicated.

Some authorities suggest that hastening larval death with anthelmintic drugs might be contraindicated given concerns over drug toxicity and the potential for exacerbation of symptoms.

The prognosis for ocular toxocariasis is more guarded and any child with suspected ocular toxocariasis should be referred to an experienced ophthalmologist. Steroids have proved beneficial in severe vision-threatening forms of this disease. Anthelmintic agents have not been demonstrated to be effective and should be used cautiously, if at all.

PREVENTION

Puppies are the principal source of infection in young children. Puppies should be wormed before they reach 2 to 3 weeks of age, and worming should be repeated every 2 weeks until the puppy is 4 months old. Thereafter, fecal examinations should be performed twice yearly with treatment as indicated. Pica should be discouraged, and good hygiene should be practiced. For young children with persistent pica, close supervision is recommended when they play outdoors in parks, backyards, or sandboxes.

Once soil is contaminated with *T. canis* eggs, it cannot be decontaminated.

CHAPTER 123
Toxoplasmosis

Adapted from Ruth Lynfield
and Nicholas G. Guerina

Toxoplasma gondii is an obligate intracellular protozoan parasite found in many animal species throughout the world. Infection is usually asymptomatic in normal hosts, but serious disease may occur in the setting of congenital infection or in an immunodeficient host. Infection with *Toxoplasma* is a life-long condition. The acute stage of infection is characterized by parasitemia. The chronic stage occurs when the parasite becomes encysted in host tissues. *Toxoplasma* may break out of host cells causing a local reactivation and systemic spread of the parasites.

LIFE CYCLE AND TRANSMISSION

Toxoplasma has a sexual cycle that occurs exclusively in felines and an asexual cycle that occurs in most warm-blooded animals (Fig. 123-1). The sexual cycle takes place in the cat intestine,

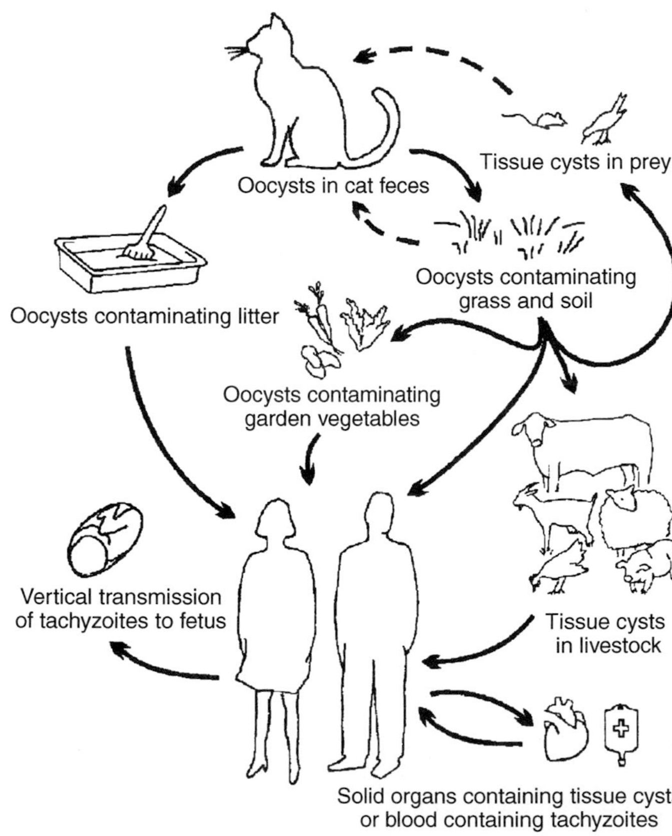

Figure 123-1. The *Toxoplasma gondii* life cycle and pathways for infection. The only source for the production of *T. gondii* oocysts is the feline intestinal tract. Acquired disease in humans occurs by direct ingestion of oocysts from contaminated sources (soil, cat litter, garden vegetables) or the ingestion of tissue cysts present in undercooked tissues from infected animals. Fetal infection most commonly occurs after acute maternal infection in pregnancy, but it can also occur after reactivation of latent infection in immunocompromised women. Pathways leading to human disease are indicated by solid arrows, and pathways leading to feline infection are indicated by broken arrows. (Reproduced from Lynfield R, Guerina G. Toxoplasmosis. *Pediatr Rev* 1997;18:75.)

where gametocytes are formed and fertilized to form zygotes, which are shed as oocysts. The oocysts sporulate and become infectious 24 hours or more after excretion. Sporulated oocysts may remain infectious in soil for more than 1 year, especially in warm, humid environments.

After an animal or human ingests *Toxoplasma* oocysts, the oocyst ruptures in the intestine and releases sporozoites. The sporozoites divide in the intestinal cells and associated lymph nodes. Tachyzoites, the rapidly dividing form characteristic of the acute stage of infection, are formed and dispersed via blood and lymph. When an effective immune response is established, the parasites become localized in tissue cysts composed of components from both the parasites and infected host cells. Within the tissue cysts are slowly dividing forms of *T. gondii* called bradyzoites. Bradyzoites within intact tissue cysts can survive for the life of the host. Occasionally, tissue cysts may rupture releasing bradyzoites. In the presence of an intact immune response, infection is usually controlled. In immunodeficient hosts, bradyzoites may be transformed into tachyzoites, which may proliferate rapidly and induce tissue damage.

The infectious cycle may be perpetuated by tissue cysts when an infected animal is ingested by a carnivore.

Outbreaks of toxoplasmosis have been linked to the ingestion of contaminated water, soil, and undercooked hamburger. Ingestion of oocysts may occur after the handling of contaminated soil or cat litter or after ingestion of contaminated water or food (e.g., unwashed garden produce). Oocysts are very hardy and can resist drying or treating with disinfectants, alcohols (95% ethanol, 100% methanol), or 10% formalin. They may be inactivated by heating (66°C).

Transmission can also occur by ingestion of tissue cysts present in undercooked meat (especially pork and mutton). The bradyzoites in tissue cysts can be destroyed by heating (66°C) or gamma irradiation. Generally, freezing meat at –20°C will also kill tissue cysts. In addition to ingestion, bradyzoites can be transmitted via transplant of an organ containing tissue cysts.

EPIDEMIOLOGY

Some of the highest rates of seropositivity have been reported for Central America, Central Africa, Tahiti, and France. In Central America, seropositivity begins at approximately age 1 year, when children begin playing in oocyst-contaminated sand and soil, and it reaches 50% to 75% by adolescence. With few exceptions, congenital infection occurs in the setting of primary maternal infection during pregnancy. Congenital toxoplasmosis is described in detail in Chapter 33.

CLINICAL MANIFESTATIONS

Clinical manifestations and the severity of disease after *Toxoplasma* infection are based on parasite and host factors such as strain virulence, size of inoculum, stage of parasite, and competence of the host immune response.

Acquired Infection in Immunocompetent Hosts (Including Pregnant Women)

Most cases of *Toxoplasma* infection are subclinical in individuals with normal immune systems, and disease is usually self-limiting. Lymphadenopathy is the manifestation recognized most frequently, and the location is most often cervical, followed by axillary and then inguinal sites. Usually, the lymph nodes are firm and movable and may initially be tender. They do not suppurate. Usually, the lymph nodes are 1 to 2 cm but may be as large as 6 cm. Most cases resolve over the course of 1 to 2 months. Occasionally, disease may persist beyond 6 months. Adenopathy may be recurrent and other causes such as leukemia or cat-scratch disease may need to be investigated. Other clinical presentations include an infectious mononucleosis-like illness with fever, malaise, and myalgia, although sore throat and hepatosplenomegaly are not typical with *Toxoplasma* infection.

Although rare, occasional presentations in normal hosts include encephalitis, ocular disease, pneumonitis, myocarditis, pericarditis, and meningitis.

Infection in Immunocompromised Hosts

Toxoplasmosis in immunocompromised hosts may be due to acute or reactivated infection. Transplant patients undergoing immunosuppressive therapies, with malignancies, or congenital or acquired immunodeficiencies are at risk. Disseminated, systemic infection may occur. Diagnosis may be difficult, because signs and symptoms are not specific to toxoplasmosis. Early treatment can improve outcome. Reactivation of infection may occur in the setting of altered immunity as well. Clinical findings may include retinal disease, encephalitis, pneumonitis, myocarditis, or multiorgan disease.

Toxoplasma encephalitis (TE) is a common opportunistic infection in adult AIDS patients (10%–50% of patients seropositive for Toxoplasma with CD4 counts of fewer than 100 cells per microliter). TE is uncommon in children with AIDS, most likely due to a low incidence of *T. gondii* infection. Generally, focal hypodense mass lesions can be seen on neuroimaging. The main differential diagnosis of TE is primary central nervous system (CNS) lymphoma, especially in the presence of a single lesion. Other possibilities include progressive multifocal leukoencephalopathy, bacterial abscess, Cryptococcus, cytomegalovirus, mycobacterium tuberculosis, and focal viral encephalitis.

Pulmonary toxoplasmosis may be seen in immunosuppressed AIDS patients. Often, diffuse bilateral interstitial pneumonitis is seen on chest radiography. The organism may be found in a bronchoalveolar lavage aspirate and in biopsy specimen, or in both, using appropriate histologic staining techniques.

Congenital Infection: See Chapter 33

Ocular Disease

Toxoplasma is the most common cause of infectious chorioretinitis in immunocompetent children. In most cases, it is thought to be due to sequelae from congenital infection. Mechanisms for new-onset retinal disease may include an inflammatory reaction to old retinal tissue cysts, a hypersensitivity reaction to *Toxoplasma* antigens localized in the retina, and invasion of the eye after recurrent parasitemia. Usually, chorioretinal disease associated with acquired disease involves one eye. Disease associated with reactivation from congenital infection may be bilateral, although many cases are unilateral.

Ocular symptoms include blurred vision, photophobia, and vision loss. Usually, the lesion of ocular toxoplasmosis is a focal necrotizing retinitis. The differential diagnosis includes CMV, herpes simplex virus, rubella, varicella, syphilis, and congenital anomalies.

DIAGNOSIS

Diagnostic tests for *T. gondii* infection include the measurement of *Toxoplasma*-specific antibodies, detection of

Toxoplasma-specific DNA by polymerase chain reaction (PCR), isolation or histologic demonstration of the organism, and detection of *Toxoplasma* antigens in tissues and body fluids. Serology is the technique used most frequently to make a diagnosis of *Toxoplasma* infection.

Enzyme-linked immunosorbent assays for IgG (IgG-ELISA) and IgM are available but may lack sensitivity and specificity outside of reference labs. Interpretation of titers requires consultation with the laboratory performing the assays. Significance of results and necessary follow-up studies should be determined in conjunction with an infectious disease expert.

Toxoplasma-specific IgG may be detected within 1 week of a primary infection, and peak titers are found 3 to 8 weeks later. In children and adults with normal antibody responses, typically IgG antibody lasts for life. *Toxoplasma*-specific IgM can also be detected within 1 week of infection, and peak titers occur 3 to 4 weeks later. Depending on the assay used, specific IgM titers may persist for months to more than 1 year after a primary infection. Other assays available are the IgA-ELISA and IgE-ELISA.

The PCR for DNA has been used to detect *T. gondii* in body fluids and tissue including amniotic fluid, CSF, blood, urine, ocular fluid, and bronchoalveolar lavage specimens.

Using special techniques, tachyzoites and tissue cysts can be visualized directly in histologic sections or cytologic preparations. The histologic findings of toxoplasma lymphadenitis are often described as a triad of reactive follicular hyperplasia, focal distension of sinuses with monocytoid cells, and irregular clusters of epithelioid histiocytes located around the margins of the germinal centers. These findings can be suggestive even in the absence of finding organisms. Isolation of *T. gondii* is cumbersome and expensive and, therefore, is available in only a few reference laboratories.

Antibody production may be impaired in certain immunodeficient states, making diagnosis more difficult. Aggressive testing, including biopsy of focal lesions, may be needed and PCR can be a useful aid in diagnosis.

Acute Maternal and Fetal *Toxoplasma* Infection in Pregnancy

Pregnant women who are seronegative on initial testing remain at risk for acute *Toxoplasma* infection for the remainder of their pregnancy. For this reason, some countries have established Toxoplasma screening programs that use repeated serologic testing at regular intervals throughout pregnancy. Once acute maternal infection has been identified, tests for fetal infection should be undertaken. Combination evaluation with ultrasonographic surveys for fetal anomalies plus fetal blood sampling (for specific and nonspecific tests for *Toxoplasma* infection) have been used successfully to test for fetal infection by experienced maternal-fetal medicine personnel in collaboration with a Toxoplasma reference laboratory. The single best test for fetal infection, however, may be the *Toxoplasma*-specific PCR on amniotic fluid as performed by a *Toxoplasma* reference laboratory.

Acute Ocular Toxoplasmosis

Postnatal *Toxoplasma* chorioretinitis can result from late sequelae of congenital infection or after acute acquired *Toxoplasma* infection. In cases of reactivated infection, *Toxoplasma* IgG may be at low levels, and *Toxoplasma* IgM is typically negative. Often, the diagnosis is made when characteristic retinal lesions are seen in a *Toxoplasma*-seropositive patient, but if the lesions appear atypical to an experienced ophthalmologist, other diagnoses should be considered.

TREATMENT

Pyrimethamine and sulfadiazine (or trisulfapyrimidines) provide synergistic activity against *Toxoplasma* when used in combination. Activity is against the tachyzoite form of *T. gondii*. Pyrimethamine is a folic acid antagonist and can cause bone marrow suppression. Usually, this suppression can be prevented by folinic acid (leucovorin), which should always be administered prophylactically. The selection of a treatment regimen including dosing should be made in consultation with an infectious disease expert.

Other drugs being investigated in the treatment of *Toxoplasma* infection include the macrolides clarithromycin, azithromycin, and roxithromycin and atovaquone. Atovaquone is attractive because it is active against both the tachyzoite and the cystic forms of *T. gondii*.

Acquired Toxoplasmosis

Most cases of acquired toxoplasmosis in immunologically normal children and nonpregnant adults are self-limiting, and specific drug therapy is reserved for the rare occurrence of severe or persistent clinical symptoms or for compromise of vital organs. Combination therapy is usually given with pyrimethamine and sulfadiazine with folinic acid rescue. Therapy is continued until symptoms resolve (approximately 2–6 weeks).

Infection in Immunocompromised Patients

In immunocompromised patients, acute or active infection should be treated regardless of symptoms, because such patients are at high risk of severe disease due to *Toxoplasma*. Combination drug therapy with pyrimethamine and sulfadiazine (or clindamycin for the sulfa drug-intolerant) plus folinic acid is given. Treatment in nonAIDS patients is given for at least 4 to 6 weeks beyond complete resolution of all signs and symptoms of disease. This treatment may be followed by chronic therapy, particularly in the case of encephalitis. Many prophylactic dosing regimens are available. In immunosuppressed patients, these regimens should be administered in consultation with an infectious disease specialist. A full description of current guidelines can be found at http://www.aidsinfo.nih.gov/guidelines/op_infections/OI_112801.pdf

Ocular Toxoplasmosis

Active chorioretinitis should be treated in both children and adults. Combination therapy with pyrimethamine and sulfadiazine (plus folinic acid) is generally preferred, especially in children. Some experts use a regimen that includes clindamycin. The duration of treatment is approximately 2 weeks after acute inflammation has resolved. Most experts also treat vision-threatening lesions with prednisone until acute inflammation resolves.

PREVENTION

Avoiding exposure to sources of *Toxoplasma* is an important way to prevent infection. This caution is particularly important for seronegative pregnant women and immunocompromised patients. Individuals should be advised not to eat undercooked or raw meat. Meat should be cooked to an internal temperature of 66°C (150°F). Hands should be washed thoroughly after handling raw meat and vegetables and fruits, and raw vegetables and fruits should be washed thoroughly before they are eaten. Kitchen surfaces, cutting boards, and utensils should be cleaned after each use. Gloves should be worn and hands should be washed thoroughly after handling potentially contaminated materials such as soil, cat litter, or sandboxes or after gardening. Cats should be kept indoors and should be fed only dry, canned, or cooked food. Cat litter should be changed daily (as oocysts do not sporulate in the first 24 hours after passage), preferably by someone not pregnant or immunocompromised. The possibility of transmission of infection via oocysts can be reduced further by soaking a cat's litter pan in near-boiling water for 5 minutes.

2

Respiratory Tract

CHAPTER 124

The Common Cold

Adapted from Sarah S. Long

Initially believed to be caused by either a single virus or a group of viruses, the common cold is now recognized to be associated with more than 200 viruses, occasional bacteria, protozoa, and *Mycoplasma*. Table 124-1 provides an abbreviated list of causative agents and their relative prevalence in children. Rhinoviruses and coronaviruses have even more importance in adults, in whom symptoms of the common cold are the classic manifestations of infection.

Although rhinoviruses are the most frequent cause of the common cold overall, the role of other agents can be suggested by consideration of factors related to the host and the setting of the illness (Table 124-2). Season (Table 124-3), age, and prior immunologic experience are the most important influences on cause. For example, disease resulting from respiratory syncytial virus and parainfluenza viruses is most common and most severe in patients who are younger than 3. Infection occurs less commonly and with milder symptoms (frequently those of the common cold) with increasing age.

TABLE 124-1. Etiologic Agents of the Common Cold in Children

Agent	Prevalence
Viruses	
Rhinoviruses	+++
Parainfluenza viruses	++
Respiratory syncytial virus	+
Coronaviruses	+
Adenoviruses	+
Enteroviruses	+
Influenza viruses	+
Reoviruses	+
Other	
Mycoplasma pneumoniae	+
Bordetella pertussis	+

+, occasional cause; ++, prevalent cause; +++, most prevalent cause.

EPIDEMIOLOGY

Peak age of occurrence is the second 6 months of life. Incidence does not fall significantly until the second decade. The number of colds increases during group child-care exposure in infancy. Exposure to viruses in schools and child-care centers serves to introduce viruses into the family. Boys have symptomatic respiratory tract illnesses more frequently than girls. Usually, adults are victims rather than sources of common cold viruses; primary caregivers and infants have the highest rates of secondary illness.

Viruses causing the common cold spread from person to person by means of virus-contaminated respiratory secretions. Studies in adult volunteers suggested that rhinoviruses are spread by small airborne particles, by inhalation or impalement of large particles when transmitters and recipients are at very close range, and through self-inoculation after direct hand contact with a transmitter's infected nasal secretions or indirect contact with contaminated objects. Direct contact is the primary means for the spread of rhinovirus infections. Compared with adults, infected children have higher concentrations of virus in secretions and longer duration of shedding. Coughing, talking, drooling, and kissing are not highly contagious behaviors. Sneezing, nose blowing and wiping, and hand transfer of secretions from paper tissues or environmental surfaces to nose or conjunctiva are more contagious behaviors.

CLINICAL CHARACTERISTICS

Symptoms

The common cold syndrome has been defined as that which most typically follows rhinovirus infection. Throat irritation, sneezing, and nasal stuffiness are the primary complaints on the first and second days of illness; rhinitis, watering eyes, and sometimes hoarseness and cough follow on the second to fourth days of illness. Fever is absent or low-grade. Chilliness, headache, and achiness can be present early in the illness. Cough and nasal discharge are the most persistent complaints. Typically, illness caused by rhinoviruses lasts for 6 to 7 days. Nasal symptoms tend to be more prominent, and throat and systemic symptoms tend to be less prominent in upper respiratory tract illness caused by rhinovirus as compared with that caused by other viruses. The large number of rhinovirus types is associated predictably with variable symptoms and degrees of discomfort.

The symptoms described are typical for older children and adults. Infants are more likely to exhibit a temperature of 38°C or 39°C, fussiness, and restlessness. Nasal obstruction can interfere with sleeping and eating.

Infection

Infection with rhinovirus and other common cold viruses can extend to cause viral otitis media, sinusitis, and pneumonia or can predispose to secondary bacterial infections. Rhinoviruses cause exacerbation of bronchitis in adults and, alone or in consort with other viruses, occasionally cause pneumonia. In children with hyperreactive airways, mild viral upper respiratory tract illnesses can incite episodes of asthma or can induce pulmonary decompensation in infants with bronchopulmonary dysplasia.

TABLE 124-2. Use of Historical Information to Differentiate Among Causes of Nonspecific Upper Respiratory Tract Illnesses

Factor	Typical for rhinovirus	Examples of factors typical for other etiologies	
Age	School-aged	Toddler	Parainfluenza viruses
		School-aged	*Mycoplasma pneumoniae*
Season	Fall, spring	Winter	RSV, influenza
		Summer	Adenoviruses
Immunization status	Any	Incomplete	*Bordetella pertussis*
		Incomplete	Mumps
Sibling	School-aged	Infant	RSV
		Adolescent	Adenoviruses
		Toddler	Parainfluenza viruses
Illness in contacts	Common cold	Bronchiolitis	RSV
		Croup	Parainfluenza viruses
		Conjunctivitis	Adenoviruses
		Exudative pharyngitis	Adenoviruses, Epstein-Barr virus
		Ulcerative enanthem	Enteroviruses
Incubation period	3–5 d	2 wk	*M. pneumoniae* , *B. pertussis*
Acquisition	Home	Hospital	RSV, influenza viruses
		Day care	All agents
Community epidemic	Common cold	Parotitis	Mumps
		Hand-foot-and-mouth disease	Enteroviruses
		Aseptic meningitis	Enteroviruses
		Febrile upper respiratory tract infection	Influenza viruses, adenoviruses

RSV, respiratory syncytial virus.

TREATMENT AND PREVENTION

Treatment of the common cold is supportive. No antiviral agent effective against rhinovirus is available. Although annual sales of proprietary cold remedies total more than $1 billion in the United States, these preparations have been shown to have no (or modest) benefit and can be harmful in children. Performing clinical trials in children is difficult, as potentially beneficial outcomes rely on subjective assessments of severity of symptoms or objective measurements that require considerable cooperation of involved subjects. On the other hand, studies of cold remedies showing benefit in adults can be misleading when symptoms are due to allergic, rather than infectious, illnesses. In blinded, placebo-controlled studies in adults, rhinorrhea and sneezing improved modestly (though statistically significantly) with use of a first-generation antihistamine, as did cough with use of an antihistamine-decongestant combination. Using objective measurements, a topical adrenergic decongestant did not improve abnormal middle-ear pressure in infants with nasal congestion during the common cold. Pharmacokinetics of orally administered cold remedies given to children have been subjected to little or no study or have been shown to vary from those in older individuals. Side effects such as sedation, hypertension, and dystonic reactions are especially common in children. Considering the data (albeit imperfect) and potential benefit versus safety of cold remedies for symptoms of the common cold, nasal or oral decongestants, and antihistamines should not be given to children younger than age 6 months and should be given infrequently and individually to older infants and children.

TABLE 124-3. Seasonal Peaks of Respiratory Tract Pathogens

Fall
Rhinoviruses
Parainfluenza viruses
Group A streptococcus
Winter
Respiratory syncytial virus
Adenoviruses
Influenza viruses
Coronaviruses
Spring
Rhinoviruses
Parainfluenza viruses
Group A streptococcus
Summer
Adenoviruses
Bordetella pertussis
Enteroviruses

Aspirin

Aspirin should not be given to children with symptoms of viral illness because of its association with Reye syndrome. Acetaminophen or ibuprofen should be used infrequently for the common cold (and rarely in children younger than age 6 months) to relieve discomfort. Hepatotoxicity, hepatic failure, and deaths have occurred from inadvertent overdosing of acetaminophen, especially in infants.

Alternative Therapies

Assessment of effectiveness of alternative therapies for colds has been controversial for decades. Although in some studies, vitamin C apparently reduced severity and duration of symptoms, the large doses used cannot be recommended for use in children; whether effective or not, zinc lozenges would not be practical for younger patients because of metallic taste; aromatic rubs cannot be subjected to placebo-controlled study; results of hot mist are conflicting; hot chicken soup may temporarily increase velocity of nasal mucus, but hypernatremia must be avoided; and adequate study of homeopathic and herbal remedies has not been performed.

Antibiotics

Antibiotics have no place in the therapy for the common cold and have been shown to be ineffective in altering the course of attendant purulent rhinorrhea. Expected changes in character of nasal secretions during uncomplicated rhinovirus infection are progression from clear to mucoid, mucopurulent (opaque white, yellow, or green) and clear over a 7- to 10-day period.

Supportive Care

The relief of nasal obstruction is the most important focus of supportive care. Comfortable environmental temperature and humidity should be maintained. Humidification soothes irritated nasopharyngeal mucosa and helps to prevent drying of nasal secretions, thus promoting their elimination. Use of isotonic saline nasal drops and gentle aspiration or, occasionally, higher-volume nasal saline flush can provide temporary relief for young infants.

Hygiene and Disinfectants

Meticulous hand washing by staff should be practiced in hospitals and other facilities where small children are located. Personal hygiene should be taught to children. Phenol-alcohol solution (Lysol) is an effective environmental disinfectant, as are tincture of iodine and povidone-iodine.

Vaccines

Interest in the development of a vaccine against the common cold viruses waned when continual antigenic drift of rhinoviruses was considered the best explanation for the multiple serotypes, conventional parenteral routes of vaccine administration did not provide protection against nasal challenge, and nasal inoculation provided only short-term benefit. The task of developing an attenuated nasal vaccine seems less formidable now that the serotypes of rhinovirus appear to be multiple but stable and the number of serotypes causing the majority of disease may be only 30.

CHAPTER 125
Sinusitis

Adapted from Ellen R. Wald

Acute infection of the paranasal sinuses is a common complication of allergic or infectious inflammation of the upper respiratory tract. Approximately 5% of upper respiratory infections are complicated by acute sinusitis. Children experience six to eight colds per year, therefore, sinusitis is a problem commonly seen in clinical practice.

Of the four paired paranasal sinuses—ethmoid, maxillary, sphenoid, and frontal—all but the frontal sinuses are present at birth. The frontal sinuses develop from the anterior ethmoid sinuses and become clinically important after the tenth birthday. The maxillary and ethmoid sinuses are the principal sites of sinus infection in young children.

ANATOMY

The anatomic relationship between the nose and the paranasal sinuses is shown in Fig. 125-1. Beneath the middle and the superior turbinates is a natural meatus that drains two or more of the paranasal sinuses. The posterior ethmoid sinus and the sphenoid sinuses drain into the superior meatus, and the anterior ethmoid sinuses, the frontal sinuses, and the maxillary sinuses drain into the middle meatus; only the lacrimal duct drains into the inferior meatus. The position of the outflow tract of the maxillary sinus, high on the medial wall of the nasal cavity, impedes gravitational drainage of secretions and accounts for the frequency of involvement of the maxillary sinuses when upper respiratory tract inflammation becomes complicated by bacterial superinfection.

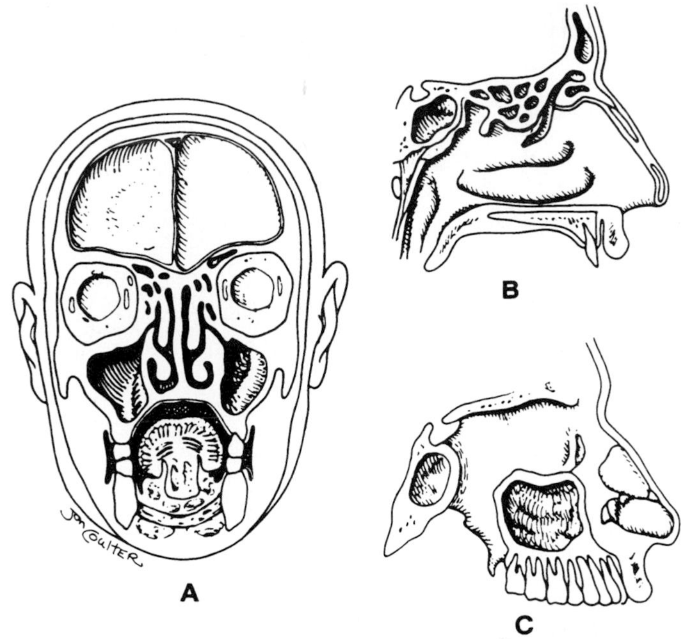

Figure 125-1. Anatomy of the paranasal sinuses. **A:** Coronal section demonstrating the relationship between the nose and the ethmoid and maxillary sinuses. **B:** Sagittal section showing the nasal turbinates as well as the frontal, ethmoid, and sphenoidal sinus. **C:** Parasaggital section shows the body of the maxillary and sphenoid sinus.

PATHOGENSIS

Three elements are important to the normal physiology of the paranasal sinuses: the patency of the ostia, the function of the ciliary apparatus and, integral to the latter, the quality of secretions. Retention of secretions in the paranasal sinuses is caused by one or more of the following: obstruction of the ostia, reduction in the number (or impaired function) of the cilia, or overproduction or change in the viscosity of the secretions.

The factors predisposing to ostial obstruction can be divided into those factors that cause mucosal swelling and those factors that result from mechanical obstruction (Table 125-1). Although many conditions may lead to ostial closure, viral upper respiratory infection and allergic inflammation are, by far, the most common and most important.

In the posterior two-thirds of the nasal cavity and within the sinuses, the epithelium is pseudostratified columnar, in which most of the cells are ciliated. Usually, the normal motility of the cilia and the adhesive properties of the mucous layer protect respiratory epithelium from bacterial invasion. However, certain respiratory viruses (influenza, adenovirus) may have a direct cytotoxic effect on the cilia. The alteration of cilia number,

TABLE 125-1. Factors Predisposing to Sinus Ostial Obstruction

Mucosal swelling
Systemic disorder
Viral upper respiratory infection
Allergic inflammation
Cystic fibrosis
Immune disorders
Immotile cilia
Local Insult
Facial trauma
Swimming, diving
Rhinitis medicamentosa
Mechanical obstruction
Choanal atresia
Deviated septum
Nasal polyps
Foreign body
Tumor

morphology, and function may facilitate secondary bacterial invasion of the nose and the paranasal sinuses.

CLINICAL CHARACTERISTICS

In most children with acute or chronic sinusitis, the respiratory symptoms of nasal discharge, nasal congestion, and cough are prominent. During the course of an apparent viral upper respiratory tract infection, two common clinical presentations suggest a diagnosis of acute sinusitis.

The first, most common clinical situation raising suspicion of sinusitis is persistent signs and symptoms of a cold. Nasal discharge and daytime cough that continue beyond 10 days and are not improving are the principal complaints. Most uncomplicated upper respiratory tract infections last for 5 to 7 days; although patients may not be asymptomatic by the tenth day, their condition has usually improved. The persistence of respiratory symptoms without appreciable improvement beyond the 10-day mark suggests that a complication has developed. The nasal discharge may be of any quality (thin or thick, clear, mucoid, or purulent) and usually the cough (which may be dry or wet) is present in the daytime, although it is often noted to be worse at night. Cough occurring only at night is a common residual symptom of an upper respiratory tract infection. When it is the only residual symptom, it is usually nonspecific and does not suggest a sinus infection; it is more likely to represent reactive airways disease. On the other hand, the persistence of daytime cough is frequently the symptom that brings affected children to medical attention. Such children may not appear ill; usually, if fever is present, it will be low-grade. Often, malodorous breath is reported by parents of affected preschoolers. The complaint of malodorous breath accompanied by respiratory symptoms (in the absence of exudative pharyngitis, dental decay, or nasal foreign body) is a clue to the presence of a sinus infection. Facial pain is rarely present, although intermittent, painless, periorbital swelling (present in the morning and resolving later in the day) may have been noted by involved parents. In this case, the persistence, not the severity, of the clinical symptoms calls for attention.

The second, less common presentation is a cold that seems more severe than usual: The fever is high (above 39°C), the nasal discharge is purulent and copious, and associated periorbital swelling or facial pain may be present. The periorbital swelling may involve the upper or lower eyelid; it is gradual in onset (evolving over hours to days) and most obvious in the morning after awakening. The swelling may decrease and actually disappear during the day, only to reappear the following day. A less common complaint is headache (a feeling of fullness or a dull ache either behind or above the eyes) reported most often in children older than 5. Occasionally, such children complain of dental pain, either from infection originating in the teeth or referred from the sinus infection.

Headache is not a common complaint in children with acute sinusitis. When headache is a symptom of acute sinusitis, it is almost always accompanied by prominent respiratory complaints. Usually, the headache is most severe on awakening and is relieved partially when affected patients are up and about. Chronic sinusitis is distinguished from acute sinusitis by persistence of respiratory symptoms (nasal discharge or cough or both) beyond 4 to 6 weeks.

DIAGNOSIS

Physical Examination

On physical examination, patients with acute sinusitis may display mucopurulent discharge in the nose or posterior pharynx. The nasal mucosa is erythematous; the throat may show moderate injection. Usually, the cervical lymph nodes are neither enlarged significantly nor tender. None of these characteristics differentiates rhinitis from sinusitis. Occasionally, as the examiner palpates over or percusses the paranasal sinuses, tenderness will be apparent, or appreciable periorbital edema will be seen (soft, nontender swelling of the upper and lower eyelid with discoloration of the overlying skin), or both may occur. Malodorous breath in concert with nasal discharge or cough suggests bacterial sinusitis.

In general, for most children younger than age 10, the physical examination is not very helpful in making a specific diagnosis of acute sinusitis. However, if the mucopurulent material can be removed from the nose and the nasal mucosa is treated with topical vasoconstrictors, pus may be seen coming from the middle meatus. The latter observation, the presence of periorbital swelling, or a combination is the most specific finding in acute sinusitis. Transillumination of the maxillary sinuses may be done in older cooperative children to look for evidence of opacification.

Radiography

Traditionally, radiography has been used to determine the presence or absence of sinus disease. Standard radiographic projections include an anteroposterior, a lateral, and an occipitomental view. The anteroposterior view is optimal for evaluation of the ethmoid sinuses, and the lateral view is best for viewing the frontal and sphenoid sinuses. The occipitomental view, taken after tilting the chin upward 45 degrees from the horizontal, allows evaluation of the maxillary sinuses. The radiographic findings most diagnostic of bacterial sinusitis are the presence of an air–fluid level in, or complete opacification of, the sinus cavities. However, an air–fluid level is an uncommon radiographic finding in children who are younger than 7 or 8 years and have acute sinusitis. In the absence of an air–fluid level or complete opacification of the sinuses, measuring the degree of mucosal swelling may be useful. If the width of the sinus mucosa is 5 mm or greater in adults or 4 mm or greater in children, the sinus aspirate will likely contain pus or will yield a positive bacterial culture. When clinical signs and symptoms suggesting acute sinusitis are accompanied by abnormal maxillary sinus radiographic findings, bacteria will be present in a sinus aspirate 70% of the time. A normal radiograph is strong evidence that a sinus is free of disease.

Computed tomographic (CT) scans are superior to plain-film radiography in the delineation of sinus abnormalities. However, such scans are not necessary in children with uncomplicated acute sinusitis and should be reserved for the evaluation of children with recurrent, chronic, or complicated sinus infections.

MICROBIOLOGY

Maxillary sinus aspiration in children with acute bacterial sinusitis has shown the microbiology of sinus secretions to be similar to that found in acute otitis media. The predominant organisms are *Streptococcus pneumoniae*, *Moraxella catarrhalis*, and nontypable *Haemophilus influenzae*. Both *H. influenzae* and M. catarrhalis may produce beta-lactamase and, consequently, may be resistant to amoxicillin. In addition, a dramatic increase has been seen in the frequency of *S. pneumoniae* isolates not susceptible to penicillin. As many as 50% of maxillary sinus isolates have a minimum inhibitory concentration of more than 0.1 μg/mL for penicillin. Anaerobic isolates and staphylococci are rarely recovered. Several viruses, including adenoviruses, influenza viruses, parainfluenza viruses, and rhinoviruses, have been isolated from maxillary sinus aspirates. Summary figures for the prevalence of various bacterial species in children with acute sinusitis are shown in Table 125-2. The performance of nasal, throat, or nasopharyngeal cultures is of no value in patients with acute sinusitis, as the results are not predictive of the bacterial isolates within the maxillary sinus cavity. The microbiology of chronic sinusitis differs slightly from that of acute sinusitis. Anaerobes of the respiratory tract, viridans streptococci and, occasionally, *Staphylococcus aureus* are found, in addition to the aerobes of acute sinusitis.

DIFFERENTIAL DIAGNOSIS

The major symptoms that prompt consideration of the diagnosis of acute sinusitis are persistent or purulent nasal discharge and persistent cough. Alternative diagnoses to consider for patients with purulent nasal discharge are simple viral upper respiratory infection, group A streptococcal infection, adenoiditis, and nasal foreign body. In simple upper respiratory infection, the purulent nasal discharge is usually accompanied by low-grade fever and other elements of upper respiratory inflammation such as pharyngitis and conjunctivitis. The symptoms commonly begin to improve after a few days. Streptococcal infection in children younger than 3 years, so-called streptococcosis, may present with such persistent respiratory symptoms as nasal discharge, low-grade fever, lassitude, and poor appetite. The diagnosis can be excluded by culturing the nasopharynx or throat for group A streptococci. Adenoiditis is suggested when purulent nasal discharge persists without improvement beyond 10 days in patients with normal sinus radiographic findings. Usually, nasal foreign body is characterized by unilateral nasal discharge, which is purulent and often bloody. Most strikingly, the nasal discharge is very foul smelling—a fact that can often be noted from the doorway of the examining room.

Patients who have persistent cough as the most troublesome symptom prompt the consideration of several diagnoses including reactive airways disease, *Mycoplasma pneumoniae* bronchitis, cystic fibrosis, whooping cough, and gastroesophageal reflux. Reactive airway disease triggered by upper respiratory infection may cause dramatic cough without accompanying wheezing. Occasionally, this condition occurs in conjunction with acute sinusitis, but it is more often a residual symptom after an upper respiratory infection and substantially prolongs the clinical course of the illness.

TABLE 125-2. Bacteriology of Acute Sinusitis

Bacterial species	Prevalence (%)
Streptococcus pneumoniae	25–30
Moraxella catarrhalis	15–20
Haemophilus influenzae	15–20
Streptococcus pyogenes	2–5
Anaerobes	2–5
Sterile	20–35

TREATMENT

Antimicrobial Agents

The relative frequency of occurrence of the various bacterial agents suggests that amoxicillin (at 40–60 mg/kg/day in two divided doses) is an appropriate drug for most uncomplicated cases of acute sinusitis in children who have not received recent antimicrobial treatment. The prevalence of beta-lactamase-positive, ampicillin-resistant *H. influenzae*, and *M. catarrhalis* may vary geographically. In areas where ampicillin-resistant organisms are prevalent, in patients with severe disease or in those with a toxic appearance, in situations in which the patient is allergic to penicillin or has mild periorbital swelling, or in instances in which there is an apparent failure to respond to amoxicillin, several alternative regimens are available (Table 125-3).

A combination of amoxicillin and potassium clavulanate (Augmentin) is a therapeutic agent for use in patients with beta-lactamase-producing bacterial species in their maxillary sinus secretions. Some experts are recommending a combination

TABLE 125-3. Antimicrobials and Dosage Schedules for the Treatment of Sinusitis in Children

Antimicrobial agent	Dose
Amoxicillin	60–90 mg/kg/d in two divided doses
Amoxicillin–potassium clavulanate	45/10 mg/kg/d in two divided doses plus amoxicillin at 45 mg/kg/d in two divided doses
Erythromycin-sulfisoxazole	50/150 mg/kg/d in four divided doses
Trimethoprim-sulfamethoxazole	8/40 mg/kg/d in two divided doses
Cefaclor	40 mg/kg/d in three divided doses
Cefuroxime axetil	30 mg/kg/d in two divided doses
Cefprozil	30 mg/kg/d in two divided doses
Cefixime	8 mg/kg/d in a single daily dose
Cefpodoxime proxetil	10 mg/kg/d in two divided doses
Loracarbef	30 mg/kg/d in two divided doses
Ceftibuten	9 mg/kg/d in a single daily dose
Azithromycin	10 mg/kg/d on day 1; 5 mg/kg/d on days 2 to 5 in a single daily dose
Clarithromycin	15 mg/kg/d in two divided doses

of amoxicillin (at 45 mg/kg/day in two divided doses) and amoxicillin–potassium clavulanate (at 45 mg/kg/day in two divided doses). This dosage will be effective against beta-lactamase-producing bacterial species and most *S. pneumoniae*, even some that are highly resistant to penicillin.

Cefuroxime axetil is another potent agent for treating most respiratory pathogens. The newer macrolides clarithromycin (Biaxin) and azithromycin (Zithromax) have received mixed reviews. Clarithromycin has weak activity against *H. influenzae*, and neither agent is consistently effective against penicillin-resistant *S. pneumoniae*. Some reports cited children who had acute otitis media caused by *H. influenzae* and whose disease failed to improve when treated with azithromycin. Additional data are necessary to determine the overall effectiveness of azithromycin for patients with acute bacterial sinusitis. Patients with acute sinusitis may require hospitalization because of systemic toxicity or inability to take oral antimicrobial agents. These patients may be treated with either cefuroxime, at a dosage of 100 to 200 mg/kg/day, or cefotaxime, at 200 mg/kg/day intravenously, in three and four divided doses, respectively.

Clinical improvement is prompt in nearly all children treated with an appropriate antimicrobial agent. Patients febrile at the initial encounter will become afebrile, and a remarkable reduction in nasal discharge and cough takes place within 48 hours. If affected patients do not improve or worsen in 48 hours, clinical reevaluation is appropriate. If the diagnosis is unchanged, sinus aspiration may be considered for precise bacteriologic information. Alternatively, an antimicrobial agent effective against beta-lactamase-producing bacterial species and penicillin-resistant *S. pneumoniae* should be prescribed. If the clinical response is poor again, aspiration of the maxillary sinus is definitely appropriate.

Usually, the antimicrobial regimens recommended to treat acute sinusitis are prescribed for 10 to 14 days. If affected patients are improved but not recovered completely by 10 or 14 days, continuing treatment for another week is reasonable. In patients with chronic sinusitis, antimicrobial therapy should be maintained for 3 to 4 weeks.

Adjuvant Therapies

The effectiveness of antihistamines or decongestants, or combinations thereof, applied topically (by inhalation) or administered by mouth in patients with acute or chronic sinus infection has not been studied adequately. Because appropriate antimicrobial therapy results in prompt clinical improvement within 48 to 72 hours, additional pharmacologic agents are not usually necessary.

Irrigation and Drainage

Irrigation and drainage of infected sinuses may result in dramatic relief from pain for patients with acute sinusitis. Usually, drainage procedures are reserved for those who fail to respond to medical therapy with antimicrobial agents, for immunosuppressed patients who may be infected with unusual microbiological species, or for those who have a suppurative intraorbital or intracranial complication. If an episode of acute sinusitis cannot be treated effectively by medical therapy alone or by medical therapy and simple sinus puncture, more radical surgery may become necessary.

Surgical Therapy

Surgical therapy in children with chronic sinusitis initially focused on creating a nasoantral window, or fistula, in the maxillary sinus to facilitate gravitational drainage. However, these fistulas proved to be relatively ineffective, in part, because the cilia that line the maxillary sinus still transport secretions toward the natural meatus.

At present, the focus of surgical therapy is the ostiomeatal unit. Most current surgical efforts involve using an endoscope to enlarge the natural meatus of the maxillary outflow tract by excising the uncinate process and the ethmoidal bullae and performing an anterior ethmoidectomy. Endoscopic surgery in children requires further systemic study. It may be helpful for patients with cystic fibrosis or for those patients with specific anatomic abnormalities. It is unclear which other patients will benefit more from surgical therapy than from medical therapy alone.

COMPLICATIONS

Complications of sinus disease may cause both substantial morbidity and occasional mortality. Major complications result from either contiguous spread or hematogenous dissemination of infection. A complete list of the major complications of sinusitis is provided in Table 125-4. Orbital complications are the most common serious complication of acute sinusitis. See Chapter 47 for a discussion of orbital and periorbital cellulitis.

Intracranial extension of infection is the second most common complication of acute sinusitis. Although the incidence of suppurative intracranial disease in patients with sinusitis is unknown, paranasal sinusitis is the source of 35% to 65% of subdural empyemas.

Intracranial Complications

CLINICAL FEATURES

Four groups of symptoms and signs may be recognized:

- Signs of pansinusitis: Approximately 50% to 60% of patients with subdural empyema secondary to sinusitis have symptoms of acute frontal sinusitis or an acute exacerbation of chronic pansinusitis. They have low-grade fever, malaise, frontal headache, and marked forehead and maxillary tenderness to digital pressure. Occasionally, subperiosteal pus overlying the anterior wall of the frontal sinus results in dramatic epicranial edema and a painful fluctuation called Pott's puffy tumor.
- Signs of increased intracranial pressure: With increased intracranial pressure, an initial headache worsens despite

TABLE 125-4. Major Complications of Sinusitis

Orbital
Inflammatory edema (preseptal or periorbital cellulitis)
Subperiosteal abscess
Orbital abscess
Orbital cellulitis
Optic neuritis
Osteomyelitis
Frontal (Pott's puffy tumor)
Maxillary
Intracranial
Epidural abscess
Subdural empyema or abscess
Cavernous or sagittal sinus thrombosis
Meningitis
Brain abscess

repeated doses of analgesic and oral antibiotic agents. Vomiting becomes intractable, and the level of consciousness deteriorates gradually. High intracranial pressure results from local cerebral edema in the area adjacent to the subdural pus, and it may progress rapidly to cause stupor and coma. With an isolated extradural empyema, cortical involvement is less extensive, and affected patients generally remain alert.

- Signs of meningeal irritation: During the stage of depressed sensorium, nuchal rigidity and photophobia are usually seen. This condition reflects an intense inflammatory response in the leptomeninges in contact with a subdural abscess, rather than septic leptomeningitis.
- Focal neurologic deficits: Focal neurologic deficits are caused by a combination of local brain compression (by the empyema), edema, and infarction. A frontoparietal convexity subdural empyema causes contralateral brachiofacial weakness, contralateral conjugate gaze palsy, and expressive dysphasia. Usually, lower-limb involvement occurs late. Focal seizures involving the arm and face occur in more than 60% of patients with dorsolateral lesions. With a parafalcine empyema, often jacksonian seizures begin in the foot and march upward and include the trunk, arm, and face. Weakness also affects primarily the leg with sparing of speech and facial musculature. Bilateral parafalcine collections may present with paraplegia simulating thoracic spinal cord compression. In the disease's terminal stage, affected patients are comatose and hemiplegic, have evidence of generalized and meningeal sepsis and, finally, show signs of uncal or tonsillar herniation.

DIAGNOSIS

Intracranial infection should be suspected if signs of systemic toxicity and headache do not improve after an adequate course of oral antibiotics has been given for the original sinusitis. Diagnostic tests must be arranged immediately if the headache becomes excruciating, if systemic toxicity worsens, or if intractable vomiting or visual blurring develops. Whenever meningeal signs develop in patients with sinusitis, attendant clinicians may be tempted to obtain cerebrospinal fluid by lumbar puncture. They must remember, however, that pure meningitis rarely occurs with sinusitis and that all the other intracranial suppurative complications are mass lesions likely to cause brain herniation with lumbar puncture. This procedure should be deferred, therefore, until the CT scan has ruled out empyema and abscess.

CT scanning is now recognized as the most definitive test for the diagnosis of intracranial suppuration secondary to sinusitis; it has virtually eliminated the need for cerebral angiography, radionuclide scanning, and electroencephalography. This noninvasive procedure defines and localizes even small purulent collections exactly, delineates associated cerebral edema, assesses the amount of brain shift, and detects concomitant brain abscess or bilateral empyema that was often missed by angiography in the era before CT.

TREATMENT AND OUTCOME

The treatment of sinusitis-related intracranial suppuration requires antimicrobial agents, drainage, and excellent supportive care. Rarely, brain abscess or highly selected cases of subdural empyema may be treated nonoperatively. More commonly, aspiration rather than excision is the operative procedure performed. Because either acute sinusitis or an acute exacerbation of chronic sinusitis may precede intracranial complications, the antibiotics selected must be appropriate to include activity against *S. pneumoniae*, *H. influenzae*, *M. catarrhalis*, respiratory anaerobes, streptococci, and *S. aureus*.

Hyperosmolar agents should be given if high intracranial pressure threatens brain herniation. Systemic steroids should be prescribed with caution because of their theoretic suppressive effect on granulocytic and immune functions. Anticonvulsant agents should be given prophylactically to protect against a high incidence of associated seizures.

Extradural and subdural empyemas should be drained through a generous craniotomy. An underlying brain abscess is handled best by intracapsular evacuation and catheter drainage to avoid unnecessary brain damage associated with radical excision of deep-seated lesions within eloquent areas of the brain. In some cases of subdural empyema, the underlying brain is so swollen that the bone flap must be left out for external decompression.

Postoperatively, intravenous antibiotics should be maintained for a minimum of 2 to 3 weeks. The shrinking of the abscess or empyema can be observed accurately by serial CT scans. Despite modern diagnostic and surgical capabilities, the mortality associated with subdural empyema and brain abscess is more than 20%. Early diagnosis remains the most effective way of improving survival.

CHAPTER 126
Pharyngitis

Adapted from Margaret R. Hammerschlag

Children and young adults visit physicians for sore throats more often than for any other problem or symptom. Technically, *pharyngitis* is an inflammatory illness of the mucous membranes and underlying structures of the throat. Although the symptom of sore throat is invariably present with pharyngitis, it should not be used as the sole criterion for diagnosis. Sore throat can be a common complaint in children with colds when no evidence of pharyngeal inflammation is present.

Pharyngitis can be subdivided into two categories: illness with and illness without nasal symptoms. This division has important etiologic implications. Almost always, nasopharyngitis has a viral cause, whereas illness without nasal symptoms (pharyngitis or tonsillopharyngitis) can have diverse causative agents, including bacteria, viruses, and fungi (Table 126-1).

ETIOLOGY

Viruses

Most often, the etiologic agents involved in nasopharyngitis are viruses with adenovirus types 7a, 9, 14, and 15 being the most common. Influenza, parainfluenza, and Epstein-Barr virus are the other major viral agents. Rhinovirus and respiratory syncytial virus infections are not often associated with objective pharyngeal findings.

Infectious Agents

Pharyngitis (including tonsillitis and tonsillopharyngitis) can be caused by a diversity of infectious agents ranging from group A beta-hemolytic streptococci to more obscure agents such as *Corynebacterium diphtheriae* and *Francisella tularensis*. As with other infections, the probability that any one agent is the cause of pharyngitis depends on the age and immune status of affected patients, the season, and the environment. In normal, healthy children, more than 90% of all cases of pharyngitis are caused by the following organisms, listed in order of decreasing

TABLE 126-1. Causes of Pharyngitis

Organism	Percentage of cases
Bacteria	
Group A streptococcus	5–20
beta-Hemolytic streptococci group C or G	6
Neisseria gonorrhoeae	Rare
Arcanobacterium haemolyticum	0.4–2.0
Corynebacterium diphtheriae	Rare
Francisella tularensis	Rare
Virus	
Adenovirus, types 7a, 9, 14, 15	19
Epstein-Barr virus	7–15
Rhinovirus	?
Respiratory syncytial virus	1
Parainfluenza virus	5
Influenza A and B virus	?
Cytomegalovirus	?
Herpes simplex virus types 1, 2	?
Human immunodeficiency virus	?
Other	
Mycoplasma pneumoniae	10–13
Chlamydia pneumoniae	?

frequency of occurrence: group A beta-hemolytic streptococci; adenoviruses; influenza viruses A and B; parainfluenza viruses 1, 2, and 3; Epstein-Barr virus; enteroviruses; and *Mycoplasma pneumoniae*. Pharyngitis and sore throat may also be present in 44% of patients with acute human immunodeficiency virus type 1 infection.

Other Streptococci

Other beta-hemolytic streptococci, especially groups C and G, have also been isolated from children and young adults with pharyngitis. *Neisseria gonorrhoeae* should be considered in adolescents who are sexually active or are known to have been exposed and possibly should be considered in abused children. Most abused children from whom *N. gonorrhoeae* has been isolated from the nasopharynx are asymptomatic, however.

Adenoviruses

Among viral causes, adenovirus is the most prevalent. One study found viruses to be responsible for 42% of all cases of pharyngitis in a group of children who were between ages 6 months and 17.9 years and had acute exudative tonsillitis. Adenovirus was responsible for 19% of the cases, followed by Epstein-Barr virus. Two children (1.8%) had infections with herpes simplex virus, and five children had infections with *M. pneumoniae*.

CLINICAL CHARACTERISTICS

Adenoviral Infections

Nasopharyngitis tends to be more common in younger children. The presentation can vary depending on the agent. Usually, fever is present. Infection with adenovirus may be associated with conjunctivitis and exudative pharyngitis, whereas infection with influenza A or B is frequently associated with more severe systemic complaints. The onset of pharyngitis can be acute with fever and the complaint of sore throat. Affected children may also have headache, nausea, vomiting and, occasionally, abdominal pain. Usually, physical examination reveals moderate to severe pharyngeal erythema and tonsillar enlargement and varying degrees of cervical adenitis. The erythema can be associated with follicular, ulcerative, and petechial lesions and with areas of exudate. Follicular tonsillitis is fairly characteristic of adenoviral infections, and ulcerative lesions are usually observed with enteroviral infections. The presence of exudate has been thought in the past to be most common or characteristic of group A streptococcal infection or infectious mononucleosis. A prospective, 1-year study of acute febrile exudative tonsillitis, however, found that 42% of the cases had a viral cause, predominantly adenovirus. The only clinical clues to the nature of the infecting agent were cough and rhinitis, both of which were observed in 45% of patients with viral disease and in only 10% of children with beta-hemolytic streptococci. Pharyngitis in children is almost entirely acute and self-limited lasting from 4 to 10 days depending on the cause.

Other Infections

Streptococcal pharyngitis can have significant suppurative complications including peritonsillar abscess and bacteremia. Postanginal sepsis is a clinical syndrome that usually occurs in adolescents or young adults after an oronasopharyngeal infection (frequently infectious mononucleosis). After a latency period of several days, contiguous or lymphatic spread of local infection, septicemia, and septic metastases can be observed. Septicemia, in these cases, is usually attributed to thrombophlebitis in small and large vessels of the face and neck. The organisms involved most frequently in this syndrome are anaerobes including Fusobacterium species and Bacteroides species.

DIFFERENTIAL DIAGNOSIS

Because of the numerous organisms that can cause pharyngitis and the significant overlap among them in clinical presentation and findings, making a specific diagnosis on the basis of physical findings alone (e.g., the presence of exudate) is difficult. The age and clinical status of affected patients and the time of year should be taken into account. Age may be the most important factor in predicting the causative agent with viral tonsillitis being most common in patients younger than age 3 and group A beta-hemolytic streptococci being found most often in children age 6 or older. The presence of rhinitis is also more suggestive of a viral infection. In adolescents and adults, viral infection or infection with *M. pneumoniae* is more likely. Although pharyngitis and sore throat are frequent in patients with lower respiratory tract infection due to *Chlamydia pneumoniae*, the role of this organism as an etiologic agent of pharyngitis is unknown.

SPECIFIC DIAGNOSIS

Available Tests

Because infection with group A streptococci can have significant suppurative and nonsuppurative complications, streptococcal disease must be excluded in all instances of acute pharyngitis. If affected children are young (less than 3 years) or have obvious viral infection such as pharyngoconjunctival fever (adenovirus) or herpangina, antibiotic therapy is not needed and, therefore, cultures are not indicated. The only way to make a definite diagnosis of group A streptococcal infection is to identify the organism in the pharynx by culture. Confirmation that early treatment of severe streptococcal pharyngitis hastens recovery has rendered rapid diagnosis of this condition desirable. A number of rapid, nonculture antigen detection kits are available for the diagnosis of streptococcal pharyngitis. The majority is based on latex agglutination or enzyme immunoassay. Although these tests appear to be very specific (95%–99%), the sensitivities range from 60% to 90%. Even in several kits in which the sensitivities appear to be high (greater than 90%), they are actually much lower because the kits were compared to less sensitive culture methods. Two approved tests using novel technology, a direct DNA probe and an optical immunoassay, reportedly have better sensitivities (greater than 93%) than those in previously available tests. However, the evaluation of any new technology is influenced by the choice of the reference method. An insensitive reference method causes a test to appear unjustifiably more sensitive. It may be postulated that those patients who have false-negative streptococcal antigen detection test results do not have significant pharyngeal infection. However, several studies have demonstrated little correlation between the degree of positivity (number of colonies) and changes in streptococcal antibody titers. In one study, 45% of the children who had false-negative throat antigen test results using a rapid test kit had significant changes in their streptococcal antibody titers. If the prevalence of infection is also low (less than 50%) in a particular population, the positive predictive value of these tests may be 56% or less.

Test Results

Some have suggested, on the basis of false-negative result rates that average 15%, that the specimen might be obtained using two swabs for the tonsillar sweep. If the rapid antigen detection test result is positive, affected patients can be treated, and the second swab can be discarded. If the test is negative, the second swab should be used for a standard culture on blood agar with a bacitracin disc. For identification of other bacteria such as *A. haemolyticum* or *N. gonorrhoeae*, the laboratory must be informed specifically so that appropriate media are used. Examination of Gram stains of the exudate does not appear to be an accurate way to identify group A streptococci, *N. gonorrhoeae*, or *C. haemolyticum*.

Rapid differentiation of infectious mononucleosis from streptococcal pharyngitis was once thought to be possible by demonstration of atypical lymphocytes in Wright–Giemsa-stained smears of the exudate. Newer tests using agglutination of red cells or latex particles to detect heterophil antibody responses are simpler, faster, and more accurate.

TREATMENT

Appropriate Therapy

Because the majority of pharyngitis episodes are viral and self-limited, specific therapy is not indicated except for a streptococcal pharyngitis. The importance of accurate diagnosis and appropriate therapy of streptococcal pharyngitis cannot be emphasized too strongly. A resurgence of acute rheumatic fever has been seen in several parts of the United States including Utah, Pennsylvania, and Ohio. In an outbreak in Akron, Ohio, the patients were not generally indigent and had good access to medical care. Approximately 80% of the patients had had an illness suggesting pharyngitis within 1 month of the onset of acute rheumatic fever; of these, 39% had either failed to receive a full 10-day course of antibiotics or had received no antibiotics at all.

Antibiotics

Intramuscular benzathine penicillin or a 10-day course of oral penicillin (amoxicillin) remains the treatment of choice for streptococcal pharyngitis because of the proven efficacy (greater than 90%), safety, narrow spectrum, and low cost. For children under age 12 years old, the dose of oral penicillin (amoxicillin) is 250 mg PO BID for 10 days. For children over 12 years, the dose is 500 mg PO BID for 10 days. Erythromycin is a suitable alternative for patients sensitive to penicillin. First- or second-generation cephalosporins are also acceptable for treating patients who do not exhibit immediate hypersensitivity to beta-lactam antibiotics. Most oral antibiotics must be administered as a 10-day course to achieve maximal eradication of group A streptococci from the pharynx. Some of the newer cephalosporins and macrolides have been reported to achieve comparable clinical and bacteriologic cure rates when these drugs were given for 5 days or less. However, data are still limited, and these shorter courses cannot be recommended unequivocally at this time. In addition, these antibiotics have spectrums much broader than those of penicillin and are more expensive. Resistance of group A streptococci to erythromycin and other macrolides can develop with extensive use of these agents. Currently, the rates of resistance to erythromycin among group A streptococci in the United States is not more than 5%. Studies have suggested that some clinical and bacteriologic treatment failures after therapy with penicillins may have been caused by the presence of alpha-lactamase-producing bacteria, especially Bacteroides fragilis and Bacteroides melaninogenicus. Subsequent treatment with an antibiotic resistant to alpha-lactamase such as clindamycin or with a cephalosporin was frequently effective.

CHAPTER 127
Herpangina

Adapted from Sarah S. Long

Herpangina is characterized by painful oral lesions caused by enteroviral agents that tend to circulate in the spring and summer. Enteroviruses have a worldwide distribution and produce disease in both sporadic and epidemic forms. Group A coxsackieviruses are probably the most common cause of herpangina. Echoviruses and group B coxsackieviruses are also associated with epidemic and sporadic cases of herpangina. Other viruses such as herpes simplex virus and polioviruses are occasional causes of nonepidemic herpangina. Humans are the only known natural host and illness is reported most commonly in children ages 1 to 4. Fortunately, the majority of enteroviral infections cause either no symptoms or mild nonspecific febrile illnesses.

CLINICAL CHARACTERISTICS

The diagnosis of herpangina is made on clinical grounds and suggested by the presence and character of lesions in the oropharynx. With no prodrome or only a few hours of anorexia or listlessness, herpangina begins suddenly with the onset of fever. Temperature varies from normal to 41°C, and onset can be accompanied by a seizure. High fever, listlessness, and vomiting are more common in children younger than age 5. Headache, backache, sore throat, and dysphagia are noted by older patients. Usually, the oropharyngeal lesions are present at the onset of fever or occur in the subsequent 24 hours. The characteristic lesion evolves from a small papule to a 1- to 2-mm vesicle with

TABLE 127-1. Features Differentiating Herpangina from Other Diseases with Enanthems

Disease	Etiology	Occurrence	Character of oral lesions	Site of oral lesions	Number of lesions	Size of lesions	Other features
Herpangina	Coxsackieviruses, echoviruses	Acute	Vesicles, ulcers with erythema	Anterior pillars, posterior palate, and pharynx	1–5	1–2 mm	Dysphagia
Herpetic stomatitis	Herpes simplex virus type 1	Acute	Vesicles, shallow ulcers	Gingival and buccal mucosa, tongue, lips	Any	>5 mm, coalescent	Drooling, lymphadenopathy
Hand-foot-and-mouth disease	Coxsackieviruses, enterovirus 71	Acute	Vesicles, shallow ulcers	Tonsillar fauces, buccal mucosa, tongue	Any	1–3 mm, coalescent	Vesicles on hands and feet, maculopapular rash
Aphthous stomatitis	Unknown	Acute, recurrent	Ulcers with rim of erythema, gray exudate	Buccal and lingual mucosa, lateral tongue	1–2	>5 mm	Pain, no fever
Behçet syndrome	Unknown	Chronic, recurrent	Ulcers with rim of erythema, gray exudate	Any	1–5	>5 mm	Ulcers of genital mucosa, uveitis
Stevens-Johnson syndrome	Many, unknown	Acute	Ulcers, hemorrhagic ulcers, pseudomembranes	All, lips	Confluent	Confluent	Systemic illness, rash, drug history
Mucositis (ulcerative gingivitis)	Neutropenia, chemotherapy, bacteria	Acute, recurrent, chronic	Ulcers, exudate, pseudomembranes	Gingival, buccal mucosa	Confluent	Confluent	Fetid breath, pain, other gastrointestinal mucosal lesions
Kawasaki disease	Unknown	Acute	Erythema, strawberry tongue	Diffuse	—	—	Prolonged fever, rash, conjunctival hyperemia, cracked lips
Toxin-mediated syndromes	*Staphylococcus aureus* and group A streptococcus toxins	Acute	Erythema, strawberry tongue	Diffuse	—	—	Erythroderma and scarlatina, conjunctival hyperemia, hypotension
Streptococcal pharyngitis	Group A streptococcus	Acute	Erythema exudates, strawberry tongue, palatal petechiae	Tonsils, pharynx	—	—	Sore threat, dysphagia, lymphadenitis
Adenoviral, pharyngitis	Adenoviruses	Acute	Follicles, erythema, exudate	Tonsils, pillars, pharynx	—	—	Dysphagia, lymphadenopathy, conjunctivitis
Epstein-Barr virus pharyngitis	Epstein-Barr virus	Acute	Exudate, palatal petechrae	Tonsils	—	—	Lymphadenopathy, fatigue, splenomegaly

surrounding erythema and then to an ulcer. Lesions enlarge to only 3 to 4 mm over 3 days and remain discrete (i.e., do not coalesce as do ulcers of herpes simplex virus infection, mucositis, and Stevens-Johnson syndrome). The average number of lesions is five with more than 20 being distinctly unusual. Characteristically, lesions involve the anterior tonsillar pillars, tonsils, soft palate, uvula, and pharyngeal wall. Occasionally, posterior buccal surfaces and the tip of the tongue are involved. The diagnosis of herpangina should be made only when the enanthem on the posterior oral cavity is obvious. Usually, other diseases associated with enanthems can be distinguished by careful attention to the number, size, and nature of the lesions involved. Features differentiating herpangina from other diseases with enanthems are shown in Table 127-1.

TREATMENT AND PREVENTION

No specific antiviral therapy is available for the treatment of herpangina due to enteroviruses. Acyclovir and ganciclovir have no role. Treatment is focused on maintaining comfort and adequate hydration and on observing patients for the involvement of other organ systems. Analgesics such as acetaminophen can be used for discomfort. In addition, children's diphenhydramine mixed 1:1 with aluminum hydroxide/magnesium hydroxide (Maalox, Mylanta) can be used as a mouthwash to maintain comfort. Dosage is based on the diphenhydramine component. Unfortunately, data on the efficacy of this intervention is lacking. The usual duration of signs and symptoms is 3 to 6 days. The prognosis is excellent, except in rare instances when herpangina is associated with hepatitis, meningitis, encephalitis, or myocarditis or with disseminated disease in the neonate.

Oral secretions and feces are infectious during acute phases of the illness, and virus can be recovered from feces for weeks after symptoms abate. Asymptomatically infected individuals are probably the primary sources for the spread of infection. Care in handling diapers, good hand-washing practices, and attention to personal hygiene limit the spread of these viruses.

CHAPTER 128

Peritonsillar and Retropharyngeal Abscesses

Adapted from Paul E. Hammerschlag and Margaret R. Hammerschlag

PERITONSILLAR ABSCESS (QUINSY)

A peritonsillar abscess is circumscribed medially by the fibrous wall of the tonsil capsule and laterally by the superior constrictor muscle. The cause of peritonsillar abscesses is not constant; the abscesses may follow any "virulent" tonsillitis with extension through the fibrous tonsil capsule. Peritonsillar abscesses are rare in young children. They are most common in late adolescence and in the early part of the third decade. There is a relatively high incidence of reported peritonsillar abscess, which raises the possibility that the decreasing rate of tonsillectomy might increase the risk of developing peritonsillar abscess.

Clinical Characteristics

Common presenting symptoms may include a sore throat with occasional unilateral pain, malaise, low-grade pyrexia, chills, diaphoresis, dysphagia, reduced oral intake, trismus, and a muffled "hot-potato" voice. Trismus results from irritation and reflex spasm of the internal pterygoid muscle. Impaired palatal motion from edema contributes to the muffled voice. Physical examination reveals minimal to moderate toxicity, dehydration, and drooling. Inspection of the oropharynx may be compromised by trismus. The soft palate is displaced toward the unaffected side, is swollen and red, and frequently contains a palpable fluctuant area. The edematous uvula is pushed across the midline. Rarely, the displaced tonsil and its crypts are coated with exudate. The breath is fetid, and ipsilateral, tender cervical adenopathy is found. Indirect laryngoscopy reveals supraglottic and lateral pharyngeal edema. The white blood cell count is elevated with a predominance of polymorphonuclear leukocytes.

Treatment

Commonly, aspiration of the fluctuant mass with an 18-gauge needle confirms the diagnosis of peritonsillar abscess, especially if the pus is located in the superior pole. Aspiration, along with intravenous antibiotics, has been found to be very effective treatment. Some clinicians prefer the time-honored method of incision and drainage under local anesthesia, which poses a slight risk of aspiration of the pus. Pus in locations other than the superior pole may not be accessible to aspiration intraorally or might not be amenable to drainage by this route. An "acute quinsy tonsillectomy," in which the medial wall of the abscess is removed, is the ideal procedure by which to provide adequate drainage. Often, bilateral tonsillectomies are advocated, although the incidence of abscess within the contralateral peritonsillar capsule varies from 2% to 24%.

Several studies have suggested that many patients with peritonsillar abscess can be treated on an outpatient basis with simple needle aspiration combined with antibiotic therapy. An extensive metaanalysis of ten previous studies conducted from 1961 through 1994 and involving 496 patients with peritonsillar abscess found an overall success rate of needle aspiration of 94% (range, 85%–100%). This figure compares favorably with the success rate reported for incision and drainage. Intraoral sonography can also be used to monitor affected patients' responses after treatment.

Preoperatively and postoperatively (in tonsillectomy, aspiration, or incision and drainage), patients should be treated with appropriate intravenous antibiotics until they are asymptomatic, then they should be switched to oral medications. Lavage with warm saline every 2 hours aids in débridement of the area, may reduce the peritonsillar edema, and provides some symptomatic relief. An untreated peritonsillar abscess may spontaneously rupture or can extend to the pterygomaxillary space with potentially fatal complications.

RETROPHARYNGEAL ABSCESS

The anterior wall of the retropharyngeal space is the middle layer of the deep cervical fascia, which abuts the posterior esophageal wall (the superior pharyngeal constrictor muscle). The deep layer of the deep cervical fascia circumscribes the posterior wall of this potential space. Inferiorly, these two fasciae fuse to limit the depth of this pocket at a level between the first and second thoracic vertebrae. A retropharyngeal abscess can erode inferiorly through the junction of these fasciae to extend posteriorly into the prevertebral space. Subsequently, pus in the prevertebral space can descend inferiorly below the diaphragm to the psoas muscles.

The retropharyngeal space contains two paramedian chains of lymph nodes that receive drainage from the nasopharynx, adenoids, and posterior paranasal sinuses. These structures are prominent in early childhood and undergo atrophy at puberty. Retropharyngeal abscesses are most common in young children. The mean ages reported in two series were 4.0 and 4.5 years. Retropharyngeal abscesses are thought to be secondary to suppurative adenitis of these retropharyngeal nodes. Other sources of infection are penetrating foreign bodies, endoscopy, trauma, pharyngitis, vertebral body osteomyelitis, petrositis, and dental procedures.

Clinical Characteristics

Frequently, the symptoms from a retropharyngeal abscess begin insidiously after a mild antecedent infection. Airway stridor from edema, cellulitis, or an obstructing mass is common. Laryngeal edema may cause dyspnea and tachypnea. Dysphagia, drooling, and odynophagia may occur. No trismus occurs, but a stiff neck secondary to muscle tenderness may be present, along with an ipsilateral tender cervical adenopathy. Chest pain may reflect mediastinal extension. Early in the course, midline or unilateral swelling of the posterior pharynx is evident. Later, gentle palpation may demonstrate a large fluctuant mass in the posterior pharynx. Vigorous palpation should be avoided, as the abscess may rupture into the upper airway.

Treatment

The administration of intravenous antibiotics combined with incision and drainage is the treatment of choice for retropharyngeal abscess. If the mass is small, a peroral incision made with the patient in Rose's position (supine, with the neck hyperextended) may provide some drainage but poses a slight risk of aspiration. If the mass is large or fever persists after peroral drainage, an external incision is preferred. A tracheostomy may be required in the event of risk of airway compromise.

Posterior mediastinitis can result from the spread of infection from the retropharyngeal area into the prevertebral space. Other complications may be seen when the abscess extends to the parapharyngeal space and involves the great vessels and cranial nerves.

CT SCANNING FOR DEEP NECK INFECTIONS

Data are now more extensive regarding the use of CT scanning in the diagnosis of deep neck infections. A 10-year retrospective study from the Massachusetts Eye and Ear Infirmary found that the intraoperative findings confirmed the CT scan interpretation in 76.3% of the patients. CT scans in five of the 38 (13.2%) patients were indicative of abscesses that were not confirmed at surgery. Exploration of the parapharyngeal or retropharyngeal space revealed cellulitis. The false-negative rate was 10.5%. The sensitivity of CT scanning for detection of parapharyngeal or retropharyngeal space abscess was 87.9%. A study from Pittsburgh showed that the sensitivity for differentiating an abscess from cellulitis using CT scanning was 91%. In three cases, the radiologist's blinded CT scan interpretation did not correlate with the operative findings. Two patients with false-positive interpretations had retropharyngeal infections and underwent needle aspiration. The positive predictive value of CT scans in detection of abscess versus cellulitis was 83%. These findings have important implications in considering whether affected patients should be managed by needle aspiration or by incision and drainage. One study reported eight of 14 patients who had deep neck infections, seen over a 9-year period, and were treated successfully by antibiotics alone. All were reported to have small abscesses on CT scan; however, some may have had only cellulitis. In the Pittsburgh study 12 (44%) of the children with retropharyngeal infections were treated with intravenous antibiotics alone, and all did well.

MICROBIOLOGY OF DEEP NECK ABSCESSES

Group A streptococci (*Streptococcus pyogenes*) and *Staphylococcus aureus* have been considered to be the organisms associated most frequently with pharyngeal space infections. Several studies, however, have demonstrated the presence of oral anaerobes in the majority of these infections. In more recent studies of peritonsillar and retropharyngeal abscesses, anaerobes were isolated from all the patients and were the only isolates in approximately 20% of the patients. This outcome is not surprising, because the main portals of entry for pharyngeal space infections are the nasopharynx, oropharynx, paranasal sinuses, mastoid, and lower molars—all of which are areas colonized with anaerobes. The predominant organisms isolated from deep neck infections are listed in Table 128-1.

Because a large variety of organisms can be found in pharyngeal space infections, obtaining adequate cultures is highly important. The optimal material for culture is an aspirate of the pus obtained at operation. Usually, throat swabs or swabs of the abscess obtained after drainage are inadequate because of contamination with normal oropharyngeal flora. The pus, when it is obtained, can be transported in a capped syringe if anaerobic transport media are not available. Most pathogenic obligate anaerobes can survive in a purulent exudate despite extended periods of air exposure. A Gram stain of the exudate provides important clues to the bacterial cause. A Gram stain showing a mixture of organisms suggests a mixed aerobic-anaerobic infection.

Because anaerobic bacteria are frequently recovered from deep neck abscesses, antimicrobial therapy should be directed at the eradication of these organisms. Antibiotic therapy is effective, however, only in conjunction with adequate surgical drainage. Resolution of some peritonsillar and retropharyngeal infections may occur without drainage when therapy is initiated at an early stage of infection, before suppuration occurs. Probably penicillin and ampicillin are adequate antibiotic therapy,

TABLE 128-1. Organisms Found in Deep Seeded Neck Infections

Common
Streptococcus pyogenes (Group A Streptococcus)
Staphylococcus aureus
Bacteroides species
Fusobacterium species
Peptostreptococci
Haemophilus species
Viridans streptococci
Rare
Escherichia coli
Klebsiella pneumoniae
Mycobacterium tuberculosis
Atypical mycobacterium
Coccidioides immitis

but the frequent presence of penicillin-resistant bacteria such as *S. aureus* and Bacteroides species may warrant the administration of antimicrobial agents that are effective against these organisms (e.g., clindamycin, amoxicillin–clavulanic acid, ticarcillin–clavulanic acid, ampicillin-sulbactam, or metronidazole in combination with an antistaphylococcic beta-lactam). The newer, expanded-spectrum oral cephalosporins such as cefixime, quinolones, and new macrolides do not have adequate gram-positive or anaerobic coverage to enable them to be used alone for these infections.

CHAPTER 129

Otitis Media

Adapted from Mark W. Kline

Otitis media is one of the most common infectious diseases of childhood. One large study revealed that 33% of pediatric office visits for illness of any kind were attributable to disease of the middle ear (*acute otitis media* or otitis media with effusion). Infants and young children are at highest risk for the development of otitis media with a peak prevalence between 6 and 36 months of age. Two of every three children have at least one episode of otitis media before their first birthday. By age 3, 80% of children have had at least one episode of acute otitis media, and nearly 50% have had three or more episodes. After an initial episode of acute otitis media, 40% of children have middle-ear effusion that persists for at least 4 weeks, and 10% have persistent effusion after 3 months. Children in whom otitis media with effusion develops early in life are at increased risk of recurrent acute or chronic middle-ear disease. The overall childhood prevalence of otitis media with effusion is estimated to be 15% to 20%. The incidence and prevalence of otitis media decline after approximately age 6.

Otitis media occurs more commonly in boys than in girls and is particularly prevalent among Eskimos and Native Americans and among children with cleft palate or other craniofacial defects. A genetic predisposition to otitis media may exist in some cases. Other implicated predisposing factors include lower socioeconomic group status, bottle-feeding in the horizontal position, bottle-feeding versus breast-feeding, day-care center attendance, and atopy. In general, the highest rates of otitis media are observed in the winter months coinciding with the peak incidence of respiratory viral infections.

Abnormal eustachian tube function underlies most cases of otitis media. Normally, the eustachian tube permits equilibration of middle-ear pressure with atmospheric pressure, protects the middle ear from reflux of nasopharyngeal secretions, and drains secretions from the middle ear into the nasopharynx. Either obstruction or abnormal patency of the eustachian tube may lead to the development of otitis media. The intrinsic type (e.g., inflammation secondary to infection or allergy) and the extrinsic type (e.g., tumor or adenoid enlargement) of mechanical eustachian tube obstruction are recognized. Functional obstruction caused by persistent collapse of an abnormally compliant eustachian tube, an abnormal active opening mechanism, or both is common in young children and individuals with cleft palate. An abnormally patent, or patulous, eustachian tube, commonly found among Native American populations, permits reflux of nasopharyngeal secretions into the middle ear. Reflux, aspiration, or insufflation of nasopharyngeal bacteria into the middle ear, on any basis, leads to mucoperiosteal inflammation and otitis media.

ACUTE OTITIS MEDIA

Clinical Manifestations

The classic description of acute otitis media is of children who have upper respiratory tract infection and suddenly develop fever, otalgia, and hearing loss. A classic presentation, however, may be the exception rather than the rule. Fever and hearing loss are inconstant features of the disease, and otalgia may not be reported. In many young children, in particular, otitis media must be inferred on the basis of nonspecific symptoms (e.g., fretfulness or irritability, anorexia, loose stools) and subtle findings suggestive of middle-ear disease (e.g., scratching or tugging at the ear).

The appearance of the tympanic membrane is key to the diagnosis of acute otitis media. All wax and debris must be removed from the external canal before examination. Usually, otoscopy reveals a hyperemic, opaque tympanic membrane with distorted or absent light reflex and indistinct landmarks. A red appearance of the drum may be noted if affected children are agitated or if inadequate illumination is provided; this condition is not evidence of otitis media in the absence of other findings. Adequate assessment of tympanic membrane mobility requires pneumatic otoscopy using an ear speculum large enough to occlude the external canal completely. Decreased mobility of the drum results from either eustachian tube dysfunction or middle-ear effusion.

Etiologies

The bacterial etiologies of acute otitis media beyond the neonatal period are shown in Table 129-1. *Streptococcus pneumoniae, Haemophilus influenzae* mostly nontypable, and *Moraxella catarrhalis* remain the three most common bacterial isolates. Eleven serotypes of *Streptococcus pneumoniae* account for approximately 85% of cases of otitis media caused by that organism, and all are included in the polysaccharide pneumococcal vaccine. An increasing percentage of *S. pneumoniae* isolates are resistant to penicillin; decreased susceptibility to other oral penicillins and cephalosporins has also been observed. Many *H. influenzae* strains and most strains of *Moraxella catarrhalis* produce beta-lactamase and, therefore, are resistant to amoxicillin and penicillin. Bacterial cultures of middle-ear fluid are sterile in approximately one-third of patients with acute otitis media. Studies assessing the role of viruses have found a low rate of isolation from middle-ear fluid with respiratory syncytial virus and influenza viruses being most common.

TABLE 129-1. Bacterial Etiology of Acute Otitis Media in Children*

Bacterial isolate	Prevalence (%)
Streptococcus pneumoniae	31
Haemophilus influenzae	22
Moraxella catarrhalis	7
Group A streptococcus	2
Enteric gram-negative bacteria	1
Staphylococcus aureus	1
Other	3
No bacterial isolate	33

*Findings based on cultures obtained by needle tympanocentesis.

Treatment

A number of agents active against the common bacterial pathogens of otitis media are available (Table 129-2). As a general rule, children younger than 1 month with otitis media should be admitted to the hospital. Cultures of blood, cerebrospinal fluid, and middle-ear fluid should be obtained, and parenteral antibiotic therapy should be initiated. If blood and cerebrospinal fluid cultures are sterile after 48 hours and affected infants appear well with disease limited to the middle ear, therapy may be completed with an oral antibiotic active against the middle-ear isolate.

The choice of an antibiotic for acute otitis media must take into account many factors including the local antibiotic susceptibility patterns of common bacterial isolates, compliance of the patient population with various antibiotic regimens, and the cost of the various antibiotics under consideration. Amoxicillin is a reasonable first choice for the treatment of otitis media in older infants and children. For children without risk factors for pneumococcal resistance, traditional dosing of 40 mg/kg/day may be appropriate. However, for children with risk factors for pneumococcal resistance such as day-care attendance and children who have received antibiotics within the last month, higher doses of amoxicillin may be needed (80–90 mg/kg/day). An alternative agent may be needed in the absence of response to therapy in 72 to 96 hours, or if a resistant organism is cultured from middle-ear fluid. Amoxicillin-clavulanate and Cefuroxime axetil can be used as second line agents for these situations, but they are considerably more expensive. A single intramuscular dose of ceftriaxone was found to be comparable in clinical efficacy to 10 days of oral trimethoprim-sulfamethoxazole for treatment of acute otitis media. The usual duration of oral antibiotic therapy in uncomplicated cases of acute otitis media is 10 days, but both longer and shorter therapy courses have been proposed. Nasal and oral decongestants, sometimes administered in combination with an oral antihistamine, have been advocated for relief of nasal and eustachian tube obstruction in children with otitis media. At present, the efficacy of these preparations is unproven, and their routine use cannot be recommended. Supportive therapy including acetaminophen and local heat may be helpful in treating children with acute otitis media.

Ideally, children with acute otitis media should be reexamined 4 to 6 weeks after they have received antibiotic therapy to document resolution of tympanic membrane inflammation and middle-ear effusion. Complete resolution of middle-ear effusion may require 2 to 3 months.

RECURRENT ACUTE OTITIS MEDIA

Recurrence of episodes of acute otitis media is common. Underlying susceptibility to middle-ear infection is important in the development of recurrent otitis media; recurrences represent reinfection more often than recrudescence or relapse. Early development of otitis media caused by *S. pneumoniae* seems particularly likely to predispose to recurrent otitis media.

Several strategies have been used for the prevention of recurrent acute otitis media. Antibiotic prophylaxis with amoxicillin (20 mg/kg once daily) or sulfisoxazole (75 mg/kg/day in two divided doses) is reasonable in children who have at least three episodes of acute otitis media within 6 months or four episodes in 1 year. Generally, prophylaxis is continued for 3 to 6 months, at which time the antibiotic is discontinued, and affected children are observed. Myringotomy with tympanostomy tube insertion is an option for patients who fail to respond to antibiotic prophylaxis. Adenoidectomy may be beneficial for selected patients.

OTITIS MEDIA WITH EFFUSION

After an episode of acute otitis media, 10% of children have middle-ear effusion that persists for 3 months or longer (chronic otitis media with effusion). Clinically, otitis media with effusion is characterized by a sensation of fullness in the ears, muffled hearing, and tinnitus. Usually, pneumatic otoscopy reveals an opaque tympanic membrane with decreased mobility. Frequent acute otitis media, catarrh, exposure to cigarette smoke, and atopy may increase the risk of persistent effusion.

Bacteria are recovered from one-third to one-half of all middle-ear fluid specimens obtained at myringotomy in cases of otitis media with effusion. The bacteriology closely mimics that of acute otitis media. Whether the bacteria have a direct pathogenic role is not known, but an initial course of antibiotic therapy similar to that used for acute otitis media seems warranted. Oral decongestant-antihistamine combinations and corticosteroids have not been found to be effective in the treatment

TABLE 129-2. Antimicrobial Therapy for Acute Otitis Media

Age of patient	Drug	Dosage
<1 mo	Ampicillin	200 mg/kg/d IM or IV in four divided doses
	and	
	Gentamicin	7.5 mg/kg/d IM or IV in three divided doses
1 mo to 15 yr	Amoxicillin	40 mg/kg/d PO in three divided doses (standard dose) 80–90 mg/kg/d PO in two divided doses (high dose)
	or	
	Trimethoprim-sulfamethoxazole	8–10 mg/kg/d trimethoprim PO in two divided doses
	or	
	Erythromycin-sulfisoxazole	40 mg/kg/d erythromycin PO in three divided doses
	or	
	Cefuroxime axetil	250–500 mg/d PO in two divided doses
	or	
	Cefixime	8 mg/kg/d PO in one dose
	or	
	Cefpodoxime proxetil	10 mg/kg/d PO in two divided doses
	or	
	Amoxicillin-clavulanate	40 mg/kg/d PO in three divided doses
	or	
	Ceftriaxone	50 mg/kg/d (max. 1 g) IM 1–3 daily doses

of persistent middle-ear effusion. Evaluation for respiratory allergy, obstructive adenoid enlargement, immune deficiency, or anatomic abnormalities such as submucous cleft palate may be necessary in patients whose disease does not respond to treatment.

For patients whose condition fails to respond to medical therapy, myringotomy with tympanostomy tube insertion may prevent subsequent accumulation of middle-ear fluid and can improve hearing. Tympanostomy tubes are also used to prevent structural middle-ear damage and cholesteatoma in selected cases. Tonsillectomy is not efficacious in the treatment of otitis media with effusion.

COMPLICATIONS

Serious complications of otitis media are uncommon when appropriate medical therapy is promptly initiated. Extracranial complications include serous or purulent labyrinthitis, mastoiditis, osteomyelitis of the temporal bone, and facial nerve paralysis. Intracranial complications are subdivided into meningeal and extrameningeal complications. Epidural and subdural abscess, meningitis, lateral sinus thrombosis, and otitic hydrocephalus are reported as meningeal complications of otitis media. Lateral sinus thrombosis is characterized by high temperature, chills, signs and symptoms of increased intracranial pressure, and septicemia with embolization. The mortality is approximately 25%. Otitic hydrocephalus may follow acute otitis media by several weeks and is usually associated with impaired intracranial venous drainage. Commonly, hydrocephalus subsides spontaneously. Extrameningeal complications of otitis media include brain abscess and petrositis.

CHAPTER 130
Otitis Externa

Adapted from Mark W. Kline

CLINICAL CHARACTERISTICS

A history of swimming or diving or of repetitive ear cleansing with soapy water and cotton-tipped swabs is often elicited. Most patients are seen for evaluation of ear pain, itching, and fullness. Pain is exacerbated by manipulation of the pinna or tragus, a feature useful in differentiating between otitis externa and otitis media. Purulent discharge may be present in the external auditory canal. The canal walls are diffusely erythematous and edematous. Ipsilateral cervical lymph node enlargement may be noted, but fever usually is absent.

DIAGNOSIS

Otitis externa is a clinical diagnosis. The historical features and physical findings are sufficiently characteristic so that most patients present no real diagnostic dilemma. On the other hand, several other conditions mimic external otitis in some cases. Furunculosis is, in a sense, a focal form of otitis externa. Symptoms and signs resemble those of the diffuse condition, but otoscopy reveals a discrete furuncle or pustule with surrounding erythema in the outer portion of the external auditory canal. Otitis media causes ear pain that is not exacerbated by manipulation of the pinna. Usually, perforation of the tympanic membrane results in symptomatic improvement, although the external canal may fill with purulent debris. Cleansing the canal permits otoscopic detection of the perforated tympanic membrane. A foreign body, usually visible in the external canal, may cause inflammation and discharge closely mimicking diffuse external otitis.

A microbiological diagnosis may help to guide antibiotic therapy for otitis externa. A nasopharyngeal calcium alginate swab can be used to obtain purulent material from the auditory canal for routine bacterial cultures and Gram stain. Special stains and cultures for fungi, mycobacteria, or viruses may be indicated under unusual circumstances. The most common causative agents are *Staphylococcus aureus*, *Pseudomonas aeruginosa*, and other gram-negative bacilli and group A streptococci. Frequently, infections are polymicrobial. Fungi such as *Aspergillus niger* and *Candida albicans* are occasionally isolated as the sole or predominant organisms. Varicella-zoster virus may produce external otitis with ipsilateral oral vesicles and facial nerve paralysis.

TREATMENT

A suspension of polymyxin B-neomycin-hydrocortisone (Cortisporin) is instilled in the canal four times daily, generally for 10 to 14 days. Initial swelling may be so severe that drops will not enter the auditory canal. In these cases, Cortisporin cream may be placed in the canal on a wick and removed in approximately 24 hours (when inflammation has subsided). Cutaneous sensitivity to neomycin with local signs and symptoms mimicking those of otitis externa is a potential complication of therapy with Cortisporin. Some authorities recommend initiating therapy with Cortisporin and then using an agent that does not contain neomycin (e.g., clindamycin or polymyxin B drops) once culture results are known. Prevention of recurrent otitis externa may be accomplished by use of 2% acetic acid eardrops after swimming.

Systemic antibiotic therapy for otitis externa is indicated if affected patients are febrile or exhibit associated cervical adenitis or cellulitis of adjacent tissues. Appropriate oral antibiotics for initial therapy include trimethoprim-sulfamethoxazole, cefuroxime axetil, or amoxicillin-clavulanate.

Generally, malignant otitis externa, a particularly aggressive form of the disease, is diagnosed in elderly patients with diabetes. It rarely occurs in immunocompromised children and is characterized by extensive destruction of soft tissues, cartilage, bone, and nerves around the external auditory canal. Granulation tissue may be seen in the canal itself. The causative organism is *P. aeruginosa.* Effective therapy combines surgical débridement with intravenous antibiotics that are active against *Pseudomonas.*

CHAPTER 131
Mastoiditis

Adapted from Mark W. Kline

CLINICAL CHARACTERISTICS

Almost invariably, children with mastoiditis have otitis media concomitantly. Classically, children with acute mastoiditis present with fever, otalgia, and postauricular swelling and redness. Typically, swelling occurs over the mastoid process pushing the earlobe superiorly and laterally; in infancy, it may occur above the ear displacing the pinna inferiorly and laterally. The clinical presentation of acute mastoiditis may be fairly subtle, particularly in children who have received oral antibiotic therapy for otitis media (so-called masked mastoiditis). Mastoiditis should be considered in patients with otitis media unresponsive to antibiotic therapy.

Generally, chronic mastoiditis develops in individuals with long-standing middle-ear disease. The clinical course is indolent. Fever and local signs referable to the mastoid may or may not be present. Chronic purulent drainage from the ear and conductive hearing loss may occur.

DIAGNOSIS

In some cases, the diagnosis of mastoiditis can be made with confidence on clinical grounds alone. Plain-film roentgenography may show coalescence of mastoid air cells and loss of normal bony trabeculations. If osteomyelitis develops, sometimes sclerosis or destruction of adjacent bone is noted. Abnormalities on roentgenography of the mastoid bone do not necessarily imply mastoiditis, however; conversely, normal study results do not exclude the diagnosis. Sometimes, computed tomography is helpful in cases in which clinical findings and plain-film roentgenography are equivocal or nonspecific.

Causative Agents

A bacteriologic diagnosis is highly desirable in cases of mastoiditis. Tympanocentesis obtained through an intact tympanic membrane yields bacteriologic information that correlates well with specimens obtained from the mastoid bone itself. Common causative agents of acute mastoiditis include *Streptococcus pneumoniae*, group A streptococcus, *Staphylococcus aureus*, and *Haemophilus influenzae*. In chronic mastoiditis, prevalent isolates include anaerobic bacteria such as *Peptococcus* species, *Actinomyces* species, or *Bacteroides* species, and aerobic gram-negative bacilli (including *Pseudomonas aeruginosa*). Frequently, chronic mastoiditis is polymicrobial. Mycobacterium tuberculosis rarely causes chronic mastoiditis today, but it should be considered in the presence of suggestive epidemiologic or historical features in the case.

In all cases of mastoiditis, specimens from the middle ear or mastoid should be cultured aerobically and anaerobically, and a Gram stain should be performed. Special fungal and mycobacterial stains and cultures may be indicated in some cases. A skin test for tuberculosis should be performed in all cases of chronic mastoiditis or with a history of exposure to tuberculosis.

TREATMENT

Usually, patients with acute onset of symptoms and no evidence of intracranial or local extracranial complications of mastoiditis are treated initially with myringotomy and parenteral antibiotics alone. Signs of increased intracranial pressure or meningeal irritation signal complications of mastoiditis such as meningitis, brain abscess, epidural abscess, subdural empyema, or venous sinus thrombosis. A postauricular fluctuant area implies subperiosteal abscess formation. Because of proximity to the mastoid bone, other local structures may be involved by infection producing facial-nerve paralysis, jugular venous thrombosis, or internal carotid artery erosion and hemorrhage. Lack of appropriate response to medical therapy or development of complications necessitates mastoidectomy and possibly other surgical interventions.

The initial selection of specific antibiotic therapy is made empirically with some guidance provided by Gram stain of specimens from the middle ear or mastoid. In acute mastoiditis, a combination of a penicillinase-resistant penicillin (e.g., nafcillin or oxacillin) and one of the third-generation cephalosporins (e.g., cefotaxime or ceftriaxone) is reasonable. In severe or complicated cases, vancomycin should be substituted for the penicillinase-resistant penicillin to provide coverage against penicillin-resistant *S. pneumoniae* and oxacillin-resistant *S. aureus*. In chronic mastoiditis, an aminoglycoside with activity against *Pseudomonas* (e.g., amikacin or tobramycin) may be used initially, usually in combination with an antipseudomonal penicillin (e.g., ticarcillin-clavulanate) that is active against many anaerobic bacteria and *S. aureus*. Eventual antibiotic therapy is determined by the bacteriology of the process. Provided complications have not occurred and if it is feasible on the basis of the organisms' susceptibility to oral agents, the course of therapy can be completed orally once signs of acute inflammation have subsided. The minimum course of therapy for mastoiditis is 21 days, and it may be longer if complications of infection have occurred. For patients discharged on oral antibiotic therapy, careful monitoring of compliance and documentation of bactericidal activity in serum are desirable.

CHAPTER 132
Acute and Chronic Bronchitis

Adapted from I. Celine Hanson
and William T. Shearer

ACUTE BRONCHITIS

Acute bronchitis is encountered commonly in children. In 1989, the National Health Interview Survey estimated that 1.8 million episodes of acute bronchitis occurred in American preschool children alone. Most clinicians describe acute bronchitis as a febrile illness with cough, rhonchi, and referred breath sounds. Infectious agents associated with acute bronchitis are shown in Table 132-1. Viral agents predominate including adenovirus, influenza viruses, and respiratory syncytial virus.

Clinical Characteristics

By definition, fever and cough are associated with acute bronchitis, almost invariably in connection with upper respiratory

TABLE 132-1. Infectious Agents Associated with Acute Bronchitis

Agent	Importance in causation
Viruses	
Adenovirus types 1–7, 12	+++
Enteroviruses	+
Coxsackievirus B	+
Echoviruses 8, 12, 14	+
Polioviruses	+
Herpes simplex	+
Influenza	+++
A	++
B	++
C	+
Measles	+
Mumps	+
Parainfluenza	+++
1	++
2	++
3	+++
4	+
Respiratory syncytial	+++
Rhinoviruses	++
Bacteria	
Bordetella pertussis	+
Bordetella parapertussis	±
Haemophilus influenzae	+
Streptococcus pneumoniae	±
Streptococcus pyogenes	±
Other	
Chlamydia psittaci	+
Mycoplasma pneumoniae	+++

+++, very common; ++, common; +, rare, ±, of questionable etiologic significance.
Modified from Cherry JD. Lower respiratory tract infections: acute bronchitis. In: Feigin RD, Cherry JD, eds. *Textbook of pediatric infectious diseases*, 4th ed. Philadelphia: Saunders, 1998:243.

congestion (predominantly nasal). Patients' temperatures can range from 37°C to 39°C (100°F–103°F). Usually, cough is dry and harsh without sputum production in young infants. Coughing can be accompanied by gagging and vomiting leading to poor oral intake and dehydration. Occasionally, older children with persistent cough will produce sputum and may complain of chest-wall pain. Usually, the clinical illness is preceded by 24 to 48 hours of lassitude or malaise. Subsequently, fever and cough develop; these findings may persist for as long as 1 week. A relatively slow recovery phase spanning 1 to 2 weeks with persistent cough is characteristic. Secondary bacterial infection can complicate the recovery period causing exacerbation of fever and other clinical findings.

On physical examination, lung auscultation reveals rhonchi and referred upper airway breath sounds. Usually, rhinitis is present and may be mucopurulent. Typically, chest radiography results are normal, unless secondary bacterial infection has occurred. The value of laboratory data is limited usually suggesting a viral process (i.e., the white blood cell count is elevated mildly, and only one-third of all cases are associated with an increased neutrophil count).

Differential Diagnosis

The differential diagnosis is somewhat limited, but acute bronchitis should be distinguished from chronic bronchitis, infectious asthma, and asthmatic bronchitis and sinusitis. More serious illnesses associated with recurrent acute upper respiratory tract infections (e.g., immunodeficiency states, immotile cilia syndrome, and cystic fibrosis) should be distinguished from acute bronchitis. Acute bronchitis is a self-limited illness, and one bout of clinical disease does not warrant additional investigation.

Treatment and Complications

Usually, acute bronchitis is a benign illness unless secondary infection occurs. Appropriate preventive therapy includes adherence to recommended immunization schedules for children. Accordingly, therapy is palliative (i.e., analgesic therapy for febrile episodes; antitussive, decongestant, and antihistamine agents for cough and rhinitis). The latter approach has not been documented to be helpful in acute bronchitis; in fact, cough suppressant therapy with codeine or dextromethorphan should be used with great care in affected children. Persistent coughing with gagging and vomiting can precipitate dehydration and serum metabolic changes. Monitoring these parameters in severely affected hosts and reconstitution of deficits by oral or parenteral rehydration are indicated. When secondary bacterial infection is suggested by exacerbation of fever or by evidence of pneumonia on a chest radiograph, broad-spectrum antibiotic therapy may be indicated. Specific antimicrobial therapy can be provided when *Haemophilus influenzae* or *Streptococcus pneumoniae* is isolated. Recurrent acute bronchitis has been associated with reactive airway disease or asthma. Complications of acute bronchitis are few; in the majority of cases, the outcome is excellent with resolution of disease and return to baseline health.

CHRONIC BRONCHITIS

Chronic bronchitis, which is described widely in the adult literature, is ill defined in children and is described less frequently. The prevalence of childhood bronchitis varies ranging from 2% to 40% in selected series. Since the late 1980s, the prevalence rates of asthma and chronic bronchitis have increased 50% and 46%, respectively.

Chronic bronchitis is often associated with bacterial agents. The predominant pathogens isolated from sputum in a group of 40 pediatric patients with chronic bronchitis are shown in Table 132-2. Usually, treatment of exacerbations of chronic bronchitis with antibiotic therapy is effective in reducing sputum volume and purulence but shows no parallel elimination of the cultured microorganisms.

Clinical Characteristics and Differential Diagnosis

Clinically, chronic bronchitis is characterized by excessive mucus production, and by cough that is present on most days for a minimum of 3 months per year. Fever can accompany the cough, and the temperature can range from 37°C to 39°C (100°–103°F). Chronic bronchitis can be a clinical manifestation of numerous disorders, some of which are listed in Table 132-3. Asthma, or reversible obstructive airway disease, can be distinguished by patients' clinical response to the administration of traditional bronchodilators. Often, recurrent episodes of acute bronchitis are interpreted as chronic bronchitis, although the intermittent nature of these episodes and the absence of a persistent cough usually distinguish acute bronchitis clinically. Persistent lower respiratory tract infections (e.g., pertussis) and *Chlamydia* and *Mycobacterium* infections can present with a similar complex of symptoms. These entities can be diagnosed by chest radiography (e.g., hilar lymph nodes being more common in *Mycobacterium* infection) and by isolation of the pathogen from nasopharyngeal secretions or sputum. In addition, serologic determinations of antibacterial antibodies assist in the diagnosis. Documentation of

TABLE 132-2. Dominant Pathogens in Washed Sputum from Patients with Chronic Bronchitis (40 Cases)

Pathogen	Number of cases (%)
Haemophilus influenzae and *Streptococcus pneumoniae*	21 (52.5)
H. influenzae	17 (42.5)
Staphylococcus aureus	2 (5.0)
Superinfection with gram-negative rods	
Pseudomonas aeruginosa	4
Klebsiella pneumoniae	2
Escherichia coli	1
Enterobacter cloacae	1

From Kubo AS, Funabashji S, Uehara S, et al. Clinical aspects of "asthmatic bronchitis" and chronic bronchitis in infants and children. *J Asthma Res* 1978;15:99.

a delayed hypersensitivity skin test response to the antigen *Mycobacterium tuberculosis* is helpful in identifying tuberculosis.

Cystic fibrosis, which is typically accompanied by steatorrhea, nasal polyps, and failure to thrive, is also manifested prominently by recurrent lower respiratory tract symptoms. The diagnosis of cystic fibrosis can be established by documentation of abnormally elevated chloride levels (greater than 60 mEq/L), as measured by sweat iontophoresis. Primary ciliary dyskinesia encompasses the immotile cilia disorders and Kartagener syndrome (rhinosinusitis, bronchitis, or bronchiectasis and situs inversus). Patients affected with these disorders exhibit a defect in mucociliary transport, as evidenced by a decrease in ciliary beat frequency. Electron microscopy of bronchial cilia classically reveals structural defects with absent dynein arms. This diagnosis is made by bronchial or (occasionally) nasal turbinate biopsy.

The immune disorders associated most frequently with recurrent sinopulmonary infection include selective IgA deficiency (serum IgA level, 10 mg/dL or less), hypogammaglobulinemia (primary and secondary), IgG subclass deficiencies, and ataxia-telangiectasia. In addition, immunodeficient patients receiving bone marrow reconstitution by transplantation have been described with graft-versus-host disease that affects the lungs and manifests clinically as a symptom complex suggestive of chronic bronchitis.

TABLE 132-3. Conditions Associated with Chronic Cough (3 Months or Longer) or Lower Respiratory Tract Illness

- Asthma
- Recurrent episodes of bronchitis infections (*Chlamydia*, pertussis, *Mycobacterium*)
- Cystic fibrosis
- Primary ciliary dyskinesia
  - Kartagener syndrome
  - Immotile cilia syndrome
- Immunodeficiency
  - Selective IgA deficiency
  - Subclass of IgG deficiency
  - Hypogammaglobulinemia (primary and secondary)
  - Ataxia-telangiectasia
  - Graft-versus-host disease after bone marrow transplantation
- Anatomic lesions
  - Foreign body
  - Previous esophageal atresia repair
  - Mediastinal tumors
  - Congenital heart disease
- Irritants
  - Milk aspiration (gastroesophageal reflux, tracheoesophageal fistula)
  - Tobacco smoke
  - Pollution
  - Occupational exposure

Modified from Morgan WT, Taussig LM. The chronic bronchitis complex in childhood. *Pediatr Clin North Am* 1984;31:853.

Anatomic lesions that lead to obstruction of the respiratory tree can mimic chronic bronchitis. Congenital heart disease should be considered in this patient population and is best evaluated with clinical examination, chest radiography, electrocardiography, and echocardiography. Mediastinal tumors, although uncommon, can produce extrinsic obstruction leading to recurrent cough and wheezing. The infant with chronic cough, poor feeding habits, and failure to thrive should be evaluated for gastroesophageal reflux or a tracheoesophageal fistula, which is identified most easily by barium swallow or pH probe monitoring.

Respiratory tract irritants have been implicated in chronic cough. Interestingly, nonindustrial, rural communities such as the forest zone of Nigeria report virtually no chronic bronchitis, whereas reports from metropolitan New York suggest that an increased risk of respiratory tract infections exist in adults and children who reside in those parts of the city having the highest ambient air levels of sulfur dioxide and particulate air pollution. The correlation between tobacco smoking and reduced ventilatory capacity in adults has been reported by many investigators. Passive smoking has also been implicated as a factor that increases the risk of developing lower respiratory tract infection in children and of impairment of lung function at the beginning of adult life. Clinicians should obtain a history of smoking not only from the patient, but also from other members of the household.

Treatment

When a specific diagnosis can be identified with chronic cough or wheezing, therapy is directed toward the primary disease entity, in addition to the clinical presentation. Hence, bronchodilators and antiinflammatory agents are used when deemed appropriate in the treatment of chronic cough associated with asthma. Cough secondary to gastroesophageal reflux can be approached with altered feeding schedules, positioning techniques (prone 30 degrees), and occasional medications. Patients with hypogammaglobulinemia or IgG subclass deficiency may be aided by replacement intravenous immunoglobulin therapy using preparations currently commercially available at appropriate doses and schedules (200–400 mg/kg per dose every 2–4 weeks).

It's imperative that patients with chronic pulmonary disease as a result of cystic fibrosis or asthma understand the pulmonary irritant effect and possibly additive reduction in pulmonary function caused by tobacco smoking, dust exposure, and air pollution. In addition, parents of such children should be made aware of the effects of passive smoking on the already compromised pulmonary function of their children and should be encouraged to stop smoking.

Antimicrobial therapy in chronic bronchitis is reserved for severely ill patients in whom the likelihood of secondary bacterial infection is great. In these instances, therapy usually consists of ampicillin (75 mg/kg/day), erythromycin (40 mg/kg/day), or (in adolescents and adults) tetracycline (25–50 mg/kg/day). In adults, newer antimicrobials such as macrolides (clarithromycin) and fluoroquinolones (ciprofloxacin) have improved clearing of acute exacerbations of chronic bronchitis. Because patients with chronic bronchitis are at risk of pneumococcal and influenza morbidity, receipt of the pneumococcal vaccine and annual delivery of the influenza vaccine are recommended. Overall, the prognosis for the chronic bronchitis complex is varied and depends on the specific diagnosis.

CHAPTER 133
Croup

Adapted from Ellen R. Wald

ACUTE INFECTIOUS LARYNGITIS

Acute infectious laryngitis is experienced primarily by older children, adolescents, and adults during the respiratory virus season. The principal symptom of infection is hoarseness, which may be accompanied by variable upper respiratory symptoms (coryza, sore throat, nasal stuffiness) and constitutional symptoms (fever, headache, myalgias, malaise). The presence of associated complaints varies with the infecting virus: Adenoviruses and influenza viruses may cause more systemic disease; parainfluenza viruses, rhinoviruses, and respiratory syncytial virus most often cause mild illness.

The diagnosis of acute laryngitis is made on clinical grounds, and laboratory evaluation is unnecessary. In febrile school-aged children who experience hoarseness, complain of sore throat, and have tender anterior cervical adenopathy, a throat culture to detect *Streptococcus pyogenes* may be appropriate. Hoarseness without any other respiratory symptoms may represent voice abuse.

Acute infectious laryngitis is virtually always self-limited. Treatment consists of symptomatic therapy with fluids and humidified inspired air. Voice rest is beneficial. Protracted episodes of hoarseness (no improvement after 7–10 days) suggest an underlying anatomic abnormality.

ACUTE LARYNGOTRACHEITIS

Acute laryngotracheitis is usually referred to as croup. It is a respiratory disease seen in children of any age but is most common between the first and third years of life; boys are affected more often than girls. The causative agents are respiratory viruses exclusively and, frequently, the illness occurs in epidemic patterns. Most frequently, the viruses implicated are parainfluenza types 1 and 3, but influenza A and B, respiratory syncytial virus, parainfluenza 2, adenoviruses, and herpes simplex virus have been cited as other causes. *Mycoplasma pneumoniae* may also cause croup. In areas in which measles is endemic, severe croup may dominate the clinical picture. In summertime croup, the enteroviruses (coxsackievirus A and B and echovirus) or parainfluenza type 3 is the usual cause.

Clinical Characteristics

The usual onset of croup is with the signs and symptoms of a common cold: coryza, nasal congestion, sore throat, and cough with variable fever. The cough becomes prominent with a barking quality (akin to that of a puppy or seal), and the voice becomes hoarse. Many children with this syndrome never visit a physician. Such children may begin to have evidence of respiratory distress, however, with the onset of tachypnea, stridor (when agitated or crying), nasal flaring, and suprasternal and intercostal retractions. The increase in respiratory distress prompts a visit to the physician or emergency department. Usually, the illness peaks in severity over 3 to 5 days and then begins to resolve. Most characteristically, the signs and symptoms worsen in the evening.

In typical cases of acute laryngotracheitis, the diagnosis is easily made on clinical grounds, and no radiography or blood tests are required. If anteroposterior radiography is performed, a so-called steeple sign may be seen as a consequence of subglottic swelling. Usually, the blood count is less than 10,000 cells per cubic millimeter with a predominance of lymphocytes. Indications for hospitalization undertaken in approximately 10% of children with laryngotracheitis include the presence of stridor, anxiety or restlessness, cyanosis, or retractions at rest. In addition, children with a history of croup or previous airway intubation may benefit from hospitalization. Children for whom close follow-up cannot be arranged or whose families cannot provide the necessary observation and care should also be admitted to the hospital.

As laryngeal inflammation increases and secretions accumulate, respiratory distress increases, and complete obstruction may occur. Almost always, this progression is gradual and is signaled by slowly increasing respiratory rate and effort, increased stridor at rest, and pallor or cyanosis. Agitation increases and air entry is poor. In approximately 5% of hospitalized patients, intubation is required to overcome the respiratory obstruction. Children who have a deteriorating respiratory status should be monitored in an intensive care unit by staff skilled in the care of pediatric patients.

Treatment

One of the most important principles of treatment of patients with croup or other upper airway problems is minimal disturbance. Any stimulus that upsets affected children will result in crying, which causes hyperventilation and an increase in respiratory distress. The parents should be encouraged to hold and comfort such children whenever possible, and invasive procedures should be kept to a minimum.

Treatment strategies for acute infectious laryngotracheitis have included mist, racemic epinephrine, and corticosteroids. Although not subjected to study until recently, mist therapy has been considered standard management. Several small investigations have suggested that mist is of no demonstrable benefit; however, this remedy is still used routinely. Racemic epinephrine is a potentially lifesaving therapy in croup patients who are in moderate to severe respiratory distress. Racemic epinephrine is an equal mixture of the D- and L-isomers of epinephrine. The dose is 0.5 mL of a 2.25% solution diluted with 3.5 mL of water (1:8), delivered via a nebulizer with a mouthpiece held in front of the child's face. Administration results in rapid clinical improvement; by its beta-adrenergic vasoconstrictive effects on mucosal edema, racemic epinephrine increases the airway diameter. The peak effect is observed in 2 hours. Accumulating evidence substantiates that patients who receive a single dose of epinephrine do not necessarily require hospitalization. Affected children may be discharged to home if, in addition to receiving epinephrine, they were treated simultaneously with dexamethasone and remain improved during a 3-hour observation period. The dosing interval for epinephrine in hospitalized patients depends on the severity of the laryngotracheitis; it can be administered every 20 to 30 minutes in the intensive care unit, where monitoring is possible, but is usually spaced 3 to 4 hours apart when such patients are in a regular hospital unit.

The use of corticosteroids in acute laryngotracheitis has been controversial for three decades. However, the efficacy of glucocorticoids for hospitalized children with croup has now been accepted as the standard of care consequent to the accumulation of a consistent body of evidence from prospective, randomized, controlled trials. Corticosteroids have shown to be effective when given by the oral route (0.15 mg/kg of dexamethasone), the parenteral route (0.3–0.5 mg/kg per dose), or as nebulized budesonide. In general, the corticosteroid dose is given only once, although it can be repeated. In addition to the acceptance of corticosteroid therapy in hospitalized patients, enthusiasm is increasing for the use of nebulized budesonide or oral dexamethasone in patients who are seen in the emergency department and for whom admission may not be necessary. Nebulized budesonide results in acute improvement in croup symptoms, shortens stays in the emergency department, and significantly reduces admission rates. Antibiotics are not indicated in the routine treatment of children with this croup syndrome.

Most patients who are hospitalized for acute laryngotracheitis are treated with supportive therapies (mist and, occasionally, oxygen and intravenous fluids) and can be discharged in a few days. Patients treated with corticosteroids recover more quickly than those patients who are not given corticosteroids; intubated children can be extubated earlier, and patients with severe disease may avoid intubation. If intubation is required, frequently the nasotracheal tube must remain in place for 3 to 4 days until an air leak develops around it reflecting subsidence of the inflammation. Hospitalization for several days after extubation is desirable to ensure respiratory stability and the reintroduction of oral feeding.

SEVERE LARYNGOTRACHEOBRONCHITIS (BACTERIAL TRACHEITIS)

Bacterial tracheitis is a recently redescribed example of upper airway obstruction that was recognized more regularly in the era before antibiotics. The consensus holds that bacterial tracheitis represents a secondary bacterial infection of viral laryngotracheitis. The specific agents that have been implicated in the etiology of the viral tracheitis include parainfluenza and influenza viruses and enterovirus. Most often, the secondary bacterial invaders are coagulase-positive staphylococci. Group A streptococci, viridans streptococci, *Haemophilus influenzae*, gram-negative enteric bacteria, and anaerobes have also been implicated. Bacterial tracheitis occurs principally during the respiratory virus season overlapping the seasonal occurrence of laryngotracheitis: fall and winter. This pathologic entity affects all age groups from young infants to school-aged children, with a predominance in 1- to 2-year-olds. Boys and girls are equally affected.

Clinical Characteristics

Some children with croup become ill acutely and have severe respiratory distress within hours of onset of the illness. Others exhibit a 1- to 5-day prodromal period of mild upper respiratory symptoms and the onset of cough, stridor, and hoarseness characteristic of typical croup; then, within just a few hours, higher temperature, a toxic appearance, and a remarkable increase in respiratory distress develop. Notably, as distress becomes apparent, such patients do not respond to the inhalation of racemic epinephrine. Typically, high temperature, prominent cough, and stridor are noted at the time of clinical presentation. Clinical differentiation of this illness from epiglottitis may be helped by the usual absence of dysphagia and drooling in bacterial tracheitis. When signs of airway obstruction escalate, however, the key issue, as in cases of suspected epiglottitis, is securing the airway.

Diagnosis

The diagnosis of bacterial tracheitis may be suspected clinically, but it is confirmed endoscopically. At the time of intubation or bronchoscopy, the epiglottis is found to be normal. The pathologic process involves the subglottic area with extension into the trachea. Abundant purulent exudate and pseudomembranes may be present. If radiographic studies have been performed, the anteroposterior radiograph will show the steeple sign and, occasionally, the detached pseudomembrane may be seen as a soft tissue shadow or shadows of irregular configuration in the upper trachea. Frequently, pneumonia is a complication in cases of bacterial tracheitis. Leukocytosis may be prominent, but blood culture results are negative.

Treatment

The appropriate treatment of bacterial tracheitis includes securing the airway and instituting antimicrobial therapy. Tracheal intubation is recommended for patients in whom bacterial tracheitis has been diagnosed. This procedure can be accomplished with nasotracheal intubation or tracheostomy. In either case, observation in an intensive care unit is essential. The copious and thick secretions may lead to blockage of the artificial airway necessitating meticulous respiratory toileting. As the bacterial species implicated most commonly has been the *Staphylococcus*, nafcillin therapy is indicated in patients in whom gram-positive cocci or no organisms have been seen at all on a smear. In patients in whom gram-negative rods or mixed flora are observed, an advanced-generation cephalosporin such as cefuroxime, cefotaxime, or ceftriaxone may be best. Parenteral therapy should be continued for the duration of intubation or for several days after the patient's fever has abated. Oral antimicrobial agents may be used to complete a 10-day course of therapy in patients in whom the clinical improvement has been prompt. Typically, the clinical course of bacterial tracheitis is longer than that of uncomplicated croup or epiglottitis and requires an average of 10 days of hospitalization.

Complications

Complications of croup occur before and after intubation. The most serious is complete respiratory obstruction leading to respiratory arrest. A number of cases of severe hypoxia and, ultimately, death have occurred in patients with bacterial tracheitis. Pneumomediastinum and pneumothorax may also be seen as complications of intubation. Pneumonia occurs in approximately 50% of cases. Rarely, a toxic shock syndrome has accompanied bacterial tracheitis due to *Staphylococcus aureus*.

SPASMODIC CROUP

Acute spasmodic croup is a clinical entity seen in exactly the same age group and during the same season, and it is caused by the same viruses as acute infectious laryngotracheitis. Typically, children experiencing an episode of acute spasmodic croup go to sleep well or with the mildest of upper respiratory infections. They awaken in the night with a barking cough, hoarseness, inspiratory stridor, and variable degrees of respiratory distress. They are always afebrile. Most patients respond to mist therapy provided by the bathroom shower or a cool-water vaporizer. Occasionally, the night air inhaled en route to the hospital is sufficient to reduce the dyspnea. Although most episodes are mild to moderate, occasionally airway support is required. Recurrences may be observed during the same evening or on the subsequent 2 to 3 nights.

Spasmodic croup may be differentiated from infectious laryngotracheitis endoscopically. Whereas examination of the mucosa in spasmodic croup reveals an erythematous, inflamed, velvety appearance, the mucosa is pale and boggy in infectious laryngotracheitis. Although viral cultures yield the same agents as those

TABLE 133-1. Differential Diagnosis of Acute Infectious Obstruction in the Region of the Larynx

Feature	Epiglottitis	Acute laryngotracheitis	Laryngotracheobronchitis	Spasmodic croup
Prodrome	Usually none or mild upper respiratory infection	Usually upper respiratory symptoms	Usually upper respiratory symptoms	None or minimal coryza
Age	1–8 yr	3 mo to 3 yr	3 mo to 8 yr	3 mo to 3 yr
Onset	Rapid (4–12 hr)	Gradual	Variable	Sudden, always at night
Fever	High (39.5°C)	Variable	Usually high	None
Hoarseness, barking cough	No	Yes	Yes	Yes
Dysphagia	Yes	No	No	No
Toxic appearance	Yes	No	Yes	No
Microbiology	Blood culture positive for *Haemophilus influenzae* type b	Viral infection	Viral infection with bacterial superinfection	Viral infection with allergic component

Adapted from Cherry JD. Croup. In: Feigin RD, Cherry JD, eds. *Textbook of pediatric infectious diseases*, 2nd ed. Philadelphia: Saunders, 1987.

found in laryngotracheitis, the mucosal appearance and clinical course suggest an allergic component of the pathophysiologic process. Usually, this group of patients benefits from racemic epinephrine if the degree of respiratory distress mandates its use. Likewise, these patients may do well with corticosteroid therapy reflecting either the allergic nature of the process or the natural history of a self-limited disease.

DIFFERENTIAL DIAGNOSIS OF UPPER AIRWAY OBSTRUCTION

The differential diagnosis in patients who have upper airway obstruction includes both infectious and noninfectious problems. The noninfectious causes are foreign-body aspiration and angioneurotic edema. Foreign-body aspiration occurs most often in children aged 2 to 4 years. If aspiration is observed, the diagnosis is straightforward. However, ambulatory preschoolers are often unobserved when such aspiration occurs. They experience an initial choking and gagging episode usually followed by a "silent" period during which they are asymptomatic. The recurrence of symptoms may include the acute onset of cough, wheezing, stridor, or dysphagia in variable combinations. Usually, such children have no upper respiratory symptoms or fever. Auscultation of the lungs may reveal differential aeration and wheezing. Most aspirated foreign bodies are vegetable matter (e.g., peanuts, carrots, corn); therefore, plain-film radiography may not reveal their presence. The sudden onset of upper respiratory tract obstruction in previously well children should always arouse concern about foreign-body aspiration. Endoscopy is diagnostic and therapeutic in this situation.

Angioneurotic edema may cause sudden respiratory obstruction in previously well children of any age. Such children may have a history of allergies or previous episodes of respiratory tract obstruction. The angioneurotic edema may be based on a hereditary C1 esterase deficiency; in these patients, a positive family history may be found. Alternatively, a sudden allergic reaction to ingested material or inhalants may cause swelling of the tongue, epiglottis, or larynx. In any case, if severe reactions do not respond to injected or inhaled epinephrine, endoscopy and airway intubation may be necessary.

In addition to laryngitis, laryngotracheitis, laryngotracheobronchitis, and spasmodic croup, the infectious causes of upper airway obstruction include laryngeal diphtheria. Currently, this infection is rare in the United States occurring in limited geographic regions. Fully immunized individuals should be immune. The remaining causes of acute infectious obstruction in the region of the larynx are contrasted in Table 133-1. Laryngitis is not included, as it rarely presents difficulty in differential diagnosis. Acute epiglottitis is a medical emergency that must be differentiated from the remaining croup syndromes to enable appropriate airway management. Severe laryngotracheobronchitis (bacterial tracheitis) may require immediate airway placement. In both situations, affected children are highly febrile, appear to be in a toxic condition, and in marked respiratory distress. Immediate endoscopy is diagnostic and allows proper airway management.

CHAPTER 134
Bronchiolitis

Adapted from I. Celine Hanson and William T. Shearer

Lower respiratory tract infection in children younger than 24 months is a common clinical occurrence. Criteria for the diagnosis of bronchiolitis include first episode of acute wheezing aged 24 months or younger, accompanying physical findings of viral infection (i.e., coryza, cough, fever), and exclusion of pneumonia or atopy as the cause of wheezing.

Table 134-1 lists the infectious agents that have been associated with the clinical entity of bronchiolitis. Viruses, particularly respiratory syncytial virus (RSV), account for the majority of pathogens isolated during clinical disease. Epidemics of bronchiolitis are almost always linked to RSV as the causative infectious

TABLE 134-1. Bronchiolitis: Etiologic Agents

Viral
Respiratory syncytial virus
Adenovirus (types 3, 7, 21)
Parainfluenza virus (type 3)
Rhinoviruses
Mumps
Influenza viruses
Miscellaneous
Mycoplasma pneumoniae

agent. RSV infection is estimated to be a very common childhood event affecting almost 60% of infants during the first year of life. The vast majority of previously healthy infants infected with RSV and other agents of bronchiolitis have a lower respiratory tract infection of mild to moderate severity that lasts for 3 to 10 days, and most do not seek medical care for their illness. Usually, the ones who do so are treated as out-patients.

CLINICAL CHARACTERISTICS

Most often, bronchiolitis affects children between ages 2 and 12 months. The clinical presentation of bronchiolitis is that of a lower respiratory tract viral illness: fever [usually 38.3°C (101°F) or less], cough, dyspnea, and rhinitis. Hypoxia with cyanosis and increased work of breathing precipitates most hospitalizations for infants with bronchiolitis, but hypoxia can frequently be documented even without clinical evidence of desaturation (i.e., cyanosis or poor peripheral perfusion). Common findings on physical examination include tachypnea with chest retractions and wheezing with rhonchi. Additionally, mild conjunctivitis and otitis can be found on exam. Often, increased respiratory effort, fever, and cough lead to poor feeding and vomiting.

Usually, radiographic abnormalities are nonspecific and may include air trapping, atelectasis, and peribronchial thickening and consolidation. A diffuse interstitial infiltration pattern has also been reported.

DIFFERENTIAL DIAGNOSIS

The differential diagnosis of bronchiolitis includes triggering of underlying reactive airway disease or asthma, other infectious lower respiratory tract diseases (e.g., pneumonia and chemical irritation, as with reflux or aspiration pneumonia), anatomic abnormalities (vascular ring, lung cysts), and extrapulmonary causes of wheezing (cardiac asthma, acidosis, poisoning). Often, chest radiography is helpful in excluding pneumonia. A barium swallow or pH probe determination can document reflux as a cause of recurrent lower respiratory tract diseases that are accompanied by wheezing. Evidence of cardiac disease may be noted by echocardiography and electrocardiography; evidence of extrinsic bronchial constriction may be identified by barium swallow.

Diagnostic Distinction

The diagnostic distinction most difficult to make in infants is between intrinsic reactive airway disease and bronchiolitis. Reactive airway disease, or asthma, is a reversible obstructive airway disease; a 20% reduction in pulmonary function—forced expiratory volume in 1 minute—may be noted after cold or methacholine challenge and is reversible with inhaled bronchodilators. Use of this diagnostic technique is limited to children who are old enough to perform pulmonary function testing (older than age 6); it is not without hazard in that marked bronchospasm can ensue. In small children, the diagnosis of asthma is more difficult; a clinical history or family predisposition, atopy, and recurrent bouts of wheezing that are responsive to bronchodilators assist in making a diagnosis. Recurrent episodes of bronchiolitis have been implicated in the occurrence of reactive airway disease in later childhood. Because the majority of children with bronchiolitis have a viral illness, the diagnosis of bronchiolitis can be made on the basis of clinical and historical findings.

Cystic Fibrosis

Children with cystic fibrosis can have bouts of bronchiolitis that manifest clinically as prolonged or unusually complicated or severe lower respiratory tract illnesses. The diagnosis of cystic fibrosis can be made by documenting elevated chloride levels (greater than 60 mEq/L) by sweat iontophoresis testing.

Allergies

IgE-mediated hypersensitivity to foods, airborne allergens, or insect stings can precipitate systemic allergic reactions including urticaria, wheezing, and hypotension. The history and physical examination can be very helpful in identifying allergies in children. Evidence that the administration of food is followed quickly by diarrhea, vomiting, angioedema, or hives and wheezing clearly suggests food allergy. Radioallergosorbent testing of serum for specific IgE response to food is helpful in confirming this clinical diagnosis. Often, wheezing with airborne allergen exposure is accompanied by symptoms of allergic rhinitis characterized by watery, clear rhinorrhea, nasal and ocular pruritus, and sneezing. Physical examination may reveal the classic stigmata of atopy (e.g., an upturned nose with a nasal crease, allergic shiners, follicular conjunctivitis, bluish boggy nasal mucosa, or a cobblestone appearance of the posterior pharynx). Allergic reactions to insect bites are common and should be suspected when physical examination reveals either typical lesions, such as vesicular skin lesions after fire ant bites, or an intact stinger still embedded in the skin after bee or wasp stings.

PATHOPHYSIOLOGY

The sites of inflammation in bronchiolitis are the small bronchi and bronchioles; the alveolar spaces are spared. Pathologic changes include necrosis and sloughing of respiratory epithelium with destruction of ciliated cells, lymphocytic infiltration of epithelium, and intrabronchiolar plugs of fibrin and mucus causing either complete or partial obstruction. Usually, 1 to 2 weeks are required before the respiratory epithelium is restored completely.

Long-Term Complications

Investigation of immunologic responses at the site of injury after viral infection and bronchiolitis has led to speculation regarding long-term complications and sequelae of bouts of bronchiolitis including subsequent reactive airway disease. Traditionally, inflammatory responses after viral infection are thought to be cell-mediated with lymphocytic infiltration and recruitment of macrophages to clear debris. Several investigators have documented immediate hypersensitivity phenomena after viral infection, particularly in patients with RSV infection; an increase in respiratory epithelial cell-bound IgE in patients with RSV infection and wheezing, as compared to those without wheezing; detection of RSV-specific IgE and eosinophil cationic protein in the nasopharyngeal secretions of patients with infection and wheezing, as compared to its absence in those without wheezing; higher nasopharyngeal concentrations of histamine in patients with RSV infection, as compared to those without this virus; and higher RSV IgA titers than those in controls. IgA and IgE antibody formation is strongly T_H2 cell-dependent and suggests that immediate hypersensitivity tissue responses play a role in the pathogenesis of wheezing in patients with bronchiolitis. Therefore, therapeutic intervention aimed at minimizing bronchospasm has been suggested in the treatment of bronchiolitis.

COMPLICATIONS

One child in 50 with RSV bronchiolitis requires hospitalization; of these, respiratory failure develops in 3% to 7%, and 1% die. Children with significant cardiopulmonary disease or immunodeficiency, however, are at much greater risk of serious sequelae from bronchiolitis. Mortality from nosocomial RSV infection can reach 20% in ill neonates and infants.

Acute Complications

Atelectasis, apnea, and respiratory failure are the most important acute complications of bronchiolitis. Immature ventilatory control and respiratory muscle fatigue lead to apnea and respiratory failure in the youngest patients with bronchiolitis. Once they are intubated and mechanically ventilated, infants with bronchiolitis are at risk for pneumothorax and pneumomediastinum. Intubated patients should be monitored for changes in the amount of tracheal secretions and for secondary fever, which may indicate superinfection and the need for antibiotic therapy. Infants who have bronchopulmonary dysplasia and have been weaned from oxygen therapy may require supplemental oxygen at the time of discharge from the hospital after a bout of bronchiolitis.

Bronchiolitis obliterans is a complication of bronchiolitis caused by adenovirus types 3, 7, and 21; influenza viruses; M. pneumoniae; and Pneumocystis carinii. This disorder is characterized pathologically by diffuse destruction of distal small airways and physiologically by hypoxia and fixed airflow obstruction. Bronchiolitis obliterans has not been described in association with RSV infection.

Recurrent Episodes

Recurrent childhood episodes of bronchiolitis in the absence of underlying pulmonary disease have been implicated as causative agents of subsequent pulmonary dysfunction and the development of asthma. Concurrent genetic and environmental factors (including hyperactive airways that are prone to episodic obstruction) and parental smoking have been implicated in the development of recurrent wheezing after bronchiolitis. Significant pulmonary dysfunction noted in affected children in adult life may be coupled to subsequent environmental exposures including adult smoking practices and pollution exposure.

TREATMENT

Progress has been made in the use of bronchodilators in bronchiolitis. In one series, 30% of infants with RSV bronchiolitis responded to nebulized albuterol with improvement in their pulmonary function. This improvement is short term and may not reduce admission rates or decrease the length of hospitalization. Nebulized epinephrine has an impact on both short-term outcome, through acute improvement in airway resistance leading to acute improvement in oxygen requirement, and long-term outcome, by decreasing the length of time in the emergency department or hospital. The role of corticosteroids in bronchiolitis remains controversial, although most clinicians report using various methods (oral, inhaled, intramuscular) of steroid use. In a study of children with RSV bronchiolitis and receiving varying treatment regimens, including nebulized salbutamol, normal saline, or corticosteroids, corticosteroids were no more effective than the nebulization therapy. In contrast, a study of hospitalized children with RSV bronchiolitis showed improvement in clinical recovery for oral corticosteroid recipients, as compared to placebo controls. No complications of corticosteroid use have been described and, in patients with severe disease, their addition is not contraindicated. Using racemic epinephrine to treat wheezing infants with bronchiolitis seems reasonable, particularly if one or more doses of epinephrine reduce tachypnea and quiet retractions.

Children with suspected bronchiolitis should be admitted to the hospital if they are tachypneic, have marked retractions, seem listless, or have a history of poor fluid intake. Immunocompromised infants and those with underlying cardiopulmonary disease should be hospitalized if bronchiolitis develops.

The inpatient evaluation may include a chest film, arterial blood gas measurements, and oxygen saturation (S_aO_2) monitoring. Nasopharyngeal washings should be obtained for viral cultures and RSV enzyme immunoassay. The infant should receive intravenous fluids at maintenance rates with additional fluids to restore normal hydration. Care to avoid overhydration should be observed. Humidified oxygen should be begun and adjusted to maintain the S_aO_2 greater than or equal to 93%. Nebulized epinephrine or beta$_2$ agonists should be given as needed. If nebulized therapy is required more often than every 2 hours (for a falling S_aO_2 level, marked retractions, or listlessness), affected children should be transferred to an intensive care unit.

Intubation and mechanical ventilation are indicated for apnea, for a rising P_aCO_2 value, and for listlessness and retractions suggesting impending respiratory failure. Corticosteroids, theophylline, and furosemide have all been used in ventilated patients with bronchiolitis. Most patients ventilated for bronchiolitis require 7 to 14 days of mechanical support before they can be weaned from the ventilator.

Ribavirin is an antiviral agent that is effective against RSV and influenza viruses A and B. It is indicated for the early treatment of RSV bronchiolitis in infants with congenital heart disease, bronchopulmonary dysplasia, lung and chest-wall anomalies, and immunodeficiency. Infants younger than 6 weeks and severely ill patients (P_aO_2 less than 65 mm Hg, rising P_aCO_2) with bronchiolitis are also candidates for ribavirin therapy. This agent is approved for use by nebulization into a hood, mask, or tent. Ribavirin should be delivered by a small-particle aerosol generator for 12 to 18 hours a day, and it should be continued for 3 to 7 days until an affected patient improves.

The role of antibiotic therapy in bronchiolitis is minimal because no bacterial agent has been described as causative. Antimicrobial therapy may be administered because of concomitant radiographic evidence of pneumonia. Traditional causative agents should be considered (*Haemophilus influenzae*, *Streptococcus pneumoniae*). If secondary bacterial infection is a consideration, nosocomial infectious agents (*Staphylococcus aureus*) should be considered.

PROPHYLAXIS

Palivizumab (Synagis) is a monoclonal antibody to RSV that has been approved as immunoprophylaxis for children who are younger than 24 months and have a history of chronic lung disease or a history of premature birth (less than 35 weeks' gestation). It is given once per month as an intramuscular injection during RSV season (October through March, however regional differences are acknowledged) and the dose is 15 mg/kg. Palivizumab is approved for children with hemodynamically significant congenital heart disease and it will not interfere with the immune response to any vaccine in the vaccination schedule.

CHAPTER 135

Nonbacterial Pneumonia

Adapted from Kenneth M. Boyer

ETIOLOGY

At least 14 different virus groups, three *Mycoplasma* species, one *Rickettsia* species, three *Chlamydia* species, and one protozoan parasite have been associated with pneumonia syndromes in children. The overall importance of these agents is not measured simply by their incidence. Some agents, although they are fairly common, generally give rise to relatively mild illness; others encountered less frequently characteristically cause serious disease. In Table 135-1, the major agents causing disease in various age groups are presented according to their overall frequency, their typical degree of severity, and their usual mode of access to the lung.

EPIDEMIOLOGY

Major Contributors

The major contributors to the overall epidemiology of nonbacterial pneumonia in children are RSV, parainfluenza viruses, *M. pneumoniae* and, to a lesser extent, influenza viruses A and B. Because of their brief incubation periods and high degree of communicability, these agents often spread through communities in well-defined waves. RSV and the influenza viruses occur almost exclusively in the winter months; usually, parainfluenza viruses 1 and 2 are seen in the spring and fall. During intervals between epidemics, *M. pneumoniae* and parainfluenza virus 3 tend to persist endemically.

Causative Agents

Annual rates of childhood pneumonia show a rough inverse correlation with age ranging from 40 in 1,000 children younger than 5 years to 7 in 1,000 adolescents aged 12 to 15 years. RSV

TABLE 135-1. Etiologic Agents in Nonbacterial Pneumonia

	Frequency[a]			Usual degree of severity[b]			
Etiologic agents	*0–3 mo*	*4 mo to 5 yr*	*6–16 yr*	*0–3 mo*	*4 mo to 5 yr*	*6–16 yr*	Mode of access to lung
Viruses							
Respiratory syncytial virus	+++	++++	+	++	++	+	Respiratory
Parainfluenza viruses							
Type 1	+	++	+	++	++	+	Respiratory
Type 2	+	+	+	++	++	+	Respiratory
Type 3	++	+++	++	++	++	+	Respiratory
Influenza viruses							
Type A	++	+++	+++	++	++	+	Respiratory
Type B	++	++	+	++	++	+	Respiratory
Adenoviruses[c]	+	++	++	+++	++	+	Respiratory
Rhinoviruses[d]	+	+	+	–	++	+	Respiratory
Enteroviruses[e]	+	+	+	++	++	+	Respiratory (hemoatogenous)
Coronaviruses	–	+	+	–	++	+	Respiratory
Measles virus	+	++	++	+++	++	++	Respiratory (hematogenous)
Rubella virus	+	–	–	++	–	–	Hematogenous
Human immunodeficiency virus	+	++	+	++	++	++	Hematogenous
Varicella-zoster virus	+	+	+	+++	+++	+++	Hematogenous (respiratory)
Cytomegalovirus	++	+	+	++	+++	+++	Hematogenous (respiratory)
Epstein-Barr virus	–	+	++	–	++	+	Hematogenous (respiratory)
Herpes simplex viruses	++	+	+	++++	+++	+++	Hematogenous (respiratory)
Mycoplasmas							
Mycoplasma pneumoniae	–	+	++++	–	++	+	Respiratory
Mycoplasma hominis	?	–	–	?	–	–	Respiratory
Ureaplasma urealyticum	?	–	–	?	–	–	Respiratory
Chlamydiae							
Chlamydia pneumoniae	?	?	+++	?	?	+	Respiratory
Chlamydia psittaci	–	+	+	–	++	++	Respiratory
Chlamydia trachomatis	++++	–	–	++	–	–	Respiratory
Rickettsiae							
Coxiella burnetii	–	+	+	–	++	++	Respiratory (hematogenous)
Protozoa							
Pneumocystis carinii	+	+	+	+++	+++	+++	Respiratory

[a]++++, most frequent; +++, frequent; ++, infrequent; +, rare; –, no reported cases; ?, uncertain.
[b]++++, often fatal; +++, severe; ++, usually hospitalized; +, home management; –, no reported cases; ?, uncertain.
[c]Types 1, 2, 3, 4, 5, 7, 8, 11, 21, and 35.
[d]Ninety or more types known.
[e]Coxsackieviruses A9, A16, B1, B4, and B5; echoviruses 9, 11, 19, 20, and 22.
Modified from Boyer KM. Nonbacterial pneumonia. In: Feigin RD, Cherry JD, eds. *Textbook of pediatric infectious diseases*, 4th ed. Philadelphia: Saunders, 1998:262.

is the most common causative agent in children younger than 5; *M. pneumoniae* is most common in older children.

In children, congenital heart disease and bronchopulmonary dysplasia are associated with viral pneumonia of greater severity, particularly that caused by RSV. Pulmonary deterioration in patients with cystic fibrosis has been shown to be associated with respiratory viral infection. Surprisingly, common respiratory viruses have an impact in patients with hematologic malignancy and immunosuppressed states only moderately greater than that in normal hosts.

Transmission

Most often, transmission of the more common agents of lower respiratory tract disease occurs by means of droplet spread resulting from relatively close contact with a source case. Direct inoculation at the alveolar level probably does not occur in most cases because of the extremely small size of aerosolized particles necessary to accomplish it. Studies of RSV infections transmitted nosocomially have shown the importance of adults with relatively trivial upper respiratory tract infection as intermediates in transmission to susceptible young infants. Often, school-aged children introduce respiratory viral agents into households resulting in secondary infections in parents and siblings. The increasing use of group day care by working parents has been associated with enhanced transmission of a number of respiratory pathogens and certainly has extended "school age" to include a group of younger children.

CLINICAL CHARACTERISTICS

Symptoms

Generally, acute nonbacterial pneumonia in infants or young children follows 1 or 2 days of coryza, decreased appetite, and low-grade fever, and generally the onset is gradual with increasing fretfulness, respiratory congestion, vomiting, cough, and fever. In very young infants, fever may be minimal, and apneic spells ("near-miss" sudden infant death syndrome or "apparent life-threatening events") are the most prominent (and frightening) presenting complaint. The most reliable physical findings of pneumonia are those of respiratory distress—tachypnea, tachycardia, nasal flaring, and retractions—but without the stridor characteristic of upper airway obstruction. Patients with diminished functional residual capacity may exhibit grunting. Generally, cyanosis accompanies apneic spells or coughing attacks, but it may be present at rest if significant ventilation–perfusion mismatch has developed.

Other physical findings are fairly variable and may be normal. Wheezing is present in infants with bronchiolitis. Hyperresonance may be noted if significant air trapping is present. Diminished local percussion or breath sounds may indicate lobar consolidation or atelectasis. In patients with interstitial pneumonia, fine crackles may be present diffusely or locally. Also important in initial assessments is an evaluation of young children' s state of hydration because increased insensible losses from fever and hyperventilation, coupled with anorexia, can result in significant fluid deficits.

The afebrile pneumonitis syndrome of young infants, in contrast to the usual acute viral pneumonias affecting this age group, is subacute to chronic in its development and is nonseasonal. Characteristic features include the absence of fever, a "staccato" cough pattern, and diffuse rales on auscultation. Usually, radiographic findings consist of interstitial infiltrates with subsegmental atelectasis. Hypergammaglobulinemia and mild eosinophilia are common laboratory abnormalities.

Nonbacterial pneumonia in older children and adolescents occurs clinically more nearly like that in an adult. Generally, premonitory complaints include such systemic symptoms as malaise, myalgia, and anorexia, in addition to upper respiratory tract symptoms. "Chilliness" may occur, but generally rigors are absent. Usually, cough is irritative and nonproductive. A temperature of more than 39°C is unusual. Although tachypnea, flaring, and retractions are generally present, they may be less apparent than in infants or young children. Findings on chest examination are more reliable than those taken of infants and may include local percussion dullness or diminished breath sounds and local or diffuse fine rales. Because apnea is rare in older patients, cyanosis is an ominous sign of impairment of gas exchange. Although mild dehydration is often present, it is not generally evident on examination.

Radiologic findings in nonbacterial pneumonia vary according to patients' age and the infecting agent. In infants and young children, bilateral air trapping and perihilar infiltrates are the most frequent findings. Patchy areas of consolidation may represent lobular atelectasis or alveolar pneumonia. In older children and adolescents, lobar involvement can be defined more often, but typically the affected areas are not consolidated completely. Although lobar consolidation may occur in patients with nonbacterial pneumonia, this finding should be distinguished from atelectasis and is more consistent with a bacterial cause of disease. Similarly, although small pleural effusions may be detected in decubitus films in patients with nonbacterial pneumonia, effusions are much more suggestive of bacterial infection.

Peripheral leukocyte counts vary but tend to be less than 15,000 cells/mm^3 in patients with nonbacterial pneumonia. Gram stains of sputum or tracheal secretions tend to show epithelial cells as the predominant cell type with a mixed bacterial population representing normal pharyngeal flora. Dominance of polymorphonuclear leukocytes and a uniform bacterial population are more consistent with bacterial infection.

DIFFERENTIAL DIAGNOSIS

In the differential diagnosis of nonbacterial pneumonia, the following factors must be considered: status of the host (normal or compromised); environment (family or school exposure); age of the patient; and season of the year. In certain epidemiologic settings, the specific cause of nonbacterial pneumonia may be guessed with relative certainty. Often, however, this category of pulmonary infection is a diagnosis of exclusion. The major conditions to be differentiated include noninfectious pulmonary diseases, bacterial pneumonias amenable to conventional antibiotics, and the more unusual bacterial, fungal, or parasitic infections that may require specialized forms of therapy.

Noninfectious Conditions

Noninfectious conditions that may simulate nonbacterial pneumonia are summarized in Table 135-2. The demarcation between infectious and noninfectious conditions is not always sharp. In children with sickle cell anemia, for example, pulmonary vasoocclusive crisis presents with fever, leukocytosis, and patchy pulmonary infiltrates. Differentiation from pneumococcal, *Haemophilus*, or *Mycoplasma* pneumonia to which the

TABLE 135-2. Noninfectious Conditions that may Simulate or Underlie Pneumonia in Children

Technical
Poor inspiratory chest radiograph
Underpenetrated chest radiograph
Physiologic
Prominent thymus
Breast shadows
Chronic pulmonary disease
Asthma
Cystic fibrosis
Bronchiectasis
Bronchiolitis obliterans
Pulmonary sequestration
Congenital lobar emphysema
Pulmonary hemosiderosis
Desquamative interstitial pneumonitis
Recurrent aspiration
Gastroesophageal reflux
Tracheoesophageal fistula
Craniofacial defect
Neuromuscular disorders
Familial dysautonomia
Pulmonary edema
Congestive heart failure
"Adult" respiratory distress syndrome
Total anomalous pulmonary venous return
Allergic alveolitis
Dusts (farmer's lung)
Molds (allergic aspergillosis)
Excreta (pigeon-breeder's lung)
Atelectasis
Cardiomegaly
Mucus plug
Foreign body
Damage by physical agents
Bronchopulmonary dysplasia
Lipoid pneumonia
Petroleum distillate ingestion
Near drowning
Smoke inhalation
Iatrogenic pulmonary damage
Fluid overload
Drugs (nitrofurantoin, bleomycin)
Radiation pneumonitis
Graft-versus-host disease
Pulmonary infarction
Sickle vasoocclusive crisis
Fat embolism
Miscellaneous
Systemic lupus erythematosus
Sarcoidosis
Neoplasms (lymphoma, teratoma, neuroblastoma)
Pleural effusion or reaction
Bronchogenic cyst
Vascular ring
Histiocytosis

Modified from Boyer KM, Pneumonia. In: Dershewitz RA, ed. *Ambulatory pediatric care*, 2nd ed. Philadelphia: Lippincott, 1992:621.

child with sickle cell anemia has increased susceptibility may be difficult or impossible. Early recognition of noninfectious conditions either mimicking or underlying pneumonia may prevent recurrence or may improve the prognosis. Recognition of the "snowman in a snowstorm" chest radiograph of total anomalous pulmonary venous return may lead to a curative open-heart procedure. Recognition and treatment of cystic fibrosis may prevent early irreversible pulmonary damage.

Causative Agents

Classically, pneumonias caused by pyogenic bacteria are lobar in distribution and exhibit consolidation on roentgenography. Atelectasis, on the other hand, is common in viral pneumonia and must be distinguished from true consolidation. Pleural effusions, circular infiltrates, consolidations with convex margins, and pneumatoceles favor a bacterial infection. Because of the association of bacteremic infection with a high fever and significant leukocytosis in young children, these clinical findings also favor a bacterial cause of pneumonia. Frequently, the results of numerous other laboratory determinations such as erythrocyte sedimentation rate, C-reactive protein level, and reduction of nitroblue tetrazolium by leukocytes are positive in patients with bacterial respiratory infection. However, these tests add little to a careful initial clinical examination, roentgenographic findings, and differential white blood cell count. Only positive results of cultures of blood, pleural fluid, or lung aspirates definitely prove the cause of bacterial pneumonia.

Among the less common causes of pneumonia, tuberculosis should never be forgotten. Tuberculin testing should be included in the initial evaluation and is especially important for children who live in urban areas, for recent immigrants, and for Native Americans. Fungal pneumonia, particularly coccidioidomycosis, blastomycosis, and histoplasmosis, should be considered in children who live in or visit endemic areas. Often, a suggestive history such as exposure to excavations (e.g., backyard swimming pools, geologic or archeologic digs), clean-up chores in old sheds and barns, and dust storms, may be elicited. Erythema nodosum and eosinophilia are common clinical clues to these entities. Other fungal pneumonias such as aspergillosis and cryptococcosis occur in the setting of immunosuppression. These conditions, coupled with the possibilities of infection with Pneumocystis, fungi, resistant bacteria, and CMV, may warrant the use of bronchoalveolar lavage or open lung biopsy as definitive approaches to diagnosis in the compromised host.

SPECIFIC DIAGNOSIS

The methods used for virologic and chlamydial isolation are available in most major medical centers and public health laboratories. With the possible exceptions of herpes simplex viruses and adenoviruses, respiratory viruses are rarely carried asymptomatically. Thus, identification of an agent in upper respiratory tract secretions is strong evidence for its causative role in pneumonia. Conventional virologic techniques provide the most sensitive and specific means of identification. Rapid diagnosis of influenza A virus, parainfluenza viruses, RSV, and Chlamydia infections by means of fluorescent antibody techniques, enzyme-linked immunosorbent assays, direct DNA probes, or polymerase chain reaction has proved useful in numerous centers. In individual cases, serologic diagnosis of respiratory viral infection is generally less satisfactory than virologic diagnosis. The difficulties associated with serology relate to the timing of specimen collection, the choice of antigens to test, and variation in the quality and specificity of available reagents. In contrast, serologic diagnosis of chlamydial pneumonitis can be very helpful. Even at the onset of illness, affected infants have high titers of specific IgG and IgM antibodies. Similarly, a positive antibody test result for HIV infection constitutes strong evidence for either pulmonary lymphoid hyperplasia or opportunistic *Pneumocystis* pneumonia in a child with pulmonary infiltrates and a compatible epidemiologic history for pediatric AIDS.

Laboratory facilities for the isolation of mycoplasmas and rickettsiae are less readily accessible to clinicians. DNA probes have become available for diagnosis of *M. pneumoniae*. However, serologic techniques are the most practical means of making a specific diagnosis. Acute-phase reactants (e.g., cold agglutinins in M. pneumoniae infection) are of greatest diagnostic help during acute illness but are not present invariably. Definitive etiologic identification requires testing of paired sera for specific antibodies. Usually, Pneumocystis infection is diagnosed by visualizing organisms in silver-stained specimens obtained by bronchoscopy or biopsy using silver impregnation stains or fluorescein-labeled monoclonal antibodies.

Because of the epidemiologic behavior of nonbacterial respiratory infections, often a reasonable guess as to a specific cause can be made on the basis of factors such as patient age, season of the year, and associated clinical features. If the presence of a particular nonbacterial agent in a community can be established by isolation or serologic means, the probability that other patients with similar manifestations have illness caused by that agent is increased greatly.

THERAPY

Therapy for nonbacterial pneumonia is primarily expectant and supportive. The course of uncomplicated viral pneumonia is not influenced by the administration of antibiotics. In the vast majority of cases in which pulmonary involvement is uncovered, however, antibiotic therapy is used because bacterial disease cannot be ruled out with certainty. In all but the mildest cases, this approach is both reasonable and practical. Nonetheless, antibiotic therapy in routine cases must be appropriate for the most common bacterial pathogens (*S. pneumoniae* and *H. influenzae*). In the immunocompromised host or when secondary infection is a possibility, S. aureus and other hospital-associated and opportunistic pathogens must be considered.

Antibiotic Therapies

In certain fulminant viral pneumonias, such as varicella in a child with leukemia, antiviral chemotherapy with acyclovir may be lifesaving, but one should recall that as many as one-half of all patients with this condition have complicating bacterial sepsis amenable to antibiotic therapy. The treatment of pneumonia caused by CMV in immunocompromised hosts now consists of the combination of ganciclovir and intravenous hyperimmune globulin. Inhalational administration of the antiviral compound ribavirin appears to shorten the courses of viral pneumonias caused by RSV and influenza. This drug is recommended particularly for the treatment of RSV infection in infants with underlying cardiopulmonary disease. The therapeutic effects of ribavirin therapy are not dramatic, which has led to revisions in recommendations for its use.

Specific antimicrobial therapy for mycoplasmal, chlamydial, and rickettsial pneumonias with erythromycin or tetracycline shortens the course of the illness but generally has a less dramatic therapeutic effect than specific antibiotic therapy for bacterial infections. The drug of choice for *Pneumocystis* pneumonia is oral or parenteral trimethoprim-sulfamethoxazole.

Supportive Therapy

The elements of supportive therapy include adequate hydration, high humidity, maintenance of oxygenation, and mobilization of lower respiratory tract secretions. Because of increased insensible fluid losses as a result of fever, hyperventilation, and anorexia, mild dehydration is frequently observed initially, and usually continuing losses occur during the acute phase of illness. Thus, restoration of deficits and adequate maintenance of fluid intake are desirable. With regard to the latter, one should remember that fluid requirements increase by approximately 12% per degree Centigrade of fever and that hyperventilation increases fluid requirements by an additional 15%.

Therapeutic Therapy

The therapeutic benefits of mist tents are debated because of the negligible amounts of nebulized water that actually reach the bronchiolar level. A high level of humidity is required to prevent the drying effects of supplemental oxygen therapy, however; by slowing evaporation, it probably also serves to reduce the viscosity of mucus secretions and the magnitude of insensible fluid losses. Mobilization of respiratory secretions by means of vibration and postural drainage is indicated in patients with nonbacterial pneumonia complicated by atelectasis, but it is not helpful in the absence of excessive secretions or mucus plugging.

Oxygen Therapy

Because of ventilation-perfusion abnormalities and alveolocapillary block, most children with nonbacterial pneumonia have some degree of hypoxemia. In children with respiratory distress, provision of supplemental oxygen reduces anxiety and ventilation rates. Increases in inspired oxygen to approximately 30% are provided easily with nasal prongs or "face tents," which are the most convenient means of administering oxygen. More severe respiratory distress or cyanosis requires documentation of patients' respiratory status by means of arterial blood gas determinations and more exact regulation of inspired oxygen administered by hood or facemask. Oximetry, capnography, or transcutaneous monitoring can reduce the need for frequent blood gas sampling and insertion of arterial lines. In patients with respiratory failure, mechanical ventilation is required to maintain oxygenation and to control carbon dioxide retention.

Viral Pneumonia

Apnea and bradycardia occur commonly in young infants with pneumonia caused by RSV, parainfluenza viruses, and influenza viruses, and there are particularly frequent complications in those patients with a history of premature birth. Although the mechanism for these episodes is unclear, continuous monitoring for apnea is prudent in young infants with viral pneumonia.

Medications

Acetaminophen or ibuprofen may be used for fever and discomfort. Although these agents are prescribed widely for upper respiratory tract infections in children and adults, expectorants and cough suppressants are not helpful in the initial treatment of nonbacterial pneumonia. Theophylline and aerosolized bronchodilators are used widely in patients with nonbacterial pneumonia complicated by apnea or bronchospasm. Controlled trials suggest a therapeutic benefit of albuterol in the emergency department setting, but trials in hospitalized infants with bronchiolitis have not shown a beneficial effect. During convalescence, a persistent irritative cough that interferes with sleep may be alleviated by judicious use of antihistamines, dextromethorphan, or codeine.

PROGNOSIS

Children with pneumonia should be reevaluated clinically 2 to 3 weeks after the condition is diagnosed. If affected children are asymptomatic, have returned to normal activities, and have benign results on physical examination, follow-up radiography is not required. Repeated chest radiography is indicated in children with complicated clinical courses, underlying cardiopulmonary disease, or prior episodes of pneumonia, or if signs or symptoms of respiratory difficulty persist at the time of follow-up. What should be recognized is that approximately 20% of patients with uncomplicated cases of pneumonia have persistent radiographic abnormalities 3 to 4 weeks after diagnosis, but a selective approach to follow-up films permits the early recognition of atelectasis or chronic disease.

PREVENTION

Person-to-Person Transmission

Nosocomial spread of respiratory viruses occurs readily in pediatric wards and involves intermediate carriage by medical personnel who have acquired mild upper respiratory tract infections. A reasonable approach to interdicting nosocomial transmission is to group patients with pneumonia and to exclude personnel with symptomatic respiratory illness from ward duties. With the exceptions of measles and varicella, mask or gown isolation has no effect on transmission. Avoiding close contact, washing hands, and wearing glasses or goggles will minimize respiratory infections of personnel. Regardless of HIV serologic status, blood and secretion precautions (universal precautions) are recommended for all hospitalized patients.

Vaccines

For the common viral causes of pneumonia, vaccines are available only for influenza viruses and adenoviruses. Annual influenza vaccination using "split product" vaccines is recommended for children with chronic respiratory disease and other conditions that predispose them to the development of pneumonia. Vaccination of adult health care personnel reduces the number of work days missed because of illness and can prevent nosocomial transmission. Adenovirus vaccines have been used widely in the military forces but are not recommended for use in the pediatric population. Attenuated, inactivated, and subunit vaccines against RSV, parainfluenza virus type 3, and *M. pneumoniae* have received considerable investigative effort but have not yet proved to be entirely satisfactory.

Passive Immunization

RSV bronchiolitis and pneumonia can be prevented in high-risk infants by passive immunization. Intravenous gamma globulin preparations with high-titer antiRSV activity are in current use. "Humanized" monoclonal antiRSV antibodies administered intramuscularly have proved highly effective in clinical trials.

Prophylactic Administration

P. carinii pneumonia can be prevented in pediatric patients with hematologic malignancy or AIDS by the prophylactic administration of trimethoprim–sulfamethoxazole. This medication has become part of the routine management of these conditions and has reduced the incidence of *P. carinii* infection dramatically. Note that prophylaxis should be started even in seropositive infants whose HIV infection status is indeterminate. Opportunistic pneumonia caused by CMV, which is a major hazard in seronegative, high-risk, premature infants and in recipients of allogeneic bone marrow transplants, can be prevented effectively by the exclusive use of CMV-seronegative blood products. In seropositive marrow transplant recipients who are, thus, at risk for reactivated disease, acyclovir, ganciclovir, and intravenous immunoglobulin have been shown to reduce rates of infection and interstitial pneumonia.

CHAPTER 136
Bacterial Pneumonia

Adapted from John F. Modlin

In the United States, recognized infection of the lower respiratory tract occurs annually in 15 to 20 of 1,000 infants younger than 1 year and in 30 to 40 of 1,000 children from ages 1 to 5. Whereas the respiratory viruses and *Mycoplasma pneumoniae* are the most common agents of lower respiratory tract disease in children and young adults, pyogenic bacteria cause a substantial minority of cases of pneumonia. For example, one study found that bacteria were responsible for 19% of pneumonia cases among ambulatory children. Bacterial pneumonia is observed most commonly in the winter and early spring and occurs almost twice as frequently in boys as in girls. In practice, distinguishing bacterial pneumonia from other forms of pneumonia may be difficult. Young children do not produce adequate sputum for Gram stain and culture, and more invasive procedures are not warranted except in a few cases of the most severely ill patients or patients with underlying immunodeficiency.

ETIOLOGY

Age and the presence or absence of underlying disease are the two most important patient characteristics determining the etiology of bacterial pneumonia. Bacterial pneumonia presenting in the first 2 days of life, which is generally considered to be acquired *in utero* or intrapartum, is caused by the same organisms responsible for generalized neonatal sepsis (i.e., group B streptococci, *Listeria monocytogenes*, *Haemophilus influenzae*, and *E. Coli*). Most cases of perinatally acquired pneumonia occur among low-birth-weight (LBW) infants and infants who have peripartum complications. Chlamydia trachomatis, a pathogen acquired from the maternal genital tract at delivery, may not cause respiratory symptoms until the second month of life.

After the neonatal period, *Streptococcus pneumoniae*, Moraxella catarrhalis, and group A streptococci are responsible for most cases of bacterial pneumonia in otherwise healthy children. *Staphylococcus aureus* pneumonia is now rarely seen in infants and toddlers, and *H. influenzae* type b (Hib) pneumonia has been eliminated in the United States and other developed countries with universal use of Hib vaccine. In patients older than 4 or 5 years, the spectrum of bacteria causing pneumonia narrows with *M. pneumoniae, Chlamydia pneumoniae,* and *S. pneumoniae* predominating. *M. pneumoniae* and *C. pneumoniae* infections are rare in young children. In contrast, they are the pathogens identified most commonly as causing pneumonia in children older than 5 years.

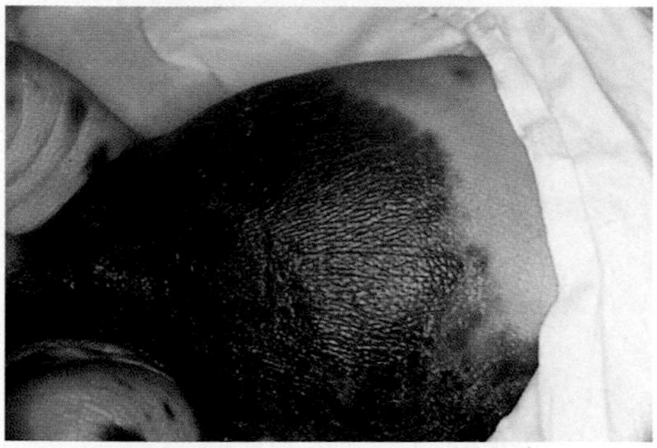

Figure 40-1. Giant congenital melanocytic nevus with atypical features including a scalloped border, irregular pigmentation, and variable thickness.

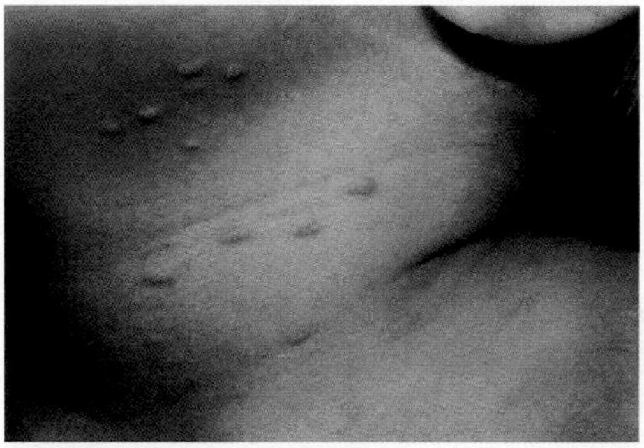

Figure 40-2. Multiple pinkish brown papules and nodules of generalized cutaneous mastocytosis.

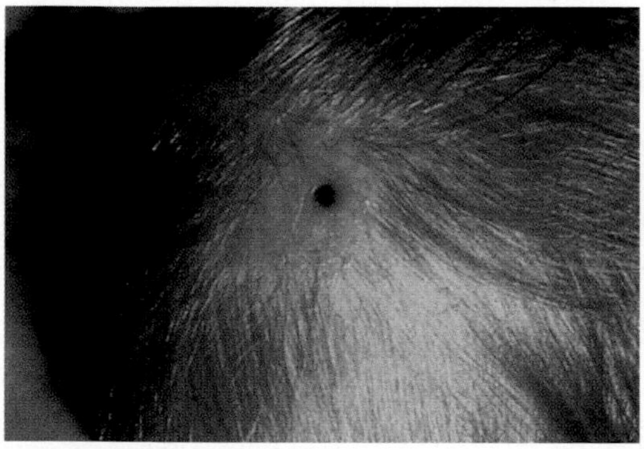

Figure 40-3. Striking yellow-orange, pebbly appearance of a typical nevus sebaceous on the scalp. Note the absence of hair within the lesion. The dark, crusted area is the site of a punch biopsy.

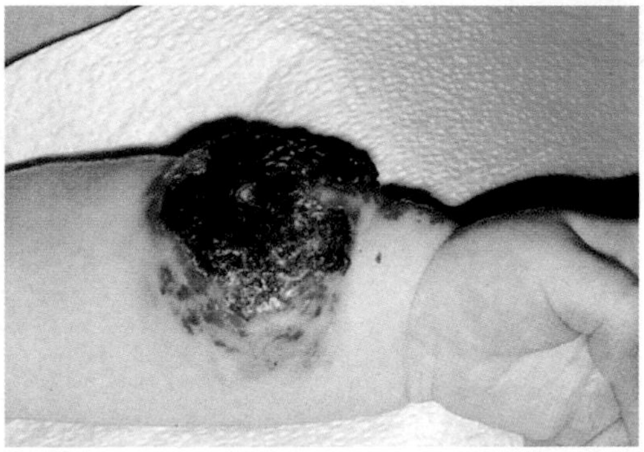

Figure 40-4. Large, mixed capillary and cavernous hemangioma on the left forearm with ulceration and crusting. The capillary component is superficial and bright red; the cavernous component is deeper and blue.

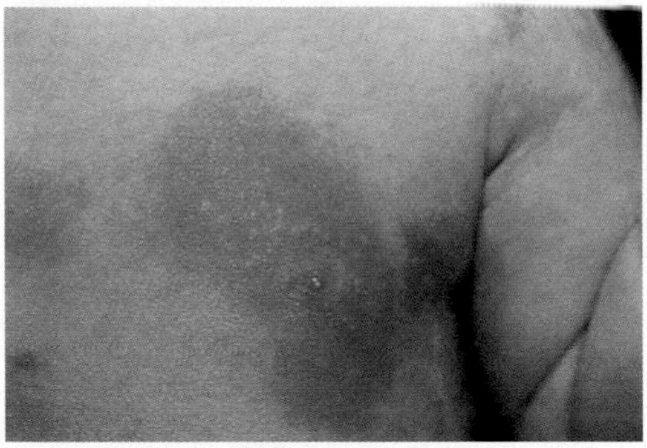

Figure 40-5. The hallmark splotchy erythema studded with small papules and pustules of erythema toxicum.

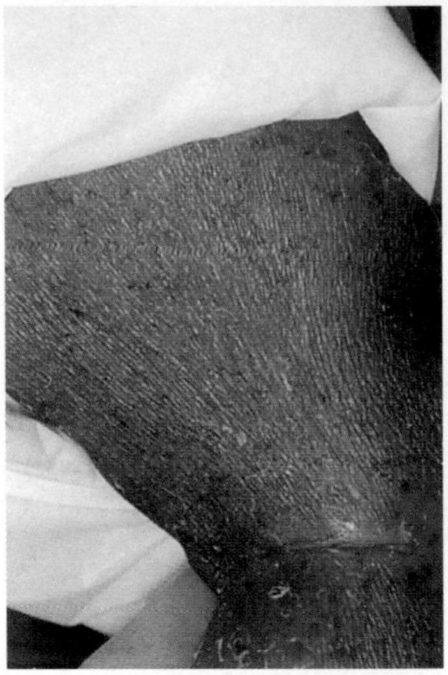

Figure 40-6. Hyperpigmented macules of transient neonatal pustular melanosis, many of which are surrounded by a collarette of scale that is the remnant of the roof of the preceding pustule.

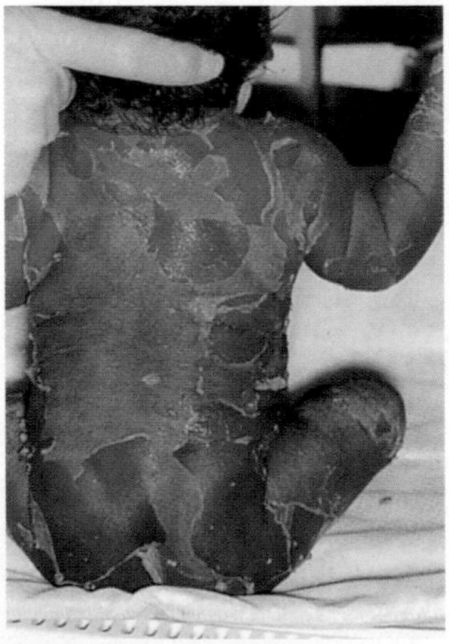

Figure 40-7. Newborn with widespread blistering of epidermolytic hyperkeratosis.

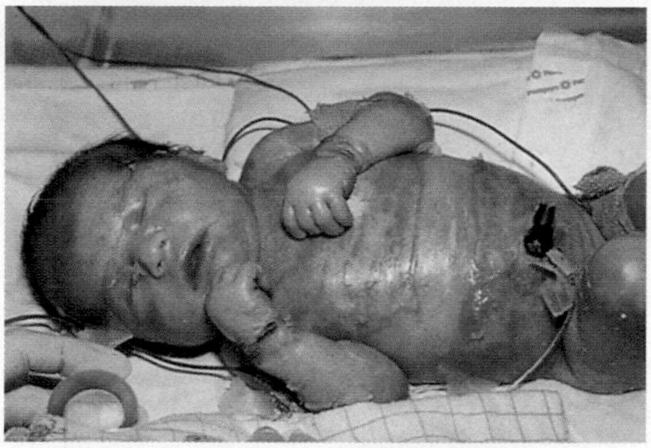

Figure 40-8. Collodion baby after partial shedding of the collodion membrane. The hands, arms, legs, and a portion of the abdomen are still encased in a tight, shiny membrane.

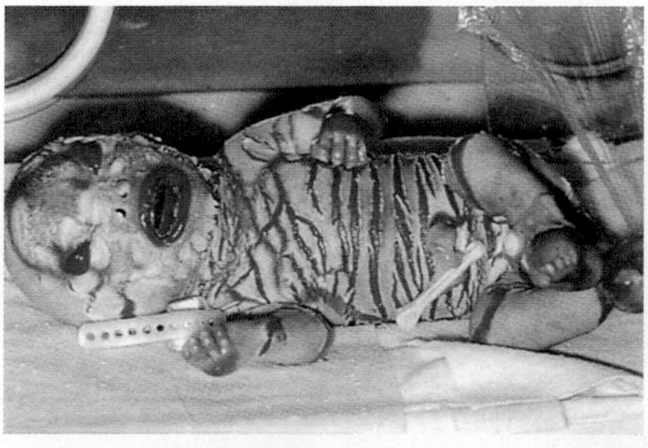

Figure 40-9. Harlequin fetus with thick yellow skin traversed by deep fissures, ectropion, eclabium, and mitten deformity of the hands and feet.

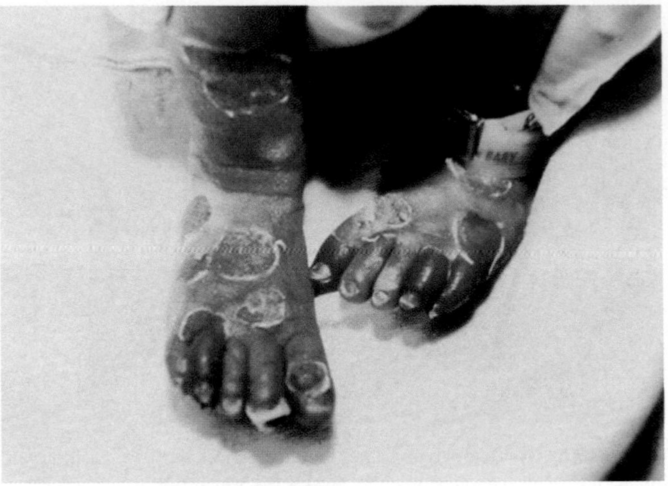

Figure 46-2. Pemphigus syphiliticus, a widely disseminated vesiculo-bullous eruption in an infant with early congenital syphilis. (Courtesy of Charles Ginsburg, M.D.)

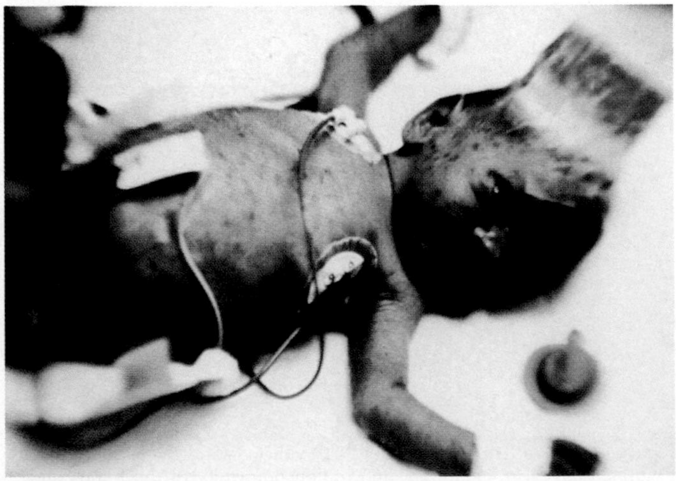

Figure 46-5. So-called blueberry-muffin spots. Extramedullary dermal erythropoiesis is observed in the most severely affected infants with congenital cytomegalovirus infection and congenital rubella.

PATHOGENESIS

Bacterial pathogens that cause pneumonia in children are transmitted person to person via close personal contact or via airborne spread. Colonization of young children's upper respiratory tract with pathogenic bacteria is relatively common; the prevalence for carriage of pneumococci is 25% to 40% during winter months and somewhat lower during other seasons. Pneumonia results from aspiration of pathogenic bacteria into the lower respiratory tract; often, the process is aided by concurrent viral infection, particularly with the influenza viruses and measles virus. Careful studies have documented the coexistence of a respiratory virus in 30% to 50% of children with bacterial pneumonia. Acute viral infection serves to disrupt the normal anatomic and physiologic barriers of the respiratory tract mucosa and may briefly suppress the activity of phagocytic leukocytes in the airways and lung.

CLINICAL CHARACTERISTICS

The signs and symptoms of bacterial pneumonia vary with affected children's age, with the organism, and with the presence or absence of underlying disease. Characteristically, older children and adolescents present with fever, chills, headache, dyspnea, productive cough, chest pain, abdominal pain, and nausea or vomiting. However, infants are likely to present with the largely nonspecific symptoms of fever, lethargy, poor feeding, vomiting, or diarrhea. Apnea may be a prominent sign among infants younger than 2 months. Tachypnea may be overlooked by the parents, and cough, if present, is not often a prominent finding in very young infants. Similarly, the physical examination findings in young infants with pneumonia are less definitive; usually, percussion and auscultation do not elicit the characteristic dullness to percussion and decreased breath sounds found in older children and adults with pneumonia, and distinguishing rales from the sounds produced by a congested upper respiratory tract may be difficult.

DIAGNOSIS

In practice, the diagnosis of pneumonia is made with the demonstration of infiltrates on anteroposterior and lateral chest radiography. Sometimes, false-negative results are attributed to dehydration. Conversely, many noninfectious diseases of the lung, including malignancy, collagen-vascular disease, congestive heart failure, pulmonary embolus, allergic alveolitis, pulmonary hemorrhage, and hemosiderosis, may mimic the radiographic appearance of pneumonia. A pattern of peribronchial or "patchy" infiltrates (bronchopneumonia) does not distinguish viral or mycoplasmal pneumonia from bacterial pneumonia, but demonstration of hyperinflation is most consistent with viral infection. The presence of lobar consolidation or pleural effusion suggests bacterial infection, whereas pneumatoceles and abscess cavities are virtually diagnostic. Roentgenograms demonstrate bilateral disease in 20% to 25% of pediatric patients. The resolution of the pulmonary infiltrates will lag behind clinical improvement of the patient. Routine follow-up radiographs contribute little to the management of the child with an uncomplicated course of pneumonia.

Computed tomography of the chest provides better resolution and, thus, is more sensitive than radiography for the detection of pulmonary infiltrates. However, the expense of computed tomographic scanning justifies its use only when complications such as adenopathy, empyema, or cavitation are suspected.

Tests and Procedures

WBC and differential cell counts and an erythrocyte sedimentation rate test are performed routinely on all pediatric patients with suspected pneumonia. An attempt to determine the etiology should be made in all cases of suspected bacterial pneumonia in hospitalized children. Cultures of blood and pleural fluid (if present) are obtained, usually from children requiring hospitalization. Gram staining of expectorated sputum may be valuable in the diagnosis of pneumonia in school-aged children or adolescents, especially when a single organism is seen in association with polymorphonuclear leukocytes; usually, culture of an adequate sputum specimen will yield the pathogenic organism. However, infants and young children are incapable of producing a spontaneous sputum specimen and, generally, efforts to induce sputum in younger children are unsuccessful. Cultures of the nasopharynx and throat are not useful and should not be attempted because of the risk of producing misleading information. Invasive procedures such as bronchoalveolar lavage or open-lung biopsy are justified in cases of pneumonia that are severe or complicated by underlying disease. Direct transthoracic needle aspiration of the lung has proved to be a very useful procedure in cases in which recovery of an organism is critical for management.

ANTIBIOTIC MANAGEMENT

The management of pneumonia depends on the severity of the illness and the presence or absence of underlying chronic disease. In practice, children with mild to moderate pneumonia are often managed as outpatients. Oral amoxicillin is used widely for outpatient management of pneumonia for infants and for children younger than age 5, although a beta–lactamase-stable drug such as amoxicillin–clavulanate (Augmentin) or a second-generation cephalosporin (e.g., cefuroxime, cefadroxil) should be given to patients incompletely immunized against *H. influenzae*. Often, a macrolide (azithromycin, clarithromycin, erythromycin) is considered the drug of choice for older children (greater than 5 years old) and adolescents because of its activity against *M. pneumoniae* and *C. pneumoniae*.

Treatment for More Serious Disease

For hospitalized children with more serious disease, antibiotics and maintenance of adequate oxygenation are the mainstays of treatment of bacterial pneumonia; chest physical therapy and intermittent positive-pressure treatments provide little additional benefit. Initial antibiotic therapy should be guided by the results of a sputum Gram stain and should be modified, if necessary, once the results of cultures of blood, sputum, or pleural fluid are reported. A variety of options, including ampicillin-sulbactam (Unasyn) and cefuroxime, are available for parenteral antibiotic management of suspected bacterial pneumonia in infants or young children. Intravenous or oral erythromycin should be added to this regimen for children older than age 5 until M. pneumoniae pneumonia is ruled out. A 3- to 4-week course of metronidazole or ampicillin combined with a beta–lactamase inhibitor (e.g., Augmentin, Unasyn) is appropriate therapy for lung abscess.

COMPLICATIONS

A parapneumonic effusion (the presence of fluid in the pleural space) may be caused by congestive heart failure, malignancy, collagen-vascular disease, and infection within the parenchyma of the lung. The composition of the parapneumonic effusion secondary to infection can vary from a thin, serous transudate with few white blood cells (WBCs), low protein content, and a pH of more than 7.2, to a thick, purulent exudate (or empyema) in which the WBC count is greater than 15,000 cells per cubic millimeter, the protein content is more than 3.0 g/dL, and the pH is less than 7.2. S. *pneumoniae, S. aureus,* and *H. influenzae* are the major causes of empyema. Parapneumonic effusions secondary to viral, mycoplasma, and chlamydia pneumonia are uncommon and are usually composed of a transudate of low volume when they occur. Parapneumonic effusions are found more commonly in young children and in male individuals. The presence of fluid in the pleural space results in continued fever, chest pain, and dyspnea and in tachycardia, dullness to percussion, and diminished breath sounds on examination. A chest radiograph with an affected patient in the lateral decubitus position will demonstrate layering of free pleural fluid. Approximately one-half of cases are unilateral. Loculation of fluid, which occurs in approximately 75% of cases of frank empyema, may inhibit dependent layering of the effusion on the lateral decubitus film. If necessary, computed tomography of the chest will demonstrate the presence of loculated pleural fluid.

Pneumatoceles are thin-walled cavities that develop in the lung in the course of bacterial pneumonia. Pneumatoceles complicate approximately 40% of cases of staphylococcal pneumonia and are unusual complications of pneumonia due to S. pneumoniae, *H. influenzae,* group A streptococci, and gram-negative enteric bacilli. Pneumatoceles are asymptomatic except when they rupture into pleural space causing a pneumothorax or pyopneumothorax. Most persist for 2 to 3 months and resolve spontaneously.

Management of parapneumonic effusions associated with bacterial pneumonia consists of antibiotic administration and drainage of the pleural fluid. Frequently, drainage can be accomplished by needle aspiration during the exudative stage, although more than one aspiration procedure may be required. Empyema requires the insertion of one or more thoracotomy tubes, which, sometimes, must be repositioned in order to drain loculated areas of purulent fluid. Generally, the tubes are withdrawn when drainage ceases, usually after a period of 2 to 5 days. Rarely, open thoracotomy and drainage procedures are required in the management of empyema in children. The clinical response to management of empyema is characteristically slow. Fever, chest pain, and irritability may persist for 1 to 2 weeks, although stabilization of vital signs and improvement of systemic oxygenation occur more rapidly. Clearing of abnormalities on chest radiography may take weeks to months. In most children, gradual improvement of pulmonary function occurs with little or no long-term restrictive lung abnormality. Surgical decortication of the organized peel is no longer performed in children, except in unusual circumstances. The overall mortality for empyema in children is 6% to 12%, but it may be higher in infants and in patients with staphylococcal empyema.

Lung abscesses arise at the site of a necrotizing pneumonia that follows aspiration of oropharyngeal secretions containing normal bacterial flora of the upper respiratory tract. Children with severe mental-motor retardation, seizure disorders, poor oral hygiene, and periodontal disease are particularly susceptible to the development of lung abscesses. Dependent segments of the lung (i.e., the posterior segment of the right upper lobe and the superior segments of the right and the left lower lobes) are the usual locations of abscess formation. Anaerobic bacteria play a prominent role in abscess formation. Usually, one or more species of oral anaerobes, with or without such other oral bacteria as streptococci, staphylococci, or gram-negative enteric bacilli, are recovered from abscess cavities. Fever, cough, tachypnea, and a fetid breath odor are the major presenting manifestations of lung abscess. Chest radiography reveals a focal infiltrate surrounding a cavity that may contain an air-fluid level. Approximately 10% of patients have more than one cavity. Fiberoptic bronchoscopy may be used to obtain a specimen directly from the abscess cavity for diagnostic purposes.

CHAPTER 137

Cystic Fibrosis

Adapted from Beryl J. Rosenstein

GENETICS

Cystic fibrosis (CF) is the most common lethal or semilethal genetic disease affecting populations of European origin. The disease's incidence for whites is 1 in 3,300 live births, American blacks (1 in 16,300), and Asian–Americans (1 in 32,100). Transmission is autosomal recessive. On the basis of incidence figures, 1 in 29 whites in the United States is estimated to be a carrier (heterozygote) of a CF mutation.

The gene responsible for CF has been localized to the long arm of chromosome 7. It encodes a protein called the cystic fibrosis transmembrane conductance regulator (CFTR). The ΔF508 mutation is present on approximately 70% of CF chromosomes. The remaining cases are explained by more than 700 mutations, none of which accounts for more than 2% of the cases. The ability to detect CF mutations by direct DNA analysis represents a major improvement in prenatal diagnosis, newborn screening, and heterozygote detection.

The CFTR protein appears to be related to a family of membrane-bound glycoproteins involved in the transport of small molecules across cell membranes. Functional expression of the CF defect reduces the ability of epithelial cells in the airways and pancreas to transport chloride in response to cAMP-mediated agonists. Abnormal transport of sodium and chloride across the airway epithelium is thought to lead to increased viscosity of airway mucus and the abnormal mucociliary clearance and lung disease seen in patients with CF.

CLINICAL CHARACTERISTICS

Table 137-1 is a summary of clinical features consistent with a diagnosis of CF.

Pulmonary System

The respiratory tract is almost always involved in CF, and pulmonary complications usually dominate the clinical picture. However, manifestations may not appear until weeks, months, or even years after birth. Autopsy studies suggest that the lungs are normal at birth. Fig. 137-1 shows a proposed mechanism for the pathophysiology of lung disease in CF.

Infection

Secondary bacterial infection, due initially to *Staphylococcus aureus* and then to *Pseudomonas aeruginosa,* initiates a cycle of obstruction, chronic infection, inflammation, tissue damage,

TABLE 137-1. Clinical Features Consistent with a Diagnosis of Cystic Fibrosis

Chronic sinopulmonary disease manifestations
Persistent colonization or infection with typical cystic fibrosis pathogens, including *Staphylococcus aureus,* nontypeable *Haemophilus influenzae,* mucoid and nonmucoid *Pseudomonas aeruginosa,* and *Burkholderia cepacia*
Chronic cough and sputum production
Persistent chest radiograph abnormalities (e.g., bronchiectasis, atelectasis, infiltrates, hyperinflation)
Airway obstruction (wheezing and air trapping)
Nasal polyps; radiographic or computed tomographic abnormalities of the paranasal sinuses
Digital clubbing
Gastrointestinal and nutritional abnormalities
Intestinal: meconium ileus; distal intestinal obstruction syndrome; rectal prolapse
Pancreatic: pancreatic insufficiency; recurrent pancreatitis
Hepatic: chronic hepatic disease manifested by clinical or histologic evidence of focal biliary cirrhosis or multilobular cirrhosis
Nutritional: failure to thrive (protein-calorie malnutrition), hypoproteinemia and edema, complications secondary to fat-soluble vitamin deficiency
Salt loss syndromes (acute salt depletion; chronic metabolic alkalosis)
Male urogenital abnormalities resulting in obstructive azoospermia

and ventilatory failure. Once established in the airways, Pseudomonas is virtually impossible to eradicate. Systemic defense mechanisms appear to be intact, and infection tends to be localized to the respiratory tract. Septicemia and extrapulmonary infections are rare. During the 1990s, the incidence of Burkholderia cepacia colonization among adolescent and adult CF patients has increased. Risk factors for colonization include increasing age and severity of underlying disease and recent hospitalization.

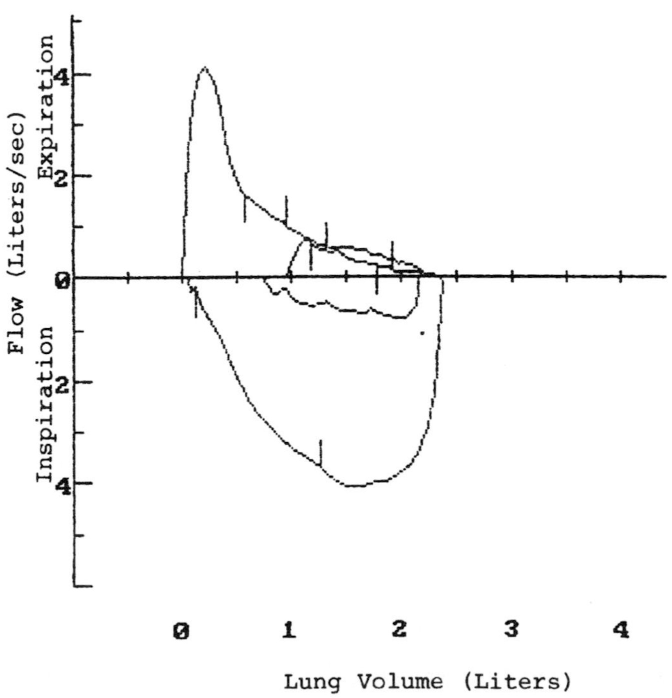

Figure 137-1. Flow-volume loop from a 23-year-old patient showing decreased flow at all lung volumes. The scooped-out appearance is indicative of small-airways disease.

Person-to-person transmission has been documented. Acquisition of this organism, especially by patients with moderate or advanced pulmonary disease, may be followed by an unexpectedly rapid decline. In some patients, the course is characterized by recurrent episodes of fever and bacteremia. If patients do not respond as expected to antimicrobial therapy, infection with unusual organisms (e.g., Mycobacterium tuberculosis, nontuberculous mycobacteria, aspergillus) should be considered.

Signs and Symptoms

One-half of patients present with pulmonary manifestations usually consisting of chronic cough and wheezing along with recurrent or chronic infections. Young infants can present with atelectasis, often involving the right upper lobe, or a severe bronchiolitic syndrome. The most prominent and constant feature of pulmonary involvement is chronic cough. Although at first, the cough may be dry, with progression, it becomes paroxysmal and productive. Older patients expectorate mucopurulent sputum, particularly in association with pulmonary exacerbations. Often, wheezing is a prominent feature, especially in association with pulmonary exacerbations, but whether it reflects inflammation and bronchial obstruction or coincidental atopy remains unclear. Up to 5% of patients develop allergic bronchopulmonary aspergillosis. Physical findings of CF include a barrel-chest deformity, use of accessory muscles of respiration, growth retardation, digital clubbing, pulmonary hypertrophic osteoarthropathy, and cyanosis. Pulmonary function tests reveal hypoxemia, as well as a reduction in forced vital capacity (FVC), forced expiratory volume over 1 second (FEV_1), and in the ratio of FEV_1 to FVC. There is an increase in residual volume and in the ratio of residual volume to total lung capacity. Airway reactivity, based on bronchoprovocative challenges, is present in 50% of patients and may be associated with accelerated progression of pulmonary disease. The response to bronchodilators is unpredictable and varies over time and with changes in underlying pulmonary status.

Clinically significant sinusitis is common and particularly troublesome in some patients. Chronic sinusitis may contribute to infection of the lower respiratory tract. Nasal polyps occur in 6% to 24% of patients. Manifestations include obstruction to nasal airflow, mouth breathing, localized infection, epistaxis, rhinorrhea, and widening of the nasal bridge. Polyps occur at a much younger age in patients with CF as compared with those with underlying atopy. There are also histologically different and tend to recur.

Radiographic Changes

Chest radiographic findings are not pathognomonic but can help to suggest a diagnosis of CF. Hyperinflation and bronchial wall thickening are the earliest findings. Subsequent changes include areas of infiltrate, atelectasis, and hilar adenopathy. With advanced disease, segmental or lobar atelectasis, cyst formation, bronchiectasis, and pulmonary artery and right ventricular enlargement are seen. Characteristic branching, finger-like opacifications representing mucoid impaction of dilated bronchi strongly suggest CF. In patients with mild disease and normal chest radiographic findings, bronchiectasis may be evident on high-resolution computed tomography (CT).

Course

The pulmonary course is characterized by chronic suppurative endobronchial infection with recurrent pulmonary exacerbations, often after viral respiratory infections. Infection with respiratory syncytial virus may be an important cause of significant respiratory morbidity in young infants. By age 10 years, 90% of patients have intermittent sputum production; by age 15 years, 90% have daily sputum production. Progressive shortness of breath and exercise intolerance occur. Other cardiopulmonary complications include pneumothorax, hemoptysis, and cor pulmonale. Pulmonary involvement advances at a variable rate, usually faster in female than in male patients, but eventually leads to respiratory failure, cardiac failure, or both.

GASTROINTESTINAL SYSTEM

Pancreatic Exocrine Deficiency

The most common gastrointestinal manifestations result from loss of pancreatic enzyme activity and consequent intestinal malabsorption of fats, proteins and, to a lesser extent, carbohydrates. Complete loss of enzyme activity is seen in 85% to 90% of patients. Loss of function may be progressive. Clinical manifestations include poor weight gain, abdominal distention, deficiency of subcutaneous fat and muscle tissue, rectal prolapse, and frequent passage of pale, bulky, malodorous, and often oily stools. Steatorrhea and azotorrhea may be pronounced. Secondary to pancreatic insufficiency, patients have low serum lipid levels and may be deficient in fat-soluble vitamins and linoleic acid. Although some patients have a voracious appetite, often caloric intake is deficient. In adolescent patients, absence of a pubertal growth spurt and delayed maturation may occur. In general, growth retardation correlates closely with the degree of pulmonary involvement. Patients with residual pancreatic function may have recurrent episodes of pancreatitis, sometimes as the presenting manifestation. Patients with pancreatic sufficiency tend to have lower sweat chloride values, less severe pulmonary involvement, better nutritional status, and better survival.

Carbohydrate Intolerance

In addition to experiencing pancreatic exocrine dysfunction, up to 40% of patients show carbohydrate intolerance that progresses to frank diabetes in 5% to 10% of cases. Average age of onset is between 18 and 21 years, but it can occur at any age. Diabetes in patients with CF is characterized by insidious onset, mild clinical course, and virtual absence of ketoacidosis. However, retinopathy, nephropathy, and neuropathy may occur. The mild diabetic course in CF patients may be due to preservation of some endogenous insulin output, decreased glucagon secretion, and compensatory enhancement of peripheral tissue sensitivity to insulin.

TABLE 137-2. Other Intestinal Complications

Distal intestinal obstruction syndrome (recurrent episodes of partial or complete obstruction of the small or large bowel)
Small bowel volvulus
Intussusception
Recurrent rectal prolapse
Gastroesophageal reflux disease
Peptic ulcer disease
Associated Disorders
Crohn's disease
Giardiasis
Celiac disease

TABLE 137-3. Additional Organ Systems Affected in CF

Hepatobiliary system
Liver
Focal and multilobular biliary cirrhosis
Portal hypertension
Fatty infiltration of the liver
Liver failure (rare)
Gallbladder
Cholelithiasis
Cholecystitis
Reproductive system
Males
Azoospermia and infertility
Increased incidence of hernia, hydrocele, and undescended testes
Delayed puberty
Females
Decreased fertility
Increased incidence of premature labor and low birth weight
Delayed puberty
Skeletal system
Pulmonary hypertrophic osteoarthropathy
Arthralgias, long bone pain, joint swelling, periostitis
Rheumatoid arthritis
Seronegative polyarthritis
Back pain and spinal deformity
Ocular system
Visual field defects
Acute hemorrhagic retinopathy (high altitude)
Optic atrophy and neuritis (chloremphenicol related)

Meconium Ileus

Meconium ileus (MI), which demonstrates obstruction of the distal ileum by inspissated, tenacious meconium, occurs in 18% of newborns with CF. With rare exception, MI is always associated with CF. Probably, it is related to *in utero* deficiency of proteolytic enzymes, along with secretion of abnormal mucoproteins by the goblet cells of the small intestine. Infants present with evidence of intestinal obstruction. Abdominal radiography shows distended bowel loops and a "bubbly" pattern of inspissated meconium in the terminal ileum. Contrast enema shows a microcolon from disuse secondary to intrauterine obstruction. Associated intestinal complications including small-bowel atresia, volvulus, and perforation peritonitis are present in 40% to 50% of cases. MI tends to recur in patients' families. A delay in the passage of meconium and distal colonic obstruction secondary to the meconium plug syndrome may also be a presenting manifestation of CF. Table 137-2 lists other intestinal complications associated with CF. The pulmonary and gastrointestinal systems are commonly associated with CF, however, many other organ systems may be affected (Table 137-3).

NUTRITION AND METABOLISM

Vitamin and Mineral Deficiencies

Secondary to pancreatic achylia, malabsorption of fat-soluble vitamins occurs. Low serum vitamin A levels are due to steatorrhea and a reduction of retinol-carrier protein and retinol-binding protein. Xerophthalmia and night blindness rarely occur, usually in association with hepatic involvement. A bulging fontanelle secondary to vitamin A deficiency may be the presenting manifestation in infants. Overt rickets is rare, but a significant reduction in vitamin D biological activity with associated secondary hyperparathyroidism, reduced bone mineral content, and delayed bone maturation is common. Significant demineralization is present in one-half of all patients. Severe bleeding in association with hypoprothrombinemia and deficiency of clotting factors II, VII, IX, and X secondary to vitamin K deficiency may occur in infants. All patients with pancreatic achylia show a marked reduction in plasma alpha–tocopherol levels. Red blood cells show a moderate decrease in survival and, on occasion, may result in hemolytic anemia. A progressive spinocerebellar syndrome consisting of ataxia, areflexia, and proprioceptive loss has been seen in patients with prolonged vitamin E deficiency. No clinical problems are associated with deficiency of water-soluble vitamins.

Symptomatic hypomagnesemia, as well as decreased plasma levels of zinc and selenium have been reported. Iron-deficiency anemia is seen in one-third of patients. Probably, it is related to inadequate iron intake, impairment of iron absorption, and effects of chronic infection.

Edema and Hypoproteinemia

The syndrome of edema and hypoproteinemia, secondary to pancreatic enzyme deficiency, may be the presenting manifestation in as many as 8% of patients with CF. Most often, it is seen in infants who are between ages 1 to 6 months and are breast-fed or receiving soy-based formula. Associated findings include hepatomegaly, elevation of liver enzymes, skin rash (acrodermatitis enteropathica), and anemia. False-negative sweat test results can be seen in the presence of edema.

Salt Loss

The sweat gland abnormality has important clinical implications. Patients may have a "salty taste" or salt crystal formation on the skin, findings that are highly suggestive of CF. Patients may also develop dehydration with massive salt depletion, especially in association with gastrointestinal losses or thermal stress. Profound hypoelectrolytemia, not accounted for by gastrointestinal losses, particularly suggests CF. In arid climates, chronic salt loss can lead to metabolic alkalosis and electrolyte depletion without appreciable dehydration and is a common presenting manifestation of CF.

DIAGNOSIS

Clinical Presentation

Overall, 18% to 20% of patients present with neonatal intestinal obstruction secondary to MI or meconium plug syndrome. In the remaining percentage of patients, the diagnosis is suggested because of pulmonary manifestations or steatorrhea, often associated with failure to thrive, a positive family history, or a variety of miscellaneous manifestations related to salt depletion or deficiencies of vitamins, protein, minerals, or calories. In some patients, a single clinical feature (e.g., electrolyte abnormalities, pancreatitis, liver disease, or sinusitis or nasal polyps) predominates. The types and severity of CF manifestations somewhat reflect genotypic heterogeneity. The spectrum of clinical features is so varied and symptoms may be so minimal that one cannot exclude the possibility of CF even with a normal growth pattern, absence of pulmonary disease, or normal pancreatic exocrine function.

Sweat Testing

The diagnosis of CF is almost always confirmed by documenting an elevated sweat electrolyte concentration. Indications for a sweat test are outlined in Table 137-4. The standard sweat test method is the quantitative pilocarpine iontophoresis sweat test (Gibson–Cooke) in which localized sweating is stimulated by the iontophoresis of pilocarpine into the skin, a sufficient volume of sweat (greater than 75 mg) is collected, and the electrolyte concentration is measured. A chloride concentration greater than 60 mmol/L is consistent with the diagnosis of CF. In infants younger than 3 months, a sweat chloride concentration greater than 40 mmol/L is highly suggestive of CF. The diagnosis of CF should not be based solely on an elevated sweat electrolyte concentration but should be made only when it is associated with pancreatic exocrine deficiency, chronic pulmonary disease, MI, or a positive family history. The sweat electrolyte abnormality is present from birth and persists throughout life. However, obtaining a volume of sweat sufficient for analysis may be difficult in the neonatal period.

TABLE 137-4. Indications for Sweat Testing

Pulmonary and upper respiratory tract
Chronic cough
Recurrent or chronic pneumonia
Wheezing*
Hyperinflation*
Tachypnea*
Retractions*
Atelectasis (especially of the right upper lobe)
Bronchiectasis
Hemoptysis
Pseudomonas colonization, especially with a mucoid strain
Nasal polyps
Pansinusitis
Digital clubbing
Gastrointestinal
Meconium ileus
Meconium plug syndrome
Prolonged neonatal jaundice
Steatorrhea
Rectal prolapse
Mucoid impacted appendix
Late intestinal obstruction
Intussusception, recurrent or at an atypical age
Cirrhosis and portal hypertension
Portal hypertension
Recurrent pancreatitis
Metabolic and miscellaneous
Acrodermatitis enteropathica
Family history of cystic fibrosis
Failure to thrive
Salty taste on skin
Salt crystals on skin
Salt-depletion syndrome
Metabolic alkalosis
Vitamin K deficiency (hypoprothrombinemia and bleeding)
Vitamin A deficiency (bulging fontanelle, night blindness)
Vitamin E deficiency (hemolytic anemia)
Obstructive azoospermia
Absent vas deferens
Scrotal calcification
Hypoproteinemia and edema

*If persistent or refractory to usual therapy.

Elevated concentrations of sweat electrolytes have been reported in other conditions including adrenal insufficiency, ectodermal dysplasia, nephrogenic diabetes insipidus, type I glycogen storage disease, anorexia nervosa, hypoparathyroidism, Mauriac syndrome, familial cholestatic syndromes, malnutrition, hypothyroidism, mucopolysaccharidoses, and fucosidosis. Most of these disorders can be differentiated by characteristic clinical features. Transient elevation of sweat electrolyte concentrations has been observed in children with evidence of abuse and neglect. In patients for whom a diagnosis is "confirmed" but whose disease does not follow a typical course, repeating the sweat test is crucial. Normal sweat electrolyte concentrations have been reported in some patients with CF in the presence of edema and hypoproteinemia. Values become abnormal with resolution of the edema. Most false-positive and false-negative results are due to technical errors including inadequate sweat collection, sample contamination, and failure to interpret test results correctly. Physiologic variables such as sweating rate, salt intake, and acclimatization may affect the concentration of sweat electrolytes, but they do not usually interfere with the diagnostic value of the test. Although sweat electrolyte concentrations increase slightly with increasing age, they remain excellent discriminants for CF in adults. The sweat test is not useful in diagnosing CF heterozygotes.

Mutation Analysis

Because of its ability to detect CF mutations, DNA testing may substitute for the sweat test in certain situations. The presence of a mutation on each CFTR gene that is known to cause CF predicts with a high degree of certainty that an individual has CF. To date, more than 700 CF mutations have been identified, but only a limited number of these are included in currently available CF mutation panels.

Nasal Potential Difference Measurement

The active transport of ions across epithelial surfaces generates an electrical potential difference (PD) that can be measured *in vivo*. Abnormalities in ion transport in the respiratory epithelia of CF patients are associated with a different pattern of nasal PD as compared to normal epithelia and provide a basis for the use of nasal PD as a diagnostic aid.

Newborn Screening

Newborn screening for CF has been possible since 1979 using blood spot analysis of immunoreactive trypsinogen (IRT). IRT is elevated both in pancreatic-insufficient and pancreatic-sufficient newborns with CF. Currently being used are IRT/DNA protocols in which an IRT assay is performed on all samples followed by direct gene analysis for F508 or a pool of common mutations on those samples with an IRT value above a predetermined cut-off level (typically, the ninety-ninth percentile). Universal screening has not been recommended in the United States and, at present, is carried out in only two states. However, accumulating evidence of the benefits of newborn screening indicates that widespread implementation may be recommended soon.

MANAGEMENT

Pulmonary

ANTIBIOTIC THERAPY

Aggressive antimicrobial therapy is a key component in the management of patients with CF, but great variation in treatment strategies exists. Options include short-term treatment of acute exacerbations with oral, aerosol, or intravenous antibiotics; chronic suppressive therapy with oral or aerosol antibiotics; and long-term intermittent treatment with quarterly courses of intravenous antibiotics. Ideally, antibiotic choice should be based on the results of respiratory tract (oropharyngeal, sputum, bronchoalveolar lavage fluid) culture and sensitivity testing. Patients with mild to moderate acute pulmonary exacerbations are usually treated with a 2- to 4-week course of oral or aerosol antibiotics or both. Coverage against *Haemophilus influenzae* and *Staphylococcus aureus* can be achieved with a beta–lactamase-stable penicillin or cephalosporin, trimethoprim–sulfamethoxazole, clarithromycin, or chloramphenicol. For patients colonized with *P. aeruginosa*, an oral fluoroquinolone or aerosol aminoglycoside (tobramycin) used alone or in combination may be effective. Patients who do not respond to oral or aerosol therapy and those with more severe exacerbations are candidates for a 10- to 21-day course of intravenous antibiotics, usually consisting of an antipseudomonal beta-lactam (ticarcillin, piperacillin, ceftazidime) in combination with an aminoglycoside (tobramycin, gentamicin) chosen on the basis of susceptibility test results. For patients who are allergic to beta–lactams, the carbapenem imipenem and the monobactam aztreonam may be useful alternatives. Patients with CF may require high doses (approximately 10 mg/kg/day) of aminoglycosides to achieve acceptable serum concentrations. Patients who have an acute pulmonary exacerbation and are otherwise clinically stable and who meet well-defined selection criteria may be candidates for home intravenous antibiotic therapy.

Chronic suppressive antibiotic therapy has been used in patients of all ages to improve quality of life, to slow decline in pulmonary function, and to increase the interval between pulmonary exacerbations. The oral agents used most commonly are trimethoprim–sulfamethoxazole, amoxicillin–clavulanate, and beta–lactamase-stable cephalosporins. In patients colonized with *P. aeruginosa*, chronic alternate-month aerosol administration of high-dose tobramycin (300 mg twice daily) has been shown to decrease sputum density of *P. aeruginosa*, decline in pulmonary function, and frequency of acute pulmonary exacerbations. Because of the rapid emergence of antibiotic-resistant isolates, the fluoroquinolones should not be used for chronic suppressive therapy.

AIRWAY CLEARANCE TECHNIQUES

Airway clearance techniques enhance the removal of bronchial secretions and are usually recommended at the time of diagnosis or at the first indication of lower respiratory tract involvement. In infants, toddlers, and young children, chest physiotherapy consisting of postural drainage, manual or mechanical percussion, vibration, and assisted coughing is carried out several times each day. A regular exercise program should be encouraged to complement, but not replace, airway clearance techniques. Exercise has no demonstrable short-term effect on lung function, but it can improve cardiorespiratory conditioning, muscle strength, exercise tolerance, sense of well-being, and self-image. Supplemental oxygen therapy may allow patients with severe disease to exercise safely and with benefit.

MUCOLYTIC AGENTS

Recombinant human DNase [dornase alfa (Pulmozyme)] enzymatically degrades DNA, which is present in high concentration in purulent airway secretions, and decreases sputum viscoelasticity. In patients older than age 5, continuous daily nebulization of Pulmozyme at a dose of 2.5 mg/day has been shown to delay decline in pulmonary function and to reduce the frequency of pulmonary exacerbations. It can be used in conjunction with all other usual CF therapies. Preliminary data suggest that daily ultrasonic nebulization of hypertonic (6%) saline after pretreatment with nebulized salbutamol leads to improvement in pulmonary function in patients with moderate to severe pulmonary disease, possibly related to enhanced mucociliary clearance. No data document the efficacy of oral expectorants or aerosolized N-acetylcysteine. Cough suppressants are contraindicated.

BRONCHODILATOR THERAPY

A number of studies have demonstrated that bronchodilators in the form of oral or intravenous xanthines (aminophylline, theophylline), aerosolized $beta_2$–adrenergic agents (albuterol, metaproterenol, terbutaline), and parasympatholytic agents (ipratropium) can improve pulmonary function and lessen wheezing in many (though not all) patients with CF. Responses tend to vary over time and with degree of illness, but the majority of patients will be bronchodilator-responsive at least some of the time. In clinical practice, the majority of patients with CF use a $beta_2$–adrenergic agonist before performing airway clearance techniques. Nebulization and metered-dose inhalation (MDI) are probably equally effective, but ease of administration using a spacer device favors MDI. In patients with moderate to severe pulmonary disease, a prudent approach is to carry out pre- and postbronchodilator pulmonary function testing to identify patients with paradoxical bronchoconstriction.

ANTIINFLAMMATORY AGENTS

Antiinflammatory agents are playing an increasingly important role in the treatment of patients with CF. Long-term daily use of ibuprofen at a dose sufficient to achieve a peak plasma concentration between 50 and 100 μg/mL has been shown to significantly slow the rate of decline in pulmonary function and to decrease the need for intravenous antibiotics in young patients (aged 5 to 13 years) with mild pulmonary involvement. In several long-term controlled trials, alternate-day glucocorticoid therapy at a dose of 1 to 2 mg/day has been shown to slow the expected rate of decline in pulmonary function and to decrease serum IgG levels. However, treatment for longer than 24 months has been associated with linear growth retardation, glucose abnormalities, and cataract formation. Systemic glucocorticoids are indicated for infants with a severe bronchiolitic syndrome, patients with severe airway obstruction unresponsive to conventional bronchodilators, patients with allergic bronchopulmonary aspergillosis, and those with evidence of hypersensitivity characterized by recurrent episodes of fever, rash, and joint pain. Some preliminary results suggest that inhaled glucocorticoids may also improve pulmonary function.

Lung Transplantation

Heart–lung and bilateral lung transplantations have been performed successfully in carefully selected patients with chronic cardiorespiratory failure. Results are similar to those seen in nonCF patients with 75% survival at 1 year, 60% at 2 years, and 55% at 3 years after transplantation. Overall, survival is comparable for children and adults.

Immunoprophylaxis

Recommended vaccination schedules should be followed, especially for pertussis, varicella, H. influenzae type b, and measles. Patients should be immunized against influenza starting at age 6 months and followed by a yearly booster. Household contacts should also be immunized. In patients who are exposed to influenza A and have not received vaccine, amantadine prophylaxis can be used until the risk of infection passes. An increase in susceptibility to or morbidity from pneumococcal infection has not been documented, and routine use of pneumococcal vaccine is not recommended. *Pseudomonas* vaccines have been used investigationally but are not available for clinical use.

Gastrointestinal Therapy

TREATMENT OF PANCREATIC EXOCRINE DEFICIENCY

Pancreatic enzyme supplements constitute the primary therapy of the pancreatic enzyme deficiency. The most effective preparations consist of capsules containing pancrelipase in pH-sensitive enteric-coated microspheres or microtablets. Powdered preparations are available for use in young infants. Enzyme supplements are given with all meals and snacks; the dosage is determined by the frequency and character of the patient's stools and the patient's growth pattern. Usually, infants are started at a dose of 2,000 to 4,000 lipase units per 120 mL of formula or per breast-feeding. Beyond infancy, weight-based dosing is used starting at 1,000 lipase U/kg per meal for children younger than age 4 and at 500 lipase U/kg per meal for those older than age 4. Usually, one-half the standard dose is given with snacks. Doses of more than 2,500 lipase U/kg per meal or 10,000 lipase U/kg/day should be avoided, because high enzyme dosages have been associated with the development of fibrosing colonopathy. Manifestations of this disorder include intestinal obstruction, bloody diarrhea, or chylous ascites or the combination of abdominal pain, ongoing diarrhea, and poor weight gain. Strictures can be suggested by contrast enema, and the diagnosis can be confirmed by biopsy. Often, development of constipation while a patient is taking enzymes is an indication for more rather than less enzyme.

Nutritional Therapy

The goal of nutrition therapy is to promote normal growth. Contrary to earlier anecdotal reports of a voracious appetite in patients with CF, most patients have a grossly deficient caloric intake. Because of incomplete correction of steatorrhea and increased metabolic demands, the recommendation is that patients receive 30% to 50% more calories than usual daily allowances, which can usually be achieved by a well-balanced, high-protein diet with liberal fat. Fat restriction is no longer recommended. Infants can be breast-fed if they are receiving enzyme supplements, but weight gain must be monitored closely.

Older patients should be provided with an unrestricted fat, high-protein, high-calorie diet consistent with food preferences and lifestyle. Supplements with medium-chain triglycerides and glucose polymers can boost caloric intake. For patients who have poor growth and inadequate caloric intake despite nutritional counseling and oral supplementation, enteral supplementation may be useful. This is accomplished by nightly infusion of high-calorie elemental formulas via a nasogastric, gastrostomy, or jejunostomy tube. This type of supplementation, when carried out over an extended period, may stabilize or even improve pulmonary function. Parenteral hyperalimentation can be used for short-term support in patients with specific problems, but it is costly and associated with complications of prolonged central-line infusions.

VITAMIN AND MINERAL SUPPLEMENTATION

Vitamin deficiencies can be prevented by daily administration of a water-miscible vitamin preparation. Patients with steatorrhea should receive a daily supplement of a water-miscible alpha–tocopherol preparation at a dose of 5 to 10 U/kg up to a maximum daily dose of 400 units. Routine supplementation with vitamin K is not recommended but may be indicated in patients with extensive liver involvement, at times of surgery, and in patients with demonstrated coagulation problems. Iron deficiency is common. Iron status should be evaluated periodically, and appropriate supplementation should be provided to patients with anemia or low serum ferritin levels. Supplementation with other trace metals should not be needed. Additional dietary salt should be provided at times of thermal stress including increased activity in hot weather. Usually, supplementation with salt tablets is not indicated.

Treatment of Distal Intestinal Obstruction Syndrome

In DIOS cases in which no evidence of complete obstruction exists, oral administration of a cleansing electrolyte solution (GoLYTELY) is the treatment of choice. On evidence of significant obstruction, enemas with isoosmolar contrast material may be both diagnostic and therapeutic. Most episodes can be managed without surgical intervention. For patients with recurrent episodes, helpful measures include optimization of pancreatic enzyme dosing, increased fluid intake, and administration of a prokinetic agent (cisapride), wetting agents, high-fiber diet, lactulose, and mineral oil. In patients with intussusception, hydrostatic reduction should be attempted, although surgery may be necessary. Surgery is indicated for episodes of volvulus.

Course and Prognosis

The course of disease varies from patient to patient, probably in relation to genetic heterogeneity, intensity of treatment, and environmental factors. Prognosis is determined largely by degree of pulmonary involvement. Some patients retain near-normal lung function over 5 to 7 years but, in general, experience an exponential decline in pulmonary function of approximately 2% per year. The FEV_1 adjusted for age and gender is the best predictor of prognosis. Early colonization with mucoid *Pseudomonas* may be associated with a more rapid decline in pulmonary function. Exposure to cigarette smoke is associated with a more rapid decline in clinical status and should be avoided. Patients who are pancreatic-sufficient have milder pulmonary disease and better survival. Other factors associated with improved longevity are male gender, absence of colonization with mucoid *Pseudomonas*, presentation with predominantly gastrointestinal symptoms, balanced family functioning and coping, and compliance with treatment regimens. Clinical scoring systems are available for longitudinal assessment of patients for prognosis counseling and for classifying patients in clinical studies.

A steady improvement in prognosis has occurred over the last four decades. Approximately one-third of all patients under care at specialized CF centers are older than 18, and survival into the fourth and fifth decades is no longer rare. For reasons that are not clear, survival of male patients is better than that of female patients, but the gap has narrowed.

CHAPTER 138
Cervical Lymphadenitis

Adapted from Carol J. Baker

Cervical adenitis is inflammation of one or more lymph nodes of the neck. In children, the most common causes of cervical lymph node enlargement exceeding 10 mm are reactive hyperplasia in response to an infectious stimulus in the head or neck and infection of the node itself. Self-limited cervical lymph node inflammation occurs in association with upper respiratory tract infection as the lymphatic channels drain proximally affected sites. In 80% of children with acute cervical adenitis, the submaxillary, submandibular, and deep cervical nodes are inflamed, because these are the routes by which much of the lymphatic drainage of the head and neck proceeds. Malignancy is the second most common cause of lymph node enlargement in children, but neoplasia and infiltrative disorders constitute a minority of neck masses. Children with malignant lesions tend to have systemic complaints and firm, nontender nodes located characteristically in the posterior triangle or supraclavicular regions.

Although patients at any age may be affected, the majority of children with cervical adenitis are 1 to 4 years old. This age restriction and the peak in incidence reflect the prevalence of infections caused by viral agents, *Staphylococcus aureus*, group A streptococci, and atypical mycobacteria. The genders are affected equally with two exceptions: Some studies indicate a female patient predominance for granulomatous lymphadenitis caused by atypical mycobacteria, and young infants with the cellulitis–adenitis syndrome caused by group B streptococci are predominantly male patients. No ethnic predilection avails for acute bacterial cervical adenitis (Table 138-1). In contrast, adenitis caused by atypical mycobacteria occurs commonly in whites, whereas that caused by *M. tuberculosis* tends to have a greater incidence in blacks and Hispanics. For children living in temperate climates, an increase in incidence occurs during the winter and spring months. A history of dog or cat contact, bite, or scratch may be a helpful clue in suggesting specific causative agents such as *Pasteurella multocida, Bartonella henselae,* or *Toxoplasma gondii*. Similarly, a history of a minor inoculation wound of the skin proximal to affected cervical lymph nodes should suggest the possibility of soil organisms such as *Nocardia brasiliensis*, atypical mycobacteria, or gram-negative enteric organisms. Finally, HIV should be added to the list of agents causing cervical adenopathy and, because most HIV-infected children are infected perinatally, the epidemiology reflects that of the mothers.

PATHOGENESIS

Some authors have stated that in considering the pathogenesis of cervical adenitis in children, physicians should consider the three Ts: tonsils, teeth, and areas of skin trauma. A microorganism must first asymptomatically infect the upper respiratory tract, anterior nares, mouth, or skin of the head or neck before spreading to the cervical lymph nodes. Overt infection of the skin, teeth, or oropharynx may occur in association with cervical adenitis, but clinically evident infection proximal to the affected nodes is not a requisite.

The increased size of lymph nodes (greater than 1.0 cm) in response to infection is the result of an increase in the number of cells. While the lymph node is filtering pyogenic microorganisms, chemoattraction of neutrophils to the lymph node may result in the formation of microabscesses and small areas of necrosis or in frank suppuration. Rapid, extensive reactions are almost always caused by pyogenic organisms, notably *S. aureus* or group A streptococci. Granuloma formation with a delayed cellular immune response that may lead over a period of weeks or months to the formation of a "cold" abscess is characteristic when the infection is caused by mycobacteria, fungi, or *B. henselae*. Once infection has resolved, destruction of nodal tissue sometimes leads to healing with fibrous tissue proliferation, most often in the submandibular group, and this may persist indefinitely.

TABLE 138-1. Differentiation of Bacterial and Mycobacterial Cervical Adenitis

Clinical characteristics	Bacteria	Atypical mycobacteria	*Mycobacterium tuberculosis*
Onset	Acute (<1 wk)	Subacute to chronic	Subacute to chronic
Age (yr)	1–4*	1–4	All
Ethnic origin	All	White	Black or Hispanic
Regional node distribution	Unilateral	Unilateral	Unilateral or bilateral
Focal tenderness	Mild to marked	Often absent	Usually absent
Exposure to adult with tuberculosis	Absent	Absent	Present
Abnormal chest radiograph appearance	Never	Never	Sometimes
Mantoux test (PPD-S) result >15 mm induration	Never	Up to 40%	Often

PPD, purified protein derivative.
*Constitutes 70% to 80% of cases.
Adapted from Butler KM, Baker CJ. Cervical lymphadenitis. In: Feigin RD, Cherry JD, eds. *Textbook of pediatric infectious diseases,* 4th ed. Philadelphia: Saunders, 1997:170.

CLINICAL CHARACTERISTICS

Causative Agents

Cervical adenitis may be classified according to its mode of presentation as *acute,* in which symptoms are of less than 2 weeks' duration, or as *subacute to chronic* (Table 138-2). The causative agents tend to fall into one of these two categories, although they may overlap. Overall, approximately three-fourths of all the infections have an acute presentation. The duration of lymph node swelling is less than 3 days in one-half of all children with acute adenitis and less than 1 week in the majority. Generally, acute bilateral cervical adenitis is associated with upper respiratory tract viral infection including EBV and CMV or with acute streptococcal pharyngitis. Lymph nodes may be tender, but no other signs of inflammation are found. The appearance of an enanthem such as gingivostomatitis or an exanthem such as scarlatina should suggest either a viral or a streptococcal cause.

Systemic Manifestations

Generally, children with acute unilateral cervical lymphadenitis have a paucity of systemic manifestations. A history of upper respiratory tract symptoms such as sore throat, earache, coryza, or impetigo can be elicited from one-fourth to one-third of patients. Usually, the diameter of an infected node (or nodes) ranges from 2.5 to 6.0 cm; the nodes are tender and exhibit varying degrees of warmth and erythema. *S. aureus* and group A streptococci are the causative agents in approximately 50% to 90% of infections. Less commonly, other bacteria residing in the oropharynx are implicated (Table 138-2). Streptococcal adenitis occurs in younger children, is accompanied more often by generalized adenopathy, has a shorter duration of symptoms (less than 5 days), and is less likely to suppurate than nodes infected by *S. aureus*. Overall, one-fourth to one-third of involved nodes suppurate, and 90% of those become fluctuant within 2 weeks of onset. Concomitant lymphadenopathy at other sites is observed in as many as one-third of children with acute unilateral cervical adenitis, most commonly in association with a generalized viral process (e.g., EBV) or a group A streptococcal infection in very young children. Hepatomegaly or splenomegaly is rare, however; if found, either should suggest a generalized process (e.g., EBV, CMV, HIV, tuberculosis, reticuloendotheliosis, lymphoma).

In infancy, *S. aureus* is the agent most commonly grown from unilaterally infected cervical lymph nodes. The presentation is similar to that in older infants and children, except that irritability and other systemic symptoms may be observed more frequently. Infants at ages 1 to 2 months with facial or submandibular

TABLE 138-2. Infectious Agents or Diseases Associated with Cervical Adenitis

Agent or disease	Frequency	Onset	Generalized adenopathy
Bacterial			
Staphylococcus aureus	+++	A	–
Group A streptococcus	+++	A	+
Anaerobes	+++	A/S	–
Bartonella henselae	+++	S	–
Atypical mycobacteria	+++	S	–
Mycobacterium tuberculosis	++	S	±
Nocardia brasiliensis	++	S	–
Gram-negative enteric organisms	++	A	–
Group B streptococcus*	++	A	–
Pasteurella multocida	++	A	+
Haemophilus influenzae	+	A	–
Yersinia pestis	+	A	+
Actinomyces israelii	+	A	–
Diphtheria	+	A	–
Tularemia	+	A	–
Brucella	+	S	+
Syphilis	+	S	+
Anthrax	+	A	–
Viral			
Epstein-Barr virus	+++	A/S	+
Herpes simplex virus	+++	A	–
Cytomegalovirus	+++	A/S	+
Adenovirus	+++	A	–
Varicella	++	A	+
Enterovirus	+++	A	+
Human herpesvirus type 6	+	S	+
Measles	+	A	+
Mumps	+	A	–
Rubella	+	A	+
Human immunodeficiency virus	+	S	+
Fungal			
Histoplasmosis	+	S	+
Cryptococcus	+	S	–
Aspergillosis	+	S	–
Candida	+	S	–
Coccidioides	+	S	–
Sporotrichosis	+	A	–
Parasitic			
Toxoplasma gondii	+	S	+

–, not found; +, rare; ++, uncommon; +++, common; A, acute onset; S, subacute to chronic onset.
*Neonates and young infants only.
Adapted from Butler KM, Baker CJ. Cervical lymphadenitis. In: Feigin RD, Cherry JD, eds. *Textbook of pediatric infectious diseases,* 4th ed. Philadelphia: Saunders, 1997:170.

adenitis, particularly male infants with ipsilateral otitis media, may have the cellulitis–adenitis syndrome that is caused by group B streptococci. In contrast to infants with staphylococcal adenitis, those with group B streptococcal infection have a high likelihood (greater than 90%) of concomitant bacteremia.

Most Common Causes

The most common causes of subacute to chronic cervical adenitis are EBV, atypical mycobacteria, cat-scratch disease caused by *B. henselae,* and *Nocardia.* Less frequently, *T. gondii,* fungal infections, or syphilis may present as subacute or chronic cervical lymphadenitis (Table 138-2). The features that aid in differentiating atypical mycobacterial adenitis from that caused by *M. tuberculosis* are found in Table 138-1.

Cat-scratch disease is a lymphocutaneous syndrome in which regional lymph nodes proximal to the subcutaneous inoculation of *B. henselae* become inflamed. The interval between the cat scratch (or bite) and the development of adenitis ranges from 1 week to 2 months. Lymph nodes of the head or neck were involved in 58% of the 548 patients described in one large series. Fever with a mean duration of 7 days occurs in 25% of children, but constitutional symptoms of malaise, anorexia, and headache are mild or absent in the majority. In approximately 25% of children, the lymph nodes suppurate. Uncommon manifestations include oculoglandular syndrome of Parinaud, encephalopathy, osteolytic lesions, and prolonged fever with hepatosplenic granulomas. Usually, adenitis resolves after 2 to 6 weeks, but it may persist for a more protracted interval in some children (up to 20%).

TABLE 138-3. Noninfectious Causes of Cervical Adenitis

Causes	Frequency	Associated with generalized adenopathy
Neoplasm		
Hodgkin's disease	++	+
Lymphosarcoma, rhabdomyosarcoma	++	–
Non-Hodgkin's lymphoma	++	+
Neuroblastoma	++	+
Leukemia	+	+
Metastatic carcinoma	+	–
Thyroid tumor	+	–
Collagen-vascular disease		
Lupus erythematosus	+	+
Juvenile rheumatoid arthritis	+	+
Miscellaneous		
Kawasaki disease	+++	+
Drug-associated disease	++	+
Sarcoidosis	+	+
Histiocytosis X	+	+
Reticuloendotheliosis	+	+
Sinus histiocytosis with massive lymphadenopathy	+	+

–, not found; +, rare; ++, uncommon; +++, common.
Adapted from Butler KM, Baker CJ. Cervical lymphadenitis. In: Feigin RD, Cherry JD, eds. *Textbook of pediatric infectious diseases,* 4th ed. Philadelphia: Saunders, 1997:170; Margileth AM. Cervical adenitis. *Pediatr Rev* 1985;7:13.

DIFFERENTIAL DIAGNOSIS

Noninfectious Causes

Cervical swellings are common in pediatric practice, and most represent lymph nodes that are infected. Noninfectious causes of cervical adenitis include a variety of benign and malignant entities (Table 138-3). Their duration is an aid to diagnosis, because most tumors and miscellaneous conditions that cause cervical adenitis are characterized by chronicity. Usually, these lymph nodes are painless, are not inflamed, and exhibit a firm consistency. Location is also a helpful distinguishing feature, because approximately one-half of all masses located in the posterior triangle are malignant tumors, whereas masses found in the anterior triangle, with the exception of those involving the thyroid, tend to be benign. Masses that extend across the sternocleidomastoid muscle and involve both the anterior and the posterior triangles should be viewed as potentially malignant. Finally, age is a discriminator to some extent, because lymphoreticular malignant tumors are more frequent in older children, in contrast to the infectious causes that predominate in children younger than age 6.

Clinical Features

Lymphoid neoplasms and neuroblastoma constitute two-thirds of all malignant neck masses seen in children (Table 138-2). Lymphomas, both Hodgkin's and nonHodgkin's types, are more common than neuroblastoma in older children, whereas neuroblastoma is the malignant lesion most common in young children. Kawasaki disease deserves special mention, as it is a common cause of unilateral anterior cervical adenitis for which the causative agent is undefined. Clinical criteria that include persistence of fever for 5 days or longer and the presence of other major features—conjunctivitis, truncal exanthem, oral manifestations, and involvement of the hands and feet—are diagnostic of this syndrome. An enlarged lymph node (greater than 1.5 cm) in the cervical chain is one clinical feature of this disease that is noted in one-half to two-thirds of affected patients.

Congenital lesions of the neck may simulate cervical adenitis. The most common of these lesions is the thyroglossal duct cyst, which may be distinguished by its midline location and movement with tongue protrusion. The existence of a pit, dimple, or draining sinus along the anterior margin of the sternocleidomastoid muscle serves to differentiate between branchial cleft cyst and cervical adenitis, although the distinction may be difficult if the cyst becomes infected secondarily. Cystic hygromas are soft masses that transilluminate aiding in their differentiation from inflammatory or malignant neck masses.

DIAGNOSIS

A detailed history to ascertain the duration of the illness (acute or subacute to chronic), the presence or absence of associated systemic symptoms, animal exposures, preceding trauma, contact with an adult with tuberculosis, the presence of maternal risk factors for HIV infection, drug usage (especially phenytoin), ingestion of unusual substances (i.e., undercooked meat, unpasteurized milk), or recent travel may yield important diagnostic clues regarding the cause of cervical adenitis. The physical examination reveals the location of the adenitis (anterior or posterior triangle), the presence of dental disease, noncervical lymphadenopathy, oropharyngeal or skin lesions, and evidence of generalized or localized involvement.

In children with acute infection, needle aspiration of the largest or most fluctuant-affected node is the best method for establishing a specific cause. In 60% to 88% of patients with acute cervical adenitis caused by aerobic agents or mycobacteria, a causative agent is recovered by this diagnostic maneuver. Gram and acid-fast bacillus stains of the aspirated material should be performed, in addition to aerobic and anaerobic cultures. If Nocardia is suspected, the laboratory should be informed and asked to hold blood agar plates for up to 7 days. If mycobacterial or fungal infection is suspected, processing of the aspirate in appropriate culture media should be requested. Cultures of infected skin lesions or exudates on tonsils (if present) should also be performed.

Biopsies

If purulent material is not obtained, cultures for aerobic bacteria fail to yield a pathogen, and an affected patient does not respond to antibiotics active against staphylococci and streptococci, the following laboratory evaluation should be considered: throat culture; Mantoux intradermal purified protein derivative test; complete blood cell count; and serologic tests for EBV, CMV, *Bartonella*, toxoplasmosis, HIV, tularemia, and *Brucella*. Mantoux testing for *M. tuberculosis* with 5 tuberculin units of tuberculin should always be performed in patients with subacute or chronic adenitis. If the foregoing evaluation does not reveal the cause of the adenopathy and it persists, enlarges, or is hard or fixed to adjacent structures, excisional biopsy should be strongly considered. Older children are more likely to be candidates for excisional lymph node biopsy. They are also the patients more likely to have lymphomas or other malignant lesions. Therefore, a biopsy of the appropriate node must be performed, and the specimen must be removed intact for proper fixation, cutting, and staining. The largest node should be chosen, and if several sites of involvement are present, specimens from the lower neck and supraclavicular area should be removed, because they have the highest diagnostic yield. Reactive hyperplasia is the final diagnosis in approximately one-half of all cases. In these children, particularly when no improvement is noted, a repeat biopsy performed at a later time may offer additional information.

TREATMENT

Antimicrobial Therapy

Many infants and children with cervical lymphadenopathy accompanying viral infections of the respiratory tract never see a physician because of the self-limited nature of these infections. In children, where the primary site of infection involves acute inflammation of cervical lymph nodes, empiric antimicrobial therapy may be given. However, if no clinical response occurs within 48 hours, needle aspiration should be considered. Empiric antibiotic therapy should be directed against *S. aureus* and group A streptococci, and it should include agents such as cloxacillin (50 mg/kg/day) or, for penicillin-allergic patients, clindamycin (30 mg/kg/day) or cefprozil (30 mg/kg/day). A combination of amoxicillin and clavulanic acid (Augmentin), 45 mg/kg/day, provides good activity for staphylococci and streptococci and for oral anaerobic bacteria, if a dental focus of infection is suspected. This expanded activity and palatability render amoxicillin–clavulanic acid a good alternative to penicillinase-resistant penicillins. Some patients have progression of local inflammation and persistence of systemic symptoms despite oral antimicrobial therapy. Such children require parenteral therapy with an antimicrobial such as nafcillin (100–150 mg/kg/day). In the penicillin-allergic patient, cefazolin (100 mg/kg/day) or clindamycin (30 mg/kg/day) may be substituted. Antimicrobial therapy should be modified once a causative agent is identified (i.e., group A streptococcal infection should be treated with penicillin G or V) and may need to be modified for an obvious primary infectious focus such as a dental abscess when therapy for anaerobes is mandatory. In the latter circumstance, penicillin V (50 mg/kg/day), clindamycin (25–30 mg/kg/day), or amoxicillin–clavulanic acid (45 mg/kg/day) is a useful agent. In children with acute suppurative cervical adenitis, surgical drainage is key to appropriate resolution.

Adenitis caused by group A streptococci should be treated for a minimum of 10 days or approximately 5 days after signs of local inflammation and systemic symptoms have disappeared. If affected children are penicillin-allergic, erythromycin ethylsuccinate (40 mg/kg/day) or cephalexin can be used. Warm, moist dressings over the inflamed area give symptomatic relief but probably do not aid in the localization process. If abscess formation occurs late in the first or early in the second week of antibiotic therapy, incision and drainage are indicated, and therapy should be continued for another 5 to 7 days.

Clinical improvement in bacterial adenitis is expected within 48 to 72 hours of the initiation of treatment, but usually the size of the node or nodes does not regress at this stage, and low-grade fever may persist. Regression of lymph node enlargement is slow. As a general guideline, significant enlargement that persists beyond 6 to 8 weeks demands exclusion of an underlying disorder and consideration of an excisional biopsy.

Specific Therapies

When organisms other than staphylococci or streptococci are involved or when lymph node enlargement is the result of noninfectious processes, rational therapy for cervical lymphadenitis depends on the cause of the condition. Disease caused by *M. tuberculosis* requires antituberculous chemotherapy and family-contact tracing for the infected adult. Disease caused by atypical mycobacteria requires complete surgical excision of affected lymph nodes without medical therapy. *Nocardia* infections are treated with trimethoprim-sulfamethoxazole orally, but therapy for as long as 3 or 4 weeks is often required for resolution. Usually, *Bartonella* infections are benign, and resolution without specific therapy occurs. In certain patients, however, ongoing local discomfort may be an indication for aspiration to hasten resolution and to relieve discomfort. Surgical excision is reserved for occasional patients who have ongoing systemic symptoms, persistence of significant adenopathy, or development of draining sinuses. Patients who are immunocompromised or healthy children with uncommon manifestations of cat-scratch disease such as hepatosplenic granulomas or osteolytic lesions may benefit from treatment with trimethoprim-sulfamethoxazole (10 mg/kg/day), rifampin (20 mg/kg/day) or, in older children, ciprofloxacin.

CHAPTER 139

Obstructive Sleep Apnea Syndrome

Adapted from Carole L. Marcus and John L. Carroll

Obstructive apnea is defined as the cessation of airflow at the nose and mouth, despite continued respiratory effort, secondary to upper airway obstruction. This disorder is distinct from central apnea in which cessation of airflow is associated with absent respiratory effort. Many children with obstructive sleep apnea syndrome (OSAS) exhibit continuous partial airway obstruction associated with hypoxemia and hypoventilation, rather than complete airway obstruction; this form of the disorder has been termed obstructive hypoventilation.

The prevalence of OSAS in the pediatric age group is estimated to be 1% to 3% of preschool children. The peak incidence is between ages 2 and 6, which is the age at which the tonsils and adenoids are the largest in relation to the oropharyngeal size. However, OSAS can occur at any age from the neonatal period through adolescence. OSAS is thought to occur equally among male and female children, although this theory has not been evaluated rigorously.

PATHOPHYSIOLOGY

OSAS results from a combination of abnormal neuromuscular control and anatomic narrowing of the upper airway. During wakefulness, patients with a narrow airway can compensate by augmenting upper airway muscle tone; thus, OSAS does not occur. During sleep, decreases in ventilatory drive and in neuromuscular tone facilitate upper airway collapse. In children, the anatomic narrowing of the upper airway is usually due to adenotonsillar hypertrophy. Other common causes of structural narrowing include craniofacial anomalies and obesity. Patients with neuromuscular disorders resulting in hypotonia (e.g., muscular dystrophy) or incoordination of the upper airway musculature (e.g., cerebral palsy) are also at increased risk for OSAS. Children with syndromes encompassing developmental delay, hypotonia, obesity, and upper airway narrowing (e.g., children with trisomy 21) are at very high risk for OSAS.

HISTORY

Symptoms

Most children present with a history of snoring and difficulty in breathing during sleep. Usually, the onset is insidious. Children with OSAS have persistent, loud snoring that can frequently be heard outside the bedroom. During sleep, such children have labored breathing, retractions, and paradoxical inward motion of the chest wall during inspiration. During periods of complete obstruction, affected children can be observed making respiratory efforts, but no snoring is heard, and no airflow is detected. Usually, obstructive episodes are terminated by gasping, movements, or arousal from sleep. Such children sleep restlessly and may adopt unusual sleeping positions such as sleeping in a seated position or with the neck hyperextended. Enuresis is common. Diaphoresis, pallor, or cyanosis may be present. The appearance of affected children during sleep can be so alarming that it is not unusual for parents to maintain bedside vigils or to stimulate or reposition them continually throughout the night. Nevertheless, many parents do not volunteer a history of their child's sleep symptoms unless specifically asked. Asking parents to mimic an affected child's snoring and breathing pattern is useful.

Nonspecific Symptoms

During wakefulness, children with OSAS breathe normally. Nonspecific symptoms of adenotonsillar hypertrophy may be present. These include mouth breathing, rhinorrhea, dysphagia, and recurrent otitis media. Excessive daytime sleepiness may be present but is unusual in young children. Often, there is a family history of snoring or OSAS.

PHYSICAL EXAMINATION

In most children with OSAS, the physical examination during wakefulness is entirely normal. However, failure to thrive or, conversely, obesity may be present. Allergic stigmata, mouth breathing, adenoidal facies, midfacial hypoplasia, retrognathia or micrognathia, or other craniofacial abnormalities may be present. The patency of the nares should be assessed. The pharynx should be evaluated for tongue size, palatal integrity, oropharyngeal diameter, redundant palatal mucosa, palatal length, tonsillar size, and uvula size. Usually, the lungs are clear to auscultation. Cardiac examination may reveal signs of pulmonary hypertension such as an increased pulmonic component of the second heart sound. A neurologic examination should be performed to evaluate muscle tone and developmental status.

DIAGNOSTIC TESTS

The diagnosis of OSAS should be established by polysomnography (sleep study). History alone is inadequate, as it cannot distinguish between OSAS and simple snoring or other causes of sleep-related symptoms. In addition, polysomnography provides objective measures of severity and provides a baseline for those affected children whose condition does not resolve postoperatively. During polysomnography, noninvasive monitoring of sleep architecture, chest and abdominal wall motion, airflow, oxygenation, and carbon dioxide tension is performed. Polysomnography should be performed in a laboratory accustomed to studying children, as both techniques and normative values differ widely between children and adults. Home video recording can be a useful screening tool. When necessary, adenoidal size can be assessed by lateral neck radiography or endoscopy. An electrocardiogram and an echocardiogram should be obtained in patients with severe OSAS.

TREATMENT

Conventional Treatment

Most children are cured by adenotonsillectomy. OSAS results from the relative size and structure of the upper airway components, rather than the absolute size of the tonsils and adenoids. Usually, therefore, both the tonsils and the adenoids should be removed, even if one or the other appears to be the primary abnormality. By the same logic, adenotonsillectomy should be the initial treatment of OSAS in children with other predisposing factors (e.g., obesity, Down syndrome), although further treatment may be necessary. Although frequently considered to be minor surgery, adenotonsillectomy can be associated with significant complications. Therefore, snoring without OSAS is not an indication for surgery. Children with OSAS are at risk for postoperative complications including upper airway edema, pulmonary edema, and respiratory failure. Perioperative deaths have been reported. High-risk patients (those younger than age 3 and those with severe OSAS, cerebral palsy, or craniofacial anomalies) should be monitored as inpatients postoperatively. OSAS may not resolve fully until 6 to 8 weeks postoperatively.

Hospitalization

Occasionally, children present with severe OSAS requiring emergency admission to the hospital. Monitoring in the hospital should include pulse oximetry, as cardiorespiratory monitors alone will not detect obstructive apnea until bradycardia occurs. Sedative drugs should be avoided, as these may aggravate OSAS. Supplemental oxygen should not be administered without simultaneous monitoring of Pco_2, as it may precipitate respiratory failure. Obstructive episodes can be terminated by awakening an affected patient, but this solution is only very temporary. Nasopharyngeal tubes can be placed to bypass the obstruction pending definitive treatment. Vigilant nursing is necessary, as the tubes frequently clog with mucus. Alternately, nasal continuous positive airway pressure (CPAP) may be administered. Occasionally, intubation is necessary.

Other Treatments

A minority of patients with OSAS do not respond to adenotonsillectomy. Nasal CPAP can be used successfully in most children provided that the parents and child are motivated and the care providers are well versed in pediatric CPAP use. Other treatments are useful in individual cases. When applicable, specific craniofacial surgery may be beneficial (e.g., lip–tongue adhesion procedures in patients with Pierre Robin sequence). Uvulopharyngopalatoplasty has been shown to be helpful in children with cerebral palsy. Obese OSAS patients should be encouraged to lose weight. With the advent of nasal CPAP, tracheotomy is rarely necessary for sleep apnea.

COMPLICATIONS

The trend to earlier diagnosis has resulted in a decrease in the rate of complications. Patients with severe OSAS can exhibit failure to thrive. Severe OSAS can cause pulmonary hypertension. This condition can progress to cor pulmonale and congestive heart failure but resolves after successful treatment of OSAS. Systemic hypertension may occur. Neurobehavioral complications result from sleep fragmentation and nocturnal hypoxemia. These complications include hyperactivity, personality changes, poor school performance, and developmental delay. Seizures, asphyxial brain damage, and coma have been reported. Enuresis, especially secondary enuresis, may result from OSAS. Respiratory arrest and sudden death have been reported.

PROGNOSIS

Most children with OSAS experience a dramatic resolution of their symptoms after adenotonsillectomy. However, the natural course and the long-term prognosis of pediatric OSAS are unknown. Some evidence suggests that children with treated OSAS are at risk for recurrence during adulthood.

3
Cardiovascular System

CHAPTER 140
Ventricular Septal Defect

Adapted from Carl H. Gumbiner

Ventricular septal defect (VSD) is the most common cardiac abnormality in children with an incidence of 1.5 to 2.5 per 1,000 live births. Approximately 20% of patients followed-up by pediatric cardiologists in the United States carry the diagnosis of VSD. The ventricular septum separates the left ventricle from the right ventricle and, to a small extent, from the right atrium. It consists of a membranous and a muscular portion and is subdivided into inflow, trabecular, and outflow regions. Defects in the septum may occur in each region (Table 140-1). The location of a defect within the ventricular septum is not of great hemodynamic consequence, but it is a critical surgical consideration and an important determinant of natural history. Defects range in size from 1 mm or less to virtual absence of the septum.

CLINICAL MANIFESTATIONS

Small VSDs seldom cause significant symptoms and usually come to the attention of a physician because of the associated heart murmur. Whereas the murmur is not present in the immediate newborn period, it may be audible as early as the second day of life and is usually heard at the routine 2-week checkup. It is characteristically a high-pitched, harsh, holosystolic murmur, well localized along the left sternal border. A small VSD may produce a murmur of lower pitch, but a high-pitched murmur strongly suggests that the defect is not large. The precordium is quiet, but a localized thrill may be palpable. The first and second heart sounds are normal, and a diastolic murmur is seldom present. Except for mild tachypnea in small infants, other physical findings are normal. Small defects do not interfere with normal growth. A significant number, estimated to be in the range of

TABLE 140-1. Types of Ventricular Septal Defects

Type	Characteristics
Perimembranous	Bounded by portions of membranous and muscular septums
Muscular	Bounded by muscle entirely, often multiple and difficult to repair, frequently close spontaneously
Subarterial Defects	Lie beneath the aortic and pulmonary arteries in the outflow portion of the muscular septum, associated with aortic regurgitation
Malalignment Defects	Crest of septum lies in different plane than the aortic root, often found in complex lesions, left ventricular outflow obstruction is common

30% to 70%, undergo spontaneous closure, usually in the child's first 2 years of life. Certain types of defects regardless of size, however, may predispose to development of secondary conditions, especially aortic regurgitation and left ventricular outflow tract obstruction. For this reason, in children with physical findings of a small VSD, echocardiographic examination should be performed to confirm the diagnosis and localize the defect.

Large Defects

Large defects may come to the attention of a physician later than small defects, because elevated pulmonary vascular resistance may delay the appearance of a murmur. When present, symptoms are those of congestive heart failure (CHF). They include irritability, increased respiratory effort, poor feeding, and poor weight gain. Recurrent respiratory infections are common, and pneumonia is often the preliminary diagnosis.

Symptoms

Signs of CHF include tachycardia, tachypnea, increased work of breathing, pallor, diaphoresis, and failure to thrive. Pulmonary rales are a late finding. The precordium is hyperactive, and a thrill is often palpable. The second heart sound is single or narrowly split. When audible, it is usually accentuated, but it is often obscured by a loud, low-pitched, harsh, holosystolic murmur. The murmur is loudest along the left sternal border, but it is much less well-localized than the murmur of a small VSD. It may radiate to the right of the sternum but radiates poorly to the back. A diastolic murmur or rumble heard at the lower left sternal border is related to increased mitral flow. Pulses may be diminished with severe CHF, but they are symmetric in the absence of aortic coarctation. The liver and sometimes the spleen are enlarged. Children with large VSDs may develop pulmonary vascular obstructive disease (PVOD) due to sustained elevated pulmonary artery pressures.

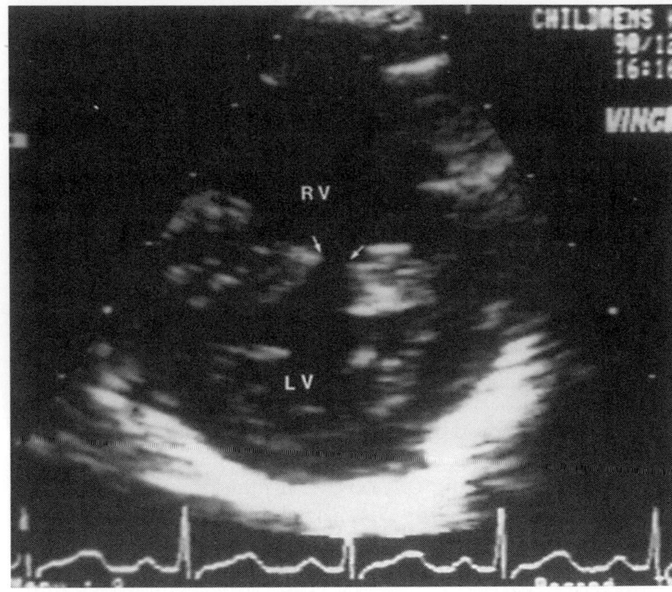

Figure 140-1. Short-axis two-dimensional echocardiographic view of a large muscular ventricular septal defect. Arrows point to margins of the defect. LV, left ventricle; RV, right ventricle.

NONINVASIVE AND INVASIVE STUDIES

Small defects may produce mild cardiac enlargement on a plain chest roentgenogram, but usually the roentgenogram is normal. Moderate defects are associated with cardiomegaly, usually of a predominant left ventricular type. The left atrium may be enlarged on lateral projection. Large defects produce a more diffuse cardiomegaly, increased pulmonary vascular markings and, often, signs of pulmonary edema. In patients with a large VSD and PVOD, only mild cardiomegaly is demonstrated on the chest roentgenogram. The main pulmonary artery segment is usually prominent, and central vascular markings are normal or diminished.

Electrocardiographic changes with a small VSD are minimal. Moderately sized defects usually produce some degree of left ventricular hypertrophy, whereas large defects commonly produce combined ventricular hypertrophy on electrocardiography. Large defects with PVOD may show more right ventricular hypertrophy than left.

Anatomic and Physiologic Assessments

Echocardiography and Doppler echocardiography are the primary modalities for anatomic and physiologic assessment of VSD. Real-time, two-dimensional echocardiographic imaging in the standard views discloses the presence, location, and size of nearly all defects (Fig. 140-1), as well as the presence of associated lesions. Color-flow Doppler investigation increases the sensitivity of standard imaging, particularly for small or multiple defects. Pulsed and continuous-wave Doppler studies facilitate assessment of right ventricular pressure and pressure gradients between ventricles. Systemic and pulmonary blood flows can be estimated indirectly by measuring semilunar valve diameter and recording flow velocity.

Cardiac catheterization and angiography is reserved for patients with unusual or complex anatomy and for patients who require precise investigation of pulmonary blood flow or vascular resistance beyond Doppler capability. Such evaluation may also entail assessment of response to intervention such as administration of oxygen or vasodilators.

Magnetic resonance imaging and cine-magnetic resonance imaging offer other methods for the anatomic assessment of these defects and are particularly useful for evaluating associated extracardiac vascular malformations such as coarctation of the aorta.

MANAGEMENT

Therapeutic Approach

The therapeutic approach to an infant or child with VSD depends on the patient's age, the size of the defect, the severity of symptoms, and the anatomy of the defect itself. Infants with small VSDs seldom require treatment. They should be evaluated during the first 6 months of life when pulmonary vascular resistance is expected to decline. Physical examinations and noninvasive studies should be employed to ascertain the expected minimal increase in pulmonary blood flow and absence of pulmonary hypertension. Many defects, especially those in the muscular septum, close spontaneously.

Conventional Therapy

Infants with moderate or large VSDs often have symptoms associated with significant left-to-right shunting. CHF caused by an isolated VSD can be treated with conventional medical therapy including diuretics, afterload reduction, and digoxin. The usual initial choice of diuretic is furosemide, 1 to 2 mg/kg twice daily, or chlorothiazide, 10 to 20 mg/kg twice daily. Afterload reduction with an angiotensin-converting enzyme inhibitor (captopril, 0.1–0.5 mg/kg three times daily, or enalapril, 0.08 mg/kg twice daily) may significantly improve symptoms, especially in patients with low pulmonary vascular resistance. Digoxin, 0.01 mg/kg/day, remains part of the therapeutic regimen in many centers, despite controversy over its efficacy in left-to-right shunts. It should not be used in lieu of afterload reduction.

Even with aggressive medical therapy, infants with excessive pulmonary blood flow may gain weight poorly. Caloric requirements often in excess of 140 kcal/kg/day, fluid restriction, and poor feeding combine to make adequate nutrition a challenge. Standard formulas can be supplemented with carbohydrates and medium-chain triglycerides and, occasionally, nasogastric feeding may be necessary.

Goals of Therapy

The goals of medical therapy are relief of symptoms and normal growth. When these goals are not achieved, early surgical repair should be strongly considered. Perimembranous defects associated with uncontrolled symptoms or failure to thrive should be repaired promptly. Large muscular defects, because of their propensity for spontaneous size reduction or closure and the difficulty associated with the surgical approach to apical or multiple defects, may be managed medically for a longer time, but they, too, may ultimately require surgical repair.

Surgical Repair

Patients in whom medical therapy is successful but pulmonary artery pressure remains elevated should undergo surgical repair before 1 year of age. When pulmonary artery pressure is normal, the decision of whether to repair the defect is largely dependent on its location. All subarterial defects, because of their high association with development of aortic regurgitation, should be repaired by the time the child reaches school age. An association between perimembranous defects and aortic valve insufficiency, subaortic obstruction, right ventricular outflow tract obstruction, and left ventricle–to–right atrial shunting, with an attendant increased risk of endocarditis, can also exist. For these reasons, many centers are now advocating repair of all perimembranous defects before the child reaches school age, regardless of the size of the defect. Small muscular defects are generally benign and require only periodic follow-up to ensure the appropriate use of endocarditis prophylaxis.

Markedly elevated pulmonary vascular resistance in the older child renders the risk of surgical repair untenable. No effective treatment for advanced PVOD exists, although occasionally, the patients benefit from oxygen administration and periodic red blood cell volume reduction. Lung transplantation may hold promise for these young people, although to date, the frequent occurrence of debilitating bronchiolitis obliterans in transplanted lungs has been discouraging.

CHAPTER 141
Defects of the Atrial Septum Including the Atrioventricular Canal

Adapted from G. Wesley Vick III and Jack L. Titus

ISOLATED ATRIAL SEPTAL DEFECTS

Pathologic Features

PATENT FORAMEN OVALE

Approximately 30% to 40% of normal adult hearts have a patent, valve-competent foramen ovale that is not usually considered an atrial septal defect (ASD). The smallest ASDs are caused by incompetence of the valve of the foramen ovale. This incompetence may be congenital or may be acquired by stretching of the right or left atrium in conditions in which those chambers are enlarged.

DEFECTS AT THE FOSSA OVALIS (SECUNDUM DEFECTS)

Typical defects in the fossa ovalis are contained within the area bordered by the limbus of the fossa ovalis. Sizes of these defects vary greatly. In addition, the floor of the fossa ovalis (valve of foramen ovale) in this region may be fenestrated, so multiple defects are possible. Secundum defects may be associated with or confluent with other defects of the atrial septum such as a sinus venosus defect or ostium primum defect.

In addition to secundum defects and patency of the foramen ovale, abnormalities in the sinus venosus and coronary sinus may result in isolated ASDs.

ASSOCIATED CARDIOVASCULAR DEFECTS

Often, ASDs occur in conjunction with other congenital cardiac anomalies. In many of these anomalies, the associated defects are the lesions of primary importance; however, the ASD may play a major role in the physiologic features of the condition. For example, in complete transposition of the great arteries, an ASD permits mixing between the pulmonary and systemic circulations necessary to sustain life. Another example is tricuspid atresia, in which the entire cardiac output must pass across the ASD.

Natural History

Isolated secundum ASDs do not cause major symptoms in most cases during infancy and childhood. In the absence of unrelated problems, more than 99% of patients with isolated secundum defects will live beyond the first year of life. As previously noted, mild to moderate cyanosis is sometimes evident during the neonatal period. Children and infants with these defects tend to be smaller than normal, but failure to thrive on the basis of the ASD alone is rare. Exercise intolerance may develop in some patients as early as the second decade of life. Others may remain asymptomatic for several more decades.

Left–to–right shunting tends to increase with age in many patients. Thus, the frequency of congestive heart failure with attendant fluid retention, hepatomegaly, and elevated jugular venous pressure increases with the age of the patient. The large shunts present in many older patients cause stretching of the atria, which presumably predisposes them to atrial arrhythmias such as atrial flutter, fibrillation, and tachycardia. These arrhythmias are a major cause of morbidity and mortality in older patients with ASDs.

Physical Examination

INSPECTION AND PALPATION

Often, the height and weight of patients with ASDs are below normal, although usually not substantially so. A precordial bulge may be present in those patients with a large left–to–right shunt, and Harrison grooves (transverse depressions along the sixth and seventh costal cartilages at the site of attachment of the anterior part of the diaphragm) may be apparent in some patients. The presence of a hypoplastic thumb, radius, or phocomelia should cause suspicion that the patient has the Holt–Oram syndrome, an autosomal dominant disorder in which an upper limb deformity is found with congenital heart disease (most often an ASD in association with prolonged AV conduction). Cyanosis may be present in infants, particularly those with right ventricular outflow obstruction of any form. In patients with a thin body habitus, an uncomplicated ASD, and a large volume of left–to–right shunting, a hyperdynamic right ventricular impulse may be observed. Palpation along the left sternal border and in the subxiphoid area will demonstrate this impulse, often termed a *right ventricular heave*.

AUSCULTATION

In patients with ASDs, the first heart sound—best heard at the apex and lower left sternal edge—is often split and the second component is intensified. ASDs with moderate to large left–to–right shunts are associated with a pulmonary systolic murmur that begins shortly after the first heart sound, peaks in early to midsystole, and ends before the second heart sound. Usually, this murmur is not associated with a thrill. When a thrill is present, either a very large shunt or pulmonic stenosis is usually present. Rapid flow through the peripheral pulmonary arteries may cause systolic crescendo–decrescendo murmurs that are most prominent at locations in the chest other than the second intercostal space.

The characteristic auscultatory finding in ASD is wide, fixed splitting of the second sound. This finding is present in patients with large left–to–right shunts and normal pulmonary artery pressure. The fixed splitting of the second sound results from a combination of factors. In normal individuals, inspiratory splitting of the second sound results primarily from increased pulmonary capacitance during inspiration. The increase causes an inspiratory increase in the "hangout" interval (the time between the descending portions of the right ventricular and pulmonary arterial pressure pulses) and a consequent delay in the pulmonic component of the second sound. With expiration in normal persons, the pulmonary capacitance decreases, the hangout interval decreases, and the splitting of the second sound decreases.

In contrast, in patients with ASD, the capacitance of the pulmonary bed is increased and its impedance is decreased. The increased capacitance causes an increase in the hangout interval with a consequent wide splitting between the first and second components of the second heart sound. Because of respiratory variation in the pulmonary capacitance, little variation in the hangout interval and splitting of the second sound occurs in patients with an ASD. When the left-to-right shunt is small or negligible, as it is in most neonates with ASDs, fixed splitting of the second sound does not occur. Because relatively wide (but not truly fixed) splitting of the second sound is common in the supine position, evaluation of the second sound is better when the patient is sitting or standing.

The diastolic murmur most commonly associated with ASD is a middiastolic murmur resulting from the high flow across the tricuspid valve. This murmur becomes apparent when the left-to-right shunt is greater than 2:1. The murmur is of low-to-medium frequency and does not increase with inspiration. Another diastolic murmur sometimes associated with ASD is a low-pitched murmur of pulmonic regurgitation, probably a consequence of dilatation of the pulmonary artery.

Because the pressure gradient across the atrial septum is seldom large, audible murmurs from flow across the ASD itself are rare, though intracardiac phonocardiography can demonstrate them.

ELECTROCARDIOGRAPHY

Sinus rhythm is customary in young patients with uncomplicated secundum ASDs. Prolongation of the PR interval is common and sometimes has a familial association. Beyond the third decade of life, patients with ASD have a high frequency of atrial arrhythmias including atrial fibrillation, atrial flutter, and supraventricular tachycardia.

Usually, patients with secundum ASDs have normal P waves. Often, the QRS complex in patients with secundum ASDs has a slightly prolonged duration and a characteristic rSr′ or rsR′ pattern. The reason for this orientation of the QRS is thought to be disproportionate thickening of the right ventricular outflow tract, which is the last portion of the ventricle to depolarize. Often, the term *incomplete right bundle branch block* is used to describe this QRS pattern, but that term is a misnomer because the pattern is a consequence of hypertrophy and not a conduction disturbance.

With increasing degrees of pulmonary hypertension, patients with secundum ASDs tend to lose the rSr′ pattern in V_1 and develop a tall monophasic R wave with a deeply inverted T wave. Left axis deviation of the QRS axis with a counterclockwise frontal plane loop suggests the presence of an AV canal defect, but such deviation can occur with uncomplicated secundum ASD.

CHEST RADIOGRAPHY

Generally, the chest radiograph in patients with secundum ASD and sizable left–to–right shunts shows cardiac enlargement and increased pulmonary vascularity. Typically, increased pulmonary vascularity extends to the periphery of the lung fields with a dilated pulmonary trunk and central branches. Although the ascending and transverse aorta are of normal diameters in these patients, enlargement of the pulmonary arteries prevents the aorta from forming the border of the cardiac shape. The consequence is the creation of a characteristic "triangular" cardiac shape. Usually, right atrial and right ventricular enlargement are present, but the sizes of the left atria and left ventricles are usually normal.

ECHOCARDIOGRAPHY

Two-Dimensional Echocardiography

Two-dimensional echocardiography enables direct noninvasive visualization of all types of ASDs (Fig. 141-1). In addition to direct visualization of the ASD, two-dimensional echocardiography may also demonstrate enlargement of the right atrium and right ventricle and pulmonary arteries, and it often shows paradoxical motion of the ventricular septum in a two-dimensional format. In many cases, the pulmonary and systemic venous connections can also be demonstrated.

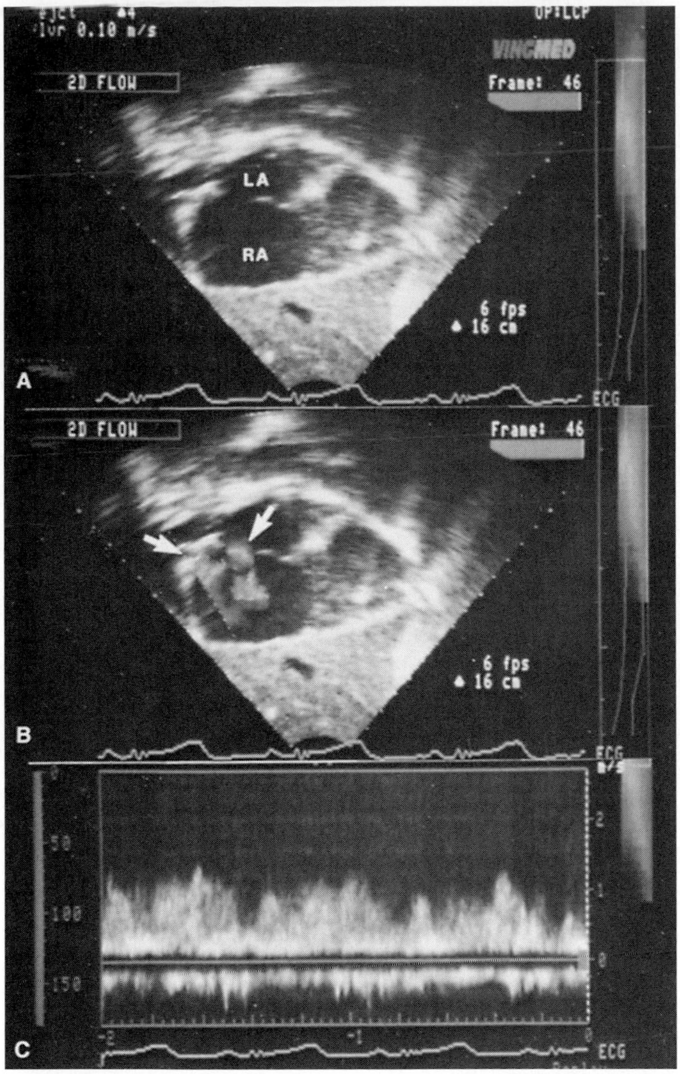

Figure 141-1. Two-dimensional echocardiogram demonstrating a fossa ovalis atrial septal defect. **A:** Note the opening in the fossa ovalis region of the septum between the left atrium (*LA*) and the right atrium (*RA*). **B:** Color Doppler study demonstrating flow across the atrial septum from left to right through the secundum atrial septal defect. **C:** Pulsed Doppler study demonstrating low-velocity flow from left to right across the defect.

Doppler Echocardiography

Abnormal flow across the atrial septum can be reliably detected by pulsed Doppler echocardiography. The accuracy of Doppler identification of flow across the atrial septum can be greatly improved by the use of two-dimensional echocardiographic direction of the Doppler sampling. Characteristically, a shunt across the ASD shows turbulent flow in the direction of the shunt and minimal flow in the opposite direction.

Transesophageal Echocardiography

Transthoracic echocardiography is limited by the ability of ultrasonography to penetrate to regions of interest. Particularly in older patients and in patients with chest wall deformities and lung disease, transthoracic echocardiographic windows may be so poor that the atrial septum cannot be clearly visualized in its entirety. In such instances, transesophageal echocardiography is often helpful. Generally, two-dimensional anatomic visualization of the atrial septum from the transesophageal approach is excellent. In addition to its diagnostic role in selected cases, transesophageal echocardiography is especially useful for guiding catheter placement of occlusion devices to close ASDs.

CARDIAC CATHETERIZATION

Sometimes, secundum ASDs can be differentiated from sinus venosus and AV canal defects because characteristic high or low catheter courses across the atrial septum are seen with the latter two defects, respectively. In secundum ASDs, the catheter passes across the middle portion of the atrial septum.

Left–to–right shunting across the atrial septum causes an increase (step-up) in oxygen saturation in the right atrium. An increase of 10% over superior vena caval blood in one oxygen saturation series or an increase of 5% in two series generally indicates the presence of a left–to–right shunt at the atrial level.

Treatment

Isolated secundum ASDs associated with a large left–to–right shunt and either symptoms or significant cardiomegaly should be electively closed in childhood. Many physicians believe that when the findings from a comprehensive noninvasive evaluation demonstrate a classic isolated secundum ASD, cardiac catheterization for diagnosis is not essential. The noninvasive studies should be of good technical quality, however, so that pulmonary hypertension can be excluded, and so that associated anatomic defects such as anomalous pulmonary and systemic venous connections can be excluded.

When pulmonary hypertension is present or the atrial shunt is small, recommendations regarding closure are more controversial. When advanced pulmonary vascular disease is present, operative mortality and morbidity are high, and closure of the ASD may worsen the prognosis. Small ASDs only cause a minimal increase in cardiopulmonary stress. Therefore, the hemodynamic gain from closing them may not be worth the hazard of the procedure. However, the risk of paradoxical embolism through a small atrial defect or valve-competent patent foramen ovale is uncertain. This risk may justify closure in selected patients such as those with a history of cryptogenic stroke. Further clinical studies are required to assess more definitely the benefits of intervention in such cases.

Successful catheter closure of secundum ASDs has been performed using occlusion devices. Although catheter occlusion of ASDs remains investigational at present, its role in the management of moderate and small defects in the fossa ovalis region may be expected to increase. Large secundum defects substantially greater than approximately 20 mm in diameter cannot be reliably closed with current catheter devices. Catheter closure has the advantage of avoiding cardiopulmonary bypass, thoracotomy, and atriotomy with their attendant potential problems. Initial and intermediate-term results with catheter ASD occlusion are promising, but long-term follow-up studies subsequent to catheter ASD closure are not yet available.

Surgical closure is usually performed with the aid of cardiopulmonary bypass. Patch closure with either pericardium or Dacron is preferred for all but small defects because closure of large defects by direct suture can distort the atrium.

PROGNOSIS

Surgical results in uncomplicated secundum ASD are good. Mortality is less than 2% in many large series. Mortality and morbidity are increased with advanced age and congestive heart failure. After operation, the left–to–right shunt and its consequent cardiac volume overload are eliminated in nearly all patients. Without closure, patients with moderate and large secundum ASDs generally do well until the third decade of life, after which they tend to become progressively more symptomatic with a substantially higher mortality than that for the general population.

PERSISTENT COMMON ATRIOVENTRICULAR (AV) CANAL DEFECTS

AV canal defects include a range of malformations, a central feature of which is usually an ASD of the primum type. In addition, such malformations generally involve the ventricular septum and one or both AV valves. There is a spectrum of AV canal defects. In this discussion, the term *complete AV canal* indicates the presence of both atrial and ventricular septal defects and a common AV orifice with a common AV valve (Fig. 141-2); all other forms that are parts of the spectrum are termed partial or incomplete forms.

Pathologic Aspects

ATRIAL SEPTUM

Most AV canal defects include an interatrial communication, usually called *ostium primum ASD*. They lie at the lowest part of the atrial septum and vary in size but are usually large in relation to cardiac size.

VENTRICULAR SEPTUM

The basal portion of the ventricular septum is deficient in most hearts with persistent common AV canal. In those hearts without interventricular communication, the AV valve tissue attaches to the crest of the deficient ventricular septum such that interventricular communication is precluded. In hearts with interventricular communication, valvular tissue does not attach to the crest of the deficient septum and interventricular communication exists between the valve tissues superiorly and the crest of the deficient septum inferiorly.

ATRIOVENTRICULAR VALVES

The hallmarks of persistent AV canal defects are abnormal AV valves. The abnormalities involve both the overall configuration and orientation of the valve apparatus and the local structure of the AV valves. Usually, partial forms of AV canal defects have two separate AV valve annuli. In this situation, the left and right AV valve leaflets are usually named according to the normal mitral and tricuspid valve components to which they correspond most closely. In complete AV canal defects, a common AV valve exists. Both an ostium primum ASD and a ventricular septal defect of the AV canal type are present and confluent. The common AV valve has anterior and posterior common leaflets that bridge across the ventricular septum and relate to both ventricles (also called *anterior and posterior bridging leaflets*).

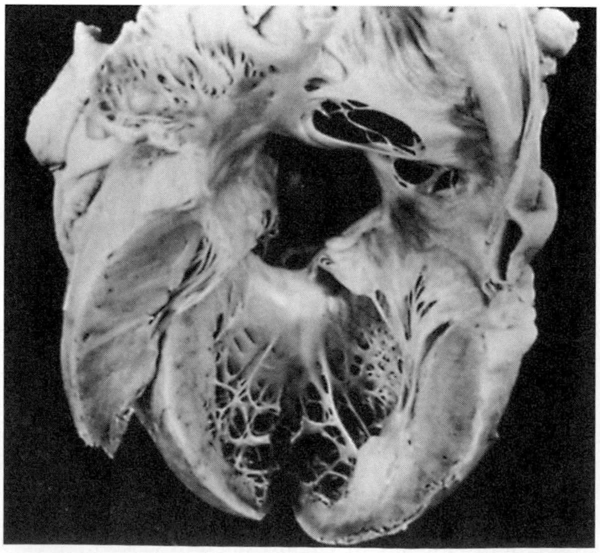

Figure 141-2. Complete atrioventricular canal defect. View is from the opened left atrium and left ventricle. Note the large cleft in the anterior mitral leaflet. (Courtesy of Debra Kearney, M.D.)

COMMON ATRIUM

An uncommon form of ASD is that in which almost the entire atrial septum is absent. Often, a band of muscular tissue crosses the atrium suggesting a vestigial atrial septum. Nearly always, these defects are associated with a cleft anterior leaflet of the mitral valve and a deficient summit of the ventricular septum.

Natural History

The natural history of AV canal defect primarily depends on the pathologic anatomy of the malformation. In patients with only an ostium primum ASD and minimal insufficiency of the left AV valve, the clinical course is similar to that for patients with a large secundum ASD. Generally, these patients do well without treatment during infancy, childhood, and adolescence. During adulthood, they have an increasing tendency to develop congestive heart failure, particularly as atrial arrhythmias develop and with the increasing mitral regurgitation that occurs with time.

Patients with ostium primum ASDs and moderate to severe left AV valve insufficiency develop congestive heart failure in early life with consequent high morbidity and mortality that primarily relate to the severity of the AV valve insufficiency.

Generally, patients with complete AV canal defects develop severe symptoms of congestive heart failure in early infancy. They have frequent respiratory infections and poor weight gain. If they survive infancy untreated, they generally develop pulmonary vascular disease with fixed pulmonary hypertension as an additional major deleterious factor.

Physical Examination

SIGNS AND AUSCULTATORY MANIFESTATIONS

Appearance

Usually, patients with partial AV canal defects and minimal mitral insufficiency appear normal in infancy and childhood. Patients with partial AV canal and substantial mitral insufficiency may manifest growth failure and other signs of chronic congestive heart failure. Usually, patients with complete common AV canal are symptomatic in early infancy, with manifestations such as poor physical development, hyperinflated thorax, bulging precordium, Harrison grooves, and mild or intermittent cyanosis. If no signs of chronic congestive heart failure are present in a patient with known complete common AV canal defect, pulmonary stenosis or pulmonary vascular obstructive disease should be suspected.

The patient with Down syndrome, which is frequently associated with endocardial cushion defects, has a characteristic physical appearance. When the Down syndrome is seen in conjunction with the physical signs of chronic congestive heart failure, the coexistence of complete common AV canal should be suspected. Other types of congenital heart disease also occur in Down syndrome.

Auscultation

Complete AV canal defects may be associated with a variety of auscultatory manifestations depending on the nature of the underlying pathologic physiology. Because one common AV valve is present, the first heart sound is usually single. When the AV conduction time is prolonged (as is often the case), the first heart sound tends to be relatively soft. Usually, constant or fixed splitting of the second sound occurs, although when severe pulmonary hypertension is present, the splitting will be narrow. Pulmonary hypertension may also be associated with a loud pulmonic component of the second sound. Frequently, a murmur of AV valve incompetence is present. Usually, this murmur is maximal at the left ventricular apex and often radiates toward the sternum rather than toward the left axilla reflecting the predominance of left ventricular–to–right atrial shunting over left ventricular–to–left atrial shunting. When the ventricular septal defect is restrictive and a substantial pressure gradient between the left and right ventricles exists, a separate murmur of ventricular septal defect may be present, most prominently heard at the lower left sternal border.

ELECTROCARDIOGRAPHY

The most characteristic ECG abnormality of AV canal defect is a superiorly oriented QRS frontal plane axis with a counterclockwise depolarization pattern. The mechanism of alteration of the frontal plane QRS axis in these patients is not caused by ventricular hypertrophy but by abnormally positioned conduction tissue, which causes abnormal sequences of cardiac activation. Often, AV conduction delay exists (as evidenced by a prolonged PR interval). Typically, electrocardiographic manifestations of right ventricular hypertrophy are also present. Electrocardiographic suggestions of biventricular or left ventricular hypertrophy may occur, particularly if mitral or AV valve insufficiency is severe.

CHEST RADIOGRAPHY

Usually, cardiac enlargement is present on chest radiography in patients with ostium primum or complete AV canal defects. In particular, right atrial and right ventricular enlargement are often present. The enlarged right heart may displace the left ventricle rendering evaluation of left ventricular size difficult.

Usually, the main pulmonary artery is prominent and, if a large left–to–right shunt is present, increased pulmonary vascular markings usually exist. With severe pulmonary vascular disease, the distal pulmonary vessels may have a lucent, pruned appearance. Severe enlargement of the pulmonary trunk and left atrium may compress the left main stem bronchus and cause atelectasis of parts of the left lung.

ECHOCARDIOGRAPHY

Two-Dimensional Echocardiography

Two-dimensional echocardiography is highly reliable in identifying AV canal defects. The hallmark of the diagnosis is demonstration of an absent AV septum. In ostium primum ASDs, the AV valve leaflets appear to originate from the crest of the ventricular septum. In complete AV canal defects, the bridging leaflets of the common AV valve are observed to cross the ventricular septum.

Doppler Echocardiography

Doppler echocardiography can substantially contribute to the evaluation of AV canal defects. Pulsed Doppler is especially useful in the detection of left and right ventricular outflow obstruction and the presence of a ductus arteriosus. Pulsed Doppler examination also facilitates identification of AV valve regurgitation and has been used to quantitate its degree. Continuous-wave Doppler is useful in quantitating pressure gradients in these patients. When a ventricular defect is present, the instantaneous pressure difference between the right and left ventricles can be determined using the modified Bernoulli formula. Similarly, pressure gradients across the left and right ventricular outflow tracts can be quantitated. Color Doppler studies are also helpful, particularly for determining the location and roughly quantitating the degree of AV valve insufficiency.

Transesophageal Echocardiography

Excellent images of the AV septum and of the AV valves and their attachments can be obtained with transesophageal echocardiography. Generally, Doppler color flow mapping of AV valve flow from the transesophageal approach is also excellent. The most extensive use of transesophageal imaging in patients with AV canal is intraoperatively to evaluate postoperative AV valve regurgitation, to check for residual atrial and ventricular septal defects, to rule out ventricular outflow tract obstruction, and to assess cardiac function.

CARDIAC CATHETERIZATION

AV canal defects can be suspected at cardiac catheterization when the catheter course across the atrial septum is low in the septum. Oxygen saturation and hemodynamic data obtained at cardiac catheterization can provide definitive assessment of pulmonary pressures, of left–to–right and right–to–left shunting, and of pulmonary vascular resistance.

Treatment

MEDICAL THERAPY

When heart failure and associated pulmonary congestion are present, anticongestive measures such as diuretics and digoxin are indicated. Generally, long periods of fluid restriction are counterproductive, because the patients in distress are usually small infants and such restriction deprives them of calories needed for growth. Hydralazine has been shown to reduce the magnitude of left–to–right shunting acutely in these patients, but no long-term experience with the drug in complete AV canal defects has been reported. Most cardiologists do not favor prolonged medical therapy in affected patients if their symptoms are refractory but, instead, refer them for surgical treatment.

SURGICAL THERAPY

Recommendations for surgical treatment depend on the anatomic characteristics of the defect and on associated anomalies. Generally, patients with an ostium primum ASD, separate AV valves, no ventricular defect, and minimal AV valve insufficiency are asymptomatic during infancy and childhood. Because repair of ostium primum ASD is associated with a substantially greater morbidity and mortality than is repair of a secundum ASD, many cardiologists do not recommend surgery at any age if cardiomegaly is absent, which is usually the case when AV valve insufficiency is mild and the pulmonary–to–systemic flow ratio is less than 2:1. Almost invariably, infants who have partial AV canal defects and are symptomatic have severe AV valve regurgitation. Generally, pulmonary artery banding does not help these patients. Therefore, corrective surgery with mitral valvuloplasty and closure of the ASD is usually recommended. Usually, asymptomatic patients with ostium primum ASDs that do exhibit substantial cardiomegaly are referred for elective surgical repair when they are near school age.

For patients with uncomplicated complete AV canal defects, most centers advocate corrective surgery in early infancy. Palliative procedures such as pulmonary artery banding may be more appropriate in patients who have AV canal defects in association with other anomalies such as hypoplasia of the left ventricle. When pulmonary pressures are near systemic, as they generally are in patients who have complete AV canal defects but do not have associated right ventricular outflow obstruction, pulmonary vascular disease usually develops after the first year of life. Therefore, either corrective surgery or a palliative procedure to protect the pulmonary circulation during infancy is recommended in such patients.

PROGNOSIS

Long-term results of surgical therapy greatly depend on the degree of preoperative pulmonary vascular disease and on the extent of residual left AV valve regurgitation. In many cases, the left AV valve regurgitation is reduced substantially and the left–to–right shunt is abolished or reduced to minimal levels by corrective surgery. However, when pulmonary vascular disease is present preoperatively, hospital morbidity and mortality are high, and little improvement occurs in the late follow-up period for those patients who survive operation. Postoperative arrhythmias including complete heart block can occur and may increase in frequency as patients grow older. With advancing age, patients may require mitral valve replacement.

CHAPTER 142
Pulmonary Stenosis

Adapted from John P. Cheatham

PULMONARY VALVE STENOSIS

Pulmonary valve stenosis constitutes approximately 7% to 12% of all congenital heart disease and up to 80% to 90% of all lesions causing obstruction of right ventricular output. The gross and microscopic features of pulmonary valve stenosis are classified into six categories (Table 142-1). The pathologic processes affecting the remaining portion of the right-sided cardiac structures involve changes secondary to the valve obstruction (i.e., right ventricular hypertrophy, fibrosis, and tricuspid valve abnormalities).

Clinical Characteristics

Clinically, pulmonary valve stenosis with intact ventricular septum is best described as mild, moderate, or severe, which is dependant upon the systolic transvalvular gradient and right ventricular pressure. Patients with mild stenosis are asymptomatic, exhibiting normal growth and development, and no cyanosis. The jugular venous pulse is normal, and no sign of congestive heart failure is present. Children with moderate stenosis and an intact ventricular septum may develop mild dyspnea with exertion, but they are frequently asymptomatic. Cyanosis with exertion may be noted occasionally if an atrial septal defect is present. Individuals with severe valvular stenosis usually demonstrate symptoms, although as many as 25% of these patients are asymptomatic. Frequently, dyspnea and fatigue with only a moderate amount of exertion are present. Central cyanosis is one of the most important signs in patients with an atrial communication; it may be present at rest or with minimal exercise. Some evidence indicates that the degree of cyanosis increases with age. When "squatting" is seen in a cyanotic child suspected of having pulmonary valve stenosis, the diagnosis of tetralogy of Fallot must be considered. Growth and development in infants with severe stenosis are usually normal without evidence of wasting. "Moon facies," in conjunction with a chubby phenotype, has been described as characteristic of children with pulmonary valve stenosis, but it is not pathognomonic and is present in fewer than 50% of infants with severe obstruction.

The cardiovascular examination aids in the diagnosis of pulmonary valve stenosis. The precordial activity is quiet with mild obstruction, but it may be increased with a palpable right ventricular tap in patients with moderate or severe stenosis. A systolic thrill over the pulmonary valve area may be present as the severity increases. The striking auscultatory feature of pulmonary valve stenosis is a prominent systolic ejection murmur. The murmur may vary in length and intensity, but it usually ends before the aortic valve closes. The maximum intensity of the murmur is at the upper left sternal border radiating to the back, but it is also heard along the precordium and the neck. As the severity increases, the systolic ejection murmur lengthens, and the peak in intensity occurs later. The murmur of pulmonary valve stenosis increases in duration and intensity after amyl nitrate inhalation, whereas the opposite is true in children with tetralogy of Fallot.

A high-pitched ejection sound or systolic click is usually audible along the left upper sternal border. The click probably originates from the sudden opening and doming of the thickened pulmonary valve leaflets. As the severity of the obstruction increases, the systolic ejection click occurs earlier until, in severe stenosis, it may be indistinguishable from the first heart sound. The second heart sound is usually split and of normal intensity in mild stenosis. The degree of splitting is directly proportional to the severity of obstruction. An inverse relationship exists between the severity of stenosis and the intensity of the pulmonary component of the second heart sound. In severe stenosis, therefore, a wide splitting of the second heart sound is present with a very soft pulmonary component that is often heard as a single second sound.

The electrocardiogram is frequently normal in mild stenosis, whereas it is normal in only 10% of children with moderate obstruction, and it is uniformly abnormal in cases of severe stenosis. Right axis deviation is frequently seen with right ventricular hypertrophy noted in the anterior precordial leads. In moderate stenosis, the magnitude of the R wave in V_1 is usually less than 20 mm, whereas an upright T wave in V_1 is present approximately 50% of the time. A qR or a pure R wave of more than 20 mm is present in patients with severe stenosis. In some children, ST or T waves may suggest ischemia.

The most consistent and distinctive radiographic feature is prominence in the main pulmonary artery segment secondary to poststenotic dilatation of the pulmonary trunk and the proximal left pulmonary artery (Fig. 142-1). The aortic arch is usually left-sided. Presence of a right arch should

TABLE 142-1. Gross and Microscopic Features of Pulmonary Valve Stenosis

Domed	42%
Dysplastic	19%
Unicommissural	16%
Bicuspid	10%
Hypoplastic annulus	6.5%
Tricuspid	6.5%

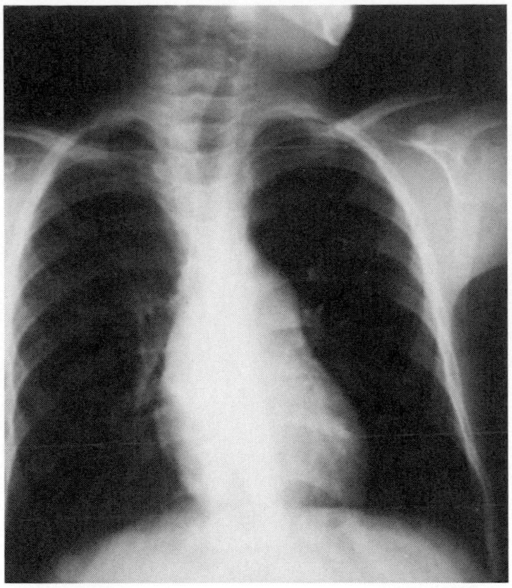

Figure 142-1. Chest roentgenogram from an 8-year-old boy with mild stenosis of the pulmonary valve. Heart size is usually normal. Pulmonary vascular markings are unremarkable. The most distinctive radiographic feature of this disease is poststenotic dilatation of the pulmonary trunk, as depicted in this chest film. The degree of dilatation is unrelated to the severity of stenosis.

lead the physician to consider the diagnosis of tetralogy of Fallot.

Doppler echocardiography with color flow mapping techniques increases both the sensitivity and specificity of the diagnosis of pulmonary valve stenosis. Two-dimensional echocardiography enables visualization of the thickened and domed pulmonary valve leaflets, pulmonary annulus, dilated pulmonary trunk, hypertrophic right ventricle, and other associated congenital heart defects. Pulsed and continuous-wave Doppler echocardiography enable accurate estimation of the location and severity of pulmonary stenosis without invasive procedures.

The role of cardiac catheterization and angiography in the diagnosis and treatment of pulmonary valve stenosis has changed significantly since the early 1980s. In the past, information obtained in the catheterization laboratory was a prerequisite for selecting patients for surgical valvotomy. Since the initial use of percutaneous, transluminal balloon pulmonary valvuloplasty in 1982, the catheterization laboratory has become the location for the "treatment" of moderate and severe pulmonary valve stenosis. The most important hemodynamic information obtained during cardiac catheterization is the measurement of right ventricular pressure simultaneously with left ventricular or aortic pressure and the systolic gradient across the pulmonary valve. Defining any associated cardiac defects at this time is also important. Angiographic features of pulmonary valve stenosis include thickening and doming of valve leaflets with poststenotic dilatation of the pulmonary trunk (Fig. 142-2).

The differential diagnosis of pulmonary valve stenosis with intact ventricular septum is shown in Table 142-2. When cyanosis is present, tetralogy of Fallot and pulmonary valve atresia with intact ventricular septum should be considered. The correct diagnosis can usually be made by physical examination, but echocardiography may help distinguish among various congenital heart defects. Pulmonary valve stenosis may be associated with various systemic diseases and syndromes (e.g., glycogen storage disease, neurofibromatosis, gout, neoplasm, carcinoid bowel disease, and Noonan, Williams, Watson, and Leopard syndromes).

The natural history of mild pulmonary valve stenosis is benign. Little improvement in severe obstruction occurs, however, and the transvalvular gradient often increases with age. A definite risk of right-sided congestive heart failure, myocardial fibrosis, and sudden death in these patients exists. The clinical course and prognosis of moderate pulmonary valve stenosis is under debate, but exercise studies demonstrating right ventricular dysfunction in adults are alarming. The risk of infective endocarditis in patients with pulmonary valve stenosis is low, but all individuals, regardless of the severity of stenosis or whether intervention has taken place, should receive selected antibiotics for infective endocarditis prophylaxis during indicated dental or surgical procedures.

Treatment

Medical treatment of children with pulmonary valve stenosis is usually confined to neonates with critical obstruction. These newborns present with cyanosis, right-sided congestive heart failure, and cardiomegaly. Because adequate pulmonary blood

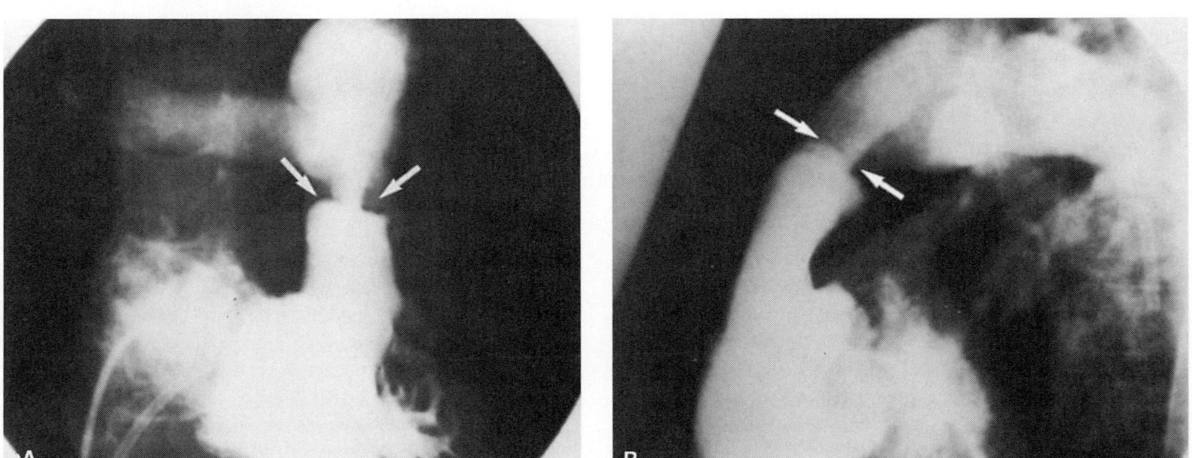

Figure 142-2. Right ventriculogram in a patient with typical features of moderate pulmonary valve stenosis. **A:** Anteroposterior view demonstrating systolic doming of the stenotic leaflets with a "jet" of contrast material noted (*arrows*). The infundibulum is widely patent, and the main pulmonary artery is dilated. **B:** Lateral projection shows the systolic jet that passes through the thickened leaflets (*arrows*).

TABLE 142-2. Differential Diagnosis of Pulmonary Valve Stenosis

Atrial septal defect (ASD)
Pulmonary artery stenosis
Ventricular septal defect (VSD)
Idiopathic dilatation of the main pulmonary artery
Straight-back syndrome
Mitral valve prolapse (MVP)
Aortic valve stenosis
Benign pulmonary flow murmurs

flow depends on patency of the ductus arteriosus, prostaglandin E_1 intravenous infusion (0.05–0.10 mg/kg/minute) is lifesaving. Anticongestive medications (e.g., digoxin, furosemide, dopamine) may also be necessary. The treatment of choice in these neonates, as well as in children with moderate to severe stenosis, is transcatheter balloon pulmonary valvuloplasty performed in the cardiac catheterization laboratory.

Since its initial description in 1982, balloon dilation of the thickened pulmonary valve has evolved into a fairly standard treatment performed by the pediatric cardiac interventionalist. After hemodynamic measurements are obtained and right ventriculography is performed, a properly sized balloon catheter is chosen (1.2–1.4 times the size of the angiographically measured annulus). The balloon catheter is positioned over a guidewire through the stenotic pulmonary valve, and the balloon is inflated (by use of a hand-held gauge) to the recommended burst pressure (measured in atmospheres) or until the balloon "waist" disappears (Fig. 142-3). The introduction of larger-diameter balloon catheters (20–40 mm) allows a single catheter to be used in most instances. Occasionally, two balloon catheters are required. In the neonate with critical pulmonary valve stenosis, the transcatheter dilation of the valve is considerably more difficult and requires operator expertise.

Balloon valvuloplasty produces relief of obstruction by commissural splitting of the valve but sometimes may cause avulsion of leaflets. Typically, immediate relief of the transvalvar gradient occurs in moderate pulmonary valve stenosis after successful balloon valvuloplasty. In patients with severe stenosis, and certainly in the neonate with critical obstruction, the right ventricular pressure falls significantly but is seldom normal. Dynamic infundibular subpulmonary stenosis accounts for the residual gradient initially, but it has a tendency to improve with time as the right ventricular hypertrophy regresses.

The response of dysplastic pulmonary valves to balloon dilation varies but, in general, is less than that of nondysplastic valves. This type of valvar stenosis is present in approximately 50% of children with Noonan syndrome. Valve leaflets are unfused and excessively thick and demonstrate little motion during the cardiac cycle. Both balloon valvuloplasty and surgical valvotomy are usually inadequate procedures to relieve the obstruction completely. Partial or total surgical valvectomy may be required to relieve the valvar gradient in these children, but balloon valvuloplasty should be attempted initially.

According to the Valvuloplasty and Angioplasty of Congenital Anomalies (VACA) Registry, the overall risk of a major complication during balloon pulmonary valvuloplasty is 0.6% percent including death (0.2%), cardiac perforation with tamponade (0.1%), and severe tricuspid insufficiency (0.2%). Minor complications occur in 1.3% of patients, whereas 2.6% experience an incident defined as arrhythmia, hypoxemia, or venous bleeding. The incidence of complications is inversely related to age, and is substantially higher in neonates who exhibit critical narrowing of the pulmonary valve.

Although surgical pulmonary valvotomy is a relatively low-risk procedure (3%–4% mortality), this procedure is seldom necessary because balloon valvuloplasty is available and effective. When surgery is required, inflow occlusion with transarterial valvotomy or "open" valvotomy with cardiopulmonary bypass is the method usually used. The incidence of pulmonary insufficiency postoperatively varies from 57% to 90%, whereas an incidence of 13% to 45% has been reported after balloon valvuloplasty. However, Doppler echocardiography and color-flow mapping are sensitive methods for detecting valvar insufficiency and suggest that a small amount of regurgitation is present in most patients after surgical or balloon valvotomy.

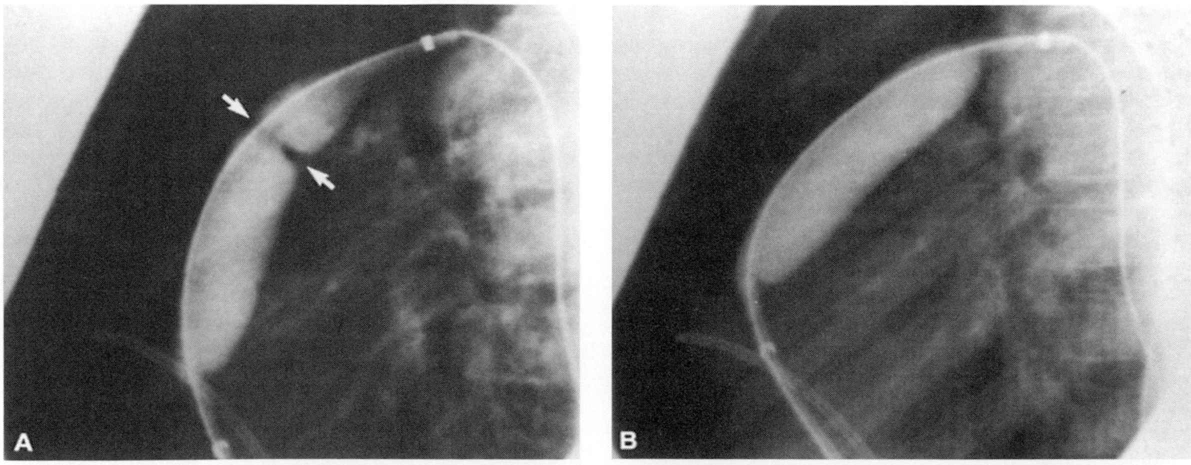

Figure 142-3. Proper positioning of the balloon catheter for pulmonary valvuloplasty via the lateral view under fluoroscopy. **A:** A guidewire passes through the catheter from the right ventricular outflow tract into the left pulmonary artery. The balloon is inflated with diluted contrast material (20%) until a "waist" is seen that corresponds to the stenotic valve leaflets (*arrows*). Attempts to maintain the waist at the mid-portion of the balloon should be made while the catheter is positioned. In this case, the waist is toward the distal one-third of the balloon. **B:** The balloon is repositioned more distally and is completely inflated using a hand-held manometer. Note that the hourglass waist has disappeared.

A special task force committee composed of members of the American Heart Association who specialize in cardiovascular diseases of the young recommends that physical activity in patients with treated or untreated mild pulmonary valve stenosis remain unrestricted. Light exercise (e.g., nonstrenuous team games, recreational swimming, jogging, cycling, and golf) is recommended for patients with moderate stenosis. Moderate limitation of physical activities (e.g., attending school but not participating in physical education classes) is recommended for children with severe pulmonary valve stenosis. A general guideline is to treat the underlying stenosis rather than restrict physical activity.

PULMONARY ARTERY STENOSIS

Obstruction of pulmonary blood flow along the pulmonary arterial tree may occur at many sites. The overall incidence of pulmonary arterial stenosis is 2% to 3% of cases of congenital heart disease. Isolated pulmonary artery stenosis occurs in one-third of the cases, but associated cardiac defects occur in two-thirds of the patients. The most common associated defects are pulmonary valve stenosis and VSD (i.e., tetralogy of Fallot). Multiple peripheral pulmonary artery stenoses are commonly present in rubella and the Williams syndrome. Several other syndromes including Noonan, Alagille, Ehlers-Danlos, cutis laxa, and Silver-Russell also have this associated defect.

Clinical Characteristics

Clinical features of pulmonary artery stenosis may be easily masked by associated defects. Close inspection and auscultation, however, reveal a systolic ejection murmur that is heard over the pulmonary area but is particularly loud in the back and lateral lung fields. A systolic ejection click is absent. A continuous murmur may be present in as many as 10% of patients indicating a significant diastolic, as well as systolic, gradient. The degree of right ventricular hypertrophy visible on the electrocardiogram depends on the severity of the obstruction. The chest roentgenogram is usually normal. Whereas the echocardiogram may be helpful in defining associated intracardiac defects, it is not reliable in imaging the sites of pulmonary artery stenosis. Therefore, cardiac catheterization and angiography are imperative for these children. Selective right ventriculography and pulmonary arteriography are necessary to precisely define the areas of stenosis.

Treatment

In isolated cases, the natural history may be benign, but progressive increase in severity with subsequent death in early infancy and childhood has been reported. Because of the poor surgical results in the treatment of isolated and complicated pulmonary artery stenosis, the use of balloon angioplasty began in 1980. Initial balloon diameters three to four times the diameter of the stenotic vessel were chosen when only low-pressure balloons (4–6 atm) were available. However, newer materials allow high-pressure balloon inflation (8–18 atm) with improved results of gradient reduction using balloon diameters of only two to three times the stenotic pulmonary artery diameter. The mechanism of successful balloon angioplasty may play a role in the potential complication of vessel disruption leading to hemorrhage. For this reason, surgical backup and blood availability are arranged when this procedure is to be performed.

The VACA Registry reports a 3% risk of death during balloon pulmonary artery angioplasty. In addition, complications such as vessel perforation, hemorrhage, and arrhythmias occur in 10% of patients. Success for dilation was arbitrarily defined as (a) an increase in stenosis diameter equal to or greater than 50% of predilation diameter, (b) an increase of more than 20% of blood flow to the affected lung, or (c) a decrease of at least 20% in the ratio of systolic right ventricular to aortic pressure. The success rate using low-pressure balloons (4–8 atm) was a disappointing 55%. However, using high-pressure balloons, the rate increased to 80% in the vessels dilated with only a 2% mortality risk and an overall 13% complication rate.

Since 1991, the use of the balloon expandable Palmaz intravascular stent has dramatically improved the results of transcatheter therapy for pulmonary artery stenosis. The intravascular stent overcomes the natural "recoil" of the artery and significantly reduces the pressure gradient and increases vessel diameter. In addition, the balloon expandable characteristic of the stent allows for future redilation to a larger diameter as the child grows. The addition of intravascular stents in the treatment of pulmonary artery stenosis has significantly improved the overall results in more than 95% of stenotic lesions.

The operator expertise and skill required to implant intravascular stents successfully in children with pulmonary artery stenosis is high. Therefore, this procedure should only be performed by appropriately trained pediatric cardiac interventionalists. The risks of the procedure are no different from those of balloon angioplasty alone, except for the possibility of stent migration or embolization. Antiplatelet therapy (aspirin, dipyridamole) is usually recommended after intravascular stent implantation to decrease the incidence of thrombosis. Regardless of therapy, infective endocarditis prophylaxis is recommended for all patients with this cardiac defect.

CHAPTER 143
Patent Ductus Arteriosus

Adapted from Charles E. Mullins

The patent ductus arteriosus (PDA) is an essential structure that occurs normally in the fetus and only becomes abnormal when it persists after birth. In the full-term infant, the persistent ductus probably represents a structural abnormality in the ductus tissues present at birth. The persistent patency of the ductus in a premature infant is a more common problem and is usually a result of immaturity of ductal tissues. Persistent PDA is the second most common congenital heart defect accounting for approximately 10% of all congenital heart defects in full-term infants.

In the fetal circulation, the ductus allows right ventricular blood to bypass the nonexpanded and nonventilated lungs. Both the low Po_2 of the blood and a high level of circulating prostaglandins in the fetus inhibit constriction of the ductus. In the normal newborn, lung expansion occurs immediately on delivery. As a result, most of the right ventricular blood and, in turn, pulmonary artery blood is diverted immediately to the now lowered-resistance pulmonary vascular bed. This obligatory flow through the lungs allows circulating prostaglandins in the fetus to be cleared by the most effective clearing system, the lungs, and permits immediate oxygenation of the blood, thereby increasing the circulating Po_2. Both the decreased prostaglandins and the increased blood Po_2 contribute to normal constriction of the ductus. Normally, the ductus of a newborn is functionally closed by, at most, 72 hours of age, and it is structurally sealed by 3 months.

Not all factors that result in persistent patency of the ductus are understood. Factors such as high altitude or severe pulmonary disease that cause persistent hypoxia predispose the infant to persistent patency of the ductus. Continued high prostaglandin levels, in the presence of a compromised or inefficient pulmonary clearing function (found in premature infants or in the case of marked decreased pulmonary flow, as occurs in some pulmonary atresia patients), contribute to the persistent patency of the ductus. Rubella and, possibly, other viral infections during the first trimester of pregnancy frequently result in patency of the ductus. Some evidence shows that a lower socioeconomic status, probably resulting in inadequate perinatal nutrition, may also be a predisposing factor.

In the usual patient with a left aortic arch, the ductus arteriosus connects the junction of the main and left pulmonary arteries to the descending thoracic aorta at a point just distal to the origin of the left subclavian artery. Clinical findings depend on the final net flow through the lungs into the left atrium, left ventricle, and aorta, and back through the ductus. The uncomplicated patent ductus places a pure volume workload on the left heart with little or no effect on the right heart.

CLINICAL FINDINGS AND DIAGNOSIS

Symptoms

Clinical histories of patients with persistent patent ductus range from florid heart failure in the young infant to an incidental murmur in an otherwise perfectly healthy child or, occasionally, even in an adult. The patient with a persistent patent ductus may present as early as the newborn period and anytime thereafter including late adulthood. The most common presentation is a heart murmur discovered incidentally in an asymptomatic young child who is being examined for some other reason. The infant or child with a moderate to large patent ductus may be more susceptible to secondary infections in the lower respiratory tract after initial upper respiratory infections, probably because of the decreased compliance of the lungs associated with significantly increased pulmonary blood flow.

The typical murmur of a patent ductus is continuous (sounding like machinery) and is maximum in the first and second left intercostal spaces in the left midclavicular line. The murmur begins with the first heart sound, then crescendos throughout systole until the second heart sound. The murmur peaks in intensity at the second sound before trailing off during diastole. Depending on the shape and size of the ductus, the intensity of the murmur varies from grade 1 to grade 6, and the quality ranges from high pitched and blowing to low frequency and rough.

Because of the increased volume of flow and the direction of this flow directly toward the pulmonary valve, the pulmonary component of the second sound is intensified and delayed. Peripheral pulses are bounding in quality, as a result of both the increased left ventricular stroke volume and the diastolic runoff into the lungs. This combination generates a wide pulse pressure. In the patient with a large persistent ductus, pulses are often visible in the suprasternal, carotid, axillary, and femoral areas.

Tests

The electrocardiogram in the uncomplicated ductus is normal or, in a large ductus, demonstrates left ventricular hypertrophy and left atrial enlargement. The chest radiograph shows cardiomegaly proportionate to the flow through the ductus with a prominent main pulmonary artery segment, large ascending aorta and arch, increased pulmonary vascular markings, and a "left ventricular" contour of the heart shadow with possible left atrial enlargement.

The diagnosis can be documented by echocardiography. The ductus can usually be seen on two-dimensional echocardiogram. Turbulent flow on Doppler interrogation in the main pulmonary artery supports the echocardiogram. Intracardiac lesions other than the persistent ductus can be ruled out, as can lesions that can be confused with the ductus. Continuous-wave Doppler studies detect very small streams of abnormal flow in the pulmonary artery. Even the very tiny ductus that is too small to be audible or visualized by echocardiogram can be detected by continuous-wave Doppler; alternatively, the flow can be seen on color Doppler.

When all clinical findings of the ductus are assimilated and are absolutely characteristic, the diagnosis is established without further study. If even one atypical feature is present in any part of the clinical assessment, the diagnosis should be established by cardiac catheterization. Catheterization definitively rules out defects that may be confused with a ductus or establishes the presence of other defects that may be incidentally associated with the ductus.

DIFFERENTIAL DIAGNOSIS

The Venous Hum

A venous hum is the murmur most often confused with a PDA; it is the most benign and easiest murmur to differentiate clinically. When carefully examined, the venous hum is continuous but usually of a softer, "more distant" quality than a PDA. Most importantly, the venous hum crescendos or peaks in diastole. It is usually maximum in the first and second right intercostal spaces. It varies in intensity, or it can be eliminated by changes in body position, respirations, or neck rotation. The venous hum can be stopped by placing the patient in the supine position and simultaneously applying light compression over the right jugular vein in the right supraclavicular area. Given the auscultatory characteristics of the venous hum and the maneuvers to eliminate it, no further diagnostic studies should be necessary.

Aortopulmonary Windows

The lesion that is potentially most difficult to differentiate from the persistent ductus is an aortopulmonary window, which is a rare occurrence. An aortopulmonary window is a window-like communication between the proximal ascending aorta and the main pulmonary artery that allows systemic blood to flow directly from the ascending aorta into the pulmonary artery. The hemodynamics are identical to those of the ductus, and the site of the abnormal communication is anatomically close to that of the ductus; thus, many clinical findings are similar, if not identical, to the patent ductus. However, patients with an aortopulmonary window usually present early in infancy with significant respiratory distress and signs of congestive heart failure. Confirmation of the diagnosis must be made by echocardiogram and usually by high-quality angiography also.

VSD with Aortic Insufficiency

A more common lesion that can be confused with a patent ductus, if the physical examination is not precise, is the combination of ventricular septal defect with associated aortic valve insufficiency. The murmur in these patients is "to and fro" rather than continuous. A plateau pansystolic murmur that ends at the second heart sound is detected from the ventricular septal defect, followed by a higher-pitched decrescendo diastolic murmur from the aortic regurgitation. Other physical findings, the electrocardiogram, and radiographs may be similar to those of a patent ductus, but the lesions should be distinguishable by astute auscultation and, if not by the physical examination, then by echocardiography and cardiac catheterization.

COMPLICATED DUCTUS

Bounding Pulses

When a ductus is present with other congenital heart lesions, it may be difficult to detect. The characteristic murmur and radiographic findings of the ductus may be overshadowed by the physical signs, radiographic appearance, and electrocardiogram of the associated lesion. In the absence of the classic continuous murmur of a persistent ductus, the one finding on physical examination that should cause the examiner to suspect a patent ductus is the presence of full or bounding pulses, which would not be expected with intracardiac shunts. Associated defects and persistent ductus should be visualized by a carefully performed echocardiogram.

Ductal Dependent Lesions

For two categories of patients with congenital heart lesions, the associated patent ductus is essential to survival of the patient and is, therefore, a ductus-dependent lesion. The first category includes those patients with severe coarctation of the aorta or interruption of the aortic arch. In these patients, the blood flow to the lower body may depend on the ductus. With the coarctation, the dilated aortic end of the open ductus allows blood flow around or adjacent to the obstruction in the aorta. With complete interruption of the aorta, the blood flow is from the pulmonary artery through the ductus into the descending aorta with the lower body blood flow emanating solely from this route. The second category includes cyanotic patients with a severely restricted or totally obstructed pulmonary valve. In these patients, the total or greatest amount of pulmonary blood flow emanates from the patent ductus. These ductus-dependent lesions must be recognized early, and efforts must be made to keep the ductus open until the appropriate surgical procedure can be performed.

Complications

Bacterial endocarditis is a potential complication in the patient with patent ductus. Since the advent of early surgical correction of the ductus and the use of prophylactic antibiotics in patients with congenital heart lesions, the incidence of this complication has decreased markedly. Its occurrence in patients with patent ductus is now the least of the isolated congenital heart defects. The prevention of this complication is now the major indication for correction of most of the small ductus.

THERAPY

Supportive

Therapy for patent ductus can be supportive or definitive. Supportive therapy involves treatment of symptoms resulting from the patent ductus. Patients with a large persistent ductus exhibit signs and symptoms of pulmonary overcirculation with shortness of breath, dyspnea, and even overt pulmonary edema. Symptoms can be treated with digoxin and vigorous diuretic therapy. Occasionally, the young infant with a large patent ductus must be intubated and ventilated with positive end-expiratory pressure to control pulmonary overcirculation. These medical measures help control symptoms, but they do not treat the underlying anatomic defect.

Surgical Repair

Definitive therapy for the ductus is complete interruption of blood flow through the ductus. Heretofore, the established definitive therapy for a persistent ductus was surgical ligation and division of the ductus. Definitive therapy is indicated when supportive therapy does not allow normal growth, development, and activity of the infant or child. When no supportive therapy is necessary or when supportive therapy is required and satisfactorily maintains the patient, then elective surgical repair is considered for the patient any time after 2 to 3 years of age but usually before the child enters school. Surgical repair of the ductus requires a thoracotomy; however, it does not require cardiopulmonary bypass. In addition to the acute risks of surgery and recovery, rare but, possibly, permanent complications can occur including vocal cord or diaphragmatic paralysis from intrathoracic nerve injury or even ligation of the wrong vessel or structure within the chest. In addition to the morbidity of the surgery, a small, finite mortality is associated with surgical repair of the patent ductus.

Recanalization

One year after the ligation and division surgery, the ductus is considered cured. By then, complete healing is ensured and risk of endocarditis is considered eliminated. After surgical ligation only, instances of "recanalization" of the ductus have occurred in as many as 10% of cases. Data accumulated from other ductus occlusion techniques and from high-resolution Doppler studies show that "recanalization" of the ductus after surgical ligation may have actually been a residual tiny ductus after an initial attempted ligation.

Nonsurgical Approaches

Alternative, nonsurgical, definitive approaches to elective correction of the patent ductus are available. William Rashkind reported closure of a patent ductus using a tiny, single-hooked umbrella in a 3.5-kg infant in 1979. The device was effective in that patient, but because of the attachment hooks, it is unsatisfactory for general use. As a result, a safer, more usable version, the Rashkind PDA Occluder (USCI Division of CA Band, Billerica, MA), was developed. The Rashkind device is a tiny spring-loaded, double umbrella that is delivered through a relatively small catheter by either the arterial or venous approach. Unfortunately, this device did not get FDA approval for use in the United States. However, the Rashkind PDA Occluder is approved and is in clinical use in most countries outside the United States. In the experience of more than 10,000 patients and with a 16-year follow-up, the device has proved effective and safe. The results show no mortality, little morbidity, and 87% total occlusion with the device. The major remaining problem with the device is the presence of tiny inaudible residual leaks in 10% to 12% of cases. These tiny leaks have no known clinical consequence, but, theoretically, they could be a site for endocarditis.

Alternative Devices

Lack of approval to use a catheter-delivered device in the United States led to the development of several effective alternatives for transcatheter repair of a PDA. The most useful alternative was a unique new application for an approved vascular occlusion device. Cambier and Moore demonstrated the safe use of a standard Gianturco coil (Cook Inc., Bloomington, IN). This relatively easy, inexpensive, effective, and safe procedure was adopted by most pediatric cardiology centers and, by 1997, had become the accepted standard therapy for closure of a patent ductus. The Gianturco coil bears the limitation of poor controllability and, as a consequence, occasional embolization of the coil. To overcome this problem, several modifications of the delivery technique have been developed. Outside the United States, the coil and delivery apparatus have been modified to include a built-in attach-release mechanism to render the procedure even safer.

Additional Devices

In addition to the Gianturco coil and its modifications, several devices have been specifically developed for transcatheter PDA occlusion. In the United States, the Gianturco–Grifka Vascular Occlusion Device (Cook Inc., Bloomington, IN) was designed and approved by the FDA for the occlusion of long tubular structures up to 9 mm in diameter. A preformed, specifically coiled wire occluder, the Duct–Occlud Device (PFM, Gmbh, Köln/Sürth, Germany), has been used outside the United States, and preliminary trials of the device have begun in this country. Additional devices designed for occlusion of other structures have been used sporadically and will be more appropriately applied in the future for the closure of a large PDA.

Transcatheter ductal occlusion with one of the occlusion devices is not only an acceptable technique but is also now the preferred procedure for elective correction of a PDA. If occlusion with one of the occlusion devices is unsuccessful, then the patient may have to undergo surgical repair of the ductus. Whereas a patent ductus in the premature infant still requires surgical closure, elective correction of a patent ductus beyond infancy should be relegated to the annals of congenital heart disease history.

CHAPTER 144
Coarctation of the Aorta

Adapted from Mary J. H. Morriss and Dan G. McNamara

Coarctation of the aorta is a congenital malformation characterized by a constriction of a segment of the aorta. Usually, an abrupt narrowing of the lumen of the vessel occurs in the thoracic descending aorta producing obstruction to blood flow (Fig. 144-1). To be clinically significant, the narrowing must be marked and must effectively reduce the diameter of the aorta by at least 50%. To maintain flow and adequate perfusion pressure to the kidneys and lower body, blood pressure proximal to the obstruction becomes elevated.

Coarctation of the aorta is a common congenital defect occurring in frequency just after ventricular septal defect and patent ductus arteriosus in most series. It has a striking male–to–female patient preponderance in excess of 2:1. Patients with the full XO Turner syndrome with ovarian agenesis and short stature have a high incidence of coarctation in 20% of cases. A more extreme anomaly with complete interruption of the aortic arch in a slightly different location, just proximal to the origin of the left subclavian artery, has a high association with DiGeorge syndrome, with deletion in a defined region of chromosome 22, and is functionally analogous to severe coarctation with a reverse ductus arteriosus.

COARCTATION IN INFANCY

Symptoms

Coarctation syndrome in infancy is characterized by a high association with other defects that result in systemic right ventricle, reversed flow from right to left through the ductus arteriosus, and more severe hypoplasia of a greater portion of the aortic arch, although discrete coarctation may be present. Infants with coarctation can appear to be well at birth, but cardiac failure, respiratory distress, and cardiogenic shock may rapidly appear as the ductus constricts. Because of the severe impairment of cardiac output, a murmur may not be detected until the infant is stabilized and treated. The pulse discrepancy may not be apparent in the infant because the widely patent ductus serves as a route for flow to the descending aorta, so coarctation is not excluded even if normal pulses are felt on a routine newborn examination. Differential cyanosis can exist potentially with shunting of the blood with a lower saturation to the lower body from the pulmonary artery via the ductus; however, the high frequency of associated defects, particularly left–to–right shunts, may allow pulmonary saturations to be only slightly lower than aortic saturations masking this difference clinically. Marked benefit can be obtained by dilating the ductus arteriosus with prostaglandin infusion, thus enabling improved renal perfusion and reversal of acidosis and cardiogenic shock.

Tests

The electrocardiogram of infants with coarctation of the aorta is normal less frequently because it reflects coexistent anatomic defects. Isolated coarctation of the aorta in infancy is accompanied by electrocardiographic evidence of right ventricular hypertrophy, but additional left ventricular hypertrophy or rare left ventricular strain can also be present.

The chest film of the ill infant generally correlates with the clinical state showing dilatation of the heart with congestive heart failure and an increase in pulmonary vascular markings caused by either an associated left–to–right shunt or passive venous congestion.

The echocardiogram helps outline additional defects of the heart, enables assessment of left ventricular function, and possibly shows the area of coarctation. However, testing may be confounded in the presence of a widely patent ductus arteriosus.

COARCTATION BEYOND INFANCY

Symptoms

Coarctation of the aorta beyond infancy is recognized clinically when blood pressure recordings are obtained from all four extremities; its hallmark is hypertension in the upper extremities and decreased blood pressure in the lower extremities. The discrepancy in blood pressure, rather than an absolute level of proximal blood pressure elevation, is the most striking event; however, evaluation of any patient with hypertension should exclude coarctation as a cause. Most individuals with isolated

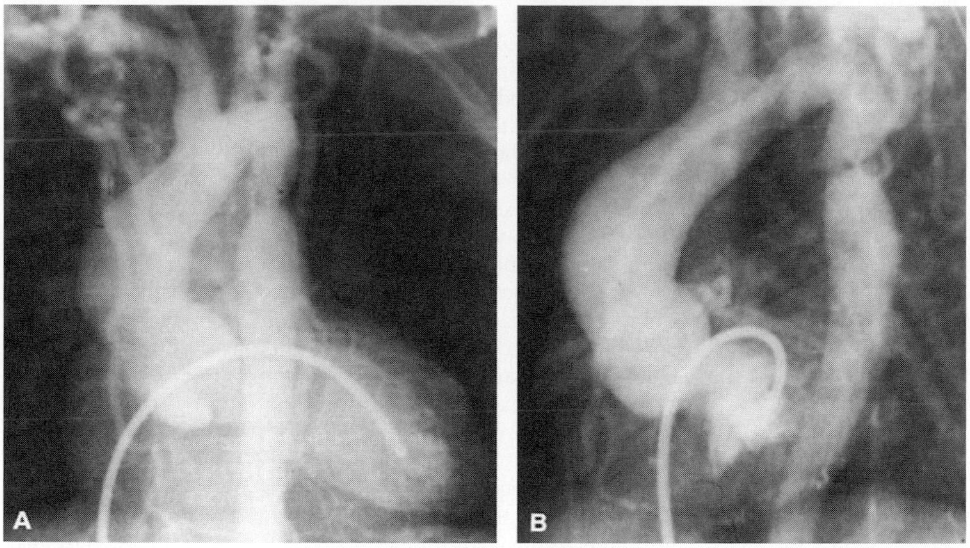

Figure 144-1. Anteroposterior (A) and lateral (B) frames from left ventricular angiography. Discrete coarctation is seen in the descending thoracic aorta. Well-developed collateral vessels are evident.

coarctation have no cardiac symptoms, although minor complaints of cold feet, leg cramps, and nose bleeds are often volunteered. Unilateral headaches, particularly of unusual severity, rarely point to an associated cerebral aneurysm, but they may be worrisome enough to prompt a full neurologic evaluation. Physical examination shows striking inequality between the strength of pulses from vessels arising proximal to the obstruction and those distal to the obstruction. Simultaneous palpation of brachial and femoral pulses is recommended; in the presence of well-developed collateral vessels, femoral pulses can be felt easily despite coarctation, and the discrepancy in timing and pulse volume should be sought. Auscultation should be performed systematically in an attempt to explain the auscultatory findings, rather than with a prejudice that a particular murmur is always found with coarctation. A systolic murmur generated from the coarctation site may be heard best in the left infraclavicular area, in the axilla, or over the left posterior chest. The murmur may seem to originate after the first heart sound, accentuate in later systole, and extend into diastole. The murmur reflects an apparent lag between cardiac systole and flow through the coarctation site, as well as the persistence of a coarctation gradient in early diastole.

True continuous murmurs may be generated by collateral vessels. Presence of an aortic ejection click and an ejection murmur in the aortic area may raise suspicion of an additional bicuspid aortic valve, which is found with high frequency in as many as 85% of patients with aortic coarctation. A thrill at the right upper sternal border or suprasternal notch may accompany significant aortic stenosis, but it can also be found with coarctation alone because of rapid ejection into the dilated proximal aorta.

Tests

Despite significant aortic coarctation, the results of the electrocardiogram may be normal in older children. When changes occur, they are manifested chiefly by voltage criteria for left ventricular hypertrophy. The rare patient with severe coarctation and left ventricular dysfunction may additionally have ST-T wave changes indicative of ischemia. The typical radiologic examination of an older child reveals normal heart size with less common findings of mild enlargement and left ventricular contour. Pulmonary vascular markings are normal in the absence of associated intracardiac defects. Dilatation of the ascending aorta may be present. In some patients, radiographic evidence of the prestenotic and poststenotic dilatations resulting from coarctation appears along the left paramediastinal shadow and is referred to as the 3 sign. Reversed 3 sign, or E sign, refers to the mirror-image prestenotic and poststenotic dilatations impinging on a barium-filled esophagus. Rib notching, if present, is pathognomonic of coarctation of the aorta, but it is related to age because erosion of the inferior portion of the ribs caused by dilated intercostal collateral vessels is a slow process, rarely seen before a patient reaches school age (Fig. 144-2). Unilateral rib notching suggests that one subclavian artery arises below the coarctation in the low-pressure zone with poor development of collaterals and rib notching on that side.

An echocardiogram, particularly when suprasternal notch and high left parasternal views are used, may enable recognition of coarctation, but difficulties in examining the entire aorta throughout its course are well described. The principal values of echocardiography are that associated defects can be assessed, left ventricular function and hypertrophy can be quantitated, and, if visualization of the coarctation site is possible, a more

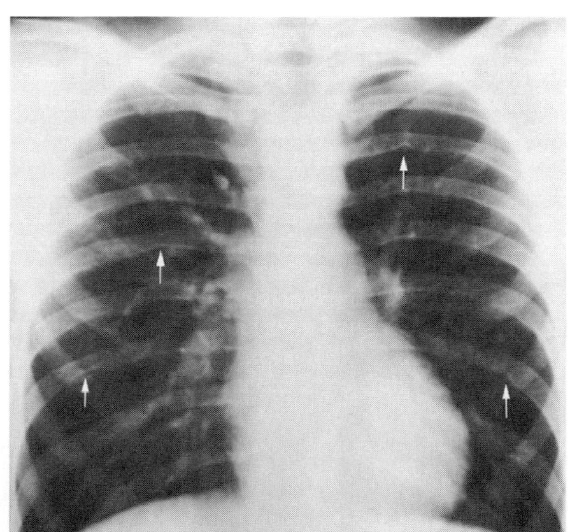

Figure 144-2. Posteroanterior chest film with rib notching (*arrows*) and "3 sign" identified in a 7-year-old child.

confident recommendation can be made to the surgeon that a typical coarctation is present. Parameters of Doppler flow including peak velocity and, in particular, striking pandiastolic flow are useful in supporting echocardiographic recognition of coarctation. Coexistence of coarctation with a persistently patent ductus in the neonate further challenges echocardiographic accuracy.

Magnetic resonance imaging has a newer application in prospective identification and follow-up of patients with coarctation of the aorta, and testing of this method's contribution is ongoing.

Catheterization and angiography, with detailed visualization of the anatomy of the coarctation area, can confirm the diagnosis directing surgical technique.

TREATMENT

Coarctation of the aorta has been considered a congenital defect amenable to surgical repair since the mid-1940s. The expected result is complete relief of the obstruction, so flow to the distal aorta remains unobstructed. Best results are obtained by elective resection and end-to-end anastomosis in a school-aged child with the single operation providing immediate and long-term relief of hypertension without the need for reoperation. Surgery is performed from a posterolateral thoracotomy incision, spreading the ribs to allow access to the thorax. No one method of repair is ideal for all patients (Fig. 144-3). Complications of surgery include injury to the recurrent laryngeal nerve

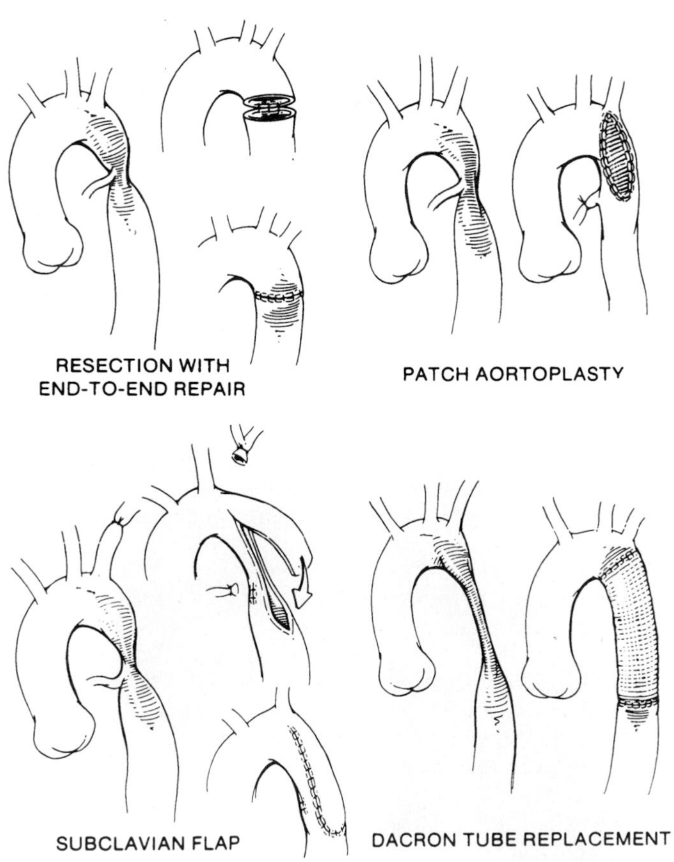

Figure 144-3. Techniques of repair commonly used for coarctation.

with resulting hoarseness; diaphragmatic injury from phrenic nerve trauma; bleeding from high-pressure suture lines; chylothorax; and, rarely, spinal cord injury, which is less likely when a well-developed collateral circulation is present.

A special postoperative syndrome of mesenteric arteritis may be related to the duration of preoperative hypertension, the presence of postoperative rebound hypertension, and the introduction of feeding too early postoperatively. Typically, this postcoarctectomy syndrome is recognized by hypertension, abdominal pain and tenderness, vomiting, and, in severe cases, a progression to bowel necrosis. The exact mechanism is unknown, but it appears to be related to vasoconstriction of mesenteric vessels reintroduced to pulsatile flow after successful repair of the coarctation. Because of this described problem, postoperative hypertension is treated vigorously and nothing-by-mouth status is continued for 72 hours with slow introduction of feeding in these patients.

An infant requiring early repair of a coarctation may also require pulmonary artery banding because of associated defects, although enthusiasm for cardiopulmonary bypass, even in very young patients, has led to a preference for complete, definitive repair.

Therapeutic Catheterization

Therapeutic catheterization using balloon angioplasty techniques has been offered enthusiastically for patients who have restenosis of coarctation sites previously treated surgically. A dilatation balloon is introduced retrograde from the femoral artery, positioned to straddle the obstruction, and inflated. Application has also been available for virgin coarctations with excellent relief of the obstruction. Concerns about a higher than acceptable rate of aneurysm formation after successful dilatation may limit use of the technique for native coarctation when surgery offers a safe alternative. These dilatation techniques have also been offered, perhaps more safely by the umbilical arterial route, as a palliative measure for selected critically ill newborns, although early restenosis is such a common sequela that operation may be preferable.

NATURAL HISTORY AND FOLLOW-UP

The former natural history of coarctation of the aorta, with an estimated 75% rate of mortality by mid-adult years, has been altered by surgical treatment. Endocarditis with the potential for mycotic aneurysm formation is a lifelong threat, and endocarditis prophylaxis should be observed by all patients, both preoperatively and postoperatively. The reversibility of hypertension is thought to be favored by repair in early childhood avoiding long-standing preoperative hypertension, as well as permitting complete relief of the obstruction. Considerations based on normal growth of the aorta and concern about reversibility of preoperative hypertension have led pediatric cardiologists to recommend elective repair of aortic coarctation for patients between the ages of 3 and 9 years.

A high incidence of congenital berry aneurysms is described, estimated at up to 10% of patients with coarctation. The likelihood of intracranial hemorrhage may be reduced by successful coarctation repair. Follow-up of patients with coarctation for restenosis, recurrent or residual hypertension, endocarditis, and surveillance of aneurysm formation at sites of repaired coarctation continues to be appropriate.

CHAPTER 145

Tetralogy of Fallot

Adapted from William H. Neches
and Jose A. Ettedgui

Tetralogy of Fallot refers to a spectrum of anatomic abnormalities that have two features in common: a large, unrestrictive ventricular septal defect and a right ventricular outflow tract obstruction. Clinical presentation varies from asymptomatic acyanotic children with a heart murmur to severely hypoxic newborn infants. Severity of presentation largely depends on the nature and degree of the outflow obstruction. The anatomic hallmark of tetralogy of Fallot is the anterocephalad deviation of the outlet portion of the interventricular septum. Apart from producing infundibular pulmonary stenosis, this deviation also accounts for the ventricular septal defect and the third feature of the tetralogy: aortic override (Fig. 145-1). The fourth feature of the tetralogy—hypertrophy of the right ventricle—is the result of the underlying anatomic and hemodynamic abnormalities. The severity of the infundibular stenosis ranges from mild to severe pulmonary stenosis and to pulmonary atresia. Further obstruction to pulmonary blood flow often occurs at other levels. Pulmonary valve stenosis is common, and stenoses are often found in the supravalvar region at the bifurcation of the pulmonary artery branches or in the distal pulmonary arteries.

The typical ventricular septal defect in tetralogy of Fallot is large and nonrestrictive and is due to malalignment of the outlet portion with the rest of the interventricular septum. Muscular ventricular septal defects, an inlet defect, or a complete atrioventricular septal defect may also be present.

Other possible associated abnormalities include an atrial septal defect (so-called pentalogy of Fallot) or coronary artery abnormalities. Approximately 25% of patients with tetralogy of Fallot have a right-sided aortic arch, an important consideration if a patient undergoes systemic–to–pulmonary artery anastomosis.

Tetralogy of Fallot occurs in some 6% of infants born with congenital heart disease. The etiology is obscure. Although tetralogy of Fallot and most other forms of congenital heart disease generally occur as isolated abnormalities, children with tetralogy of Fallot are afflicted with additional major extracardiac malformations significantly more often (15.7%) than patients with other congenital heart defects (6.8%). In addition, the extracardiac malformations may be more serious in patients with tetralogy of Fallot and include cleft lip and palate, hypospadias, and skeletal malformations. Although tetralogy of Fallot is not commonly part of specific hereditary malformation syndromes or chromosomal abnormalities, it is often found in a number of malformation associations including cardiofacial, VACTERL (*v*ertebral, *a*nal, *c*ardiac, *t*racheal, *e*sophageal, *r*enal, and *l*imb), and CHARGE (*c*oloboma, *h*eart anomaly, *c*hoanal *a*tresia, *r*etardation, and *g*enital and *e*ar anomalies) associations, as well as DeLange, Goldenhar, and Klippel-Feil syndromes.

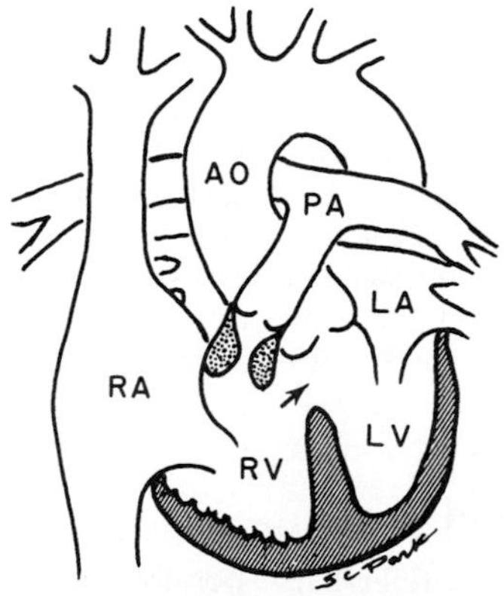

Figure 145-1. Anatomic abnormalities in tetralogy of Fallot. Note the ventricular septal defect (*arrow*), the infundibular pulmonary stenosis (stippled area), and the overriding aorta. AO, aorta; LA, left atrium; LV, left ventricle; PA, pulmonary artery; RA, right atrium; RV, right ventricle.

CLINICAL AND DIAGNOSTIC CHARACTERISTICS

Symptoms

Cyanosis may be mild or undetectable at rest in patients with tetralogy of Fallot, but it usually becomes apparent or increases with physical activity. With exercise, increased cardiac output and decreased systemic arteriolar resistance result in a considerable increase in the degree of right–to–left shunting. Although effective cardiac output is maintained, right–to–left shunting produces a rapid decrease in systemic arterial oxygen saturation and results in exertional dyspnea and decreased exercise tolerance. In contrast to episodes of paroxysmal hypoxemia (tetralogy spells), the systemic desaturation is limited by the duration of exercise and improves as soon as activity ceases.

Squatting

Squatting is a common posture in patients with tetralogy of Fallot, particularly in young children who easily assume the more comfortable knee-chest position. Squatting is often seen in children after exercise. Also, they are frequently seen to assume this position while playing quiet games with their peers who are sitting. Likely, squatting results in an increase in systemic arterial resistance caused by kinking and compression of the major arterial circulation to the lower extremities. This increase in peripheral resistance, in the presence of relatively fixed pulmonary outflow resistance, decreases the degree of right–to–left shunting and increases pulmonary blood flow. The result is an immediate increase in systemic arterial oxygen saturation.

Tetralogy Spells

Episodes of paroxysmal hypoxemia, also called hypercyanotic or tetralogy spells, are often seen in infants and children with tetralogy of Fallot and other cardiac malformations with similar physiology. Usually, these spells are self-limited and last less than 15 to 30 minutes, although they may be longer. The spells occur more often in the morning, but they may occur during the day and may be precipitated by activity, sudden fright, or injury, or they may occur spontaneously without any apparent cause. The spell is characterized by increasing cyanosis and an increased rate and depth of respiration. The physiologic change that produces a hypoxemic spell is an increase in right–to–left shunting and concomitant decrease in pulmonary blood flow. The exact mechanism by which this occurs is unknown.

Clubbing

Clubbing may be present on physical examination of children with tetralogy of Fallot. An increased left parasternal impulse indicating right ventricular hypertrophy may be present. Usually, the first heart sound is normal, whereas the second sound is single, because the pulmonary closure sound is very soft. An ejection systolic murmur is heard at the middle to upper-left sternal border and may radiate toward the back. Loudness of the murmur depends on the volume of blood crossing the right ventricular outflow tract. As infundibular stenosis becomes more severe, less blood flows through the right ventricular outflow, and the murmur becomes softer and shorter. In children having a hypoxemic spell, antegrade flow into the pulmonary arteries is much less, and the murmur disappears.

Tests

The chest radiograph in older children with tetralogy of Fallot exhibits the classically described "boot-shaped" heart. It is caused by mild enlargement of the right ventricle and concavity of the upper left heart border resulting from absence of the main pulmonary artery segment. In infants, the chest radiograph may be normal or may show only decreased pulmonary vascular markings.

The anatomic features of tetralogy of Fallot are identified by echocardiography. The large ventricular septal defect is easily visualized, and the aorta overriding the ventricular septal defect is apparent. Usually, the infundibular narrowing of the right ventricular outflow tract or a thickened and abnormal pulmonary valve can be demonstrated. Doppler echocardiography demonstrates an increased velocity of blood flow in the main pulmonary artery and is useful in estimating the gradient across the right ventricular outflow tract.

Cardiac catheterization and angiocardiography are important in the evaluation of the patient with tetralogy of Fallot. In the preoperative patient, important steps are to define the levels and severity of stenosis in the right ventricular outflow tract and pulmonary artery and to predict whether the repair is likely to be successful. Associated abnormalities such as multiple ventricular septal defects or coronary artery abnormalities that might adversely affect the success of surgical repair can also be demonstrated. In the postoperative patient with residual defects, cardiac catheterization provides an assessment of the hemodynamic result, ventricular function, severity of residual anatomic abnormalities, and electrophysiologic status.

MEDICAL MANAGEMENT

Although many patients with tetralogy of Fallot are acyanotic in early infancy, the subpulmonary stenosis tends to be progressive and usually results in the appearance of cyanosis during infancy or early childhood. Before the development of systemic–to–pulmonary artery anastomoses in the mid-1940s, approximately 50% of patients with tetralogy of Fallot died in the first year of life, and for a patient to survive past the third decade was unusual. Generally, mortality was a consequence of hypoxia, secondary hematologic changes, or problems such as infectious endocarditis or brain abscess. With palliative surgical procedures and complete repair, which is possible even during infancy and early childhood, 90% or more of patients with tetralogy of Fallot are expected to survive to adulthood.

Treatment

Treatment of significant resting hypoxia or hypercyanotic spells is surgical. Medical management in patients with tetralogy of Fallot is, therefore, directed toward treating associated noncardiac abnormalities, avoiding problems associated with anemia or polycythemia, preventing infectious complications such as infectious endocarditis or brain abscess, and acutely managing paroxysmal hypoxemic spells. Usually, hypoxemic spells are self-limited and last less than 15 to 30 minutes, but they can be prolonged. The patient should be comforted during one of these episodes and should be encouraged to assume the knee-chest position. Such squatting may cause increased peripheral resistance in the lower extremities that, in turn, promotes increased pulmonary blood flow. In a hospital situation, oxygen is administered by facemask during a hypoxemic spell. Combined with the foregoing physical maneuvers, it is often sufficient management for a short spell. If this approach is not successful and the patient's hypoxemic episode does not appear to resolve, morphine sulfate can be administered intramuscularly, subcutaneously, or intravenously in a dose of 0.1 mg per kilogram of body weight. The effectiveness of morphine sulfate in treating hypoxemic spells has been known for many years. Its exact mechanism of action is unclear, but it helps to relieve agitation and hyperpnea that can be exacerbating factors. Because this drug can be administered intramuscularly, the use of morphine is valuable for initial management of a hypoxemic spell when an intravenous route is unavailable. Once an intravenous line is placed, the dose of morphine sulfate can be repeated. Because metabolic acidosis appears quickly after the onset of a hypoxemic spell, sodium bicarbonate in a dose of 1.0 mEq/kg can be given empirically as soon as intravenous access is available. If these measures are unsuccessful, a beta–adrenergic blocking agent such as propranolol is valuable in managing a hypoxemic spell. This drug is given intravenously to a maximum total dose of 0.1 mg/kg. The total calculated dose should be diluted with 10 mL of fluid in a syringe, and no more than one-half the calculated dose should be given initially as an intravenous bolus. The remainder can be given slowly over the next 5 to 10 minutes, if necessary. Propranolol has also been used in the long-term nonoperative management of paroxysmal hypoxemic spells. It is administered orally in a dose of 1 to 4 mg/kg/day in four divided doses.

SURGICAL MANAGEMENT

Procedures

Surgical management of patients with tetralogy of Fallot consists of either palliative systemic–to–pulmonary artery anastomoses (shunts) or complete repair. Palliative procedures do not require cardiopulmonary bypass and, thus, can be performed in very small infants or in patients with anatomy that is unfavorable for complete repair. In most centers, primary repair is performed electively during infancy or early childhood, if the anatomy is suitable.

Surgical palliation became possible in the 1940s with the development of the Blalock–Taussig shunt, an end-to-side anastomosis between the subclavian artery and the pulmonary artery. Currently, a modified Blalock–Taussig shunt is popular. It consists of interposition of a synthetic tube between the subclavian artery and the pulmonary artery, thereby preserving blood flow to the arm.

Total Correction

Total correction is preferred, if possible, and consists of patch closure of the ventricular septal defect and relief of the right ventricular outflow tract obstruction. Occasionally, infundibular resection alone relieves the subpulmonary stenosis, but placement of a patch of synthetic material, or pericardium, to widen the right ventricular outflow tract further is generally necessary. In patients with severe pulmonary stenosis, this patch may have to be extended across the pulmonary valve annulus onto the main pulmonary artery and even out onto the branches when pulmonary artery hypoplasia is present. In some affected patients, homograft conduits rather than patch material are used. When reconstruction of the right ventricular outflow tract is not possible such as when an anomalous coronary artery crosses this area, a palliative procedure may be performed initially, thus delaying definitive repair until the patient is older and surgery is technically easier.

LATE RESULTS

In most centers, more than 90% of patients who undergo complete repair of tetralogy of Fallot will survive to adulthood and have a good functional long-term result. Postoperative hemodynamic abnormalities such as residual ventricular septal defects, some degree of right ventricular outflow tract obstruction, and pulmonary regurgitation are often present, but usually, further treatment is not required. Arrhythmias, particularly ventricular ectopy, are of concern in patients who have undergone repair of tetralogy of Fallot. Sudden, unexpected death occurs in a small percentage of postoperative patients and may be caused by a ventricular arrhythmia.

After complete repair, patients with tetralogy of Fallot are still at risk of infectious endocarditis and should receive appropriate antibiotic prophylaxis for dental or surgical procedures. Preservation of good right and left ventricular function and the possible effects of coronary artery disease in a heart with a repaired congenital defect are potential long-term problems.

CHAPTER 146
Total Anomalous Pulmonary Venous Connection

Adapted from Kent E. Ward

Total anomalous pulmonary venous connection (TAPVC) affects 2% to 5% of all patients with congenital heart disease. In all cases, systemic blood flow is maintained by way of right–to–left shunting through an interatrial communication, usually a patent foramen ovale. The male–to–female patient ratio is equal in most types of TAPVC, except for a strong male patient predominance (3:1) in infants with TAPVC of the infradiaphragmatic type. In the group of patients with this abnormality, approximately one-third have other significant major cardiac malformations including single ventricle, atrioventricular canal defect, hypoplastic left heart, patent ductus arteriosus, and transposition of the great vessels. Many patients in this group have been found to have abnormalities of atrial and visceral situs associated with the heterotaxy syndromes (asplenia and polysplenia). Most cases of TAPVC are sporadic and are not associated with syndromes or chromosomal abnormalities.

TAPVC can be classified according to the site of insertion of the anomalous channel. The four types and their frequency of occurrence are type 1, supracardiac connection (55%); type 2, cardiac connection (30%); type 3, infracardiac (infradiaphragmatic) connection (13%); and type 4, mixed connection (2%) (Fig. 146-1).

CLINICAL CHARACTERISTICS

Total Anomalous Pulmonary Venous Connection with Obstruction

Infants born with obstruction in the anomalous pulmonary venous channels develop symptoms shortly after birth and demonstrate severe cyanosis and respiratory distress. Physical examination reveals a prominent right ventricular impulse, accentuation of the second heart sound, and, at times, a gallop rhythm over the left lower sternal border. Murmurs are infrequent. Hepatomegaly is usually present and is often dramatic in anomalous pulmonary venous connection to the portal venous system. The electrocardiogram may demonstrate right ventricular hypertrophy and a paucity of left ventricular forces.

The chest radiograph, at times, is diagnostic in TAPVC with obstruction. The cardiac size is usually normal. Pulmonary vascular markings are striking, characterized by a diffuse, linear reticular pattern radiating from the hilar regions (Fig. 146-2). Overt pulmonary edema with Kerley B lines may be present. Hyperinflation of the lungs may be seen, which should differentiate this cardiac anomaly from early hyaline membrane disease. Increased pulmonary vascularity helps distinguish this entity from persistent fetal circulation syndrome.

Total Anomalous Pulmonary Venous Connection with a Restrictive Interatrial Communication

Infants born with a restrictive interatrial communication are usually asymptomatic at birth and during the first few weeks of life; then they develop respiratory distress, feeding difficulties, and poor weight gain. Physical examination reveals tachypnea with perioral duskiness, a hyperdynamic precordium, and hepatomegaly. Auscultation demonstrates a pulmonary systolic murmur, fixed splitting of the second heart sound, and, often, a diastolic murmur over the left lower sternal border. Occasionally, a continuous venous hum may be detected in an area overlying the anomalous venous connection. The electrocardiogram demonstrates right axis deviation, right atrial enlargement, and right ventricular hypertrophy. The chest roentgenogram reveals cardiomegaly, dilatation of the pulmonary artery, and increased pulmonary vascularity. Distinctive radiographic features may be observed reflecting the course of the anomalous pulmonary venous channel (Fig. 146-3).

DIAGNOSTIC STUDIES

Echocardiography and cardiac catheterization are the diagnostic procedures of choice in patients with TAPVC. Cine-magnetic resonance imaging has been shown to be comparable in diagnostic accuracy, especially in the older infant. Although surgery may be performed based on two-dimensional and color Doppler echocardiography alone, catheterization and selective angiography are often required to delineate the anatomy in patients with complex cardiac defects or in mixed-type TAPVC. In

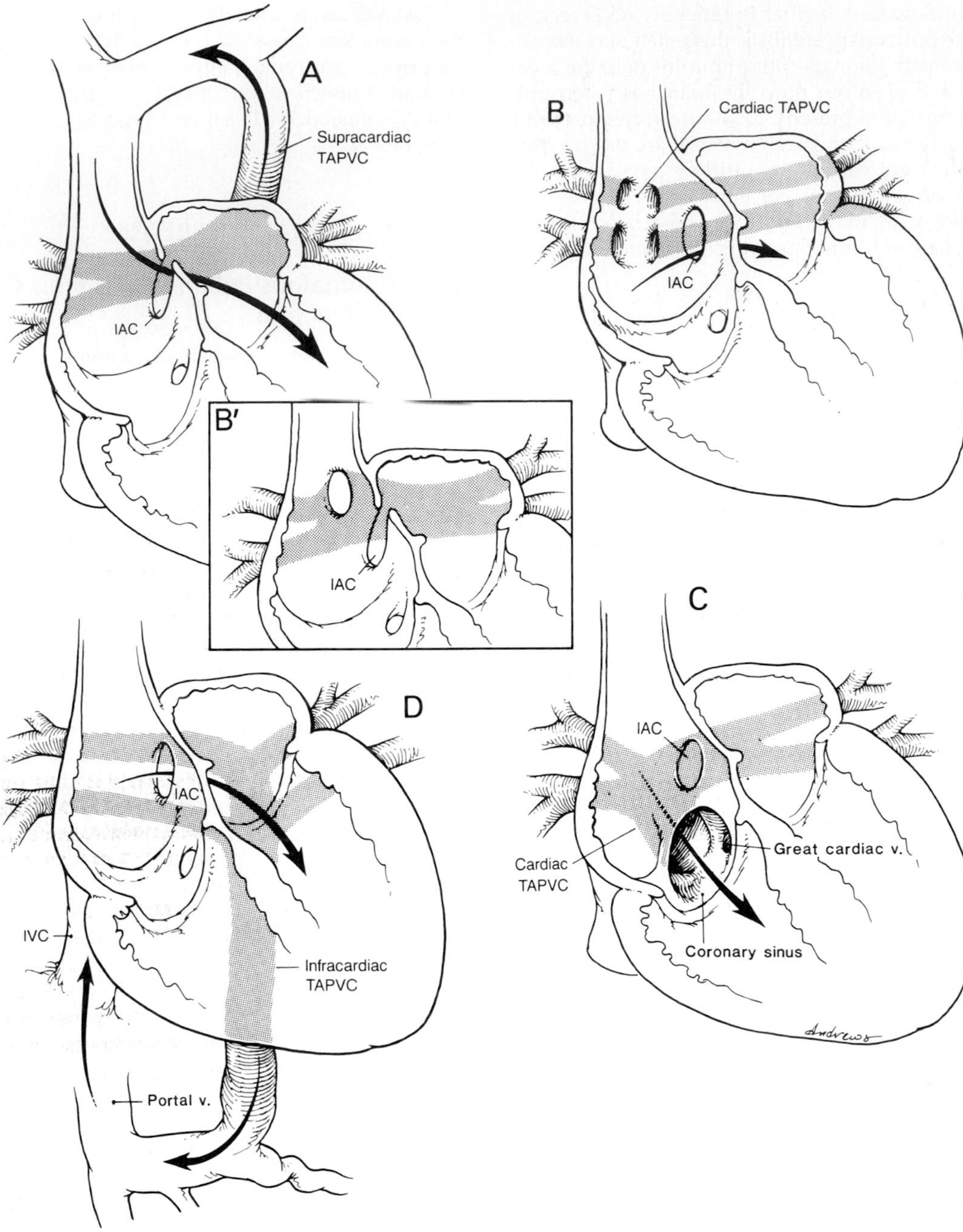

Figure 146-1. Types of total anomalous pulmonary venous connection (TAPVC). **A:** Supracardiac connection to left innominate vein. **B:** Cardiac connection via four separate veins. **B′:** Cardiac connection via single common orifice. **C:** Cardiac connection to coronary sinus. **D:** Infracardiac (subdiaphragmatic) connection to portal system. IAC, interatrial communication. (Adapted from Ward KE, Mullins CE. Anomalous pulmonary venous connections. In: Garson A Jr, Bricker JT, Fisher DJ, Nelsh SR, eds. *The science and practice of pediatric cardiology.* Baltimore: Williams & Wilkins, 1998:1442.)

addition, atrial septostomy can be performed during catheterization if surgery is to be delayed until the patient is older.

TREATMENT

In infants with TAPVC who present with marked cyanosis, respiratory distress, and cardiovascular collapse in the first few days of life, severe obstruction in the extracardiac pulmonary venous channels must be assumed. Surgery should be undertaken immediately after diagnostic studies are performed. Alternatively, extracorporeal membrane oxygenation has been used in some infants to rapidly stabilize their cardiovascular system before surgical repair. Prostaglandin E_1 has been reported to dilate the ductus venosus in patients with TAPVC below the diaphragm to enhance pulmonary venous return and relieve severe obstruction. Operative mortality has improved to as low as 14%, but it still remains relatively high in these patients when compared with patients without obstruction.

Infants without obstruction are treated somewhat differently. Some cardiac centers prefer to operate soon after the diagnosis is established, whereas others elect to use medical therapy

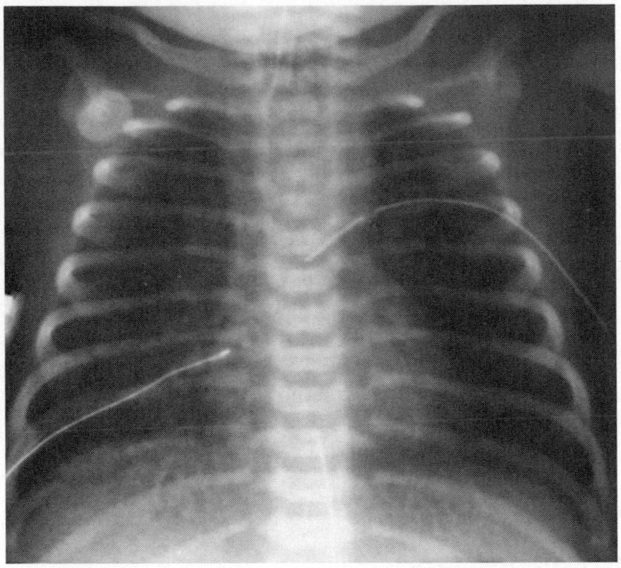

Figure 146-2. Total anomalous pulmonary venous connection with obstruction. Heart size is normal and lungs are hyperinflated. Pulmonary vascularity demonstrates a diffuse, linear reticular pattern radiating from the hilum representing pulmonary venous engorgement.

after an adequate atrial septostomy to delay surgery for weeks or months to allow for growth and adequate weight gain. The two approaches are equally successful resulting in operative mortality of less than 10%. The surgical technique involves anastomosis of the pulmonary venous confluence to the left atrium with ligation of the anomalous channel.

The long-term outlook after surgery is excellent, although a few patients may require reoperation for obstruction because of inadequate growth of the pulmonary venous confluence and left atrial anastomosis.

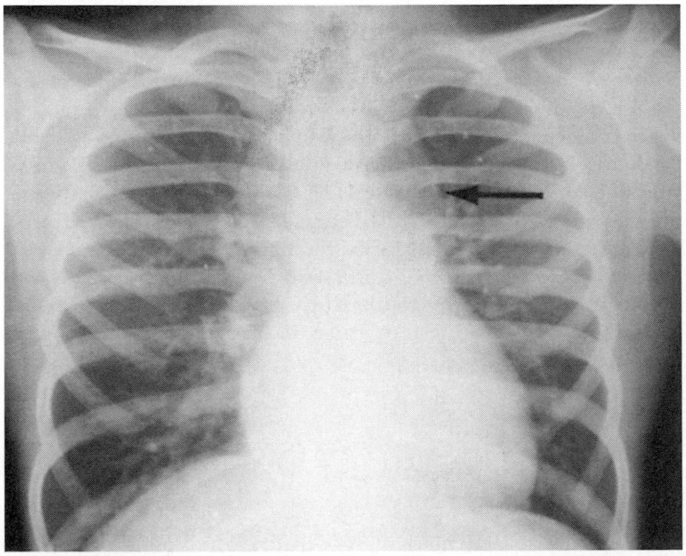

Figure 146-3. Supracardiac total anomalous pulmonary venous connection. Chest radiograph in a child with connection to the left innominate vein demonstrating figure-of-eight or "snowman" appearance. Arrow points to anomalous vertical vein. (Courtesy of Dr. Teresa Stacy.)

CHAPTER 147

Transposition of the Great Arteries

Adapted from William H. Neches, Sang C. Park and Jose A. Ettedgui

Transposition of the great arteries, or complete transposition, is a common form of cardiac abnormality found in approximately 5% of all patients with congenital heart disease. The distinguishing anatomic feature of transposition is the discordant ventriculoarterial connection of the great arteries, whereby the aorta originates from the morphologic right ventricle and the pulmonary artery originates from the morphologic left ventricle (Fig. 147-1). The consequence of this anatomic arrangement is that unoxygenated systemic venous blood returning to the heart passes through the right atrium and right ventricle and is ejected into the aorta. Similarly, oxygenated pulmonary venous blood reaches the left side of the heart and is returned to the pulmonary artery. The clinical situation that results from this cardiac anomaly is characterized by severe, life-threatening hypoxemia early in life. There are three main categories of patients with transposition (Table 147-1).

PHYSIOLOGY AND HEMODYNAMICS

Intact Interventricular Septum

In the neonate with transposition of the great arteries and an intact interventricular septum, usually a foramen ovale or atrial septal defect is present and facilitates exchange of blood at the atrial level. A patent ductus arteriosus enhances this exchange.

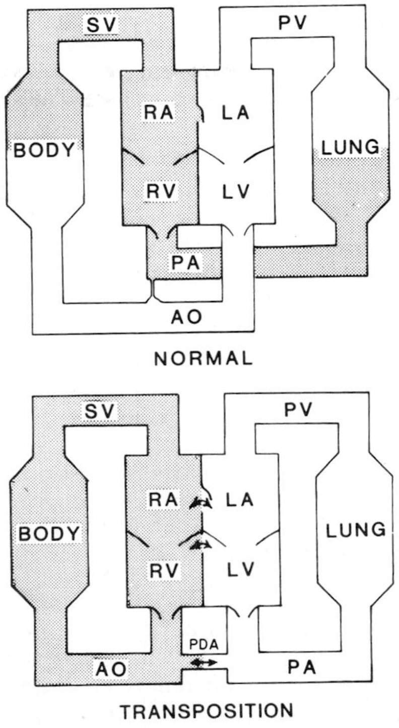

Figure 147-1. Circulatory pathways in transposition of the great arteries. AO, aorta; LA, left atrium; LV, left ventricle; PA, pulmonary artery; PDA, patent ductus arteriosus; PV, pulmonary veins; RA, right atrium; RV, right ventricle; SV, systemic veins.

TABLE 147-1. Categories of Patients with Transposition

- Transposition with an intact interventricular septum (complete transposition)
  Affected patients may or may not have left ventricular outflow tract obstruction (subpulmonary stenosis)
- Transposition with ventricular septal defect
  No narrowing in the left ventricular outflow tract
- Complex transposition
  There are varying degrees of left ventricular outflow tract obstruction. Usually, affected patients have significant subpulmonic stenosis and equal right and left ventricular pressures. This category includes patients with pulmonary atresia.

Usually, the ductus arteriosus is a transient neonatal structure, however, and tends to close physiologically within a few days after birth. Closure of the duct precipitates a dramatic change in clinical appearance of an apparently healthy newborn to one with intense cyanosis.

Ventricular Septal Defect

Patients with transposition of the great arteries and a ventricular septal defect of significant size present an entirely different clinical picture. Often, such patients have adequate exchange of blood with a combination of mixing at atrial and ventricular levels. As a result, only mild cyanosis is present in the early neonatal period; therefore, a significant cardiovascular anomaly may not be suspected until a few weeks later. As a result of this large ventricular septal defect, patients may present with congestive heart failure toward the end of the first month of life and are at risk for subsequent development of pulmonary vascular disease.

Complex Transposition

The physiology in patients with complex transposition (transposition with ventricular septal defect and pulmonary stenosis) differs from either of the other two clinical forms. In patients with complex transposition, a large ventricular septal defect is present, and the balance between pulmonary and systemic blood flow depends on the degree of pulmonary stenosis. When severe pulmonary stenosis or pulmonary atresia is present, patients present with cyanosis and reduced pulmonary blood flow early in life. If pulmonary stenosis is less severe, clinical presentation is due to the presence of cyanosis or detection of a heart murmur and may occur even later in infancy.

DIAGNOSIS

Most Common Presenting Manifestations

Cyanosis, with or without associated heart murmur, is the most common presenting manifestation of transposition of the great arteries. As stated, associated lesions may temporarily provide adequate blood mixing, so affected infants may be only mildly cyanotic or may exhibit significant cyanosis only during exercise (feeding or crying). Patients with transposition and an intact interventricular septum often have no murmur; other than cyanosis, the only abnormalities on physical examination may be a loud, single second heart sound and a prominent right ventricular impulse. In other patients, a murmur may be related to a ventricular septal defect or patent ductus arteriosus or may be caused by pulmonary stenosis.

Tests

The electrocardiogram from such patients shows right axis deviation and right ventricular hypertrophy, which is a normal pattern in newborns. Although the classic "egg-on-a-string" radiographic pattern may be seen in some one-third of patients, usually the chest roentgenogram is normal in the first few days of life.

Cross-sectional echocardiography has had a dramatic impact on the noninvasive diagnosis of transposition of the great arteries. The atrioventricular and ventriculoarterial connections can be demonstrated reliably, thus enabling the diagnosis of transposition of the great arteries. All the echocardiographic modalities—cross-sectional, Doppler, and color flow mapping—are important in demonstrating the associated lesions and physiologic derangements that occur in these patients.

MANAGEMENT

Interventional Procedures

Introduction of balloon atrial septostomy was the single most important factor influencing survival of infants with transposition of the great arteries. This was the first interventional procedure used in the cardiac catheterization laboratory. Surgical interventions have evolved tremendously since the 1940s and 1950s. Various types of partial and complete atrial redirection operations such as the Senning operation were suggested but had little success before the description of the atrial baffle repair by Mustard in 1964. The goal of both the Mustard and the Senning atrial baffle procedures was to redirect the venous inflow to the heart so that systemic venous drainage was channeled to the mitral valve, then into the pulmonary circulation, while the pulmonary venous drainage was channeled to the tricuspid valve and, eventually, out into the aorta.

Arterial Switch Repair

Concerns about long-term systemic ventricular function, along with problems of atrial baffle obstruction and electrophysiologic abnormalities that are present with both types of atrial baffle repair, led surgeons to consider arterial switch repair. Technically, dividing the transposed great arteries and reanastomosing the vessels to provide a concordant ventriculoarterial connection is relatively easy. The problem is that the coronary arteries arise from the sinuses of the semilunar valve that is connected to the right ventricle. Thus, if only the transposed great arteries were switched, the coronary arteries would be perfused with low-pressure, unoxygenated systemic venous blood, which is invariably fatal. In 1976, Jatene et al. reported survival after an arterial switch repair that included transplantation of both coronary arteries into the reconnected aorta. Although this procedure was associated with high mortality during its initial use, the subsequent mortality is quite low, and this anatomic repair is now a worldwide standard.

LATE RESULTS

Atrial Baffle Procedures

Although most patients have good functional results, numerous long-term problems have been identified in patients who have undergone atrial baffle procedures. Approximately 10% to 20% of patients who underwent a Mustard operation developed systemic venous obstruction and 5% to 10% developed pulmonary venous obstruction postoperatively. Generally, systemic venous obstruction was uncommon in patients who underwent a Senning operation. However, pulmonary venous obstruction occurred with a frequency similar to that found after the Mustard operation.

Atrial Arrhythmias

Atrial arrhythmias such as atrial flutter, supraventricular tachycardia, and sick-sinus syndrome were important problems in patients who underwent either a Mustard or a Senning operation. Modification of the operative technique to avoid injury to the sinoatrial node or its artery were successful in reducing the incidence of early postoperative rhythm disturbances. However, the incidence of atrial arrhythmias continues to increase in frequency with increasing length of postoperative follow-up. Also, sudden death has been seen in the young adult population and is believed to be caused by ventricular arrhythmias.

Tricuspid valve incompetence has also been reported to occur after atrial baffle operations. Possibly, it is caused by inability of the tricuspid valve to function as the systemic atrioventricular valve over a long period. Another major concern is the ability of the right ventricle to function as the systemic ventricle over a patient's lifetime.

Atrial Baffle Repair

These problems, which are present with both types of atrial baffle repair, led to development of the arterial switch procedure. Because this operation results in both an anatomic and a physiologic correction, this procedure is believed to provide a better functional result over many years. Long-term results of patients who underwent an arterial switch repair for transposition of the great arteries are still unknown. Maintenance of normal coronary artery blood flow is of major importance, and long-term effects related to growth are unknown. Another concern is the site of anastomosis for reconnection of the great arteries. Stenosis at the site of anastomosis of the great arteries, particularly the pulmonary artery, is fairly common, and some patients have required balloon angioplasty or reoperation to correct this problem. Aortic regurgitation is also seen but much less commonly, and it is usually mild. Despite these concerns and the lack of long-term follow-up, the results of this operation over a decade of widespread use are excellent. Today, the arterial switch repair is the preferred procedure for surgical management of the patient with transposition of the great arteries.

CHAPTER 148

Tricuspid Atresia

Adapted from David J. Driscoll

Tricuspid atresia, the third most common form of cyanotic congenital heart disease, consists of complete agenesis of the tricuspid valve and absence of direct communication between the right atrium and the right ventricle. The prevalence of tricuspid atresia in clinical series of patients with congenital heart disease ranges from 0.3% to 3.7%. The prevalence rate in autopsy series is 2.9%. Tricuspid atresia occurs in 1 in 10,000 to 1 in 17,857 live births.

PATHOLOGY

Tricuspid atresia is divided into three types on the basis of the great artery relationship (Table 148-1). An opening in the atrial septum allows egress of blood from the right atrium. The interatrial communication can be (or can become) restrictive. Additional cardiovascular abnormalities occur in 18% of patients with normally related great arteries and in 63% of patients with transposed great arteries. These abnormalities include coarctation of the aorta, patent ductus arteriosus, and right aortic arch. Extracardiac anomalies occur in 20% of cases.

In tricuspid atresia, the left bundle of the cardiac conduction system originates early from the bundle of His and is unusually posterior and short. Presumably, this anatomic malformation of the conduction system accounts for the leftward or superior frontal plane axis of the electrocardiogram in patients with tricuspid atresia.

CLINICAL FINDINGS

History

Because of the presence of cyanosis, congestive heart failure, or growth failure, tricuspid atresia is usually detected in infancy. Cyanosis is the prominent feature in patients whose pulmonary blood flow is limited by pulmonary atresia or pulmonary stenosis. Symptoms of pulmonary edema and congestive heart failure predominate in patients with unobstructed pulmonary blood flow; cyanosis can also be apparent. If pulmonary blood flow depends on the patency of the ductus arteriosus and that vessel closes, the degree of cyanosis and arterial hypoxemia may increase dramatically. If pulmonary atresia is present, closure of the ductus can produce profound hypoxemia, acidosis, and death. For patients with unobstructed pulmonary blood flow, as pulmonary vascular resistance decreases and pulmonary blood flow increases, signs and symptoms of congestive heart failure and pulmonary edema can increase.

Bacterial endocarditis and brain abscess are relatively common complications of tricuspid atresia. Neurologic complications can also result from cerebrovascular accidents secondary to polycythemia or to intravascular thrombosis or embolic phenomena.

TABLE 148-1. Classifications of Tricuspid Atresia

		Relative frequency (%)	
Type	Description	*Clinical*	*Autopsy*
I	Normally related great arteries	70	69
I-A	No VSD; pulmonary atresia		9
I-B	Restrictive VSD; pulmonary stenosis		51
I-C	Large VSD; no pulmonary stenosis		9
II	D-Transposition of great arteries	23	28
II-A	VSD; pulmonary atresia		2
II-B	VSD; pulmonary stenosis		8
II-C	VSD; no pulmonary stenosis		18
III	L-Transposition of great arteries	7	3

VSD, ventricular septal defect.
Adapted from Rosenthal A, Dick M, Tricuspid atresia. In: Adams FH, Emmanouilides GC, eds. *Moss's heart disease in infants, children, and adolescents,* 3rd ed. Baltimore: Williams & Wilkins, 1983:271.

Physical Examination

Cyanosis is the most common clinical feature of tricuspid atresia. Infants with tricuspid atresia and normally related great arteries may have excessive pulmonary blood flow and little cyanosis, but the degree of cyanosis may increase as the ventricular septal defect becomes progressively restrictive causing subpulmonary stenosis and decreasing blood flow.

The intensity of the second heart sound usually is normal if the great arteries are related normally (i.e., pulmonary artery anterior) and the pulmonary artery pressure is normal. Because the aorta is nearer to the anterior chest wall when great arteries are transposed (i.e., the aorta is anterior to the pulmonary artery), the second heart sound may be more intense despite normal pulmonary artery pressure.

Cardiac murmurs are present in 80% of patients with tricuspid atresia. A low-frequency holosystolic (or, at times, a crescendo–decrescendo) murmur is produced by the flow of blood through the ventricular septal defect. A systolic mid-frequency crescendo–decrescendo murmur is present in patients with pulmonary stenosis. Patients with pulmonary atresia and a systemic-to-pulmonary collateral blood supply and patients who have had a surgical systemic arterial-to-pulmonary arterial anastomosis have a continuous murmur. A diastolic mitral murmur may be audible in patients who have excessive pulmonary blood flow.

Electrocardiography

First-degree atrioventricular block occurs in 15% of cases and is presumably caused by prolonged atrial conduction, because atrioventricular node function is usually normal. Because of early origin of the left bundle from the common bundle, the frontal plane QRS axis is usually leftward or superior, and the frontal plane electrocardiographic loop is counterclockwise. Rarely, the frontal plane QRS axis is normal, which suggests the presence of transposed great arteries. The right ventricular electrocardiographic forces are diminished, and left ventricular hypertrophy is evident, as are frequently discordant QRS and T waves.

Chest Radiography

Usually, the heart is enlarged. The right border of the heart may be prominent reflecting enlargement of the right atrium. The pulmonary vascular markings are increased when the pulmonary blood flow is excessive. In 80% of patients with tricuspid atresia, however, the pulmonary blood flow is diminished, and the pulmonary vascular markings are decreased.

Echocardiography

Basic anatomy, size of the atrial septal defect, size of the ventricular septal defect, ventricular function, great artery relationships, and valvular function can be ascertained by using M-mode, two-dimensional, Doppler, and color flow echocardiography.

Cardiac Catheterization

In infants, cardiac catheterization is used mainly to determine sources and reliability of pulmonary blood flow. Administration of prostaglandin E_1 to maintain ductal patency has improved the safety of cardiac catheterization for babies with decreased or duct-dependent pulmonary blood flow. Cardiac catheterization may be necessary in infants (2–6 months old) to measure pulmonary artery pressure and resistance. This information can serve as a guide to the need for pulmonary artery banding to prevent development of pulmonary vascular obstructive disease. In adolescents and adults, cardiac catheterization and angiography define anatomic and hemodynamic details important in surgical management.

CLINICAL MANAGEMENT

Infants

Three major considerations should guide the management of infants with tricuspid atresia:

- The need for manipulating the amount of pulmonary blood flow, either to decrease hypoxemia and polycythemia by increasing pulmonary blood flow or to decrease symptoms of congestive heart failure by decreasing pulmonary blood flow
- The need to preserve myocardial function, pulmonary vascular integrity, and the pulmonary vascular bed to optimize conditions for future Fontan operation
- The need to reduce risks of associated cardiovascular complications such as bacterial endocarditis and thromboembolism

Babies with severe hypoxemia and acidosis should be treated promptly with an infusion of prostaglandin E_1 to maintain patency of the ductus arteriosus, thus improving pulmonary perfusion. Cardiac catheterization and angiography establish sources of pulmonary blood flow and provide help in planning for the type of surgical systemic–to–pulmonary artery anastomosis.

Infants with transposed great arteries and unrestricted pulmonary blood flow have signs and symptoms of pulmonary edema and congestive heart failure. Such infants benefit from treatment with digitalis and diuretics. Traditionally, these patients have had a pulmonary artery band surgically placed to decrease the pulmonary blood flow. Some investigators suggest, however, that pulmonary artery banding might accelerate ventricular septal defect closure. In patients with tricuspid atresia with transposed great arteries, this procedure would create subaortic obstruction and might lead to marked ventricular hypertrophy. Because marked ventricular hypertrophy is an adverse risk for a subsequent successful Fontan operation, surgical procedures to reduce pulmonary blood flow and to bypass potential areas of subaortic obstruction have been recommended. Advantages of these more complicated and riskier palliative procedures have not been established.

The Fontan Procedure

Before 1971, palliative procedures to control pulmonary blood flow (pulmonary artery banding, systemic–to–pulmonary artery anastomoses, or superior vena cava–to–pulmonary artery anastomoses) were the mainstay of surgical treatment for patients with tricuspid atresia. In 1971, Fontan et al. described a unique procedure for separating the systemic and pulmonary venous returns to eliminate the right–to–left intracardiac shunt and thereby reduce the volume of ventricular overload. They constructed a Glenn anastomosis to direct superior vena caval systemic venous return to the right lung and directed inferior vena caval systemic venous return to the pulmonary artery with a valve-containing conduit connecting the right atrium and the pulmonary artery. They also inserted a valve into the inferior vena cava, closed the interatrial communication, and obliterated the connection between the pulmonary artery and the ventricle. Since its original description, the procedure has been modified considerably, but the concept of directing systemic venous return directly to the pulmonary artery retains the eponymic label *modified Fontan procedure*.

TABLE 148-2. Criteria of Choussat and Fontan for Low-Risk Operation

Age at operation: 4–15 yr
Sinus rhythm
Normal systemic venous return
Normal right atrial volume
Mean pulmonary artery pressure $\leq$15 mm Hg
Pulmonary arteriolar resistance <4 U/m^2
Pulmonary artery/aorta diameter ratio >0.75
Left ventricular ejection fraction $\geq$0.60
Competent mitral valve
Absence of pulmonary artery distortion

Adapted from Choussat A, Fontan F, Bosse P, et al. Selection criteria for Fontan's procedure. In: Adams RH, Shinebourne EA, eds. *Paediatric cardiology 1977.* Edinburgh: Churchill Livingstone, 1978:559.

Ten guidelines for relatively low-risk operations described by Choussat et al. are listed in Table 148-2. Additional criteria include the absence of ventricular hypertrophy, more recent calendar year of operation, absence of subaortic obstruction, shorter operative ischemic time, and absence of incorporation of prosthetic valves into the repair. Although most of these criteria are relative, clearly, as more of them are violated, operative mortality increases, and the chances of excellent long-term results decrease.

In a follow-up study of 125 patients who underwent a modified Fontan operation between 1973 and 1985, the 30-day, 6-month, and 1-, 5-, and 10-year survival rates were 90%, 84%, 84%, 80%, and 70%, respectively. Quality of life and tolerance for exercise improved after the operation. Preliminary data suggest that the operation prolongs life. However, a relatively high incidence of atrial arrhythmias occurs in survivors of the Fontan operation. In addition, 5% to 10% of survivors may develop protein-losing enteropathy, a complication that has a 5-year 50% mortality.

CHAPTER 149

Truncus Arteriosus

Adapted from Robert Lee Williams

Persistent truncus arteriosus may be defined as a single great artery arising from the base of the heart and giving origin to the coronary, pulmonary, and systemic arteries. The incidence of truncus arteriosus is low: It occurs in approximately 2% of patients with congenital heart defects. It has no apparent gender predilection. Without treatment, truncus arteriosus is usually fatal; the mean age of death is 2.5 months, and 80% of affected children die by 1 year of age.

EMBRYOLOGY AND ANATOMY

Classifications

Collett's and van Praagh's classifications of truncus arteriosus are shown in Fig. 149-1. Persistence of truncus arteriosus usually occurs in the presence of a ventricular septal defect. The truncal root straddles the ventricular septal defect equally in approximately 60% of cases with 20% of the remaining cases having either a dominant right or a dominant left ventricular override.

Associated Abnormalities

Usually, the truncal valve leaflets are abnormal and frequently appear to be thick, fleshy, soft, and polypoid. The number of leaflets varies. Approximately 65% of patients have tricuspid valves, 23% have quadricuspid valves, and 9% have bicuspid valves. In 2% of cases, five or more valves may occur. Truncal valve regurgitation is present in approximately 50% of patients and is moderate to severe in one-half of these cases. Truncal valve stenosis may be seen in approximately one-third of affected patients. The arch is right-sided in approximately one-third of cases. In approximately 12% of interrupted aortic arch anomalies, an associated truncus arteriosus is present. Noncardiac anomalies are present in approximately 20% of cases with DiGeorge syndrome being one of the more common associated anomalies. Conversely, in patients who have DiGeorge syndrome, which may be an autosomal dominant inheritance, approximately 9% have truncus arteriosus; in those who have DiGeorge syndrome with interrupted arch, 33% have truncus arteriosus. DiGeorge syndrome may be screened in patients with truncus arteriosus by fluorescence *in situ* hybridization (FISH) study, which will demonstrate the deletion of chromosome 22q11.

CLINICAL FEATURES

Cardiac Abnormalities

With the advent of fetal ultrasonography, cardiac abnormalities may be suspected before birth, and fetal echocardiography can demonstrate truncus arteriosus. Before delivery, affected patients can be scheduled for neonatal evaluation and potential correction. Usually, patients with truncus arteriosus not diagnosed prenatally present with severe congestive heart failure during the first few months of life. Cyanosis is not usually visible clinically because increased pulmonary blood flow produces a greater mixing of saturated than of desaturated blood volume, which obfuscates clinical cyanosis. Increased pulmonary flow, which is caused by the perfusion of lungs at systemic pressure from the truncus, is augmented because pulmonary resistance tends to decrease in early infancy. The severity of congestive-heart failure not only depends on pulmonary blood flow volume but also may be aggravated by truncal valve regurgitation.

Physical Exam

Frequently, a systolic murmur that is usually holosystolic can be heard at the left sternal border. It is accompanied by an ejection click, followed by a single-second heart sound. Palpable peripheral pulses may become quickened and sharp in contour secondary to the pulmonary artery run-off. Tachypnea, decreased feeding, and irritability may be the first clinical symptoms. Although symptoms usually occur within the first few days of life, they may be delayed for several weeks, secondary to the delay in the decrease in pulmonary vascular resistance.

Tests

Usually, the electrocardiogram shows biventricular hypertrophy. Isolated right or left ventricular hypertrophy is less common. Occasionally, left ventricular ischemic changes caused by coronary insufficiency are noted. The chest roentgenogram shows cardiomegaly after the first day or two of life. Heart size continues to increase as pulmonary overcirculation occurs with regression of fetal pulmonary vascular resistance.

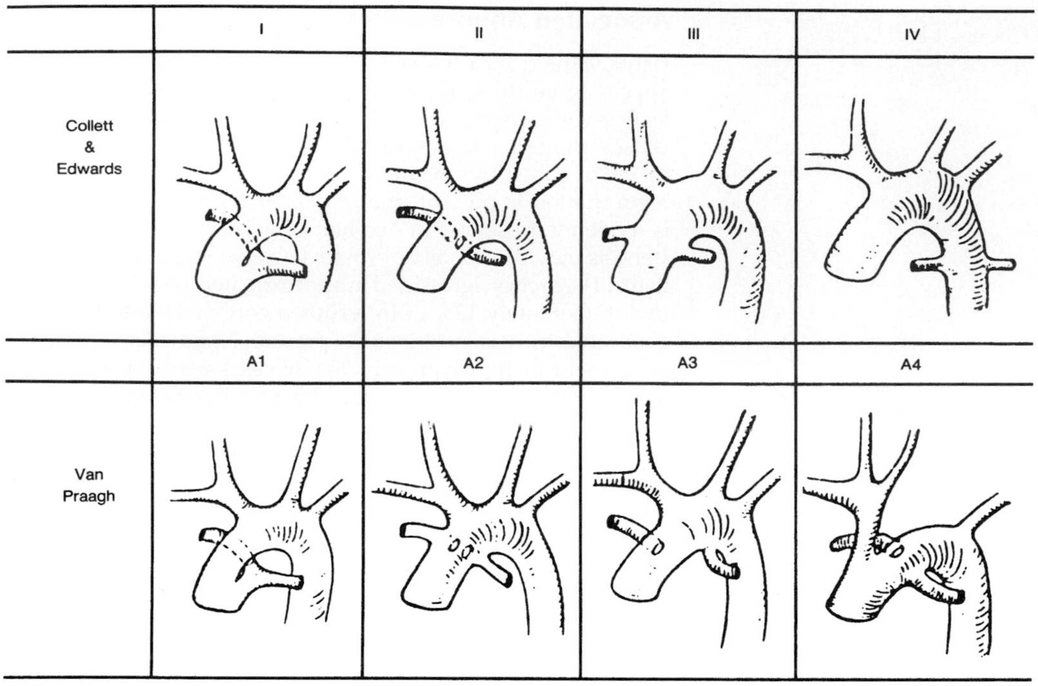

Figure 149-1. Classic Collett and Edwards classification of truncus arteriosus compared with the van Praagh classification. Type I is the same as A1. Types II and III are grouped as a single type, A2. Type A3 denotes unilateral pulmonary artery atresia with collateral supply to the affected lung. Type A4 is truncus associated with an interrupted aortic arch. Type IV is commonly known as *pseudotruncus.*

The position of the aortic arch should always be identified. The finding of a right aortic arch with increased pulmonary vascularity gives an extremely high probability of truncus arteriosus.

ECHOCARDIOGRAPHIC AND DOPPLER FEATURES

Usually, echocardiogram evaluation is the first noninvasive test that can corroborate clinical suspicion of truncus arteriosus. The *sine qua non* of persistent truncus arteriosus is the demonstration of the pulmonary arteries originating from a common trunk and semilunar valve. Doppler evaluation can accurately indicate the competency of the truncal valve, and color Doppler evaluation can better demonstrate the flow pattern across the truncal valve and the competency of the valve. With parasternal, subcostal, and suprasternal views, differentiation of truncus arteriosus and ventricular septal defect can be made with a high degree of accuracy, but problems may arise in differentiating between truncus arteriosus and pulmonary atresia with ventricular septal defect. An echocardiographic diagnosis, which is complete in children younger than 3 months, is sufficient as a presurgical workup except in infants with type A3 (unilateral pulmonary artery atresia or truncus arteriosus with interrupted aortic arch). Infants older than 3 months may require cardiac catheterization to evaluate the pulmonary resistance.

CARDIAC CATHETERIZATION AND ANGIOGRAPHIC FEATURES

Cardiac catheterization and angiography have long been the definitive way to evaluate the anatomic detail and physiologic variables in truncus arteriosus. In the past, before surgical repair was considered, evaluation of pulmonary arterial resistance was extremely important for patients older than 2 years. Surgery was considered not feasible if the pulmonary arteriolar resistance was greater than 8 U/m^2. The present policy of performing corrective surgery by 6 months of age, however, should prevent the steady increase of pulmonary arteriolar resistance from becoming persistent pulmonary vascular disease.

Performing truncal angiography is imperative, and an assessment of the valve can be made from the selective truncal angiograms. If the aorta is significantly smaller than the pulmonary artery portion of the truncus, an interrupted aortic arch is expected. Frequently, the aortic arch is right-sided, and a persistence of the ductus arteriosus may be present. The ventriculograms can delineate the anatomy and physiology of the truncus arteriosus. Other imaging methods may be used more widely in the future to detect truncus arteriosus. Magnetic resonance imaging can delineate the vessels and chambers in truncus arteriosus accurately without the use of contrast material or exposure of the patient to ionizing radiation, and ultrafast computed tomography may eventually be a useful imaging technique in diagnosing truncus arteriosus. Neither one is used routinely in the workup of truncus arteriosus.

TREATMENT

Initial Treatment

The ultimate treatment for truncus arteriosus is surgical. The initial treatment, however, is medical and should be aimed at cardiac decongestive therapy. In neonates, diagnosis of classic truncus arteriosus is sufficient to instigate cardiac decongestive therapy, even without signs or symptoms of congestive heart failure. As pulmonary vascular resistance decreases, congestive heart failure occurs requiring digitalization and aggressive diuretic therapy. Before 1968, the only surgical palliation available for truncus arteriosus was pulmonary artery banding. Evolution of radical corrective surgery for truncus arteriosus began with the demonstration that the right ventricular outflow tract in tetralogy of Fallot could be enlarged with a patch. Rastelli et al. (1965) used an artificial, valveless pulmonary artery conduit made of pericardium. In 1967, they used an experimental aortic homograft with a valve conduit for right ventricular pulmonary flow. McGoon et al. (1968) used this method for the first successful correction of truncus arteriosus. Homografts were found to calcify and become stenotic, and Bowman et al. (1973) used an artificial pulmonary trunk of Dacron containing a valve xenograft. Ebert et al. (1976) championed the use of pulmonary artery conduits in infants younger than 6 months, with modification of the conduit when the child was older, and reported a resultant mortality of 11%. Some physicians suggest the use in neonates of valveless conduits as a primary repair. In most patients who have returned for conduit change, repairs were made without the use of a valve conduit.

The alternative to early repair is palliative banding of the pulmonary artery, with complete repair a second stage. Banding of the pulmonary artery in truncus arteriosus frequently requires bilateral banding and is extremely difficult with a mortality approaching 50%. The overall mortality for banding with repair later is 75%.

Surgical Intervention

After diagnosis of truncus arteriosus, the challenge to the cardiologist is determining the optimum time for surgical intervention. Stabilization of the hemodynamics and maturation and growth of the infant must be balanced with the potential for rapid cardiac deterioration or potential for pulmonary hypertension. To prevent persistent pulmonary hypertension, surgical correction should be performed in neonates and in all infants younger than 6 months. With surgical correction in infants at age 6 months or younger, persistent pulmonary hypertension can be prevented. The exception may be infants with a single pulmonary artery, but the only chance for these infants to avoid persistent pulmonary hypertension is surgery performed before the child reaches 6 months. Not only is the cardiologist challenged by timing the initial corrective surgery, but also close follow-up and deliberation are needed to determine optimal timing for conduit replacement.

CHAPTER 150
Congenital Mitral Valve Disease

Adapted from Janette F. Strasburger

The left atrioventricular valve (mitral valve) includes the anterior and posterior mitral valve leaflets separated by their commissures, the chordae tendineae, and the anteromedial and posterolateral left ventricular papillary muscles. The annulus, or skeletal support of the mitral valve, is fibromuscular and contracts with the heart. Abnormalities in the development of the mitral valve apparatus can result in hemodynamic and physiologic alterations in blood flow, which can present with either congestive heart failure or pulmonary edema during fetal, neonatal, or later development.

Most abnormalities of the mitral valve, even in the pediatric age group, are acquired as the result of rheumatic carditis, myocardial ischemia or infarction, hypertension, Marfan syndrome, mitral valve prolapse syndrome, bacterial endocarditis, myocarditis, or cardiomyopathy. Congenital mitral valve abnormalities are much more rare. Because of the severity of obstruction of flow across the valve, valvular regurgitation, or associated cardiac defects, patients with congenital mitral abnormalities often present during infancy. Congenital lesions of the mitral valve are listed in Table 150-1.

TABLE 150-1. Congenital Abnormalities of the Mitral Valve Apparatus

Congenital mitral stenosis
Parachute mitral valve
Double orifice mitral valve
Mitral valve stenosis or hypoplasia
Congenital mitral insufficiency
Cleft mitral valve
Congenital mitral valve regurgitation
Double orifice mitral valve
Ruptured chorda tendineae or papillary muscle

CONGENITAL MITRAL STENOSIS

Clinical Manifestations

Mitral valve stenosis presents clinically with right-sided cardiac failure and pulmonary hypertension. The age at presentation depends on the degree of obstruction of left atrial emptying. Because exercise demands greater cardiac output, initial symptoms are often related to exercise. In infants, feeding requires increased cardiac output, and babies often present with dyspnea or cyanosis during feeding and with failure to grow. Because of pulmonary edema, infants and children are at risk for recurring respiratory infections. Tachypnea, hemoptysis, respiratory distress, low cardiac output, and atrial fibrillation can be associated findings of mitral stenosis. Atrial fibrillation and left atrial thrombi are relatively uncommon in children; however, if atrial fibrillation is observed, the presence of intracardiac thrombi must be excluded before cardioversion.

Physical Exam

The physical examination in mitral stenosis is characterized by a right ventricular lift and by an increased pulmonary component of the second heart sound caused by pulmonary hypertension. A fourth heart sound is sometimes audible secondary to enhanced atrial systolic contraction. A long pandiastolic murmur is often audible at the cardiac apex.

Tests

The chest radiograph usually shows left atrial enlargement with widening of the angle between the left and right main bronchi. In older children, a redistribution of blood flow can be seen with increased flow to the upper lobes. Kerley B lines and pulmonary edema are also present. Generally, the electrocardiogram shows left atrial or biatrial enlargement during sinus rhythm, and, rarely, atrial fibrillation is present. Right ventricular hypertrophy with right-axis deviation is generally seen. Two-dimensional and Doppler echocardiography determine the presence of mitral stenosis and detect structural abnormalities of the mitral valve or supporting apparatus. The left atrial size is often enlarged, but the left ventricular volume is usually 70% to 100% of normal. Transesophageal echocardiography, which allows excellent imaging of the left atrium and mitral valve when the patient is under sedation or general anesthesia, is frequently used during catheterization and surgical valvuloplasty procedures or before cardioversion. Cardiac catheterization demonstrates elevation in pulmonary arterial pressure and right ventricular systolic pressure. A gradient between the left atrial A wave and the left ventricular end-diastolic pressure exists. Often, estimating the left atrial pressure using a pulmonary capillary wedge pressure or entering the left atrium via a transseptal puncture is necessary. Injections in the pulmonary artery or left atrium usually demonstrate abnormalities of the mitral valve or adjacent structures.

Treatment

Mild or moderate mitral stenosis can be managed by diuretic therapy, supplemental nutrition, and aggressive management of respiratory infections. Usually, digoxin is not helpful for right ventricular failure, although it is sometimes used for arrhythmias. Generally, transesophageal echocardiography is indicated before cardioversion of atrial fibrillation to exclude atrial thrombi that might not be evident on precordial echocardiography. Acute anticoagulation before cardioversion is necessary when thrombi are suspected. Long-term anticoagulation with warfarin (Coumadin) is indicated in patients for whom recurrence of atrial fibrillation is likely. The addition of quinidine, procainamide, sotalol, or amiodarone to digoxin therapy is rarely necessary to maintain sinus rhythm.

Balloon mitral valvuloplasty to enlarge the mitral valve orifice during cardiac catheterization has been successful in pediatric patients with both congenital and post-rheumatic mitral stenoses. The procedure is technically possible in most patients and is relatively safe. Improvement in exercise tolerance is seen in approximately 80% of patients initially. Greatest experience with this technique has been gained in the adolescent patient. Five-year follow-up after balloon mitral valvuloplasty has shown that restenosis rates vary from 2% to 30%, depending on the technique used. Complications have included thromboembolism, endocarditis, atrial septal injury, and mitral regurgitation.

Surgery is indicated for children with low cardiac output, severe symptoms with exercise, and severe pulmonary hypertension who are refractory to or ineligible for balloon mitral valvuloplasty. The preferred treatment is surgical commissurotomy, which is open heart surgery consisting of incision along the mitral commissure. The operation must be considered palliative because either annular hypoplasia or abnormalities in the supports of the mitral valve are often present. Whenever possible, mitral valve replacement should be avoided in young children, because anticoagulation is necessary for metallic prosthetic valves in the mitral position. Replacement of the valve is often required in later childhood or adulthood.

Unlike isolated mitral stenosis, parachute mitral valve, double orifice mitral valve, and mitral hypoplasia usually occur with other cardiac defects, not as isolated defects. These defects can cause mitral stenosis, mitral regurgitation, or both. Because of the complexity of associated defects, they are less amenable to surgical repair. Shone complex consists of parachute mitral valve, subaortic stenosis, and coarctation of the aorta with or without a ventricular septal defect.

CONGENITAL MITRAL REGURGITATION

Clinical Manifestations

Clinical symptoms of mitral regurgitation are related to the severity of the regurgitation, associated cardiac defects, left ventricular function, pulmonary artery pressure, and rate of development of the regurgitation. Acute mitral regurgitation of moderate or severe degree is poorly tolerated and rapidly leads to acute pulmonary edema and low cardiac output. Chronic mitral regurgitation of mild or moderate degree may be asymptomatic. With increasing severity, symptoms in infants and children include diaphoresis, recurrent respiratory infections, tachypnea, exercise intolerance, and failure to grow because of high caloric requirements.

Children with mitral regurgitation generally have a diffuse left ventricular lift and a palpably enlarged heart. The first heart sound is normal or decreased, and the pulmonary component of the second heart sound is either normal or increased. Mitral regurgitation causes a high-pitched, blowing, apical pansystolic murmur; it must be differentiated from the murmur of a ventricular septal defect, which is usually audible near the left sternal border rather than at the apex. During diastole, the increased flow across the mitral valve results in a low-pitched diastolic flow rumble and sometimes a third heart sound at the apex.

Tests

The radiographic appearance of mitral regurgitation consists of cardiomegaly of moderate degree with increased pulmonary vascular markings. Enlargement of the left atrial and left ventricular contours of the heart is present. The electrocardiogram generally shows left atrial enlargement and left ventricular hypertrophy. Atrial fibrillation is uncommon. Two-dimensional echocardiography detects abnormalities of valve appearance, motion, and attachments. The left ventricular systolic function is normal or increased because of Starling forces. Decreased left ventricular contractility, especially in the presence of cardiomegaly, suggests cardiomyopathy in association with mitral regurgitation. Color-flow mapping is useful in qualitative assessment of the amount of regurgitation. Severe regurgitation occurs over a broad area of the annulus and refluxes far into the left atrium, whereas in mild mitral regurgitation, only a small jet is noted near the valve. Reversal of flow velocities in the pulmonary veins is also indicative of severe regurgitation.

Treatment

Mild or moderate mitral insufficiency can generally be managed by diuretic and digoxin therapy. Afterload reduction with nitroprusside has been lifesaving in acute mitral regurgitation. Oral afterload-reducing agents such as captopril and enalapril are used as adjuvant therapy in patients with congestive heart failure or cardiomyopathy associated with mitral regurgitation.

Surgical intervention is necessary for congestive heart failure and pulmonary edema secondary to mitral regurgitation, which is poorly controlled by medical management, or for progressive left ventricular dysfunction and cardiomegaly. The surgical treatment of choice is mitral valvuloplasty (repair of the mitral valve) or annuloplasty (plication of the mitral annulus). Often, however, a damaged valve must be replaced, so mitral valve surgery should be delayed whenever possible. Because calcification develops on bioprosthetic valves, generally a low-profile tilting disk valve must be implanted in the mitral position. This procedure requires long-term anticoagulation therapy. An International Normalized Ratio of 3.0 to 3.5 is recommended. The smallest valve available is a 17-mm valve that can be implanted in a child at a minimum age of 1 to 2 years. Surgical correction of other lesions such as double orifice mitral valve and parachute mitral valve is also difficult and depends on associated cardiac defects.

Pulmonary hypertension secondary to either mitral regurgitation or mitral stenosis is generally relieved by surgery because venous congestion does not commonly result in irreversible pulmonary vascular disease. The mortality for valvuloplasty surgery is approximately 4% for patients in stable condition, but it may exceed 10% when a child has low cardiac output, systemic infection, multiple cardiac defects, or severe pulmonary edema, or requires more than one valve replacement.

CHAPTER 151
Mitral Valve Prolapse

Adapted from Victoria E. Judd

Mitral valve prolapse (MVP) is the most common cardiac disorder diagnosis. On the basis of auscultatory evidence only, the overall incidence of MVP in children is 5%. Evaluation of the presence of MVP solely by echocardiography estimates the prevalence at 13% in children aged 5 days with up to 35% prevalence in the 10- to 18-year range. With more stringent echocardiographic criteria, prevalence drops from 13.0% to 0.5%. The true incidence of MVP probably lies in the range of 4% with a 2:1 female–to–male patient ratio present at all ages. Why MVP is more common in female patients is not clear, although smaller left ventricular size and lower body weight may contribute. The primary cause of MVP is uncertain. MVP may occur as an autosomal dominant trait or as an isolated case.

CLINICAL CHARACTERISTICS

Symptoms

Most children with MVP are asymptomatic and are initially referred for cardiac evaluation because of a click or a murmur detected during a routine examination. Numerous studies report a high incidence of symptoms with MVP, but these may be due to selection bias. Small subgroups of patients may be highly symptomatic. Symptoms may include chest pain, fatigue, weakness, palpitations, dyspnea, dizziness, near syncope, syncope, anxiety, and orthostatic hypotension.

Abnormalities on Physical Exam

Abnormalities on physical examination include thoracic and skeletal abnormalities such as a tall slender habitus, pectus excavatum, pectus carinatum, scoliosis, or kyphosis. A high arched palate, increased joint laxity, or abnormal dermatoglyphics patterns may also be present.

Characteristics

MVP is characterized by a midsystolic click or a late systolic murmur. The click and murmur vary depending on an affected patient's position and may vary in auscultatory findings at different times in different patients. The change in the click and murmur is caused by alterations in left ventricular end-diastolic volume. Such maneuvers as moving from a sitting to a supine position or from a standing to a squatting position, passive leg raising, and maximal isometric exercise increase left ventricular volume and decrease the degree of MVP and mitral regurgitation. The click and murmur move toward the second heart sound, and the murmur is shorter.

Auscultation

Left ventricular size and left ventricular volume are decreased by administration of amyl nitrate; a Valsalva maneuver; sudden change from a supine to a sitting position, from a sitting to a standing position, and from a squatting to a standing position; and inspiration. MVP and mitral valve regurgitation increase; thus, the click and murmur move toward the first heart sound, and the murmur becomes longer. Because of the changing intensity or timing with different body positions, auscultation should be performed with the patient in many positions.

The high-pitched, low-intensity, nonejection midsystolic click is best heard at the apex of the heart. It may occur from just after the first heart sound to just before the second heart sound. Multiple clicks may be present in certain patients. Usually, the crescendo, late systolic murmur of MVP is preceded by a click and is heard best at the apex. Occasionally, the murmur is described as having a honking or whooping quality and may be heard without a stethoscope.

The murmur of MVP may be confused with the murmur of hypertrophic cardiomyopathy. During the strain of the Valsalva maneuver, the murmur of hypertrophic cardiomyopathy increases in intensity and the murmur of MVP becomes longer but not louder.

Tests

Usually, the chest radiograph is normal unless associated cardiac defects are present. If a routine chest roentgenogram shows thoracic spine and chest wall abnormalities such as scoliosis, pectus excavatum, or straightened thoracic spine, an evaluation for MVP is indicated.

The electrocardiogram is usually normal. Three types of abnormalities are reported: T wave inversion in leads II, III, and aV_F; prolongation of the QT interval; and arrhythmias. Usually, the ST segments are normal at rest, but ST changes may be induced during standing or exercise.

Usually, the exercise test is normal. Arrhythmias and ST-T wave changes have been reported.

Echocardiography is useful in defining MVP. M-mode echocardiography alone should not be used to diagnose MVP; two-dimensional echocardiography should be used as well. M-mode echocardiography may over diagnose or under diagnose MVP. The apical four-chamber view in two-dimensional echocardiography is sensitive but not specific for the diagnosis of MVP. Many patients who have a normal auscultatory examination may have MVP as documented by the apical four-chamber view. The mitral valve annulus is not flat but is saddle-shaped. The four-chamber view may show superior displacement of the mitral valve leaflets, but it may not be true of MVP. The long axis view seems to be the most specific view to determine the presence or absence of MVP.

Echocardiographic evaluation of patients with possible MVP should include evaluation for mitral annulus dilatation, dysplasia of the mitral valve, mitral valve regurgitation, presence or absence of ruptured chordae and vegetations, and coexistent cardiovascular abnormalities. Prolapse of the tricuspid valve and aortic valve occurs more often in patients with MVP.

Stress radionuclide scintigraphy aids in the differential diagnosis between MVP (associated with atypical chest pain and electrocardiogram abnormalities) and primary coronary artery disease associated with MVP. A negative test may confirm the diagnosis of primary MVP without coronary artery disease. A false-positive test, however, may occur in patients with MVP without associated coronary artery disease.

Diagnostic cardiac catheterization with angiography is rarely needed in patients with isolated MVP. If needed, it is used to assess the severity of associated cardiac abnormalities.

ASSOCIATED CONDITIONS

MVP occurs in increased frequency in patients with Marfan syndrome, Ehlers–Danlos syndrome, and other heritable disorders of connective tissue disease that increase the size of mitral valve leaflets and apparatus. It is also seen with higher frequency in patients with myotonic dystrophy, hyperthyroidism, Turner syndrome, fragile X syndrome, anorexia nervosa, systemic lupus erythematosus, polyarteritis nodosa, and adult polycystic kidney disease. It is seen in patients with thoracic abnormalities such as straight-back syndrome.

Chest Pain

If patients with MVP have symptoms, the most common presenting symptom is disabling chest pain. The exact mechanism of chest pain is unknown. In some patients with MVP, esophageal motility disorders account for chest pain.

Infective Endocarditis

Patients with MVP and mitral regurgitation have an increased incidence of infective endocarditis. Antibiotic prophylaxis should only be used in the presence of a systolic murmur.

Thromboembolism

Acute hemiplegia, transient ischemic attacks, cerebellar infarcts, amaurosis fugax, and retinal arteriolar occlusion appear to be more frequent in patients with MVP syndrome. They may result from thrombosis formation on the valve or abnormalities in the platelet coagulant activities, shortened platelet survival time, and plasma hyperactivity.

Arrhythmias

All types of arrhythmias are reported. Premature ventricular contractions are reported to be present in as many as 50% of children with MVP, and complex ventricular arrhythmias are reported in as many as 18.5%. Twenty-four-hour Holter monitoring may be more sensitive than ECG for detecting arrhythmias.

Sudden Death

Sudden death is a rare complication postulated to be secondary to a lethal arrhythmia. Patients who may be at increased risk of sudden death may have complex ventricular arrhythmias, severe mitral regurgitation, left ventricular dysfunction, prolonged QT interval, dysplastic mitral valve, a history of syncope, presyncope, palpitations, chest pain, or a family history of sudden death.

Mitral Regurgitation

Progressive mitral regurgitation is a rare complication. It occurs in approximately 15% of patients over a 10- to 15-year period. In many patients, it is related to rupture of the chordae tendineae or to infective endocarditis. Severe mitral valve regurgitation occurs more frequently in men who are older than 50 and have MVP.

Mitral Valve Prolapse Syndrome

MVP syndrome is an association of symptoms: syncope, presyncope, chest pain, fatigue, dyspnea, palpitations, exercise intolerance, and neuropsychiatric symptoms with autonomic dysfunction or neuroendocrine abnormalities. The pathogenesis of symptoms in MVP syndrome is not well understood.

MANAGEMENT

Examinations

Evaluation of an affected patient for presence of MVP is first performed by a thorough physical examination that includes maneuvers to elicit the click and murmur, a two-dimensional echocardiogram, and a Doppler study.

Tests

A resting electrocardiogram is recommended in all patients to look for evidence of ST-T wave changes, prolonged QT interval, or an arrhythmia. If coexisting cardiac defects are not present, a chest roentgenogram is not needed in patients with isolated MVP. A 24-hour Holter monitor or exercise treadmill is indicated in patients with palpitations, lightheadedness, dizziness, syncope, arrhythmias on resting electrocardiogram, family history of sudden death, complaints of chest pain, or a prolonged QT interval on resting electrocardiogram. Angiography may be indicated if other cardiac defects coexist.

Follow-Up

An asymptomatic patient with an isolated midsystolic click, no evidence of mitral regurgitation, or dysplastic mitral valve should be reassured of the benign nature of MVP and should be followed-up every few years.

Mitral Valve Replacement

Indications for mitral valve replacement are severe mitral regurgitation, severe life-threatening arrhythmias, and uncontrollable chest pain, all unresponsive to medical management.

Therapy

Prophylactic treatment of patients for cerebral ischemia is not indicated. Patients who have MVP with transient ischemic attacks should receive prophylaxis with antithrombotic and antiplatelet therapy.

Evaluation for Competitive Athletics

Patients with MVP should not participate in competitive athletics if they have a history of syncope or near syncope, a history of disabling chest pain, complex ventricular arrhythmias, significant mitral regurgitation or left ventricular enlargement or dysfunction, prolongation of the QT interval, Marfan syndrome, or a family history of sudden death. Patients who are asymptomatic and are found to have isolated uniform premature ventricular contractions may participate in competitive athletics if no mitral insufficiency or family history of sudden death exists. Patients who have MVP and are asymptomatic should be evaluated before they are cleared for competition.

CHAPTER 152
Anomalous Origin of the Left Coronary Artery

Adapted from David J. Driscoll

CLINICAL CHARACTERISTICS

Anomalous origin of the left coronary artery (ALCA) from the pulmonary artery may be the most common important coronary anomaly with which pediatricians and pediatric cardiologists must deal. Usually, the anomalous coronary artery arises from the left sinus of the pulmonary artery.

Signs and Symptoms

A patient with ALCA may present with signs and symptoms of myocardial infarction and congestive heart failure in infancy, or the condition may be unassociated with myocardial infarction or symptoms of heart disease until detected serendipitously in adulthood or at autopsy. The patient's age at presentation depends on the degree of collateral circulation between the right (RCA) and left (LCA) coronary artery systems. Subjects with well-developed collateral connections may not develop myocardial infarction and may do well, but subjects with poor collateral circulation may have myocardial infarction, which is apparent at an early age.

In the immediate newborn period, pulmonary artery resistance and pressure are increased, flow through the anomalously arising LCA is antegrade from the pulmonary artery, and myocardial perfusion is adequate. As pulmonary artery resistance and pulmonary pressure decrease, antegrade flow of blood from the pulmonary artery through the LCA decreases. If collateral circulation between the RCA and LCA is inadequate, myocardial infarction probably occurs at this time. If collateral circulation exists, myocardial infarction may occur depending on (a) the degree of retrograde flow from the right coronary system through the collateral circulation (bypassing the distribution of the LCA) and into the pulmonary artery (i.e., coronary steal phenomenon) and (b) the degree of antegrade flow along the distribution of the LCA (i.e., myocardial perfusion).

Clinical Features

Clinical features of ALCA in infancy are similar to those of myocarditis and cardiomyopathy, and the diagnosis of ALCA must be considered in the differential diagnosis of unexplained congestive heart failure in infancy. In teenagers and adults, the presence of ALCA may be suspected in the presence of unexplained cardiomegaly, mitral insufficiency, or continuous cardiac murmur. Angina may occur secondary to a coronary steal phenomenon.

TREATMENT AND OUTCOME

The ideal treatment of ALCA is to detect the presence of the anomaly before myocardial infarction occurs and to establish a coronary system that prevents myocardial infarction. However, all cases in infancy come to medical attention only after myocardial ischemia and infarction have occurred. Older data indicated that infants with ALCA and poor left ventricular function (ejection fraction less than 20%) do poorly regardless of surgical or medical management at a young age, whereas infants with ALCA and good left ventricular function do well regardless of their age at the time of operation. Infants who do poorly occasionally have spontaneous improvement. More recently, the overall survival for 42 patients who had dual coronary artery repair for ALCA was 86%. All six patients who died were younger than 1 year. Increasing severity of mitral regurgitation preoperatively was associated with increased mortality, but age and left ventricular shorting fraction were not. In another study of 39 patients, survival was 84%. After a mean follow-up period of 40 months, left ventricular shortening fraction was normal in 86%, but left ventricular dilation persisted in 73% of the patients, and 39% had regional wall-motion abnormalities.

Attempts to establish a two-coronary-artery system for patients with ALCA seem warranted. Because no procedure is deemed superior, surgeons should use the technique with which they are most comfortable. Patients with ALCA and evidence of congestive heart failure benefit from treatment with digitalis and diuretics. Infants with evidence of acute myocardial infarction should be treated with oxygen, sedation, rest, digitalis, and diuretics while awaiting definitive operation.

CHAPTER 153
Abnormalities of Cardiac Rate and Rhythm

Adapted from Arthur Garson, Jr.

ABNORMALITIES IN SINUS RHYTHM: WOLFF-PARKINSON-WHITE SYNDROME AND LONG QT INTERVAL

The normal values for heart rate are shown for different ages in Table 153-1. On any routine electrocardiogram (ECG) or rhythm strip taken in the office or emergency department, the tracing should be examined for indications of two abnormalities: Wolff–Parkinson–White syndrome and long QT interval.

TABLE 153-1. Heart Rates in Normal Infants and Children*

Age (yr)	Awake: Low	Awake: High	Asleep (low)
<1	90	200	70
1–9	60	180	45
10	50	180	35

*Rates are approximate and may vary with clinical situation (e.g., fever may elevate heart rate).

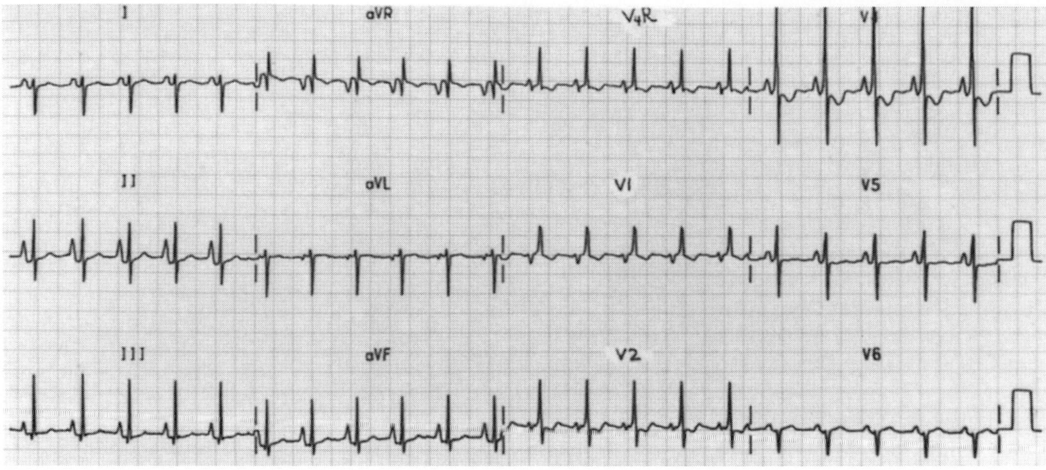

Figure 153-1. Electrocardiographic evidence of Wolff–Parkinson–White syndrome in a baby is seen on this strip. In the limb leads, no delta wave is apparent. In lead V_4 and in the short PR interval (0.075 seconds), the delta wave and the bizarre QRS morphology are seen most easily. The P waves are tall and broad indicating atrial enlargement. This patient had just undergone conversion from supraventricular tachycardia to sinus rhythm. Frequently, the P waves show atrial enlargement immediately after conversion.

Unfortunately, both may be missed by automated pediatric ECG analysis programs. In Wolff–Parkinson–White syndrome, the PR interval is short for the age of the patient, the QRS complex (i.e., delta wave) has a slurred upstroke, and usually changes as the ST or T waves occur. These findings may not be found in all leads, and the midchest leads (V_2 to V_4) may be the most sensitive (Fig. 153-1). A prolonged QT interval is diagnosed when the corrected QT interval (i.e., QT interval in seconds per square root of the RR interval in seconds) is longer than 0.44 (Fig. 153-2). Because both of these problems can cause syncope or seizures in a previously well child, an ECG should probably be part of the workup of a patient who presents with his or her first nonfebrile seizure and definitely in the child who presents with atypical syncope. Atypical syncope occurs during exercise or without the typical circumstances associated with vasodepressor syncope such as a hot, crowded room. It frequently occurs without any warning and, therefore, may result in injury; it may last longer than the 60 seconds associated with the usual faint.

Vagal Arrhythmias

The arrhythmias that appear with increasing amounts of vagal tone are sinus arrhythmia, wandering pacemaker, and junctional rhythm.

In sinus arrhythmia, the P wave axis remains normal (i.e., isoelectric or positive in leads I and aVF), but the interval between P waves increases with inspiration and decreases with expiration. This variation in rate rarely exceeds 100% [e.g., from a rate of 50 to a rate of 100 beats per minute (bpm)]; if it does, it may signify pathology. In sinus arrhythmia, a QRS complex follows every P wave.

In wandering pacemaker, the P wave axis and morphology may change such that the P wave varies from positive to negative in lead aVF. Rarely does the wandering pacemaker wander to the left atrium making the P wave negative in lead I. A QRS complex follows every P wave.

In junctional rhythm, the P wave occurs within or after the QRS complex.

In most patients, these arrhythmias are entirely normal. Excessive variation in the rate, constant sinus bradycardia below the normal limits for age, or constant junctional rhythm may indicate an underlying abnormality. The most common disorder is the *athletic heart*, a condition that may cause bradycardia in adolescents and requires no further workup if the patient is asymptomatic. Other reasons for excessive vagal arrhythmias are increased intracranial pressure, pharyngeal stimulation, gastric distention, upper airway obstruction, asthma, and drugs that potentiate

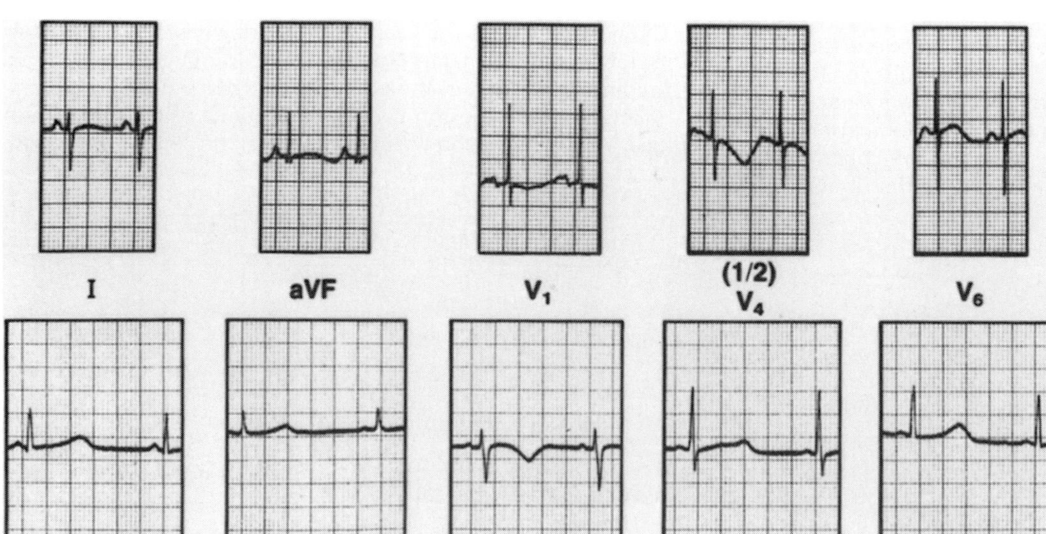

Figure 153-2. Congenital prolongation of the QT interval. The top tracings are from a 9-day-old infant with a history of ventricular tachycardia and ventricular fibrillation at the age of 4 days. All the T waves are abnormal; the T waves in lead V_4 are especially bizarre. The QT interval is 0.43 seconds, and the RR interval is 0.58 seconds; the corrected QT interval (QT/square root of RR) is 0.56 seconds. The bottom tracings are from a 12-year-old child who had his first episode of syncope at 10 years of age. He was being treated for a "familial seizure disorder," although the actual cause of the seizures was ventricular tachycardia. The terminal portion of the T wave in lead V_4 is greater in amplitude than the initial portion. The corrected QT interval is 0.55 seconds.

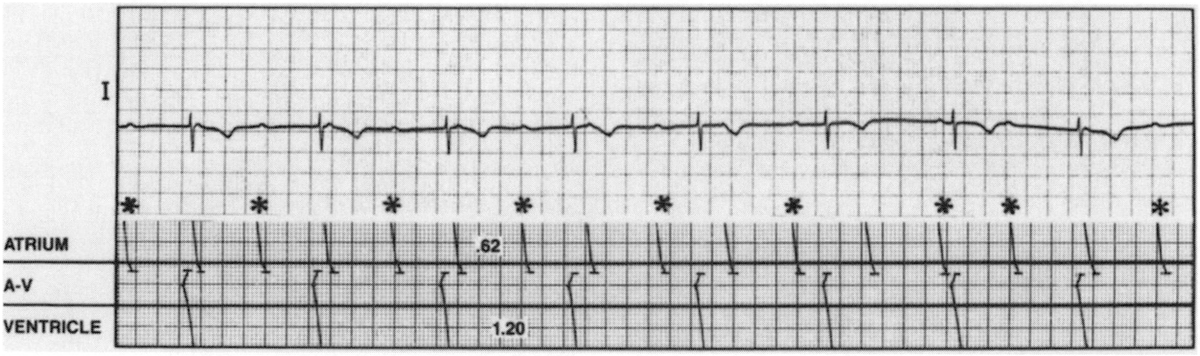

Figure 153-3. A complete atrioventricular (AV) block in a 1-month-old child is demonstrated on this strip. The atrial rate is 97 beats per minute (cycle length of 0.62 seconds), and the ventricles are controlled by a junctional, narrow QRS rhythm at a rate of 50 beats per minute (cycle length of 1.2 seconds). The P waves with asterisks should conduct to the ventricles; they occur beyond the end of the preceding T wave, and they do not change the ventricular rate. Complete AV dissociation is seen with no relation of the P waves to the QRS complexes.

bradycardia such as digoxin, propranolol, verapamil, and morphine.

Complete Atrioventricular Block

In complete atrioventricular (AV) block, the P waves are entirely dissociated from the QRS complexes (Fig. 153-3). The QRS complexes are usually extremely regular; a variation in the PP interval (i.e., superimposed sinus arrhythmia) may occur. In awake newborns with congenital complete AV block, the ventricular rate is usually between 60 and 80 bpm. Commonly associated with congenital complete AV block are congenital heart disease (most often corrected transposition of the great arteries) and maternal collagen vascular disease.

Mothers with collagen vascular disease are frequently asymptomatic, although some may have systemic lupus erythematosus or a similar disease. Women with clinical or subclinical disease have a high titer of antiRo or antiLa antibodies that cross the placenta and preferentially attack the AV node. The infants do not usually have other signs of collagen vascular disease. Despite a low antibody titer, the complete AV block does not reverse in these infants. Some infants born with second-degree AV block may develop complete AV block in the first year or two of life, which implies that *congenital* complete AV block may be an evolving process.

Some of these children also have a prolonged QT interval. Patients with the combination of long QT with second- or third-degree AV block are at high risk for sudden death.

Children with complete AV block may not require immediate pacemaker therapy. As long as the ventricular rate is consistently greater than 55 bpm and no symptoms of congestive heart failure exist, these infants and children fare quite well. If coexistent congenital heart disease exists, especially with a physiologic abnormality such as a ventricular septal defect (frequently associated with corrected transposition), pacing may be instituted earlier. The development of syncope, presyncope, or even sudden death appears to be more common in patients with extremely low ventricular rates (i.e., consistently in the 40s), prolonged QT interval, or complex ventricular ectopy. Consideration should be given to earlier pacing in these patients.

As children with congenital complete AV block grow, they may exhibit subtle symptoms such as frequent naps, mild growth failure, night terrors, and lack of full participation in sports. If these subtle symptoms occur, pacemakers are usually implanted. Pacemakers that sense the atrium and pace the ventricle can correct the situation physiologically returning normal variation to the ventricular rate.

SUPRAVENTRICULAR ARRHYTHMIAS

Premature Atrial Contractions

A premature atrial contraction (PAC) is defined as a premature P wave. In most instances, it has a different morphology and axis from those of the sinus P waves. If a P wave has a similar morphology and axis to the sinus P wave, a regular underlying sinus rhythm and a P wave occur obviously early. This condition may be classified as a PAC, most of which are conducted to the ventricles with a normal QRS. As the premature P wave occurs earlier and earlier, conduction to the ventricles with a different QRS (i.e., aberrant PAC) from that of the sinus beat may occur, simulating a premature ventricular contraction (PVC). For any early QRS that has a morphology different from that of the sinus, the preceding T wave should be examined carefully for a hidden P wave. In children, the presence or absence of a compensatory pause is not helpful in differentiating an aberrant PAC from a PVC. Occasionally, a premature P wave may occur so early that it does not conduct to the ventricles at all, and it may simulate sinus bradycardia because the premature P wave may conduct into the sinus node, delaying the next expected sinus impulse. In many cases of paroxysmal bradycardia, especially those in which conducted PACs are on the same tracing, the T wave should be searched carefully for the presence of hidden P waves. This phenomenon is especially common in newborn infants. Many tracings similar to the one in Fig. 153-4 are interpreted as multiform PVCs with PACs and sinus bradycardia, but most of these infants have only PACs, some conducted aberrantly and some not conducted at all. PACs apparently do not predispose to supraventricular tachycardia, and treatment is not necessary.

Supraventricular Tachycardia

Supraventricular tachycardia is defined as an abnormally rapid rhythm that originates proximal to the bifurcation of the bundle of His, which is caused by an abnormal mechanism (specifically excluding sinus tachycardia), and does not have flutter waves on the surface ECG. In most cases of supraventricular tachycardia, the onset is paroxysmal and the rate is faster than 230 bpm; in infants, the most common rate is 300 bpm. In approximately

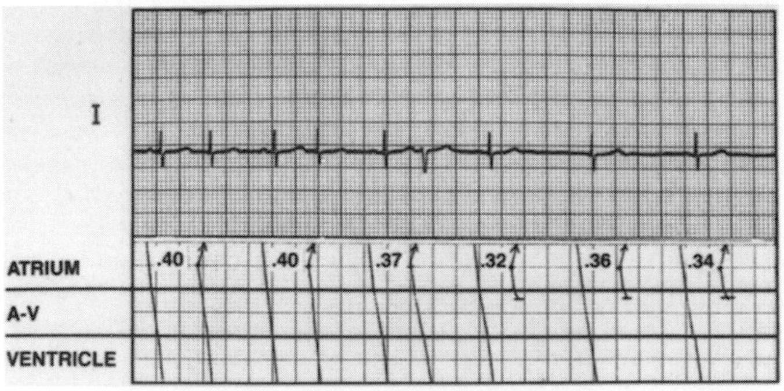

Figure 153-4. Blocked premature atrial contractions are demonstrated in this tracing taken from a 1-day-old infant. The first beat is of sinus origin, and it is followed by a premature atrial contraction. The baseline is completely flat immediately after the sinus T wave, after which a slight change in the baseline occurs indicating a premature P wave (i.e., premature atrial contraction). This conducts to the ventricles normally. The premature atrial contraction occurs 0.40 seconds after the preceding P wave. This sequence is repeated in the next two beats. The premature P wave that occurs 0.37 seconds after the preceding sinus P wave conducts with a different QRS indicating QRS aberration. In the last three beats, the sinus T wave has a different shape than the other sinus T waves, which indicates that a P wave is buried in the T wave. The premature P wave occurs 0.32 seconds after the preceding sinus P wave. Because this is too early for conduction to the ventricles to occur, the premature P wave is not followed by a QRS complex. This "blocked premature atrial contraction" simulates sinus bradycardia.

one-half of patients, P waves may be found, but they are not as obvious as they are in sinus tachycardia.

In 98% of the children with supraventricular tachycardia, the QRS complex during tachycardia (after the first 5–10 beats) is identical to the QRS complex during sinus rhythm (Fig. 153-5). Rarely, supraventricular tachycardia may occur with aberration; infants younger than 6 months appear slightly more likely to have supraventricular tachycardia with aberration when it occurs. Left bundle branch block morphology is more likely than right bundle branch block. It remains that most infants and children with a wide QRS tachycardia have ventricular tachycardia.

The major problem in the differential diagnosis of supraventricular tachycardia in children is with sinus tachycardia, because both rhythms usually have a normal QRS complex. If the rate is faster than 230 bpm, the rhythm is virtually always supraventricular tachycardia; if the rate is slower, the disorder could be supraventricular tachycardia or sinus tachycardia. If the P waves are clearly visible and positive in leads I and aVF, it is likely sinus tachycardia. The condition of the patient may be helpful. Most infants or children with very rapid sinus tachycardia have fever, sepsis, hypovolemia, aminophylline intoxication, or another reason for this finding. Most of the children with supraventricular tachycardia are otherwise well.

Three major predisposing causes of supraventricular tachycardia exist: Wolff–Parkinson–White syndrome (Fig. 153-1), congenital heart disease, and sympathomimetic drugs (e.g., decongestants). Rarely does a child develop a tachyarrhythmia associated with the ingestion of caffeine-containing compounds. Because children vary in their responses to the conditions triggering supraventricular tachycardia, we try not to restrict them from any drug or situation, unless it is known to lead to arrhythmia in that particular patient.

The initial treatment of paroxysmal supraventricular tachycardia involves assessing whether the patient has a compromised cardiac output (e.g., decreased peripheral pulse volume, decreased capillary refill, diaphoresis). Many infants with less severe circulatory embarrassment present with mild irritability, decreased feeding, tachypnea, and hepatomegaly. If the infant is judged to be compromised, the following steps should be undertaken to stop the supraventricular tachycardia: The diving reflex should be initiated by placing a wet washcloth in crushed ice or filling a rubber glove with crushed ice and placing it on the infant's face for as long as 30 seconds (this should always be done with ECG monitoring, and the team should be prepared for cardiopulmonary resuscitation because of asystole or ventricular fibrillation, both of which have been reported, although rarely). Other vagal maneuvers such as Valsalva and carotid sinus massage may be attempted, but they are less effective for patients younger than 4 years. We do not recommend eyeball pressure because dislocated lenses have been reported. Intravenous bolus administration of adenosine, 100 to 300 μg/kg, should be attempted next with constant ECG monitoring and equipment available for defibrillation. If the drug and vagal maneuvers fail, we then use DC cardioversion, which must be synchronized to the QRS; the dose is 0.5 to 1.5 watt-seconds/kg.

If the patient is not compromised hemodynamically and if the diving reflex, vagal maneuvers, and adenosine are ineffective, procainamide, 15 mg/kg intravenous drip over 1 hour, may be used. During procainamide infusion, the ECG should be monitored for QT prolongation and appearance of ventricular arrhythmias. To avoid possible hemodynamic deterioration, intravenous propranolol or intravenous verapamil should probably not be used.

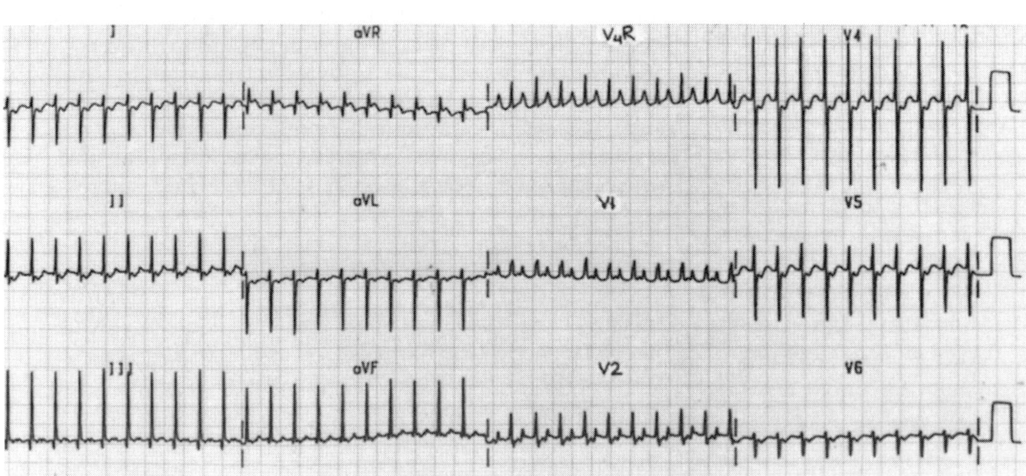

Figure 153-5. This tracing was taken from the patient whose tracing was shown in Figure 153-1. The ventricular rate is 250 beats per minute. In this patient who has Wolff–Parkinson–White syndrome demonstrated during sinus rhythm, the QRS complex during supraventricular tachycardia is normal. P waves occur after the QRS complex, seen best in lead V_2.

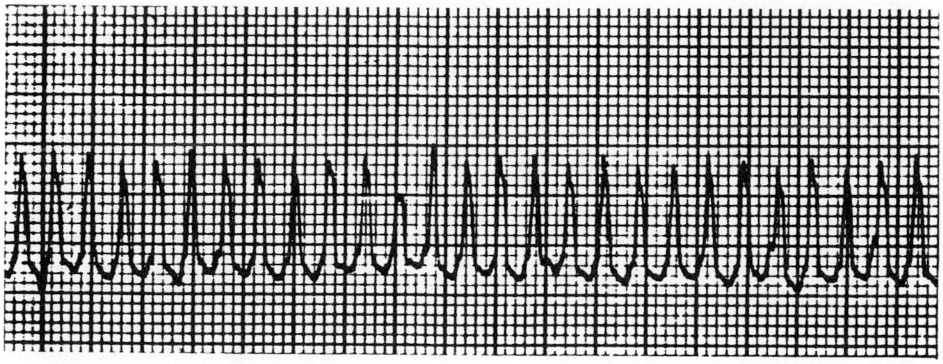

Figure 153-6. This strip demonstrates ventricular tachycardia in an infant. The ventricular rate is 500 beats per minute, and the QRS duration is only 0.045 seconds. This may be mistaken for supraventricular tachycardia. However, the notched morphology of the QRS complexes and the discordance between the QRS complexes and the T waves (i.e., QRS pointing upward and T waves pointing downward) suggests ventricular tachycardia, even though the QRS duration is normal. In sinus rhythm, this infant had a QRS duration of 0.025 ms with a completely different QRS morphology.

VENTRICULAR ARRHYTHMIAS

Premature Ventricular Contractions

A PVC is recognized as a premature QRS complex that does not have the same morphology as the sinus complex and is not preceded by a premature P wave. Especially in infants, PVCs may not have a broad QRS complex, but they may have a morphology different from that of the sinus QRS. If PVCs all have similar shapes, they are referred to as uniform, and if they have more than one morphology, they are called multiform. A couplet is two PVCs in a row, and bigeminy is an alternating rhythm in which every other beat is a PVC.

Most children with PVCs have a normal heart. Occasionally, PVCs are associated with long QT syndrome, mitral valve prolapse, hypertrophic cardiomyopathy, congestive cardiomyopathy, and congenital heart disease before or after surgery. If the heart is completely normal, the prognosis for the child with uniform PVCs (even those frequent enough to present as bigeminy) is good, and the condition is entirely benign. For the child with a normal heart and multiform PVCs or couplets, less data are available. Because the prognosis may be serious (including sudden death in some children with PVCs and abnormal hearts), it is important to assess whether the heart is normal. In the child with uniform PVCs, if the history, physical examination, ECG (other than the rhythm), and chest radiograph are normal, echocardiography is probably not necessary. Further workup is probably indicated for multiform PVCs and couplets.

Ventricular Tachycardia

Ventricular tachycardia is defined as three or more PVCs in a row at a rate faster than 120 bpm; slower rates are referred to as *accelerated ventricular rhythms*. The QRS complex in ventricular tachycardia is different from that of the sinus QRS complex, although it may not be broad. In our series of 22 infants younger than 2 years with ventricular tachycardia, the QRS duration ranged from 0.06 to 0.11 seconds. The rate may be as rapid as 400 or 500 bpm (Fig. 153-6). Although ventricular tachycardia is an unusual diagnosis for an infant or a child, it must be suspected in any case in which the QRS complex does not appear to be similar to the sinus QRS complex. We have found that ventricular tachycardia in young infants may be associated with a small ventricular tumor or with the long QT syndrome. In older children, ventricular tachycardia is associated with mitral valve prolapse, various forms of cardiomyopathy, and congenital heart disease before and after surgery. In most series, it is uncommon for a child with sustained ventricular tachycardia to have an entirely normal heart; even if no known history of heart disease exists, some of these children have early cardiomyopathy.

The initial management of ventricular tachycardia consists of intravenous lidocaine (1 mg/kg every 5 minutes for three doses). If the lidocaine is not effective and the patient is hemodynamically unstable, synchronized DC electrical cardioversion should be used (0.5–1.5 watt-second/kg). Because most infants and children with ventricular tachycardia have abnormal hearts, additional diagnostic studies should be performed.

CONCLUSION

Most arrhythmias in children with an entirely normal heart are benign; for a child with an abnormal heart, these arrhythmias may be lethal. In the case of a tachyarrhythmia, the patient should be evaluated for hemodynamic stability. If the patient is hemodynamically stable, the physician should take time to analyze the ECG, not mistaking supraventricular tachycardia for sinus tachycardia or ventricular tachycardia for supraventricular tachycardia. If the patient is unstable, synchronized DC electrical cardioversion should be performed.

CHAPTER 154
Cardiomyopathy

Adapted from Brian D. Hanna and Marc Paquet

The term *cardiomyopathy* refers to any structural or functional abnormality of the ventricular myocardium not associated with disease of the coronary arteries, high blood pressure, valvular or congenital heart disease, or pulmonary vascular disease. It can be divided into two categories: primary, or heart muscle disease of known cause associated with disorders of other systems, and secondary (Table 154-1). This chapter is limited to primary cardiomyopathies grouped into four types: dilated, hypertrophic, restrictive, and arrhythmogenic.

IDIOPATHIC DILATED CARDIOMYOPATHY

Idiopathic dilated cardiomyopathy (IDC) is a disease of infancy. More than 50% of patients present before age 2 years. Incidence is equal in both genders. Etiology is unknown. Familial incidence is 600 to 700 times that of the general population and, in some cases, a hereditary basis has been documented. Histologic examination of endomyocardial biopsy obtained from adult patients with IDC has shown a high incidence of myocardial inflammation, but

TABLE 154-1. Classification of Cardiomyopathy in Children

Primary
Dilated
Idiopathic dilated
Cardiomyopathy
Endocardial fibroelastosis
Hypertrophic
Obstructive
Nonobstructive
Restrictive
Endomyocardial fibrosis
Löffler eosinophilic endomyocardial disease
Hemochromatosis
Fabry disease
Pseudoxanthoma elasticum
Arrhythmogenic
Arrhythmogenic right ventricular dysplasia
Oncocytic cardiomyopathy
Secondary
Infection
Metabolic
General system disease
Heredofamilial
Sensitivity and toxic reactions

these findings have not been duplicated in children. Reports have shown an increase in structural abnormalities of mitochondrial DNA in a high percentage of patients with IDC. Clinical and experimental reports suggest that an immunologic abnormality may be implicated in the pathogenesis of the disease.

Since the late 1980s, numerous reports have described various cardiovascular abnormalities including dilated cardiomyopathy in children infected with the human immunodeficiency virus (HIV). Usually, the pathologic process involves the myocardium of both ventricles in a uniform fashion producing generalized cardiac dilatation. The myocardium is pale, and the endocardium is thin and translucent. Microscopical examination shows interstitial fibrosis, myofiber hypertrophy, degeneration, and necrosis.

Clinical Characteristics

In one-third to one-half of reported cases, the initial presentation is preceded by a respiratory or gastrointestinal illness. Symptoms of congestive heart failure—tachypnea, fatigue during feedings, excessive perspiration and, occasionally, failure to thrive—are usually dominant at the initial presentation. Some patients initially present with ventricular or supraventricular arrhythmias.

Usually, physical examination reveals an ill-appearing child in moderate to severe respiratory distress. Cyanosis is unusual, but pallor of the skin is common. Peripheral pulses are often weak, blood pressure is low with a narrowed pulse pressure, and pulsus alternans is a common finding. Thoracic overdistention and, rarely, prominence of the left hemithorax are apparent on examination of the chest. Often, auscultation of the lungs reveals decreased air entry at the base, but inspiratory rales are rare. On palpation of the precordium, the heart is usually quiet, and localizing the apex may be difficult. On auscultation, heart sounds are muffled, but careful auscultation usually reveals the presence of a gallop rhythm. Often, murmurs are absent at the time of initial presentation, but the soft apical pansystolic murmur of mitral regurgitation often appears after a few days, once the cardiac function improves. Usually, the liver edge is palpable well below the right costal margin, and it is rounded as a result of passive congestion. Neck vein distention and peripheral edema are rarely found in infants but are not unusual in older children and young adults.

Laboratory Findings

Chest radiography shows cardiomegaly secondary to dilatation of the left atrium and left ventricle and evidence of pulmonary venous congestion that can progress to frank pulmonary edema (Fig. 154-1). Electrocardiography shows sinus tachycardia with ST-T wave abnormalities and left ventricular hypertrophy in most patients (Fig. 154-2). The echocardiographic features include dilatation of the left atrium and the left ventricle and reduction of the shortening fraction (percentage of change in left ventricular dimension). Usually, two-dimensional echocardiography shows global left ventricular dysfunction and is essential in the early detection of intracavitary thrombi. Often, Doppler examination demonstrates the presence of mitral regurgitation before it can be detected clinically. Indices of diastolic function are abnormal. Radionuclide angiographic studies confirm dilatation of both ventricles and permit noninvasive measurement of the ejection fraction, which is always decreased.

Treatment

During the acute phase of illness, treatment is directed at controlling congestive heart failure and includes bed rest, fluid restriction, and use of agents that decrease the cardiac load or improve myocardial contractility. Infants with severe congestive heart failure should be given nothing by mouth but should receive intravenous hydration up to 75% to 80% of their calculated maintenance.

Infants and children with less severe congestive failure can be fed orally on demand without restriction. Because it renders food unpalatable, sodium restriction usually results in reduced caloric intake in infants and children; thus, low-sodium diets should be avoided. Instead, diuretic agents should be used to handle the sodium load. Usually, furosemide or ethacrynic acid,

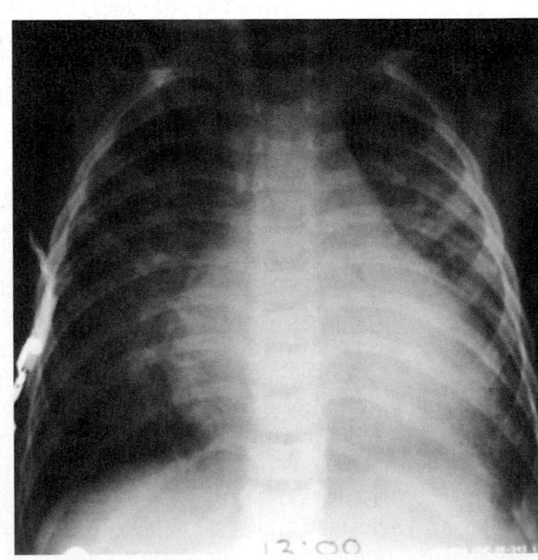

Figure 154-1. This chest radiograph of a 12-month-old boy with idiopathic dilated cardiomyopathy shows cardiomegaly and pulmonary venous congestion.

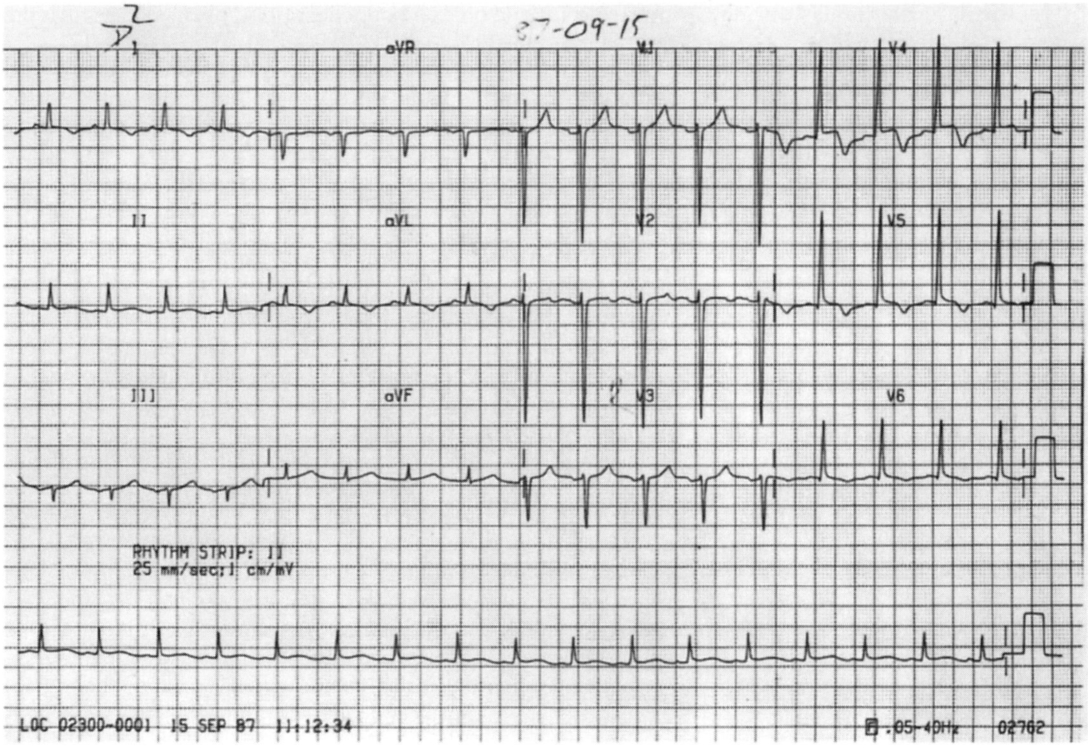

Figure 154-2. This 12-lead electrocardiogram from a 12-month-old boy with idiopathic dilated cardiomyopathy shows left ventricular hypertrophy and diffuse ST-T wave abnormalities.

1.0 to 2.0 mg/kg/day, is effective. Serum electrolytes and renal function tests should be obtained before institution of diuretic therapy. If potassium or chloride depletion occurs, a potassium-retaining agent such as spironolactone (1.5–3.0 mg/kg/day) may be added to the regimen. Frequently, supplementation of chloride may be necessary because loop diuretics are less effective with chloride levels lower than 90 to 95 mEq/L. Oral or intravenous KCl or NH_4Cl is effective in maintaining the chloride and the diuretic response. Oral digitalization (20–30 μg/kg over 16–24 hours) should be initiated soon after the diagnosis is made. Twelve hours after digitalization is completed, oral maintenance therapy using 7.5 to 10.0 μg/kg/day divided into two doses should be started. This medication should be continued for many months after the clinical and laboratory evidence of myocardial impairment regresses.

For patients who present with severe congestive heart failure and pulmonary edema, nasotracheal intubation and mechanical ventilation may be lifesaving. Sedation with morphine sulfate often improves the overall condition of these patients. In these acutely ill infants, the sympathomimetic amines dopamine and dobutamine have a faster onset of action and a shorter half-life than digitalis. Also, the type III phosphodiesterase inhibitor milrinone should be used to improve contractility and to reduce afterload to both ventricles.

The role of afterload-reducing agents in the treatment of patients with IDC is well established. During the acute phase of illness, intravenous sodium nitroprusside or hydralazine is the best agent; for long-term therapy, hydralazine (0.25–1.00 mg/kg four times daily), prazosin (50–100 μg/kg four times daily), and captopril (1–2 mg/kg three times daily) are used orally. At least one clinical study suggested that the addition of the calcium antagonist diltiazem to conventional therapy (digitalis, diuretics, and vasodilators) significantly reduces mortality and improves myocardial function and clinical status in a group of adult patients with IDC; this drug may prove to benefit infants and children as well. Although significant atrial or ventricular arrhythmias should be treated according to accepted principles, the question of such arrhythmias representing an independent prognostic factor remains unanswered.

The role of corticosteroids and other immunosuppressive agents such as azathioprine is unclear and controversial in the treatment of children with IDC. Because of the high risk of serious side effects such as growth retardation, bone marrow suppression, and infection, use of corticosteroids, and immunosuppressive agents should be restricted to those patients in whom myocardial inflammation is documented by endomyocardial biopsy.

Patients with atrial fibrillation, intracavitary thrombus demonstrated by two-dimensional echocardiography, or suspected or confirmed arterial embolization should be anticoagulated. Anticoagulation is achieved with heparin, 100 U/kg intravenously, followed by constant infusion of 10 to 20 U/kg/hour adjusted to maintain the partial thromboplastin time at 1.5 times that of the control. After 1 or 2 weeks of this regimen, oral warfarin (0.05 mg/kg/day) should be started, and the heparin should be discontinued over the next 48 to 72 hours. Oral warfarin should be continued for the duration of predisposing factors to thromboembolic episodes (atrial fibrillation or left ventricular dilatation with shortening fraction of less than 20%). Subcutaneously administered low-molecular-weight heparins are also effective in this realm, and monitoring is much simpler in the small child.

Patients who fail to respond to medical therapy and whose condition rapidly deteriorates are candidates for cardiac transplantation. Indications for cardiac transplantation are New York Heart Association class IV symptomatology and a life expectancy of less than 6 months. Patients who present after age 2 years and those who present before age 2, but have persistent cardiomegaly or develop significant atrial or ventricular arrhythmias during follow-up, may be candidates for transplantation.

Prognosis

The prognosis for infants with IDC is poor with mortality ranging from 35% to 63%, although in one retrospective study, the 5-year survival was close to 80%. Most deaths occur during the first year after diagnosis. Few parameters, if any, are useful in predicting the survival of a patient, but reports strongly suggest that patients who present before age 2 years have a better chance of survival than do those who present after age 2. Other factors suggestive of poor outcome include persistent congestive heart failure or cardiomegaly and development of significant arrhythmias (i.e., atrial fibrillation or flutter or complex ventricular ectopy) during follow-up. The most common cause of death is intractable congestive heart failure, followed by sudden death secondary to an arrhythmia. Approximately one-half of survivors recover completely, whereas the other half continues to present clinical or echocardiographic evidence of myocardial dysfunction.

HYPERTROPHIC CARDIOMYOPATHY

Hypertrophic cardiomyopathy (HC) is characterized by a disproportionate increase in the myocardial mass in the absence of cavity dilatation. The size of the left ventricular cavity may be either normal or small. The presence or absence of obstruction to left ventricular ejection can distinguish the two types of HC: obstructive and nonobstructive. HC is rare in children accounting for 20% to 30% of pediatric primary myocardial disease.

Etiology

Most authors believe that the hypertrophy manifests itself in response to altered intramyocardial wall stress that, in turn, is the result of the primary lesion; myofibril disarray. No definite explanation for the myocardial disarray exists. One suggestion is that it is the result of an arrest in the maturation of the normal myocardial architecture. Although ample evidence supports the possibility of an autosomal inheritance pattern with variable penetrance, the disease manifests itself differently in relatives of patients. Molecular genetic analysis of members from a large kindred has determined that genes linked to familial HC are located on chromosome 14. Approximately 45% of patients are considered sporadic cases.

Clinical Characteristics

In children, diagnosing HC by clinical findings alone is difficult. Clinical presentation is different in infants younger than aged 1 year as compared to those who present after age 1. In general, affected infants present with congestive heart failure. More than 60% have right and left ventricular gradients and die in the first year of life. Children, on the other hand, are often asymptomatic and have predominantly left ventricular gradients; their symptom complex tends to be nonprogressive, but they are more prone to sudden death. In general, symptoms tend to be more severe in young patients. Thirty-five percent of infants and 50% of children are referred for evaluation of a systolic ejection murmur or for screening after the detection of an affected family member. In infants, the most common symptoms are tachypnea, tachycardia, and poor feeding, whereas children usually complain of dyspnea and fatigue on exertion, chest pain, presyncope, syncope, and palpitations.

On physical examination, the peripheral pulses present an initial brisk upstroke, followed by a reduction in amplitude in midsystole as the ventricular ejection is impeded. On palpation of the precordium, the apex may be displaced inferiorly and toward the left, and its impulse may be sustained. In some cases, a systolic thrill is felt at the lower left sternal border. On auscultation, S1 is normal, and S2 is normally split in most patients but, with significant left ventricular outflow tract obstruction, paradoxical splitting occurs. Early (S3) and late (S4) diastolic filling sounds are heard in 37% and 50% of patients, respectively. Systolic ejection murmurs of grade 3 (of 6) or higher are common. Usually, the murmur begins well after S1 and is loudest between the mid-retrosternal region and the apex; it radiates widely but not to the carotids. At the apex and into the left axilla, it is often holosystolic marking the presence of mitral regurgitation. Quality of the systolic murmur varies with the physiologic state of the patient. Maneuvers and agents that increase contractility or decrease preload or afterload (i.e., exercise, standing, the straining phase of Valsalva maneuver, digitalis, isoproterenol, amyl nitrate, and nitroglycerin) can be used to augment the gradient and the murmur. On the other hand, the gradient and the murmur are decreased by the following interventions: Müller maneuver, the overshoot phase of Valsalva maneuver, squatting, handgrip, alpha-adrenergic stimulation, beta–adrenergic blockade, or general anesthesia.

Laboratory Findings

Almost all infants and most children demonstrate cardiomegaly on the chest radiograph. Pulmonary vascular markings are usually normal. Usually, the electrocardiogram (Fig. 154-3) shows left ventricular hypertrophy with ST segment and T wave abnormalities and abnormal Q waves. In some patients, evidence of right ventricular hypertrophy is present.

Often, the diagnosis is made on the basis of echocardiography. The M-mode examination reveals asymmetric septal hypertrophy with systolic anterior motion of the anterior leaflet of the mitral valve and midsystolic closure of the aortic valve. Two-dimensional echocardiography (Fig. 154-4) shows the extent of hypertrophy and the presence or absence of obstruction, and it permits assessment of left ventricular systolic and diastolic function. In general, the presence of systolic anterior motion of the anterior mitral leaflet, combined with prolonged contact with interventricular septum, is predictive of a left ventricular outflow tract gradient of more than 30 mm Hg. The disease must be differentiated from other causes of myocardial hypertrophy. In infants younger than 1 year, the most common cause of myocardial hypertrophy is maternal diabetes or steroid use in infants with bronchopulmonary dysplasia. In older children, causes include Pompe disease, Friedreich ataxia, and lentiginosis.

Treatment

The first-line drug in the treatment of symptomatic children is propranolol, which reduces heart rate, left ventricular contractility, and wall stress. Approximately one-third of symptomatic patients obtain complete relief of symptoms with standard doses of oral propranolol. However, this drug has no effect on the extent of hypertrophy, does not reduce the incidence of ventricular arrhythmia and, more important, does not eliminate the risk of sudden death. Calcium channel blockers such as verapamil and nifedipine are effective in the treatment of HC, even in patients who do not respond to propranolol. Verapamil decreases the

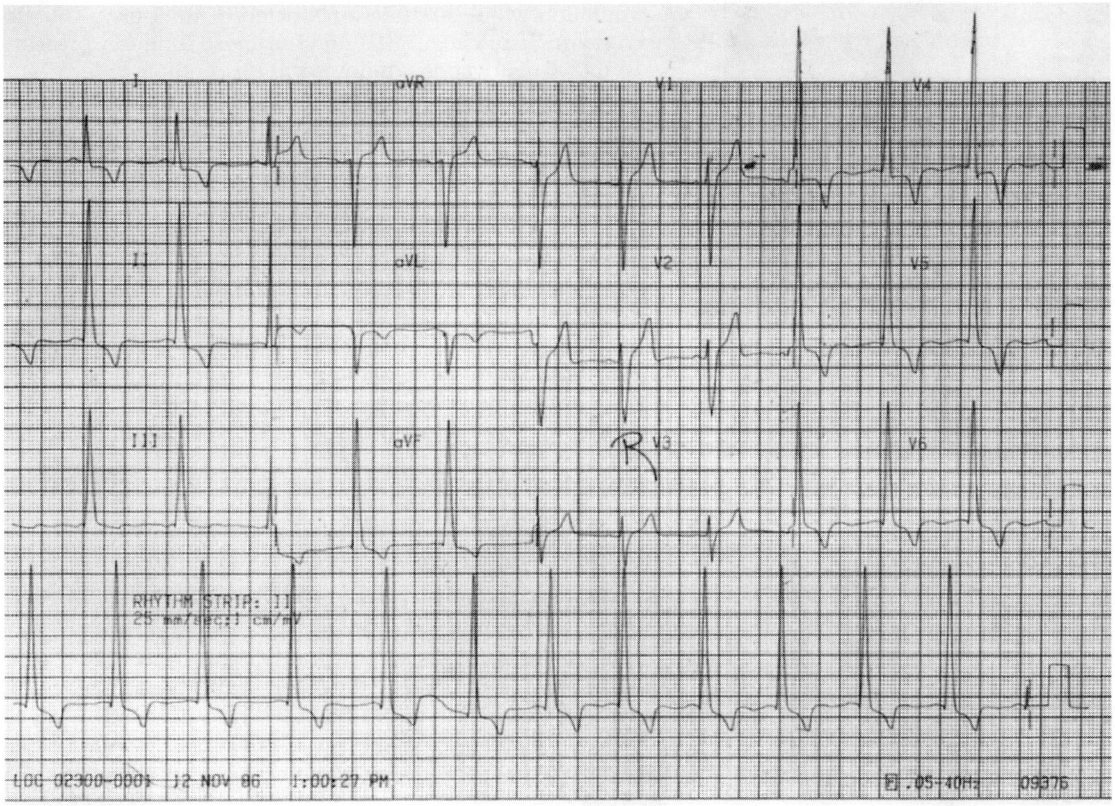

Figure 154-3. Electrocardiogram from a 12-year-old with hypertrophic cardiomyopathy. Voltage criteria for left ventricular hypertrophy and inverted T waves are evident in the left precordial derivations and in leads I, II, aV_L, and aV_F.

systolic gradient, improves diastolic filling, and may be effective in decreasing the amount of hypertrophy. The role of amiodarone in the treatment of infants and children with HC is unclear, and its use should be reserved for patients with refractory and potentially lethal arrhythmias. Positive inotropic agents such as digoxin must be used with caution. Increasing contractility may produce an increase in systolic gradient and a concomitant deterioration in clinical status. Likewise, by decreasing preload, diuretic agents may worsen the outflow obstruction. Nonspecific therapy includes prophylaxis against bacterial endocarditis at the time of at-risk procedures. General anesthesia and pregnancy carry increased risk. Active sports participation is not recommended, because sudden deaths in adolescents with HC occur during or after exercise.

Dual-chamber cardiac pacing with optimization of the atrioventricular interval has decreased the outflow tract obstruction and improved symptoms in HC. However, not all patients will respond with improvement in symptoms despite a significant gradient reduction; such patients probably have a significant reduction in diastolic function.

Surgical intervention is indicated when medical therapy fails to alleviate symptoms. Studies show that, in selective patients, myectomy–myotomy provides symptomatic relief, reduces the gradient, and prolongs life. Mitral valve replacement is recommended only in patients whose septum is too thin to allow adequate resection, in those patients in whom previous resections have not reduced the obstruction, or in those patients for whom mitral regurgitation is severe.

Prognosis

The prognosis for infants who present at younger than 1 year is dismal, especially for those who initially present with congestive heart failure or cyanosis. If the initial presentation is that of an asymptomatic murmur, chances of survival to 1 year are greater than 50%. Of those patients alive at 1 year, 40% to 50% improve, 30% to 40% die, and 10% to 20% have residual disease. If a strong family history of sudden death exists, children are at increased risk for such an event. Mortality is twice as high in children as in adults. No predictive variable to help to identify patients at risk for sudden death exists. One study demonstrated that nonsustained ventricular tachycardia (more than three beats) increases the risk for sudden death from 8% to 10% per year, whereas in another study, the absence of ventricular arrhythmia during ambulatory electrocardiogram monitoring did not correlate with a low risk of sudden death.

RESTRICTIVE CARDIOMYOPATHY

Restrictive cardiomyopathy (RC) is characterized by impairment of diastolic filling secondary to scarring of the endocardium. Usually, the left ventricular end-diastolic volume is normal or reduced, and the ejection fraction is only slightly decreased. The primary physiologic anomaly is decreased ventricular compliance. The major diagnostic challenge is to distinguish RC from constrictive pericarditis. The two conditions present similar clinical and hemodynamic features and, in a significant number of patients, the definitive diagnosis requires endomyocardial biopsy or exploratory thoracotomy.

Endomyocardial fibrosis and Löffler disease are the same disease at different stages of evolution. The term hypereosinophilic syndrome describes the disease, and the presence of cardiac involvement is described as endomyocardial disease with or without eosinophilia. Endomyocardial fibrosis affects adolescents and young adults of both genders more often, whereas Löffler

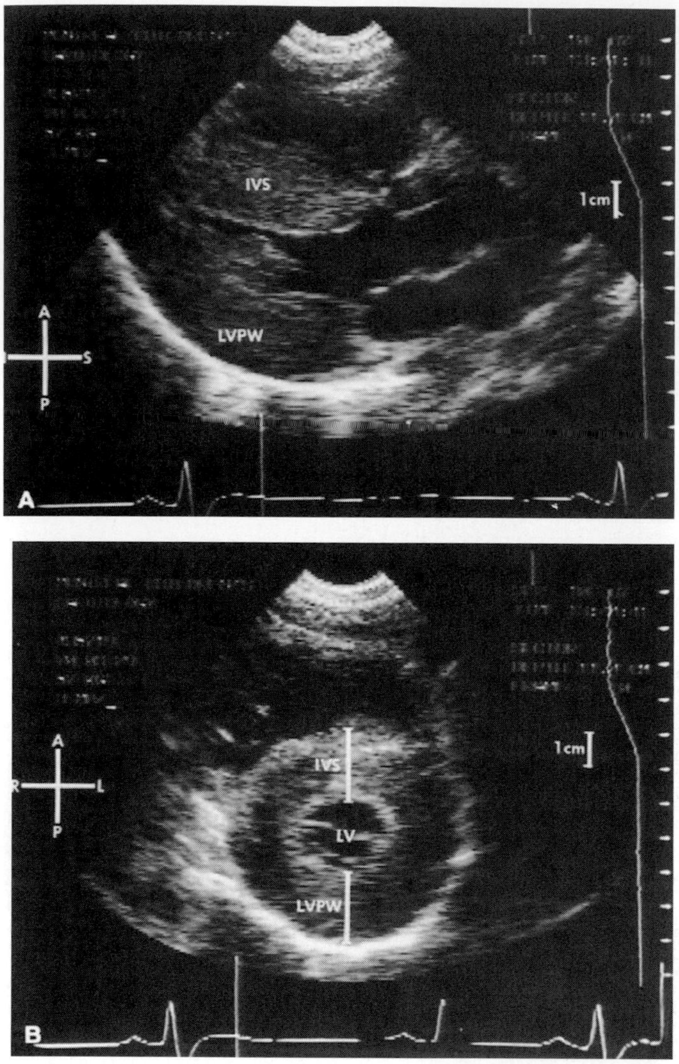

Figure 154-4. Two-dimensional echocardiogram of a 17-year-old boy with nonobstructive hypertrophic cardiomyopathy. Systolic frames in parasternal long axis (**A**) and parasternal short axis (**B**) views show concentric hypertrophy of left ventricular wall and nearly complete cavity obliteration. IVS, interventricular septum; LV, left ventricle; LVPW, left ventricular posterior wall.

disease presents at any age and affects boys three times more often than girls. Although the disorder's exact etiology is not identified, the consensus is that it results from an immunologic reaction involving the eosinophil itself.

The disease is characterized by layers of fibrosis of variable thickness over the endocardium occurring predominantly in three areas: the left ventricular apex, the mitral valve apparatus, and the right ventricular apex. The histologic picture is characterized by the absence of elastic fibers in the areas of fibrosis. The process can be restricted to either the left or the right ventricle, or both ventricles may be involved simultaneously. In Löffler disease, intracavitary thrombus and acute myocarditis are more common than in endomyocardial fibrosis; often, eosinophilic infiltration of extracardiac organs occurs.

Clinical and Laboratory Findings

The clinical picture depends on whether one or both ventricles are involved. Involvement of the left ventricle results in mitral regurgitation, whereas disease restricted to the right ventricle produces tricuspid regurgitation. The most common presenting symptom is dyspnea, followed in descending order of incidence by chest pain. Physical findings include nonspecific systolic ejection murmur, holosystolic murmur at the apex, third and fourth heart sounds, jugular venous distention, and peripheral edema.

Often, chest radiography shows cardiomegaly secondary to dilatation of the atria, hypertrophy of the ventricular walls, and pericardial effusion. Electrocardiographic features include nonspecific ST-T wave changes, small QRS voltage, first-degree atrioventricular block, and variable degrees of atrial dilatation and ventricular hypertrophy. Characteristic echocardiographic features include apical obliteration, preserved contractile function of the ventricle, involvement of the papillary muscle and posterior leaflet of the mitral or tricuspid valve, and normal or small ventricles with dilated atria. Frequently, intracavitary thrombi are identified on two-dimensional echocardiography.

Treatment and Prognosis

Because of the low incidence of RC in infants and children, determining the natural history in this age group is difficult. However, because most cases reported in children were taken from necropsy studies, the overall prognosis seems poor. No specific treatment exists. Medical treatment with diuretics, venous vasodilators, digitalis glycosides, or arteriolar vasodilators is either ineffective or may be detrimental. In some cases, surgical resection of the subendocardial fibrosis or atrioventricular valve replacement has resulted in hemodynamic and symptomatic improvement.

ARRHYTHMOGENIC RIGHT VENTRICULAR DYSPLASIA

Since the disorder was first described in 1978, arrhythmogenic right ventricular dysplasia has been reported in multiple case studies of infants and children. The American Heart Association nomenclature calls this entity right ventricular cardiomyopathy so as to include cases with similar pathology but without the arrhythmia. The clinical presentation is one of abrupt onset of syncopal episodes, palpitations, or ventricular tachycardia. Boys are affected four times more often than girls. Usually, the cardiovascular examination is normal. Symptoms are secondary to episodes of ventricular tachycardia of left bundle branch block morphology (Fig. 154-5). Patients also exhibit a spectrum of right ventricular impairment ranging from normal function in some to severe dysfunction in others. Arrhythmias originate in areas of localized dysplasia limited to the right ventricular free wall. On histology, these areas show variable reduction in myofibril number and interstitial infiltration by lipoid cells, histiocytes, and lymphocytes. The disorder's etiology is unknown, but familial occurrence is widely recognized. Studies have reported genetic linkage to the long arm of chromosome 2 in some familial clusters. Usually, electrocardiography shows frequent ventricular premature depolarizations of left bundle branch block morphology with inversion of the T waves in leads V_1 to V_4; "epsilon waves" are found in the ST segments in the right precordial leads in 30% of patients. Often, evidence of right ventricular dysfunction can be identified on two-dimensional echocardiography and radionuclide angiography. However, of current imaging techniques, magnetic resonance imaging identifies the dysplasia with the highest accuracy.

Frequently, combinations of antiarrhythmic drugs are required to control episodes of ventricular tachycardia. Surgical

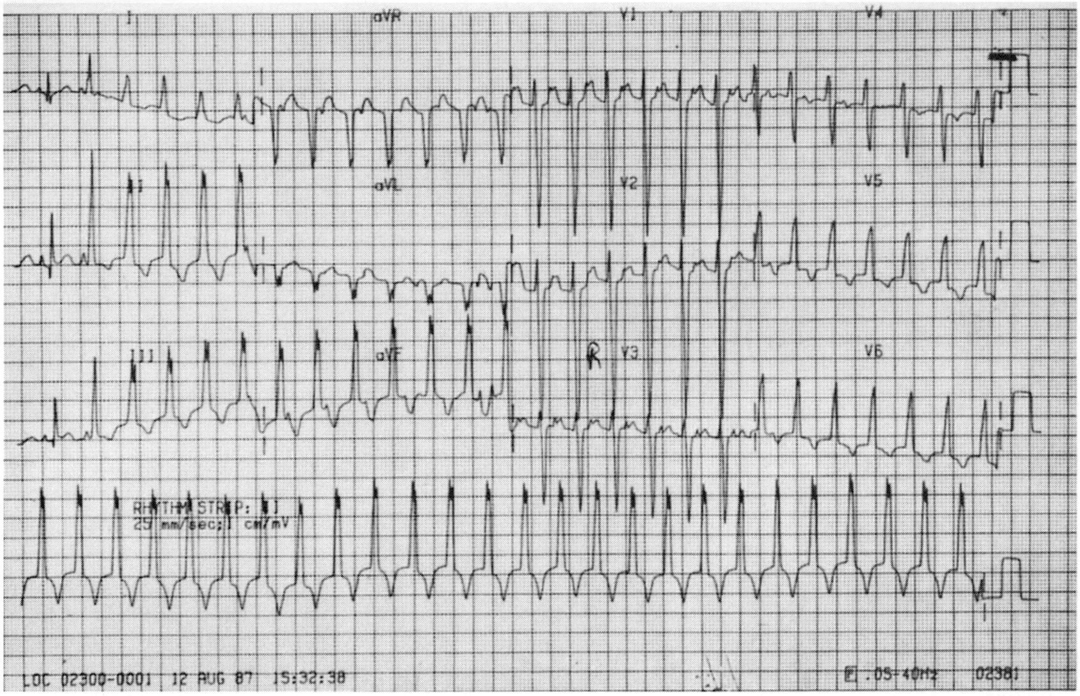

Figure 154-5. Twelve-lead electrocardiogram showing ventricular tachycardia with left bundle branch block morphology at a rate of 155 beats per minute. The first and second complexes in leads I, II, and III represent a sinus beat and a fusion beat, respectively.

treatment ranging from simple ventriculotomy to total disconnection and resuturing of the right ventricular free wall has been successful in some cases. The disorder's usual course is one of slow deterioration in right ventricular function and a reduction in efficacy of antiarrhythmic treatment.

CHAPTER 155
Infective Endocarditis

Adapted from Richard A. Friedman
and Jeffrey R. Starke

Infective endocarditis (IE) refers to a condition in which an organism or organisms infect the endocardium, valves, or related structures that have been previously injured by surgery, trauma, or disease. The infecting organism may be bacterial, fungal, chlamydial, rickettsial, or viral. In the first half of the twentieth century, many patients with IE had had prior rheumatic heart disease. In the latter part of the century, most children with IE have complex congenital heart defects.

Virtually any congenital defect may predispose to the development of IE. In a large, cooperative study of the natural history of aortic stenosis, pulmonic stenosis, and ventricular septal defect, the risk of developing endocarditis by 30 years of age was determined to be 9.7% for unoperated patients; if the patient had undergone surgical repair, the incidence of IE was much lower. In other studies, tetralogy of Fallot accounted for the largest percentage of patients with CHD who developed IE. Ventricular septal defect was the second most common lesion, followed by atrial stenosis (8%), patent ductus arteriosus (7%), and transposition of the great vessels (4%).

IE associated with prosthetic materials, especially valves and valved conduits, is likely to increase in the future. Prosthetic valve endocarditis has been categorized as early onset (i.e., within 3 months of implant) or late onset. The incidence of infection ranges from less than 1% to 10% after implantation. Neither the type of valve nor the site of implant significantly affects the incidence of prosthetic valve endocarditis.

CLINICAL CHARACTERISTICS

The clinical characteristics of IE depend on the underlying pathophysiologic processes of the disease. The extent of local involvement of the myocardium or valves, embolization from vegetations, and activation of immunologic mechanisms play essential roles in clinical expression. Patients with acute IE may present in shock and with clinical pictures consistent with overwhelming sepsis. In some cases, confirmation of endocarditis may be found only at autopsy. The subacute form of the disease may follow an indolent course, and a diagnosis may not be established for weeks or months. Because endocarditis frequently occurs in children with underlying heart disease, subtle changes in their physical examination may be missed, unless the examiner is discerning and alert. Table 155-1 lists the major clinical manifestations of IE and their relative frequency of occurrence in children.

The most common finding in IE is fever, although approximately 10% of patients have no fever. Fever is usually low grade and shows no specific pattern, especially in the subacute form. Other nonspecific complaints include malaise, anorexia, weight loss, fatigue, and sleep disturbances. Involvement of the large joints with arthralgias or arthritis occurs in 24% of patients. Nausea, vomiting, and nonspecific abdominal pains are found in 16% of patients. Chest pains, which are usually related to myalgias but are sometimes secondary to pulmonary embolism, especially with tricuspid valve involvement, occur in as many as 10% of older children.

Specific skin lesions associated with IE are more common in adults than in children. Petechiae are seen in approximately one-third of the children, especially in those with a more chronic course. Common sites of involvement are the mucous

TABLE 155-1. Symptoms and Physical Findings in Infective Endocarditis

Symptom/finding	Incidence (%)
Fever	56–100
Anorexia/weight loss	8–83
Malaise	40–79
Arthralgias	16–38
Gastrointestinal problems	9–36
Chest pain	5–20
Heart failure	9–47
Splenomegaly	36–67
Petechiae	10–50
Embolic events	14–50
New/changing murmur	9–44
Clubbing	2–42
Osler's nodes	7–8
Roth's spots	0–6
Janeway lesions	0–10
Splinter hemorrhages	0–10

membranes of the mouth, the conjunctivae, and the extremities. Petechiae are the most common skin manifestation in IE occurring in as many as 40% of patients; purpura is rare. Osler's nodes, which have also been described in systemic lupus erythematosus and in extremities distal to the sites of prolonged arterial catheterization, are exquisitely tender lesions. They are found most commonly on the pads of the fingers and toes, the thenar and hypothenar eminences, the sides of the fingers, and the skin on the lower part of the arm. Much controversy exists regarding whether they represent an immunologic response to infection manifesting as a vasculitis or are septic emboli. Janeway lesions are nontender, hemorrhagic plaques that occur frequently on the palms and the soles and represent septic emboli with bacteria, neutrophils, and subsequent necrosis with subcutaneous hemorrhage. Roth's spots are small, pale retinal lesions with areas of hemorrhage that are usually located near the optic disc.

Infants and neonates may present with a clinical picture less specific than that seen in older children. The onset is more acute and clinically mimics overwhelming sepsis. The diagnosis is rarely suspected before death. The use of indwelling vascular catheters has increased the incidence of endocarditis in neonates. Persistent bacteremia associated with a deterioration in pulmonary function, coagulopathies, thrombocytopenia, and the appearance of murmurs should arouse suspicion of possible endocarditis in a neonate.

The clinical presentation of IE in intravenous drug abusers has several distinctive features. Previous underlying heart disease is found in one-third of these patients. The tricuspid valve is the site most commonly affected, and these patients often have pulmonary complications including infarction, abscess formation, and signs and symptoms of pleural effusion. Extracardiac sites of infection are found in approximately two-thirds of these patients. Tricuspid insufficiency with findings of a murmur of tricuspid regurgitation, a pulsatile liver, and a gallop rhythm are found in 33% of patients.

DIAGNOSIS

Laboratory Investigation

Table 155-2 summarizes the most common laboratory findings in children with IE. Blood cultures are the single most important diagnostic tool for establishing the diagnosis of IE. Because bacteremia is usually continuous and low grade, the timing and site of collection do not affect the yield. In approximately 66% of all cases of IE, the blood cultures grow the infecting organism and, in 90%, the results of the first two blood cultures are positive. If a patient has received antibiotics before the culture is tried, the chance of obtaining a positive culture may be reduced from between 95% and 100% to 64%. If pretreatment has occurred, placing the blood sample in hypertonic media may enhance the chance of isolating the organism. Patients with fungal endocarditis may have only intermittently positive blood culture results, and the organism may take a week or longer to grow in culture.

TABLE 155-2. Laboratory Findings in Infective Endocarditis

Finding	Incidence (%)
Elevated erythrocyte sedimentation rate	71–94
Positive rheumatoid fever	25–55
Anemia	19–79
Positive blood culture result	68–98
Hematuria	28–47

Ideally, three to five sets of blood cultures should be obtained within the first 24 hours. These specimens should be taken from different sites and contain 3 to 5 mL of blood. Thioglycolate broth should be used, and the bottles should be kept for 3 weeks to detect slow-growing organisms. Blood culture results may be negative in 10% to 15% of cases of suspected endocarditis because of prior administration of antibiotics; endocarditis caused by rickettsiae, chlamydiae, or viruses; slow-growing organisms (e.g., Candida species, Haemophilus species, Brucella species) or nutritionally variant streptococci; infections caused by anaerobic organisms; nonbacterial thrombotic vegetation endocarditis; mural endocarditis; right-sided endocarditis; fungal endocarditis (especially Aspergillus species); or an incorrect diagnosis. Additional sites including urine, sputum, cerebrospinal fluid, synovial fluid, bone marrow, and lymph nodes may be infected concomitantly, and cultures of these additional sites should be included if blood culture results fail to demonstrate an infecting agent.

Necessary adjunctive laboratory tests include measurement of the erythrocyte sedimentation rate, which is elevated in as many as 90% of patients and correlates with the hypergammaglobulinemia found in this disease. The erythrocyte sedimentation rate should decrease toward normal if therapy has been successful, and serial measurements may be helpful in monitoring therapy.

Echocardiography

Two-dimensional (2D) echocardiography uses multiple echo beams and provides a cross-sectional moving image of the heart, which can be recorded from several angles. Some areas of the heart such as the pulmonary valve are better visualized using 2D imaging, and the increased sensitivity of this technique in detecting pulmonary valve endocarditis has been documented. Adjunctive use of the Doppler technique to diagnose prosthetic valve regurgitation before it becomes clinically apparent may aid in earlier diagnosis. The sensitivity of echocardiography in detecting vegetative lesions in suspected endocarditis in adults ranges from 13% to 83%.

Transesophageal echocardiography (TEE) has become important in evaluating patients for vegetations. TEE takes advantage of the proximity of the heart, especially the left atrium to the esophagus. This technique also eliminates the inability to image transthoracically in some patients who do not have good "echo windows" from that approach. The quality of the image is better making diagnosis more certain.

A negative echocardiographic study result does not rule out the presence of vegetations. The resolution on most equipment limits the detection of vegetations to those larger than 2 to 3 mm. Rheumatic heart disease with preexisting valve disease, mitral valve prolapse (MVP) with thickened leaflets, marantic vegetations, Löffler endocarditis, Chiari networks in the right atrium, and valve ring abscesses pose interpretive problems to the echocardiographer. After a vegetation is detected, it may show no significant change during therapy, and a recurrence of disease cannot be diagnosed unless a noticeable increase in size occurs or a new vegetation appears. Continued growth of a vegetation coexistent with persistent bacteremia or evidence of further endocardial infiltration may indicate a treatment failure or the need for surgical intervention. An echocardiographic examination at the time of hospital discharge of a patient after an apparently successful course of antibiotic therapy can be used as a baseline for further evaluation.

Prophylaxis

The use of antibiotics before and during any procedure that induces a transient bacteremia has become standard medical practice for the prevention of IE. Numerous failures with subsequent development of endocarditis have been reported. Although failure is often related to inappropriate drug regimens, infection occasionally develops despite adherence to published guidelines. In 1997, significant revisions were made in the guidelines for endocarditis prophylaxis. This report emphasized that, in fact, most cases of endocarditis are not attributable to an invasive procedure. Cardiac conditions were stratified into high, moderate, and negligible risk categories to help the clinician assess risk based on potential morbidity and mortality. These conditions are summarized in Table 155-3. In addition, further elaboration on the types of procedures that are associated with a relatively higher risk of bacteremia is given. Two doses of antibiotics are no longer recommended for oral procedures. Rather, only one dose with a maximum of 2 g (50 mg/kg) is given, and either cephalexin (50 mg/kg, maximum dose of 2 g) or, for patients with immediate-type hypersensitivity reactions to penicillins, azithromycin or clarithromycin (15 mg/kg, maximum 500 mg) should be given 1 hour before the procedure. Finally, prophylaxis for genitourinary and gastrointestinal procedures was simplified. These changes are shown in Tables 155-4, 5, and 6.

The use of antibiotic prophylaxis in patients with mitral valve prolapse (MVP) is controversial. This condition exists in approximately 5% of the population in the United States. A case-control study comparing persons with MVP with normal controls found that the odds for the association of IE with MVP was 8.2; it increased to 15.2 when a murmur of mitral regurgitation was present. Unfortunately, reports on the natural history of MVP in children that address the risk of developing IE are sparse. Until data for the exact incidence of mitral regurgitation associated with MVP in children are available, the safest course is probably to prescribe routine subacute bacterial endocarditis prophylaxis for all children who have documented MVP.

Microbiology

Many different organisms have been associated with IE in humans. Table 155-7 lists the most common causative agents responsible for the development of IE. Gram-positive cocci are the etiologic agents in 90% of cases in which an organism is isolated.

TABLE 155-3. Cardiac Conditions Associated with Endocarditis

Endocarditis prophylaxis recommended
High-risk category
Prosthetic cardiac valves, including bioprosthetic and homograft valves
Previous bacterial endocarditis
Complex cyanotic congenital heart disease (e.g., single ventricle states, transposition of the great arteries, tetralogy of Fallot)
Surgically constructed systemic pulmonary artery shunts of conduits
Moderate-risk category
Most other congenital cardiac malformations (other than those listed previously of that follow)
Acquired valvar dysfunction (e.g., rheumatic heart disease)
Hypertrophic cardiomyopathy
Mitral valve prolapse with valvar regurgitation, thickened leaflets (men older than 45 even without regurgitation, exercise-induced regurgitation), or both
Endocarditis prophylaxis not recommended
Negligible-risk category (no greater risk than general population)
Isolated secundum atrial septal defect
Surgical repair of atrial septal defect, ventricular septal defect, or patent ductus arteriosus (without residua beyond 6 months)
Previous coronary artery bypass graft surgery
Mitral valve prolapse without regurgitation
Physiologic, functional, or innocent heart murmurs
Previous Kawasaki disease without valvular dysfunction
Previous rheumatic fever without valvular dysfunction
Cardiac pacemakers (intravascular and epicardial) and implanted defibrillators

TABLE 155-4. Dental Procedures and Endocarditis Prophylaxis

Endocarditis prophylaxis recommended[a]
Dental extractions
Periodontal procedures, including surgery, scaling and root planing, probing, and recall maintenance
Dental implant placement and reimplantation of avulsed teeth
Endodontic (root canal) instrumentation or surgery only beyond the apex
Subgingival placement of antibiotic fibers or strips
Initial placement of orthodontic bands but not brackets
Intraligamentary local anesthetic injections
Prophylactic cleaning of teeth or implants where bleeding is anticipated
Endocarditis prophylaxis not recommended
Restorative dentistry[b] (operative and prosthodontic) with or without retraction cord[c]
Local anesthetic injections (nonintraligamentary)
Intracanal endodontic treatment; postplacement and buildup
Placement of rubber dams
Postoperative suture removal
Placement of removable prosthodontic or orthodontic appliances
Taking of oral impressions
Fluoride treatments
Taking of oral radiographs
Orthodontic appliance adjustment
Shedding of primary teeth

[a] Prophylaxis is recommended for high- and moderate-risk cardiac conditions.
[b] This includes restoration of decayed teeth (filling cavities) and replacement of missing teeth.
[c] Clinical judgment may indicate antibiotic use in selected circumstances that may create significant bleeding.

TABLE 155-5. Other Procedures and Antibiotic Prophylaxis

Endocarditis prophylaxis recommended
Respiratory tract
Tonsillectomy, adenoidectomy, or both
Surgical operations that involve the respiratory mucosa
Bronchoscopy with a rigid bronchoscope
Gastrointestinal tract[a]
Sclerotherapy for esophageal varices
Esophageal stricture dilation
Endoscopic retrograde cholangiography with biliary obstruction
Biliary tract surgery
Surgical operations that involve the intestinal mucosa
Genitourinary tract
Prostatic surgery
Cystoscopy
Ureteral dilation
Endocarditis prophylaxis not recommended
Respiratory tract
Endotracheal intubation
Bronchoscopy with flexible bronchoscope, with or without biopsy[b]
Tympanostomy tube insertion
Gastrointestinal tract
Transesophageal echocardiography[b]
Endoscopy with or without gastrointestinal biopsy
Genitourinary tract
Vaginal hysterectomy[b]
Vaginal delivery[b]
Cesarean section
Infected tissue caused by urethral catheterization, uterine dilation and curettage, therapeutic abortion, sterilization procedures, insertion or removal of intrauterine devices
Other
Cardiac catheterization, including balloon angioplasty
Implanted cardiac pacemakers, implanted defibrillators, and coronary stents
Incision or biopsy of surgically scrubbed skin
Circumcision

[a]Prophylaxis is recommended for high-risk patients and is optional for medium-risk patients.
[b]Prophylaxis is optional for high-risk patients.

Streptococci, especially of the viridans group, remain the bacteria most frequently isolated. Because of the increasing role of surgery and prosthetic material in the correction and palliation of CHD, the percentage of cases caused by staphylococci, gram-negative bacilli, and fungi have increased. Identification of the causative agent is the single most important procedure involved in confirming the diagnosis, directing therapy, and predicting outcome and possible complications.

TREATMENT

Several general principles provide the basis for treatment of IE. The preferable route of antibiotic administration is intravenous. Oral antibiotics may be absorbed poorly or erratically, especially in infants, which may result in treatment failure. A course of at least 4 and up to 6 weeks or longer is required to sterilize vegetations and prevent relapse. Bacteriostatic agents are contraindicated and may lead to failure or relapse if used. Synergism between certain agents may produce a rapid bactericidal effect and allow smaller doses of each drug to be administered, thereby reducing possible toxic side effects. However, certain drug combinations such as penicillin and chloramphenicol may be antagonistic.

After initiation of therapy, daily blood cultures should be obtained. Although negative blood culture results may not necessarily correlate with therapeutic success, continued positive blood culture results usually indicate a need for investigation of the serum concentration of the drug in the patient, for the addition of another agent, or for a change in therapy. If the patient has not responded clinically to initial antibiotic therapy within several days, more blood cultures should be obtained. In addition, attention to the patient's clinical course is essential. Patients usually begin to improve within a few days of the initiation of appropriate therapy, although persistent fever may occasionally occur in patients who eventually have a good outcome.

Electrocardiographic monitoring should be performed in the early stages to assess for the presence of arrhythmias or the development of conduction disturbances that may require immediate attention. If second-degree atrioventricular block develops during an episode of endocarditis, temporary transvenous pacing should be considered. Pacing should always be instituted for third-degree atrioventricular block. Physical examination to assess for development of regurgitant murmurs or embolic events is also mandatory.

Current recommendations for optimal therapy in pediatric IE are largely based on studies from adult patients. These regimens are usually more successful and less toxic in children than in adults (Table 155-8).

Fungal endocarditis presents the clinician with several difficult problems. The overall survival rate is only 20%, and only rarely is medical therapy reported to be successful in eradicating the disease. A delay in making the diagnosis is frequently encountered because of slow growth in blood culture media. Embolic events are often the first serious sign of fungal endocarditis that may necessitate immediate surgical intervention. The primary antifungal agent used is amphotericin B, alone or in

TABLE 155-6. Prophylactic Regimens for Surgical Procedures

Situation	Agent[a]	Regimen[b]
Dental, oral, respiratory tract, or esophageal procedures		
Standard general prophylaxis	Amoxicillin	Adults: 2 g; children; 50 mg/kg Orally 1 hour before procedure
Unable to take oral medications	Ampicillin	Adults: 2 g IM or IV; children: 50 mg/kg IM or IV Within 30 minutes before procedure
Allergic to penicillin	Clindamycin *or*	Adults: 600 mg; children: 20 mg/kg Orally 1 hour before procedure
	Cephalexin or cefadroxil *or*	Adults: 2 g; children: 50 mg/kg Orally 1 hour before procedure
	Azithromycin or clarithromycin	Adults: 500 mg; children: 15 mg/kg Orally 1 hour before procedure
Allergic to penicillin and unable to take oral medications	Clindamycin *or*	Adults: 600 mg; children: 20 mg/kg IV Within 30 minutes before procedure
	Cefazolin	Adults: 1 g; children: 25 mg/kg IM or IV Within 30 minutes before procedure
Genitourinary/gastrointestinal procedures (excluding esophageal)		
High-risk patients	Ampicillin plus gentamicin	Adults: ampicillin, 2 g IM or IV, plus gentamicin, 1.5 mg/kg (not to exceed 120 mg), within 30 minutes of starting procedure; 6 hours later, ampicillin, 1 g IM or IV, or amoxicillin, 1 g orally Children: ampicillin, 50 mg/kg IM or IV (not to exceed 2 g), plus gentamicin, 1.5 mg/kg, within 30 minutes of starting procedure; 6 hours later, ampicillin, 25 mg/kg IM or IV, or amoxicillin, 25 mg/kg orally
High-risk patients allergic to ampicillin/amoxicillin	Vancomycin plus gentamicin	Adults: vancomycin, 1 g over 1 to 2 hours, plus gentamicin (as previously mentioned); complete injection/infusion within 30 minutes of starting procedure Children: vancomycin, 20 mg/kg IV over 1 to 2 hours, plus gentamicin (as previously mentioned); complete injection/infusion within 30 minutes of starting procedure
Moderate-risk patients	Amoxicillin or ampicillin	Adults: amoxicillin, 2 g orally 1 hour before procedure, or ampicillin, 2 g IM or IV, within 30 minutes of starting procedure Children: amoxicillin, 50 mg/kg orally 1 hour before procedure, or ampicillin, 50 mg/kg IM or IV within 30 minutes of starting procedure
Moderate-risk patients allergic to ampicillin/amoxicillin	Vancomycin	Adults: vancomycin, 1 g IV over 1 to 2 hours; complete infusion within 30 minutes of starting procedure Children: vancomycin, 20 mg/kg IV over 1 to 2 hours; complete infusion within 30 minutes of starting procedure

[a]Total children's dose should not exceed adult dose.
[b]No second dose of vancomycin or gentamicin is recommended.

TABLE 155-7. Causative Agents in Pediatric Infective Endocarditis

Organism	Incidence (%)
Streptococci	
Viridans	17–72
Enterococci	0–12
Pneumococci	0–21
beta-Hemolytic	0–8
Staphylococci	
S. aureus	5–40
S. epidermidis	0–15
Gram-negative aerobic bacilli	0–15
Fungi	0–12
Miscellaneous	0–10
Culture negative	2–32

combination with 5-fluorocytosine. Amphotericin B is given at a dose of 0.5 to 1.0 mg/kg/day. Although usually less severe in children than in adults, toxic reactions may necessitate altering the usual regimen. Fevers, chills, phlebitis, anemia, nephrotoxicity, renal tubular acidosis, hypocalcemia, and thrombocytopenia are the toxic effects most commonly reported. Although the optimal dose of amphotericin B is unknown, total doses of 20 to 50 mg/kg are usually used. Therapy usually continues for at least 8 weeks and, over a long time, evidence of recurrence must be looked for, because relapses have been observed as long as 2 years after a presumed cure. Most physicians agree that the combination of antifungal agents and surgery is the treatment of choice in fungal endocarditis.

In patients with culture-negative endocarditis, empiric therapy with two or more agents is used for 6 weeks, during which time continuing efforts to identify an organism are pursued. Surgery has been a valuable adjunct to medical therapy for IE in certain circumstances.

TABLE 155-8. Recommended Antimicrobial Therapy for Infective Endocarditis in Children

Alternate agent in infecting organism	Length of antibiotic agent*	Alternate agent in allergic patients*	Length of therapy (wk)
Streptococci			
Susceptible viridans (MIC <0.2 μg/mL penicillin G)	Aqueous penicillin G + streptomycin or gentamicin	Vancomycin ± streptomycin or gentamicin	2–4
Resistant viridans (MIC <2.0 μg/mL penicillin G) and enterococci	Aqueous penicillin G + gentamicin	Vancomycin + gentamicin	4–6
Staphylococci			
S. aureus (methicillin susceptible)	Nafcillin or methicillin ± gentamicin	Cephalothin or vancomycin	6–8
S. aureus (methicillin resistant)	Vancomycin	Same	6–8
S. epidermidis	Vancomycin ± rifampin	Same	6–8
Gram-negative organisms			
Enteric bacilli	Ampicillin + gentamicin (based on *in vitro* susceptibilities)		6–8
Pseudomonas aeruginosa	Ticarcillin + gentamicin		6–8
Haemophilus	Ampicillin ± gentamicin		4–6
Culture negative			
Postoperative	Vancomycin + gentamicin		6–8
Nonoperative	Nafcillin or methicillin + gentamicin ± aqueous penicillin G		6–8

MIC, minimal inhibitory concentration.
*All daily doses for children with normal renal function are as follows: aqueous penicillin G, 200,000 to 250,000 U/kg in divided doses q4–6h; streptomycin, 20 to 40 mg/kg in divided doses q12h; gentamicin, 60 to 90 mg/m^2 in divided doses q8h; vancomycin, 40 to 60 mg/kg in divided doses q6h; nafcillin, 100 to 200 mg/kg in divided doses q4–6h; methicillin, 100 to 200 mg/kg in divided doses q4–6h; cephalothin, 100 mg/kg in divided doses q6–8h; rifampin, 15 to 30 mg/kg in divided doses q12h; ampicillin, 200 to 300 mg/kg in divided doses q6h; ticarcillin, 200 to 400 mg/kg in divided doses q6h.

CHAPTER 156
Myocarditis

Adapted from Richard A. Friedman

The term *myocarditis* refers to inflammation of the muscular walls of the heart. Generally, it is thought to be a sporadic disease, although epidemics have been reported. Until the early 1990s, coxsackievirus B, an enterovirus, was the most frequently reported cause of epidemics in children. Infections secondary to coxsackieviruses are common throughout the general population. Target organs include the upper respiratory tract, gastrointestinal tract, liver (hepatitis), lung (pneumonia), central nervous system (meningoencephalitis), lymph nodes (infectious mononucleosis-like syndrome), kidney (hemolytic uremic syndrome), and heart (carditis). The coxsackievirus B organisms use receptors that are not shared with other enteroviruses to attach to their target cells. These receptors are believed to be an element essential for viral replication and may help determine tissue tropism. Infections caused by coxsackievirus B or other enteroviruses are subclinical in 50% of cases. During an outbreak of coxsackievirus B in Europe in 1965, cardiac manifestations were noted in 5% of patients. Whereas myocarditis is associated with coxsackievirus B serotypes 1 to 6, the most serious disease is attributed to types 3 and 4. Although much less common, enteroviruses such as coxsackievirus A and echovirus are suspected etiologic agents of myocarditis.

Rubella virus, a teratogen present during the first trimester of pregnancy, is also implicated in myocarditis. Persistence of the virus in the fetus has been shown to produce severe cases of myocarditis. A significant reduction in the number of cases of congenital rubella has occurred because of aggressive immunization programs, and only 28 cases were recorded in 1975.

More recently, adenovirus has emerged as a major cause of this disease in children. The identification of this agent has been greatly aided using modern molecular biologic techniques including in situ hybridization and polymerase chain reaction (PCR). PCR has been used to examine autopsy specimens of patients with myocarditis and a previously unidentified etiology. In those cases, adenovirus emerged as the major organism placing it second in importance to the enteroviruses as the etiologic agent responsible for myocarditis. Other viruses such as herpes simplex virus, varicella, and influenza have also been implicated in myocarditis cases.

The prognosis for acute myocarditis in newborns is poor. A 75% mortality was found in 25 infants with suspected coxsackievirus B myocarditis. The highest rate of mortality occurred in the first week of illness. The six infants who survived showed no apparent sequelae, although long-term follow-up was not reported. Older infants and children have a better prognosis with a mortality between 10% and 25% in clinically recognizable cases. Adult patients who recover may be asymptomatic at rest or with light exertion, but they may demonstrate a reduced working capacity with exercise stress testing.

CLINICAL CHARACTERISTICS

Host Factors

The clinical presentation of myocarditis varies in response to host factors including age and immunocompetence. Although the majority of cases are probably not noticed, with no apparent clinical illness, a rapidly fatal illness may occur. Newborn infants are susceptible to infection with coxsackievirus B, which may result in the severe form of myocarditis. Infections with rubella, herpes simplex, and toxoplasmosis may also result in a severe form of illness in infants.

Symptoms

Myocarditis may be merely one component of a more severe generalized illness with coexisting hepatitis or encephalitis. Myocardial involvement may be only a mild clinical disturbance in these cases. One study found a nursery epidemic of coxsackievirus B5 infection in preterm infants during a virologic survey in one institution. The disease was unnoticed clinically and discovered by chance during this survey. No instance of severe myocarditis was seen, and all infants recovered fully from infection. The major symptoms were lethargy, failure to gain weight, and aseptic meningitis. In a review of 25 infants with myocarditis caused by coxsackievirus B, other symptoms of lethargy and anorexia heralded the onset of severe disease. Fever was recorded in more than 50% of the cases, although hypothermia was also noted. Cyanosis, respiratory distress or tachycardia, cardiomegaly, or electrocardiographic changes were present in 19 of 23 infants; vomiting was noted in four. Initial symptoms in infants include irritability and periodic episodes of pallor, which may precede sudden onset of cardiorespiratory symptoms.

Clinical manifestations of myocarditis are generally less severe in older infants and children than in newborns. Rapidly fatal illness has been reported in association with myocarditis of unknown etiology, enteroviruses, adenoviruses, mumps, varicella, cytomegalovirus, and diphtheria. The usual clinical picture is either an acute or a subacute illness, often beginning with a mild respiratory infection and low-grade fever.

Physical examination usually shows the child to be anxious and apprehensive, although some children appear apathetic and listless. Pallor and mild cyanosis may be present with the skin cool to the touch and mottled in appearance. Respirations are usually rapid and sometimes labored; grunting may be prominent. The pulse is thready, although blood pressure may be normal or slightly reduced unless the patient is in shock. Palpation of the chest demonstrates a quiet precordium. Tachycardia is usually present. Heart sounds may be muffled, especially in the presence of pericarditis, and a gallop rhythm is frequently heard. With severe ventricular dysfunction, mitral regurgitation with a pansystolic murmur at the apex may be heard. Auscultation of the lungs reveals scattered rhonchi and fine crepitations in the lung bases. Peripheral edema is rare, but hepatomegaly is found almost uniformly. Some infants may have only mild congestive heart failure without evidence of peripheral circulatory compromise, whereas others have such a mild illness that the only abnormal finding may be a conduction disturbance visible on surface electrocardiography.

DIAGNOSIS

The diagnosis of myocarditis is often difficult to establish but should be suspected in any infant or child who presents with unexplained congestive heart failure. Fever is a common occurrence in children, and the frequency of viral illness may be so high as to invalidate the causal relationship in the history of recent illness in the child who presents with congestive heart failure. If this relationship is found, however, it should be documented for epidemiologic purposes.

A sinus tachycardia out of proportion to the level of fever and in association with a quiet precordium and a gallop rhythm should strongly suggest the diagnosis. A third heart sound, which is a common finding in healthy children, is usually associated with a relatively hyperdynamic precordium with heart sounds that are increased or crisp. When a prominent third heart sound exists without these findings, a significant disturbance in ventricular compliance is usually present and deserves further investigation by chest radiography, electrocardiography, and echocardiography. Children with myocarditis and congestive heart failure usually show cardiomegaly and pulmonary edema on chest radiography.

In newborn infants whose first sign of illness is acute circulatory collapse, the cardiac size may be normal. This may also be true in children who present with an arrhythmia secondary to myocarditis. Stokes–Adams attacks secondary to complete atrioventricular block may also be a presenting sign of myocarditis in children.

Other Signs of Disease

When an arrhythmia occurs after a febrile illness, the clinician should suspect the diagnosis and look for other signs of disease. Paroxysmal atrial tachycardia has been reported in patients with viral myocarditis. Atrial ectopic-focus tachycardia may mimic sinus tachycardia and should be suspected in a child with persistent sinus tachycardia and congestive heart failure. Careful inspection of the P wave axis and morphology in a 15-lead electrocardiogram and a 24-hour Holter monitor to observe the variance in rate are essential in establishing the diagnosis. Complete atrioventricular block secondary to idiopathic myocarditis, rubella, coxsackievirus, and respiratory syncytial virus has been described. Some of these patients developed permanent atrioventricular block and required permanent pacing, whereas the finding was transitory in others.

Ventricular tachycardia, when present, is usually poorly tolerated and should be treated aggressively. Our initial approach is to use lidocaine and, if unsuccessful, administer amiodarone intravenously. Despite this, infants who present with hemodynamically unstable ventricular tachycardia have a mortality rate exceeding 50%.

Tests

The electrocardiographic pattern classically described in myocarditis is that of low-voltage QRS complexes (less than 5 mm of total amplitude in all limb leads), with low-amplitude or slightly inverted T waves and a small or absent Q wave in leads V_5 and V_6. The low voltage may also be present in the precordial leads.

Echocardiography is essential in establishing the diagnosis. Pericardial effusion, as a cause of cardiomegaly, can be determined using either single-crystal or two-dimensional techniques. Depressed ventricular function with dilatation of one or more chambers in the absence of any structural abnormality helps establish the diagnosis.

Acutely ill patients with myocarditis should be stabilized before undergoing cardiac catheterization. Infants may require study to exclude anomalous origin of the left coronary artery, although advances in two-dimensional echocardiography have helped to determine origins of the coronary arteries.

Biopsy

Since the 1980s, endomyocardial biopsy has become a relatively safe and effective means of sampling heart muscle. The widest application for endomyocardial biopsy is in patients who have undergone cardiac transplantation and who require repeated samples to assess the degree of allograph rejection. Endomyocardial biopsy helps to establish the diagnosis of myocarditis and possibly to classify the phase of disease (acute, healed, chronic). A new technique of gene amplification using PCR may aid in the diagnosis of myocarditis, especially in borderline cases that have significant inflammatory cells but no concomitant myocyte destruction. Gene amplification leads to identification of the target

DNA with a specific viral agent. Several reports link the presence of viral RNA in patients with dilated cardiomyopathy, thus implicating viral myocarditis as a precursor illness.

LABORATORY TESTS

Although rarely successful, an attempt should be made to identify the offending organism for each child with the suspected diagnosis of myocarditis. Early in the course of illness, isolating the virus from the stool, throat washings or, rarely, blood is possible. Active infection is diagnosed when a fourfold increase is found in antibody titer to the isolated virus.

Even when a diagnosis of myocarditis is likely, blood cultures should be obtained in any infant with fever and signs of compromised cardiovascular function. A complete blood count should be ordered; a leukemoid reaction may be noted. The erythrocyte sedimentation rate is usually elevated during acute myocarditis, although a normal value does not exclude the diagnosis. Elevated levels of serum glutamic–oxaloacetic and glutamic–pyruvic transaminase can occur as the result of a generalized viral infection, although they may also be seen during episodes of diphtheritic myocarditis. Creatine phosphokinase and lactate dehydrogenase enzymes should also be measured. One study found elevation of isozyme 1 of lactate dehydrogenase was a specific finding in patients with idiopathic myocarditis.

DIFFERENTIAL DIAGNOSIS

Any cause of acute circulatory failure may mimic the presentation of acute myocarditis. Hypoxia, hypoglycemia, and hypocalcemia in newborns may be seen with heart failure. Circulatory collapse with shock frequently occurs in cases of overwhelming sepsis in this age group. Serum measurements of glucose and calcium, as well as blood cultures should be obtained in infants presenting with heart failure if sepsis is suspected.

Many infants with significant structural defects of the heart (e.g., hypoplastic left-heart syndrome, critical aortic valve stenosis) have no audible murmur when severely ill because of extremely low cardiac output. When cardiac function is improved, however, murmurs may be apparent, as may be hyperactive precordium and clear, not muffled, heart sounds. Echocardiographic diagnosis is essential in the evaluation of these patients to rule out structural abnormalities.

Other Etiologies

Beyond the immediate neonatal period, many other etiologies are possible. Anomalous left coronary artery arising from the pulmonary artery should be investigated by echocardiography and angiography. Endocardial fibroelastosis, type II glycogen storage disease (Pompe disease), medial necrosis of the coronary arteries, and left atrial myxoma are among the many diseases that can present a clinical picture similar to that of myocarditis. Murmurs may be audible with anomalous left coronary artery or endocardial fibroelastosis. They are usually apical in location, rarely more than grade 3 (of 6), and usually secondary to mitral insufficiency. Endocardial fibroelastosis is impossible to differentiate from myocarditis by clinical presentation. Endomyocardial biopsy and angiographic changes of the left ventricle help make this diagnosis. Electrocardiography in the anomalous left coronary artery may show a pattern of myocardial infarction with abnormal q waves in the anterolateral precordial leads. A qR pattern with inverted T waves in limb leads I and aVL may also be noted.

Pericarditis, which may be secondary to viral illness, usually occurs in children rather than infants. The clinical history may be similar to that in patients with myocarditis. Cardiovascular function, however, is usually less severely compromised for the degree of apparent cardiomegaly because of the amount of pericardial effusion. Cardiac tamponade may occur in severe cases and present with circulatory collapse. When pericarditis and myocarditis coexist, perimyocarditis results, and a clinical picture consistent with both diseases may be found. Echocardiography establishes pericardial effusion and left ventricular size and function. Perimyocarditis may be seen with rheumatic fever, collagen vascular disease, other autoimmune diseases, and coxsackievirus B disease. Myocarditis has also been described with rheumatoid arthritis, systemic lupus erythematosus, and ulcerative colitis.

TREATMENT

Level of Care

The level of care for the patient presenting with a clinical picture and history strongly suggestive of myocarditis depends on the severity of myocardial involvement. Many patients present with a relatively mild disease (i.e., minimal or no respiratory compromise and mild signs of congestive heart failure). These patients require close monitoring to assess whether the disease will progress to worsening heart failure and require intensive medical care. Experimental studies in animals suggest that bed rest may prevent an increase in intramyocardial viral replication during the acute stage; therefore, it is prudent to place patients under this restriction at the time of diagnosis.

Specific Therapy

Although no specific therapy aimed at reversing myocardial injury is recommended widely, maintenance of cardiac output at levels that supply adequate tissue perfusion and prevent metabolic disturbance is essential. In cases of congestive heart failure, digitalis may be used and has effected dramatic improvement in some instances. Diuretics are frequently administered in conjunction with digitalis. Although no direct beneficial effect on the myocardium is achieved, removal of excess extracellular fluid volume may help improve cardiac function.

Newborn infants may initially present in shock. Blood pressure is usually maintained at or near normal levels until late in the course and is not a sensitive indicator of the severity of illness. Rather, close attention to the adequacy of peripheral perfusion, heart rate, and urine output gives the clinician a better picture of the hemodynamic status of the infant. Although the hearts of these infants and children generally respond poorly to volume loading, selected patients may respond temporarily to boluses of 5 mL/kg of 5% albumin in Ringer lactate or a transfusion of packed red blood cells if a concomitant anemia exists. High central venous filling pressures of 12 to 18 mm Hg may be required to sustain adequate cardiac output, in contrast to 5 mm Hg in a child with a normally functioning heart.

Inotropic Agents

When these measures fail to reestablish an adequate cardiac output, a positive inotropic agent is administered. Dopamine in doses of 2 to 10 $\mu g/kg/minute$ is recommended to support blood pressure and effect some degree of dilation of the renal vasculature. As the dose increases toward 20 μg/kg/minute, dopamine exerts an increasingly dominant alpha–adrenergic effect and may increase systemic peripheral vasculature resistance; therefore, avoiding doses of more than 15 μg/kg/minute is usually wise. Dobutamine, a sympathomimetic amine that stimulates $beta_1$–, $beta_2$–, and alpha–adrenergic receptors, is frequently used in combination with dopamine. This agent exerts significant positive inotropy while reducing left ventricular filling pressure. Its chronotropic response is not as positive as dopamine's, and it seems to result in less ventricular ectopy during administration. When used in combination with dopamine at low doses (more than 10 μg/kg/minute), dobutamine, in doses of 10 μg/kg/minute or more, may result in a significant increase in ventricular contractility while avoiding a sinus tachycardia that may compromise cardiac output. For this reason, isoproterenol is best avoided in these patients because the resultant sinus tachycardia, which in other patients may improve cardiac output, may be affected adversely in this circumstance.

Because of its afterload-reducing effects, sodium nitroprusside has been used extensively in children. Cardiac output is improved by reduction of systemic arterial resistance and, thus, ventricular filling pressure. In patients with myocarditis, this agent may be used in conjunction with dopamine or dobutamine if hypotension does not coexist. When chronic oral therapy is possible, an afterload-reducing drug such as captopril, an angiotensin-converting enzyme inhibitor, may be used with digitalis and diuretics.

Arrhythmias should be treated vigorously. Supraventricular tachyarrhythmias are often suppressed with digitalis, which has usually been administered previously for the treatment of congestive heart failure. Ventricular arrhythmias may be responsive to lidocaine given in a loading dose of 1 mg/kg (up to 50 mg total bolus dose), followed by a continuous infusion adequate to maintain a therapeutic serum concentration (1–5 mg/mL). If lidocaine fails to adequately control the ventricular tachycardia, then amiodarone is administered intravenously. If complete atrioventricular block occurs, a temporary transvenous pacemaker should be inserted. The patient must be observed over 10 to 14 days (in an intensive care unit) for the return of normal atrioventricular conduction. A permanent pacing device should be implanted if complete atrioventricular block persists beyond that time. Implantation can be done as an elective procedure when the patient's condition is stable.

Antibiotic agents should not be given unless a bacterial infection is suspected and cultures are obtained before initiating therapy.

Immunosuppressive Agents

The use of immunosuppressive agents in suspected or proven viral myocarditis remains controversial. Some animal studies suggest an exacerbation of virus-induced cytotoxicity in the presence of immunosuppressive drugs, possibly caused by interference with interferon production. Studies in humans have demonstrated mixed results. Complications of immunosuppressive therapy including opportunistic infections and a cushingoid state should be considered before administration of these drugs. Controlled studies are under way in the adult population to address the usefulness of immunosuppressive therapy including use of cyclosporine; a similar study in children should be undertaken before firm recommendations can be given to clinicians.

A promising therapy that deserves a more in-depth study is the use of intravenous immunoglobin in children with myocarditis. The initial study reported in 1994 showed that 21 of 46 children treated with this agent soon after initial presentation had better left ventricular performance at 1-year follow-up and a trend to better survival. A larger multicenter study is drastically needed to help further analyze whether this promising therapy is worthwhile.

CHAPTER 157
Rheumatic Heart Disease

Adapted from Galal M. El-Said

RHEUMATIC MITRAL INSUFFICIENCY

Mitral insufficiency is the most common cardiac defect in children and adolescents with rheumatic heart disease (RHD). As the left ventricle (LV) contracts, part of its stroke volume regurgitates into the left atrium (LA) through the incompetent mitral valve. Because of the pressure difference between the LV and LA, regurgitation starts during the isometric contraction phase.

Compensation begins with dilation of the LV to accommodate the increased blood volume. In chronic mitral insufficiency, the increase in LV end-diastolic volume is not usually accompanied by increased end-diastolic pressure because of increased LV compliance. The increase in LV end-diastolic volume (i.e., increased preload) brings the Frank–Starling mechanism into play, which permits a large stroke output. Because the regurgitant mitral orifice is in parallel with the aortic orifice, the resistance to LV emptying is reduced (i.e., decreased afterload) (Fig. 157-1).

The compensatory mechanisms of increased compliance, increased preload, decreased afterload, and increased wall thickness are not sufficient to overcome persistent mitral insufficiency. Myocardial contractility becomes impaired because of the chronic volume overload. Symptoms of low cardiac output are followed by symptoms of lung congestion caused by left ventricular failure (Fig. 157-1).

Clinical Characteristics

Because symptoms do not usually develop until the LV is compromised, the interval between acquiring rheumatic fever (see Chapter 95 for a complete discussion of rheumatic fever) and the development of symptoms of mitral insufficiency tends to be longer than for mitral stenosis, often exceeding two decades. Unlike mitral stenosis, symptoms of low cardiac output (e.g., weakness, fatigue) are more prominent and appear before symptoms of lung congestion (e.g., exertional, nocturnal, or resting dyspnea; recurrent chest infections; hemoptysis).

The cardiac impulse is diffuse, forceful, and displaced downward and laterally. The first heart sound is usually diminished. A loud apical third heart sound is usually audible and caused by the increased transmitral volume flow during the rapid filling phase. The characteristic murmur of mitral insufficiency is a high-pitched holosystolic murmur beginning with the soft first sound and continuing to the second sound. The second heart sound is sometimes obscured by the murmur. The murmur is loudest at the apex with radiation to the axilla and left infrascapular area.

Laboratory Findings

In chronic mitral insufficiency, the electrocardiogram exhibits evidence of LV and LA enlargements. Radiologically, the cardiac

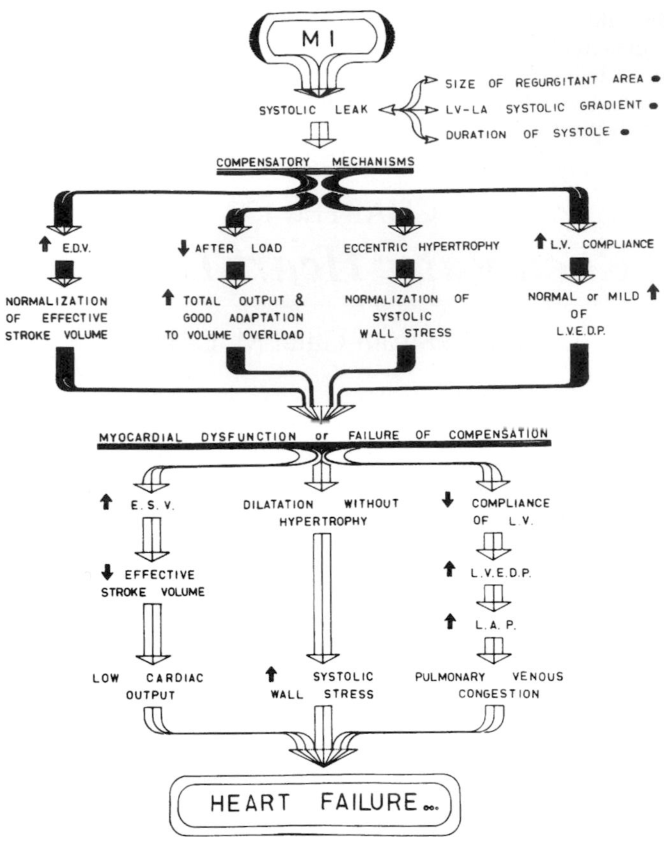

Figure 157-1. The diagram depicts factors that determine the degree of regurgitation, compensation, and decompensation in mitral insufficiency. EDP, end-diastolic pressure; EDV, end-diastolic volume; ESV, end-systolic volume; LA, left atrium; LAP, left atrial pressure; LV, left ventricle; MI, mitral insufficiency.

shadow is normal early in the course of the disease; later, LA and LV enlargements become evident.

Echocardiography is useful for identifying the cause and degree of mitral insufficiency and for evaluating LV function. M-mode echocardiography can show an increase in the LV diastolic dimension and a significant decrease in LV diameter during the preejection phase. The two-dimensional (2D) echo criteria for the diagnosis of rheumatic mitral insufficiency include thickened mitral valve leaflets, incomplete closure of the mitral valve, a relatively immobile posterior mitral leaflet, a dilated LA with systolic expansion, and a dilated LV with hyperdynamic septal and posterior wall motion. The degree of mitral insufficiency can be assessed using echo Doppler, determining the extension and intensity of the Doppler signal of the regurgitant jet in the LA. Color-flow Doppler and pulsed techniques correlate well with angiographic methods of estimating the severity of mitral insufficiency. Transesophageal echocardiography (TEE), especially color mapping, is superior to transthoracic echocardiography in assessing the degree of mitral regurgitation. Although slight overestimation may occur, TEE is also useful in delineating the anatomy of the mitral valve and, thus, is useful for determining whether the mitral valve can be repaired or whether mitral valve replacement will be necessary.

Cardiac catheterization demonstrates elevated LA pressure (particularly the v wave). The diagnosis can be established by left ventriculography. Mitral insufficiency is indicated by the appearance of contrast material in the LA after LV injection through a retrograde aortic catheter.

RHEUMATIC MITRAL STENOSIS

Stenosis of the mitral valve is usually secondary to rheumatic carditis. Other causes include congenital mitral stenosis, atrial myxoma, infective endocarditis with bulky vegetations, and mucopolysaccharidosis of the Hunter–Hurley phenotype. The combination of mitral stenosis and secundum atrial septal defect is frequently referred to as Lutembacher syndrome, but the mitral stenosis is almost always rheumatic, and the association is fortuitous.

Rheumatic fever causes mitral stenosis through fusion of the commissures, cusps, or chordae tendineae of the mitral valve apparatus (Fig. 157-2). Obstruction of flow across the narrowed mitral valve produces a diastolic gradient between the LA and LV. Serious circulatory disturbances with consequent clinical symptoms occur when the area of the mitral opening is less than 1 cm^2. As narrowing proceeds, the LA pressure increases, as does the pressure in the pulmonary veins and capillaries, leading to lung congestion. Pulmonary arteriolar vasoconstriction occurs to protect the lungs against congestion, but the protection is at the expense of developing pulmonary hypertension, which produces RV hypertrophy and possible RV failure (Fig. 157-3).

Clinical Characteristics

The symptoms of mitral stenosis may appear insidiously within 3 to 4 years after the attack of acute rheumatic fever, or they may be delayed for as long as 50 years. The onset of symptoms is sometimes abrupt, and acute pulmonary edema, systemic embolism, or atrial fibrillation may be the initial manifestations. The symptoms depend on the state of the disease. No symptoms may be present in mild cases. If the lungs are congested, dyspnea, orthopnea, nocturnal dyspnea or pulmonary edema, recurrent chest infections, and hemoptysis occur. As pulmonary hypertension develops, symptoms caused by lung congestion decrease, and low cardiac output symptoms (mainly exertional fatigue) begin to appear. Symptoms caused by systemic congestion appear if the RV fails.

In a patient with mitral stenosis, the pulse is usually normal unless atrial fibrillation supervenes. The apical impulse is felt at the normal location as a "hurried, slapping" impulse. A characteristic diastolic or presystolic thrill ending in a palpable

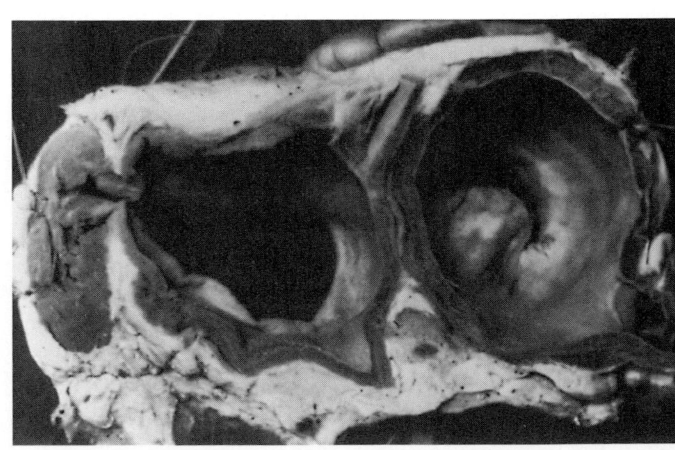

Figure 157-2. The cross section shows a stenosed mitral valve (*right*) giving a buttonhole appearance. The tricuspid valve on the left is grossly insufficient. Insufficiency occurs in the later stages of mitral stenosis after long-standing, severe secondary pulmonary hypertension. (Courtesy of Dr. Soheir Mahfouz, Pathology Department, Cairo University.)

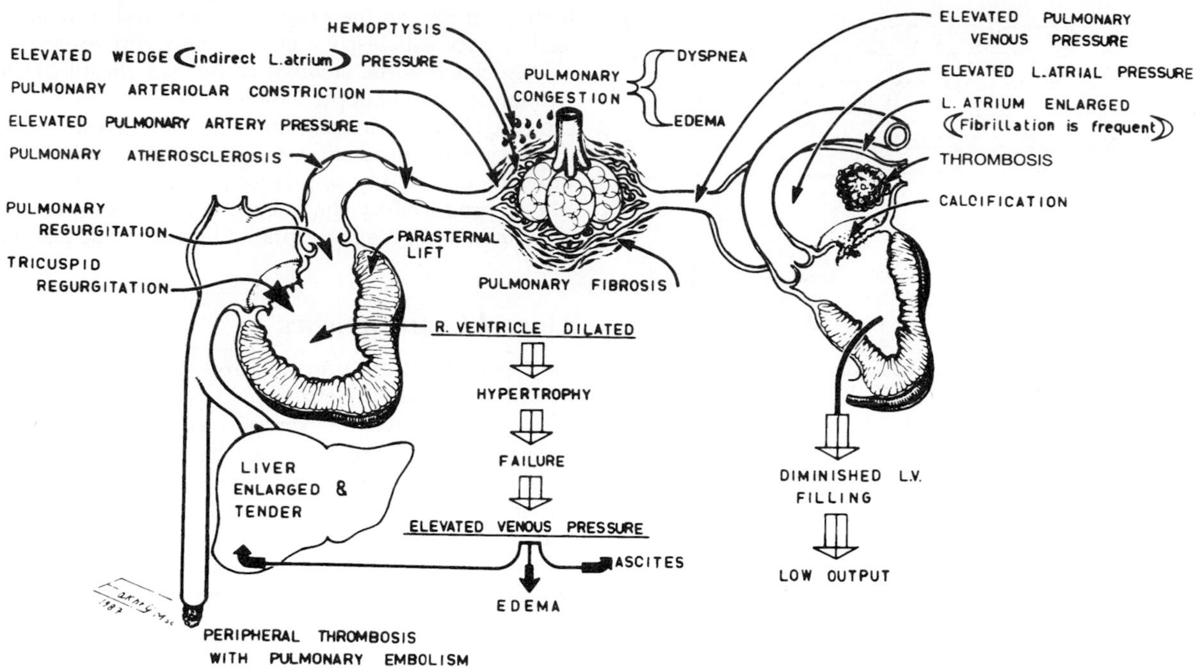

Figure 157-3. The diagram depicts the hemodynamic alterations and complications that occur because of mitral stenosis. LV, left ventricle.

accentuated first sound can be detected over the apex. The first mitral sound is loud, short, and snappy. The accentuation of the first sound is caused by the open position of the cusps in the LV at the end of diastole as a result of the high LA pressure and the incomplete emptying of the LA. An opening snap occurs, which is a sharp, clicky sound separated from the second sound by the isovolumic relaxation phase. The snap is caused by the sudden opening of the rigid mitral valve by the high LA pressure. The murmur characteristic of mitral stenosis is a middiastolic or presystolic murmur. Developing pulmonary hypertension produces an accentuated pulmonary second sound.

Laboratory Findings

The electrocardiographic and cardiac silhouettes are normal in mild cases. In patients with moderate or severe obstruction, the principal feature is LA enlargement. RV hypertrophy is seen when pulmonary hypertension develops.

The M-mode echo criteria for the diagnosis of mitral stenosis include a reduced ejection fraction slope of the anterior mitral leaflet (reflecting elevated left atrial pressure) and diastolic anterior movement of the posterior mitral leaflet. The latter results from commissural fusion and is considered to be the main diagnostic hallmark of mitral stenosis in M-mode echo studies. The feature diagnostic of mitral stenosis in a 2D echo study is doming of the anterior leaflet in diastole (i.e., the body of the leaflet separates more widely than the edges). The posterior leaflet is frequently immobile or severely restricted in diastolic movement. The 2D echo-derived mitral valve area often compares favorably with that measured directly at surgery. A Doppler echo study provides information about the flow of blood across the mitral valve and can estimate the gradient and the mitral valve area reasonably well. TEE, which provides images superior to those seen by transthoracic echocardiography, can show a detailed anatomy of the mitral valve apparatus and, thus, is useful in evaluation before balloon valvuloplasty in determining the presence of a left atrial thrombus, the thickness of the interatrial septum, and the degree of associated mitral regurgitation.

Cardiac catheterization and angiography are usually unnecessary for evaluating isolated mitral stenosis, but they may be performed for atypical cases. Pressure measurements show elevated LA and pulmonary wedge pressures. In patients with severe stenosis and those in whom the pulmonary vascular resistance is increased, the pulmonary arterial pressure is elevated.

RHEUMATIC AORTIC VALVE DISEASE

Aortic valvulitis, which may develop during rheumatic carditis, may cause aortic insufficiency or stenosis. Aortic insufficiency, which results from damage of the aortic leaflets, may occur relatively early in the course of the disease and may be exaggerated over time by fibrosis, thickening, and contracture of the aortic leaflets. Aortic stenosis, which results from fusion of the commissures, takes a long time to develop. As a result, in children and adolescents, aortic valve disease caused by rheumatic conditions usually presents as isolated or dominant aortic insufficiency with mild or no stenosis. Dominant stenosis at a young age, with or without insufficiency, is usually congenital.

The inability of the scarred and shortened aortic leaflets to coapt and close the aortic orifice completely during ventricular diastole causes diastolic regurgitation of blood from the aorta to the LV, because the normal aortic diastolic pressure approximates 80 mm Hg, and the normal LV diastolic pressure is 0 to 12 mm Hg.

With chronic aortic insufficiency, the LV dilates with an increasing volume of blood for many years. The increased LV diastolic volume is not accompanied by an increase in end-diastolic pressure, probably because of an increase in the LV diastolic compliance. The increased LV end-diastolic volume, according to the Frank–Starling principle, results in increased stroke volume (i.e., preload reserve). The stroke volume is also maintained by reduced aortic impedance, which occurs with peripheral vasodilation (i.e., decreasing afterload) (Fig. 157-4).

The increased LV stroke volume, with consequent elevation in the systolic blood pressure accompanied by a decrease in the

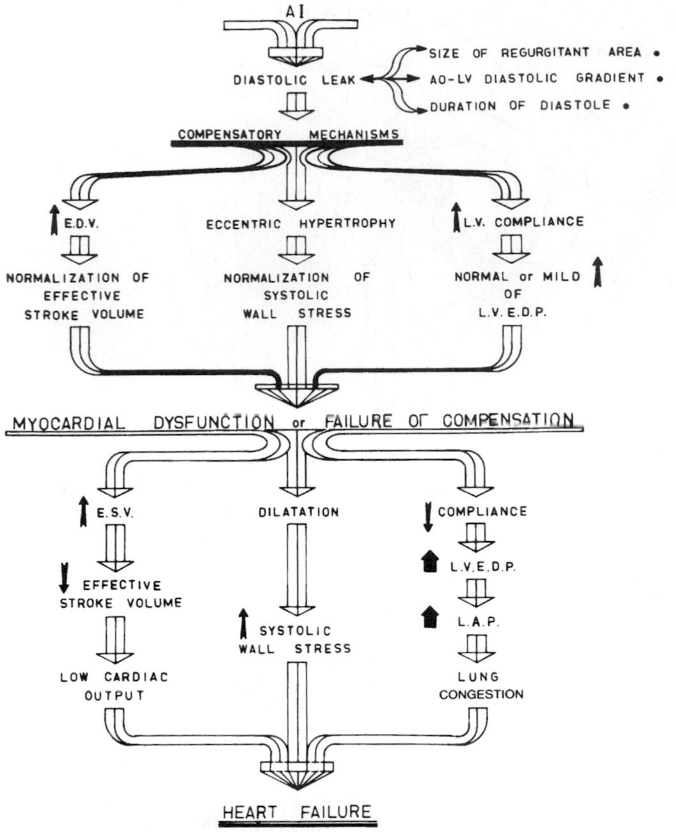

Figure 157-4. The diagram depicts factors that determine the amount of regurgitation, compensation, and decompensation in aortic insufficiency. AI, aortic insufficiency; AO, aorta; EDP, end-diastolic pressure; EDV, end-diastolic volume; ESV, end-systolic volume; LAP, left atrial pressure, LV, left ventricle.

diastolic blood pressure (caused partly by regurgitation of a part of the stroke volume and partly by peripheral arteriolar vasodilation), increases the pulse pressure. The classic peripheral arterial pulses of aortic insufficiency have a rapid increase to a high peak with a collapsing descending limb and a low diastolic pressure.

Because the major portion of coronary flow occurs during diastole, when arterial pressure is lower than normal, coronary perfusion may be reduced. The increased oxygen demand caused by hypertrophy in the presence of reduced coronary flow may lead to myocardial ischemia, especially with exercise.

Associated aortic stenosis causes significant deleterious alterations in the pathophysiology. The increased stroke volume produced by aortic insufficiency causes a corresponding increase in the pressure gradient across the stenotic valve. At the same time, the decreased compliance of the LV secondary to hypertrophy produced by the aortic stenosis prevents the LV from accommodating the regurgitant blood of aortic insufficiency.

Clinical Characteristics

Early symptoms are unusual, except with gross aortic insufficiency. Patients may complain that they are aware of their hearts' beating, especially with exercise, because of the large stroke volume and forceful contractions. Chest pain may be a prominent symptom during exertion. Disturbing anginal pains may occur at night accompanied by tachycardia, sweating, and paroxysmal hypertension. The major symptoms, especially breathlessness, are caused by LV disease. Symptoms are exaggerated and occur earlier if aortic insufficiency is associated with aortic stenosis.

The characteristic peripheral signs of aortic insufficiency are produced by the combined large pulse volume and peripheral vasodilation. The sharp rise of the pulse gives it a characteristic "water hammer" quality. The visible, jerky arterial pulsations in the neck are known as Corrigan's sign. The blood pressure is normal in patients with very mild aortic insufficiency. With increasing severity of aortic insufficiency, the systolic pressure increases and the diastolic pressure decreases. The apical impulse in aortic valve disease is diffuse and hyperdynamic, and it may be displaced laterally and inferiorly.

The typical murmur of aortic insufficiency is an early diastolic, high-pitched, blowing, decrescendo murmur over the base, which begins with the second sound. The murmur is heard best with the diaphragm of the stethoscope in full expiration while the patient is sitting and leaning forward. The duration, rather than the quality or the loudness, of the aortic diastolic murmur correlates with the severity of the aortic insufficiency. An ejection systolic murmur at the base, caused by increased blood flow across the aortic valve in systole, is heard in almost all cases of aortic insufficiency of more than mild degree. The diagnosis of associated aortic stenosis cannot be based merely on the presence of this systolic murmur. A middiastolic or presystolic rumble over the mitral area, the Austin Flint murmur, is usually heard in patients with moderate or severe aortic insufficiency

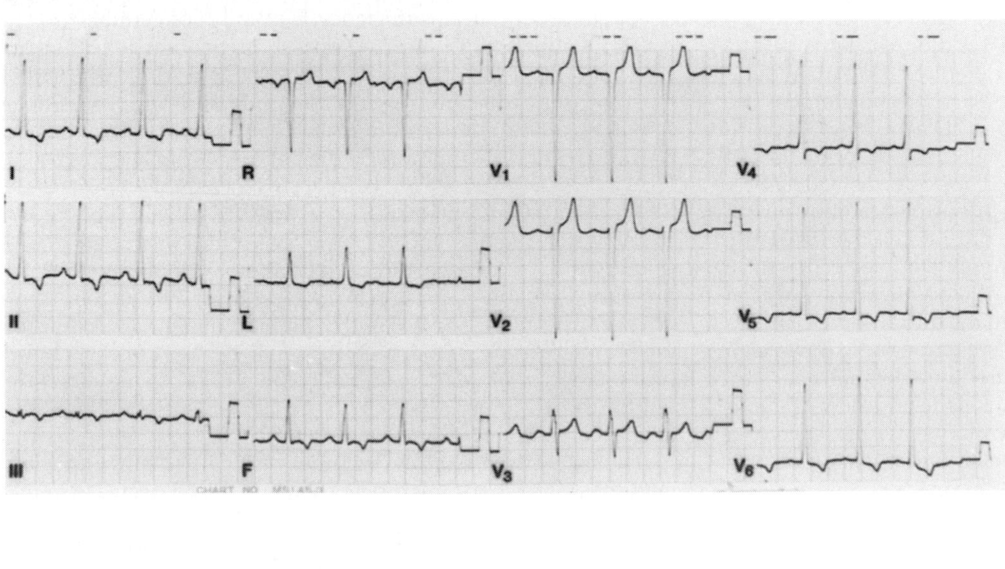

Figure 157-5. The electrocardiogram shows severe left ventricular hypertrophy and strain in a patient with gross aortic insufficiency.

without associated organic mitral stenosis. The Austin Flint murmur may be caused by relative mitral stenosis secondary to improper opening of the anterior leaflet of the mitral valve by the regurgitant bloodstream or by the high LV diastolic pressure. Echocardiography is the most sensitive way to differentiate an Austin Flint from an organic apical diastolic murmur.

Laboratory Findings

The electrocardiogram is normal in mild cases of aortic insufficiency. Left ventricular hypertrophy develops in severe cases (Fig. 157-5). As the severity of aortic insufficiency increases, more dilation and enlargement of the LV occur radiologically. Typically, the LV enlarges in an inferior and leftward direction and can be seen below the diaphragmatic level.

The most common and characteristic M-mode echocardiographic finding in chronic aortic insufficiency is fine diastolic fluttering of the mitral valve, more frequently, the anterior leaflet. The echo study has an important role in the clinical assessment and evaluation of changes in LV function in patients suffering from aortic insufficiency. Serial echo studies can reveal early changes in LV functions. Deterioration is indicated if a progressive increase in end-systolic and end-diastolic dimensions accompanied by gradual reduction in LV shortening is present. Doppler is the most sensitive noninvasive method for detecting aortic insufficiency. Color Doppler flow mapping of the regurgitant jet offers a more precise approach to quantitation of the severity of the aortic insufficiency. Aortography enables diagnosis of aortic insufficiency and grading of its severity, but it is rarely needed.

RHEUMATIC TRICUSPID VALVE DISEASE

Rheumatic tricuspid valve disease develops in 5% to 10% of patients with RHD and is associated almost invariably with mitral or mitral and aortic valve disease. Organic tricuspid insufficiency can occur alone or with organic tricuspid stenosis as a result of rigidity of the valve edges, shrinkage of leaflet tissue, annular dilation, or a combination of these abnormalities. Functional tricuspid incompetence is the result of annular dilation and malalignment of papillary muscles secondary to RV failure complicating pulmonary hypertension.

Tricuspid insufficiency permits blood to regurgitate into the right atrium diminishing the forward flow by the same amount. The larger volume of blood in the right atrium increases the right atrium pressure. When the RV relaxes, it is subjected to a higher filling pressure and dilates more to accommodate this extra blood. RV dilation intensifies the leak and magnifies the heart failure.

Clinical Characteristics

Symptoms of tricuspid valve disease are dominated by the associated, more severe left-sided lesions. Systemic venous pressure is elevated because of tricuspid valve obstruction or incompetence. The murmur of tricuspid insufficiency is audible at the lower left sternal border, is pansystolic, is usually followed by a third sound, and may radiate laterally. The diastolic murmur of tricuspid stenosis mimics that of mitral stenosis, but it is usually heard best at the lower left sternal border and has a higher pitch. Tricuspid murmurs tend to increase with inspiration, but this is usually difficult to elicit because of gross heart failure and because lung expansion during inspiration interferes with auscultation.

TREATMENT OF RHEUMATIC HEART DISEASE

Effective prevention of RHD includes prophylaxis against rheumatic fever and its recurrence and against the occurrence of infective endocarditis. For asymptomatic patients with mild or moderate valvular disease and with normal heart size or insignificant cardiomegaly, normal school activity should be encouraged. Restriction of activity is unnecessary. For symptomatic patients, activities should be limited to those that do not produce symptoms of fatigue, dyspnea, or excessive palpitation. Weight lifting and other isometric exercises should be discouraged. Competitive sports are not encouraged because individuals tend to ignore symptoms in the excitement of a contest.

Anemia and Infections

Patients with chronic RHD have diminished cardiac reserves. Cardiac decompensation can be precipitated by anemia or minor infections, which should be promptly and aggressively treated. Because chest infections may be precipitated by pulmonary congestion, a diuretic is usually needed.

Arrhythmias

In rheumatic mitral valve disease, frequent atrial premature contractions often presage atrial fibrillation, and the administration of antiarrhythmic drugs may be effective in preventing this complication. Atrial fibrillation, flutter, and tachycardia can complicate these cases. The immediate treatment for atrial fibrillation should be directed toward reducing the ventricular rate and, if possible, reestablishing sinus rhythm by pharmacologic treatment and cardioversion singly or in combination. After reversion to the sinus rhythm, administration of quinidine or a similar antiarrhythmic agent should be continued indefinitely to diminish the likelihood of recurrence.

Thromboembolic Complications

If surgery is not performed, oral anticoagulants should be administered to patients with mitral valve disease who have had systemic emboli and to patients who are at high risk of embolization such as those who are in atrial fibrillation, have a greatly enlarged LA, or have LA thrombus demonstrated by transthoracic echocardiography and TEE.

Heart Failure

Digitalis should be administered to patients with significant valvular lesions who begin to develop effort fatigue or dyspnea with or without frank evidence of left-sided or right-sided heart failure. However, if a patient with isolated mitral stenosis does not have right-sided heart failure or atrial fibrillation or flutter, little hemodynamic benefit can be expected from the use of digitalis. Fluid retention in such conditions responds well to treatment with diuretics. A low-sodium diet is advisable, especially if the diuretics are not completely effective. The measures designed to reduce pulmonary venous pressure including sedation, assumption of upright posture, and aggressive diuresis are used to treat the hemoptysis of lung congestion. Patients with overt cardiac failure are treated in the usual way. Uncontrollable heart failure in children suggests the possibility of severe valvular afflictions, rheumatic activity, infective endocarditis, or electrolyte imbalance.

For patients with isolated mitral stenosis, beta-blocking agents may increase exercise tolerance by reducing the heart rate and increasing the diastolic time.

The response to vasodilator therapy, which diminishes the afterload, is impressive in patients with mitral and aortic insufficiency. Reducing the impedance to ejection in the aorta reduces the volume of regurgitating blood. Hemodynamic studies have shown beneficial effects of intravenous sodium nitroprusside in acute mitral insufficiency and oral angiotensin-converting enzyme inhibitors and prazosin in chronic cases. This therapy may be helpful in stabilizing patients who are waiting for surgery. Agents such as sublingual nitroglycerin may be effective in relieving dyspnea brought on by exercise and may permit the same exercise to be undertaken with the pulmonary artery pressure lowered because of venous dilatation, arteriolar dilatation, or both.

Catheter Balloon Valvuloplasty

Dilation of a stenosed mitral valve by a balloon valvuloplasty catheter can relieve mitral obstruction. This procedure is used in patients who have pliable, noncalcified mitral leaflets. Left atrial thrombi must be excluded. The best way to determine this is by TEE studies, especially in patients with atrial fibrillation. The balloon technique is an ideal way for children (who usually have pliable, noncalcified leaflets) to avoid thoracotomy. The patients should be symptomatic [functional class (FC) II or more] with moderate to severe mitral stenosis (with a mitral valve area of 0.8 cm^2/m^2 of body surface area).

Surgery

The following list presents indications for surgery for the different valve diseases.

- Mitral stenosis: symptomatic mitral stenosis and moderate to severe mitral stenosis, as mentioned previously, with nonpliable or severely calcified mitral leaflets or those with a left atrial thrombus.
- Mitral regurgitation: symptomatic mitral regurgitation (FC II or more); asymptomatic mitral regurgitation, but with an end-systolic volume greater than 50 mL/m^2 of body surface area, or an end-systolic diameter greater than 45 mm; deterioration of left ventricular function by serial echocardiography.
- Aortic regurgitation: symptomatic aortic regurgitation; asymptomatic aortic regurgitation with deterioration of left ventricular function by serial echocardiography, left ventricular end-systolic diameter greater than 55 mm, left ventricular end-systolic volume greater than 55 mL/m^2 of body surface area, and ejection fraction less than 50%.

Although the only direct therapy for cardiac valve disease is surgical (i.e., valvotomy for severe mitral stenosis, replacement for severe mitral insufficiency and aortic insufficiency), the management of children with rheumatic valve disease should conserve the natural valve if possible. No prosthesis is totally free of thromboembolic and anticoagulation problems and has an effective orifice that will not be outgrown by a small child. Tissue heterografts are prone to calcification and early failure, and they cannot be recommended for children except under unusual circumstances. Mechanical aortic and mitral valves should be used for children, and anticoagulant therapy should be used with all types of mechanical valve prostheses, even though the incidence of thromboemboli in children is much lower than in adults.

CHAPTER 158
Aortic Arch and Pulmonary Artery Abnormalities (Vascular Rings and Slings)

Adapted from W. Robert Morrow

Anomalies of the aortic arch and pulmonary arteries constitute a diverse group of malformations. The range of possible deviations from normal morphology of the aortic arch and pulmonary artery is broad. Vascular rings are formed when one or more aortic arch anomalies, with or without a patent ductus arteriosus or ligamentum, produce a ring that completely encircles the trachea and esophagus leading to symptoms of tracheal or esophageal constriction. A vascular sling, produced by an abnormal origin and course of the left pulmonary artery or left ductus arteriosus, does not encircle the trachea and esophagus completely but usually produces severe symptoms of tracheal and bronchial compression.

AORTIC ARCH ANOMALIES

Left Aortic Arch with Anomalous Right Subclavian Artery

Left aortic arch with anomalous origin of the right subclavian artery is the most common aortic arch malformation noted on postmortem examination. The incidence of this abnormality in the general population is approximately 0.5%. The left arch has a normal course to the left and anterior to the trachea, but the right subclavian artery arises as the last branch of the arch and courses posterior to the esophagus. Most patients with anomalous right subclavian artery are asymptomatic, and the abnormality is discovered incidentally at esophagography or at catheterization. Often, an anomalous right subclavian artery is seen in patients with tetralogy of Fallot and left aortic arch and, therefore, has a significant bearing on which systemic–to–pulmonary artery shunt is chosen for palliation of cyanosis. In addition, anomalous right subclavian artery may be present in patients with coarctation of the aorta and often arises distal to the site of coarctation. In these patients, blood pressure in the right arm and legs does not reflect the coarctation gradient. What is necessary, then, is to determine blood pressure in both arms and in the legs during examination of patients with suspected coarctation.

Although most patients with an anomalous right subclavian artery are asymptomatic, some older children and adults may experience dysphagia. Routine chest radiography does not demonstrate this anomaly, but barium esophagography is diagnostic. The oblique course of the anomalous vessel posterior to the esophagus in the anteroposterior projection and the posterior indentation of the esophagus in the lateral or left anterior oblique projection are usually diagnostic (Fig. 158-1). The diagnosis of anomalous right subclavian artery may be made with two-dimensional echocardiography when the first branch of the aorta is to the right but the normal bifurcation into a right carotid artery and right subclavian artery cannot be demonstrated. An anomalous right subclavian artery may be noted incidentally when aortography is performed in patients with congenital heart disease.

If symptoms of a vascular ring (e.g., stridor, wheezing, cough) are present in a patient with an anomalous right subclavian

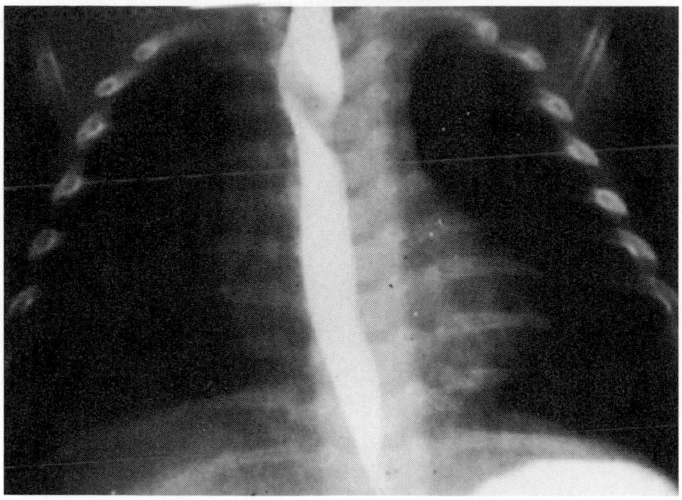

Figure 158-1. Anteroposterior projection of a barium esophagogram obtained from a patient with tetralogy of Fallot, left aortic arch, and anomalous right subclavian artery. The retroesophageal course of the anomalous right subclavian artery produces an oblique indentation of the esophagus. (Courtesy of Dr. Michael Nihill, Baylor College of Medicine, Houston, TX.)

artery, an alternative diagnosis such as laryngomalacia or tracheomalacia should be considered. Rarely, an anomalous right subclavian artery in association with a left aortic arch, retroesophageal descending aorta, and right ductus arteriosus or ligamentum produces a symptomatic vascular ring. The retroesophageal descending aorta in these patients results in a large, rounded, posterior indentation on barium esophagogram, which is usually distinguished readily from the more shallow indentation produced by an anomalous right subclavian artery without a retroesophageal descending aorta. The diagnosis should be confirmed by magnetic resonance imaging (MRI).

Double Aortic Arch

Double aortic arch is the most common clinically recognized form of vascular ring. The ascending aorta divides anterior to the trachea into left and right arches, which then pass on either side of the trachea. Usually, the right arch is larger than the left and passes posterior to the esophagus to join the descending aorta to the left of the midline. Uncommonly, the left arch is atretic. A complete vascular ring is formed by the arches on each side of the trachea and esophagus with the ascending aorta anterior and the retroesophageal arch or descending aorta posterior. Usually, the ductus arteriosus is left-sided and is not an essential component of the vascular ring, but the length of the ductus arteriosus or ligamentum may significantly affect the severity of symptoms. Usually, associated congenital heart disease is not present, but it may occur in as many as 22% of patients. Cyanotic congenital heart disease including tetralogy of Fallot and transposition of the great arteries predominates.

Usually, patients with double aortic arch are severely symptomatic in infancy with stridor, dyspnea, cough, and recurrent respiratory infections. Infants feed poorly because of severe respiratory distress and may prefer to assume an opisthotonic posture. Life-threatening episodes of apnea with cyanosis may occur. The diagnosis of double aortic arch, like almost all vascular rings, is often suggested by the presence of a right aortic arch on routine chest radiography. In patients with double aortic arch, both arches are sometimes seen, and evidence of hyperinflation of either or both lungs caused by obstruction of the lower trachea and main stem bronchi may be present.

Barium esophagography often demonstrates bilateral indentations of the esophagus in the anteroposterior projection (Fig. 158-2) but may only show a prominent right-sided indentation. When two indentations are seen, the right arch usually produces the larger and more superior indentation. In the lateral or left anterior oblique projection, a large posterior indentation is seen and represents the retroesophageal component of the arch. Also present is anterior and more inferior indentation of the arch

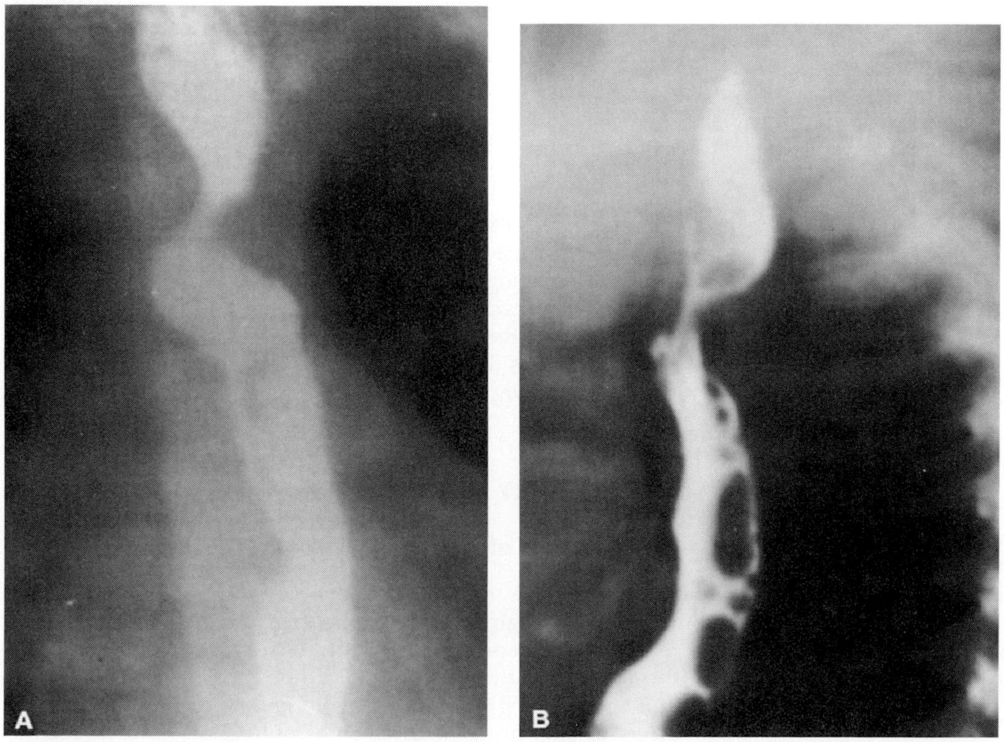

Figure 158-2. In double aortic arch, bilateral indentation of the esophagus is characteristic in the anteroposterior projection (**A**), with a deep posterior indentation on the lateral projection produced by the retroesophageal portion of the arch (**B**). The larger and more superior indentation in the anteroposterior projection—in this case, on the right of the esophagus—is usually produced by the dominant arch. (Courtesy of Dr. Michael Nihill, Baylor College of Medicine, Houston, TX.)

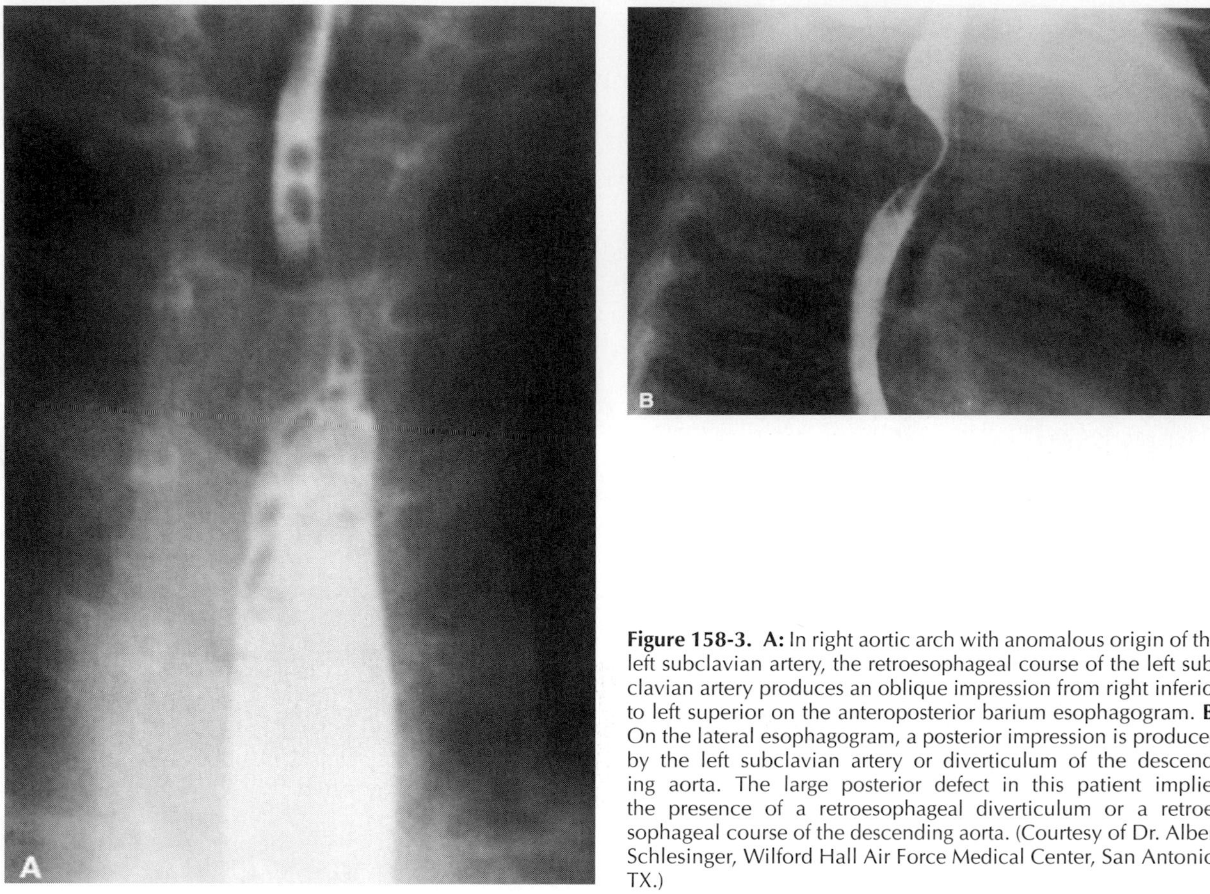

Figure 158-3. A: In right aortic arch with anomalous origin of the left subclavian artery, the retroesophageal course of the left subclavian artery produces an oblique impression from right inferior to left superior on the anteroposterior barium esophagogram. **B:** On the lateral esophagogram, a posterior impression is produced by the left subclavian artery or diverticulum of the descending aorta. The large posterior defect in this patient implies the presence of a retroesophageal diverticulum or a retroesophageal course of the descending aorta. (Courtesy of Dr. Albert Schlesinger, Wilford Hall Air Force Medical Center, San Antonio, TX.)

produced by posterior deviation of the trachea. Although surgery may be performed without additional imaging studies, confirmation of the diagnosis can be obtained by MRI, echocardiography, or angiography.

Usually, stridor and respiratory distress are severe, and affected infants will die without early surgical intervention. The mortality from surgery is low, and eventual long-term relief of symptoms is usually achieved. However, short-term postoperative tracheal obstruction is the rule, and some infants require prolonged intubation and aggressive attention to pulmonary toilet in the early postoperative period. Stridor may persist to some degree for months after surgery.

Right Aortic Arch with Anomalous Left Subclavian Artery

Right aortic arch with anomalous left subclavian artery and left ductus arteriosus is the most common type of aortic arch anomaly that produces an anatomic vascular ring. Usually, this group of abnormalities is asymptomatic and, therefore, ranks as the second most common cause of symptomatic vascular ring. The essential pathologic features include course of the arch to the right of the trachea with the first branch being the left carotid artery. The left subclavian artery arises from the descending aorta, and the ductus arteriosus, which originates from a retroesophageal diverticulum of the descending aorta, courses to the left and connects to the pulmonary artery. Unlike the condition in double aortic arch, the presence of a left ductus arteriosus or ligamentum is an essential component of the vascular ring. In patients with right aortic arch and anomalous branching, associated congenital heart disease is uncommon.

Although patients with right aortic arch, anomalous left subclavian artery, and left ductus arteriosus are usually asymptomatic, symptoms of tracheal or esophageal obstruction, when they occur, are similar to those encountered with double aortic arch. In these patients, however, symptoms are milder and often lead to presentation later in infancy or childhood. Nonetheless, affected patients present with stridor, cough, and recurrent respiratory infections. Older patients may complain of dysphagia and may have a history of stridor or wheezing. Anteroposterior chest radiographs demonstrate deviation of the trachea to the left, which is produced by the density of the right aortic arch. Barium esophagography demonstrates an oblique indentation from right to left (Fig. 158-3) in the anteroposterior projection and a large posterior indentation of the esophagus in lateral views. Anatomic features can also be demonstrated with echocardiography and angiography. Surgery is indicated for patients with symptomatic tracheal or esophageal compression. As for double aortic arch, the surgical mortality is low, and long-term relief of symptoms is the rule. Symptoms may persist for weeks or months after surgical correction.

PULMONARY ARTERY ANOMALIES

Anomalous Left Pulmonary Artery–Pulmonary Artery Sling

Anomalous origin of the left pulmonary artery is a rare congenital anomaly that produces severe tracheobronchial obstruction in most affected patients. A normal left pulmonary artery is absent, and the left lung is supplied by an anomalous left pulmonary artery arising from the distal right pulmonary artery. Tracheal and bronchial compression are produced as this artery courses posterior and caudal to the right main stem bronchus and then to the left, posterior to the trachea and anterior to the esophagus. The course of the vessel to the right of the trachea produces deviation of the lower trachea to the left. The resulting compression of the right main stem bronchus and lower trachea leads to airway obstruction, primarily affecting the right lung. However, obstruction of the lower trachea and left main stem bronchus may occur resulting in bilateral obstruction.

Associated congenital anomalies are common and are present in 58% to 83% of patients. Anomalies of the trachea, bronchi, and lung parenchyma are common and include complete cartilaginous rings, tracheomalacia, abnormal pulmonary lobulation, and bronchus sinus. Congenital heart defects are present in approximately 40% to 50% of patients and include persistent left superior vena cava, atrial septal defect, patent ductus arteriosus, and ventricular septal defects, among others.

Symptoms caused by anomalous left pulmonary artery occur early in most patients. Two-thirds of affected infants are symptomatic by age 1 month. Symptoms include severe respiratory distress with stridor, wheezing, cyanosis, and recurrent pneumonitis. Obstructive apnea may occur and can be fatal. Unlike aortic vascular rings, dysphagia is rare because the anomalous left pulmonary artery passes anterior to the esophagus without significant esophageal compression. Although the majority of patients are severely symptomatic, asymptomatic and mildly affected patients have been observed.

On anteroposterior chest radiographs, hyperinflation of the right or left lung caused by tracheal and bronchial compression is often observed. Obstruction of the left bronchus may also produce varying degrees of volume loss (atelectasis) of the left lung (Fig. 158-4). Usually, barium esophagography demonstrates a characteristic anterior indentation of the esophagus on the lateral projection. The diagnosis of anomalous left pulmonary artery and of associated cardiac defects is made readily with two-dimensional echocardiography.

Although the presence of a vascular sling can be established noninvasively, pulmonary artery angiography is necessary to delineate the anatomic detail necessary for surgical correction. Catheterization is also indicated to assess the severity of associated cardiac defects. Survival of symptomatic infants is unlikely without early surgical intervention; surgery should be performed early in infants suffering from severe respiratory obstruction. Although many reports have described successful treatment of this anomaly by surgery, the mortality after surgical procedures is high at 40% to 50%. Coexisting tracheal or bronchial stenosis is disproportionately prevalent and severe in nonsurvivors and undoubtedly is a major contributing factor in postoperative death.

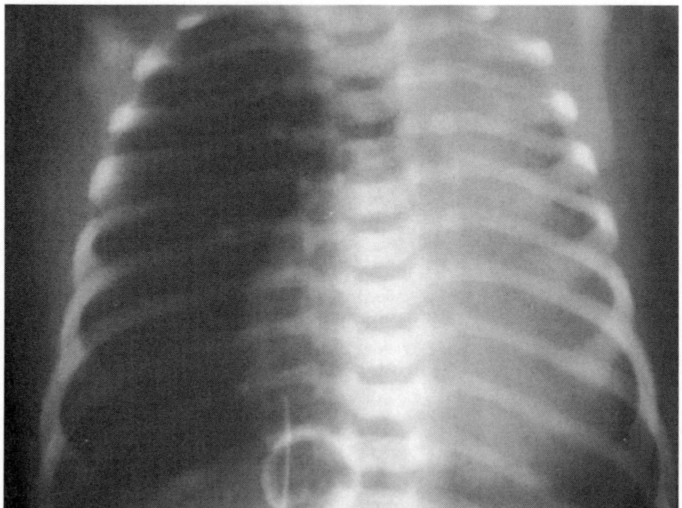

Figure 158-4. Posteroanterior radiograph demonstrating loss of volume (atelectasis) with opacity of the left lung field in a patient with a pulmonary artery sling. Often, the course of the left pulmonary artery posterior to the trachea and left bronchus produces compression with resulting atelectasis of the left lung or hyperinflation of the right. (Courtesy of Dr. Gary Hedlund, The Children's Hospital, Birmingham, AL.)

4

Diseases of the Blood

CHAPTER 159
Nutritional Anemias

Adapted from Michael Recht
and Howard A. Pearson

IRON DEFICIENCY ANEMIA

Iron deficiency anemia is defined as anemia caused by inadequate availability of iron to sustain bone marrow erythropoiesis. During the first years of life, when relatively small quantities of iron-rich food are ingested, it is difficult to maintain a positive iron balance. By 6 months of age, an infant's diet should include iron-fortified foods such as cereals or iron-supplemented formulas.

Clinical Characteristics

Anemia solely caused by inadequate dietary iron is unusual during the first 4 to 6 months of life, but it becomes more common from 9 to 24 months of age. The usual dietary pattern of infants with iron deficiency anemia is the consumption of large amounts of milk and carbohydrates not supplemented with iron. Pallor is the most frequent sign of iron deficiency anemia. In mild to moderate deficiency (i.e., hemoglobin level of 7–10 g/dL), few symptoms of anemia are seen. As the anemia progresses, tachycardia, cardiac dilation, and systolic murmurs occur. The spleen is palpable in 10% to 15% of patients. The child with iron deficiency anemia may be obese or overweight. Often other evidence of under nutrition is present.

Some children with iron deficiency anemia have pica. Iron deficiency anemia and even iron deficiency without significant anemia may adversely affect the attention span, behavior, and performance of affected children.

Laboratory Findings

Because iron is essential for hemoglobin synthesis, erythrocyte production is among the first casualties of iron deficiency. *Prelatent* iron deficiency occurs when stores are depleted without a change in hemoglobin or serum iron levels. This stage is rarely detected. *Latent* iron deficiency occurs when the serum iron level decreases and the total iron-binding capacity increases without a change in the hemoglobin. The level of serum ferritin provides a biochemical estimate of body iron stores. Serum ferritin levels in the range of 10 to 20 ng/mL indicate depletion of iron stores; levels of less than 10 ng/mL are diagnostic of iron deficiency. Frank iron deficiency anemia is associated with serum iron levels of less than 30 ng/dL, an increased serum iron-binding capacity, and the resulting serum transferrin saturation becoming less than 15%. As iron deficiency progresses, the erythrocytes become smaller than normal with decreased hemoglobin content (microcytic and hypochromic) and have abnormal shapes (poikilocytosis). The mean corpuscular volume (MCV) decreases to less than normal for age. The reticulocyte count is normal or minimally elevated, and the leukocyte counts are normal. Elevated platelet counts (greater than 600,000 per microliter) are often seen, although occasionally thrombocytopenia may be present.

Iron deficiency must be differentiated from other hypochromic, microcytic anemias. In lead poisoning, the erythrocytes are morphologically similar, but coarse basophilic stippling is prominent. Evaluation reveals elevations of blood lead and marked elevation of free erythrocyte protoporphyrins. As described previously, many children with lead poisoning have concomitant iron deficiency anemia. Thalassemia trait (alpha- or beta-thalassemia) is sometimes confused with iron deficiency anemia. Alpha-thalassemia trait occurs in approximately 3% of blacks and in many people of Southeast Asian origin. Beta-thalassemia major with its organomegaly, erythroblastosis, and hemolytic component is usually clinically apparent. Beta-thalassemia trait is common in individuals of Mediterranean descent. The erythrocyte morphology of chronic inflammatory or infectious conditions may be microcytic. In these conditions, the serum iron and iron-binding capacity is reduced, and the serum ferritin levels are normal or elevated.

Treatment

The response of iron deficiency anemia to adequate amounts of iron is an important diagnostic and therapeutic feature. Oral administration of simple ferrous salts is satisfactory therapy. Four to 6 mg/kg of elemental iron in three divided doses is optimal; larger doses do not result in a more rapid hematologic response.

Within 4 days after administration of iron, peripheral reticulocytosis is seen. The magnitude of the reticulocytic response is proportional to the severity of the anemia. After the hemoglobin level increases to normal, iron supplementation should be continued for 2 to 3 months to replenish iron stores. Poor response to oral iron therapy is most frequently because of poor compliance.

Because rapid hematologic response can be predicted confidently in typical iron deficiency anemia, blood transfusion is indicated only when the anemia is severe or if infection may interfere with response. Packed red blood cells should be administered to increase the hemoglobin to only approximately 7 g/dL, rather than attempting complete correction of the anemia. Often, it is advisable to split the packed red blood cell transfusion into two aliquots with a dose of diuretic between the administrations of each aliquot to avoid fluid overload in the patient. For frank congestive heart failure, exchange transfusion with packed red blood cells may be indicated.

Folic Acid Deficiency

Because folic acid is absorbed throughout the small intestine, diffuse inflammatory or degenerative disease of the intestine may impair folate's absorption. Both tropical and nontropical sprue, chronic infectious enteritis, or enteroenteric fistulas may lead to folic acid deficiency. Many patients have low serum levels of folic acid during therapy with anticonvulsant drugs because malabsorption of folic acid appears to be induced by these drugs. Drugs such as methotrexate prevent the use of folic acid by inhibiting reduction to its active coenzymatic forms. Megaloblastic anemia can be seen in some adolescent girls and women taking oral contraceptives. Deficiency of folate can also occur for the following reasons: defects of absorption (inherited defects of absorption, infiltrative diseases of the small bowel), inadequate nutrition (insufficient diet, maternal deficiency affecting the fetus and breast-fed infant), and inherited defects in folate metabolism (methylenetetrahydrofolate reductase deficiency and methionine synthase deficiency) and folate transfer.

A rare megaloblastic anemia of infancy is caused by a deficient intake or malabsorption of folic acid often aggravated by infection. Goat's milk and powdered cow's milk are poor sources of folic acid. The presence of an allergy to cow's milk can also cause malabsorption of folic acid. Vitamin C deficiency impairs folic acid absorption. This megaloblastic anemia has a peak incidence at 4 to 7 months of age. In addition to being pale, these children are irritable, fail to gain weight, and often have chronic diarrhea.

Vitamin B_{12} Deficiency

To be absorbed, dietary vitamin B_{12} must combine with intrinsic factor that is secreted by the parietal cells of the gastric fundus. The vitamin B_{12}–intrinsic factor complex passes to the terminal ileum, where specific absorptive receptors exist. Vitamin B_{12} deficiency can result from inadequate dietary intake, lack of secretion of intrinsic factor, disruption of the vitamin B_{12}–intrinsic factor complex, or abnormalities or absence of the receptor sites in the terminal ileum. Vitamin B_{12} deficiency can also be caused by a variety of other factors including defects in absorption, gastritis, total gastrectomy, intrinsic factor gene mutations, diseases of the small intestine, surgical resection or bypass of the terminal ileum, Crohn's disease, competition by parasites, or transcobalamin II deficiency. In children with transcobalamin II deficiency, cobalamin is malabsorbed leading to a severe megaloblastic anemia that occurs within the first few months of life.

Vitamin B_{12} is present in many foods. Pure dietary deficiency is rare. Deficiency may be seen in children eating diets containing no milk, eggs, or animal products (i.e., vegans). It is also reported in breast-fed infants whose mothers are deficient in vitamin B_{12} because of a vegan diet or pernicious anemia. Because the vitamin occurs in so many foods, most cases of vitamin B_{12} deficiency are a consequence of a failure to absorb the vitamin.

CHAPTER 160
Hemoglobinopathies and Thalassemias

Adapted from Paul L. Martin
and Howard A. Pearson

SICKLE CELL DISEASE AND TRAIT

In sickle cell disease, a valine residue is substituted for the usual glutamic acid in the chains of the hemoglobin molecule forming hemoglobin S (Hb S). When Hb S becomes deoxygenated, polymerization occurs with the formation of long, crystalline tactoids. These ultimately form elongated, sickled erythrocytes. Sickled erythrocytes have markedly shortened survival, and they can obstruct small blood vessels and cause distal tissue ischemia and necrosis.

Heterozygosity for a sickle gene has a benign clinical course. Approximately 8% of African-Americans have the trait. The sickle gene is thought to confer a degree of resistance in areas endemic for falciparum malaria in infancy. The erythrocytes in sickle trait contain only 30% to 40% Hb S, and sickling does not occur under physiologic conditions. Anemia or hemolysis should not be attributed to the sickle trait.

In persons homozygous for the sickle gene, sickle cell anemia is a severe, chronic hemolytic anemia. The clinical course is marked by episodes of pain caused by occlusion of small blood vessels by the spontaneously sickled erythrocytes.

Clinical Characteristics

Manifestations of sickle cell disease do not usually appear until the second 6 months of life, coincident with the postnatal decrease in fetal hemoglobin (Hb F) and increase in Hb S. The hemolytic process is evident by 6 months of age.

The painful or vasoocclusive crises are the most frequent clinical symptoms. Symmetric, painful swelling of the hands and feet (i.e., hand–foot syndrome) caused by infarction of the small bones of the hands and feet may be the initial manifestation of sickle cell anemia in infancy. Older patients may have painful involvement of the larger bones and joints and severe abdominal pain resembling acute surgical conditions. Strokes may leave permanent paralysis. Extensive pulmonary consolidation occurs, and it is difficult to differentiate infarction from pneumonia. Vasoocclusive crises are not usually associated with changes in the usual hematologic picture.

A second type of crisis, seen only in young infants and children, is called the *sequestration crisis*. Large amounts of blood become pooled in the abdominal organs. The spleen becomes massively enlarged, and signs of circulatory collapse rapidly develop. If volume replacement is given, much of the sequestered blood is remobilized. The sequestration crisis is an important cause of death in infants with sickle cell disease.

The third well-characterized type of crisis is the aplastic crisis. In addition to these acute crises, a variety of clinical signs and symptoms result from chronic severe hemolytic anemia and vasoocclusive disease. Impairment of liver function contributes to the jaundice of these patients. Gallstones can occur in children as young as 3 years. Renal function is progressively impaired by diffuse glomerular and tubular fibrosis resulting in hyposthenuria and polyuria.

As many as 30% of children with sickle cell anemia develop pneumococcal sepsis during the first 5 years of life. The increased risk is a result of functional hyposplenia and low levels of specific serum antibodies. Increased susceptibility to salmonella osteomyelitis is also a feature of sickle cell disease.

By mid-childhood, most patients are underweight and puberty is delayed, particularly in boys. Chronic leg ulcers are common in adolescence and early adult life.

Laboratory Findings

Hemoglobin levels range from 5 to 9 g/dL. Peripheral blood smears show irreversibly sickled cells, a finding almost diagnostic of homozygous sickle cell disease. The reticulocyte count ranges from 5% to 15%, and nucleated erythrocytes and Howell–Jolly bodies are usually observed. The total leukocyte count is elevated (12,000–20,000 per microliter) with a predominance of neutrophils. The platelet count is increased and the sedimentation rate is slow. Other changes include abnormal liver function test results, hyperbilirubinemia, and diffuse hypergammaglobulinemia. The bone marrow shows erythroid hyperplasia.

Diagnostic studies to demonstrate Hb S include the sickle cell preparation and hemoglobin solubility studies. However, hemoglobin electrophoresis is more conclusive and is necessary for a precise diagnosis. After infancy, the erythrocytes of patients with sickle cell anemia contain approximately 90% Hb S, 2% to 10% Hb F, and a normal amount of Hb A2; they do not contain Hb A.

Treatment

For mild or moderately painful crises, analgesics are indicated. Parenteral narcotics are often necessary for severe pain. Dehydration and acidosis should be corrected. Bacterial infections require appropriate antibiotic therapy. The risk of sepsis from encapsulated organisms is high enough to justify the use of prophylactic penicillin in all sickle cell patients from 6 months to at least 6 years of age, as well as immunization with pneumococcal vaccine. The value of prophylaxis after 6 years of age is being studied. Blood transfusions are unnecessary for the usual painful crises but are indicated for prolonged or extreme pain, for extensive involvement of lungs or central nervous system, and as preparation for general anesthesia. When the homozygous patient's circulating Hb SS erythrocytes can be diluted to less than 40% by transfusions of normal blood, vasoocclusive symptoms usually abate. Partial exchange transfusion can be done to rapidly lower the percentage of Hb SS erythrocytes.

Investigational treatments for sickle cell anemia include the use of hydroxyurea to cause "stress" erythropoiesis, which can increase the percentage of Hb F. Bone marrow transplantation from HLA-identical siblings has been performed in at least 21 children with sickle cell disease. The risk of death from toxicity of the transplant and the risk of chronic graft–versus–host disease appear to be 5% to 10%. Until the toxicity of bone marrow transplantation can be reduced, parents and physicians will face the difficult task of weighing the risk of early death from transplantation with the risk of death from long-term complications of sickle cell disease.

Newborn screening for sickle hemoglobinopathies is mandated in 38 states. Medical counseling of affected families and initiation of prophylactic penicillin for affected infants have been effective in decreasing early mortality from sickle cell disease.

THALASSEMIAS

The thalassemias are a group of hereditary hypochromic anemias associated with defective synthesis of one of the polypeptide chains of hemoglobin. In the United States, thalassemias chiefly affect persons of Mediterranean and Southeast Asian ethnic backgrounds. In the heterozygous state, thalassemia genes produce mild anemia. In the homozygous form, they are associated with severe hematologic disease.

Clinical Characteristics

Heterozygous thalassemia of the beta-chain variety (i.e., thalassemia minor) is a mild familial hypochromic microcytic anemia. Hemoglobin levels are 2 to 3 g/dL less than age-appropriate normal values. The mean corpuscular volume averages 68 fL (range, 58–75 fL). The erythrocytes are hypochromic and microcytic with target cells, ovalocytes, and basophilic stippling. Elevation of Hb A2 levels (greater than 3.5%) establishes the diagnosis. No therapy is effective or necessary.

Homozygous beta-thalassemia (i.e., thalassemia major, Cooley anemia) usually becomes symptomatic in the first year of life. The anemia is so profound that regular blood transfusions are necessary to sustain life; if untreated, the life expectancy is only a few years. However, approximately 10% of homozygous patients are able to maintain hemoglobin levels of 6 to 8 g/dL without regular transfusions (i.e., thalassemia intermedia). In the untransfused or poorly transfused patient, massive splenomegaly and progressive bone changes become evident during the first few years of life.

Laboratory Findings

The erythrocyte changes of thalassemia major are extreme. In addition to severe hypochromia and microcytosis, many poikilocytes and target cells are seen. Large numbers of nucleated erythrocytes circulate, especially after splenectomy. Typically, the hemoglobin level decreases progressively to less than 5 g/dL unless transfusions are given. The unconjugated serum bilirubin level is elevated. The serum iron level is high with increasing saturation of iron-binding capacity. Lactate dehydrogenase activities are very high reflecting ineffective erythropoiesis. Large amounts of fetal hemoglobin are contained in the erythrocytes. The level of Hb F exceeds 70% during the early years of life but tends to decline with increasing age.

Treatment

Transfusions of packed erythrocytes are given to maintain the hemoglobin level at more than 10 g/dL. This hypertransfusion has a striking clinical benefit: It permits normal activity with comfort and prevents progressive marrow expansion and its attendant cosmetic problems and osteoporosis. Transfusions are necessary every 4 to 5 weeks.

Hemosiderosis is an inevitable and fatal consequence of prolonged transfusion therapy, because each 200 mL of erythrocytes contains approximately 200 mg of iron that cannot be physiologically excreted. The iron burden can be reduced with iron-chelating agents, especially desferoxamine, which must be given parenterally, administered subcutaneously at night over 8 to 12 hours using a battery-driven pump. In many patients, a negative iron balance is possible. A chronic chelation program can reverse the poor prognosis of this disease if the patient complies with the demanding regimen. Iron-chelating drugs, especially those that can be taken orally, are undergoing clinical testing. If efficacious and safe, these new drugs will improve compliance with chelation therapy and significantly reduce the incidence of hemosiderosis in chronically transfused patients.

Splenectomy is often necessary because of the size of the organ or because of secondary hypersplenism, but it has no effect on the basic hematologic disease. Immunization with pneumococcal vaccine is indicated, and prophylactic penicillin therapy is advocated by some authorities.

Bone marrow transplantation from HLA-identical and partly mismatched siblings has been performed in more than 400 children with thalassemia. Early death from toxicity and graft–versus–host disease is low (less than 10%) in young patients without hepatic dysfunction. The risk of death is considerably higher for older patients, especially if liver function is already compromised by hemosiderosis. If an HLA-matched, healthy sibling is available, bone marrow transplantation should be considered, especially in a patient without symptoms of hemosiderosis. Introduction of abnormal beta-globin gene using gene therapy remains an area of active research.

Alpha-Thalassemias

A group of diseases, especially prevalent in Southeast Asians, results from genetic deletions of alpha-chain genes. Typically, four alpha-chain genes are described. Five percent of African-Americans have an alpha-thalassemia trait associated with deletion of two alpha-chain genes. Clinically, the disorder is characterized by microcytic anemia that is unresponsive to iron. Three and four alpha-chain deletions are rare among African-Americans. The diagnosis is made by excluding other causes of anemia. Hemoglobin electrophoresis is not helpful after the immediate postnatal period. In the newborn period, hemoglobin electrophoresis shows 3% to 6% Hb Barts. Patients are asymptomatic but should be counseled so that they may prevent well-meaning health providers from prescribing iron for presumed iron deficiency or from performing a workup for anemia.

In Asians, the four distinct alpha-thalassemia syndromes are the silent carrier state, alpha-thalassemia trait, Hb H disease, and fetal hydrops syndrome. These result from increasing numbers of alpha-thalassemia gene deletions from one to four. Deletion of four alpha-thalassemia genes produces the clinical picture of hydrops fetalis *in utero*. The predominant hemoglobin is Barts (γ_4). This variant has abnormal oxygen dissociation properties that make oxygen unavailable to the tissues causing fetal death.

Deletion of three alpha-thalassemia genes causes the less severe Hb H disease, which is a moderately severe anemia that resembles thalassemia major or intermedia. It is characterized by 5% to 10% of unstable Hb H (γ_4).

CHAPTER 161
Hemolytic Anemias

Adapted from Michael Recht
and Howard A. Pearson

INTRINSIC HEMOLYTIC ANEMIAS

Hereditary Spherocytosis

Hereditary Spherocytosis (HS) occurs predominantly in people of Northern European ancestry, although it has been found in patients of many ethnic groups. The typical features are a familial hemolytic anemia of various degrees of severity, splenomegaly, and spherical erythrocytes found on the blood smear.

Pathophysiology

A deficiency or abnormality of the erythrocyte membrane structural protein spectrin appears to affect most patients with HS. This deficiency is associated with an accelerated loss of the erythrocyte membrane, which reduces the erythrocyte surface area. Because no concomitant loss of cellular volume occurs, the erythrocytes assume a spherical shape.

The spleen is intrinsically involved in the hemolytic process. The splenic circulation imposes a metabolic stress on spherocytic cells. The spherocyte is relatively rigid and passes with difficulty through the splenic cords and sinuses. This results in their sequestration and destruction. The hemolytic process regresses after splenectomy, although biochemical and morphologic abnormalities persist.

Clinical Characteristics

The disease may present in the neonatal period with anemia and hyperbilirubinemia that may require phototherapy or exchange transfusion. The anemia varies considerably in severity but tends to be similar within the same family. The patient usually has slight jaundice. Expansion of the marrow cavity occurs to a lesser extent than in thalassemia. The spleen is almost always palpably enlarged after 2 or 3 years of age. Pigmentary gallstones have occurred as early as 4 years of age. Aplastic crises associated with parvovirus infections are the most serious complications during childhood. Other complications have been reported and are less common including gout, leg ulcers, and growth retardation.

Laboratory Findings

Indicators of hemolysis include reticulocytosis, anemia, and hyperbilirubinemia. The hemoglobin level ranges from 6 to 10 g/dL and the reticulocyte count from 5% to 20% (average, 10%). Abnormality of the erythrocyte can be demonstrated by osmotic fragility studies. This test measures the ability of red blood cells to swell and increase their volume when subjected to varying degrees of hypotonic environments. Because of their decreased surface-to-volume ratio, spherocytes have a limited capability of doing so and will be lysed at a higher salt concentration than normal cells.

HS must be differentiated from other congenital hemolytic states. Family history, blood smear, and osmotic fragility studies offer the most diagnostic value. Acquired spherocytosis of the erythrocytes is seen in autoimmune hemolytic anemias in which the spherocytosis is often more pronounced than in HS, and the direct Coombs test result is positive. It may be difficult to differentiate HS from hemolytic disease caused by ABO incompatibility in the newborn infant. A period of observation may be necessary to clarify the diagnosis.

Therapy

Splenectomy almost invariably produces a clinical cure, although in a few instances of severe HS with recessive transmission, the operation is not curative. Splenectomy should be deferred if possible until the patient is at least 5 or 6 years of age. If anemia is severe enough to impair growth or normal activity, the operation can be considered earlier, after a period of observation. Splenectomy prevents further gallstone formation and eliminates the threat of aplastic crises.

After splenectomy, jaundice and reticulocytosis disappear. The hemoglobin level becomes normal, although the spherocytosis and osmotic fragility abnormalities become more pronounced. Overwhelming sepsis after splenectomy occurs infrequently if the surgery is delayed until the child is 5 or 6 years of age, but the febrile child must be carefully evaluated for sepsis. Polyvalent pneumococcal, Haemophilus influenzae type b, and perhaps meningococcal vaccines should be given before splenectomy. Prophylactic penicillin therapy after splenectomy is mandatory if the operation is done before the child is 6 years of age.

HEREDITARY ELLIPTOCYTOSIS

Some oval or elliptical erythrocytes may be seen in a number of conditions, especially thalassemia and iron deficiency; however, they occur in much larger numbers as a dominantly inherited trait in hereditary elliptocytosis (HE; hereditary ovalocytosis). Fifteen percent to 50% of the circulating erythrocytes of these patients are elongated. In most patients, no associated hemolysis occurs and the hematologic values including reticulocyte counts are normal. However, in approximately 10% of patients with elliptical cells, evidence of hemolysis exists with hemoglobin levels averaging 8 to 10 g/dL and reticulocytes comprising 5% to 15% of the cells.

Clinical Characteristics

HE with hemolysis may be associated with neonatal jaundice, but characteristic elliptocytosis may not be evident at birth. The blood smear instead shows bizarre poikilocytes and pyknocytes. The usual features of chronic hemolytic process including anemia, jaundice, splenomegaly, and osseous changes may be seen later. Cholelithiasis occurs in later childhood, and aplastic crises have been reported.

Laboratory Findings

The morphology of the erythrocytes is the most important diagnostic feature. Elliptical cells characterized by a length more than 1.5 times the diameter account for 15% to 70% of the erythrocytes. In hemolytic HE, the reticulocyte count is increased.

Therapy

If significant hemolysis exists, splenectomy is usually beneficial. Erythrocyte morphology is not changed after the operation, and it may become even more abnormal.

HEMOLYTIC ANEMIAS RESULTING FROM ABNORMALITIES OF ERYTHROCYTE GLYCOLYTIC ENZYMES

Glucose-6-Phosphate Dehydrogenase (G6PD) Deficiency

Thirteen percent of black men and 2% of black women have a mutant enzyme called G6PD A^- that is unstable and associated with reduced erythrocyte enzyme activity (5%–15% of normal). Affected persons of Mediterranean, Arabic, and Asian ethnic groups have relatively high frequencies of G6PD deficiency because of a variant designated G6PD B^-. The enzyme activity of the homozygous female or the hemizygous male subject is less than 5% of normal.

G6PD, the rate-limiting enzyme of the pentose phosphate pathway, is crucial for protection of the erythrocytes from oxidant stress. In G6PD deficiency, oxidant metabolites of a number of drugs produce denaturation and precipitation of hemoglobin causing erythrocyte injury and rapid hemolysis. Hemolysis occurs only if the patient is exposed to oxidant drugs such as antipyretics, naphthalene, sulfonamides, antimalarials, and naphthaquinolones or to the fava bean. The degree of hemolysis varies with the drug's antioxidant effect, the amount ingested, and the severity of the enzyme deficiency in the patient.

Laboratory Findings

Hemoglobinemia and hemoglobinuria occur 24 to 48 hours after the ingestion of an oxidant substance. The hemoglobin level may decrease to as low as 2 to 5 g/dL. Heinz bodies are not visible on stained blood smears. They can be demonstrated initially on supravital preparations, but they disappear after 3 or 4 days. Spontaneous recovery is usual and is heralded by reticulocytosis and an increase in hemoglobin concentration starting 4 or 5 days after the acute hemolytic episode.

Diagnosis depends on direct or indirect demonstration of reduced G6PD activity in erythrocytes. By direct measurement, enzyme activity in affected persons is less than 15% of normal. The reduction of enzyme activity is more extreme in whites and Asians than in G6PD-deficient blacks. Shortly after a hemolytic event, G6PD activity may be normal, secondary to a reticulocytosis. A repeat examination several weeks later may be necessary to prove the diagnosis.

Therapy

Prevention of hemolysis by avoiding oxidant drugs is important. Men and boys belonging to ethnic groups in which a significant incidence of G6PD deficiency occurs should be tested for the defect before drugs that are known to be potent oxidants are given. After hemolysis has occurred, supportive therapy is indicated including blood transfusions if the anemia is severe and the patient symptomatic.

EXTRINSIC HEMOLYTIC ANEMIAS

Autoimmune Hemolytic Anemias

In the autoimmune hemolytic anemias (AIHAs), the patient's antibodies are directed against the patient's own erythrocytes. The factors evoking such an autoimmune response are unknown but include viral infections and occasionally specific drugs.

Clinical Characteristics

AIHAs occur in two clinical patterns. The first type, a fulminant variety that occurs in infants and young children, is frequently preceded by a respiratory infection. The onset is acute with pallor, jaundice, and hemoglobinuria. The spleen is enlarged. A consistent response to corticosteroid therapy, low mortality, and complete recovery are characteristic. No underlying disease is found. A second type of AIHA has a prolonged course and a significant mortality. Underlying diseases are frequently found.

Laboratory Findings

The anemia may be severe with hemoglobin levels of less than 6 g/dL. Spherocytosis and polychromasia are prominent. Reticulocytosis and nucleated erythrocytes are found and leukocytosis is common. The platelet count is usually normal; occasionally, concomitant immune thrombocytopenic purpura occurs (i.e., Evans syndrome).

The direct and indirect Coombs test results are positive indicating the presence of antibodies attached to the erythrocytes or free in the serum. These antibodies belong to the IgG class. They are often nonspecific panagglutinins, but they may have specificity for ubiquitous antigens of the Rh system (e.g., E, LW). Because of spontaneous erythrocyte agglutination, the patient may be mistakenly typed as blood group AB, Rh^+. In acute, transient cases, only complement is found on the erythrocytes, chiefly the C3 and C4 components. In chronic AIHA, a pure IgG Coombs test result is often found.

Treatment

Transfusion may be required, but it offers only transient benefit. Completely compatible blood is difficult to find and giving blood that is "incompatible" as judged by the cross-match is often necessary. Prednisone should be administered in a dosage of 2 to 4 mg/kg every 24 hours. Treatment should be continued until hemolysis decreases. The dose can then be gradually reduced. The acute form of the disease usually remits spontaneously within a few weeks or months, but the Coombs test result may remain positive for an extended period. Splenectomy may be beneficial in several refractory cases. Immunosuppressive agents have been used in patients refractory to conventional therapy. In AIHA secondary to lymphoma or lupus erythematosus, the disease tends to be chronic and the course of the underlying disease determines the ultimate prognosis.

CHAPTER 162
Hypoplastic and Aplastic Anemias

Adapted from Paul L. Martin and Howard A. Pearson

CONGENITAL HYPOPLASTIC ANEMIA

At the 1938 meeting of the American Pediatric Society, Diamond and Blackfan described four children with severe aregenerative anemia that developed during the first year of life and required regular transfusions for survival. Only approximately 300 cases of congenital hypoplastic anemia (CHA) have been described in the literature, but many more cases have been recognized.

Clinical Characteristics

Anemia at or shortly after birth is the presenting manifestation of CHA. Approximately one-fourth of the patients are pale at birth. Sixty-five percent are anemic by 6 months of age, and almost all are anemic by 1 year of age. CHA described in older infants, particularly those reported before 1970, must be viewed with some skepticism because the cases may have represented transient erythroblastopenia of childhood.

Laboratory Findings

At the time of diagnosis, hemoglobin levels may be as low as 2.5 g/dL. The erythrocytes are macrocytic and have biochemical properties of fetal erythrocyte [i.e., increased levels of fetal hemoglobin for the patient's age, presence of the i erythrocyte antigen, and increased levels of age-dependent erythrocyte enzymes such as glucose-6-phosphate dehydrogenase (G6PD)]. These findings may be of limited diagnostic value in early infancy when fetal cells are still present.

The reticulocyte count is characteristically very low, even in the presence of severe anemia. The remainder of the peripheral blood count is usually normal, although elevated platelet counts and modest neutropenia have been occasionally found. Serum bilirubin levels are normal. Serum iron levels are usually elevated with increased transferrin saturation. Plasma and urinary levels of erythropoietin are elevated.

The most important diagnostic features are found in the bone marrow. The marrow in patients with CHA is normally cellular with normal numbers of megakaryocytes, lymphocytes, and myeloid precursors. However, erythrocyte precursors at every level of development are absent or markedly reduced.

Therapy

The degree of anemia is often so profound at presentation that erythrocyte transfusions are necessary. Approximately 10% to 20% of patients are refractory to therapy and continue to require regular transfusions. Transfusions with packed, leukocyte-poor erythrocytes are given to maintain a hemoglobin level compatible with normal activity and comfort, usually more than 8.0 g/dL.

When chronic transfusion therapy is necessary, transfusional hemosiderosis inevitably occurs. Serum ferritin levels should be monitored periodically, and chelation therapy should be begun when evidence exists of tissue iron.

Between 60% and 70% of patients respond to corticosteroid therapy. The mechanism of corticosteroid action may involve an enhancement of the effect of erythropoietin on CFU-E proliferation and maturation. Corticosteroids such as prednisone are administered at an initial dose of 2 mg/kg. Response is heralded by the appearance of erythropoietic precursors in the bone marrow within 1 to 2 weeks, followed by reticulocytosis and an increase in the hemoglobin level. The full dose of prednisone is continued until the hemoglobin attains a normal level. The dose can then be gradually decreased until a minimal effective dose is attained, which is often as little as 0.5 to 1.0 mg/day. In many instances, corticosteroids can be administered on alternate-day schedules that further decrease corticosteroid side effects. Some patients do not respond to the usual dose of corticosteroids and should be given a trial with larger doses (4–6 mg/kg). Approximately 20% to 30% of these children are nonresponsive to corticosteroids and require regular blood transfusions.

Children refractory to corticosteroids have not usually responded to other forms of therapy including androgenic and immunosuppressive agents. Bone marrow transplantation has been effective for a few patients.

TRANSIENT ERYTHROBLASTIC ANEMIA OF CHILDHOOD

Transient erythroblastic anemia of childhood (TEC) is a striking syndrome of temporary failure of erythropoiesis, which is increasingly encountered in clinical practice. TEC is characterized by moderate to severe aregenerative anemia in an otherwise healthy child. The condition is self-limited and does not usually recur.

Pathophysiology

TEC seems to have an autoimmune basis. A circulating immunoglobulin that inhibits growth of CFU-E or BFU-E in tissue culture has been found in most of these patients. The stimulus that evokes this antibody has not been defined, and the inhibitor disappears from the serum as recovery occurs. TEC has not been associated with parvovirus infection.

Clinical Characteristics

TEC occurs in children older than 1 year, but it has been seen as early as 4 months of age. Pallor and symptoms of anemia are the usual presenting manifestations. Because the anemia reflects a complete cessation of erythropoiesis without increased hemolysis, the anemia develops very slowly.

If a patient has a hemoglobin level of 5 g/dL on presentation, it can be assumed that erythrocyte production has been minimal for at least 2 months. Because the anemia develops insidiously, pallor or symptoms may not be noticed by the parents. Except for the features of anemia, the remainder of the physical examination is normal.

Laboratory Findings

The degree of anemia may be severe, as low as 2.5 g/dL, with a low reticulocyte count. The leukocyte count is normal. The platelet count is usually normal but may be elevated. Other laboratory findings include a high serum iron level reflecting decreased use. The bone marrow shows a paucity of erythrocyte precursors with a high M:E ratio. The other marrow elements are normal.

Recovery occurs spontaneously within a few weeks and is accompanied by a brisk reticulocytosis and rapid increase in hemoglobin level.

The major differential diagnosis of TEC is CHA, particularly in the infant younger than 1 year. In contrast to CHA, in TEC the erythrocyte population at presentation has age-appropriate characteristics; a mean corpuscular volume of 70 to 80 fL; fetal hemoglobin less than 2% to 5%; normal levels of erythrocyte age-dependent enzymes (G6PD); and the usual adult I erythrocyte antigen. Erythrocyte adenine deaminase levels are not elevated.

A patient first seen in the recovery state of TEC may be erroneously considered to have a hemolytic process because of the concomitant low hemoglobin and high reticulocyte count. Observation can clarify the diagnosis.

Therapy

No specific therapy is necessary. Corticosteroid therapy is not indicated. If the anemia is severe, a small erythrocyte transfusion may be considered to sustain the child until recovery occurs. Most children have no recurrence of this disease.

APLASTIC ANEMIAS

The aplastic anemias have diverse causes whose common features are varying degrees of peripheral pancytopenia accompanied by marked hypocellularity of the bone marrow. Many drugs, infections, and environmental factors have been associated with the development of acquired aplastic anemia. Chloramphenicol has been the drug most frequently associated with acquired aplastic anemia. It has been estimated that only approximately 1 in 20,000 to 50,000 persons taking chloramphenicol develops aplastic anemia, but in as many as 50% of the cases of drug-related aplastic anemia, chloramphenicol has been implicated. A particularly serious form of aplastic anemia occurs in the wake of viral hepatitis. In approximately one-half of these patients, no causative factor can be implicated, and their disease is designated idiopathic, although an environmental factor cannot be excluded.

Congenital Aplastic Anemia

Congenital aplastic anemia (CAA; Fanconi syndrome, constitutional aplastic anemia) was first described by Professor Fanconi in Switzerland in 1927. More than 600 cases have been reported in many ethnic groups. Although CAA is genetically determined and transmitted as an autosomal recessive disorder, it is not usually hematologically evident during infancy and early childhood. Clinical CAA is characterized by severe pancytopenia, hypoplasia of the bone marrow, and a constellation of physical abnormalities. Some patients do not have obvious physical anomalies.

CLINICAL CHARACTERISTICS

Short stature and generalized hyperpigmentation affect most patients. Approximately one-half of the patients with CAA have congenital skeletal anomalies. The most striking of these anomalies includes bilateral absence or hypoplasia of the thumb, sometimes accompanied by abnormalities of the radii. Approximately one-third of patients have renal abnormalities including unilateral aplasia and horseshoe kidney. Approximately 50% of patients have no gross anatomic abnormalities.

The onset of progressive bone marrow failure is initially manifested by petechiae and ecchymosis secondary to thrombocytopenia between 2 and 22 years of age (mean age, 7). Anemia and neutropenia develop somewhat later than thrombocytopenia.

LABORATORY FINDINGS

Disordered erythropoiesis is manifested by macrocytosis (mean corpuscular volume greater than 90 fL) and elevated levels of fetal hemoglobin before the onset of marrow failure. Ultimately, severe pancytopenia develops. Serial bone marrow examinations show progressive hypocellularity and, ultimately, frank aplasia. The peripheral blood lymphocytes, when cultured in the presence of diepoxybutane, an alkylating agent, consistently show chromosomal abnormalities. This is a useful test when the physical stigmata of Fanconi anemia are absent.

TREATMENT

Supportive therapy including transfusions of erythrocytes and platelets offers only temporary benefit. In the past, approximately three-fourths of these patients died within 2 years of the onset of marrow failure.

Therapy with pharmacologic doses of androgenic hormones produces a hematologic improvement in more than two-thirds of patients. The response to these agents may be sustained for several years, but maintenance therapy is usually necessary. Complications of androgen therapy including masculinization and liver dysfunction are common. Ultimately, most patients become refractory to androgens and again require transfusions. Bone marrow transplantation using HLA-compatible siblings who do not themselves have CAA has been successful in many patients.

Long-term complications of the disease and its therapy include androgen-associated hepatic disease and tumors and an increased risk of acute myeloid leukemia and other malignancies.

CHAPTER 163
Disorders of Coagulation

Adapted from James F. Casella, Daniel C. Bowers, and Maria A. Pelidis

QUANTITATIVE CONGENITAL ABNORMALITIES OF THE PLATELETS

Thrombocytopenia with Absent Radius Syndrome

The thrombocytopenia with absent radius (TAR) syndrome is perhaps the most striking and most easily recognized of the congenital thrombocytopenias. Clinical recognition of the disorder occurs soon after birth in the infant with purpura and characteristic limb deformities. Although absence of the radius is the most consistent finding in this condition, cardiac, renal, and other skeletal malformations (e.g., complete or partial agenesis of other bones or joints, bony synostoses) may also occur. Leukoerythroblastic responses, often associated with severe diarrhea, are often observed in the neonatal period and infancy. The inheritance pattern appears to be autosomal recessive. Bone marrow specimens exhibit reduced numbers of megakaryocytes, which often appear dysplastic. Transfused platelets survive normally, and with the use of HLA-matched platelets, many patients can be maintained on weekly platelet transfusions for long periods. The thrombocytopenia tends to remit spontaneously in the second and third year of life.

QUALITATIVE CONGENITAL ABNORMALITIES OF THE PLATELETS

Glanzmann Thrombasthenia

Glanzmann thrombasthenia is a prototype of the qualitative platelet disorders. This abnormality is inherited as an autosomal recessive trait. Although the number and morphology of the platelets are normal, life-threatening hemorrhagic complications may be encountered. The spectrum of severity of bleeding symptoms is broad ranging from mild to severe. Platelets from patients with Glanzmann disease do not aggregate *in vitro* in response to adenosine diphosphate, collagen, epinephrine, and thrombin, but they do agglutinate in the presence of ristocetin and vWF. Clot retraction may be abnormal. These abnormalities are caused by the partial or complete absence of a cytoadhesive protein, glycoprotein IIb/IIIa (the platelet fibrinogen receptor), from platelet membranes. The ability of these platelets to agglutinate in the presence of ristocetin and vWF can be attributed to the presence of normal amounts of another cytoadhesive membrane protein, glycoprotein Ib, the major vWF receptor. Transfusion of platelets is the only effective therapy for severe bleeding but may result in the development of antibodies directed against the glycoprotein IIb/IIIa complex and resistance to further platelet transfusions. Larger than predicted platelet transfusions may be required, presumably because of the interference of abnormal platelets with the transfused platelets. Epsilon–aminocaproic acid can be extremely helpful for oral or nasal hemorrhage. Patients with Glanzmann thrombasthenia are at high risk for iron deficiency anemia secondary to frequent bleeding episodes; in particular, iron supplementation should be considered for infants and adolescent female patients with Glanzmann thrombasthenia.

Numerous mutations in both glycoprotein IIb and IIIa have been described that result in Glanzmann phenotypes.

QUANTITATIVE ACQUIRED ABNORMALITIES OF PLATELETS

Idiopathic (Immune) Thrombocytopenic Purpura

Idiopathic thrombocytopenic purpura, sometimes referred to as *immune* or *autoimmune thrombocytopenic purpura* (ITP or ATP), is perhaps the most commonly encountered acquired platelet disorder of childhood.

ETIOLOGY AND PATHOGENESIS

Although abundant evidence indicates an immunologic basis for this disease, in most cases, the cause of the immunologic aberration is not clear, and the term idiopathic is preferred. Clinically, the disease is recognized in acute and chronic forms, and a multitude of pathogenic mechanisms are probably involved. Many studies have demonstrated an immunologic basis for the observed thrombocytopenia. The reticuloendothelial system of the spleen is the major site of destruction of platelets in ITP with a less important contribution from the reticuloendothelial system of the liver, bone marrow, and lungs.

Although the concept that an immunologic basis exists for ITP is well accepted, the inciting cause for antibody production often remains obscure. Acute ITP in childhood is often preceded by a viral illness, and it has been postulated that viral antigens may trigger the production of antibodies that cross-react with the platelet membrane. Studies have shown decreased production of platelets in otherwise classic cases of ITP suggesting that the thrombocytopenia may be the consequence of decreased production and increased destruction in some cases.

CLINICAL AND LABORATORY FEATURES

The acute and chronic ITPs tend to vary considerably in their initial presentations. In acute ITP, preceding viral illnesses are common, and the onset of purpuric symptoms is typically abrupt, so much so that parents can often recount the exact hour that they became aware of the problem. In chronic ITP, antecedent illnesses are less common, and the onset of purpura is often much more insidious. Acute ITP most often presents in previously healthy children, whereas chronic ITP is more common in patients with other underlying immunoregulatory abnormalities such as systemic lupus erythematosus, IgA deficiency, autoimmune endocrinopathy, common variable immunodeficiency, or autoimmune hemolytic anemia (i.e., Evans syndrome) or with family histories of these disorders. Immunologic destruction of platelets associated with human immunodeficiency virus (HIV) infection is often chronic as well. Acute ITP tends to occur equally in both genders, whereas chronic ITP is more common in female patients. Acute ITP is predominately a disease of early childhood. Chronic ITP is much more common in children older than 10 years.

In acute and chronic ITP, purpura and mucosal bleeding are the most prominent symptoms. The fact that the children generally appear well, except for the purpuric lesions, is helpful in excluding other illnesses associated with severe thrombocytopenia. Large submucous hemorrhages in the mouth are thought to be associated with an increased risk for serious hemorrhage. Hepatomegaly, splenomegaly, and lymphadenopathy are notably absent, and their presence should initiate an investigation for other possible underlying illnesses associated with thrombocytopenia. Gastrointestinal and renal hemorrhage sometimes occurs. Central nervous system bleeding is the most feared complication of ITP, but it occurs in less than 1% of these patients, usually early in the course of the illness. Such hemorrhages are often, but not invariably fatal.

Platelet counts vary from normal (in a compensated phase) to undetectable, but they tend to be lower in acute ITP than in chronic ITP. The rest of the complete blood count should be normal, unless bleeding sufficient to cause anemia has occurred. A careful review of the peripheral blood smear should be performed. Eosinophilia and atypical lymphocytosis may be seen, but other abnormalities including immature white blood cells must be excluded. Particular attention should be given to identifying red cell morphology consistent with microangiopathic hemolysis, which occurs in thrombotic thrombocytopenic purpura, a much more serious disorder that can be associated with severe thrombocytopenia. The PT and aPTT should be normal. However, no definitive test exists for ITP. The diagnosis remains one of exclusion.

ITP in young children frequently has a benign course with an excellent prognosis. More than 50% of untreated children with ITP recover within 4 weeks without treatment, and more than 80% spontaneously recover within 6 months. The resolution of symptoms and the thrombocytopenia occur in a variety of patterns from abrupt to slow with frequent relapses. ITP is not generally considered chronic unless symptoms persist for more than 6 months. Relapses are common in chronic ITP. Acute ITP tends not to recur, but relapses have been reported. Improvement of symptoms often precedes a detectable increase in the platelet count.

TREATMENT

The incidence of serious complications of ITP is very low. Mortality and morbidity are most often associated with intracranial hemorrhage. Given the low incidence of intracranial hemorrhage, no prospective, randomized trials have been carried out that can truly estimate the likelihood that this complication can be prevented. The goal of treatment for most practitioners is to reduce the likelihood of bleeding during periods of maximal risk. Because the spontaneous remission rate for acute ITP is extremely high, a waiting period is usually warranted before attempting therapy at presentation if the disease is mild (i.e., platelet count greater than 20,000 per microliter, no bleeding other than purpura). Platelet counts of less than 20,000 per microliter and extensive mucosal hemorrhage indicate a higher risk for internal hemorrhage, and treatment should be considered. If serious complications are present or suspected or if a protective environment cannot be guaranteed, treatment should be initiated. Historically, corticosteroid administration has been the most commonly used therapy. Prednisone is usually administered at an initial dosage of 2 mg/kg/day orally, but higher or intravenous dosages up to 30 mg/kg/day of prednisolone for very short periods may be more effective.

Intravenous gamma globulin is a useful modality in the treatment of ITP. The mechanism of action of this agent is not clear, but the best evidence to date suggests that it may act by causing a reticuloendothelial blockade, as evidenced by the reduced splenic clearance of sensitized erythrocytes after administration. Antiidiotypic or antiFc receptor antibodies may be involved. Modulation of T- or B-cell function has been postulated, and it has been speculated that the clearance of infection or antigenemia may play a role. Commonly used treatment regimens vary from 0.8 to 2.0 g/kg divided over 1 to 5 days. The most commonly used dose is 1 g/kg in a single administration. Responses are usually rapid and transitory and should not be expected in all patients. Although this therapy is quite efficacious, up to 34% of patients may experience transient complications manifested by severe headache, nausea and, rarely, aseptic meningitis. Premedication with corticosteroids or acetaminophen and diphenhydramine may decrease the frequency of these side effects. As with all plasma-derived products, some risk of transmission of infection exists, although modern products appear to be quite safe. In addition, intravenous IgG therapy is extremely expensive.

AntiD immunoglobulin is a relatively new, but useful, therapy for ITP. Although the mechanism of action is incompletely understood, antibody-coated red cells are hypothesized to compete with antibody-coated platelets for destruction in the reticuloendothelial system. Patients who are Rh-negative have no response to antiD immunoglobulin. Splenectomized individuals may respond suboptimally, but responses have been seen. Treatment regimens vary from 25 μg/kg per dose on 1 or 2 consecutive days to 50 to 100 μg/kg intravenously in a single administration and can be infused within half an hour. Intramuscular use has also been reported. Response rates appear to be similar to that of intravenous IgG with perhaps a slightly longer delay in response; however, this finding may be dose related. The major toxicity associated with antiD immunoglobulin is a predictable decrease in hemoglobin (mean hemoglobin decrease, 1.3 g/dL). Severe anemia as a result of therapy with antiD immunoglobulin appears to be rare. However, this therapy is not recommended for patients with significant anemia. Given its ease of use, the outstanding safety record of antiD for other indications and its significantly lower protein load and expense, use of this therapy is rapidly becoming more widespread. As with all plasma-derived products, caution is indicated in its use because of potential infectious risks and the possibility of allergic reactions.

Platelet transfusions are generally eschewed in ITP because of the shortened survival of transfused platelets. However, platelet transfusions may be effective in immediately reducing serious bleeding. Splenectomy is effective in resolving the thrombocytopenia in approximately two-thirds of patients but is generally used only in emergencies or in extremely resistant cases. Other therapeutic approaches such as Vinca-loaded platelets or vincristine infusions, immunosuppressive agents such as azathioprine, cyclosporine, and cyclophosphamide, and miscellaneous agents such as interferon, ascorbic acid, or danazol have been used in chronic ITP. Success rates tend to be low and, in general, these therapies should be used after more conventional modes of therapy have failed.

Neonatal Immune Thrombocytopenia

Severe thrombocytopenia in the neonatal period may occur because of transplacental transfer of antibody from a mother who has ITP (i.e., passive autoimmune thrombocytopenia). In these cases, PAIgG can usually be detected on the mother's platelets (i.e., direct PAIgG test) and often in the mother's serum (i.e., indirect PAIgG test). The mother's platelet count is not an absolute predictor of thrombocytopenia in the infant. Mothers with normal platelet counts, especially those who have undergone splenectomy for ITP, may deliver severely thrombocytopenic infants. However, thrombocytopenic mothers with ITP often deliver infants with normal platelet counts. In some cases, the platelet count may decrease over the first few days of life. The thrombocytopenia may persist for days to months paralleling the disappearance of maternal antibody from the infant's circulation.

Neonatal thrombocytopenia may occur in mothers who have been sensitized to antigens on the infant's platelets that are absent from her platelets (i.e., alloimmune or isoimmune thrombocytopenia). Five well-known human platelet alloantigen systems (HPA 1 through 5) exist, each a result of a single amino acid substitution in the gene for the glycoprotein on which the antigen resides. The frequency of the platelet antigens varies among different ethnic groups. The most common platelet antigen incompatibility involves the Pl^{A1} system, or HPA 1. In this system, three phenotypes are possible: HPA(1a/1a) (i.e., homozygous Pl^{A1} positivity), HPA(1a/1b) (i.e., heterozygous Pl^{A1} positivity), and HPA(1b/1b) (i.e., homozygous Pl^{A1} negativity). Approximately 98% of the population is HPA(1a/1a) or HPA(1a/1b). If the mother is HPA(1b/1b), the father is likely to be HPA(1a/1a) or HPA(1a/1b), and the infant will be a candidate for alloimmune disease. A number of platelet antigens belonging to systems HPA 2 through 5 [e.g., Bak, Pen (Yuk), Ko, Pl^t, Br] less commonly implicated as a cause of alloimmune thrombocytopenia have been described, as well as a number of other minor platelet antigens that are capable of causing alloimmune disorders. The mother's platelet count is normal in these disorders. *In vitro* testing should demonstrate that the direct test result for PAIgG on the mother is negative. However, her serum should increase the amount of PAIgG on the father's or the infant's platelets and control antigen-positive platelets (i.e., indirect test). Alloimmune thrombocytopenia most often resolves within a few weeks but can persist for a longer period. As with erythrocyte sensitization, a high risk of recurrence exists with future pregnancies.

Cesarean section should be considered for any delivery in which the child is at risk for passive immune thrombocytopenia, because the risk of intracranial hemorrhage at the time of delivery is high. Platelets should be available in the delivery room. Neonatal immune thrombocytopenia has been treated successfully with transfusion of platelets and exchange transfusion. Corticosteroids may be useful if administered to the mother before delivery or to the infant after delivery. In some infants, intracranial hemorrhages may occur *in utero*. Several therapies have been proposed to prevent them, and what constitutes optimal therapy is still controversial. A corticosteroid preparation that is not inactivated by the placenta such as dexamethasone is often used. The administration of intravenous gamma globulin to mothers prenatally appears to reduce the incidence of intracranial hemorrhage. Postnatally, intravenous gamma globulin for autoimmune thrombocytopenia appears to be equally effective as in other forms of ITP, although the experience is much less extensive. Intravenous gamma globulin may also increase the platelet count in alloimmune thrombocytopenia; however, transfusion of mother's platelets represents optimal therapy postnatally, because they do not possess the sensitizing antigen and, therefore, have normal survival. *In utero* transfusions of maternal platelets have been used to prevent intracranial hemorrhage in alloimmune disease in selected cases.

Nonimmune Causes of Thrombocytopenia

INFECTIOUS THROMBOCYTOPENIA

Thrombocytopenia may be associated with a variety of infections, viral infections being the most common offenders. The thrombocytopenia may occur during the active infection or as a postinfectious manifestation of the illness. In congenital rubella, for example, the thrombocytopenia can persist for months and often follows a course similar to that of ITP. Viral infections associated with thrombocytopenia include varicella, Epstein-Barr virus, cytomegalovirus, other herpesviruses, and measles. In some cases, thrombocytopenia may be caused by generalized marrow suppression that sometimes occurs after Epstein-Barr viral infections and hepatitis. The mechanism of the thrombocytopenia is not always clear, but in the case of rubella and cytomegalovirus, the virus can be cultured from the marrow. Thrombocytopenia may accompany a number of other systemic infections including toxoplasmosis, ehrlichiosis, malaria, syphilis, tuberculosis, and overwhelming bacterial or rickettsial sepsis.

Infection with HIV is an increasingly common cause of thrombocytopenia. Features of immune and nonimmune causes of thrombocytopenia are encountered. Thrombocytopenia can be seen early in the course of HIV infection as the only hematologic abnormality in patients who are otherwise asymptomatic or later in the disease as part of a more generalized bone marrow suppressive process associated with overt acquired immunodeficiency syndrome. The opportunistic infections of these patients, or the administration of antiviral therapy, can cause thrombocytopenia. HIV infection has been postulated to cause thrombocytopenia by a variety of mechanisms including immune destruction of platelets, direct viral invasion of megakaryocytes, and inhibition of stem cells. Increased levels of PAIgG often occur with normal numbers of megakaryocytes producing a clinical syndrome compatible with ITP. Syndromes mimicking hemolytic uremic syndrome (HUS) or thrombotic thrombocytopenic purpura (TTP) have been reported.

Administration of intravenous gamma globulin or antiD immunoglobulin is often effective in reversing thrombocytopenia in HIV infection. In many cases, corticosteroids and splenectomy are effective in elevating the platelet count but are less preferred therapies. Antiviral therapy may improve the platelet count. This result may be mediated by direct antiviral effects or an effect on the underlying aberrant immune response. Attention should be directed toward treatment of possible associated opportunistic infections. Therapies specific to the particular disorder should be considered if the symptoms suggest HUS or TTP.

DISORDERS OF COAGULATION FACTORS

Congenital Abnormalities of Coagulation Factors

FACTOR VIII DEFICIENCY

Etiology and Pathogenesis

Factor VIII deficiency (i.e., hemophilia A) is a sex-linked disorder occurring in approximately 1 per 5,000 male newborns. The disease results from a deficient or abnormal factor VIII procoagulant molecule (factor VIII:C). More than 200 discrete mutations or deletions in the factor VIII gene that result in hemophilia A have been described. However, inversions at the end of the X chromosome appear to be responsible for 35% to 45% of the cases of severe factor VIII deficiency. Spontaneous mutations are common and occur at "hot spots" in the factor VIII gene that structurally favor mutations. Factor VIII levels in affected persons vary from less than 1% to approximately 25% of normal activity. Levels of vWF are normal. Female carriers of the disease are usually asymptomatic and generally have factor VIII levels between 25% and 75% of normal with normal vWF assays. However, a carrier may have factor VIII:C activity levels higher than 100% of normal (normal range, 50%–200%); thus, the carrier state cannot be identified in all women by use of functional assays of factor VIII:C alone. However, measurements of factor VIII:C and vWF with determinations of DNA polymorphisms among family members can detect more than 95% of the carriers of the abnormal X chromosome. Clinical severity of the disease varies with the degree of deficiency of factor VIII activity and tends to be consistent among affected male subjects in a given kindred. Significant variations in factor VIII activity between siblings with the same mutation have been reported, however, suggesting that the severity of the disease can be modified by other genetic factors.

Clinical and Laboratory Features

Factor VIII deficiency is characterized by a lifelong tendency toward serious and often life-threatening hemorrhage. Whereas surface bleeding and purpura can occur, deep soft tissue bleeding and hemarthrosis are the hallmarks of the disease. Hemophiliacs can be divided into three groups based on clinical severity of the disease and the level of factor VIII activity: severe (less than 1% factor VIII activity), moderate (1%–5% factor VIII activity), and mild (5%–25% factor VIII activity). Hemophiliacs with severe disease are subject to spontaneous bleeding into joints or soft tissue sites. Hemophiliacs with moderate disease classically develop severe bleeding only after trauma, but hemophiliacs with mild disease may be symptomatic only after surgery or major trauma. Life-threatening bleeding can occur in all groups. Hemophiliacs with severe disease may not bleed excessively immediately after small lacerations or venipunctures because of lack of impairment of platelet function. However, delayed bleeding at such sites is common, particularly if sutures have been placed.

Although bleeding may occur at virtually any anatomic site, the most common serious bleeding encountered in hemophiliacs is hemarthrosis, with knees, elbows, and ankles representing the most commonly affected joints; shoulders, wrists, and hips are less frequently involved. The onset of hemarthrosis is often marked by development of pain without other objective findings, followed by acute swelling, warmth, and tenderness of the joint, sometimes accompanied by erythema or discoloration. Bleeding into soft tissues and bursae around the joint may occur. Repeated bleeding into the same joint results in synovial damage and hypertrophy producing secondary cartilaginous and bony abnormalities. The development of muscular atrophy and contraction of ligamentous structures around such target joints is common. The combination of soft tissue, bony, and cartilaginous abnormalities results in an anatomically abnormal joint that is more susceptible to successive bleeds. Disruption of the epiphyseal structures may result in growth abnormalities. The development of bony cysts represents a late complication of hemarthrosis. Rarely, erosive pseudotumors of bone may be seen.

Central nervous system bleeding is one of the most feared complications of hemophilia. Central nervous system bleeding is usually the result of trauma. Symptoms may be minimal immediately after the traumatic event, and the seriousness of the bleeding may not become evident until several days after the initial incident. Even minor episodes of head trauma may be followed by intracranial bleeding, and spontaneous intracranial hemorrhage may occur.

The diagnosis of hemophilia A requires the demonstration of low factor VIII:C activity in the presence of a normal vWF assay. The aPTT is usually prolonged, and the PT is normal. However, in some mild forms of factor VIII deficiency, the aPTT result may be normal. Test results of platelet function are usually normal, although abnormal template bleeding times have been observed in some hemophiliacs. A family history may reveal a sex-linked pattern of inheritance. However, the family history may be negative because of a predominance of females in successive generations or the high rate of spontaneous mutations.

Treatment, Prevention and General Care

Prevention of bleeding should be a major goal of treatment with care taken to avoid over protecting the patient. Infants should be provided with padded cribs and playpens. The beneficial effects of regular exercise in strengthening muscles and protecting joints from injury should be stressed. Most practitioners recommend against contact sports, but nontraumatic sports such as swimming should be encouraged. How restrictive recommendations about sports should be is a subject of considerable debate. Blanket recommendations are often of little use, and family and patient lifestyle preferences and acceptance of risk should be taken into account in these decisions. Platelet-inhibitory substances such as aspirin should be avoided. Immunizations should be administered after replacement with factor VIII or be given intradermally rather than intramuscularly to avoid hemorrhagic complications. Immunization against hepatitis B should be given as early as possible. Prophylactic dental treatment should be encouraged. Invasive procedures such as lumbar puncture should be performed only under coverage with factor VIII.

Replacement therapy with factor VIII remains the most important part of the care of the hemophiliac. Home therapy has gained widespread acceptance and offers the opportunity for earlier treatment of bleeding episodes and increased autonomy for the hemophiliac. Such programs require close physician supervision. Prophylactic therapy has gained wider acceptance and should be offered to all hemophiliacs. The goal of this therapy is to provide replacement therapy frequently enough to maintain a trough level of factor VIII greater than 1% at all times (as discussed in a following section) and reduce long-term joint morbidity. Although expensive, this therapy can result in a significant improvement in quality of life.

VON WILLEBRAND DISEASE

The term von Willebrand disease encompasses a heterogeneous group of disorders involving primary defects or deficiencies in the vWF portion of the factor VIII complex with variable deficiencies of factor VIII:C, the procoagulant component of the factor VIII molecule. The abnormalities of vWF result in decreased platelet adhesiveness, impairment of agglutination of platelets in the presence of ristocetin, and prolongation of the bleeding time. Abnormalities of factor VIII procoagulant activity contribute to the coagulation disturbance. Unlike hemophilia A, von Willebrand disease is usually transmitted as an autosomal dominant trait. Compound heterozygotes (i.e., patients who are heterozygotes for two forms of von Willebrand disease) have been described. In rare instances, transmission may be autosomal recessive. Studies suggest that 0.8% to 1.6% of the general population show biochemical abnormalities consistent with von Willebrand disease, making this disease the most common of the inherited coagulation disorders.

Most patients with von Willebrand disease have a mild to moderate bleeding tendency, usually involving mucocutaneous surfaces. Epistaxis, increased bruisability, and hemorrhage after dental extraction are common manifestations. Melena and menorrhagia may occur. Excessive bleeding after trauma or surgery can develop. Hemarthroses are unusual, except in type 3 disease or after significant trauma. Many persons with biochemical abnormalities consistent with von Willebrand disease report no bleeding symptoms.

The diagnosis of von Willebrand disease is complicated by the fact that results of laboratory testing sometimes vary, not only within families, but also for the same person on repeated determinations. Bleeding times are abnormal at some time for most persons. The aPTT results may be abnormal. The reason for the prolongation of the aPTT is not always clear. In many cases, the factor VIII:C level is low and may be the cause. In others, this prolongation occurs despite normal levels of VIII:C. Types 1 and 2 can usually be differentiated by measuring antigenic vWF (vWF:Ag) and factor VIII:C in conjunction with crossed-immunoelectrophoresis or multimer analysis. Both vWF:Ag and factor VIII:C should be proportionately reduced in type 1 disease with normal crossed-immunoelectrophoresis (a technique that combines immunologic and electrophoretic techniques to assess multimer structure) or size distribution on multimer analysis by gel electrophoresis and immunoblotting. In type 2 disease, vWF:Ag and factor VIII:C may be reduced, but crossed-immunoelectrophoresis or multimer analysis should show abnormal variants or lack of high-molecular-weight multimers of vWF. Assessment of platelet aggregation in response to ristocetin *in vitro* should define the persons with qualitative abnormalities who show hyperresponsiveness to low doses of ristocetin and are, therefore, at risk for *in vivo* platelet aggregation and thrombocytopenia. In type 3 von Willebrand disease, vWF:Ag and factor VIII:C are markedly, and usually proportionately, reduced.

Cryoprecipitate contains intact vWF of all molecular weights and is effective in treating most subtypes. The bleeding time is corrected for only a few hours after administration of cryoprecipitate despite the prolonged increase in factor VIII:C. Some intermediate-purity factor VIII concentrates contain a nearly normal complement of vWF multimers and can be effective in correcting the bleeding time in von Willebrand disease. Because these concentrates receive antiviral treatment, their infectious risk is lower than cryoprecipitate. Hence, the use of concentrates is preferred when plasma support is required. The treatment of choice for mild to moderate bleeding episodes in type 1 von Willebrand disease is 1-deamino-(8-D-arginine) vasopressin (DDAVP). This therapy is often sufficient for surgical procedures, but adjunctive therapy with plasma products may be required for extensive surgery or serious hemorrhagic episodes. DDAVP should not be given to patients who show increased responsiveness to ristocetin in platelet aggregation studies, unless they have been studied and demonstrated to benefit from this therapy, because they may be at risk for significant thrombocytopenia. It may lack effectiveness in some patients with type 2 disease. The effect of DDAVP on bleeding time is transient, approximately 3 to 4 hours, and tachyphylaxis may occur. DDAVP can be administered intravenously (0.3 μg/kg per dose) or, in some cases, intranasally (2–4 μg/kg per dose). Patients should be tested for efficacy before DDAVP is used as a therapeutic agent. In very mild cases of von Willebrand disease, specific treatment is not often required.

FACTOR IX DEFICIENCY

Like factor VIII deficiency, factor IX deficiency (i.e., hemophilia B, Christmas disease) is inherited as a sex-linked trait of variable severity. Clinically, factor IX deficiency is virtually indistinguishable from factor VIII deficiency. The diagnosis is made in the same way as factor VIII deficiency, except that a factor IX assay is used to confirm the diagnosis. Very low levels of factor IX are occasionally seen in female carriers of factor IX deficiency, in some cases, caused by abnormality of the chromosomal homologue such as a deletion in the region of the factor IX gene. Inhibitors occur much less frequently than in factor VIII deficiency. A relationship between anaphylaxis with administration of factor IX and the development of inhibitors to factor IX has been observed.

Treatment with plasma is effective, but larger doses are required than in hemophilia A to achieve the same level of replacement. Commercial concentrates containing factor IX are used more commonly than plasma. Previously, intermediate-purity concentrates contained all of the other vitamin K-dependent factors at variable levels. Higher purity products containing only factor IX, similar in purity to those used for factor VIII deficiency, have supplanted the use of vitamin K-dependent factor concentrates. Recombinant factor IX has become available. This product is produced in the absence of human or animal proteins and functions in coagulation in a manner that is indistinguishable from factor IX and is effective and safe in the treatment of factor IX deficiency. Clinical studies have demonstrated that the recovery of recombinant factor IX is reduced compared with monoclonal plasma-derived products; however, the availability of this safe and potentially infection-free product provides an important therapeutic option for patients with factor IX deficiency.

A dose of 1 unit of plasma-derived factor IX per kilogram of body weight generally increases factor IX levels by 1.0% to 1.5%, as opposed to the approximate 2% increase seen with factor VIII. This difference is compensated for by a relatively longer biological half-life of factor IX when compared with factor VIII. After an initial loading dose, a subsequent dose is usually given in 4 to 12 hours to account for the shorter initial half-life and every 24 hours thereafter. Approximately 20% higher doses of recombinant factor are recommended by the manufacturers. Individual patients should be studied to assess recovery and half-life of factor IX before relying on this product for routine use.

Inherited Coagulation Abnormalities Resulting in Hypercoagulability

The contribution of genetic risk factors to the occurrence of thrombosis has become increasingly clear. This discovery has been driven by advances in the understanding of the molecular basis of thrombosis. A high proportion of children who develop thrombosis have definable genetic abnormalities; in fact, the occurrence of multiple genetic or acquired risk factors in children with thromboses is more the rule than the exception. The discovery of the anticoagulant properties of protein C was a key step in these developments.

Protein C is a vitamin K-dependent factor, which is converted to its activated form by thrombin in the presence of protein S. This reaction is catalyzed by a surface receptor, thrombomodulin, which binds thrombin and increases its affinity for protein C. Protein C is the most potent anticoagulant protein known. Inherited protein C deficiency has been described in heterozygous and homozygous states. Homozygotes usually have no protein C activity and the condition is detected shortly after birth. Purpura fulminans is usually the first recognized symptom. Venous thromboses in the central nervous system and kidneys are common. Thrombosis of the retinal vessels tends to occur early in the illness, followed by secondary vitreous bleeds resulting in fibrosis and blindness. The disease is fatal if untreated. Patients with apparently homozygous protein C deficiency presenting later in life have been described, but they have detectable levels of protein C activity. Transmission of the disease appears to be autosomal recessive in most kindred with homozygous protein C deficiency.

Treatment with heparin is not effective, but sufficient protein C can be administered with fresh-frozen plasma to reverse the clinical symptoms. Long-term management can be achieved with warfarin (Coumadin) administration by at least partially restoring the balance between procoagulant and anticoagulant forces. Infusions of purified protein C concentrates have been used to treat this disorder. Successful correction of homozygous protein C deficiency by hepatic transplantation has been accomplished in one patient.

Heterozygous protein C deficiency can be associated with thrombotic disease. Heterozygotes typically manifest levels of activity between 35% and 65% of normal. Patients with levels of antigenic protein C higher than their activity levels have been described indicating a qualitative defect of protein C. Most heterozygotes in the best-studied kindred do not become symptomatic until the third decade of life, but children with symptomatic disease in the first and second decades are being recognized with increasing frequency. Symptomatic individuals with heterozygous protein C deficiency commonly have other associated genetic or acquired risk factors.

Deep venous thrombosis and central nervous system thrombosis are among the most common findings. Patients with heterozygous protein C deficiency may manifest skin necrosis shortly after Coumadin administration. This unusual reaction to Coumadin is attributed to the short half-life of protein C relative to some of the vitamin K-dependent procoagulant proteins. Because all of the vitamin K-dependent proteins are reduced after Coumadin therapy, very low levels of protein C may develop quickly in patients with lower than normal levels of protein C at the initiation of therapy resulting in a procoagulant–anticoagulant imbalance favoring thrombosis.

The transmission of symptomatic heterozygous protein C deficiency appears to be autosomal dominant, but asymptomatic heterozygotes are detected commonly in the families of homozygous patients. Asymptomatic heterozygotes have been detected by random screening of blood bank donors. Protein C deficiency is caused by a variety of molecular defects. Numerous differing mutations in the protein C gene have been associated with protein C deficiency, but the clinically dominant and recessive forms of the disease cannot be segregated on the basis of these mutations. In many cases, protein C deficiency is found in association with a second genetic abnormality that contributes to the expression of the disease (e.g., factor V Leiden or protein S deficiency). Symptomatic heterozygous patients can be treated with Coumadin, but it should be administered simultaneously with heparin until adequate anticoagulation with Coumadin is achieved.

A single-point mutation in the coagulation factor V gene (position 1691, Arg506 to Gln) has been identified as the most common known genetic risk factor for thrombosis. This mutation results in the production of a mutant factor V protein, factor V Leiden. Factor V Leiden has normal procoagulant activities; however, the mutation renders the factor V protein resistant to inactivation by activated protein C. In addition, normal factor V serves as a cofactor for activation of protein C; factor V Leiden performs this function inefficiently. The combination of these effects (resistance to inactivation and reduced protein C activation) produces a hypercoagulable state. Factor V Leiden is quite prevalent and has been found in 2% to 11% of the general population. This mutation is most commonly found in white people and less commonly in those of African or East Asian origin. Screening for the factor V Leiden mutation can be performed by testing for the relative resistance of the abnormal factor V molecule to inactivation by activated protein C (activated protein C resistance). In addition, this mutation can be detected using polymerase chain reaction (PCR) assays. Up to 60% of adults with venous thrombosis and a family history of thrombosis are heterozygotes for this mutation. Although few in number, similar pediatric studies have reported that up to 30% of children with venous thrombosis are heterozygotes for the factor V Leiden mutation.

Heterozygous protein S deficiency results in recurrent thromboses with a pattern similar to heterozygous protein C deficiency.

Antithrombin III deficiency is inherited as an autosomal dominant trait. The occurrence of thromboses begins in the second decade of life. Heparin resistance can be a feature of antithrombin III deficiency, because antithrombin III is a cofactor for heparin. Anticoagulation can be achieved with Coumadin.

Acquired Abnormalities of Coagulation Factors

VITAMIN K DEFICIENCY

Vitamin K is an essential substrate for the synthesis of procoagulant and anticoagulant proteins including factors II, VII, IX, X, protein C, and protein S. Identical clinical states can be produced by absence of vitamin K or interference with its action by pharmacologic means. Dietary vitamin K consists mainly of vitamin K_1, a fat-soluble naphthaquinone found in leafy vegetables. Intestinal bacteria also synthesize vitamin K compounds. Therapeutically and physiologically, the fat-soluble forms of vitamin K appear to be most useful, and toxicity has resulted from the administration of water-soluble analogues. True dietary deficiency of vitamin K appears to be unusual, except in early infancy or in the setting of prolonged intravenous feedings without supplemental administration of vitamin K. Most cases of apparent dietary insufficiency in older children are caused by malabsorptive syndromes such as pancreatic insufficiency, biliary obstruction, prolonged diarrhea affecting absorption of vitamin K in the upper small intestine, or the administration of drugs. Drugs that antagonize or interfere with the metabolism of vitamin K include phenobarbital, diphenylhydantoin, some cephalosporins, rifampin, isoniazid, and coumarin. Vitamin K deficiency caused by antibiotic suppression of intestinal flora appears to be unusual without a dietary deficiency of vitamin K. However, vitamin K deficiency has been noted in thriving infants after relatively brief bouts of diarrhea, particularly if they are breast-fed. These reports have led the American Academy of Pediatrics to recommend that "breast-fed infants who develop diarrhea of longer than several days' duration should be given one intramuscular injection of vitamin K."

Uncomplicated vitamin K deficiency is characterized by bleeding symptoms (e.g., bruising, oozing from puncture sites of the skin, visceral hemorrhage) with an acquired prolongation of the PT and aPTT and a normal fibrinogen level. Often, a disproportionate prolongation of the PT occurs, which can be helpful in diagnosis. Other clotting factors that are produced in the liver but are not vitamin K-dependent (e.g., factors V, VIII, XI, XII) are normal. However, the clinical and laboratory picture is often affected by a primary disorder that produces liver disease and malabsorption or decreased utilization of vitamin K such as biliary atresia, cystic fibrosis, hemolytic anemia with obstructive jaundice, hepatitis, $alpha_1$–antitrypsin deficiency, or abetalipoproteinemia. In the absence of severe hepatic disease or antagonists, the response to vitamin K is rapid, usually occurring within 6 hours. Anaphylactoid reactions may occur with parenteral administration of vitamin K, but they are unusual. Infusion of plasma is effective in emergent situations.

Hemorrhagic disease of the newborn appears to represent a special case of vitamin K deficiency. As classified by Hathaway, hemorrhagic disease of the newborn can occur in early, classic, and late forms. Early hemorrhagic disease of the newborn often occurs in the setting of maternal ingestion of vitamin K antagonists (e.g., anticonvulsants, antituberculous drugs) but may be unassociated with known risk factors. Early disease presents in the first 24 hours of life, often with catastrophic bleeding. Classic hemorrhagic disease of the newborn occurs after the first day of life, usually within the first week. Purpura, oozing from the umbilical cord or circumcision site, hematemesis, hematuria, and gastrointestinal and vaginal bleeding are common symptoms, but intracranial hemorrhage is rare. Premature infants are at increased risk for developing hemorrhagic symptoms. Late-onset disease occurs 1 to 3 months after birth and is associated with a high incidence of central nervous system hemorrhage and mortality. Exclusive breast-feeding without vitamin K supplementation and failure to administer parenteral vitamin K at birth appear to be at least contributing, and probably causative, factors in classic and late disease. Some cases of early disease may not respond to parenteral vitamin K at birth, and some question exists about whether all cases of late disease can be prevented by a single early dose of parenteral vitamin K alone. The trends toward decreased use of parenteral vitamin K as prophylactic treatment for hemorrhagic disease of the newborn do not appear to be justified, and routine prophylactic treatment of all infants is still recommended.

Disseminated Intravascular Coagulation

DIC describes a constellation of clinical and laboratory abnormalities indicative of a combination of accelerated fibrinogenesis and fibrinolysis. Rather than being considered a disease in and of itself, DIC should be thought of as a secondary phenomenon that occurs in response to a variety of stimuli. DIC may be triggered by local or systemic factors. Examples of local problems that can result in systemic DIC include hemangiomas (i.e., Kasabach–Merritt syndrome), in which a localized vascular lesion results in consumption of fibrinogen and platelets and in which elevations of fibrin degradation products can be massive, and brain injury, in which release of thromboplastic substances may initiate systemic clotting. Abruptio placenta and massive pulmonary emboli may also produce systemic signs of DIC. Systemic causes of DIC include sepsis, shock of any cause, transfusion of incompatible blood, and injection of snake venom. DIC is encountered in toxemia of pregnancy, respiratory distress syndrome, malignancies, burns, hypothermia, heat stroke, postoperative states, and any situation in which massive tissue damage is encountered. The severity of DIC varies widely from transient and insignificant to overwhelming. Patients with DIC manifest purpura, and oozing from incisions or venipuncture sites is common. Circulatory collapse may occur.

Purpura fulminans represents a special systemic form of DIC. This rare disorder is characterized at its onset by purpura and DIC, usually in association with viral (e.g., varicella), bacterial (e.g., meningococcal, streptococcal), or rickettsial infections or severe hypernatremia. Pathologically, this disease is characterized by widespread microthrombi in the vascular bed of a variety of organs. Renal failure is common. The purpuric lesions are often symmetric and show sharply demarcated borders with a surrounding inflammatory reaction. Scarring of the skin and loss of extremities is common, and the fatality rate is high. Rarely, purpura fulminans may be seen as a manifestation of protein C deficiency, which was discussed previously.

Laboratory findings in DIC include thrombocytopenia, prolongation of the PT and aPTT, and a reduction of clotting factors, particularly fibrinogen and factors II, V, and VIII. Protein C levels are reduced. Microangiopathic changes in the erythrocytes may be seen in the peripheral blood smear. Plasma levels of fibrin degradation products are usually elevated and may play a pathogenetic role by inhibiting clotting and platelet function. Measurement of fibrinopeptide A, a cleavage product of fibrinogen, and fibrinogen turnover studies increase the diagnostic sensitivity, but these assays are not routinely available.

Treatment of DIC should be aimed primarily at correcting the inciting cause. Concern has been raised about the possibility of "feeding the fire" by administering clotting factors and platelet concentrates. However, the risks of allowing severe thrombocytopenia or hypofibrinogenemia to develop are not warranted on the basis of what are mostly theoretical concerns, and replacement therapy should be given if the consumption has been severe. Heparin may be helpful in some cases if the underlying defect cannot be corrected, but its usefulness is still a matter of debate. Some authors believe that heparin is an effective therapy for purpura fulminans if initiated early in the illness. Protein C concentrates may be beneficial in the treatment of this devastating condition. A few reports exist of successful treatment of purpura fulminans with recombinant tissue plasminogen activator, and the usefulness of antithrombin III replacement is being investigated. Epsilon–aminocaproic acid may be helpful in cases of DIC with low levels of alpha$_2$–antiplasmin caused by hypergranular promyelocytic leukemia, but it is not considered useful in other forms of DIC.

5
Neoplastic Diseases

CHAPTER 164
General Considerations

Adapted from C. Philip Steuber

Cancer in children is a rare disease accounting for approximately 6,000 cases annually among children younger than 18 years in the United States. Nevertheless, cancer remains the leading cause of death from disease in children between 1 and 18 years of age. The disparity in numbers between childhood and adult cancers reflects the significant role of chronic environmental exposures in adult cancer. The most common cancers in children are the acute leukemias (30%) and central nervous system tumors (18%), not carcimonas, which are predominant adult malignancies. Environmental factors do play a role in pediatric carcinogenesis, but the associations are different for pediatric patients than for adults. Many pediatric neoplasms are associated with developmental defects, anomalies, or cytogenetic or molecular aberrations. Environmental factors may play a role by triggering neoplastic transformation of preexisting defects. Some tumors in children can be anticipated on the basis of preexisting immunologic deficiency states, genetic and chromosomal disorders, and congenital anomalies (Tables 164-1 through 164-4).

TABLE 164-1. Immune Deficiency Diseases Predisposing to Neoplastic Disease

X-linked lymphoproliferative disease
Bruton agammaglobulinemia
Severe combined immunodeficiency
Wiskott-Aldrich syndrome
IgA deficiency
Common variable immunodeficiency
DiGeorge syndrome
Ataxia-telangiectasia
Chédiak-Higashi syndrome

TABLE 164-2. Genetic Instability and DNA Repair Disorders Associated with Childhood Cancer

Disorders	Cancers
Xeroderma pigmentosum	Basal, squamous cell carcinoma, melanoma
Bloom syndrome	Leukemia, lymphoma, gastrointestinal cancers
Fanconi anemia	Leukemia, hepatoma, squamous cell carcinoma
Ataxia-telangiectasia	Lymphoma, leukemia, Hodgkin's disease, brain, gastric, ovarian, other epithelial cancers

DIAGNOSIS

Symptoms

Early diagnosis of childhood cancer is often delayed because of the nonspecific nature of the initial signs and symptoms. Warning signs in children can include fever, persistent headache, pain, a mass, purpura, pallor, and changes in gait, balance, personality, and the eyes (e.g., squint, retinal reflections), all of which may evolve insidiously. Some of these are common nonspecific pediatric complaints with common explanations, but the alert primary physician can quickly sort out the unusual from the usual problems. For example, morning headaches, especially associated with morning vomiting, suggest increased intracranial pressure possibly caused by brain tumor. Unusual irritability may be a symptom of intracranial disease in the very young child. Persistent pain in any joint or bone is a common complaint of children with leukemia or neuroblastoma.

Other Abnormalities

Changes in gait or balance or other neurologic abnormalities such as head tilt are common complaints in children with posterior fossa tumors. A variety of neurologic problems can

TABLE 164-3. Constitutional Chromosome Disorders Associated with Childhood Cancers

Disorders	Cancers
Down syndrome	Leukemia, testicular, retinoblastoma
Turner syndrome	Neurogenic, gonadal, endometrial
Klinefelter syndrome	Leukemia, germ cell tumors
Other sex aneuploidy	Retinoblastoma
XY gonadal dysgenesis	Gonadoblastoma, dysgerminoma
Trisomy 13	Teratoma, leukemia, neurogenic
Trisomy 18	Neurogenic, Wilms tumor
XYY, XYY mosaic	Osteosarcoma, medulloblastoma

TABLE 164-4. Congenital Malformations Associated with Tumors

Malformations	Tumor
Aniridia	Wilms tumor
Hemihypertrophy	Wilms tumor
Cryptorchidism	Testicular tumors
Gonadal dysgenesis	Gonadoblastoma
Enchondromatosis (Ollier disease)	Chondrosarcoma

result from brain tumors, and some of them may be subtle such as personality changes in children with supratentorial tumors. Fortunately, imaging studies of the head (computed tomography and magnetic resonance imaging) are widely available, are of tremendous diagnostic value, and have enhanced the ability of physicians to make an early diagnosis of intracranial lesions. These modalities have proven invaluable not only in diagnosing, but also in monitoring the course of these patients.

Management

Once a malignant neoplasm is identified, ideal management involves a team approach, which can include surgeons, pediatric oncologists, radiologists, pathologists, radiotherapists, and other specialists depending on the diagnosis and the complications at the time. Knowledge of the precise histologic diagnosis and extent of the disease (i.e., staging) is essential before planning any type of intervention. Children with probable or proven cancer must be immediately referred to the proper pediatric facility for complete diagnosis and therapy assignment.

Therapy

In general, pediatric tumors are much more responsive to therapy than adult cancers. Progress since the early 1970s has resulted in a dramatic improvement of the overall 5-year survival rate, which is approximately 70% for all children with cancer. Therapy for childhood cancer should be focused not only on cure, but also on minimization of late effects. Although for some specific entities such as Wilms tumor, therapy is close to being standardized; most therapies for newly diagnosed childhood cancer are not standardized and are administered in the setting of a clinical trial program. Participation in such trials is considered to be the standard of care in pediatric oncology.

CHAPTER 165

Acute Lymphoblastic Leukemia

Adapted from Donald H. Mahoney, Jr.

EPIDEMIOLOGY AND ETIOLOGY

Acute leukemia is the most common malignancy diagnosed in children. An estimated 2,000 cases of leukemia in children younger than 15 years occur in the United States each year. Approximately three-fourths of the cases are acute lymphoblastic leukemia (ALL). In the United States, childhood ALL has a peak incidence between 2 and 6 years in white populations but not in blacks. The reason for this difference is unexplained. Childhood ALL occurs more frequently in boys than in girls.

TABLE 165-1. Chromosomal Translocations in Childhood Acute Lymphoblastic Leukemia

Translocation	Genes	Frequency (%)	Features
t(12;21)(p13;q22)	*TEL/AML1*	21–25	B-cell lineage; favorable prognosis
t(1;19)(q23;p13)	*E2A/PBX1*	5–6	Pre–B cell; increased white blood cells
t(4;11)(q21;q23)	*MLL/AF4*	4–8	Mixed lineage; CD10$^-$; infants
t(9;22)(q34;q11)	*BCR/ABL*	3–4	B-cell lineage; older age; poor prognosis
t(1;14)(p34;q11)	*TAL1/TCR*	3	T cell; male; increased white blood cells
t(8,14)(q24;q32)	*MYC/IGH*	1	B cell; FAB L3 morphology

FAB, French-American-British classification.

Leukemia is thought to arise from a damaged progenitor cell that has the propensity for unlimited self-renewal or has lost the ability to differentiate along the lines of normal committed progenitor cells (lines such as erythroid, myeloid, megakaryocytic, eosinophilic, and monocytic–macrophage). Proposed molecular mechanisms for leukemic induction include activation of a protooncogene or the creation of a fusion gene with oncogenic properties or the loss or inactivation of genes whose proteins suppress leukemia.

A variety of environmental, genetic, viral, and immunologic factors may contribute to the development of disease. Of the possible environmental factors, ionizing radiation has been the most extensively studied. The increased incidence of leukemia in survivors within 1,000 meters of the atomic bomb explosions during World War II has been well documented.

A viral cause for leukemia has been sought for several years. A small number of RNA viruses, classified as retroviruses, have direct oncogenic potential. These viruses such as the Rous sarcoma virus and the feline leukemia virus have caused oncogenic transformations in a variety of animal species but have not been associated with cross-species transmission and cancer in humans.

An unusual susceptibility to leukemia has been associated with certain heritable diseases, chromosomal disorders, and constitutional syndromes. Children with trisomy 21 (i.e., Down syndrome) have at least a ten- to 15-fold increased risk for developing leukemia compared with normal children. Increased chromosomal fragility may predispose these patients to leukemic transformation. Cases of childhood leukemia have been associated with several other heritable syndromes such as Klinefelter syndrome and neurofibromatosis.

Several immunodeficiency states have an associated increased risk for lymphoma and leukemia (Table 165-1). The loss of cellular immune surveillance capability for tumor antigens and the inability to self-regulate lymphoproliferative processes may contribute to malignant transformation in these patients.

CLASSIFICATION AND CYTOGENETIC ASPECTS

Childhood leukemia is a heterogenous disease. Morphologic, immunologic, biochemical, and cytogenetic features are used to characterize the disease, estimate prognosis, and develop therapeutic strategies. Under normal conditions, less than 5% of the nucleated marrow is composed of blast forms. Blasts are primitive, undifferentiated-appearing precursor cells not normally seen in the peripheral circulation.

In 1976, a French–American–British (FAB) cooperative group developed a system for morphologic classification of acute leukemias. The acute lymphoblastic leukemias were divided into three classes:

- L1: Lymphoblasts are small with scant cytoplasm and indistinct nucleoli.
- L2: Lymphoblasts are larger, more heterogeneous in size, and have more abundant cytoplasm, prominent nucleoli, and reniform nuclear membranes.
- L3: Lymphoblasts are large with a deep cytoplasmic basophilia, prominent vacuolation, and one or more nucleoli.

Approximately 85% of the children with ALL have lymphoblasts of L1 morphology. Less than 15% of the patients have lymphoblasts of L2 morphology. Lymphoblasts with L3 morphology are identical to Burkitt lymphoma cells. This FAB classification may have some prognostic value. Childhood ALL with L1 morphology has a high remission induction rate and more prolonged survival, whereas patients with L3 disease have a worse prognosis.

Immunologic marker analysis has allowed lineage assignment and maturational staging of the lymphoid leukemias and has offered some insight into the pathology of these diseases. Approximately 65% of the children with ALL have early preB lymphoblasts. PreB-cell ALL represents approximately 18% to 20% of the new cases of ALL. B-cell ALL (B-ALL) is rare in children representing 1% of all cases. The lymphoblasts are characterized by their Burkitt-like appearance and express surface immunoglobulin.

T-cell phenotypes represent 13% to 15% of childhood ALL. Approximately 1% to 3% of patients fails to react with any antigen test system and is classified as undifferentiated, null, or stem cell leukemias.

These immunologic subtypes may be important for predicting response to conventional therapy. Patients with early preB-ALL experience an increased remission induction rate and prolonged remission and survival. Patients with T-cell disease are frequently older (average age, 8–12 years) and are boys (male–to–female ratio, 4:1). They frequently present with a leukocyte count of more than 100,000 per microliter, a mediastinal mass, normal hemoglobin concentration, hepatosplenomegaly, and adenopathy. This disease is more difficult to treat and cure than other forms. Infants (less than 1 year of age) frequently fail to express reactivity to any lymphoid antigens and have a poor prognosis.

Approximately two-thirds of the patients with ALL have karyotypic abnormalities involving the leukemic cell. These alterations are broadly defined as changes in chromosome number (i.e., ploidy) or chromosome structure (i.e., translocations, deletions, inversions). Prognostic significance has been suggested for certain cytogenetic subgroups. For example, patients with hyperdiploidy (more than 53 chromosomes per cell) without structural abnormalities and patients with trisomy of chromosomes 4 and 10 have a more favorable prognosis with conventional therapy than other groups.

Several specific chromosome translocations have been recognized in childhood ALL and have significance for disease ontogeny and clinical outcome (Table 165-1). For example, the t(12;21)(p13;q22) translocation produces the *TEL/AML1* fusion gene and is the most common genetic rearrangement in childhood ALL accounting for up to 25% of all cases.

The t(8;14), t(2;8), and t(8;22) are immunophenotype-specific translocations observed in B-ALL. These translocations produce a rearrangement of the myc protooncogene located on chromosome 8 with the immunoglobulin heavy chain genes located on chromosome 14 or the immunoglobulin light chain genes located on chromosomes 2 and 22. The aberrant expression of these translocated genes is postulated as a critical mechanism in the malignant transformation of B-ALL.

DIAGNOSIS AND PROGNOSIS

Clinical Presentation and Initial Laboratory Findings

The presenting signs and symptoms are typically a reflection of bone marrow failure. The most common presenting symptoms are fever, pallor, purpura, and pain (particularly bone and joint pain). At first, symptoms may be nonspecific and may mimic other nonmalignant conditions. Fever, although a nonspecific complaint, can be a significant symptom in the child with ALL. Anemia is gradual in onset, normocytic, and children may not be symptomatic but for an elevated resting heart rate. Petechiae and bruising are frequently noticed on physical examination due to thrombocytopenia. Epistaxis can also occur.

Symptoms include anorexia and vague abdominal pains, bone, hip, or joint pain. Arthralgias and refusal to walk may reflect leukemic infiltrations of the bony cortex or the joint compartment. Lymphadenopathy is common, and some degree of hepatosplenomegaly occurs in more than one-half of the patients.

Approximately 20% of children present with leukocyte counts greater than 50,000 per microliter. Approximately 44% of children have leukocyte counts less than 10,000 per microliter. Leukemic blasts may or may not be seen on peripheral smears.

The diagnosis of ALL cannot be established from peripheral blood examination alone. A bone marrow examination is needed. The normal bone marrow contains less than 5% blasts. A minimum of 25% lymphoblasts on differential examination of the bone marrow aspirate is necessary for the diagnosis of ALL. Most children with ALL have hypercellular marrow with 60% to 100% of the cells as blasts. The presenting characteristics of childhood ALL are outlined in Table 165-2.

Differential Diagnosis

Idiopathic thrombocytopenic purpura (ITP) is a common cause of bruising and petechiae in children. Anemia, leukocyte disturbances, and significant hepatosplenomegaly are not typical findings. Children with infectious mononucleosis (i.e., EBV) or other acute viral illnesses may present with fever, malaise, adenopathy, splenomegaly, rash, and lymphocytosis. In the young child with EBV, lymphocytosis may be extreme (80,000–100,000 per microliter) and thrombocytopenia and immunohemolytic anemia may further confuse the diagnosis. Specific viral serologies can establish the diagnosis, but a bone marrow examination is sometimes necessary.

Leukemoid reactions may be observed in disorders such as bacterial sepsis and granulomatous diseases. A bone marrow aspirate usually reveals myeloid hyperplasia and the leukemoid reaction resolves as the underlying disease is successfully managed.

Children with ALL presenting with fever, arthralgias, arthritis, or a limp may frequently be confused with juvenile rheumatoid arthritis (JRA). Pancytopenia and fever are presenting symptoms for both aplastic anemia and ALL in children; however, lymphadenopathy and hepatosplenomegaly are unusual

TABLE 165-2. Presenting Characteristics of Children with Acute Lymphoblastic Leukemia

Characteristic	Frequency (%)*
Age (yr)	
<1.5	6–8
>1.5–10	72–80
>10	15–22
Gender (male)	54–57
Race (white)	80–89
Leukocyte count	
<10,000/μL	44
10,000–50,000/μL	34
>50,000/μL	22
Platelets	
<20,000/μL	20
20,000–100,000/μL	51
>100,000/μL	29
Hemoglobin	
<7.5 g/dL	46
7.5–10 g/dL	30
>10 g/dL	24
Hepatomegaly (below umbilicus)	8–13
Splenomegaly (below umbilicus)	11–14
Lymphadenopathy	
None/minimal	73
Moderate/marked	28
Mediastinal mass	8
CNS symptoms	4
Immunoglobulin abnormalities (1 or more)	9
FAB	
L1	82
L2	17
L3	1
Karyotype abnormality	70–75

CNS, central nervous system; FAB, French-American-British classification.
*Percentages are estimates based on accumulated data from large numbers of patients treated by the Pediatric Oncology Group and the Children's Cancer Study Group.

findings in aplastic anemia. The bone marrow aspirate and biopsy usually clarify the diagnosis. Patients with aplastic anemia have a hypocellular marrow with cellularity usually less than 10%, no normal marrow precursors, and only small lymphocytes seen on smears.

Other malignancies can present in childhood and may produce bone marrow invasion. Neuroblastoma is the most common pediatric solid tumor associated with a high frequency (70%) of bone marrow invasion in children older than 2 years at diagnosis. Other tumors that may produce bone marrow infiltration include rhabdomyosarcoma, nonHodgkin's lymphoma, retinoblastoma, medulloblastoma, and Ewing sarcoma.

Prognostic Factors

The single most important prognostic factor in childhood ALL is effective therapy. Some clinical factors such as the patient's age at diagnosis and the initial leukocyte count can indicate response to therapy. Risk classification schemes exist to place children in high-risk or low-risk groups. Biological factors associated with favorable prognosis include leukemic DNA hyperdiploidy, leukemic trisomy 4 and 10, and t(12;21) with the *TEL/AML1* fusion gene. Biological features associated with poor prognosis include the presence of t(9;22) Philadelphia chromosome, the 11q23/MLL gene rearrangement, and leukemic hypodiploidy.

TREATMENT

The treatment of childhood ALL is complex. Curative therapy for ALL has not been established, and investigational therapy is the treatment of choice. Ongoing therapeutic trials are needed to further define factors such as optimal scheduling and delivery of effective chemotherapeutic agents. Consequently, the best therapy for the child newly diagnosed with ALL is offered by pediatric cancer centers participating in ongoing clinical therapeutic trials.

Combination chemotherapy is the principal therapeutic modality for childhood ALL. The therapy can be divided into four phases:

- Remission induction and consolidation (i.e., intensification)
- Presymptomatic central nervous system (CNS) therapy (i.e., prophylaxis)
- Maintenance
- Elective discontinuation of therapy and long-term, late-effects follow-up

Induction and Consolidation Therapy

The objectives of remission induction are to eliminate as many leukemic cells as biologically tolerable and to reestablish a normal clinical and hematologic state for the patient. Most pediatric cancer centers use three to four drugs to achieve remission: vincristine, prednisone, and L-asparaginase, with or without doxorubicin or daunorubicin. Rapid cytoreduction is associated with a decreased likelihood of emergence of resistant leukemic clones and increased relapse-free survival. Therapy is tailored for those with biologically more aggressive leukemias. The estimated remission induction rate with aggressive therapy is 98%. Patients who fail to achieve a remission at the end of 4 weeks of induction therapy have a shorter survival even if remission is obtained eventually.

The consolidation (intensification) phase of treatment delivers multiple chemotherapeutic agents in a short period to further reduce residual leukemia and minimize the development of cross-resistance. This approach has resulted in overall disease-free survival rates of 70% to 85% at 5 to 7 years.

Central Nervous System Therapy

Presymptomatic CNS prophylaxis therapy has decreased the incidence of CNS leukemia as a primary site of relapse from 50% to between 3% and 6%. Several regimens have been investigated and include, among others, intrathecal methotrexate and cranial irradiation (2,400 cGy). Cranial irradiation may have delayed effects such as growth failure, intellectual impairment, and occasional brain tumors. When it is used, using the lowest possible dose may decrease these effects.

Maintenance Therapy

The rationale for extended treatment during remission is based on historic evidence that patients discontinuing therapy after less than 6 months, after achieving remission, relapsed rapidly. The common element in all maintenance or continuation schedules has been the use of weekly methotrexate and daily 6-mercaptopurine.

Cessation of Therapy

The standard duration of therapy is 2 to 3 years. For children who remain in continuous complete remission for 2 to 3 years on therapy, it has been the practice to discontinue therapy and to observe them closely during the first 1 to 2 years off therapy for evidence of relapse. Because of the risk for late recurrence, these children require periodic monitoring indefinitely.

Complications of Therapy and Supportive Care

Hyperleukocytosis in leukemia can be associated with early morbidity and mortality. Life-threatening metabolic complications may result from spontaneous or chemotherapy-induced leukemic cell lysis. Hyperuricemia, hyperkalemia, and hyperphosphatemia with secondary hypocalcemia may develop within hours of the diagnosis and treatment. Careful hydration, alkalinization of the urine, and allopurinol are useful for managing hyperuricemia. A progressive increase in blood urea nitrogen and creatinine, phosphorous, or potassium levels requires early intervention with hemodialysis.

Hemorrhage in children with ALL is usually caused by thrombocytopenia. Intracranial hemorrhages are rare but life-threatening events. Patients with platelet counts of less than 20,000 per microliter are at the greatest risk for hemorrhage. The condition of the patient, evidence of active bleeding, and anticipated course of therapy should be used as guidelines for platelet transfusion.

Infection associated with granulocytopenia is a potentially life-threatening complication for the child with ALL. Any break in the skin, insect bite, blister, sore, gingival or mucous membrane irritation, or perianal fissure may serve as a portal for bacterial penetration with resulting overwhelming bacterial sepsis. Any child who presents with fever of 101°F or higher and an absolute granulocyte count of less than 500 per microliter must be assumed to have sepsis. This is a medical emergency. These children should be hospitalized immediately; cultures of blood, urine, and respiratory secretions obtained; and broad-spectrum intravenous antibiotics initiated without delay. The principal pathogens include Pseudomonas, Escherichia coli, and Staphylococcus. With increased use of central venous catheters, cutaneous types of organisms (i.e., skin contaminants such as Staphylococci) may be the pathogens.

A variety of nonbacterial, opportunistic infections can cause devastating illness in these patients. Varicella–zoster, herpes zoster, and herpes simplex may cause serious systemic complications including pneumonitis, hepatitis, and cerebritis. In a patient who is not taking prophylaxis with trimethoprim–sulfamethoxazole, Pneumocystis carinii may cause a life-threatening interstitial pneumonitis in those who are severely immunosuppressed. Invasive fungal infections can be seen due to Candida and Aspergillus.

Bone Marrow and Extramedullary Relapse and Transplantation

The most serious complication of ALL treatment is bone marrow relapse. Although reinduction of remission is possible, most patients relapse again and eventually succumb to their disease. Patients who relapse while receiving continuation therapy have the worst prognosis. This event usually signals the emergence of resistant leukemic clones.

Bone marrow transplantation (BMT) is the treatment of choice for patients with hematologic relapse. Allogeneic-matched BMT is the optimal approach. The procedure is risky with increased mortality and morbidity associated with nonallogeneic approaches. Acute and chronic graft–versus–host disease, interstitial pneumonitis, and relapse of leukemia are some of the many significant complications that may follow the transplantation procedure.

Although less than 10% of the children with ALL have CNS leukemia at diagnosis, it remains the most common site of extramedullary relapse. The clinical signs and symptoms of CNS leukemia may include headache, nausea, and vomiting secondary to increased intracranial pressure. The diagnosis is established by lumbar puncture and analysis of cerebrospinal fluid cytopreparations for leukemic blasts.

Isolated testicular leukemic relapse occurs in less than 5% of male subjects receiving modern therapy. Patients usually present with a painless swelling; ultrasound examination may be helpful in excluding other causes of testicular swelling. Testicular infiltration may be occult. The diagnosis is confirmed by bilateral testicular wedge biopsies.

LONG-TERM SURVIVAL, LATE EFFECTS, AND THERAPEUTIC DIRECTIONS

With prolonged survival, monitoring for late effects of antileukemic therapy assumes increasing importance. The areas of interest include monitoring for specific organ dysfunction, impaired genetic or immunologic mechanisms, and second malignancies. Several long-term problems have been associated with CNS prophylaxis. Current leukemia protocols are seeking to reduce or eliminate some of these complications by the use of high-dose systemic chemotherapy and intrathecal therapy without irradiation.

Delayed sexual maturation may be observed in children receiving irradiation to gonadal tissue such as boys with testicular leukemia. Male adolescents may be at risk for spermatogenic dysfunction after cyclophosphamide therapy. Successful parenthood in long-term survivors has been reported, but the progeny of survivors of childhood leukemia are few.

CHAPTER 166
Acute Myeloid Leukemia

Adapted from C. Philip Steuber

EPIDEMIOLOGY

The incidence of childhood acute myeloid leukemia (AML) is one-fifth to one-sixth that of acute lymphocytic leukemia (ALL) with 350 to 500 new cases diagnosed in children annually. Due to small numbers of cases, much of the approach to childhood AML has been taken from investigations on adults with this disease. The therapy for childhood AML has not reached the degree of success achieved for childhood ALL.

PATHOPHYSIOLOGY

AML is the result of a clonal proliferation of a primitive marrow cell line with the myeloid subtype designated by the cell of origin (granulocytic, monocytic, erythrocytic, or megakaryocytic). Like ALL, classification is determined using the French–American–British (FAB) guidelines (Table 166-1).

TABLE 166-1. The FAB Classification System

FAB type	Morphologic designation	Myeloperoxidase or Sudan black	Nonspecific esterase/sodium fluoride inhibition[c]
M0	Myeloblastic leukemia[a]	−	−/−
M1	Myeloblastic leukemia without differentiation	+	−/−
M2	Myeloblastic leukemia with differentiation	+	−/−
M3	Promyelocytic leukemia	+	−/−
M4	Myelomonocytic leukemia (minor component ≥20%)	+	+/+
M5	Monocytic	−	+/+
M6	Erythrocytic	−	±
M7	Megakaryocytic[b]	−	±

FAB, French-American-British.
[a]Immunophenotypically defined.
[b]Recognized by ultrastructural presence of platelet peroxidase activity or immunohistochemical evidence of platelet glycoprotein.
[c]+, shows activity; −, lacks activity; ±, positive by nonspecific esterase stain, negative by sodium fluoride inhibition.

Subtypes

Many subtypes of AML have chromosomal aberrations; these are listed in Table 166-2. The numbers of malignant cells with abnormal chromosomes at diagnosis may indicate the responsiveness of the disease; higher percentages of cells demonstrating the abnormality carries a poorer prognosis.

Individuals with specific hereditary or congenital syndromes demonstrate an increased occurrence of AML. These rare predisposing conditions are listed in Table 166-3.

MORPHOLOGIC CLASSIFICATION

Eight categories (i.e., M0–M7) of AML are defined as represented in Table 166-1. The combined M1 and M2 morphologies account for approximately 45% of childhood AML cases, and the M4 and M5 subsets account for another 45%. The remaining subgroups—M3, M6, and M7—comprise 10% to 15%.

Alternatives

Alternatives or supplements to morphologic classifications have been investigated. Flow cytometry reveals high RNA content in myeloid blast cells and can differentiate AML from ALL. Immune phenotyping uses monoclonal antibodies directed against surface antigens to identify cell type and may indicate the stage at which cell differentiation was arrested in leukemogenesis.

Acute erythrocytic leukemia (M6) demonstrates bizarre erythroblast forms. This entity frequently evolves into one of the other myeloid leukemias, usually M1 or M2. The diagnosis of acute megakaryocytic leukemia (M7) can be confirmed using immunohistochemical techniques. Often, marked fibrosis occurs in the marrows of these M7 patients.

TABLE 166-2. Associations of Nonrandom Karyotypic Abnormalities and Leukemic Subtype

Abnormality	Leukemic subtype (FAB classification)
−7	Acute myelogenous (M1 or M2)
t(8;21) t(6;9)	Acute myelogenous (M2)
+8, −5	Acute myelogenous in general
t(15;17)	Acute promyelocytic (M3)
t(4;11)	Acute myelocytic (M1)
t(1;11) t(9;11)	Acute monocytic (M5)
t(1;11) t(9;11) inv or del (16)	Acute monomyelogenous (M4)
t(6;9)	Acute myelogenous (M2), acute monomyelogenous (M4)
t(1;22)	Acute megakaryocytic

PRESENTING FEATURES AND DIAGNOSIS

Symptoms

Children with AML manifest symptoms of bone marrow infiltration and failure. Pallor, bone pain, fever, and bleeding are common complaints. Enlargement of the liver and spleen affects approximately 50% of children, particularly younger children with M4 or M5 subtypes. Lymphadenopathy and testicular involvement are not prominent features. Leukemia cutis is a common finding in affected infants. Gingival hyperplasia can develop in those patients whose disease has a monocytic component (i.e., M4, M5).

Studies

Cerebrospinal fluid studies demonstrate leukemic involvement (often asymptomatic) in 10% of patients at diagnosis. CNS

TABLE 166-3. Conditions Associated with an Increased Incidence of Childhood Acute Myeloid Leukemia

- Blackfan-Diamond syndrome
- Bloom syndrome
- Chemotherapy for previous malignancy
- Down syndrome
- Familial myeloproliferative syndromes
- Fanconi anemia
- Klinefelter syndrome
- Kostmann syndrome
- Neurofibromatosis
- Radiation exposure
- Wiskott-Aldrich syndrome

leukemia in childhood AML is responsive to therapy and does not adversely affect outcome. An exception is the infant (younger than 2 years) with monocytic leukemia and CNS disease at diagnosis who do not respond well to therapy. The initial leukocyte count is usually less than 50,000 per microliter. Extreme leukocytosis (greater than 100,000 per microliter) occurs in 20% and is an adverse prognostic factor.

Coagulation studies may indicate a consumptive coagulopathy, particularly in patients with acute promyelocytic leukemia (APL).

THERAPY

The therapeutic concepts of induction, consolidation, maintenance, and CNS prophylaxis that are used in treating ALL cannot be applied directly to childhood AML. The initial management for ALL and AML is similar: deliver a drug or combination of drugs that in 3 to 4 weeks reduces blast forms to below the detectable level and reestablish normal marrow function.

Induction regimens are more toxic for AML than ALL, and creating transient marrow aplasia is necessary to achieve a complete remission in AML. The therapeutic index for such regimens is narrow with 5% to 15% mortality. Currently, complete remissions in AML are being obtained in 70% to 85% of newly diagnosed patients. Agents such as anthracyclines (e.g., daunorubicin) and cytosine arabinoside are used to achieve these results.

At the present time, multiple therapeutic strategies for postremission therapy are being evaluated. The 5-year event-free survival rate for children with AML is approximately 35% to 40% with approximately 50% of initial responders expected to remain in remission. The median disease-free survival is 12 to 18 months.

Patients with trisomy 21 have an increased incidence of AML, particularly acute megakaryocytic leukemia. Their response to therapy appears to be exceptionally good.

Postremission therapies using allogeneic bone marrow transplantation or autografting with purged and nonpurged marrows are being compared to chemotherapy regimens. Although data supports the use of allogeneic grafts as therapy for the majority of patients with AML during first remission, continuing improvements in chemotherapy regimens may alter that recommendation.

CNS therapy, when indicated, can be accomplished using radiation therapy or intrathecal therapy with single or multiple agents.

CHAPTER 167
Hodgkin's Disease

Adapted from Kenneth L. McClain

BIOLOGY AND EPIDEMIOLOGY

Hodgkin's Disease (HD) is a malignancy of B lymphocytes as defined by studies using immunophenotype and molecular studies. The histologic types of HD include nodular sclerosis (46% of patients), mixed cellularity (31%), lymphocyte predominance (16%), and lymphocyte depletion (7%). HD rarely occurs in children younger than 7 years and is diagnosed equally in boys and girls. The incidence increases until the age of 25 and then decreases until the mid-30s.

Because more patients are from better socioeconomic conditions, delayed exposure to a common infectious agent such as EBV may be relevant. Patients with HD have a higher titer against the viral capsid antigen than most children after years of infectious mononucleosis, but finding may be secondary to abnormalities of the immune system in HD. Recent studies have reported molecular evidence of EBV in 58% of all HD cases at one institution.

CLINICAL FEATURES AND DIAGNOSIS

Presenting Signs and Symptoms

Most children present with painless lymphadenopathy, usually of the cervical, supraclavicular, axillary, or inguinal nodes. Splenic or hepatic enlargement is infrequently found in early stages of HD. Fewer than 20% of patients have the classic fever and night sweats that adults with HD demonstrate. A mediastinal mass may be seen on chest films in about 25% of patients and is found more often in children older than 12 years.

Staging

Evaluation and treatment of HD should be undertaken at a center where a team of pediatric oncologists, pathologists, surgeons, radiotherapists, nurses, and social workers are experienced in the diagnosis and care of children with cancer.

Routine evaluation of a patient with suspected HD should include a complete history to include information such as family history of cancers and exposure of the patient to toxins. Next, a complete physical examination with assessment of general health, height and weight, size and location of lymphadenopathy, liver and spleen size, skin infiltrations, pulmonary findings, and neurologic signs should be done. Laboratory evaluation should include a complete blood count, erythrocyte sedimentation rate, renal and liver function tests (including lactate dehydrogenase levels), urinalysis, anteroposterior and lateral chest radiographic films, and computed tomographic (CT) scans of the abdomen and chest with oral and intravenous contrast. Bone marrow biopsies may be indicated.

Staging has two aspects: clinical and pathologic. Clinical staging refers to an assessment of the disease extent based on history, physical examination, and radiologic tests. Pathologic staging is accomplished by histologic examination of tissues removed at a staging laparotomy and by the bone marrow biopsy. Table 167-1 outlines the Ann Arbor staging system for HD in children or adults.

TREATMENT

In the past, patients with pathologically staged I through IIA disease were treated primarily with irradiation to involved areas plus an extended field to contiguous regions that are frequently sites of relapse. For a child with a cervical node involvement, this meant the neck, supraclavicular, and axillary (mini-mantle) regions were irradiated. A mediastinal mass required a special boost of radiation if the mass was greater than one-third of the chest diameter. Historically, this approach provided disease-free survival rates of more than 80% for stage I and II HD. Some centers routinely added extended-field irradiation to paraaortic nodes and to splenic or hepatic regions, even for limited supradiaphragmatic disease. This helped improve survival when B symptoms or extensive mediastinal disease suggested a worse prognosis, but the price paid for this

TABLE 167-1. Ann Arbor System for Staging of Hodgkin's Disease

Stage I	Involvement of a single lymph node region (I) or a single extralymphatic organ or site (I_E)
Stage II	Involvement of two or more lymph node regions on the same side of the diaphragm (II), or extension to an extralymphatic site and one or more lymph node regions on the same side of the diaphragm (II_E)
Stage III	Involvement of lymph node regions on both sides of the diaphragm (III), localized involvement by extension to an extralymphatic organ or site (III_E), or involvement of the spleen
Stage IV	Diffuse or disseminated involvement of one or more extralymphatic organs or tissues with or without associated lymph node enlargement

All stages are further classified as A or B to indicate the absence or presence, respectively, of systemic symptoms: unexplained fever, night sweats, or weight loss greater than 10% of normal body weight. It laparotomy and histologic review show that disease is limited to spleen, splenic, celiac, or portal nodes, the classification is substage IIIA1. Involvement of the lower abdominal nodes, such as paraaortic, iliac, and inguinal nodes, designates substage IIIA2.

Reprinted with permission from Carbone PP, Kaplan HS. Report of the committee on Hodgkin's disease staging classification. *Cancer Res* 1971;31:1860.

extra therapy was toxicity in the form of musculoskeletal growth problems.

Most centers in the United States and Europe are now using graded amounts of radiation therapy (based on age) and chemotherapy for early- and late-stage disease.

Patients with stages I to IIIA HD are currently treated with doxorubicin, bleomycin, vincristine, and etoposide (VP-16) for two courses and then involved field radiotherapy (2,550 cGy) if they are in complete remission. If residual disease exists, two additional courses of chemotherapy are given, then radiotherapy. Advanced stages (IIIB to IV) receive the same four agents plus prednisone and cyclophosphamide plus radiation.

LATE EFFECTS

All patients undergoing treatment have alopecia, weight loss, transient pancytopenia, and extreme susceptibility to infections while on therapy. When high-dose radiation therapy is applied to the spinal area, growth is stunted. Post-radiation thyroid dysfunction is common.

Extensive radiation therapy can cause pneumonitis, pericarditis, and enteritis. Sterility in male patients was a frequent complication, particularly after older chemotherapy regimens. For female patients, delay and alteration of menstrual cycles was reported, especially after pelvic irradiation. However, this problem can be prevented by moving the ovaries out of the radiation field (i.e., oophoropexy) at the time of the staging laparotomy.

Cardiotoxicity from doxorubicin has been identified as a major long-term sequela for patients with HD. The majority of patients are asymptomatic, but sensitive diagnostic techniques identify defective wall motion in many patients, years after having received chemotherapy.

Infections have been one of the main concerns for patients with HD because of their underlying immune deficiency, splenectomy, and the toxicity of therapy.

CHAPTER 168

Non-Hodgkin's Lymphoma

Adapted from Kenneth L. McClain

Non-Hodgkin's lymphomas (NHLs) represent 10% of all tumors in the pediatric age group. The peak incidence occurs among children 7 to 11 years of age, and a male patient predominance exists. Three major histologic varieties exist—lymphoblastic, Burkitt, and large cell lymphomas—the majority of which are considered high grade. Patients with congenital or acquired immunodeficiency (including human immunodeficiency virus infection and posttransplant patients) are at higher risk for developing lymphomas than the normal population.

TYPES OF NON-HODGKIN'S LYMPHOMA

Lymphoblastic Lymphoma

Most children present with cervical lymphadenopathy, a mediastinal mass, and moderate hepatosplenomegaly. The small lymphoblast of the lymphoblastic lymphomas is morphologically similar to the lymphoblast of acute lymphoblastic leukemia. When a bone marrow aspirate is done on a child suspected with leukemia or lymphoma, less than 25% lymphoblasts existing in the marrow with malignant cells found on lymph node biopsy make the diagnosis of lymphoma. The lymphoblastic lymphomas make up 28% of childhood NHLs.

A high incidence exists of central nervous system (CNS) involvement and leukemic transformation in patients with lymphoblastic lymphoma.

Burkitt Lymphoma

Burkitt lymphoma is the most common (39%) type of NHL in childhood. Children usually present with an abdominal mass that may originate in the bowel, kidneys, or gonads and be accompanied by ascites. Enlargement of the tonsils, thyroid gland, and CNS disease may be evident. Occasionally, the enlargement of the tonsils is misdiagnosed as benign chronic tonsillitis.

Surface marker studies of Burkitt lymphoma show a mature B cell with surface immunoglobulin. The B lymphoblast is the fastest growing human tumor cell with doubling times of less than 24 hours. The disease can change from a barely palpable node to massive tumor in a matter of days.

Although the cell of origin and clinical behavior is similar to the African variety originally named after Dr. Denis Burkitt, association with Epstein–Barr virus is lacking.

Molecular analysis has shown correlations with the frequent chromosome translocations t(8;14), t(8;22), and t(2;8). The movement of DNA in these translocations brings the myc oncogene on chromosome 8 into juxtaposition with active immunoglobulin gene-regulating elements on the other chromosomes.

Large Cell Lymphoma

The third type of childhood NHL is the large cell lymphomas, previously called *histiocytic lymphomas*. This disease often presents in lymphoid tissue of the tonsils, adenoids, Peyer's patches, or anterior mediastinum. Extranodal disease in the skin and bone may be found, but bone marrow and CNS involvement is less frequent than other NHL. The cells of origin in these diffuse lymphomas are usually B or T lymphocytes, although indeterminate immunophenotypes are identified.

TABLE 168-1. Staging of Childhood Non-Hodgkin's Lymphoma

Stage I	Single tumor in node or extralymphatic site, excluding the mediastinum or abdomen
Stage II	Single extranodal tumor with regional node positive Two or more nodal areas on same side of diaphragm Two extranodal tumors on same side of diaphragm regardless of nodal involvement Primary gastrointestinal tract tumor with or without associated mesenteric nodes, grossly completely excised
Stage III	Two single extranodal tumors on opposite sides of diaphragm Two or more nodal areas above and below the diaphragm All tumors originating in mediastinum, pleura, or thymus All extensive primary intraabdominal disease (usually many implants, not totally resectable); often ascites
Stage IV	Any of previously mentioned stages with initial central nervous system, bone marrow, or both central nervous system and bone marrow involvement

Adapted from Murphy SB. Childhood non-Hodgkin's lymphoma. *N Engl J Med* 1978;299:1446.

PATIENT EVALUATION AND DIAGNOSIS

Evaluation of patients with NHL begins with a thorough history and physical examination. Laboratory investigations should include a complete blood count, urinalysis, chest radiography, lumbar puncture, and bone marrow biopsy and aspirate with samples sent for chromosome and cell marker analysis. Requisite blood chemistry evaluation includes serum electrolytes including calcium and phosphate; liver function tests and blood urea nitrogen; and creatinine, uric acid, and serum lactate dehydrogenase (LDH) levels. If the LDH levels are greater than 1,000, massive disease and a poor outcome are indicated. The renal tests are especially important because of frequent kidney involvement in lymphoblastic and Burkitt lymphomas.

The complication of tumor lysis syndrome is possible (see Chapter 166, p. 473).

Chest radiographic and abdominal computed tomographic examinations are necessary for determining the extent of intracavitary disease.

Biopsy of mediastinal nodes or other abnormal masses is required to make the diagnosis, but extensive surgery is not indicated. A staging laparotomy such as the one performed for Hodgkin's disease is unnecessary for NHL. The clinical staging categories are listed in Table 168-1.

TREATMENT

Lymphoblastic Lymphoma

Localized diffuse NHL (i.e., stages I and II) responds well to a short induction and consolidation with vincristine, doxorubicin, prednisone, cyclophosphamide, and intrathecal medications. Regimens with mercaptopurine, methotrexate, and intrathecal injections may also be used.

For stages III and IV NHL lymphoblastic lymphomas, a 12-drug regimen lasting 2 to 3 years, has resulted in a 76% disease-free survival rate. Multiple other therapies area available depending on the immunologic identification of cell type.

Burkitt Lymphoma

Stages I and II Burkitt lymphoma patients have been treated with vincristine, doxorubicin, cyclophosphamide, prednisone, and intrathecal medications as induction and consolidation. A 94% complete remission rate has been reported. Very aggressive chemotherapy treatments now cure disease in 80% of stage III and 50% of stage IV patients. These patients are at high risk for tumor lysis syndrome.

Large Cell Lymphoma

The standard therapy for large cell lymphomas includes induction treatment with doxorubicin (Adriamycin), prednisone, methotrexate, and vincristine (Oncovin), followed by maintenance therapy with vincristine, mercaptopurine, doxorubicin (to a maximum dose of 300 mg/m^2), and prednisone. Intrathecal methotrexate is given as prophylaxis for CNS disease. Radiation therapy is used only if the lymphoma is resistant to initial chemotherapy or for CNS disease. The disease-free survival rate for patients treated with these therapies is greater than 80%.

CHAPTER 169
Malignant Bone Tumors

Adapted from Murali M. Chintagumpala and Donald H. Mahoney, Jr.

The two most common malignant-bone tumors in children and adolescents are osteogenic sarcoma and Ewing sarcoma.

OSTEOGENIC SARCOMA

Incidence and Epidemiology

Osteogenic sarcoma, or osteosarcoma, is the most common primary malignancy of bone in children. It is a malignant spindle cell sarcoma of bone in which the tumor cells directly form neoplastic osteoid. The estimated incidence is 11 cases per 1 million adolescents. The male–to–female patient ratio is approximately 1.5:1.0. The peak incidence occurs within the second decade.

The etiology of osteosarcoma is unknown. Patients who have the germinal mutation for retinoblastoma and who survive the ocular tumor have a 2,000-fold increased risk for osteosarcoma in irradiated craniofacial bones. These patients have a 500-fold increased risk for osteosarcoma at any site regardless of prior radiation exposure. This risk appears to be linked to the expression of the retinoblastoma gene located on chromosome 13 at band q14. Radiation-induced osteosarcoma is also being diagnosed with increased frequency in long-term survivors of childhood cancer. Two recessive oncogenes, p53 and RB, appear to be involved either individually or in cooperation in both osteosarcoma development and progression.

Signs, Symptoms, and Diagnostic Studies

The metaphyseal portion of the long bone is the typical site of involvement. The most common sites are the distal femur, proximal tibia, and proximal humerus. Pain and swelling of the extremity are the cardinal symptoms. Pathologic fractures are uncommon.

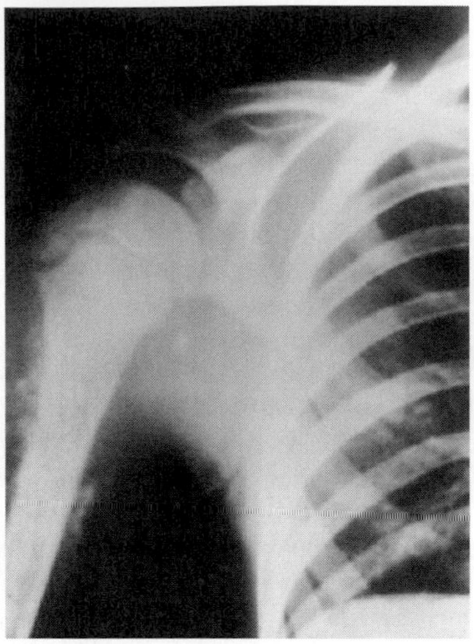

Figure 169-1. A large permeating lesion of the proximal right humerus representing osteosarcoma beginning at the metaphyseal plate with soft tissue extension and calcifications caused by osteosarcoma.

On radiographs, tumors may appear lytic, sclerotic, or mixed. Irregular periosteal new bone formation in the metaphysis may be seen early. In more advanced cases, cortical destruction, sclerosis, a sunburst pattern of periosteal new bone formation, and contiguous, calcified soft tissue extensions may be noted (Fig. 169-1).

The diagnosis is best made by incisional biopsy or a carefully performed needle biopsy. Incorrectly guided needle biopsies can create a tract that complicates consideration for limb salvage therapy. Staging should include chest radiography and computed tomography of the chest. MRI scans accurately assess intraosseous extension of tumor and are necessary for patients undergoing limb salvage procedures

Osteosarcoma may spread to lungs or bone. Approximately 2% to 3% of all cases of osteosarcoma are multifocal and carry a poor prognosis.

Treatment

Historically, osteosarcoma carried a dismal prognosis. Currently, multimodal treatment strategies have reversed this trend, and approximately 65% of patients with nonmetastatic disease of the extremities are surviving their disease. Both surgery and high-dose chemotherapy play a significant part in current therapy.

Surgery has an established role in the treatment of osteosarcoma. Ablative amputation should be 7 cm beyond the most proximal limits of the lesion to minimize the risk for local recurrence.

More effective chemotherapy has made limb salvage surgery an option. This entails en bloc tumor excision and endoprosthetic replacement. Candidates considered eligible for the limb salvage procedure are generally selected on the basis of the following criteria:

- Attainment of complete or nearly complete physical growth for patients with lesions of the lower extremities
- Anatomic site of the lesion such that no sacrifice of major arteries or nerves is involved
- Absence of metastases at diagnosis or isolated metastasis that responded to preoperative treatment
- Full understanding by the patient and parents of the nature and complications of the procedure with reasonable expectations for functional outcome.

Chemotherapy (neoadjuvant) may be given before the en bloc resection. Among other potential advantages, this allows time for acquisition of a custom prosthesis. Disease-free survival is similar for patients who undergo amputation at the time of diagnosis or have limb-salvage surgery after several courses of chemotherapy.

High-dose adjuvant chemotherapy increases relapse-free survival for patients with nonmetastatic osteosarcoma of the extremities. Several chemotherapy regimens exist with disease-free survival rates in excess of 65%. Common features of these programs include the use of high doses of methotrexate, doxorubicin, ifosfamide, or cisplatin. All patients will require extensive rehabilitation support to resume normal activities.

EWING SARCOMA

Incidence and Epidemiology

Ewing sarcoma (named after James Ewing) is an uncommon primary sarcoma of nonosseous origin that usually arises in children or adolescents. Ewing sarcoma represents approximately 1% of all cancers reported in children but approximately 30% of all bone tumors in this age group. The etiology for Ewing sarcoma is unknown. Unlike osteosarcoma, ionizing radiation exposure does not represent a significant risk factor.

Pathology

Ewing sarcoma is a small round cell tumor and, thus, can be confused with other undifferentiated round cell tumors. The diversity of light microscopical patterns in Ewing sarcoma makes the diagnosis a challenge for even the most experienced pathologist. Some investigations have demonstrated a cytogenetic abnormality [t(11;22) (q24;q12)] within tumor cells that may assist in the confirmation of the diagnosis. This cytogenetic abnormality is present in 88% to 95% of Ewing sarcoma and peripheral primitive neuroectodermal tumors, neuroepitheliomas, and Askin tumors. Other round cell tumors to be considered in the differential diagnosis include non-Hodgkin's lymphoma, rhabdomyosarcoma, neuroblastoma, small cell osteosarcoma, metastatic medulloblastoma, and the acute leukemias of all types.

Clinical Presentation and Diagnostic Evaluation

Pain is the most common first symptom in Ewing sarcoma. Swelling associated with a soft tissue mass may become evident weeks to months thereafter. Fever may be present. Pathologic fractures are uncommon.

The femur is the bone most commonly involved, but any bone of the body may be involved (Fig. 169-2). The classic radiographic feature is a diffuse, mottled, lytic lesion affecting the medullary cavity and cortical bone. Tumor that penetrates the cortex and extends into the periosteum may produce elevations characterized by multiple layers of reactive new bone formation creating an onion-skin appearance on radiographic examination. A soft tissue mass may be associated with the primary bone tumor. Several other conditions can produce similar radiographic features including acute and chronic osteomyelitis, eosinophilic granuloma, osteosarcoma, metastatic sarcomas, and lymphoma. An MRI scan of the affected bone gives the best assessment of intramedullary tumor extension.

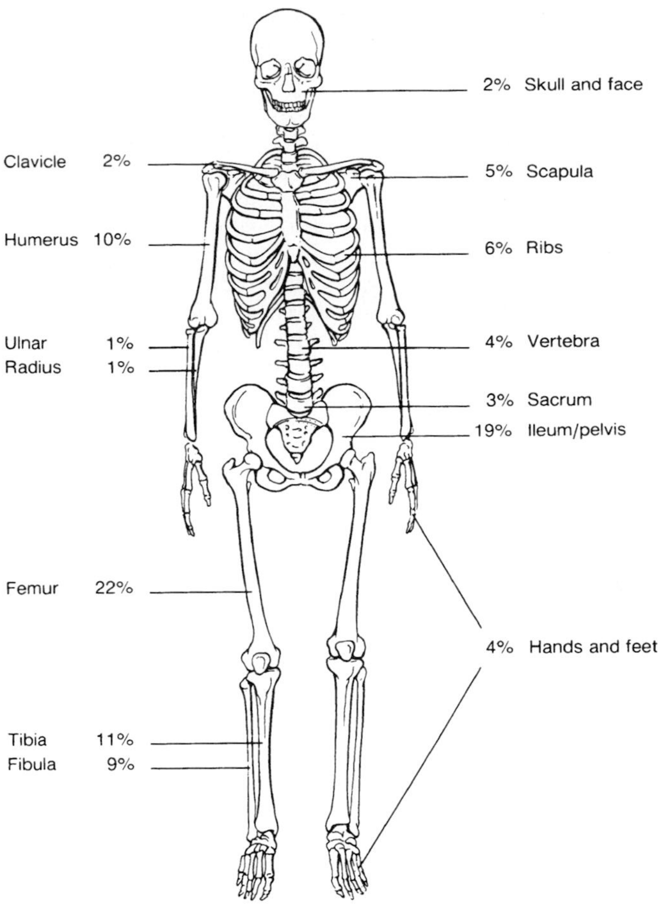

Figure 169-2. Anatomic distribution of Ewing sarcoma based on 836 cases. (After Nesbit ME, Robison LL, Dehner LP. Round cell sarcoma of bone. In: Sutow WW, Fernbach DJ, Vietti TJ, eds. Clinical pediatric oncology. St. Louis: Mosby, 1984:710.)

An open biopsy is the best procedure to establish the diagnosis of Ewing sarcoma. In any patient, if a malignant bone tumor is suspected, referral to a pediatric cancer center ensures the most experienced surgeons for optimal biopsy procedures.

Clinical staging is essential in those with confirmed disease. This should include chest radiography, CT of the chest, MRI of the bone, radionuclide bone scanning, and bone marrow aspiration and biopsy. The lungs and bones are the most common sites of metastases (90% of the cases).

Treatment and Prognosis

Historically, Ewing's sarcoma had a dismal prognosis due to a propensity for metastatic spread before diagnosis. Today, multidisciplinary treatment approaches allow survival of greater than 70% after 2 years. Tumor size, location, and metastases at diagnosis are prognostic factors. Metastatic disease at diagnosis has been reported in 14% to 35% of patients and is associated with a poor prognosis. The most favorable primary sites are distal lesions, usually in expendable bones such as those of the foot, the fibula, ribs, forearm bone, clavicle, or scapula.

Most treatment regimens include initial chemotherapy, followed by local disease control measures (surgery, radiation or both), followed by further chemotherapy. Amputation may be recommended for extremity lesions with destructive components or pathologic fractures.

Radiation therapy, when coupled with adjuvant chemotherapy, will achieve local control in more than 90% of patients with extremity lesions. A risk for the development of second malignancies exists when radiation therapy is used.

Adjuvant chemotherapy plays an important role in the treatment of patients with Ewing sarcoma. Agents established values include vincristine, dactinomycin, cyclophosphamide, doxorubicin, ifosfamide and VP-16.

For survivors of Ewing sarcoma, several late consequences of treatment such as pathologic fractures at primary tumor sites, retarded bone growth, and limb-length discrepancy may result. Due to radiation and chemotherapy, the estimated rate for second cancers is 70 times the expected value in the normal population. Other potential complications include sterility (due to cyclophosphamide) and cardiotoxicity associated with doxorubicin.

CHAPTER 170
Malignant Brain Tumors

Adapted from Murali M. Chintagumpala and Donald H. Mahoney, Jr.

Primary brain tumors are the second most common type of cancer in children with approximately 1,200 new cases in the United States each year in children younger than 15 years. Children with brain tumors should be referred to a pediatric cancer center for definitive diagnosis and treatment.

SYMPTOMS ON PRESENTATION

Early symptoms of central nervous system (CNS) tumors can be nonspecific. In infants, increasing head circumference, irritability, head tilt, and loss of developmental milestones may be seen. Older children may present with headache and early morning vomiting. Headaches can be progressive and most of these children eventually develop an abnormal neurologic exam. Specific abnormalities such as ataxia, somnolence, hemiparesis, and seizures may develop.

The differential diagnosis for CNS tumors in children includes brain abscesses, hemorrhage, nonneoplastic hydrocephalus, arteriovenous malformations or aneurysm, and indolent virus infections.

CLASSIFICATION

In children ages 4 to 11 years, infratentorial (posterior fossa) tumors such as cerebellar and brainstem tumors predominate. Supratentorial tumors are more frequent during the first years of life and during late adolescence. Of the 45% of the brain tumors that arise in the cerebellum, Cerebellar astrocytomas and medulloblastomas are the most common. Ependymomas represent between 3% and 14% of all childhood tumors.

Cerebral tumors such as astrocytomas, glioblastomas, and ependymomas account for 20% to 25% of all brain tumors. Brainstem neoplasms account for 9% to 15% of intracranial neoplasms, most in patients younger than age 10. Midline tumors such as germ cell tumors craniopharyngiomas, pinealomas, optic gliomas, and pituitary adenomas account for another 10%.

The practice of classifying CNS tumors based on location is being reevaluated. Newer classification systems classify tumors on the basis of histopathologic features alone regardless of where the tumor arises in the brain. This system recognizes the heterogeneity of tumors arising within a single site.

DIAGNOSTIC EVALUATIONS

Cranial CT scans, with and without contrast, have a sensitivity of more than 94% for primary brain tumors, but certain limitations of resolution exist. Small lesions within the posterior fossa, especially within the brainstem, and small cystic structures near the skull base may escape detection.

MRI scans have become the standard of care, particularly in the detection of low-grade glial tumors and lesions at the vertex within the posterior fossa (especially within the brainstem) and at the base of the skull. MRI's can also detect spinal cord tumors and delineating leptomeningeal tumor invasion.

Newer methodologies such as the positron emission tomography (PET scan) are gaining a role in diagnosis.

Electroencephalography and brainstem auditory-evoked potential may be useful at diagnosis and in the management of complications of the disease or treatment (e.g., seizures). The tumor markers, alpha–fetoprotein and beta–chorionic gonadotropin, are useful markers of malignant germ cell tumors. New technologies such as cytogenetics and monoclonal antibody characterization of specific tumor antigens are becoming important aspects of diagnosis and treatment. Baseline neuropsychological and endocrine testing is important for long-term management.

TREATMENT

Cerebellar Astrocytomas

Cerebellar astrocytomas account for approximately 20% of all brain tumors in children. The juvenile pilocytic type of astrocytoma accounts for 80% to 85% of the cases. With complete surgical excision, 10-year survival rates of 80% to 95% have been reported. For diffuse astrocytomas, the role of radiation therapy in treating incompletely resected tumors is under investigation. Those with residual tumor after surgery can be candidates for chemotherapy.

Medulloblastomas

Medulloblastomas are highly malignant primitive neuroectodermal tumors, which primarily affect children between 4 and 8 years of age and account for 20% of all brain tumors in children. Therapy includes surgery, irradiation, and chemotherapy in selected cases. Complete tumor excision is achievable in 50% of the patients and may offer a survival advantage. Some clinical staging scales have shown prognostic value.

Medulloblastoma is radiosensitive and chemosensitive. Five year disease-free survival rates with radiation therapy alone range from 45% to 60%. Adjuvant chemotherapy after surgery and irradiation increases the survival of children with medulloblastoma. Some protocols have demonstrated a 5-year disease-free survival rate of 88% for children treated with lomustine (CCNU), vincristine, and cisplatin. For patients with "standard risk" medulloblastoma (based on clinical staging systems), adjuvant chemotherapy has not been clearly established as beneficial.

Brainstem Tumors

Brainstem gliomas have the worst prognosis of all pediatric CNS tumors with an estimated 5-year disease-free survival rate of 15% to 18%.

Cranial nerve dysfunctions, gait disturbances, and a brainstem mass as demonstrated by neuroimaging are the hallmarks of this disease (Fig. 170-1). Surgery can be hazardous, and patients with inoperable lesions involving the pons or medulla or with malignant histology have a poor prognosis. Patients with operable lesions, lower grade histology, or higher brainstem lesions may experience longer survival.

High-dose corticosteroids and local irradiation generates a 50% response, but the tumor invariably recurs. Adjuvant chemotherapy offers no advantage.

High-Grade Astrocytomas

High-grade astrocytomas (i.e., anaplastic astrocytoma or glioblastoma) represent approximately 25% of childhood tumors. These tumors develop in the cerebral hemisphere (51%), brainstem (37%), and cerebellum.

Management consisting of surgical excision, if possible, and radiation therapy offers a 5-year disease-free survival rate of less

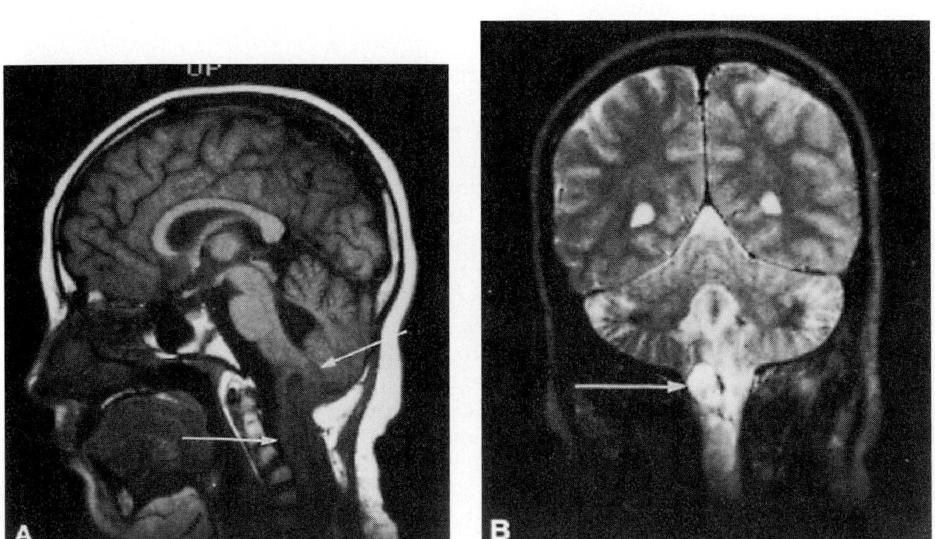

Figure 170-1. Magnetic resonance imaging study of a brainstem and cervical tumor. **A:** Sagittal view (T1-weighted) reveals enlargement of the caudal brainstem extending below the foramen magnum to the level of C5 to C6 (*arrows*). **B:** Coronal view (T2-weighted) reveals an increased signal intensity highlighting the cystic component of this lesion as it extends into the cervical cord (*arrow*).

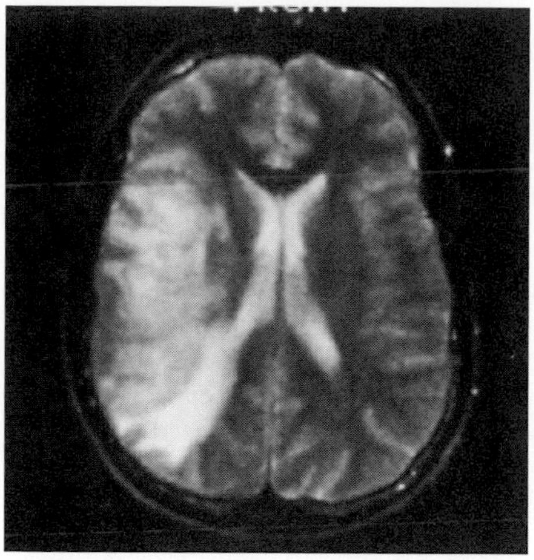

Figure 170-2. A T2-weighted magnetic resonance imaging scan in the axial projection reveals a large right frontal-parietal mass with the central component representing neoplasm (ependymoma) and the peripheral component probably representing edema.

than 25%. Adjuvant chemotherapy offers some benefit, but the extent of surgical excision has, perhaps, the most important influence on outcome.

Ependymomas

Ependymomas represent 9% of all brain tumors in children. These tumors are locally invasive, may be cystic, and are histologically diverse. Intracranial lesions typically occur in children between the ages of 2 and 6 years, but spinal tumors occur more during the teenage years. In children, most ependymomas arise in the posterior fossa near the fourth ventricle. Large supratentorial tumors in paraventricular regions may also occur (Fig. 170-2). The incidence of spinal cord seeding at diagnosis has been reported as 10% to 11%. Conventional treatment includes aggressive surgery followed by radiation therapy. The choice of radiation fields (e.g., cranial versus craniospinal) is the subject of investigation. Overall, the estimated 5-year disease-free survival rate with surgery and radiation therapy is 45% to 65%. Chemotherapy trials have been limited and inconclusive.

CHAPTER 171
Wilms Tumor

Adapted from Murali M. Chintagumpala and C. Philip Steuber

Wilms tumor is a malignant embryonal neoplasm of the kidney with incidence reported annually of 8.1 cases per 1 million white children younger than 15 years. Eighty percent occur by age 5 years, and 98% occur by age 7 years. Peak incidence is between the ages 3 and 4 years. The tumors associated with congenital anomalies and synchronous bilateral tumors occur at an earlier age.

ETIOLOGY

Wilms tumor occurs in hereditary and nonhereditary forms. The hereditary form is autosomal dominant, may be multifocal, and can be associated with other congenital anomalies.

Children with Wilms tumor, aniridia, genitourinary abnormalities, and mental retardation (WAGR syndrome) have a constitutional deletion at chromosome 11p13 where the Wilms tumor gene *WT1* has been located. These patients have a 30% probability of developing Wilms tumor. A second Wilms tumor gene (*WT2*), located at 11p15.5, was strongly suggested by tumor-specific loss of heterozygosity and linkage studies in familial Beckwith–Wiedemann syndrome. This syndrome carries a risk of Wilms tumor of 3% to 5%.

Most patients with sporadic isolated aniridia have some degree of 11p13 deletion with a significant risk of Wilms tumor. Isolated hemihypertrophy is also associated with an increased risk for the development of Wilms tumor. Other syndromes that have an increased risk of Wilms tumor include the Denys–Drash syndrome. Genitourinary abnormalities such as hypoplasia, fusion and ectopia of the kidney, duplicated collecting systems, hypospadias, and cryptorchidism can be associated with Wilms tumor.

PATHOLOGY

Persistent metanephric blastemal cells in the postnatal period are termed nephrogenic rests and are regarded as precursor lesions for Wilms tumor. The terms favorable and unfavorable are used. Favorable histology tumors are triphasic with blastemal, epithelial, and stromal elements.

Of the three unfavorable histologies identified by the National Wilms' Tumor Study (focal or diffuse anaplastic tumors, clear cell sarcomas, and rhabdoid tumors), the rhabdoid histologic type and clear cell sarcoma are no longer considered to be Wilms tumor variants.

CLINICAL AND DIAGNOSTIC FEATURES

A hard, smooth, silent mass confined to the flank or one side of the abdomen is noted in two-thirds of patients. The tumor may be accidentally detected by parents or incidentally during the course of a physical. Abdominal pain occurs in approximately one-third of the patients. Sudden hemorrhage into the tumor can occur and patients can present with rapid abdominal enlargement and anemia. Hematuria and hypertension may be noted in 10% to 25% of cases.

Wilms tumor must be suspected in any child with an abdominal mass. The evaluation includes blood counts, liver and kidney function studies, a skeletal survey, chest radiography and CT scan, ultrasonography, and a CT scan of the abdomen. If the abdominal CT does not show a renal lesion, neuroblastoma should be considered. Areas of hemorrhage and calcification are less common than in neuroblastoma.

The differential diagnosis includes neuroblastoma, rhabdomyosarcoma, leiomyosarcoma, renal cell sarcoma, fibrosarcoma, hypernephroma, polycystic kidneys, adrenal hemorrhage, renal vein thrombosis, dysplastic kidney, and renal carbuncle—almost anything that can cause a mass in the upper abdomen.

STAGING

Surgical exploration includes samples of hilar, periaortic, and other lymph nodes. Biopsies should be done of any hepatic

TABLE 171-1. Staging System Developed by the Third National Wilms' Tumor Study

Stage I	Tumor limited to kidney and is completely excised. Capsular surface intact; no tumor rupture; no residual tumor apparent beyond margins of excision
Stage II	Tumor extends beyond kidney but is completely excised. Regional extension of tumor; vessel infiltration; tumor biopsied or local spillage of tumor confined to the flank. No residual tumor apparent at or beyond margins of excision
Stage III	Residual nonhematogenous tumor confined to the abdomen. Lymph node involvement of hilus, periaortic chains, or beyond; diffuse peritoneal contamination by tumor spillage; peritoneal implants of tumor; tumor extends beyond surgical margins microscopically or macroscopically; tumor not completely removable because of local infiltration into vital structures
Stage IV	Deposits beyond stage III (e.g., lung, liver, bone, brain)
Stage V	Bilateral renal involvement at diagnosis

lesions. Exploration of the opposite kidney is essential to rule out synchronous bilateral disease.

A staging system was developed by the National Wilms' Tumor Study (NWTS) as shown in Table 171-1. The major factors in staging are distal metastatic disease, involvement of the lymph nodes or other residual disease, and histologic type of tumor (i.e., favorable or unfavorable). Favorable histology and early stage indicate a good prognosis.

For inoperable tumors based on size or invasion, or in patients with bilateral tumors, pretreatment with chemotherapy after initial biopsies of the unilateral or bilateral tumors (to establish diagnosis and local staging) can produce successful results.

TREATMENT

Wilms tumor is sensitive to chemotherapy and radiation therapy. The first line of therapy, however, is complete surgical excision of the tumor whenever possible. Combinations of doxorubicin, vincristine, and dactinomycin are used for chemotherapy.

Postoperative radiation is unnecessary in patients with stages I and II favorable histology and stage I anaplasia when treated with chemotherapy postoperatively. Patients with stage III favorable histology benefit from doxorubicin therapy, in addition to vincristine and dactinomycin (actinomycin D), and do not require more than 1,000 cGy to the abdomen. The addition of cyclophosphamide to the standard three drugs appears to benefit patients with stages II through IV anaplastic histology. With these regimens, 4-year survival rates range between 80 to 95% for favorable histology tumors and near 100% for patients with focal anaplastic disease. Those patients with diffuse anaplastic disease have a less favorable prognosis.

Combination chemoradiotherapy and surgical or multiple surgical procedures has improved the survival rates of children with bilateral Wilms tumor. The need to perform bilateral nephrectomies with subsequent dialysis and eventual renal transplantation is rare.

In patients with metstatic disease, pulmonary irradiation plus chemotherapy has achieved survival rates of more than 50%. Liver or lung metastases may be excised before administering chemotherapy or combined chemoradiotherapy.

The most prominent late effects of treatment are bone and muscle changes secondary to radiation therapy. Vertebral bone growth can be affected with a high incidence of scoliosis. The incidence of second malignancies is low and is dose-dependent to radiation. Cardiac, renal, and hepatic dysfunction can occur due to radiation, chemotherapy, or both.

CHAPTER 172
Neuroblastoma

Adapted from Douglas R. Strother and ZoAnn E. Dreyer

The neuroblastic tumors, neuroblastoma, ganglioneuroblastoma, and ganglioneuroma, develop from neural crest tissue. The behavior of the most malignant type, neuroblastoma, is different in infants compared with histologically identical disease in older children. Particularly in infants, regression of primary and metastatic disease may occur spontaneously. When neuroblastoma is recognized in the older child, it is usually metastatic and, despite sensitivity to chemotherapy and radiation therapy, it is usually fatal.

ETIOLOGY

Neuroblastoma is the most common malignancy in the first year of life. Approximately 550 new cases of neuroblastoma are diagnosed each year in the United States. The cause of neuroblastoma is unknown, but genetic predisposition through mutation of a germinal cell may play a role in 20% of cases.

PATHOLOGY

Derivatives of neural crest tissue include the adrenal medulla and sympathetic nervous system ganglia. The histologic patterns of neuroblastoma, ganglioneuroblastoma, and ganglioneuroma correlate with normal patterns of differentiation of these tissues.

Neuroblastoma is one of the small, round, blue cell tumors. Differentiation is lacking or present in less than one-half of neuroblastoma cells. Ganglioneuroblastomas are characterized by more than 50% of cells showing differentiation. Ganglioneuromas, the benign form of neuroblastic tumors, are comprised of mature ganglion cells, neuropil, and Schwann cells.

CLINICAL FEATURES

Neuroblastic tumors can arise from anywhere in the sympathetic nervous system. In two-thirds of cases, tumors arise in the abdomen from either the adrenal glands or paraspinal sympathetic ganglia. Tumors in the chest and neck are more common in infants. Tumor may metastasize to lymph nodes, liver, bone, bone marrow, and skin, and it is common for neuroblastoma to be widely disseminated at the time of diagnosis. Symptoms of metastatic disease include fever, pain, abdominal distention, lymph node enlargement, pallor, weight loss, and failure to thrive. Metastatic skin nodules are palpable, nontender, bluish subcutaneous modules.

Nonmetastatic disease may present with a palpable mass. Intrathoracic disease may be seen incidentally on a chest radiograph. Mass effect can lead to Horner syndrome, obstruction of the superior or inferior vena cava, proptosis, and periorbital ecchymoses. Compression of the spinal cord or obstruction of the gastrointestinal tract can occur. Although uncommon, symptoms may occur secondary to production of catecholamines.

Opsoclonus-myoclonus ("dancing eyes, dancing feet" syndrome) is a paraneoplastic syndrome that may include random eye movements, ataxia, developmental delay, and abnormal behavior. Despite complete resection of primary disease, these neurologic symptoms may persist indefinitely. Intractable diarrhea with secondary hypokalemia and dehydration is another paraneoplastic syndrome. This is caused by secretion of vasoactive intestinal peptide.

DIAGNOSIS AND STAGING

Although neuroblastoma is usually suspected on clinical presentation, histologic confirmation is required by biopsy of primary or metastatic lesions.

More than 90% of neuroblastomas produce the urinary catecholamines homovanillic acid (HVA) and vanillylmandelic acid (VMA). Levels of HVA and VMA can be measured in a random urine specimen.

Evaluation of patients for the presence of metastatic disease should include computed tomography (CT) or magnetic resonance imaging (MRI) of the abdomen, plain chest radiography or CT of the chest, bone radiography, and technetium bone scan. Bone marrow aspirates and biopsies should also be done.

The International Neuroblastoma Staging System is the accepted staging system (Table 172-1).

TABLE 172-1. International Neuroblastoma Staging System[a]

Stage 1	Localized tumor with complete gross excision, with or without microscopic residual disease; representative ipsilateral lymph nodes negative for tumor microscopically (nodes attached to and removed with the primary tumor may be positive)
Stage 2A	Localized tumor with incomplete gross resection; representative ipsilateral nonadherent lymph nodes negative for tumor microscopically
Stage 2B	Localized tumor with or without complete gross excision, with ipsilateral nonadherent lymph nodes positive for tumor; enlarged contralateral lymph nodes must be negative microscopically
Stage 3	Unresectable unilateral tumor infiltrating across the midline,[b] with or without regional lymph node involvement; or localized unilateral tumor with contralateral regional lymph node involvement; or midline tumor with bilateral extension by infiltration (unresectable) or by lymph node involvement
Stage 4	Any primary tumor with dissemination to distant lymph nodes, bone, bone marrow, liver, skin, and/or other organs (except as defined for stage 4S)
Stage 4S	Localized primary tumor (as defined for stage 1, 2A, or 2B) with dissemination limited to skin, liver, and/or bone marrow[c] (limited to infants less than 1 year of age)

[a]Multifocal primary tumors (e.g., bilateral adrenal primary tumors) should be staged according to the greatest extent of disease, as defined, and followed by a subscript M (e.g., 3_M).
[b]The midline is defined as the vertebral column. Tumors originating on one side and crossing the midline must infiltrate to or beyond the opposite side of the vertebral column.
[c]Marrow involvement in stage 4S should be minimal (i.e., less than 10% of total nucleated cells identified as malignant on bone marrow biopsy or marrow aspirate). More extensive marrow involvement would be considered to be stage 4. The ^{131}I-meta-iodobenzylguanidine scan result (if performed) should be negative in the marrow.
From Brodeur GM, Pritchard J, Berthold F, et al. Revisions of the international criteria for neuroblastoma diagnosis, staging, and response to treatment. *J Clin Oncol* 1993;11:1466.

TUMOR BIOLOGY

Clinical indicators such as patient age at diagnosis and stage of disease are helpful in assigning prognosis, but inherent tumor biology has independent prognostic value for the patient. The most important biological factors include tumor cell DNA content, N-myc protooncogene amplification, and tumor histopathology.

In infants with neuroblastoma, increased DNA content (DNA index) is associated with favorable outcome. In children older than 1 year, it is not prognostically useful. Amplification of N-myc number is associated with aggressive, advanced-stage disease and a poor prognosis regardless of clinical indicators. Favorable and unfavorable histologies can be classified and directly relate to prognosis.

TREATMENT

Both clinical and biological factors are used to assign a risk of relapse to patients and to tailor therapy accordingly. Within the three defined risk categories, surgery, chemotherapy, and radiation therapy are variably used.

The patient's clinical status must always be assessed. Neuroblastoma can present as a variety of oncologic emergencies. For example, respiratory failure can occur due to airway compression from intrathoracic disease.

For patients with low-risk disease, the majority of patients need only surgery. Chemotherapy is reserved for patients who present with emergent disease or for those patients with unresectable recurrence of disease. Survival rates exceed 95% with this approach.

Intermediate risk disease is treated with surgery and multiagent chemotherapy with or without radiation therapy. Platinum compounds, epipodophyllotoxins, cyclophosphamide, and doxorubicin, are among the most active agents. Radiation therapy may be useful in controlling disease that remains unresectable after chemotherapy. Treatment results in a survival rate of more than 90%.

The long-term survival for high-risk disease remains less than 20%. However, short-term survival rates have been improved with newer intensive multiagent chemotherapy regimens. Rescue with autologous bone marrow or peripheral blood stem cells has allowed intensified therapy for patients with high-risk disease.

CHAPTER 173
Retinoblastoma

Adapted from Donald H. Mahoney, Jr.

INCIDENCE, LATERALITY, AND MORTALITY

Retinoblastoma is a rare, malignant tumor of the retina. The worldwide incidence of retinoblastoma is 1 case per 18,000 to 30,000 live births with no racial or gender predilection. The average age at presentation ranges between 13 and 18 months; more than 90% of the cases are diagnosed by age 5 years. Retinoblastoma usually remains confined to the eye for months or even years. With early diagnosis, the overall 5-year survival rate exceeds 90%.

Retinoblastoma occurs unilaterally in 70% to 75% of cases. In more than 70% of cases, the tumor originates from a single focus. Multifocal involvement is more common with bilateral disease with the multiple tumor foci presenting simultaneously or developing within weeks to months after the original diagnosis. Bilateral disease is detected at an earlier age (median, 13 months) than unilateral disease (median, 24 months) and carries a worse prognosis due to an increased incidence of nonocular malignant tumors.

GENETICS

Retinoblastoma occurs in both hereditary (germinal) and nonhereditary (nongerminal) forms. A postulated "two-hit" mutational event is necessary for the development of disease. The retinoblastoma gene locus resides on human chromosome 13 at band q14. This retinoblastoma gene is a prototype tumor suppressor gene in which a loss of activity of both normal alleles is associated with tumor development. Similar gene mutations have been found in some osteosarcomas, soft tissue sarcomas, and other cancers.

Germinal Mutations

Most patients (85%–90%) have no family history of retinoblastoma and represent the first mutational event within the family. All patients with bilateral retinoblastoma and approximately 15% of the patients with unilateral retinoblastoma harbor a germinal mutation. According to the "two-hit" hypothesis, a somatic mutation after the germinal mutation is necessary for malignant transformation to occur. Approximately 85% of sporadic unilateral cases are nongerminal; according to the "two-hit" hypothesis, two somatic mutations are required to produce the disease in these patients. When patients with either bilateral or unilateral retinoblastoma have the germinal mutation, 50% of their offspring will be affected by the disease, and 1 in 100 will harbor a gene but not express the disease.

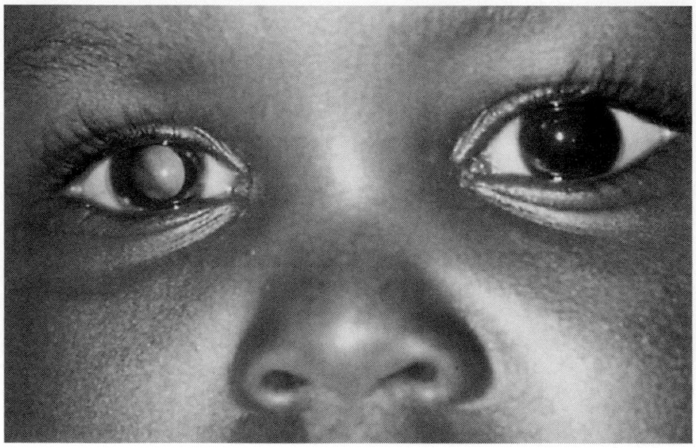

Figure 173-1. Abnormal white reflex, leukokoria, in a 7-month-old child with unilateral retinoblastoma.

SIGNS AND SYMPTOMS

The most common presenting sign (60% of patients) is a white pupillary reflex called leukokoria (Fig. 173-1) due to a centrally located tumor. The second most common sign is strabismus, present in 20% of patients. With retinoblastoma, both esotropia and exotropia may occur indicating tumor involvement of the macular area. Other signs include a red, painful eye with glaucoma (7%), poor vision (5%), unilateral dilated pupil, heterochromia (different-colored irises), or nystagmus. Children with advanced stages of disease may present with signs of lethargy, anorexia, failure to thrive, neurologic defects, orbital mass, proptosis, or blindness.

DIAGNOSIS AND DIFFERENTIAL DIAGNOSIS

During the first 2 years of life, the well-child examination should always include an assessment for strabismus and demonstration of a normal red reflex as a screen for retinoblastoma or other intraocular pathology. Any abnormal findings should be referred to an ophthalmologist.

Clinical classification systems exist to describe the intraocular extent of disease with the most widely used being the Reese–Ellsworth system. Massive tumors with extensive retinal detachment, or vitreous seeds (group V in the Reese–Ellsworth system), are associated with a poor prognosis for salvage of the affected eye.

Metastatic extension into the orbit or directly through the optic nerve tract into the central nervous system can occur. Sites of metastases include the orbit, central nervous system, bone, bone marrow, and, occasionally, the lung.

TREATMENT

The priorities in treatment for retinoblastoma are to preserve life, retain vision, and ensure favorable cosmetic results. Modalities in current use are enucleation, radiation, photocoagulation, cryotherapy, and systemic chemotherapy.

Most children with unilateral retinoblastoma present with advanced disease with little hope of vision preservation. External beam radiation (with three dimensional planning) has been the mainstay of treatment for retinoblastoma and can produce regression in virtually all tumors. Radioactive applicators, surgically attached to the sclera, have also been used.

Photocoagulation can be used to treat small tumors that appear after radiation or for treating tumors unresponsive to irradiation.

Several chemotherapy agents including vincristine, etoposide, carboplatin, and cyclosporin A have produced responses in more than 50% of patients. Together with focal treatment, tumor reduction sufficient to avoid enucleation, external beam radiation, or both may now be possible for patients with advanced-stage disease.

SECOND TUMORS

Patients who have the germinal mutation for retinoblastoma and who survive the ocular tumor have a high risk for developing other malignancies. The incidence increases with time and has been estimated to range from 30% to 50% at 20 years from diagnosis and up to 90% at 30 years from diagnosis. Tumors within the field include osteogenic sarcoma, fibrosarcoma, soft tissue sarcoma, neuroblastoma, and meningioma. Osteosarcoma of the skull occurs 2,000 times more frequently in survivors of bilateral retinoblastoma than in the general population (Fig. 173-2). The most common tumor outside the radiation field is also osteosarcoma. The mortality associated with advanced second malignancies is high.

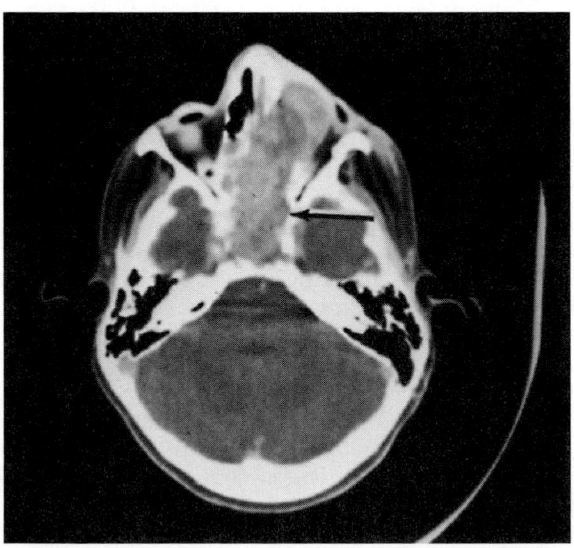

Figure 173-2. Computed tomographic scan of face, sinuses, and orbits of a 14-year-old child with bilateral retinoblastoma treated 12 years before. Note the large destructive osteosarcoma involving the left ethmoid and sphenoid area.

CHAPTER 174
Histiocytic Proliferative Diseases

Adapted from Kenneth L. McClain

LANGERHANS CELL HISTIOCYTOSIS

The term *Langerhans cell histiocytosis* (LCH) has replaced original terminology for the various syndromes in the "histiocytosis-X" category (Letterer–Siwe disease, Hand–Schüller–Christian syndrome, and eosinophilic granuloma). Common to all of these syndromes is the dendritic histiocyte, the *Langerhans cell.* These cells contain Birbeck granules and stain with monoclonal antibodies to the CD1a antigen and a neuroprotein stain, S-100.

The Langerhans cell diseases are not malignancies but are likely caused by immunologic dysregulation. The Langerhans cell is a member of the antigen-processing cells. It produces stimulating factors for T lymphocytes and other histiocytes including tumor necrosis factor–alpha, granulocyte–macrophage colony-stimulating factor, interleukin-1, interferon–gamma, and other cytokines necessary for the activation and response of T cells. Somewhere in the interactive cycle, a regulatory element is lost such that the histiocytes proliferate locally or diffusely.

Clinical Syndromes

Clinical syndromes of LCH are identified according to the degree or number of organ systems involved (e.g., LCH, solitary skull lesion).

SOLITARY LESIONS

Solitary lesions are the most benign form of LCH and can present as one or more well-circumscribed lesions in the bone. The patient presents with pain, swelling and, often, an easily palpable defect. Any bone may be involved, but the most common sites are the skull, femur, pelvis, vertebra, and mandible. Most children present between 1 and 9 years of age.

Treatments used include curettage or low-dose radiotherapy; some centers treat with chemotherapy. Most patients show sclerosis or more than 75% filling of the defect by 5 months after beginning therapy. Complete healing may take years.

MULTIPLE LESIONS

Multiorgan involvement is more prevalent in children younger than 5 years. Prognosis depends on the age of presentation (younger than age 2 have a worse prognosis) and whether any organ system function is impaired. Survival rates are 50% to 80%.

Organ dysfunction includes evidence of hepatic failure with hypoproteinemia, hyperbilirubinemia, edema, and ascites. Hematologic dysfunction includes anemia, leukopenia, neutropenia, and thrombocytopenia. Pulmonary dysfunction can manifest tachypnea, cough, pneumothorax, or pleural effusion.

Many children present with a seborrheic rash of the scalp and periauricular regions that mimic "cradle cap" or eczema. Chronic draining ears may first appear to be a chronic otitis externa. Diabetes insipidus, growth retardation, hyperprolactinemia, hypogonadism, and panhypopituitarism can occur.

Evaluation should include a complete history and physical with complete blood count, bone marrow aspirate and biopsy (when an abnormal blood count is found), complete skeletal

X-rays, bone scan, and lumbar puncture (when central nervous system symptoms are present). Even with the abnormal signs, symptoms and laboratory values, the diagnostic cell type (CD1a antigen +) must be confirmed by biopsy.

Treatment

Therapy for disseminated LCH includes prednisone and vinblastine with or without etoposide, typically for 6 weeks. Continuation of therapy with a combination of drugs is often continued for a total of 24 weeks. Patients with diffuse disease who do not respond to treatment by the sixth week have a bad prognosis. A few such patients have been treated with bone marrow transplant.

NONLANGERHANS HISTIOCYTOSES

A term given to this group is the *hemophagocytic lymphohistiocytoses*. These diseases are characterized by aggressive proliferation of macrophages and histiocytes in tissues, often accompanied by hemophagocytosis of red blood cells, other white blood cells, or platelets. The macrophages in hemophagocytic lymphohistiocytosis do not have the cellular atypia assigned to malignant histiocytes.

Hemophagocytic syndromes can be viral-associated or familial. Familial disorders include hemophagocytic lymphohistiocytosis, erythrophagocytic lymphohistiocytosis, and erythrophagocytic reticulosis. Although the laboratory findings are mostly the same as in viral-associated hemophagocytic syndromes, the familial syndromes may be recognized by a high rate of parental consanguinity, occurrence in identical twins, presence of central nervous system disease, and hypertriglyceridemia.

Diagnosis

Both forms will have significant abnormalities on peripheral blood analysis or bone marrow aspirate. Often, serum ferritin levels are very high (more than 10,000 ng/mL). Evidence for viral infections may be difficult to obtain due to multiple transfusions before titers are drawn, and, thus, it is helpful to probe leukocyte DNA for the presence of viral genomes.

Therapy

Therapy with steroids and chemotherapy for infection-associated histiocytic proliferations has been mostly ineffective. Up to 75% of the patients die from their coagulopathy or secondary infections. Allogeneic bone marrow transplantation, however, may cure more than 60% of patients.

6 Genitourinary System

CHAPTER 175
Urinary Tract Infection

Adapted from Edmond T. Gonzales, Jr. and David R. Roth

Urinary tract infection is predominantly a problem in girls. However, for the first few months after birth, the incidence of urinary tract infection in boys exceeds that of girls. A boy has approximately a 1% chance of developing an infection during childhood. In newborn boys, the incidence of urinary tract infection in those boys who have not been circumcised is approximately ten times that of boys who have been circumcised. This observation, though, is not thought to be an indication for routine circumcision in the newborn because complications from circumcision potentially negate the benefit of reducing the incidence of urinary tract infections. At this time, no data exist to suggest that remaining uncircumcised increases the risk of urinary tract infection in older boys. A girl's chance of developing an infection during childhood is close to 3%. The incidence peaks in girls between 2 and 3 years, the age that coincides with toilet training, and then returns to a baseline value between 1% and 2%.

CLINICAL CHARACTERISTICS

The signs and symptoms of urinary tract infection in an older child are the same as those seen in the adult population, namely voiding dysfunction, dysuria, hematuria, incontinence, suprapubic or flank tenderness, lethargy, and fever. However, in younger children, particularly girls under age 2 years and boys under 6 months, a urinary tract infection may present only as fever without a documented source. Young infants may present with weight loss, irritability, fever, lethargy, and cyanosis. Thus, nonspecific complaints or problems should raise the suspicion of a urinary tract infection in a newborn, although fewer than 20% of infants with nonspecific complaints and only 18% of children with specific voiding complaints actually have a urinary tract infection.

LABORATORY DATA

Documentation of urinary tract infection requires that a specimen be properly obtained. Of the several ways to collect an aliquot of urine from a child, the easiest, once a child has been toilet trained, is the midstream clean catch specimen. Before toilet training is complete, three methods remain, each with its advantages and disadvantages. The simplest, but least reliable, is an adhesive external collection bag, sometimes called a U-bag. A negative culture result from such a specimen is meaningful, but if the culture result is positive, the bacterium is possibly a contaminant from the rectum, skin, or prepuce. Therefore, whenever this method produces a positive specimen, the culture should be repeated using a more accurate method.

Two other procedures are available that should provide an uncontaminated aliquot of bladder urine. The first is a percutaneous bladder tap. In the neonate and infant, the bladder occupies an intraabdominal position making suprapubic needle access easier than in older persons. Occasionally, hematuria can result after a bladder tap, and if the bladder is not full, it can be difficult to locate.

The second method is urethral catheterization. In a small girl, visualization of the urethra may be difficult, but with practice, the procedure can be easily mastered. A small feeding tube (5 or 8 Fr.) is most appropriate for catheterization. Little risk of urethral trauma or introduction of bacteria into the bladder exists if standard care and antisepsis are used. Whereas routine urinalysis can strongly suggest that urinary tract infection is present, any treatment program should be based on an accurate culture and sensitivity. The culture is considered positive if more than 10^5 cfu/ml of one organism is growing from a catheterized specimen or if any growth of a gram-negative organism is found from a bladder tap specimen. Obtaining the culture before antibiotics are started is imperative because a single dose of medication can give a false-negative result.

CYSTITIS VERSUS PYELONEPHRITIS

Urinary tract infections are often described based on the presumed location of the infection. Cystitis is a urinary tract infection that is confined to the bladder, whereas pyelonephritis involves the kidney. Accurate delineation between the two is difficult; clinical signs and symptoms offer the most meaningful clues. High fever, nausea, vomiting, flank pain, and lethargy are usually associated with acute pyelonephritis, whereas dysuria, frequency, urgency, enuresis, suprapubic pain, and a low-grade fever are more common with cystitis. However, crossover of symptoms is common and determining whether a patient with a positive bladder urine result also has bacteria in the renal pelvis or parenchyma is difficult. Recurrent bouts of pyelonephritis may lead to renal scarring and loss of function. Currently, radionuclide renal imaging with dimercaptosuccinic acid (DMSA) is the most accurate study to demonstrate acute pyelonephritis. The decreased parenchymal uptake of the isotope has been clearly shown to correlate with areas of experimental infection in animals. In the clinical situation, however, focal decreased uptake noted during a febrile urinary tract infection could also represent an old parenchymal scar and is not necessarily a new lesion. Nonetheless, DMSA renal scanning remains the most sensitive and least invasive technique available to distinguish cystitis from apparent pyelonephritis.

TREATMENT AND FOLLOW-UP

Antibiotics

Most urinary tract infections can be treated adequately on an outpatient basis with a 7- to 10-day course of antibiotics. If shorter courses are used, the recurrence rate is higher. Initial treatment should begin after a urine specimen for culture and sensitivity has been obtained. The most common organism isolated from urine cultures has traditionally been Escherichia coli. Amoxicillin (20–50 mg/kg/day in three divided doses) or trimethoprim–sulfamethoxazole (8–10 mg/kg/day of the TMP component in two divided doses) can be started empirically. Recently, there has been an increase in ampicillin resistant E. coli, therefore, it is important to review the culture and sensitivity results and adjust therapy as needed. Some authors recommend a repeat culture to confirm eradication of the infection approximately 1 week after completion of treatment. A child with severe symptoms accompanying pyelonephritis often requires hospitalization for parenteral antibiotics and control of nausea and vomiting. For the child with frequently recurring infections (at least for a year), a long-term, low-dose daily prophylactic antibiotic (usually nitrofurantoin or trimethoprim–sulfamethoxazole at one-fourth to one-half of the therapeutic dose) is appropriate. Usually the medications are given for 6 to 12 months. Subsequent follow-up should include regular urinalyses and cultures when indicated.

Diagnostic Studies

All children with a documented urinary tract infection should undergo adequate studies to evaluate the anatomy of the urinary tract. Generally, studies to evaluate both the lower tract (the urethra and bladder) and upper tracts are suggested. This recommendation is based on the clinical observation that children most likely to sustain renal parenchymal damage from infection are those who have an anatomic defect of the urinary tract. For the older girl with symptoms of simple cystitis, performance of only an upper tract study may be sufficient because it will reveal any significant pathology. The positive yield from these evaluations is age- and gender-dependent and ranges up to 50% in young girls with pyelonephritis (primarily from discovery of vesicoureteral reflux). If an anatomic anomaly such as obstruction or reflux is discovered, it must be addressed.

The diagnostic studies available to evaluate the lower tract include either a voiding cystourethrogram (VCUG) or a nuclear cystogram. The VCUG provides optimal anatomic detail, allows for grading of reflux that may be present, and is the only study that delineates the male urethra. The nuclear cystogram is a sensitive test to identify the presence of reflux and results in less radiation exposure than the VCUG. Nuclear cystogram is the optimal test to follow reflux over the long term. Imaging of the upper tracts is nearly always begun with the renal ultrasound. This study provides excellent anatomic detail, is independent of renal function, has no untoward biological effects, and is painless. Radionuclide renal scanning with DMSA is more sensitive at identifying focal scarring, but it is not routinely used in the initial evaluation of a urinary tract infection.

CHAPTER 176
Enuresis

Adapted from Richard O. Carpenter

DIAGNOSIS

A definition of functional enuresis can be found in the *Diagnostic and Statistical Manual of Mental Disorders*, Fourth Edition (DSM-IV), of the American Psychiatric Association (Table 176-1). Primary functional enuresis refers to the situation in which the child has not been continent of urine in the past. Secondary

TABLE 176-1. *Diagnostic and Statistical Manual of Mental Disorders,* Fourth Edition, Diagnostic Criteria for Enuresis

A. Repeated voiding of urine into bed or clothes (whether involuntary or intentional)
B. The behavior is clinically significant as manifested by either a frequency of twice a week for at least 3 consecutive months or the presence of clinically significant distress or impairment in social, academic (occupational), or other important areas of functioning
C. Chronologic age is at least 5 years (or equivalent developmental level)
D. The behavior is not due exclusively to the direct physiologic effects of a substance (e.g., a diuretic) or a general medical condition (e.g., diabetes, spina bifida, seizure disorder)

Specify type:
Nocturnal only
Diurnal only
Nocturnal and diurnal

Reprinted with permission from *Diagnostic and statistical manual of mental disorders,* 4th ed. Washington, DC: American Psychiatric Association, 1994.

functional enuresis occurs when the child becomes incontinent after a period of urinary continence lasting at least 1 year. An exclusionary criterion of functional enuresis in the DSM-IV is that the urinary incontinence not be caused by the direct physiologic effects of a substance (e.g., diuretics) or a general medical condition (e.g., diabetes, sleep apnea, spina bifida, or a seizure disorder). Nocturnal enuresis refers to incontinence of urine during sleep time only. Diurnal enuresis refers to urinary incontinence during waking hours.

PREVALENCE

Enuresis is a common childhood condition that has been estimated to occur in 5 to 7 million children in the United States. The prevalence of the disorder decreases as age increases. Studies by Michael Rutter in the Isle of Wight showed that at age 5, 13.4% of boys and 13.7% of girls wet their beds at night at least once per month; by 14 years, the prevalence of nighttime enuresis decreased to 3% among boys and 1.7% among girls. After 18 years, investigators report that approximately 1% of young men have enuresis. Persistent enuresis in women after age 18 years is exceedingly rare. The spontaneous remission rate for enuresis is estimated to be 15% per year. Family studies show a strong genetic predisposition for enuresis. A study by Bakwin in 1973 showed that if both parents were enuretic as children, 77% of their children developed enuresis; 43% of children with one enuretic parent were enuretic. Concordance rates of enuresis among monozygotic twins were also greater compared with dizygotic twins (68% versus 36%, respectively). More recently, Eiberg and colleagues in Denmark have suggested a genetic linkage of primary nocturnal enuresis to chromosome 13q. In 11 families, primary nocturnal enuresis followed an autosomal dominant mode of inheritance with penetrance of more than 90%.

ETIOLOGY

Multifactorial Etiology

Investigations into various conditions predisposing to or maintaining enuresis in children have yielded a large body of literature indicating that the disorder has a multifactorial etiology. Clearly, physical and psychological factors play a role. Ideas that a child is enuretic as a means of expressing anger toward parents or to attract parental attention have been disproved. Instead, children with enuresis are recognized as emotionally sensitive to their condition and are likely to suffer loss of confidence, loss of self-esteem, and embarrassment if they are thought to be intentionally incontinent.

Most Common Factors

Physiologic and neuromaturational factors appear to be the most common etiologic factors predisposing to enuresis. Constitutional and genetic factors are suggested by the usual strong family history of childhood enuresis in other family members. Although not universal and comprehensive in scope, studies of age-matched enuretic and nonenuretic children suggest that some enuretic children suffer from a mild neuromuscular maturational delay in bladder function that results in a smaller functional bladder capacity compared with controls. These enuretic children have the same total bladder capacities as age-matched controls, yet they retain less urine in their bladders and are more prone to accidental incontinence.

Sleep Arousal Disorders

Sleep arousal disorders have attracted much interest. Theories of bedwetting resulting from failure of arousal from deep sleep have been tempered by new understanding that urinary incontinence occurs in all phases of the sleep cycle, as documented by electroencephalography. Frequency of incontinence is proportional to time spent in each sleep phase. Research has not ruled out that deep sleep and delayed arousal from sleep are factors in nighttime incontinence, but functional bladder capacity and time in each sleep phase are important.

Organic Causes

Incontinence can be the result of organic causes including anatomic defects of the genitourinary system (e.g., epispadias, posterior urethral valves), constipation with a large fecal mass decreasing bladder capacity, urinary tract infections, or systemic illness such as diabetes mellitus or insipidus, sleep apnea, and seizure disorders. These conditions are discoverable with a careful history, physical examination, and laboratory evaluation.

Psychological Factors

Psychological factors associated with enuresis are more difficult to categorize. Significant emotional disturbance occurs in a minority of enuretic children. The cause–and–effect relationship between emotional disturbance and enuresis is often unclear. A number of studies have shown that with effective treatment of the enuresis, the child's emotional disturbance resolves. On the other hand, studies of children during World War II indicated a relationship between high levels of fear and anxiety and higher prevalence rates of childhood enuresis. John Werry has pointed out that situational stress such as hospitalization of a young child, separation from the mother, birth of a sibling, or parental divorce is the most common cause of secondary enuresis. Charles Schaefer notes that parental toilet training procedures conducted in a high-stress and demeaning manner impede the child's ability to master the necessary skills for the maintenance of continence and set up a cycle of escalating anxiety and failure.

ASSESSMENT AND TREATMENT

Health practitioners have developed a wide range of treatment strategies for enuresis. Prevalence and etiologic information on childhood enuresis suggests that prevention of emotional difficulties in a child with enuresis may be possible by early education of parents and caregivers about the role of familial inheritance, developmental maturational issues, the role of anxiety, and the importance of patient, supportive toilet-training practices. For these interventions to be effective, such discussions should occur with the child's caregivers around the 12-month well-child visit and continue as needed through the early school years. The goal of preserving the child's self-esteem and confidence during the struggle to master continence is of paramount importance.

ORGANIC FACTORS

It is estimated that 97% of children do not have an organic cause for their nocturnal enuresis. Comprehensive medical assessment for possible organic factors combined with empathic listening to child and family concerns over the enuretic episodes often leads to a good understanding of the child's problem and lays the groundwork for the formulation of effective treatment strategies.

Pediatric History and Examination

A careful pediatric history that includes detailed information about the onset of difficulties with urinary incontinence (primary or secondary enuresis), frequency of accidents, precipitating circumstances, associated emotional or behavioral disturbance, and the motivation of child and caretakers to achieve change helps to guide the practitioner in ruling organic etiologies in or out. Physical examination of the oropharynx can help to rule out possible predisposing factors to nocturnal enuresis caused by sleep apnea. Dietary measures in an obese child and adenoidectomy in obligatory mouth breathers can be curative. Examination of the abdomen can reveal bowel or bladder fullness suggesting fruitful avenues of investigation including studies to rule out urinary tract obstruction (e.g., voiding cystourethrography), neurogenic bladder (e.g., bladder ultrasonography), or bowel distention due to fecal impaction (e.g., abdominal flat plate radiography). Examination of the external genitalia for physical defects (e.g., meatal strictures, ectopic placement of genitourinary structures, adhesions, signs of trauma) can further rule out physical problems that might contribute to enuresis.

Tests

Laboratory testing of electrolytes and serum glucose, urinalysis with a specific gravity, and urine culture alert the practitioner to possible difficulties with bladder infection, significant renal disease, or diabetes mellitus or insipidus. Barton Schmitt has repeatedly emphasized the importance of determining a child's bladder capacity in the laboratory assessment of enuresis. Schmitt teaches that normal bladder capacity in ounces for children is age plus 2, with adult bladder capacity in the 12- to 16-oz range. Schmitt's rule of thumb is that if bladder capacity is normal, the enuretic problem yields to simple motivational techniques. If bladder capacity is reduced from normal, the problem is more challenging to treat, often requiring behavioral techniques (e.g., nighttime wakening to void, reduced fluid intake several hours before bedtime), medication management, or both.

EDUCATION AND BEHAVIORAL TREATMENTS

Frustrated parents and caregivers burdened by their child's repeated episodes of incontinence can develop the belief that their child's behavior stems from laziness or a desire to anger or get back at the caregiver. This frustration can lead to mutual resentment, higher levels of anxiety and, occasionally, abusive situations. Clinicians are wise to intervene in these situations and to help the family and child understand that enuresis is a developmental condition that resolves with time and is amenable to treatment. Enuresis is not a product of willful misbehavior.

Toilet Training

The implementation of a behavioral reward system enhances toilet training procedures, structures parent and child interactions related to toileting, and effectively decreases episodes of urinary incontinence. A calendar can be hung in the child's room with stickers or stars used to record successful voids in the toilet during the day or to record dry nights. This emphasizes and encourages the child's success. The calendar can be taken to visits with the treating clinician so that the child's progress can be monitored over time.

Bladder Training

Another form of behavioral treatment involves bladder training. One method, retention-control training, advocates increasing the child's daily intake of fluid and encouraging him or her to hold urine in the bladder until the point of discomfort. As the bladder stretches to full capacity, the child may squirm and complain of discomfort. At this point, the child is helped by caregivers or teachers to link these feelings of bladder fullness with the need to go to the bathroom to void. Over time, this conditioning process allows the child to gain voluntary control over continence. This method can be particularly helpful with children suffering from attention-deficit hyperactivity disorder and enuresis because it helps the child pay attention to bladder signals.

A second method of bladder training that is particularly helpful in developmentally delayed or mentally retarded individuals uses the behavioral approach of clock training. In this treatment, parents or caretakers place the child on the toilet at regular intervals throughout the day. The time intervals start at a point where the chances are maximized that the child will successfully void in the toilet (e.g., an initial schedule consists of trips to the toilet every 30 minutes throughout the day with 10-minute sits on the toilet each time). Successful voids on the toilet are reinforced with praise or an opportunity to play with a favorite toy for several minutes. Once daytime continence is achieved and maintained on a particular clock interval schedule, intervals between trips to the toilet may be systematically lengthened by increments of half an hour to 1 hour. A goal of intervals of 3 to 4 hours between trips to the toilet may be reasonable in older children.

Behavioral Rewards and Enuresis Alarms

The most successful treatment for nocturnal bed-wetting involves the combination of behavioral rewards with an enuresis alarm. As miniaturization technology has advanced, alarm devices have become smaller, lighter, and more effective. The treatment involves the attachment of a moisture-sensing device to the pajama bottoms in the child's genital area and the placement of a buzzer alarm attached to a Velcro strip on the clothing over the child's shoulder. When the sensor device becomes wet, the alarm sounds. With the device, the child is awakened from sleep quite quickly after the initiation of micturition. Once awake, the child should get out of bed and finish voiding in the toilet. Bed clothing should be changed and the child should return to sleep. Over time, the child is classically conditioned to awaken from sleep when the bladder is full and before voiding. Numerous clinical studies have shown that approximately two-thirds of children respond favorably to this treatment. Subsequent relapse rates after this treatment is low. Children at least 8 years old are typically developmentally ready and have enough motivation to use enuresis alarms.

MEDICATION TREATMENT

Two types of medications have been used for the management of enuresis. In general, studies in the literature have demonstrated that these pharmacologic treatments are less effective than the behavioral treatments described previously. Furthermore, after discontinuing the medication, relapse rates are quite high. Most clinical experience has been accumulated with two drugs: the tricyclic antidepressant imipramine and desmopressin (DDAVP), the synthetic analogue of vasopressin.

Imipramine

Imipramine is typically used at a treatment dose of between 25 and 50 mg given by mouth as a single dose in the evening. Studies indicate that imipramine treatment stops enuresis in up to 80% of individuals within the first 2 weeks. Thereafter, however, continued treatment success may drop to less than 50% of treated individuals. Long-lasting remission of nocturnal enuresis with imipramine treatment occurs in roughly 25% of patients. The mechanism of imipramine's therapeutic action is unknown. Proposed mechanisms include altered sleep rhythms or altered sleep architecture and anticholinergic effects on bladder musculature. The risk of death from accidental imipramine overdose, particularly with younger siblings in the household, is significant because of the degree of cardiac toxicity of high blood levels of this tricyclic compound. The potentially serious side effects of imipramine treatment for enuresis must be carefully weighed against the morbidity associated with this nonlife-threatening condition.

DDAVP

Recently, intranasal and then oral 1-deamino-8-D-arginine vasopressin (DDAVP), the synthetic analogue of antidiuretic hormone, has been used for treatment of nocturnal enuresis. Studies of DDAVP in humans have demonstrated enhanced antidiuretic potency, diminished pressor activity, and a prolonged half-life and duration of action compared with treatment with antidiuretic hormone. The theoretic rationale for the use of DDAVP in children with nocturnal enuresis centers on the hypothesis that some children may not have the ability to concentrate urine and, thereby, decrease urine volume production at night because of dysregulation of the circadian release of antidiuretic hormone or to reduced sensitivity of receptor sites on renal distal tubules. A number of controlled studies in children treated for periods up to 4 to 12 weeks with the intranasal form have demonstrated improvement in up to two-thirds of patients. Common adverse side effects include complaints of rhinitis, nasal congestion, headaches, abdominal cramps and, rarely, epistaxis. Several reports have shown significant difficulties with electrolyte imbalance, hyponatremia, and subsequent seizures. Desmopressin is contraindicated in patients with habit polydipsia, hypertension, or heart disease. Because of a high relapse rate with DDAVP, many authors prefer behavioral interventions such as enuresis alarms. However, some authors have more recently acknowledged that a role for shorter-term use of desmopressin may exist in situations in which children spend nights at friends' homes or attend summer camp.

CHAPTER 177
Glomerulonephritis

Adapted from Eileen D. Brewer and Phillip L. Berry

OVERVIEW OF GLOMERULONEPHRITIS

Glomerulonephritis (GN), a heterogenous group of diseases, is the result of immune processes that injure the glomeruli. GN appears to be mediated primarily by immune mechanisms that invoke inflammatory reactions causing alteration of glomerular structure and function throughout both kidneys. Impairment of tubular function, which may be present but is not predominant, results from either glomerular injury itself or from direct immunologic injury similar to that affecting the glomeruli.

Pathogenesis

Although the pathogenesis of GN has been studied actively since the 1950s, it is not understood fully. Injury induced by nephritogenic immune complexes, coagulation factors (platelet activating factors and fibrin), and reaction to exogenous toxins (D-penicillamine, trimethadione, probenecid, captopril, mercury, and gold) may all contribute to the complex pathology of these disorders.

Clinical Presentations

GN may present clinically in various ways. Classification by clinical presentation (Table 177-1) is helpful in narrowing the differential diagnosis and in directing the diagnostic evaluation. The acute nephritic syndrome is the sudden onset of hematuria, either gross or microscopic; proteinuria; decreased GFR; occasionally oliguria; and retention of salt and water, which may be associated with edema, circulatory volume overload, and hypertension. The hallmark of this syndrome is hematuria and red blood cell casts in the urine with only minimal to moderate proteinuria. Acutely decreased GFR may result from decreased filtration surface area caused by cellular proliferation, endothelial swelling, and neutrophil infiltration; from inflammation-mediated local vascular changes that decrease net filtration pressure; and from obstruction of Bowman's space by fibrin

TABLE 177-1. Clinical Presentation of Glomerulonephritis

Acute nephritis syndrome
Chronic glomerulonephritis
Asymptomatic hematuria or proteinuria
Chronic renal failure
Rapidly progressive glomerulonephritis
Nephrotic syndrome

deposition and crescent formation. The mechanism for salt and water retention is poorly understood. It may occur without changes in serum albumin concentration and is often out of proportion to the decrease in GFR. Volume overload leads to suppression of aldosterone and impaired potassium and hydrogen ion excretion, which contribute to the hyperkalemia and acidosis observed in some acutely nephritic patients.

Patients with chronic GN may have few overt symptoms. Asymptomatic hematuria or proteinuria discovered on routine urinalysis may be the only presenting sign. Likewise, malaise, fatigue, anemia, and failure to grow normally may be the only signs of slowly progressive chronic GN with chronic renal failure.

If the clinical course is one of nephritis with rapid renal function decline to uremia and (often) permanent loss of renal function, the presentation is termed rapidly progressive GN. Frequently, renal biopsies from affected patients show glomerular crescent formation alone or in addition to identifying characteristics of a specific histopathologic type of GN.

Patients with the nephrotic syndrome (NS) have massive proteinuria (greater than 40 $mg/m^2/hour$ in children), hypoproteinemia, hyperlipidemia, and edema. Hematuria, either gross or microscopic, may be present but is not the prominent feature (see Chapter 178).

This chapter discusses the many kinds of GN of children and adolescents under the major headings of these clinical presentations. Because most of the disease entities that present with the acute nephritic syndrome may also have an insidious onset characteristic of chronic GN, acute and chronic GN are grouped together.

ACUTE AND CHRONIC CHILDHOOD GLOMERULONEPHRITIS

The disorders that may present primarily with hematuria and red blood cells casts, whether in an acute or chronic fashion, include IgA nephropathy, Henoch–Schönlein purpura (HSP) nephritis, lupus nephritis, the nephritis of chronic bacteremia, and membranoproliferative GN (MPGN). Because patients with MPGN usually present with the NS, this disease entity is discussed in detail (see Chapter 178, Nephrotic Syndrome). Patients with acute poststreptococcal GN (APSGN) always present acutely, although occasionally the signs and symptoms may be so mild that patients do not seek medical attention.

ACUTE POSTSTREPTOCOCCAL GLOMERULONEPHRITIS (APSGN)

APSGN is the most common form of immune–mediated nephritis in children. It is by far the most common form of postinfectious nephritis, although infection with various other bacterial, viral, parasitic, rickettsial, and fungal agents may be followed by an acute nephritic syndrome similar to that experienced after infections with nephritogenic strains of group A beta-hemolytic streptococci. Historically, most cases of APSGN were related to type 12 group A streptococci, but the current list of nephritogenic types has been expanded to include types 1, 2, 3, 4, 18, 25, 49, 55, 57, and 60 and, perhaps, 31, 52, 56, 59, and 61. In contrast to "rheumatogenic" strains of group A streptococci, which cause acute rheumatic fever associated with pharyngeal infection, nephritogenic strains of group A streptococci may cause either pharyngeal or skin infections. APSGN may occur in epidemics but is more often encountered sporadically. The attack rate in epidemics has been estimated at approximately 10% to 12%. However, incidence figures are extremely unreliable because many cases of APSGN are mild and do not come to medical attention. In fact, APSGN may occur without any accompanying identifiable urinary abnormalities.

Susceptibility to APSGN may be determined genetically and may depend on favorable host factors. Most often, the disease occurs in elementary school children (mean age, 7 years), affects twice as many male as female individuals, and is fairly rare before age 3. An episode of group A streptococcal throat or skin infection precedes all cases of APSGN. In most instances, the interval between the infection and the onset of clinical GN is about 8 to 14 days, although both longer and shorter intervals have been reported.

Proof of the previous infection by culture is seldom available, but serologic evidence of streptococcal infection (i.e., an elevated specific antibody titer) is present at the time of presentation. Serum antistreptolysin O (ASO) titer is elevated in 80% of cases associated with antecedent pharyngitis. The characteristic rise in the ASO titer is blunted by antimicrobial therapy, and the ASO titer is seldom elevated after skin infection. When antihyaluronidase (AHT) and antideoxyribonuclease B (antiDNase B) titers are also measured, proof of preceding infection nears 100%. The latter titers are particularly important if the preceding infection was a pyoderma. Elevation of serum antistreptococcal titers is essential to diagnose APSGN with certainty, but the magnitude of the titers holds no prognostic significance. The absence of serologic confirmation of a recent streptococcal infection renders the diagnosis of APSGN suspect, and other forms of nephritis should be considered (see Differential Diagnosis).

Clinical Characteristics

The clinical expression of APSGN is fairly variable and extends from a completely asymptomatic form to the most severe manifestations of acute renal failure including edema, oliguria, congestive heart failure, hypertension, and encephalopathy. The most common presenting symptoms are hematuria, proteinuria, and edema, often accompanied by rather nonspecific findings of lethargy, anorexia, vomiting, fever, abdominal pain, or headache.

Gross hematuria is present in only 30% to 50% of children with APSGN. Usually, the urine is described as smoky, tea-colored, cola-colored or, occasionally, dirty green. At least two-thirds of hospitalized patients have edema, which is initially mild and may be noted only periorbitally but can become fairly marked, especially if normal fluid intake occurs over several days at the height of the disease. Such evidence of circulatory congestion as orthopnea, dyspnea, cough, auscultatory rales, and gallop rhythms are apparent on physical examination in many children with edema. Usually, chest radiography shows cardiomegaly and pulmonary edema of varying degrees. Severe congestive heart failure is very rare. Hypertension is fairly common in inpatients (50%–90%), but hypertensive encephalopathy, characterized by headache, somnolence, convulsions, coma, confusion, aphasia, transient blindness, agitation, or combativeness, occurs in only a few (5%).

Laboratory Features

Laboratory investigation should begin with a careful analysis of the urine. The specimen may be yellow, slightly discolored, or grossly bloody and usually has a high specific gravity and a low pH. Microscopic hematuria with predominantly dysmorphic erythrocytes in the centrifuged urinary sediment is present in virtually all cases, and leukocyturia is almost as common. Red blood cell casts are found very often (60%–85%) in centrifuged specimens in which the resuspended sediment is freshly examined and exhibits an acidic pH. Often, leukocyte casts, in addition to hyaline and granular casts, are seen. The presence of leukocytes and leukocyte casts should not be considered evidence of superimposed urinary tract infection but rather of glomerular inflammation. Proteinuria occurs in most cases and correlates qualitatively with the amount of blood in the urine reaching nephrotic proportions in fewer than 5% of patients.

A laboratory evaluation for streptococcal infection is mandatory. Serum ASO, AHT, and antiDNase B titers (as described) are most helpful for confirming previous recent infection. AHT determinations have been discontinued in many laboratories because of difficulties in interpreting the test (which may be positive in other diseases). Throat and skin lesion cultures may also be positive at the time of nephritis and should be treated with appropriate antibiotics. Because asymptomatic family members may also produce positive cultures, family screening for subclinical streptococcal disease and nephritis has been recommended.

One of the most important diagnostic laboratory findings in APSGN is a depressed serum concentration of C3. Activation of the alternate pathway of complement occurs in most cases resulting in reduced serum C3 levels in at least 90% of patients examined in the early phase of their nephritis. Occasionally, serum C4 is also depressed. In most cases, serum C3 returns to normal concentrations 10 days to 8 weeks after the onset of the nephritis. If the serum C3 is not measured within the first few days of presentation of the nephritis, the concentration may have already returned to normal and its depression will have been missed. Because prior treatment of the streptococcal infection with penicillin may attenuate the period of depression of serum C3, the serum C3 may appear normal at the time of presentation of the nephritis. The degree of serum C3 depression bears no relationship to the severity of the disease. A follow-up serum C3 must be obtained 6 to 8 weeks after the onset of the acute episode to document the return of a normal concentration. If the concentration remains low, other kinds of nephritis such as MPGN or lupus are more likely, and renal biopsy confirmation of the diagnosis should be sought. Notably, this traditional approach may be tempered by further observation in patients who have resolving symptoms but complement levels that have not entered the normal range within 8 weeks.

Usually, GFR is depressed in hospitalized patients during the acute stage of moderate to severe nephritis. Serum urea nitrogen may be elevated disproportionately to serum creatinine. Even when GFR is normal or only slightly decreased, severe salt and water retention may occur. Usually, urine volume is reduced, but severe oliguria is uncommon. Urine-concentrating ability is well preserved. Usually, the fractional excretion of sodium is less than 1%, even in the presence of reduced GFR. The acutely inflamed kidney of APSGN retains sodium, even in the face of acute renal failure, unlike the high fractional excretion of sodium that occurs in acute tubular necrosis. If a child with APSGN is allowed free access to fluids, dilutional hyponatremia may develop. When acidosis and hyperkalemia occur, they are the results of aldosterone suppression caused by extracellular volume expansion and of reduced GFR, if severe.

Pathogenesis

On the basis of morphologic, serologic, and clinical parameters, APSGN is widely accepted to be immune complex–mediated, although its precise mechanism is unknown. Immune complexes containing IgG and C3 have been identified in the serum of these patients; however, attempts to identify streptococcal antigens within these complexes, either in the circulation or fixed in glomeruli, have been negative or inconclusive, and repetition is difficult. Possibly, streptococcal antigens bind to the glomerular capillary wall forming the nidus for in situ immune complex formation. Additionally, streptococci themselves possibly produce glomerular injury and set the stage for inflammatory changes, or streptococci may induce autologous IgG/antiIgG complexes through neuraminidase desialation of host IgG and neoantigen formation.

Differential Diagnosis

At their onset, many renal disorders may mimic APSGN, but only a few do so commonly and with great synonymy. The absence of proof of preceding streptococcal infection or the simultaneous occurrence of infection plus nephritis tends to discount the diagnosis of APSGN. GN caused by infectious agents other than streptococci (staphylococci, viruses) is usually coincident with the infection and often lacks the telltale sign of hypocomplementemia. Usually, the course of other infection-associated GN depends on the natural history of that infection rather than the renal manifestations.

Other disorders frequently confused with APSGN include benign hematuria, IgA nephropathy, hereditary nephritis, idiopathic hypercalciuria, and resolving episodes of previously undiagnosed postinfectious GN. Episodic hematuria coincident with an upper respiratory tract infection and normal serum complement levels help to distinguish these disorders. In contrast, MPGN may present as an acute nephritic syndrome during a streptococcal infection but with hypocomplementemia that, when reassessed at a later date, does not resolve.

The nephritis of HSP may precisely mimic APSGN if associated with mild extrarenal manifestations and an evanescent rash. A careful history and physical examination may uncover the true diagnosis in such cases. Preceding streptococcal infection and hypocomplementemia are rare.

The exacerbation of a chronic previously unrecognized GN must also be excluded. Affected patients may exhibit episodic gross hematuria, hypertension, or azotemia at the time of an intercurrent infection. A prior history of renal symptoms or features of chronic renal failure such as growth retardation or renal osteodystrophy should be carefully sought to help to distinguish them from APSGN.

Treatment

No specific or general therapy is effective in ameliorating the inflammatory lesion of APSGN. All therapy is supportive and directed toward treating the clinical manifestations of acute nephritis. Hypertension is usually only mild to moderate in severity, however, it may be severe requiring emergency treatment. Severe hypertension with encephalopathy demands immediate treatment. Fast-acting vasodilators such as intravenous diazoxide (3–5 mg/kg per dose), intravenous hydralazine (0.15 mg/kg per dose), or sublingual nifedipine (0.25–0.50 mg/kg per dose) are suitable choices for initial therapy. If multiple doses are required, maintenance antihypertensive therapy should be started. Loop diuretics and fluid restriction are important adjunct therapies and usually suffice alone for mild hypertension and for relieving edema and circulatory congestion. Restricting fluid intake to an amount equal to insensible water loss may obviate the need for diuretic therapy. On the other hand, the use of diuretics may allow affected patients to have a more palatable diet and to avoid the psychological tension associated with severe fluid restriction. Patients with oligoanuria may respond poorly to diuretics and, thus, require strict fluid restriction for control of edema and hypervolemia. In such patients, hyperkalemia should be anticipated and treated with dietary potassium restriction, binding resins, or dialysis as needed.

All patients should receive a course of penicillin or other antistreptococcal antibiotic if evidence of ongoing throat or skin infection is present. This therapy in no way influences the course or prognosis of the nephritis. Unless the disease is particularly severe and the affected child chooses to rest, bed rest is no longer recommended during the course of APSGN. Dietary limitations of sodium, potassium, and water may be necessary during hospitalization but are usually liberalized before affected patients are discharged from the hospital. Patients who require maintenance antihypertensive therapy should continue on dietary sodium restriction at home.

Prognosis

Overall, the prognosis of APSGN is excellent with full recovery expected in more than 98% of affected children. The resolution must be documented at follow-up office visits over time. Most children spend no more than 5 days in the hospital, but the disease resolves fairly slowly over many months. Few children develop chronic renal failure. Usually, hypertension resolves within 3 weeks, as does gross hematuria. The latter may be exacerbated by exercise or intercurrent infections, but its reappearance holds no prognostic significance. Microscopic hematuria persists for many months and has been documented for as long as 3 years in a few patients. Proteinuria resolves within a few months; its persistence should raise concern regarding the possibility of an incorrect diagnosis or chronicity. The serum C3 concentration must be measured again 6 to 8 weeks after the acute episode. Failure of C3 to increase into the normal range during this period, especially with persistent symptoms such as hypertension, gross hematuria, or heavy proteinuria, strongly suggests the diagnosis of MPGN, and a renal biopsy should be performed for confirmation.

IgA NEPHROPATHY

Currently, IgA nephropathy is considered the most common glomerular disease worldwide. It is characterized histologically by the presence of mesangial IgA deposits and clinically by chronic hematuria and normal renal function early in the course. Once considered a benign disease, IgA nephropathy is now known to progress to chronic renal failure in adulthood in as many as 40% of patients.

Clinical Characteristics

Almost three-fourths of the children who present with IgA nephropathy are boys. The mean age of presentation in childhood is 9 years. The prevalence is very high among Native Americans in the southwestern United States and very low among blacks. Hematuria is the most common initial sign occurring microscopically in 100% and macroscopically in 85% of the children with biopsy-proven IgA nephropathy. Gross hematuria may be a constant feature or it may occur episodically, usually in association with a febrile illness unrelated to the urinary tract. Proteinuria unrelated to gross hematuria occurs in approximately 40% to 50% of affected children reaching the nephrotic range in some. Isolated proteinuria is not a sign of IgA nephropathy in children. Patients with moderate to severe proteinuria are at greater risk of developing renal insufficiency. Hypertension, found in approximately 10%, is not a prominent feature, even when patients are followed for many years; usually its occurrence coincides with the development of chronic renal failure. Approximately 20% of the patients experience a mild decrease in GFR during episodic gross hematuria. Complaints of fever, malaise, and loin or abdominal pain are also common at that time. Usually, renal function returns to normal after an acute episode.

Laboratory Features

Laboratory studies, other than a renal biopsy examination, will not confirm the diagnosis of IgA nephropathy. Serum IgA levels are elevated in no more than one-half of affected patients and appear to bear no relationship to disease severity or activity. Serum IgG, IgM, and C3 concentrations are seldom abnormal.

Pathogenesis

The pathogenesis of IgA nephropathy remains uncertain after three decades of investigation. The serum IgA immune response of patients with IgA nephropathy is increased in both antigen-specific and nonspecific assays. The presence of IgA in the mesangium, the recurrence of IgA nephropathy in renal allografts, and the observations that serum IgA concentrations are increased in some patients and that IgA-containing circulating immune complexes are found in nearly one-half the patients studied strongly suggest that systemic IgA plays a role in the pathogenesis of this disease. The predominant form of IgA found in renal biopsies from affected patients is polymeric IgA1 reflecting the increased serum concentration of polymeric IgA1. Serum IgA1 has been found to have abnormal O-glycosylation in patients with IgA nephropathy and HSP nephritis but not with other glomerulonephritides. A combination of polyclonal stimulation of IgA plus structural abnormalities of IgA may lead to mesangial deposition of IgA1 and glomerular injury. Secretory IgA (IgA2) does not appear to play a major role in the immunogenesis of IgA nephropathy.

A genetic predisposition of some patients to IgA nephropathy is suggested by the white male preponderance; by the association of HLA-types BW35, B27, DR1, and DR4 with IgA nephropathy; and by the occurrence of the disease in multiple members of the same family and in HLA-identical twins.

Differential Diagnosis

Microscopic hematuria with or without mild proteinuria between episodes of gross hematuria also occurs in hereditary nephritis (Alport syndrome), in benign hematuria, and in idiopathic hypercalciuria. It is occasionally seen in MPGN and rarely in MGN. Hereditary nephritis can be distinguished from IgA nephropathy clinically if evidence of a positive family history or associated deafness is present. Usually, MPGN is associated with a decreased serum C3 level and heavier proteinuria, whereas MGN is associated with the NS and with microscopic and (less often) gross hematuria. Benign hematuria occurs without proteinuria or other signs or symptoms of renal disease. Proteinuria is also absent in idiopathic hypercalciuria, which can be diagnosed by the presence of abnormally high calcium excretion in a 24-hour urine collection.

IgA nephropathy is confused easily with APSGN, especially if the initial presentation is an episode of gross hematuria and mild systemic complaints. Unlike APSGN, IgA nephropathy demonstrates no latent period between the infection and the onset of hematuria, and the serum C3 concentration is normal. Gross hematuria persists for only a few days in patients with IgA nephropathy, usually resolving when the associated fever remits.

Distinguishing the nephritis of HSP from IgA nephropathy is even more difficult. If the rash is transient and not obviously purpuric and if the extrarenal manifestations of HSP are mild, the clinical syndrome is identical to that of IgA nephropathy. Furthermore, the renal biopsy findings of HSP nephritis are virtually identical to those of IgA nephropathy. These similarities have led some investigators to speculate that IgA nephropathy is a monosymptomatic form of HSP.

Therapy

No specific therapy is available for IgA nephropathy. The potential for progression of IgA nephropathy to chronic renal failure and end-stage renal disease has led to uncontrolled trials of prednisone, cytotoxic drugs, platelet inhibitors, angiotensin-converting enzyme inhibitors, antioxidants, plasma exchange, and combination therapies. Studies have been performed mainly with patients exhibiting severe symptoms or signs of progressive disease, which include advanced renal biopsy lesions, heavy proteinuria, or already apparent renal failure. Prednisone therapy appears to improve urinary findings in some children, a few of whom have also had improvement or stabilization of histopathologic lesions in subsequent renal biopsies. In adult patients, daily fish oil supplementation for 2 years retarded the progression of renal failure in one controlled trial but not in others. No children were studied. Multicenter controlled therapeutic trials for prednisone, fish oil, vitamin E, and other therapeutic agents are in progress for both children and adults and must be completed before specific drug therapy can be recommended. Attention should always be paid to controlling hypertension. Angiotensin-converting enzyme inhibitors are the antihypertensive drugs of choice because of their additional antiproteinuric effects.

TABLE 177-2. Disorders Associated with Rapidly Progressive Glomerulonephritis and Usually Glomerular Crescent Formation

Primary renal disorders
IgA nephropathy
Membranoproliferative glomerulonephritis type I and type II
Membranous glomerulonephritis
Alport syndrome (hereditary nephritis)
Idiopathic
Type I (anti-GBM disease without pulmonary hemorrhage)
Type II (immune complex disease)
Type III (no immune complexes, ANCA-associated)
Disorders associated with infection
Poststreptococcal glomerulonephritis
Bacterial endocarditis
Hepatitis B
Other infection (pulmonary, sinus, or intraabdominal abscess)
Disorders associated with systemic disease
Systemic lupus erythematosus
Henoch-Schönlein syndrome (anaphylactoid purpura)
Goodpasture syndrome (anti-GBM disease with pulmonary hemorrhage)
Wegener granulomatosis, polyarteritis nodosa, and other ANCA-associated vasculitides
Mixed cryoglobulinemia
Neoplasm (lymphoma, carcinoma)

ANCA, antineutrophil cytoplasmic autoantibodies; GBM, glomerular basement membrane.

Prognosis

Most children with IgA nephropathy have either a very slowly progressive or a completely benign course until adulthood. Predicting the 5% to 10% who will develop end-stage renal disease in childhood or adolescence is difficult. Heavy proteinuria, hypertension, and a renal biopsy showing glomerular proliferative lesions with crescents, sclerosis, or GBM alterations suggest a poor prognosis.

RAPIDLY PROGRESSIVE GLOMERULONEPHRITIS

Rapidly progressive GN (RPGN) is a designation given to the group of disease processes clinically characterized by a rapid deterioration in renal function to uremia and, often, end-stage, irreversible renal failure within a few weeks to months (Table 177-2). The term *rapidly progressive glomerulonephritis* has also been used to describe the pathologic lesion of diffuse glomerular extracapillary crescent formation common to many disorders that cause clinical RPGN. The terms crescentic GN and extracapillary proliferative GN, which describe the usual (but not invariable) pathologic lesion of clinical RPGN, are now used by many physicians instead of the term *rapidly progressive glomerulonephritis*. Other pathologic lesions such as the necrotizing GN of Wegener granulomatosis can also result in clinical RPGN. The term RPGN in this section includes all forms of clinical RPGN. The discussion of pathology and pathogenesis will focus only on crescent formation, the most common histopathologic lesion associated with clinical forms of RPGN.

Clinical and Laboratory Features

RPGN, either idiopathic or associated with any of the disorders in Table 177-2, rarely occurs. It affects adolescents more often than young children and adults more often than adolescents. Usually, RPGN presents with symptoms of acute GN, often gross hematuria, edema, hypertension, and oliguria–anuria. Most patients have severe anemia out of proportion to their degree of azotemia or the apparent duration of their symptoms. Other symptoms may be the same as those of the associated disorder such as the purpuric rash of HSP or hemoptysis from the pulmonary hemorrhage associated with Goodpasture syndrome or Wegener granulomatosis. Goodpasture syndrome includes the triad of nephritis (usually RPGN), pulmonary hemorrhage, and antiGBM antibody formation demonstrable in the circulation or in renal or lung tissue. Wegener granulomatosis is a systemic necrotizing vasculitis that involves the kidney, nasal mucosa, tracheobronchial tree, and lungs. Vasculitic skin lesions, sinusitis, serous otitis media, epistaxis, saddle-nose deformity, cough, eye lesions, and cardiac and neurologic symptoms may be present.

Antineutrophil cytoplasmic autoantibodies (ANCA), either cytoplasmic staining (C-ANCA) or perinuclear or nuclear staining (P-ANCA), are important serologic markers useful for differentiating the underlying disease and assessing the activity of many forms of RPGN. When ANCA are present in the serum, the glomerular lesion is always pauciimmune necrotizing and crescentic GN. Ninety percent of patients with untreated active Wegener granulomatosis are C-ANCA-positive, and 80% of the patients with pauciimmune polyarteritis nodosa are either C-ANCA- or P-ANCA-positive, whereas patients with immune complex–mediated polyarteritis are ANCA-negative. Usually, patients with the pauciimmune subtype of idiopathic RPGN (type III) are P-ANCA-positive.

Pathogenesis

Glomerular crescents are believed to derive from proliferation and epithelioid transformation of blood-borne monocytes (macrophages) that migrate from the glomerular capillary into the urinary space through breaks or gaps in an injured GBM. Leakage of fibrinogen and other intravascular contents through the pathologic gaps leads to fibrin polymerization, which probably acts as a nidus for the crescent formation. The increasing size of the proliferating crescent compresses the functional glomerulus to a smaller and smaller mass. Eventually, fibroblasts from the renal interstitium may migrate into the crescent and may convert the crescent into a sclerotic or fibrous scar. Predominance of fibrous crescents, global glomerular sclerosis, interstitial fibrosis, and tubular atrophy in a renal biopsy specimen portends a poor clinical prognosis. Unpredictably, some crescents may resolve without permanent injury. The latter outcome is more common in RPGN associated with infectious disorders such as poststreptococcal GN.

Therapy

Therapy for RPGN has been aimed at stopping glomerular injury to prevent progression of crescent formation. If indicated, therapy should be started as early as possible after diagnosis if it is to be of any value. Because RPGN is rare and is associated with many disorders of diverse etiology, no good or large controlled therapeutic trials have been or ever may be performed to document the efficacy of a given drug regimen. High-dose steroids alone or in combination with cytotoxic agents such as cyclophosphamide have not significantly altered the clinical outcome in small controlled studies. Anticoagulant therapy (heparin, warfarin, or dipyridamole) has theoretical appeal in preventing fibrin polymerization as a nidus for crescent formation. However, such therapy is dangerous in uremic patients, especially in those at risk for pulmonary hemorrhage, and not even a small controlled study has been performed to confirm its efficacy. At present, anticoagulant therapy alone or in combination cannot be recommended. Plasmapheresis in combination with high-dose steroids and cytotoxic agents is recommended for severely affected adults and also appears to be advantageous in the treatment of pediatric patients with antiGBM disorders or vasculitis (ANCA-associated such as Wegener granulomatosis or lupus), especially in the presence of pulmonary hemorrhage. Children with RPGN associated with poststreptococcal GN may need only supportive care, as often they will improve with or without drug therapy.

Prognosis

Hospitalization may be prolonged for children with RPGN. Most require dialysis and have complications such as severe hypertension. Approximately one-half the children with RPGN and crescents in more than 50% of their glomeruli by renal biopsy will progress to end-stage renal disease and will require chronic dialysis or a renal transplant. The recurrence rate of RPGN in the transplanted kidney is 10% to 30% depending on the underlying disorder.

CHAPTER 178
Nephrotic Syndrome

Adapted from Eileen D. Brewer and Phillip L. Berry

Nephrotic Syndrome (NS) is a clinical condition resulting from the loss of large amounts of protein from the blood into the urine. Usually, the amount of proteinuria is sufficient to cause hypoproteinemia and consequent edema. Hyperlipidemia and lipiduria are also part of the fully expressed NS.

The NS may be a feature of any form of childhood glomerulonephritis (GN) or may be secondary to other systemic diseases, nephrotoxins, or allergic reactions (Table 178-1). The discussion in this section concentrates on GN, specifically those histopathologic types that occur in children whose clinical presentation is primarily that of the NS itself and not of the nephritic syndrome. In this chapter, we have chosen to use the term primary NS instead of idiopathic NS or any of the other names to avoid confusion between clinical NS and the variety of pathologic entities associated with it. The specific disorders discussed are minimal-change disease (MCNS), diffuse mesangial proliferative glomerulonephritis, focal segmental glomerulosclerosis (FSGS), Membranoproliferative glomerulonephritis (MPGN), Membranous glomerulonephritis (MGN), and the NS of infants.

TABLE 178-1. Causes of the Nephrotic Syndrome

Primary nephrotic syndrome
Minimal-change disease
Diffuse mesangial proliferative glomerulonephritis
Focal segmental glomerulosclerosis
Membranoproliferative glomerulonephritis
Membranous glomerulonephritis
Secondary nephrotic syndrome
Other renal diseases
Hemolytic-uremic syndrome, anti-GBM disease, IgA nephropathy, idiopathic RPGN, diffuse mesangial sclerosis
Infectious diseases
Bacterial (poststreptococcal, infective endocarditis, shunt nephritis, leprosy, syphilis), viral (hepatitis B, cytomegalovirus, Epstein-Barr, varicella, human immunodeficiency virus), protozoal (malaria, toxoplasmosis), parasitic (schistosomiasis, filariasis)
Neoplasia
Lymphoma leukemia, Wilms tumor, pheochromocytoma, others
Medications
Mercurials, gold, penicillamine, trimethadione, mephenytoin
Systemic diseases
Systemic lupus erythematosus, Henoch-Schönlein purpura, polyarteritis nodosa, Takayasu syndrome, dermatitis herpetiformis, sarcoidosis, Sjögren syndrome, amyloidosis, diabetes mellitus
Allergic reactions
Insect stings, poison oak and ivy, serum sickness
Familial disorders
Alport syndrome, Fabry disease, nail-patella syndrome, sickle cell disease, Finnish nephrosis
Circulatory disorders
Constrictive pericarditis, congestive heart failure, renal vein thrombosis
Miscellaneous
Chronic renal allograft rejection, preeclampsia, malignant hypertension

GBM, glomerular basement membrane, RPGN, rapidly progressive glomerulonephritis.

MINIMAL-CHANGE DISEASE (MCNS)

MCNS is characterized by the onset of NS without systemic disease, hypocomplementemia, or other serious signs of renal disease. Although nephritic features (hematuria, azotemia, and hypertension) occur in 10% to 30% of children with MCNS, these signs seldom occur together and are almost never severe or persistent. Notably, patients with MCNS are young: Two-thirds of them present between ages 2 and 6. For this reason, preadolescents who have NS without nephritic signs, hypocomplementemia, or signs of systemic disease do not need a kidney biopsy before the initiation of therapy. Steroid therapy effectively induces a remission in most patients. Prompt and sustained remissions correlate well with minimal changes of glomerular morphology. Clinical and laboratory features and pathophysiology are the same as those of NS described earlier.

Pathogenesis

In 1974, Shalhoub hypothesized that MCNS may be caused by an abnormal clone of T cells that produces a lymphokine that damages the GBM. His hypothesis was based on four well-recognized clinical observations indicative of T-cell activity: Remissions of NS are induced by rubeola infection, patients with NS have increased susceptibility to pneumococcal infection, remissions of NS are induced by steroids and cyclophosphamide, and MCNS occurs in some patients with Hodgkin's disease. Many studies have investigated a potential role of lymphocytes in the pathogenesis of MCNS. Although no consistent abnormalities of T- or B-cell numbers have been found, abnormalities of lymphocyte function are present in patients with MCNS.

Serum from patients in relapse, but not those in remission, inhibits lymphocyte growth *in vitro*, either because it contains inhibitory substances or because it lacks certain factors necessary for growth. This finding may not be specific for MCNS, however, because serum from patients with FSGS and MGN also inhibits *in vitro* lymphocyte growth. Several experiments have shown that products of stimulated lymphocytes from nephrotic patients reduce the glomerular polyanionic charge of rat glomeruli. Foot process effacement was induced in some of the animals. Consistent production of proteinuria in these animals did not occur. Cellular immunity is altered in relapse, so that affected patients have markedly reduced response to tuberculin and other skin tests.

Although not specific for MCNS and apparently unrelated to glomerular injury, consistent abnormalities of immunoglobulins are found in NS. Serum IgG concentrations are decreased in relapse but usually return to normal in remission. Often, serum IgM concentration is increased in relapse and may continue to be high or may return to normal in remission. Low serum levels of IgG result, in part, from urinary loss, but decreased production and increased catabolism have also been demonstrated. The mechanisms controlling the observed abnormalities of serum IgG and IgM are unknown.

Differential Diagnosis

Differentiating MCNS from other disorders causing primary NS (Table 178-1) has been made easier by reports of the International Study of Kidney Disease in Children (ISKDC). By examining clinical and laboratory features of patients with biopsy-proven primary NS, these investigators identified certain clinical patterns suggesting the underlying renal histopathology. Usually, patients with MCNS present before age 6; those with MPGN rarely present before age 8. Hypertension is less common in MCNS (13%) than in FSGS (33%). Hematuria is transient and uncommon in MCNS (25%), but it occurs in more than one-half the patients with other diseases. Decreased serum C3 concentration occurs in three-fourths of patients with MPGN, but serum C3 is almost always normal in other forms of primary NS. Patients with MCNS almost always respond to steroid therapy, so when the diagnosis of MCNS is suspected clinically but no remission of the NS is induced after 8 weeks of steroid therapy, another diagnosis is likely, and a diagnostic renal biopsy should be performed.

Therapy and Outcome

Usually, the diagnosis of NS is suspected first in the outpatient setting. Hospitalization for a patient with newly diagnosed NS is strongly recommended for dietary and, if needed, diuretic management of edema, for initiation of steroid therapy, and for parent and patient education about the disease. At least 24 hours before starting steroid therapy, a tuberculin skin test should be obtained; if the result is negative, treatment may be started safely.

Recommendations for steroid therapy have been made by the ISKDC and others. Usually, an adequate steroid regimen consists of prednisone, 60 mg/m^2/day in three equally divided doses for 4 weeks, followed by 40 to 60 mg/m^2/day as a single dose given every other day in the morning for an additional 4 to 12 weeks. A maximum dose of 80 mg of prednisone per day is advisable. This standard approach was challenged by the German collaborative study, which showed that an initial 6-week course of daily prednisone followed by 6 weeks of alternate-day therapy resulted in a 50% reduction in the number of patients who relapsed during the subsequent 12 months, as compared with the relapse rate of patients treated with a shorter course of steroids. Typically, responsive patients lose the proteinuria within the first 3 weeks of therapy. During the period of alternate-day prednisone, the dose of prednisone is decreased gradually and then discontinued approximately 3 to 4 months after initiation of therapy.

Relapses occur in 80% of affected children, often during the period of slow prednisone tapering. During this time, the urine should be checked routinely at home for protein using a dipstick daily or at least three times weekly to screen for early signs of relapse before the onset of edema. Patients who have fewer than two relapses in a 6-month period may be treated as described for each relapse. Those who have more than two relapses in a 6-month period are called frequent relapsers and may do well on longer courses of alternate-day prednisone. Patients who cannot tolerate cessation of steroid therapy without a relapse are called steroid-dependent. Steroid toxicity may become a major problem for either frequent relapsers or steroid-dependent patients who receive high doses of daily steroids for a long period.

Frequent relapsers and steroid-dependent patients may require a diagnostic renal biopsy. If the biopsy shows MCNS and additional therapy to control the NS is desirable, a 2-month course of chlorambucil (0.2 mg/kg/day) or cyclophosphamide (2.5 mg/kg/day) may produce a sustained remission. Patients with frequently relapsing NS have more prolonged remissions than steroid-dependent patients after cytotoxic therapy. During therapy, patients should have a weekly complete blood cell count to monitor for signs of bone marrow depression that might require altering or stopping the drug dosage. Before beginning therapy with cytotoxic drugs, patients and parents should also be warned of other potential drug side effects such as sterility in male patients after long-term cyclophosphamide therapy. Cyclosporine has also been effective in inducing a remission in steroid-dependent patients, but the relapse rate after discontinuation of this drug has been substantial.

Most patients with MCNS are hospitalized for no more than a week at the time of diagnosis, and most never require hospitalization again. When feeling well, patients should attend school as usual without any special physical restrictions. A sodium-restricted diet is mandatory during relapses and while the patient is taking prednisone. Maintaining a low-sodium diet during remissions may be psychologically helpful if the child is a frequent relapser. Usually, immunizations are withheld until the child is in remission and has been off steroids for at least 3 months. No live-virus vaccine should be given to a patient or the parents or sibling(s) while the patient is taking high-dose daily steroids or cytotoxic drugs.

The long-term prognosis for MCNS is excellent. Most patients (80%) enter a sustained remission during adolescence. The overall mortality in a large group of patients with MCNS followed by the ISKDC for 5 to 17 years was 2.5%.

TABLE 178-2. Etiology of Focal Segmental Glomerulosclerosis

Primary renal
Idiopathic, with or without mesangial hypercellularity
Secondary
Reflux nephropathy
Reduced renal mass (single kidney, partial nephrectomy)
Heroin abuse nephropathy
Analgesic abuse nephropathy
Sickle cell disease
Alport syndrome
Late stage of nephritis of chronic bacteremia
Chronic rejection of renal transplant
Human immunodeficiency virus–associated nephropathy

DIFFUSE MESANGIAL PROLIFERATIVE GLOMERULONEPHRITIS

A few children, probably less than 3%, presenting with primary NS have diffuse mesangial hypercellularity with or without mesangial electron-dense deposits on renal biopsy. By immunofluorescence, the deposits are frequently identified as IgM, are occasionally associated with C3, and are located in the mesangium and rarely in the capillary loop. Biopsies with predominantly IgM deposits have been classified by some physicians as IgM mesangial nephropathy, but patients with this lesion have been found to have no distinguishing clinical features compared with other children with idiopathic NS. The significance of IgM deposits, like the pathogenesis of diffuse mesangial proliferation, is unknown. Some patients who have had serial biopsies have been noted to develop FSGS, which usually heralds a poor prognosis.

Clinically, children with NS and diffuse mesangial proliferative GN are more likely to have microscopic hematuria (90%), hypertension (50%), reduced renal function (25%), and poor initial response to steroid therapy (35%–70%). Despite their steroid resistance, patients generally have good prognoses with some undergoing spontaneous remission of NS and less than 10% progressing to severe renal failure. For those who do progress to end-stage renal disease, the recurrence rate of diffuse mesangial proliferative GN in a renal transplantation patient has been reported to be as high as 40%.

FOCAL SEGMENTAL GLOMERULOSCLEROSIS (FSGS)

FSGS is the pathologic description of a lesion that results from several etiologies (Table 178-2). Most likely, the idiopathic form also represents several different etiologic insults to the kidney, but our current knowledge does not allow differentiation into distinct types.

Clinical and Laboratory Features

Approximately 10% of the children presenting with primary NS are found on renal biopsy to have FSGS, but not all patients with FSGS present in this manner. Twenty percent of cases are diagnosed after asymptomatic proteinuria has been found; usually, these patients develop NS at a later date. Microscopic hematuria occurs in more than one-half the affected children at presentation, but gross hematuria is rare. Renal tubular defects including renal glucosuria, generalized ammoaciduria, renal tubular acidosis, partial or complete Fanconi syndrome, and concentrating defects occur occasionally and portend future progression to renal failure. Patients who are hypertensive at presentation (40%) do not have a significantly worse prognosis for progression to renal failure.

Clinical Course and Therapy

Regardless of whether the diagnosis of FSGS is made on the initial renal biopsy or a subsequent biopsy, affected children have a similar clinical course. Only 20% of children with FSGS initially respond to prednisone with a complete remission. Most of such patients relapse, and some progress to end-stage renal disease. Cyclosporine, tacrolimus, and mycophenolate mofetil have been used alone or in combination with steroids by some clinicians with varying degrees of success in selected patients in attempts to control severe NS. Pulse intravenous methylprednisolone therapy for 8 to 12 weeks in conjunction with alternate-day oral prednisone with or without an alkylating agent, either cyclophosphamide or chlorambucil, has been used successfully in numerous pediatric patients. In one series, 80% of patients attained a sustained remission of NS and maintained normal renal function over 1 to 12 years of follow-up. However, each treatment regimen used has had untoward side effects. Whether the pulse methylprednisolone regimen or other treatment combinations such as cyclosporine plus steroids may be the preferred modality of therapy for FSGS still requires comparative controlled trials that have not been accomplished to date.

Initially, renal failure is present in almost one-half of affected children. Progression to end-stage renal disease occurs in 20% to 30% within 5 years and in almost 60% within 10 years. Persistent NS and an increase in globally sclerotic glomeruli in follow-up biopsies have been associated with progressive disease. No other clinical or pathologic markers of progressive disease have been confirmed. FSGS recurs frequently (25%) in renal transplants, sometimes with massive proteinuria and NS within the first 24 hours and renal allograft loss within days to weeks. NS has remitted without allograft loss in many children treated with high-dose cyclosporine.

MEMBRANOPROLIFERATIVE GLOMERULONEPHRITIS (MPGN)

MPGN, a chronic disease of children and adults, may be idiopathic or occasionally associated with other systemic diseases. The age of onset in most patients is between 8 and 20. The male–to–female gender ratio is equal. A genetic predisposition to MPGN is suggested by the association of MPGN with an inherited deficiency of several complement components; an association with the extended haplotype HLA-B8, DR3, SC01, GL02; the occurrence of the disease in some siblings; and the rarity of the disease in blacks.

Clinical Characteristics

Approximately 10% of the cases of primary NS in childhood are caused by MPGN, but approximately only one-half of children with MPGN present with NS. Another one-fourth present with the acute NS, and approximately one-fourth present with asymptomatic proteinuria or hematuria. Gross hematuria, hypertension, and azotemia each occur in 30% of patients. When these signs appear together, MPGN is easily confused with APSGN. Most patients have microscopic or gross hematuria at onset, and almost all have proteinuria. In those presenting without proteinuria, a low serum C3 may be the only clue to the diagnosis.

Laboratory Features

Laboratory features of primary NS occur in most patients. In such patients and in those with nonnephrotic proteinuria, the urine is usually positive for blood and often contains cellular casts. Anemia is common and often disproportionate to the degree of renal failure. Serum C3 concentrations are decreased in 60% to 75% of patients at the time of diagnosis. Thus, the absence of this abnormality does not rule out the diagnosis of MPGN.

Pathogenesis

The morphologic diversity of renal biopsies from patients with MPGN suggests heterogeneity of pathogenesis. Immune complex deposition is a prominent feature of all types of MPGN. Circulating immune complexes have been measured in patients with all types of MPGN, but the presence of these complexes does not correlate with the severity of disease activity or the degree of hypocomplementemia. The stimulus for immune complex formation is unknown.

Complement activation occurs by at least two mechanisms in MPGN. In type I MPGN, immune complexes stimulate the classic pathway depleting serum concentration of C1q, C2, and C4 along with C3 and C5. Low serum C3 levels may retard the normal clearing of immune complexes from the circulation. As mentioned, inherited deficiencies of complement have been associated with MPGN type I and type III. In type II disease, alternate pathway activation by C3 nephritic factor (NF_a) reduces the serum concentration of C3, whereas C4 remains normal, and C5 is normal or minimally depressed. This type of C3 nephritic factor is an IgG autoantibody that increases alternate pathway degradation of C3. The presence of C3 nephritic factor does not appear to affect the outcome of patients with MPGN. Another recently described nephritic factor, NF_t, causes complement activation in type III MPGN and results in markedly depressed serum C3 and C5 levels with normal C4 concentration.

Course and Therapy

A few patients have spontaneous NS remissions that may last for years. The only evidence of disease activity during this "silent phase" may be persistent hypocomplementemia. The natural history of patients with MPGN is to progress slowly toward end-stage renal disease. Approximately one-half of affected patients reach end-stage disease 10 years after diagnosis. If the serum creatinine exceeds 2 mg/dL at presentation, dialysis will probably be required within 3 years. Hypertension, gross hematuria, and unremitting NS with edema portend a poor prognosis.

Historically, many treatments for MPGN including steroids, other immunosuppressants, anticoagulants, and nonsteroidal antiinflammatory agents have been tried. A double-blind, prospective, controlled trial of daily aspirin and dipyridamole therapy was associated with maintenance of a higher GFR, but the therapy had no effect on proteinuria in affected adults followed-up for many years. The ISKDC showed beneficial results of long-term alternate-day prednisone for maintaining renal function in children with all types of MPGN, but aggressive management of steroid-induced hypertension was required in some cases.

Renal transplantation is successful in patients with MPGN, although type I and type II may both recur in the allograft. The recurrence rate may be as high as 50% in type II MPGN. However, graft loss to recurrent disease is insufficient to consider withholding transplantation.

MEMBRANOUS GLOMERULONEPHRITIS

MGN is a rare disorder of children accounting for less than 6% of the cases presenting with primary NS. The frequency of occurrence increases in adolescence (10%–20%), and the disorder is common in adults with NS (20%–40%). MGN occurs as a primary renal disease (idiopathic MGN) in approximately 65% of affected children but is associated with systemic diseases or exposure to drugs and toxins in the rest (Table 178-3). The presentation of MGN may antedate the appearance of associated disorders such as SLE, hepatitis B infection, or neoplasm by months or years and may be confused with idiopathic MGN. MGN rarely recurs in renal transplants, but it does often arise de novo for reasons that are unclear, unless its occurrence is facilitated by glomerular changes of rejection.

TABLE 178-3. Etiology of Membranous Glomerulonephritis

Primary renal disease
Idiopathic (no identifiable associated condition)
Associated with infectious disorders
Hepatitis B (chronic presence of hepatitis B surface antigen)
Syphilis (congenital or secondary)
Poststreptococcal disease
Hydatid disease
Leprosy
Malaria
Associated with systemic disorders
Systemic lupus erythematosus
Thyroiditis (with thyroglobulin antibodies)
Fanconi syndrome (with antitubular basement membrane or antirenal tubular epithelial antibodies)
Sickle cell disease
Neoplasm (carcinoma, leukemia, Wilms tumor)
Other (Sjögren syndrome, Gardner-Diamond syndrome, Kimura disease, celiac disease, diabetes mellitus)
Associated with drugs or toxins
Heavy metals (gold, mercury, bismuth, silver)
D-Penicillamine
Trimethadione
Probenecid
Captopril
***De novo* in renal transplantation**

Clinical and Laboratory Features

Usually, onset of MGN symptoms is gradual. Approximately one-third of cases are discovered on routine screening urinalysis by the presence of proteinuria. The other two-thirds present with edema and NS. Proteinuria may be either selective or nonselective. Hypertension occurs in 30% or fewer cases. Microscopic hematuria is common in children with MGN (roughly 80% in some series), and gross hematuria occurs in up to 20%. Usually, renal function is normal at presentation. Serum C3 is normal, except in lupus and hepatitis B–associated MGN, in which it is usually low. Usually, patients with hepatitis B–associated MGN are younger than 10, male subjects, often black or Asian, and without overt clinical manifestations of hepatitis. Their serum aspartate aminotransferase is mildly to moderately elevated. Liver biopsies have shown evidence of chronic hepatitis. Hepatitis B antigen has been demonstrated in glomerular immune deposits in 90% or more of these patients and in the circulation of all. Usually, serum hepatitis B surface antibody is negative. Appearance of hepatitis B core antibody in the serum has correlated with remission of NS in a few patients.

Pathogenesis

The pathogenesis of MGN in humans is poorly understood, although it has been studied extensively in laboratory models. A likely possibility suggested by experimental models is that circulating antibodies react with intrinsic GBM antigens (or extrinsic antigens with an affinity for deposition in the GBM) resulting in formation of in situ immune complexes and the evolution of the events described. Alternately, deposition of preformed circulating immune complexes with an affinity for the GBM may be the initial event. Such deposits might be formed from various stimuli, either endogenous (tissue antigens) or environmental (infectious agents, drugs, toxins). The rarity of measurable circulating immune complexes in affected patients, however, makes this possibility unlikely. Genetic factors may also be important. Association of HLA-DRW3 and DQA1 allele has been demonstrated for adults with MGN.

Prognosis and Therapy

The course of idiopathic MGN is slowly progressive over years resulting in chronic renal failure within a decade in approximately only 10% of presenting children younger than 10 years and in 20% of adolescents. Remissions of proteinuria are spontaneous in up to 30% of patients. Whether any treatment should be given for children is uncertain, but for those with unremitting NS, a trial course of 8 weeks of alternate-day high-dose prednisone, followed by a tapering dose for a few weeks, seems to have little risk of toxicity. Currently, no criteria can identify children who are at risk of developing renal failure and might benefit from therapy, and no studies are able to suggest what treatment might be effective with the fewest side effects. Adults with MGN fare worse, so they are usually treated. What treatment, if any, should be given remains controversial. A well-controlled randomized trial of 6 months of alternate-day, moderately high-dose prednisone therapy showed no benefit of treatment during 4 years of follow-up in 158 Canadian adults with MGN, NS, and near-normal renal function before therapy. In contrast, another study of 81 similar adults in Italy followed for 10 years, after a well-controlled randomized trial of 6 months of high-dose daily methylprednisolone alternating monthly with daily chlorambucil, showed a significant remission of NS and better preservation of renal function for treated patients. However, 60% of untreated patients also did well, raising the issue that if all patients were treated, unneeded exposure to potentially toxic drugs might occur in many. More studies must be completed to identify risk factors predictive of progressive disease to help determine who needs aggressive therapy.

Treatment of patients with MGN and associated disorders is dictated by the underlying disorder. In children with MGN associated with congenital or secondary syphilis, early treatment with penicillin leads to rapid recovery. Usually, MGN associated with drugs or toxins is diagnosed after 6 to 12 months of exposure. Withdrawal of the inciting agent usually leads to recovery after several more months.

NEPHROTIC SYNDROME IN INFANTS

Onset of NS within the first year of life must be considered separately because a group of underlying disorders occurring in infants differs from that in children and adolescents. The most common disorder presents at birth or in the first few weeks of life, often in infants of Finnish ancestry, leading to the designation of congenital NS (CNS) or CNS of the Finnish type. Various other diseases, both primary renal and secondary to other disorders, either congenital or acquired, present in early infancy and may be confused with CNS (Table 178-4).

Primary Renal Disorders

The primary renal disorders are not easily separated by either clinical presentation or pathologic appearance of the kidney. All patients have proteinuria, hypoalbuminemia, hyperlipidemia, hypogammaglobulinemia, and normal renal function. Edema may not initially occur but appears within a few weeks. Hematuria is uncommon. Renal biopsies show effacement of foot processes, diffuse epithelial cell proliferation, mesangial cell proliferation, increased mesangial matrix, no electron-dense or immunofluorescent-positive deposits, persistence of fetal glomeruli, and microcysts. The microcysts represent dilated proximal tubules once thought to be a diagnostic feature of CNS but are now known to be a nonspecific finding of infants with NS. Focal segmental sclerosis progressing to global sclerosis with tubular atrophy and interstitial fibrosis occurs with advancing age in patients with CNS, diffuse mesangial sclerosis (DMS), and FSGS.

CNS is the most common form of NS in infants. With or without Finnish ancestry, CNS is transmitted genetically in an

TABLE 178-4. Causes of Nephrotic Syndrome in Infants

Primary renal diseases
Congenital nephrotic syndrome (with or without Finnish ancestry)
Diffuse mesangial sclerosis
Minimal-change nephrotic syndrome
Focal segmental glomerulosclerosis
Secondary to other disorders
Congenital infection (syphilis, toxoplasmosis, cytomegalovirus, rubella, hepatitis B, malaria)
Toxins (mercury, drugs)
Systemic lupus erythematosus
Neoplasm (Wilms tumor)
Denys-Drash syndrome (ambiguous genitalia, Wilms tumor, nephropathy)
Nephropathy associated with congenital brain malformation
XY gonadal dysgenesis
Lowe syndrome
Nail-patella syndrome
Hemolytic-uremic syndrome

autosomal recessive fashion. The incidence in Finland is approximately 1.2 cases per 10,000 births. Most cases seen in North America have no apparent Finnish ancestry but are not otherwise different from the Finnish cases. The abnormal gene has been localized to the chromosome 19q13.1 region in Finnish and nonFinnish kindred. Normally, the gene encodes for a transmembrane protein called nephrin, which is part of the immunoglobulin family of cell adhesion molecules and is expressed on the glomerular podocyte. The pathogenesis of CNS may be related to defects in the genes controlling GBM heparin sulfate–rich proteoglycan synthesis or degradation. Decreased synthesis or increased degradation could account for the decreased number of heparin sulfate–rich anionic sites observed in the lamina rara externa of the GBM of infants and children with CNS. The lack of anionic sites diminishes the effectiveness of the GBM as an electrostatic barrier. Proteinuria then occurs, and progressive glomerular damage ensues with time, as suggested by other experimental models of NS.

CNS may be identified *in utero* by elevation of amniotic fluid and maternal serum alpha–fetoprotein and in fetal renal tissue by foot process effacement with diffuse epithelial proliferation. In pregnancies known to be at risk, prenatal diagnosis is possible. A normal amniotic fluid alpha–fetoprotein does not exclude the presence of the disease in the fetus. Linkage and haplotype analysis of affected families may provide more precise prenatal diagnosis in the future.

Usually, infants with CNS are small for gestational age and are born prematurely. Often, umbilical hernias are prominent. Usually, the placenta is fairly large, often weighing more than 25% of the infant's birth weight. Edema is present at birth in at least one-half of patients. Even when edema is not present, proteinuria sufficiently significant to cause hypoalbuminemia and hypoimmunoglobulinemia is present. The infants are rendered immunocompromised and highly susceptible to severe bacterial infections; these infections may occur in more than 85% of patients and should be treated with supplemental immunoglobulins and specific antibiotics. Thyroxine (T4) is lost in the urine and usually leads to hypothyroidism that requires supplemental therapy. Newborn thyroid screening may detect low blood levels of T4 before the clinical diagnosis of CNS. Thyroid-stimulating hormone concentration may still be normal at that time, but a decreased serum thyroid-binding globulin concentration (owing to its urinary loss) will suggest the correct diagnosis. Later in infancy, sufficient loss of transferrin and iron or protein–bound 25–hydroxyvitamin D may cause iron deficiency anemia or vitamin D deficiency, respectively. Thromboembolic complications may occur from the hypercoagulability associated with severe chronic NS.

Renal function is normal initially but deteriorates progressively to end-stage renal disease, usually by the time children reach ages 3 to 8. Delayed growth and development and malnutrition from excessive protein losses, anorexia, and poor feeding occur in all affected infants. Untreated infants die before age 4. Good survival (80%) has been attained only by early aggressive medical therapy with dialysis and early renal transplantation. Catch-up growth and development are common after transplant. CNS does not recur in the renal transplant. Aggressive medical management should include nutritional supplementation, diuretics to control edema, anticoagulants (aspirin or dipyridamole) if indicated to control thromboembolism, and prophylactic penicillin to prevent infection. Bilateral nephrectomy and dialysis may be indicated before the onset of end-stage renal disease, even when renal function remains greater than 50% of normal, to treat severe growth failure, malnutrition, and other unresponsive complications of chronic NS. The diagnosis of CNS should be certain before nephrectomy, dialysis, and renal transplantation are contemplated.

NEPHROTIC SYNDROME SECONDARY TO OTHER DISORDERS

Secondary causes of NS in infancy (Table 178-4) may be identified by signs and symptoms of the underlying disorder such as the stigmata of congenital syphilis or nail-patella syndrome; by a history of exposure to toxic drugs (mercury teething solution); or by specific diagnostic laboratory tests. Renal vein thrombosis, once thought to be a secondary cause of NS, is now known to result from severe NS. The renal pathologic lesions of secondary NS vary from classic membranous nephropathy associated with congenital syphilis to immune complex proliferative GN associated with other congenital infections and lupus to the unique GBM nephropathy associated with nail–patella syndrome. Therapy is directed at the underlying disorder. Recovery may be rapid in congenital syphilis treated with penicillin and in lupus treated with corticosteroids. Denys–Drash syndrome, a rare genetic disorder associated with mutations of the WT1 gene on chromosome 11 and characterized by ambiguous genitalia, gonadoblastomas, Wilms tumor, and progressive nephropathy, has no specific therapy. The proteinuria is unresponsive to steroids, and renal failure occurs early reaching end stage between ages 1 and 3.

CHAPTER 179

Benign Familial Hematuria

Adapted from David R. Powell

The syndrome of benign familial hematuria (BFH) has been termed *benign, essential, primary, idiopathic, recurrent,* or *persistent hematuria*. Affected individuals usually present with persistent or intermittent microscopical hematuria noted on routine urinalysis or with gross hematuria brought on by a febrile illness. Significant proteinuria is absent. Physical examination is normal, and no abnormalities are noted with audiometric and ophthalmologic examinations. Laboratory studies reveal normal renal function and platelet count. Family history is negative for deafness, renal failure, and significant proteinuria. Screening typically identifies hematuria in other family members from multiple generations, but these individuals fail to demonstrate hearing loss, renal failure, or proteinuria.

Renal biopsies from affected individuals are normal by light microscopy and immunofluorescence; segmental glomerular sclerosis, interstitial foam cells, and fetal glomeruli are not found. Electron microscopy reveals the characteristic finding of focal or widespread thinning of the glomerular basement membrane; however, these thin segments are not interspersed with segments of thick and split glomerular basement membrane, as is typical of Alport syndrome.

The inheritance pattern of BFH is autosomal dominant in some kindred. In one such kindred, individuals from three generations had microscopical hematuria but no other abnormalities; two affected males were older than 75 years and had normal renal function. Linkage analysis implicated the COL4A3 and COL4A4 type IV collagen gene locus on chromosome 2, and the responsible mutation was found in the coding region of the *COL4A4* gene. *COL4A3* and *COL4A4* mutations are also linked to both autosomal dominant and autosomal recessive forms of Alport syndrome (Chapter 328, in Oski's Pediatrics, 3rd edition). Thus, in this and perhaps many BFH kindred, affected individuals may, in fact, be asymptomatic (but hematuric) carriers of autosomal recessive Alport syndrome.

The diagnosis and differential diagnosis of BFH are the same as for progressive hereditary nephritis (Chapter 328, in Oski's Pediatrics, 3rd edition). BFH is still a diagnosis of exclusion, especially because mutation of a single *COL4A3/COL4A4* allele can cause BFH or autosomal dominant Alport syndrome depending on the mutation. Affected male patients in some Alport syndrome kindred do not develop chronic renal failure until 50 years of age; because these individuals may not have electron-microscopical findings typical of Alport syndrome at a young age, their syndrome may be misdiagnosed as BFH. Presently, the best way to establish the diagnosis of BFH in a kindred is to obtain a characteristic renal biopsy from one affected family member (preferably an adult male family member) and to document that affected male patients live a long life free of chronic renal failure; this may prevent unnecessary future studies in affected family members. In kindred for whom the diagnosis of BFH is less clear, affected individuals should be regularly screened for development of proteinuria, renal failure, hearing loss, and hypertension. The appearance of chronic renal failure in any family member requires careful reevaluation of the original diagnosis.

CHAPTER 180
Renal Tubular Acidosis

Adapted from L. Leighton Hill
and Myra L. Chiang

Renal tubular acidosis (RTA), a biochemical syndrome characterized by a persistent hyperchloremic (nonanion gap) metabolic acidosis, is caused by abnormalities in the renal regulation of bicarbonate concentration. The abnormality can be in the reabsorption of filtered bicarbonate or in the production of new bicarbonate by hydrogen ion secretion. The glomerular filtration rate is usually normal but may be mildly depressed. RTA is traditionally classified as proximal or distal, based on the nephron segment that is thought to have an abnormal function (Table 180-1).

RTA can be caused by a variety of disorders, most of which are rare (Tables 180-2–3). Hereditary RTA is most common in children. Mutations in the red cell HCO_3/Cl exchanger gene AE1 have been shown to cause autosomal dominant distal RTA type 1. Proximal RTA can occur as an isolated abnormality, either sporadically or as an inherited disorder. However, much more commonly, proximal RTA is seen as part of the Fanconi syndrome with associated glycosuria, aminoaciduria, hyperphosphaturia, and so forth.

CLINICAL CHARACTERISTICS

RTA is usually suspected during the workup of patients with failure to thrive or unexplained acidosis. Children may have histories of repeated episodes of dehydration and anorexia.

TABLE 180-1. Pathophysiologic Classification of Renal Tubular Acidosis (RTA)

Type	Pathophysiology
Proximal RTA (type 2)	Impaired proximal tubular HCO_3 reabsorption
Distal RTA (type 1)	Impaired distal tubular H^+ secretion
Secretory defect ("classic distal RTA")	H^+ pump failure
Gradient defect	Increased back-leak of secreted H^+
Voltage-dependent defect	Reduced luminal electronegativity
Hyperkalemic distal RTA (type 4)	Impaired ammoniagenesis Voltage-dependent defect
Hypoaldosteronism	
Primary	
Secondary	
Pseudohypoaldosteronism	
Total	
Partial	
Chloride shunt	Increased NaCl reabsorption in ascending loop of Henle

TABLE 180-2. Disorders Associated with Renal Tubular Acidosis Type 2

Isolated defect
Sporadic
Hereditary
Use of carbonic anhydrase inhibitors
Fanconi syndrome
Primary, secondary
- Inherited
  - Cystinosis
  - Tyrosinemia
  - Lowe syndrome
  - Hereditary fructose intolerance
  - Wilson disease
  - Glycogen storage disease
  - Metachromatic leukodystrophy
  - Osteopetrosis with carbonic anhydrase deficiency
  - Cytochrome-*c* oxidase deficiency
- Defect in calcium metabolism
  - Hyperparathyroidism
    - Primary
    - Secondary
- Dysproteinemic states
  - Multiple myeloma
  - Light-chain diseases
  - Monoclonal gammopathy
  - Amyloidosis
- Interstitial renal disease
  - Sjögren disease
  - Medullary cystic disease
  - Renal transplant rejection
  - Chronic renal vein thrombosis
  - Balkan nephropathy
- Drugs and toxins
  - Outdated tetracycline hydrochloride
  - Maleic acid
  - Cadmium
  - Lead
  - Mercury
- Miscellaneous
  - Malignancy
  - Chronic nephrotic syndrome
  - Congenital heart disease

TABLE 180-3. Disorders Associated with Distal Renal Tubular Acidosis Type 1

Primary
Sporadic
Hereditary
Secondary (acquired)
Genetic diseases
Ehlers-Danlos syndrome
Wilson disease
Hereditary elliptocytosis
Fabry disease
Sickle cell nephropathy
Osteopetrosis with carbonic anhydrase deficiency
Medullary cystic disease
Hereditary hypercalciuria
Marfan syndrome
Sensorineural deafness
Disorders causing nephrocalcinosis
Idiopathic hypercalciuria
Medullary sponge kidney
Primary hyperparathyroidism
Hyperthyroidism
Vitamine D intoxication
Autoimmune diseases
Sjögren syndrome
Systemic lupus erythematosus
Chronic active hepatitis
Fibrosing alveolitis
Primary biliary cirrhosis
Hyperglobulinemic purpura
Thyroiditis
Cryoglobulinemia
Tubulointerstitial diseases
Obstructive uropathy
Balkan nephropathy
Chronic pyelonephritis
Leprosy
Transplant rejection
Drugs and toxins
Amphotericin B
Lithium
Toluene
Miscellaneous
Hepatic cirrhosis
Malnutrition

Others may present with clinical manifestations of hypokalemia such as polyuria, constipation, and profound weakness. In distal RTA type 1, signs and symptoms of kidney stones may precede the diagnosis of RTA. The physical examination may reveal only growth retardation or signs of dehydration. In some cases, the physical examination may suggest a secondary cause of proximal RTA such as the finding of cystine crystals in cystinosis, mental retardation in Lowe syndrome, or evidence of liver involvement in Wilson disease. Sensorineural deafness has been reported in the autosomal recessive form of distal RTA type 1.

LABORATORY EVALUATION

Proximal Renal Tubular Acidosis Type 2

As with all types of RTA, the acidosis in proximal RTA is a hyperchloremic (nonanion gap) metabolic acidosis. Usually, at presentation the patient is in a reasonably steady-state condition; the extent of lowering of the plasma bicarbonate is determined by the severity of the proximal tubular defect in bicarbonate reabsorption. This steady state has been reached because the filtered load of bicarbonate (glomerular filtration rate × plasma bicarbonate) has decreased to a point at which the amount that escapes reabsorption by the impaired proximal tubule is small enough to be completely reabsorbed by the distal nephron. Therefore, on presentation, no bicarbonate is usually present in the urine and, because the distal acidification mechanisms are intact in proximal RTA, the urine is acid (pH less than 5.5). If the patient is then treated with sufficient base, the plasma bicarbonate increases and the amount of bicarbonate filtered increases, which overwhelms the impaired proximal tubules with bicarbonate resulting in a large increase in delivery of bicarbonate to the distal nephron. The urine, therefore, contains increasing amounts of bicarbonate as the plasma level increases, and the urine becomes alkaline, even though the plasma bicarbonate may still be below normal.

In summary, patients with proximal RTA type 2 have severe bicarbonate wasting when plasma bicarbonate levels are normal, but during the untreated or acidotic state, their bicarbonaturia ceases, urinary pH becomes acid, and urinary net acid excretion approximates net acid production. At this point, a steady state is reached, and the acidosis does not become more severe. Patients with proximal RTA type 2 often have hypokalemia, but serum potassium levels may be normal. The low potassium levels have been attributed to increased delivery of sodium to the distal nephron, where, under the stimulus of aldosterone (aldosterone increases because of the sodium losses and mild volume depletion), sodium is reabsorbed in exchange for potassium ions, which are then excreted. Treatment with alkali may worsen hypokalemia by raising the filtered bicarbonate load. Patients with proximal RTA type 2 do not usually have hypercalciuria, and urinary citrate excretion is normal. Patients with this form of RTA seldom manifest the complications of nephrocalcinosis, nephrolithiasis, or rickets, which are common manifestations in patients with untreated distal RTA type 1.

Distal Renal Tubular Acidosis Type 1

The urine pH in distal RTA type 1 is never very acid (pH of 5.5 or greater), the total acid excretion is always abnormally low, and the urine anion gap is positive despite the degree of acidosis. Hypokalemia is common and may be severe or life-threatening. Hypercalciuria is also common, and urinary citrate excretion is low. These abnormalities, along with the persistently alkaline urine, are instrumental in the development of nephrocalcinosis and nephrolithiasis. Acidemia enhances proximal citrate reabsorption leading to low citrate excretion. Citrate is a potent inhibitor of stone formation. Proximal tubular functions in patients with RTA type 1 are normal.

Hyperkalemic Distal Renal Tubular Acidosis Type 4

Hyperkalemic distal RTA (type 4) is thought to be the most common type of RTA in both children and adults. It represents an abnormality of distal tubular function in regard to the renal handling of hydrogen and potassium ions. Hyperkalemia is the most distinctive clinical characteristic of this type of RTA when compared with types 1 and 2. Patients with RTA type 4 can usually make an acidic urine (pH less than 5.5), but total acid excretion is low because of very low rates of ammonia excretion. The urine anion gap is positive, and the renal excretion of potassium is inappropriate to the serum concentration of potassium. The defects in urinary potassium and hydrogen ion excretion appear to be secondary to hypoaldosteronism or to end-organ resistance to aldosterone (pseudohypoaldosteronism). Hypoaldosteronism can be primary or secondary Table 180-4).

TABLE 180-4. Clinical Spectrum of Distal Hyperkalemic Renal Tubular Acidosis Type 4

Mechanism designation	Plasma renin activity	Aldosterone	Plasma: *Blood volume*	Plasma: *Blood pressure*	Salt wasting
Hypoaldosteronism					
Primary mineralocorticoid deficiency, no intrinsic renal disease	Increase	Decrease	Normal or decreased	Normal or decreased	Yes
Primary hyporeninemic, secondary hypoaldosteronism due to intrinsic renal disease	Decrease	Decrease	Normal or increased	Normal or increased	No
Pseudohypoaldosteronism, end-organ resistant to aldosterone					
Total resistance	Increase	Increase	Decrease	Normal or decreased	Yes
Partial resistance associated with renal immaturity	Normal or increased	Normal or increased	Normal	Normal	No
Chloride shunt or Gordon syndrome	Decrease	Decrease	Increase	Increase	No

Modified from McSherry E. Renal tubular acidosis in childhood. *Kidney Int* 1981;20:799.

Primary hypoaldosteronism is seen in patients with acute adrenal insufficiency, Addison disease, and salt-losing congenital adrenal hyperplasia. Patients may show all the signs of adrenal insufficiency including salt wasting, tendency to low blood volume and low blood pressures, metabolic acidosis, hyponatremia, and hyperkalemia. Peripheral renin activity is increased, but circulating aldosterone is virtually absent. Renal function in these patients including renal tubular function is within normal limits.

Secondary hypoaldosteronism results from decreased production or release of the active form of renin caused by destruction of the cells of the juxtaglomerular apparatus, as seen in patients with intrinsic renal disease such as lupus nephropathy, diabetic nephropathy, obstructive uropathy, and interstitial nephritis. Reduction in overall renal function can be demonstrated, but the hyperkalemia and metabolic acidosis are out of proportion in severity to the degree of renal insufficiency. These patients do not demonstrate salt wasting.

Pseudohypoaldosteronism resembles primary hypoaldosteronism, except that the aldosterone level is either normal or elevated. The aldosterone resistance may be total or partial. Total resistance to aldosterone results in salt wasting, hyponatremia, and hyperkalemia. Patients have a marked tendency to develop low blood volume and hypotension, as do patients with true hypoaldosteronism; however, the peripheral renin activity and plasma aldosterone levels are markedly elevated. The severity of the renal salt wasting and potassium ion retention diminishes after infancy in most patients permitting discontinuation of salt supplements. However, the disordered renal handling of sodium and potassium appears to persist, although less severely. Partial resistance to aldosterone may occur in infants and young children. These patients have hyperkalemia and metabolic acidosis but not salt wasting. The peripheral renin activity and plasma aldosterone levels may be normal or only slightly elevated. The abnormalities are transient in many patients leading to the postulation that renal immaturity may be a factor.

Another form of RTA type 4 occurs in both children and adults and is associated with salt retention. Its pathogenesis has been attributed to an abnormally increased reabsorption of sodium chloride in the thick ascending limb of Henle (chloride shunt), which causes salt retention, tendency to increased blood volume, and hypertension. This entity has also been called Gordon syndrome and seems to be in many ways a mirror image of Bartter syndrome. Short stature is common, and most patients appear to have inherited the syndrome via an autosomal dominant mode of transmission. The peripheral renin activity and plasma aldosterone levels are both reduced.

DIAGNOSIS

Patients with all forms of RTA have a hyperchloremic metabolic acidosis. This type of acidosis must be differentiated from the high–anion gap type of acidosis by measuring the plasma undetermined anion gap (Fig. 180-1). Once a hyperchloremic (nonanion gap) metabolic acidosis has been demonstrated, other causes of this type of acidosis must be ruled out. The chief differential diagnosis is usually diarrhea with bicarbonate loss in the stools because it is, by far, the most common cause of hyperchloremic metabolic acidosis. For patients with consistently alkaline urine, considering the possibility of a urinary tract infection with a urea-splitting organism is wise. If any suspicion of a urinary tract infection exists, a urine culture should be performed. The plasma pH, partial pressure of carbon dioxide (Pco_2), and total carbon dioxide must be measured several times to document the persistence of the acidosis. All urine passed should be tested for pH; at least some of these tests should be performed with a pH meter, which is more accurate than a dipstick.

Although the ability to acidify is very important, very little hydrogen ion is actually excreted as free hydrogen ion. Most hydrogen ion is excreted as titratable acid or as ammonium, both components of the total acid excretion. Ammonium excretion is, by far, the more important of the two, principally because it is the one that increases so significantly in chronic metabolic acidosis. Many clinical laboratories do not provide the measurement of urinary ammonium, so indirect means of predicting ammonium excretion have been used. Measurement of the urine anion gap and urine osmolal gap provides an estimate of urinary ammonium excretion. The urine anion gap is calculated from the difference between the measured cations (Na + K) and the measured anion (Cl): urine anion gap = urine (Na + K – Cl). If the chloride concentration exceeds the sum of sodium and potassium concentrations, the urine anion gap is said to be negative. If the chloride concentration is less than the sum of the sodium and potassium,

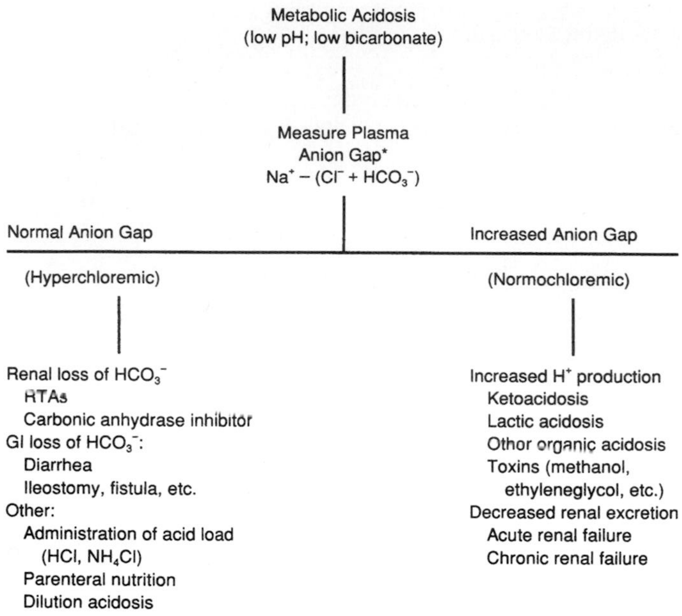

Figure 180-1. The differentiation of metabolic acidosis into hyperchloremic and normochloremic types. GI, gastrointestinal; RTAs, renal tubular acidoses. *Normals: neonates, 18 or less; older infants and children, 16 or less; adolescents, 14 or less.

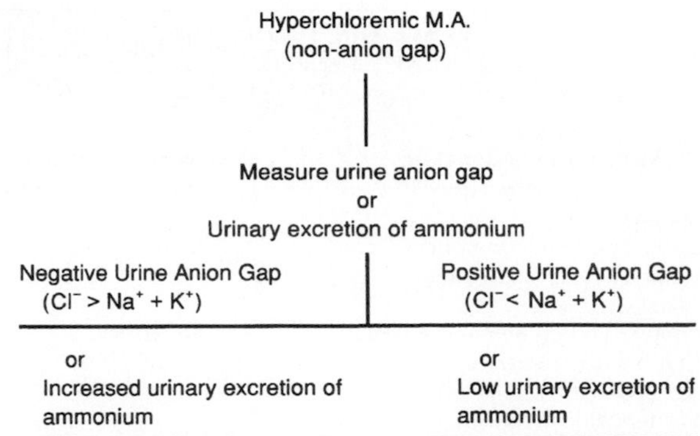

Figure 180-2. First step in the workup of a patient with hyperchloremic (nonanion gap) metabolic acidosis (*M.A.*). Ammonium can be measured directly or indirectly using the urinary anion gap. A negative urine anion gap indicates adequate urinary ammonium excretion. A positive urine anion gap indicates low excretion of ammonium and suggests a distal tubular acidification defect. Urine osmolal gap can be used in addition to or instead of the urine anion gap to estimate urinary excretion of ammonium.

the urine anion gap is said to be positive. The urine anion gap has a negative value in most patients with hyperchloremic metabolic acidosis because of the appropriate increase in urinary ammonium in an attempt to excrete the excess acid. Ammonium is an unmeasured cation and, as a result, an increase in its excretion as NH_4Cl leads to a rise in the urine chloride concentration and a negative urine anion gap. However, in two settings, the urine anion gap may not be an accurate reflection of ammonium excretion. The first is that in which the patient is volume depleted with a urine sodium concentration below 20 mEq/L and the concurrent rise in chloride reabsorption minimizes the excretion of ammonium as NH_4Cl giving an impression of a distal acidification defect. The second setting is that in which an increased excretion of unmeasured anions such as beta-hydroxybutyrate and acetoacetate in ketoacidosis occurs. In this situation, the excretion of sodium and potassium with the unmeasured anions to maintain electroneutrality may lead to a positive urine anion gap, even though ammonium excretion is increased.

In contrast to the urine anion gap, the urine osmolal gap detects all ammonium salts in the urine. This calculation requires measurement of the actual urine osmolality and the urine sodium, potassium, urea nitrogen, and—if the dipstick is positive—glucose concentrations. The calculated urine osmolality can then be estimated as follows: calculated urine osmolality $= 2 \times (Na + K) + urea$.

The gap between the measured and the calculated urine osmolalities should largely represent ammonium salts. A value below 20 mOsm/L indicates an impairment in ammonium excretion. The values of the urine anion gap and urine osmolal gap provide a rapid distinction between proximal and distal RTA (Fig. 180-2). Definitive diagnosis of proximal RTA is made by the demonstration of an acidic urine (pH less than 5.5) during periods of acidosis but only a mildly acidic or alkaline urine (pH greater than 6.0) with partial correction of acidosis. The total acid excretion (principally accounted for by ammonium) is in the normal range during the untreated period of acidosis but drops to abnormally low levels with partial correction of the acidosis. Bicarbonate is virtually absent from the urine during the period of maximal untreated acidosis but is present in large amounts with partial correction demonstrating a low threshold for bicarbonate excretion (Fig. 180-3). The $F_E HCO_3$ is low during acidosis, but with partial correction (e.g., to the 17–19 mEq/L range), the $F_E HCO_3$ is probably found to exceed 10% to 15% and certainly exceeds 10% to 15% if the plasma bicarbonate is brought to normal levels by treatment (Fig. 180-3). The urine minus blood P_{CO_2} is normal (greater than 20 mm Hg) in proximal RTA indicating intact distal

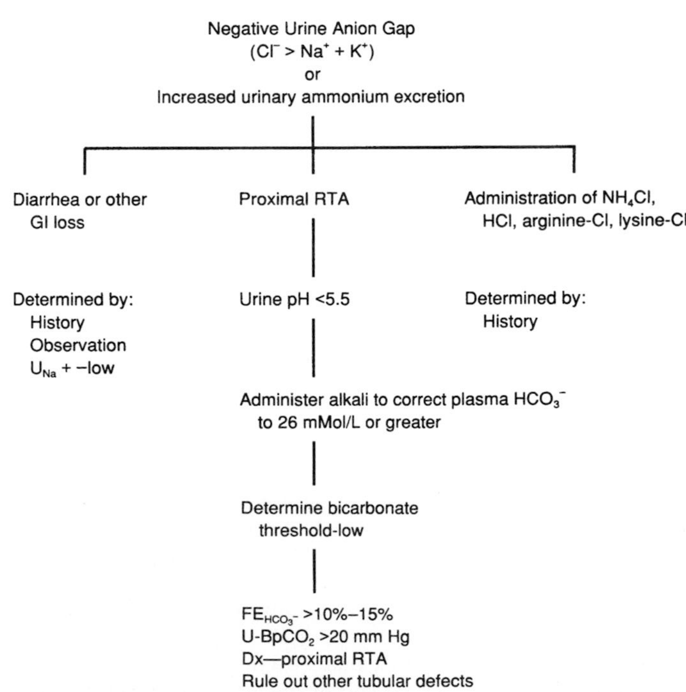

Figure 180-3. Workup of an untreated patient with hyperchloremic metabolic acidosis and a negative urine anion gap or a high urinary ammonium excretion. Dx, diagnosis; GI, gastrointestinal; RTA, renal tubular acidosis. (Modified from Rodriguez-Soriano J, Vallo A. Renal tubular acidosis. Pediatr Nephrol 1990;4:268.)

acidification mechanism. Any patient shown to have proximal RTA should have other proximal tubular functions assessed because this type of RTA is most often found as a component of Fanconi syndrome.

The patient with a positive urine anion gap (i.e., the urine chloride concentration is less than the sum of concentrations of sodium and potassium) or low urine osmolal gap (less than 20) or with abnormal total acid excretion (titratable acid plus ammonium minus bicarbonate) probably has a distal type of RTA (Fig. 180-4). The next step is to measure the plasma potassium concentration (Fig. 180-4). Normal or low potassium level, along with inability to acidify properly and a positive urinary anion gap, indicates that a diagnosis of distal RTA type 1 is appropriate. Other supporting evidence for this type of RTA includes a urine minus blood P_{CO_2} value of less than 20 mm Hg, increased urinary calcium excretion (greater than 4 mg/kg/day), and low urinary citrate level.

Urine minus blood P_{CO_2} remains a controversial test in assessing acidification mechanisms, but it is often low in distal RTA type 1. This measurement is performed by first loading the patient with bicarbonate until the plasma bicarbonate exceeds 24 mEq/L and the urine pH exceeds 7.6 and then measuring the P_{CO_2} in spot urine and blood specimens obtained nearly simultaneously. A measurement (urine minus blood P_{CO_2}) of less than 20 mm Hg strongly suggests distal RTA type 1. This test is a reliable evaluation of the exchange of hydrogen ions for sodium ions in the distal nephron because of the absence of carbonic anhydrase on the luminal surface of the collecting tubules. The carbonic acid formed in the lumen after the exchange of the sodium ion in $NaHCO_3$ for a hydrogen ion is not immediately broken down to carbon dioxide and water. Because the carbon dioxide remains hydrated, it cannot diffuse back into the cells and blood and, therefore, is delivered to the urinary bladder as H_2CO_3; the voided urine can then be measured for P_{CO_2}.

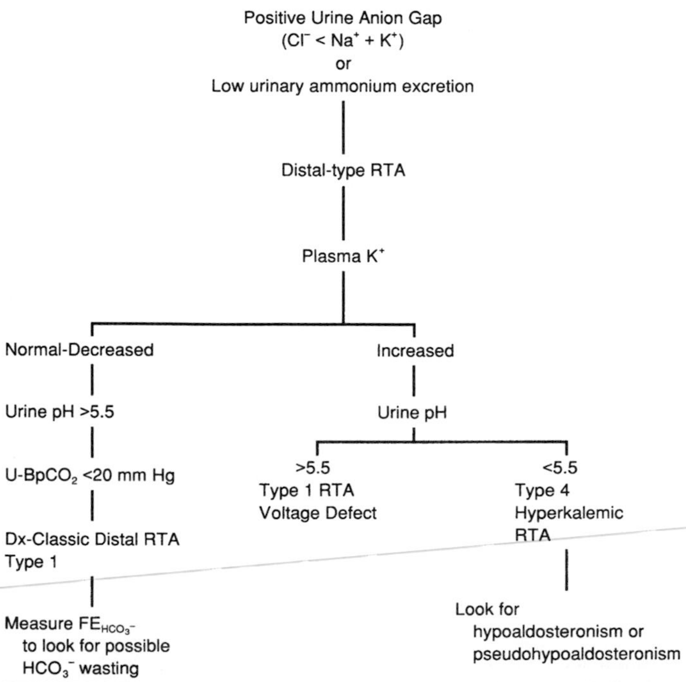

Figure 180-4. Outline of the approach to a patient with hyperchloremic metabolic acidosis who has a positive urine anion gap or low urinary ammonium excretion and, presumably, a distal renal defect. Dx, diagnosis; RTA, renal tubular acidosis.

Patients with distal RTA type 4 have a positive urine anion gap and low total acid excretion (less than 60 μEq/1.73 m^2/minute) similar to those of distal RTA type 1. However, the presence of hyperkalemia and acid urine pH (less than 5.5) distinguishes type 4 from type 1 distal RTA (Fig. 180-4).

Once the diagnosis of distal hyperkalemic RTA type 4 is established, the underlying pathophysiology should be determined if possible. At least some of the clinical determinants are shown in Table 180-4. A careful physical examination in regard to the status of the extracellular and blood vascular volume is essential, as are repeated measurements of the blood pressure. In addition, measurements of peripheral renin activity and plasma aldosterone are indicated in most instances. On the basis of these tests plus a detailed history, measurement of serum creatinine levels, ultrasound studies of the kidneys, and routine urine examinations, a diagnosis of the particular variety of RTA type 4 can usually be made (Table 180-4).

Some patients such as those with partial RTA do not have plasma bicarbonate levels that are clearly low. In those instances, provocative tests such as ammonium chloride loading, a furosemide challenge, or a sodium sulfate infusion may be needed for clarification.

THERAPY

General

Administration of alkali is common therapy for almost all types of RTA. The alkalis used most frequently are sodium bicarbonate tablets (each gram provides 12 mEq) and sodium citrate in liquid form available commercially as Bicitra. Each milliliter of Bicitra provides 1 mEq of sodium citrate. Liquid citrate is also available as Polycitra (each milliliter provides 1 mEq of Na, 1 mEq of K, and 2 mEq of citrate) or Polycitra K (each milliliter provides 2 mEq of K^+ and citrate). The latter two preparations are particularly helpful for patients with a hypokalemic type of RTA. Serum electrolyte studies should be performed every 2 to 4 days during alkali dosage adjustment. After correction of the acidosis, electrolytes should be measured monthly for several months. Ultimately, these determinations are done three to six times a year depending on the difficulty encountered in controlling the metabolic acidosis. Normal stature can usually be attained if the metabolic acidosis is well controlled over a prolonged period.

Proximal Renal Tubular Acidosis Type 2

Most patients with proximal RTA require a higher dose of alkali beginning with 4 to 6 mEq/kg/day and, occasionally, require up to 20 mEq/kg/day. The doses should be spread out over as much of the day as possible (four to six divided doses). Patients with Fanconi syndrome may require that a significant portion of the alkali be given as potassium citrate. Patients requiring very large amounts of base for correction of the acidosis may benefit from the administration of chlorothiazide (10–20 mg/kg/day), dietary sodium chloride restriction, or both. The thiazide diuretics tend to increase the proximal tubular reabsorption of bicarbonate by inducing a mild contraction of the extracellular fluid space.

Distal Renal Tubular Acidosis Type 1

In patients with distal RTA type 1, alkali therapy is usually initiated at a dose of 1 to 2 mEq/kg/day if no evidence of bicarbonate wasting exists and at 4 to 6 mEq/kg/day if bicarbonate wasting exists. Type 1 patients with particularly severe problems with potassium homeostasis may require that up to 50% of the total base be given as potassium citrate. Successful correction of the acidosis results in normal urinary calcium and citrate excretions and greatly lessens the chances of complications such as nephrolithiasis, nephrocalcinosis, and rickets.

Hyperkalemic Distal Renal Tubular Acidosis Type 4

For RTA type 4, doses of base in the range of 1 to 5 mEq/kg/day are usually sufficient to correct the acidosis and may also correct the hyperkalemia. Obviously, potassium-containing alkali should be avoided. Furosemide is also effective in returning serum potassium levels to normal but should not be used in patients with salt wasting. Temporarily resorting to the use of exchange resins (sodium polystyrene sulfonate, or Kayexalate) to control the hyperkalemia is rarely necessary. RTA type 4 has many etiologies, and often the principal therapeutic efforts are directed toward the underlying disease causing the RTA. If the problem results primarily from mineralocorticoid deficiency, hormonal replacement therapy is commonly quite effective. If the patient has pseudohypoaldosteronism, large supplements of sodium chloride may be required for successful therapy. On the other hand, patients with the chloride shunt (Gordon syndrome) usually benefit greatly from salt restriction and the use of loop diuretics. Antihypertensive drugs may also be necessary to control the hypertension.

CHAPTER 181
Nephrogenic Diabetes Insipidus

Adapted from L. Leighton Hill and Arundhati S. Kale

Nephrogenic diabetes insipidus (NDI) is a hereditary or acquired disorder characterized by renal tubular resistance to the antidiuretic hormone arginine vasopressin (AVP). The inability to concentrate the urine because of this tubular disease leads to marked polyuria with compensatory polydipsia. Two different hereditary forms of NDI exist: X-linked and autosomal recessive. In the X-linked cases, female patients usually show a limited tubular response to vasopressin. Even in male patients, variations in the degree of severity of the defect occur; most male patients are diagnosed in early infancy because of a severe defect, but some have a mild enough disease to escape detection until the second or third decade of life. The defect in hereditary NDI, at least in male patients with the severe defect, is usually more severe than that seen in the acquired type, which have two general causes. The first is the loss of the concentration gradient in the medullary interstitial tissues as a result of the tissue destruction occurring with obstructive uropathy, vesicoureteral reflux, sickle cell nephropathy, cystic disease, pyelonephritis, interstitial nephritis, or nephrocalcinosis. The second cause is decreased responsiveness to AVP of the distal tubules and collecting ducts, although the concentration gradient in the medullary interstitial tissues remains intact. Conditions that cause this alteration include hypokalemic states, hypercalcemia, amyloidosis, sarcoidosis, and various drugs that interfere with the action of AVP such as lithium, demeclocycline hydrochloride, cisplatin, vinblastine sulfate, methoxyflurane, amphotericin B, and colchicine. NDI associated with this second group of conditions more closely resembles hereditary NDI than NDI associated with the first group. NDI can also be seen as part of Fanconi syndrome, most likely because of the chronic hypokalemia that often occurs.

CLINICAL CHARACTERISTICS

The most common clinical manifestations of NDI are shown in Table 181-1. Polyuria is constant, even during periods of dehydration. Elevated body temperature, a consequence of the dehydration, often leads to multiple investigations that attempt to identify possible bacterial, viral, or parasitic infections. The large fluid ingestion may interfere with attaining adequate caloric intake; this inadequate caloric intake, along with the deleterious effects of the chronic hypernatremia, leads to failure to thrive. The constant need for intake of liquids interferes with normal sleep patterns. Chronic severe constipation is another result of the constant tendency toward negative water balance that characterizes NDI. When a child with NDI is well hydrated, a dramatic reversal in the condition is seen: the signs and symptoms of dehydration disappear, the fever abates, and the vomiting, irritability, and other manifestations disappear until dehydration recurs.

LABORATORY FINDINGS

Hypernatremia and hyperchloremia are commonly seen when the patient has been in negative water balance. The urinalysis is usually normal, except that the urine is inappropriately dilute (i.e., specific gravity less than 1.006 and urine osmolality less than 200 mOsm/kg) despite evidence of dehydration. Small amounts of protein and a few red blood cells may be found in the urine, and the blood urea nitrogen (BUN) may be elevated during dehydration. With rehydration, the sodium, chloride, BUN, and creatinine levels return to normal, and although the urine remains dilute, the protein and red blood cells disappear. When the patient is in water balance, the glomerular filtration rate and all other renal function tests are normal, aside from the inability to conserve water. In the infant with NDI, the serum sodium level is often elevated early in the morning because of insufficient fluid intake during the night but may return to normal during the day with adequate fluid intake. Ultrasound examination may reveal marked dilatation of the urinary tract in NDI because of extremely high water turnover. This condition is usually minimal at the time of diagnosis in very young infants, but it may be found to be massive later if control of water balance

TABLE 181-1. Clinical Manifestations of Nephrogenic Diabetes Insipidus

Polyuria and polydipsia
Growth and developmental failure
Recurrent bouts of dehydration
Unexplained fever
Thirst
Vomiting
Constipation
Onset during infancy
Positive family history
Irritability

is not good. Marked dilatation of the urinary tract may also be seen in patients not identified as having NDI until later in childhood.

DIAGNOSIS

Symptoms

The diagnosis of NDI is suspected when polyuria, polydipsia, bouts of dehydration, hypernatremia, dilute urines, and a positive family history are noted. The differential diagnosis includes other causes of polyuria such as central (AVP-deficient) diabetes insipidus, diabetes mellitus, psychogenic water drinking, and chronic renal insufficiency. Patients with diabetes mellitus have elevated blood and urine sugars and seldom have hypernatremia. Patients with primary polydipsia have normal to low-normal serum sodium concentrations. Patients with chronic renal insufficiency have azotemia even when hydrated, usually demonstrate isosthenuria rather than hyposthenuria, and generally have a much milder degree of polyuria than patients with diabetes insipidus. The chief differential is often between central diabetes insipidus and NDI (vasopressin-resistant). Assessment and documentation of the magnitude of the polyuria and polydipsia by measuring intakes and outputs are essential. The most important test is a well-controlled water deprivation or concentration test performed in the hospital during the day under close medical supervision (Table 181-2). The patient should not be allowed to lose more than 5% of body weight before the study is terminated. Careful weighings are essential, as are periodic observations of vital signs and urine and serum osmolalities and sodium levels. A urine–to–plasma osmolality ratio of 2.0 or more is sufficient to rule out both NDI and central diabetes insipidus. If the polyuria continues and the urine is not concentrated despite a 4% to 5% body weight loss or the completion of the whole time course of the water deprivation test, then these two diagnoses remain strong possibilities.

TABLE 181-2. Water Deprivation Test

1. Conduct the test in the hospital, during the day with close observation.
2. Give breakfast or formula feeding early (e.g., 5:45 a.m.) with usual liquids.
3. At starting time (e.g., 6 a.m.) have the patient void and discard. With an infant, record time of spontaneous voiding and use this as starting time.
4. Weigh the patient carefully at starting time and record.
5. Allow nothing by mouth from start time.
6. Obtain serum sodium and osmolality in vicinity of starting time.
7. Measure each urine voided for volume, specific gravity, and osmolality. Record time of each voiding.
8. Weigh, take temperature, and measure pulse rate every 2 hours × 3, then every hour × 6.
9. Repeat serum sodium and osmolality after 4 hours and then every 2 hours × 4 and also at conclusion of test.
10. Terminate the test when one or more of the following conditions is met:
    a. The specific gravity is 1.020 or more and urine osmolality is 600 mOsm/kg or more.
    b. The patient has lost 4–5% of body weight or has definite clinical signs of dehydration.
    c. The period of water deprivation reaches 6 hours for a young infant (<6 months), 8 hours for the child between 6 months and 2 years, and 12 hours for the child older than 2.
11. It is crucial to make the following observations at the time the test is stopped: body weight and vital signs, including temperature, serum sodium, serum osmolality, and urine specific gravity, osmolality, and volume.

Antidiuretic Response

The next step in the diagnostic process is to test the renal tubular response to antidiuretic substances. The testing substance of choice is desmopressin acetate (DDAVP), a synthetic analogue of 8-arginine vasopressin. The DDAVP should be given intranasally at a dosage of 10 μg in infants and 20 μg in older children. Urines should be measured for volume and for concentration (specific gravity and osmolality) at 1- to 2-hour intervals after administration. If no response (decrease in volume of urine and increase in osmolality of the urine) occurs, then a second dose should be given and additional urine samples collected and tested for volume and concentration. Serum sodium level and osmolality should be tested before and 4 hours after the administration of the DDAVP. The infant is allowed to take in fluid during this test. An alternative test is to give aqueous vasopressin USP (Pitressin) at a dosage of 2 U/m^2 body surface area intravenously over a 1-hour period in 20 mL of isotonic saline. Urines should be obtained during the aqueous vasopressin infusion, at the conclusion of the infusion, and 1 hour and 2 hours after the infusion for measurement of volume, specific gravity, and osmolality. With either of these stimulation tests (DDAVP or aqueous vasopressin), a urine-to-plasma osmolality ratio of 1.5 or greater would indicate an adequate tubular response to antidiuretic substances. If the patient fails to concentrate the urine with the water deprivation test and also after DDAVP or aqueous vasopressin stimulation, then a diagnosis of NDI is indicated. If the patient fails to concentrate with the water deprivation test but does respond to DDAVP or aqueous vasopressin stimulation by decreasing urine volume to less than 20 mL/m^2/hour and by raising the urine–to–plasma osmolality ratio to at least 1.5, then a diagnosis of central (AVP-deficient) diabetes insipidus is indicated.

Hereditary or Acquired

Once a diagnosis of NDI is made, whether the defect is hereditary or acquired must be determined. Onset at an early age, a family history of polyuria, and bouts of dehydration in infancy strongly suggest that the defect is hereditary. Gene analysis can be performed in newborns with a strong family history of NDI and also in all patients with a definitive diagnosis of NDI. Early identification of newborns with the disease allows prevention of dehydration episodes, and early treatment with unrestricted water intake, low-sodium diet, and hydrochlorothiazide therapy may ensure normal physical and mental development. The workup should also include a thorough drug exposure history; ultrasound studies of the kidneys and urinary tract; measurement of serum electrolyte, BUN, creatinine, and serum calcium levels; and possibly cystography. These studies should be sufficient to rule in or rule out the causes of secondary or acquired NDI mentioned above.

TREATMENT

Water Requirements and Diet

The daily water turnover of infants and children with NDI can be enormous equaling one-half or more of the patient's total body water each day. The intake of volumes of this magnitude may be very difficult to achieve purely from a mechanical point of

TABLE 181-3. Water Turnover Related to Inability to Concentrate Urine

Disease	Solute load (SL)[a]	Maximum ability to concentrate (C)	V = SL/C[b]	Obligatory renal water in liters (V)	Degree of polyuria
None	600	1,200 mOsm/kg	V = 600/1,200	0.5	None
Chronic renal failure	600	300 mOsm/kg	V = 600/300	2.0	Mild
NDI	600	100 mOsm/kg	V = 600/100	6.0	Severe
NDI	300	100 mOsm/kg	V = 300/100	3.0	Moderate

NDI, nephrogenic diabetes insipidus.
[a]Average diet might yield 600 mOsm of solute/m^2 to be excreted by kidney (principally urea, electrolytes, and other nitrogenous products).
[b]V = SL/C where V = obligatory urine volume in liters, SL = 24-hour renal solute load, and C = concentration of urine in mOsm/kg of water.

view. Fluid intake as high as 300 to 400 mL/kg/day may be required just to maintain water balance. This high free water intake should be spaced fairly evenly over the 24-hour period; water should be ingested even at night to prevent early-morning dehydration and hypernatremia. A diet that results in a low renal solute load is of major importance in reducing the obligatory renal water requirement. Such a diet is reasonably low in protein and sodium chloride. In the infant, breast milk is preferable, but if it is unavailable, a low-protein, low-electrolyte commercial formula suffices. Roughly 6% of the total calories should come from protein, and the daily sodium intake should not exceed 1 mEq/kg of body weight. In older children, the daily protein intake should be approximately 2 g/kg and the total daily sodium content should be in the range of 1 to 2 g. The importance of a low renal solute load in determining the volume of obligatory urine water is shown in Table 181-3. Two disease states, chronic renal insufficiency and NDI, are compared with the normal state. The same diet is assumed for each of these three conditions (i.e., a diet yielding approximately 600 mOsm of solute for renal excretion per day). The normal child should be able to concentrate up to 1,200 mOsm/L of urine water, the patient with chronic renal failure can usually concentrate up to approximately 300 mOsm/L, and the patient with NDI can concentrate in the vicinity of 100 mOsm/L. The obligatory urine volume is determined by dividing the total solute load for excretion by the maximum ability to concentrate. As can be seen in this theoretic example, the person with no disease would have an obligatory renal water requirement of 0.5 L; the patient with chronic renal insufficiency would have a mild polyuria with an obligatory water excretion of 2 L/day; and the patient with NDI would have severe polyuria with an obligatory renal water excretion of 6 L/day. If the diet of the patient with NDI were reduced in protein and sodium chloride content so that the renal solute load was decreased to 300 mOsm/day, the obligatory renal water excretion would be only 3 L/day instead of 6 L/day, a dramatic decrease.

Diuretics

The thiazide diuretics can be used to further diminish the polyuria. The thiazide diuretics increase sodium excretion, thereby producing a borderline low blood volume. As a result, increased proximal tubular reabsorption of salt and water occurs, and delivery of water to the concentrating sites in the kidney is less. With a slower flow rate through the collecting ducts, some water diffuses from the collecting duct lumen to the medullary interstitial tissues despite the lack of effect of AVP. The thiazide may decrease urine volume by as much as 20% to 40%. Therefore, these drugs are valuable in the very young infant who has a great physical problem in taking in the volume of free water required to stay in water balance. The decrease in urine volume also prevents or lessens dilatation of the urinary tract, which is almost inevitable at the high water turnover rates these patients experience when untreated. Because the effect of the thiazide is almost completely nullified by a high sodium intake, sodium restriction to the level previously recommended is vital.

Other Agents

The other agents that appear to be helpful in the management of NDI are prostaglandin synthetase inhibitors (e.g., indomethacin). The effects of prostaglandins on renal function are quite complex and appear to vary with the particular prostaglandin involved and the particular situation under which it is tested. In general, however, prostaglandin synthetase inhibitors usually inhibit water excretion. Obviously, treatment of the acquired types of NDI varies depending on the therapy necessary to address the underlying disease causing the secondary tubular defect. However, many of the principles outlined for the therapy of hereditary NDI also apply to treatment of patients with the acquired variety. In particular, these patients benefit from the provision of extra free water and a diet that yields a low renal solute load. With the identification of specific genes involved in hereditary NDI, gene therapy is being investigated. Experimental transfer of adenovirus-mediated genes either by direct perfusion into the renal artery or by retrograde infusion into the renal pelvis in rats resulted in expression of the gene in renal tissue. This result shows the promise of gene transfer therapy as a treatment modality in the future.

CHAPTER 182
Renal Vascular Thrombosis

Adapted from L. Leighton Hill

RENAL VENOUS THROMBOSIS

Renal venous thrombosis (RVT) may be unilateral (most common) or bilateral. It is a rare condition in children past the neonatal period.

Etiology

In neonates and young infants, RVT is seen with dehydration, shock, increased tonicity of body fluids, and polycythemia. Infants with RVT have frequently experienced perinatal asphyxia, prenatal or postnatal stress, or septicemia. A high incidence of preceding diarrhea is present. Not uncommonly, these infants have been exposed to radiographic contrast media. Additional predisposing factors in the newborn period include congenital renal anomalies, congenital nephrosis, severe pyelonephritis, and maternal diabetes. RVT can be primary, first involving the veins of the kidney, or secondary, extending into the renal veins from a thrombus in the inferior vena cava.

RVT seen after infancy is usually associated with the nephrotic syndrome or with cyanotic congenital heart disease (either spontaneously or after angiography). RVT does not cause the nephrotic syndrome; rather, patients with the nephrotic syndrome have a predisposition for the development of RVT because plasma proteins involved in the coagulation pathways are lost in the urine.

Pathogenesis

During conditions of hypovolemia, hemoconcentration, hyperviscosity, hyperosmolarity, sepsis, and asphyxia, local microthrombi may occur peripherally in venous radicals, and the thrombus formation may then progress through the arcuate and interlobular veins toward the main renal vein. More rarely, the clotting process moves in the opposite direction. RVT causes renal congestion and occasionally infarction.

Clinical Characteristics

Sudden enlargement of one or both kidneys may occur. Approximately 60% of the patients with RVT have a palpably enlarged renal mass. Most patients have hematuria, which may be gross but is more often microscopical; hematuria may also be absent. Renal enlargement may occur without other symptoms but, more often, associated symptoms and signs are present including one or more of the following: pallor, tachypnea, vomiting, abdominal distention, shock, fever, and oliguria or anuria. Many of the signs and symptoms noted are due to the underlying disorder causing the RVT rather than the vascular catastrophe itself. Hypertension is uncommon.

Laboratory Findings

Proteinuria is common, although in some instances it may be caused by the physical presence of gross blood in the urine. More than 50% of the infants with RVT demonstrate evidence of a microangiopathic hemolytic anemia with red blood cell fragmentation; thrombocytopenia; low levels of fibrinogen, factor V, and plasminogen; and an increase in fibrin degradation products. These findings may reflect the presence of an active disseminated intravascular coagulation. Depending on the severity and whether the thrombosis is unilateral or bilateral, azotemia and other biochemical evidence of acute renal failure may be present.

Intravenous urography should not be performed. The most useful imaging studies include sonography of the urinary tract, which may reveal enlarged size, altered echogenicity, loss of corticomedullary definition, and a decrease in the size of the central sinus echo; and Doppler evaluation of renal arterial and renal venous blood flow. Isotope renography may also be useful. Selective venography may provide precise delineation of the vascular thrombosis but must be considered risky and is usually unnecessary.

Differential Diagnosis

The many causes of hematuria must be considered. The common presence of a microangiopathic hemolytic anemia in RVT makes hemolytic–uremic syndrome an important differential diagnosis. Other causes of renal enlargement such as perirenal hematoma, abscess, hydronephrosis, cystic renal disease, and renal tumors should also be considered in the differential diagnosis.

Treatment

For the most part, therapy should be conservative and supportive. Correction of underlying pathophysiologic abnormalities should be attempted. If oliguria and azotemia occur, medical management of acute renal failure may be required; in some instances, dialysis is needed. The efficacy of anticoagulant therapy (heparin sodium) has not been documented by controlled studies and should be considered only if laboratory evidence of continuing intravascular coagulation exists. A surgical approach in the acute phase is rarely indicated. The mortality rate is substantial and relates more to the underlying disease process itself than to the RVT. Recovery of function in affected kidneys may occur, but progressive atrophy may result in small, scarred kidneys. Hypertension may be a late complication. Chronic renal failure can be the outcome in some patients who have bilateral RVT. Other patients may show predominantly tubular dysfunction as the sequela of RVT.

RENAL ARTERIAL THROMBOSIS

Renal arterial occlusions are more common than RVT in the neonate, probably because of the extensive use of umbilical artery catheters. Many of the same etiologic and pathogenic factors at play in RVT are also important in renal artery thrombosis.

Obstruction of the renal arterial system may result from an embolus, and the ensuing renal infarction may be unilateral or bilateral, total or segmental, depending on the number and distribution of the emboli. Obstruction of the renal artery may also result from a large thrombus of the lumen of the aorta. The kidney is usually enlarged, and abdominal distension and vomiting are common. Renin-related hypertension may be severe and difficult to control despite aggressive pharmacologic therapy. Congestive heart failure may occur. Hematuria and proteinuria are frequently seen, and the presence of renal failure often depends on whether the thrombosis is unilateral or bilateral. Color Doppler ultrasonography may demonstrate a decrease in renal blood flow, but diethylenetriaminepentaacetic acid (DPTA) renography is the method of choice to estimate renal blood flow and demonstrate perfusion defects. It is also useful in predicting outcome with regard to renal function.

Treatment is largely supportive and frequently directed at the underlying pathophysiologic abnormalities. Heparinization, thrombolysis, or both may be considered in patients with massive thrombosis. Attempts at thrombectomy are usually contraindicated but may be entertained in unstable patients who are not responding to medical treatment. Acute or chronic management of renal failure including dialysis may be necessary. The renovascular hypertension may persist requiring continued therapy; fortunately, in many instances the hypertension resolves.

CHAPTER 183
Urolithiasis

Adapted from L. Leighton Hill
and Arundhati S. Kale

Marked variation exists in the incidence of urinary tract stones in children worldwide. In some countries such as Turkey and Thailand urolithiasis is endemic; bladder stones predominate, and dietary factors are postulated to play a causative role. In contrast, stones are uncommon in children in the United States, where less than 1% of all renal stones occur in children younger than 10 and less than 3% occur in children younger than 19; most stones have a metabolic origin. In the United States, boys with stones outnumber girls by 2:1; stones are very uncommon in black children; and bladder stones are much less common than upper urinary tract stones. A distinction should be made between urolithiasis (stones in the urinary tract) and nephrocalcinosis (an increase in the calcium content of the renal tissue itself), although the two conditions may coexist.

CLINICAL CHARACTERISTICS

The presentation in children, especially young children and infants, may be very nonspecific. Gross or microscopical hematuria may be the only manifestation, or hematuria may be accompanied by nonspecific abdominal pain or by fever, pyuria, and abdominal pain. Signs and symptoms might be those of a urinary tract infection (UTI). Typical renal colic is unusual in small children, but it can be present in older children. In some instances, the stone or gravel has already been passed spontaneously. Frequently, the patient has a family history of stones. Urinary stones can cause obstruction of the urinary flow, dilatation of the urinary tract, and, ultimately, renal parenchymal damage. Stones can predispose to UTIs; conversely, UTIs can be important in the formation of stones.

TABLE 183-1. Urolithiasis Classification Based on Stone Composition

- **I. Calcium stones (calcium oxalate and calcium phosphate)**
  - A. Hypercalciuria
    - 1. Hypercalcemic hypercalciuria
      - Hyperparathyroidism
      - Thyrotoxicosis
      - Vitamin D intoxication
      - Idiopathic infantile hypercalcemia
      - Sarcoidosis
      - Neoplastic deposits in bones
      - Immobilization
    - 2. Normocalcemic hypercalciuria
      - Idiopathic or familial hypercalciuria
      - Absorptive
      - Renal
      - 1,25-Dihydroxycholecalciferol induced
      - Distal renal tubular acidosis type 1
      - Acetazolamide use
      - Loop diuretic use
      - Immobilization
      - Vitamin D excess
      - Cushing syndrome
  - B. Hyperoxaluria (calcium oxalate)
    - 1. Primary hyperoxaluria types I and II
    - 2. Secondary hyperoxaluria
      - Inflammatory bowel disease
      - Pyridoxine deficiency
      - Massive doses of vitamin C
  - C. Hyperglycinuria (calcium oxalate stones)
  - D. Idiopathic urolithiasis
- **II. Magnesium ammonium phosphate (struvite) plus basic calcium phosphate (apatite)**
  - A. Urinary tract infection with urea-splitting organisms (mostly *Proteus* species)
  - B. Foreign body plus urinary stasis plus infection
- **III. Uric acid stones***
  - A. Hyperuricosuria
    - 1. Gout
    - 2. Lesch-Nyhan syndrome
    - 3. High purine diet
    - 4. Glycogen storage disease type I
    - 5. Leukemia-lymphoma
    - 6. Leukemia-lymphoma cytotoxic prescription
- **IV. Xanthine stones***
  - A. Primary xanthinuria
  - B. Allopurinol therapy
- **V. Dihydroxyadenine stones***
- **VI. Cystine stones**
  - A. Cystinuria

*Disorders of purine metabolism.

CLASSIFICATION

Calcium Stones

HYPERCALCIURIA

Hypercalcemia may be caused by a diverse set of conditions (Table 183-1). Hypercalcemia is more apt to cause nephrocalcinosis than urolithiasis. The normocalcemic hypercalciurias include distal renal tubular acidosis type 1; they are discussed in Chapter 180. The use of acetazolamide can cause a picture identical to that of renal tubular acidosis type 1. Loop diuretic administration, especially in preterm infants, has caused nephrocalcinosis and urolithiasis. Immobilization can cause hypercalciuria, whether or not the serum calcium is elevated.

IDIOPATHIC OR FAMILIAL HYPERCALCIURIA

One of the most common causes of stones at any age is idiopathic or familial hypercalciuria, a normocalcemic form of hypercalciuria. Familial hypercalciuria may account for up to 50% of stones in children. Urinary calcium excretion exceeds 4 mg/kg/day, or the calcium–to–creatinine ratio exceeds 0.21 in a child older than 2 years. Calcium excretion is greater in infancy; normal calcium–to–creatinine ratios are as high as 0.8 mg/mg in infants up to the age of 6 months and 0.6 mg/mg in children between 6 months and 1 year of age. At least three mechanisms have been invoked to explain the familial normocalcemic type of hypercalciuria. The first—absorptive hypercalciuria—is a primary intestinal epithelial defect that permits excessive intestinal absorption of calcium. Parathyroid hormone (PTH) function is normal or suppressed, and urinary calcium excretion returns to normal during fasting. A second type of hypercalciuria is called renal hypercalciuria because of apparently defective calcium reabsorption by the renal tubules. The renal loss of calcium temporarily results in a lower serum calcium level, which stimulates PTH production bringing the serum calcium back to normal. Renal hypercalciuria is characterized by elevated PTH levels, which stimulate increased production of 1,25-dihydroxycholecalciferol, which then enhances the intestinal absorption of calcium and increases the filtered load of calcium in the kidney. Children with renal hypercalciuria continue to put out calcium in abnormal amounts (more than 4 mg/kg/day) during fasting. A third type of hypercalciuria—1,25-dihydroxycholecalciferol-induced hypercalciuria—is recognized by some investigators. The defect may be a renal tubular leak of phosphate. The ensuing hypophosphatemia is thought to stimulate the renal synthesis of 1,25-dihydroxycholecalciferol, which then enhances intestinal absorption of calcium; this in turn provides extra calcium for renal excretion. Many experts in calcium physiology argue that dividing the hypercalciurias into several pathogenetic entities is unjustified. They offer instead a unifying hypothesis that the various forms of hypercalciuria result from the same generalized defect, possibly a disordered regulation of 1,25-dihydroxycholecalciferol production. Children with idiopathic hypercalciuria may also have hematuria (either gross or microscopical), even though no stones have been detected, possibly from crystalluria. Hypercalciuria should also be in the differential diagnosis of isolated hematuria. Patients with hypercalciuric hematuria may later develop stones. Many patients with biochemical evidence of hypercalciuria never experience problems with stone formation.

HYPEROXALURIA

Primary hyperoxaluria is a general term for two rare genetic disorders that result in recurrent calcium oxalate urolithiasis and nephrocalcinosis. Nephrocalcinosis is a greater problem than is urolithiasis because the deposition of calcium oxalate in the renal parenchyma ultimately leads to tissue destruction, fibrosis, and chronic renal failure. The renal calculi are extremely radiopaque and homogenous. Secondary hyperoxaluria with stone formation can also occur, most often caused by chronic inflammatory bowel disease such as Crohn's disease or by ileal bypass. Apparently, an increase in intestinal oxalate absorption occurs in enteric types of secondary hyperoxaluria.

Struvite Stones

Struvite (magnesium ammonium phosphate) stones occur as a result of UTIs with urease-containing bacteria. These organisms, most commonly Proteus species, can split urinary urea into ammonia ions, which buffer hydrogen ions to form ammonium molecules, thereby producing a strongly alkaline urine loaded with ammonium compounds. The persistently alkaline urine favors the crystallization of calcium phosphate (apatite), and the increase in ammonium concentration raises the magnesium ammonium phosphate product. Seventy-five percent of struvite stones in children are seen before age 5, and 80% are in boys. Children with struvite stones frequently have vesicoureteral reflux or other urologic abnormalities. The UTIs associated with struvite stones can be quite resistant to therapy, and organisms have been cultured from the interior of the stone. Complete removal of these stones is mandatory.

CYSTINURIA

Cystinuria is a hereditary disorder of amino acid transport affecting the epithelial cells of both the renal tubule and the gastrointestinal tract. The gastrointestinal defect apparently causes no clinical problems. However, the renal tubular abnormality results in hyperexcretion in the urine of the neutral amino acid cystine and the cationic amino acids lysine, ornithine, and arginine. The diagnosis is proved by demonstrating abnormal quantities of these amino acids in a timed urine specimen. The only clinical expression of cystinuria is urolithiasis; otherwise, individuals with this disorder can live a normal life. Whether urolithiasis eventually develops in every person with cystinuria is unknown.

Uric Acid Stones

Uric acid stones resulting from primary gout are extremely rare in children. Hyperuricemia with uric acid calculi is seen as part of Lesch–Nyhan syndrome, a rare inborn error of metabolism. Uric acid stones may also occur as a consequence of the hyperuricosuria of glycogen storage disease type I. Hyperuricemia with uric acid stones or gravel in the urinary tracts of both kidneys is occasionally the presenting feature of leukemia. More commonly, the calculi occur after cytotoxic chemotherapy for leukemia or lymphoma (tumor lysis syndrome). Urine flow may be blocked resulting in acute renal failure. High uric acid levels can also be nephrotoxic and directly produce renal parenchymal damage.

DIAGNOSIS

A high index of suspicion is frequently required to make the diagnosis of urolithiasis. Demonstration of the stone can be accomplished by imaging techniques such as a plain radiography of the abdomen, intravenous urography, ultrasound study of the urinary tract, or, more recently, computed tomography (CT). All stones containing calcium are radiopaque. Cystine stones are slightly radiopaque because of the sulfur present in cystine. Struvite stones are also radiopaque. The stones that are most frequently radiolucent are those resulting from disorders of purine metabolism (Table 183-1). The diagnosis of urolithiasis can also be made by the proven passage of a stone, gravel, or sludge. Whenever urolithiasis is considered, any passed material must be saved, and the urine must be strained, whether at home or in the hospital, in an attempt to obtain a stone. The formation of a stone within the urinary tract is not a specific disease but, instead, a complication of many highly varied disorders. The next step must be to determine which of the disorders caused the stone. Therefore, all passed stones or stone-like material must be tested completely for composition. The stone should be solubilized and analyzed qualitatively and quantitatively for its main contents. This analysis should be performed in a laboratory with personnel experienced in stone analysis. Children with the diagnosis of urolithiasis should have radiologic investigation of the urinary tract to evaluate for a possible anatomic abnormality of the genitourinary tract, to assess for the presence of and degree of obstruction caused by the stone, to search for other stones, and to determine if nephrocalcinosis is also present. This investigation usually includes either an ultrasound study of the urinary tract or an intravenous urogram and, occasionally, a cystourethrogram. The laboratory workup is suggested in Table 183-2. The metabolic evaluation of stone formers should begin 4 to 6 weeks after stone diagnosis and passage because passage itself may cause transient changes in urinary chemistry. The patient would then also be free of the effects of obstruction and infection. The serum calcium level determines the possible presence of hypercalcemia. Serum phosphorus level may be low in hyperparathyroidism, in one type of hypercalciuria, and in renal tubular acidosis, and it may be elevated in the tumor lysis syndrome. Serum creatinine estimates glomerular function.

Electrolyte levels, pH, P_{CO_2}, and urine pH are used to investigate the possibility of renal tubular acidosis. All children with stones should have a spot chemical urine test for cystine to rule out cystinuria and a quantitative amino acid analysis if the spot test is positive. A timed urine sample (preferably 24 hours) is collected for quantitative measurement of calcium and uric acid. Because of the present difficulty in measuring oxalate, it is not quantified routinely. Quantitative urinary calcium excretion or a

TABLE 183-2. Laboratory Workup for Urolithiasis

Blood determinations
Calcium; repeat two or three times
Phosphorus
Alkaline phosphatase
Creatinine
Electrolytes
pH and Pco_2
Uric acid
Urine studies
Urinalysis, repeat two or three times
Urine culture
Spot urine for cystine (cyanide-nitroprusside test)
Urine pHs, repeat four to six times
Spot urine for calcium-to-creatinine ratio
24-hour urine for calcium, creatinine, oxalate, and uric acid: Add xanthine if patient has hypouricemia and quantitative amino acids if spot test for cystine is positive.
Other studies
Ammonium chloride loading test may be necessary to assess renal ability to acidify.

spot urine test for calcium–to–creatinine ratio provides information regarding the possible presence of hypercalciuria. Several determinations may be necessary. Hyperuricosuria can occur without hyperuricemia. These mostly routine tests frequently provide a diagnosis as to the cause of the stone. Sometimes leads from the routine tests may suggest more sophisticated studies. An accurate chemical analysis of the stone itself greatly enhances the possibility of a correct diagnosis. PTH measurement may be indicated in some cases.

TREATMENT

One of the most important measures in preventing the formation or further growth of any stone regardless of etiology is to increase urine volume, which reduces the urinary concentrations of calcium, phosphorus, oxalates, cystine, uric acid, and other possible constituents of stones. This dilution of the urine can be accomplished by raising the fluid intake to 1.5 to 2.0 times normal (2,400 mL/m^2/day or more). The high fluid intake should be distributed as much as possible throughout the 24 hours including at bedtime and during the night if the patient awakens. Early morning urines should be kept at a specific gravity of less than 1.014. UTI, if present, must be treated, and a search for anatomic abnormalities completed. Any urologic abnormalities predisposing to infections or stones should be corrected.

Stone Removal

Many stones pass through and out of the urinary tract spontaneously. Others (e.g., uric acid stones) may dissolve slowly or at least not grow as a result of medical treatment. Some stones must be removed: struvite stones, stones causing prolonged blockage with obstructive nephropathy, and stones causing significant chronic pain or resistant UTI. In the past, the traditional surgical management of patients with calculus disease consisted of endoscopic manipulation with stone baskets or loops for stones in the lower part of the ureter (below the pelvic brim) or open surgical procedures for calculi higher in the urinary tract. These traditional methods of stone removal are being replaced by a variety of new modalities including extracorporeal shock-wave lithotripsy, percutaneous nephrostolithotomy, and the use of percutaneously placed endoscopes to fragment calculi with ultrasonic waves or lasers. These techniques, used first in adults, are now finding widespread application in children and represent a dramatic advance in medical therapy. With new-generation lithotriptors, infants as young as 3 to 4 months have benefited from extracorporeal shock-wave lithotripsy with minimal side effects.

Specific Therapeutic Measures

The treatment for pediatric hypercalciuria and stones due to hypercalcemia is elimination of the cause of the hypercalcemia; that is, parathyroidectomy (for patients with hyperparathyroidism), treatment of thyrotoxicosis or Cushing disease, withdrawal of vitamin D therapy, at least partial mobilization of immobilized patients, and so on. Distal renal tubular acidosis, a form of normocalcemic hypercalciuria, can be treated with appropriate amounts of sodium bicarbonate or sodium citrate plus potassium citrate in an effort to keep the serum bicarbonate concentration in the range of 22 to 28 mEq/L (see Chapter 180). Treatment of urolithiasis caused by familial or idiopathic hypercalciuria is controversial. Trying to distinguish the various types of hypercalciuria for purposes of therapy is probably no longer necessary; rather, all patients with stones from idiopathic or familial hypercalciuria should be treated similarly with increased fluid intake and reduced calcium intake and sodium intake. Thiazide diuretics, which enhance renal tubular reabsorption of calcium, are quite effective in reducing calcium excretion and preventing recurrent stone formation. Because high sodium chloride intakes tend to negate this effect of thiazides, restriction of sodium intake to a maximum of 2 mEq/kg/day is indicated. The addition of potassium citrate to this regimen (1–2 mEq/kg/day) is advised. Whether thiazide drugs should be used for long-term therapy depends on the number of recurrences of stones and the complications encountered. Dietary calcium restriction can be tried but must be used cautiously in a growing child. The use of phosphate compounds (cellulose phosphate, orthophosphate) in children is poorly tolerated and has generally been abandoned. Of these therapies for familial hypercalciuria, the thiazide diuretics have been the most successful, but long-term use of a thiazide would be considered only in patients with recurrent stones. The treatment of familial hypercalciuria is not completely clear at this time. Thiazides reduce stone formation in patients with recurrent idiopathic urolithiasis, even though urinary calcium before treatment was normal.

No effective therapy for the primary hyperoxalurias exists. A few patients with type I appear to respond partially to pyridoxine therapy. Salts of phosphate, citrate, and magnesium, aimed at increasing the solubility of calcium oxalate, have been administered with some success. All fragments of struvite stones must be removed because failure to do so may result in persistent infection and recurrence of stones. Complete eradication of infection and the correction of any anatomic abnormality causing urinary stasis is essential. Allopurinol therapy is very effective in patients with uric acid and dihydroxyadenine stones. A high urine output is also valuable in treating these two types of stones. Alkalinization of the urine to a pH of 6.5 with sodium bicarbonate or sodium citrate is important in treating and preventing uric acid calculi. Hemodialysis may be necessary to control the extreme hyperuricemia seen in patients with the tumor lysis syndrome. Dilution of the urine decreases the saturation of cystine, and alkalinization increases the solubility of cystine. The alkali therapy must be divided over the entire day and night to ensure a pH above 7 (ideally above 7.4). Of these two treatments, increasing the fluid intake is much more important. Administration of penicillamine is another effective therapy, but it is seldom used because the drug is expensive and has many side effects.

CHAPTER 184

Hemolytic–Uremic Syndrome

Adapted from Penelope Terhune Louis

The hemolytic–uremic syndrome (HUS), first described in 1955, is characterized by the triad of nephropathy, thrombocytopenia, and microangiopathic hemolytic anemia. HUS is a heterogeneous group of disorders that have a common end result. To differentiate the pathogenesis and clinical outcome, the following classification has been proposed:

- *Classical:* presents in infants or small children after a prodrome of bloody diarrhea that may involve the verotoxin-producing strain of *Escherichia coli.*
- *Postinfectious:* associated with an identified infectious agent such as *Shigella* or *Salmonella* or with endotoxemia.
- *Hereditary:* recognized to have both autosomal dominant and recessive modes of inheritance. Affected patients probably lack a plasma factor necessary for prostacyclin production or have a prostacyclin inhibitor.
- *Immunologically mediated:* characterized by low plasma C3 and activation of the alternative pathway; also may be familial.
- *Secondary:* related to known predisposing conditions such as lupus, scleroderma, chemotherapy, malignant hypertension, and renal irradiation.
- *Pregnancy- or oral contraceptive–related:* characterized by arterial microangiopathy.

PATHOGENESIS

Mechanisms of Injury

The pathogenesis of HUS can be explained by several mechanisms. The anemia is characterized by negative direct and indirect Coombs tests, a falling haptoglobin, and a reticulocyte response. Strong evidence indicates that hemolysis is secondary to mechanical destruction of erythrocytes by fibrin strands in small renal vessels. Other evidence shows that the redox state of the red blood cell is altered leading to increased oxidation of the red blood cell membrane.

Thrombocytopenia is present universally and is secondary to peripheral destruction. The mechanisms implicated are increased platelet activation and enhanced platelet aggregation as a result of prostaglandin imbalance. The degree of thrombocytopenia does not predict morbidity or length of illness.

Nephropathy

The nephropathy of HUS is characterized by glomerular capillary endothelial injury. The endothelium separates, and the subendothelial space is littered with debris such as fibrin strands and erythrocyte fragments. As a result of the thickening of the endothelial space, the capillary narrows predisposing to capillary thrombosis. Fibrin is demonstrated with immunofluorescent techniques. No consistent existing evidence can show that immune complexes are involved with renal injury because usually immunoglobulin deposits are not found using immunofluorescent techniques.

Role of Prostaglandins

The role of prostaglandins in HUS has been studied with increased interest. Prostacyclin I2 is a potent depressor of platelet aggregation. Prostacyclin production may be decreased by damage to endothelial cells, or a circulating inhibitor to prostacyclin may be present. The platelet aggregator thromboxane may be elevated in HUS with the imbalance of decreased prostacyclin and increased thromboxane leading to enhanced platelet aggregation.

EPIDEMIOLOGY

Geography and Predilection

HUS is largely a disease of infants and children. The syndrome is endemic in Argentina, southern Africa, and the western United States. It has no predilection for either gender. In southern Africa, it is more common in white children. Age of onset is between 2 months and 8 years in most cases and is usually less than 5 years. Postdiarrheal HUS occurs more frequently during warmer months. The summer disease incidence peak correlates with the higher incidence of positive enterohemorrhagic *E. coli* fecal cultures in cattle during the warmer months.

Etiologic Agents

No single causative factor is implicated, and etiologic agents may be viral (coxsackieviruses, echoviruses, influenza viruses, Epstein–Barr virus), bacterial (*Shigella, Salmonella, Streptococcus pneumoniae, E. coli* O157:H7), or drugs (oral contraceptives and cyclosporin A) and complement abnormalities. It seems to have a genetic predisposition. Familial illness with the typical prodrome has a low mortality. If no typical prodrome is present, the mortality is high and the predisposition seems to be autosomally transmitted.

CLINICAL CHARACTERISTICS

Prodrome

Typically, the syndrome has a prodrome of diarrhea or an upper respiratory illness. The diarrhea may be bloody. The prodrome occurs 5 days to 2 weeks before the onset of the classic syndrome.

Symptoms

At initial examination, affected children are pale and irritable exhibiting petechiae and edema. Dehydration may be present if severe diarrhea occurs. Hypertension is also common.

Mildly affected patients may have only anemia, thrombocytopenia, and azotemia. Severely affected patients have the complications of metabolic derangement including hyperkalemia, metabolic acidosis, hypocalcemia, and hyponatremia or hypernatremia. Neurologic dysfunction will be manifested by seizures, coma, and stroke. Infection may be either primary or nosocomial. Cardiac failure may result from hypertension, volume overload, or severe anemia. Bleeding may also be present in severely affected patients.

Laboratory Features

Laboratory features include hemoglobin concentrations of 2 to 10 g/dL, platelet counts of fewer than 100,000 cells per cubic millimeter, and an increased prothrombin time caused by consumption of factors II, VII, IX, and X. A decrease in fibrinogen and an increase in fibrin split products also appear early in the illness.

TREATMENT

Management and Therapy

Management of patients with HUS is mainly supportive. The mainstay of therapy is meticulous control of fluid and electrolyte balance, control of hypertension, careful use of red blood cell transfusions, and early initiation of dialysis for hyperkalemia, metabolic acidosis, severe uremia, or volume overload. The aim of red blood cell transfusions during the period of hemolysis should be to prevent heart failure and to prevent the return of the hematocrit to normal. Thrombocytopenia may be severe, but it only rarely results in significant bleeding; therefore, platelets should not be given unless clearly needed to stop bleeding or in anticipation of invasive procedures. Fluid restriction to 400 mL/m^2/day is standard. The difficulty in management is distinguishing between mild disease, which responds to the therapy mentioned previously, and severe disease, which requires more aggressive treatment.

Other therapies include heparin, streptokinase, aspirin, dipyridamole, vitamin E, intravenous immunoglobulin G (IgG), and plasmapheresis. The use of heparin and streptokinase has declined because of hemorrhagic complications. Aspirin and dipyridamole have been used because of their effects on prostaglandin synthesis. Dipyridamole interferes with phosphodiesterase, which results in the slower metabolism of cyclic adenosine monophosphate. Aspirin inhibits cyclooxygenase leading to decreased platelet-aggregating thromboxane. In general, studies report little benefit from the use of heparin, fibrinolytics, and antiplatelet therapy. Vitamin E therapy has been proposed after reports of abnormal lipid peroxidation and low vitamin E activity in HUS patients, but controlled studies have shown no benefit at present. Intravenous IgG infusions have received attention on the basis of studies performed in adults showing that IgG can inhibit platelet aggregation, which presumably would diminish thrombotic microangiopathy and would reduce the period of time of thrombocytopenia. Controlled studies have not been completed, and preliminary data suggest that the period of thrombocytopenia is shortened, but that morbidity is not altered. Fresh-frozen plasma infusions have been suggested because of findings that serum from HUS patients cannot generate normal amounts of prostaglandin or does not demonstrate normal amounts of antithrombotic and antiplatelet function. Anecdotal reports describe experiences with plasmapheresis in the treatment of childhood HUS but, because no prospective clinical trials have been conducted, plasmapheresis remains untested and is not recommended.

PROGNOSIS

The prognosis for the most common forms of HUS is good. Most studies report 3% to 5% mortality, and another 3% to 5% of patients experience chronic renal disease.

CHAPTER 185
Syndrome of Inappropriate Secretion of Antidiuretic Hormone

Adapted from Penelope Terhune Louis and James D. Fortenberry

PATHOPHYSIOLOGY AND DIAGNOSIS

The Role of Antidiuretic Hormone

Fluid management in acutely ill children may be complicated by alterations in the regulatory mechanisms of sodium and water homeostasis. Antidiuretic hormone (ADH) plays an important role in responding to changes in extracellular volume by altering the renal clearance of free water to maintain appropriate serum tonicity. ADH release from the posterior pituitary gland is influenced primarily by changes in plasma osmolality and effective circulating blood volume. Hypothalamic osmoreceptors maintain osmolality over a narrow range with 1% to 2% changes altering ADH secretion. The response to volume changes by the carotid body and left atrial stretch receptors is less sensitive requiring 10% difference to stimulate or suppress ADH release.

ADH Excretion and Secretion

Many disease states, medications, and pathophysiologic processes can alter ADH excretion and secretion (Table 185-1). In some of these entities, ADH release may be an appropriate response to the alterations sensed by body receptors, as in the decreased venous return produced by positive pressure ventilation. However, if ADH release is excessive or inappropriate in relation to either normal osmolality or volume status, the typical findings of the syndrome of inappropriate ADH secretion (SIADH) ensue. Often, SIADH is recognized in children and is established by five classic clinical criteria: hyponatremia with corresponding serum hypoosmolality; urine osmolality greater than appropriate for concomitant serum osmolality (i.e., less than maximally dilute); continued urine sodium excretion that is excessive for the degree of hyponatremia with elevated urine sodium concentrations; normal renal, adrenal, and thyroid function; and absence of volume depletion.

Urine has to be only submaximally diluted to establish a diagnosis of SIADH. Normally, the kidneys can dilute urine up to 50 to 150 mOsm/kg. With urine hypotonic to plasma, the tonicity of serum can possibly fall below normal and can be maintained at subnormal levels producing hyponatremia. Hyponatremia may not be present early in the process and develops only when fluid retention occurs.

Sodium Excretion

The associated increase in urinary sodium excretion is an interesting finding. Typically, aldosterone secretion is normal and the filtered sodium load does not increase; therefore, a third factor—possibly atrial natriuretic peptide—that has been proposed may suppress proximal tubular reabsorption of sodium in response to expanded extracellular volume.

TABLE 185-1. Disorders and Agents Associated with the Syndrome of Inappropriate Antidiuretic Hormone Secretion

Central nervous system
Meningitis
Encephalitis
Head trauma
Tumor
Hypoxia-ischemia
Guillain-Barré syndrome
Subarachnoid hemorrhage
Acute intermittent porphyria
Cavernous sinus thrombosis
Anatomic abnormalities
Vasculitis
Brain abscess
Hydrocephalus
Acute psychosis
Rocky Mountain spotted fever
Spinal fusion
Craniopharyngioma (triphasic postoperative response)
Drugs
Enhancement of antidiuretic hormone release
Morphine
Vincristine
Beta-adrenergic agonists
Cyclophosphamide
Carbamazepine
Barbiturates
Halothane
Clofibrate
Nicotine
Phenothiazines
Adenine arabinoside
Potentiation of antidiuretic hormone action
Chlorpropamide
Indomethacin
Intrathoracic processes
Tuberculosis
Viral, bacterial, fungal pneumonia
Mycoplasmal pneumonia
Empyema
Asthma
Pneumothorax
Cystic fibrosis
Positive-pressure ventilation
Positive end-expiratory pressure
Tumor
Patent ductus arteriosus ligation
Miscellaneous
Pain
Stress (postoperative)
Nausea, vomiting
Bacterial endocarditis
Malignancy
Infant water intoxication (postulated)
Idiopathic

Adapted from Kaplan SL, Feigin RD. SIADH in children. *Adv Pediatr* 1980;27:247.

Tests

SIADH must be differentiated from the many clinical conditions that cause hyponatremia in children. Physical examination and evaluation of simultaneous urine and serum sodium concentrations and osmolalities, urine specific gravity, and serum electrolytes will help to exclude disorders such as hyponatremic dehydration, congestive heart failure, and renal insufficiency. Serum cortisol levels are recommended because patients with adrenal insufficiency may demonstrate a component of inappropriate ADH secretion and might present a similar picture if well compensated. Thyroid function tests should also be considered. Water-loading procedures are dangerous and unnecessary for diagnosis.

Physical Findings

Physical findings in SIADH are related to the associated disease process. Despite mildly increased total body water, edema formation is not typically seen. Symptoms are related to the presence and duration of hyponatremia. Anorexia, nausea, mental status changes, and convulsions are more likely to occur with a serum osmolality of less than 240 mOsm/kg H_2O and a serum sodium concentration of less than 120 mEq/L of acute onset.

ASSOCIATED DISORDERS

In children, SIADH occurs most often in association with central nervous system (CNS) disorders. Laboratory evidence of SIADH was noted in almost 60% of children presenting with bacterial meningitis. ADH levels in patients with meningitis were also significantly elevated in comparison with normal and febrile controls. The duration and degree of hyponatremia were shown to correlate significantly with subsequent development of seizure and subdural effusions. A leak of endogenous ADH across inflamed meninges has been suggested to explain these findings, but laboratory markers of inflammation did not show a correlation with arginine vasopressin (AVP) levels. SIADH occurs with other CNS infections including brain abscesses and encephalitis and with Rocky Mountain spotted fever, most likely secondary to hypothalamic involvement from rickettsial vasculitis. CNS disturbances such as head trauma, perinatal hypoxia, brain tumors, subarachnoid hemorrhage, anatomic defects, and Guillain–Barré syndrome may produce SIADH.

Intrathoracic Disturbances

Intrathoracic disturbances are less common causes in children. Pulmonary tuberculosis is well recognized, but viral, fungal, bacterial, and mycoplasma pneumonias have also been cited. Disorders that lead to decreased left atrial pressure such as positive-pressure ventilation or pneumothoraces can induce excessive ADH release by diminishing venous return. This condition is perceived inappropriately by stretch receptors as evidence of decreased circulating blood volume. ADH levels are probably elevated by a similar mechanism in status asthmaticus leading one to reconsider the vigorous use of intravenous fluids often recommended in initial management.

Role of Drugs and Other Agents

Many drugs have been implicated in the production of SIADH, acting either by increasing endogenous central ADH release or by enhancing its renal tubular effects (Table 185-1). Frequently used agents include chemotherapeutic agents, morphine, beta–adrenergic agonists, and indomethacin. Reportedly, carbamazepine-induced SIADH was reversed by concomitant use of phenytoin, which inhibits ADH secretion. Phenytoin may minimize SIADH while treating seizures associated with CNS insult.

Other Disorders

Many other disorders can induce SIADH. Ectopic production of ADH may occur in adults with bronchogenic carcinoma, leukemia, and thymoma. Transient increases in ADH secretion also occur as part of the triphasic ADH response after resection of craniopharyngiomas. ADH secretion caused by the effects of increased epinephrine is released from pain or stress, nausea and vomiting, the use of morphine, or the surgical procedure itself may be excessive in the general postoperative setting; posterior spinal fusion for scoliosis is a common association. A syndrome of hyponatremia with water intoxication has been described in otherwise normal infants receiving dilute formula at home; AVP levels that were increased inappropriately were found in some of these infants.

MANAGEMENT

Fluid Restriction

Appropriate treatment of the underlying disease process is essential to the resolution of SIADH. However, fluid restriction remains the cornerstone of acute therapy and prevention of symptoms in patients at risk. Intake should be limited to insensible losses (800–1,000 mL/m^2/day) with appropriate sodium content to allow the slow excretion of excess fluid diminishing extracellular volume and, thus, decreasing urinary sodium excretion.

Fluid Management of Meningitis

The fluid management of meningitis patients has undergone increasing scrutiny. Although SIADH may occur in this setting, many affected patients may be volume-depleted and may have associated hyponatremic dehydration. In a study by Powell et al., children with meningitis were randomly assigned to receive either fluid restriction (two-thirds maintenance) or maintenance fluid therapy plus estimated deficit replacement during the initial 24 hours of therapy. Initially, plasma AVP concentrations were elevated in both groups but returned to normal after 24 hours of therapy in patients who received maintenance and deficit therapy; levels were unchanged in fluid-restricted patients. ADH reduction was presumed to be secondary to correction of hypovolemia and sodium deficits. Fluid restriction in an animal model of bacterial meningitis also produced decreased cerebral flow and increased cerebrospinal fluid lactic acidosis. Therefore, an appropriate approach is probably to give maintenance plus replacement fluids to meningitis patients who initially do not demonstrate laboratory evidence of SIADH. Close monitoring of electrolytes should continue during the first 24 to 48 hours of therapy, and the presence of hyponatremia should prompt the evaluation of urine osmolality and sodium concentration to rule out SIADH.

Other Agents

Hypertonic (3%) saline infusion should be used only in patients whose hyponatremia has induced seizures or coma. Concomitant use of furosemide can act to increase free water excretion relative to sodium excretion and can diminish the volume expansion induced by hypertonic saline. The use of furosemide alone with replacement of measured urine electrolyte losses has also been suggested. Corticosteroids have been used in combination to increase sodium retention, but their use remains controversial. Lithium carbonate and demeclocycline inhibit ADH effects on the renal tubule and can correct hyponatremia, but significant complications limit their use in children.

CHAPTER 186

Chronic Renal Failure

Adapted from Edward C. Kohaut

The incidence of chronic renal disease in children is unknown, but current data suggest that 1.5 to 3.0 children per 1 million population per year develop end-stage renal disease (ESRD). Children with chronic renal disease present in a different manner from similarly affected adults (Table 186-1). The most common finding that should alert the pediatrician to the possibility of chronic renal disease is growth impairment. Short stature, particularly if associated with other symptoms such as polyuria, frequent bouts of dehydration, salt craving, bone deformities, abnormal tooth development, or anemia should suggest that the affected patient may have chronic renal disease. A previous history of urinary tract infections or glomerulonephritis adds further support to this suspected diagnosis. The currently accepted definitions for the stages of chronic renal disease are listed in Table 186-2.

ETIOLOGY

The etiologies of chronic renal failure (CRF) in children are listed in Table 186-3. The different forms of obstructive uropathy (including reflux and dysplasia) account for almost 50% of the etiologies of renal failure in children. Other relatively common causes of ESRD in children that are rare in adults include renal hypoplasia and dysplasia, hereditary nephritis, infantile polycystic disease, cystinosis, and uremic medullary cystic disease. Focal glomerulosclerosis is the most common glomerulopathy leading to renal failure in young children (accounting for 14.8% of all children with ESRD), but older children may suffer from many forms of chronic glomerulonephritis.

ABNORMALITIES ASSOCIATED WITH LOSS OF RENAL FUNCTION

Metabolic Changes

With progressive loss of renal function, many metabolic changes occur (Table 186-4). The level of blood urea nitrogen (BUN) is a

TABLE 186-1. Symptoms of Renal Failure

Symptoms seen in adults and children with chronic renal failure
Hypertension
Edema
Nocturia, polyuria
Lethargy
Itching
Nausea, vomiting
Peripheral neuropathy
Encephalopathy
Symptoms unique to children with chronic renal failure
Growth failure
Bone deformities
Abnormal tooth development
Unexplained dehydration
Salt craving

TABLE 186-2. Stages of Chronic Renal Disease

Stage	Residual renal function (%)	Symptoms or metabolic abnormality
Impaired renal function	40–80	None
Chronic renal insufficiency	25–50	Asymptomatic; short stature, increased parathyroid hormone
Chronic renal failure	<30	Acidosis, anemia, hypertension, lethargy
End-stage renal disease	Usually <10	Dialysis needed to maintain quality of life

function of dietary protein intake and renal clearance. Therefore, if protein intake remains constant as renal function declines, the BUN level increases and uremic symptoms occur. Uremia may lead to anorexia with a subsequent reduction in protein intake and a decrease in BUN. This change can lead less experienced physicians to think that the patient is improving when actually he or she is becoming malnourished, a condition that further complicates the disease process. The BUN level at which uremic symptoms occur depends on the patient's age, nutritional status, state of hydration, and the presence or absence of other metabolic abnormalities.

Phosphorus and Calcium

With further loss of renal function, phosphorus excretion decreases and may cause transient hyperphosphatemia and secondary hypocalcemia. The kidney produces 1,25-dihydroxycholecalciferol, the most active metabolite of vitamin D. Its synthesis is reduced in patients with renal insufficiency resulting in reduced intestinal calcium absorption and hypocalcemia. Hyperphosphatemia associated with reduced calcium absorption results in low serum calcium. The relative contribution of these two is unknown; however, the net result of both is a lowered level of serum calcium, which then stimulates secretion of parathyroid hormone. Increased serum parathyroid hormone suppresses proximal tubular reabsorption of phosphorus and normalizes serum phosphorus, but it also causes reabsorption of calcium and phosphorus from bone. This effect, coupled with decreased calcification of bone caused by reduction in vitamin D activity, leads to renal osteodystrophy. Renal osteodystrophy in children is a combination of the pathologic changes seen with rickets and secondary hyperparathyroidism. Rickets occurs only in growing bone; hence, the ricketic component of renal osteodystrophy is present only in children.

As reduction in renal function progresses, the hydrogen ion balance becomes positive and the phosphate balance becomes disrupted. As a result buffering capacity diminishes leading to acidosis.

TABLE 186-3. Etiology of Chronic Renal Failure in Children in Order of Frequency

Obstructive uropathy, including reflux nephropathy or renal dysplasia secondary to obstruction
Renal hypoplasia/dysplasia
Glomerulopathy/glomerulonephritis (all forms)
Hereditary disease, including hereditary nephritis or renal cystic diseases

TABLE 186-4. Metabolic Abnormalities Associated with Chronic Renal Failure

Elevated blood urea nitrogen and protein intolerance
Decreased phosphate excretion
Decreased sodium excretion
Reduced ability to conserve sodium
Decreased hydrogen ion excretion
Decreased potassium excretion
Reduced production of 1,25-dihydroxycholecalciferol
Reduced production of erythropoietin

Sodium

Sodium intolerance in patients with CRF is well recognized. However, some children with CRF secondary to obstructive uropathy or cystic diseases may not be able to conserve sodium. Children with loss of renal function must maintain sodium intake within a narrow range. A normal adult may tolerate a dietary sodium intake of 2 to 1,000 mEq/day. A patient with CRF and only 10% residual renal function may become depleted of sodium if dietary intake is less than 40 mEq/day. Conversely, the same patient may become hypertensive if sodium intake exceeds 80 mEq/day.

Potassium

Potassium balance can become positive in patients with CRF. Hyperkalemia is not usually seen until residual renal function is well less than 10% of normal. Hyperkalemia may be seen earlier in the course of CRF if the patient is depleted of sodium. Hyperkalemia may occur with greater than 10% residual function in the rare patient who has defective renin release secondary to renal damage. Hypokalemia can occur in some patients with CRF because of renal potassium wasting, but it usually results from anorexia, emesis, and inadequate potassium intake.

Anemia

Anemia, a well-known consequence of CRF, is the result of defective erythropoietin production by the damaged kidney. Patients with renal failure also have reduced gastrointestinal absorption of iron. Therefore, when evaluating these patients, iron deficiency as a cause for anemia must be considered. Exogenous erythropoietin is now available; through its use and avoidance of iron deficiency, the anemia of CRF can be reversed. Many of the symptoms that were previously thought to be from uremia have been reversed by using erythropoietin and iron therapy to correct the anemia associated with CRI.

Neuropathy

Neuropathy is a recognized part of the uremic syndrome. In children, especially infants, this consequence of CRF is of special importance. CRF early in life may delay brain development and lead to permanent neurologic impairment. Careful neurologic and frequent developmental evaluation of these children is required. Decisions concerning the timing of dialysis or transplantation may depend on the results of these examinations.

TREATMENT

Once CRF is recognized and the physiology of lost renal function is understood, treatment is required. The nondialytic

TABLE 186-5. Nondialytic Therapy of Chronic Renal Insufficiency or Chronic Renal Failure

Diet
Provide at least 100% recommended daily allowance of caloric intake
Protein intake controversial; range 0.5–1.5 g/kg/d
Renal osteodystrophy
1,25-Dihydroxycholecalciferol (dose variable)
Calcium carbonate (as a calcium supplement and PO_4 binder)
Anemia
May require iron
Erythropoietin
Hypertension
Control sodium intake
If hyperreninemic, consider angiotensin-converting enzyme inhibitor
Acidosis
May improve with reduced protein intake
Sodium citrate or $NaHCO_3$, 2–4 mEq/kg/d

treatment of a child with renal insufficiency is in a state of flux. Numerous changes in recommended therapy have been made over the past few years and will continue to be made as more information becomes available about the metabolic abnormalities and the requirements for growth in these children (Table 186-5).

GROWTH FAILURE

Growth failure is a common and often untreatable consequence of CRF in children. Growth failure is particularly severe in children who develop renal insufficiency in the first year of life. Infants with CRF grow poorly between birth and age 2 years. Even if normal growth velocity can be achieved from age 2 onward, so much growth potential has been lost that dwarfism is the result. Growth retardation could be avoided if catch-up growth were achieved after successful renal replacement therapy. However, accelerated growth only rarely occurs after a successful renal transplant. To affect growth in this population, early recognition of CRF is essential.

To correct growth failure, one must attempt to correct all the metabolic abnormalities mentioned. Adequate dietary intake is important, especially in infants with renal failure. Several infants with CRF were identified early in life, and aggressive nutritional therapy was initiated. Dietary intake was given by tube feedings (either nasogastric or transpyloric) in an amount to provide at least 100% of the RDA for calories and 1 to 2 g/kg/day of protein. Although data are sparse, near-normal growth has been achieved in some patients. Providing adequate nutrition to older dialysis patients also has affected growth favorably.

Therapy

Many children with CRF cannot conserve sodium. If sodium is restricted in these patients, poor growth may result; conversely, greater intake of sodium by these patients improves growth. Acidosis is often a complication of CRF, and correction and control of the acidosis are essential to normal growth in this population. Early and aggressive therapy of renal osteodystrophy with vitamin D metabolites and calcium carbonate is required for optimal growth in these children.

The anemia seen secondary to CRF may slow growth in these patients. Growth potential can be improved by careful attention to maintaining acid–base, electrolyte, and water balances in these patients. Treating renal osteodystrophy and providing adequate nutrition are essential in maintaining normal growth velocity. Although children with CRI and ESRD have growth hormone resistance, they respond favorably to supraphysiologic doses of growth hormone. Administration of recombinant human growth hormone has become the standard of care for the treatment of growth failure secondary to CRI and ESRD. However, its effect will be maximal only if all the other metabolic abnormalities associated with renal failure are addressed.

CHAPTER 187
Hypertension

Adapted from J. Timothy Bricker, L. Leighton Hill, and Stuart L. Goldstein

EFFECTS OF ELEVATION OF SYSTEMIC ARTERIAL BLOOD PRESSURE

The differential diagnosis of hypertension in children is shown in Table 187-1.

Neurologic Complications

Neurologic abnormalities caused by hypertension can include lethargy, headache, confusion, stupor, focal motor deficits, vision loss, seizures, and coma. In a retrospective study of hypertension with neurologic complications, convulsions were the initial feature in 42% of the children. Two of the patients had altered consciousness alone, and two had cranial nerve findings. Nausea and vomiting may be present in the early stages.

Physical findings often include advanced hypertensive retinopathy with papilledema, retinal hemorrhages, and retinal exudates, as well as abnormalities on neurologic examination.

Evidence of cerebral edema is likely on computed tomographic scanning. If features such as a stiff neck and fever mandate a lumbar puncture, both the cerebrospinal fluid pressure and protein content will probably be elevated. Most cases of hypertensive encephalopathy can be managed without a lumbar puncture, and the risk of lumbar puncture in the presence of an elevation in intracranial pressure is increased.

Treatment of the hypertension typically results in rapid improvement in the neurologic signs and symptoms, although some findings may require several days to resolve. Pathologic features include brain swelling, hemorrhages (punctate to massive), and microinfarctions. In some cases, swelling of the brain may be sufficient for herniation to be apparent.

The specific diagnosis of hypertensive encephalopathy (Table 187-2) is important to pursue because treatment for hypertensive encephalopathy (i.e., abruptly lowering the blood pressure to normal) can be detrimental in some patients with chronic hypertension. For example, the patient with severe renal artery stenosis may have diminished flow distal to the obstruction, which may result in renal ischemia if the arterial pressure is lowered abruptly by a systemic arteriolar dilator.

TABLE 187-1. Differential Diagnosis of Hypertension in Children

Iatrogenic, factitious, accidental
- Acute Na overload: $NaHCO_3$, glucose and electrolyte mixtures, Scholl's antibiotics (Na-penicillin or Na-carbenicillin), sodium polystyrene sulfonate (Kayexalate), phosphate replacements, contrast media (Hypaque = 786 mEq/L), intravenous fluids
- Licorice and related compounds (similar to aldosteronism)
- Exogenous corticosteroids
- Nonsteroidal antiinflammatory drugs: mineralocorticoidlike effect, probably mediated by prostaglandins
- Antidepressant drugs: monoamine oxidase inhibitors (with other drugs), tricyclics, lithium
- Other sympathomimetics (direct and indirect): phenylephrine eye or nose drops, appetite suppressants, cold medicines, thyroid medications
- Drug abuse: cocaine, amphetamines
- Immunosuppressive agents
- Erythropoietin
- Anesthetics: ketamine, cyclopropane, local anesthetics, pancuronium, narcotics [especially naloxone (Narcan)]
- Ergot alkaloids (for migraines, in obstetrics, from plants)
- Antihypertensive drug therapy (beta blockers, saralasin, clonidine, postganglionic blockers, methyldopa) with catecholamine excess or rebound
- Poisons: heavy metals, spider bites, drugs, plants
- Accidents: burns, orthopedic accidents, trauma

Cardiovascular etiology
- Coarctation of the aorta: preoperative, acute postoperative, residual, recurring
- Causes of *diastolic runoff* (systolic hypertension with a wide pulse pressure): patent ductus arteriosus, arteriovenous fistula, aortic regurgitation, anteroposterior window, ruptured sinus of Valsalva aneurysm, large aorticopulmonary anastomosis
- Infective endocarditis (renal mechanism)
- Arteritis (radiation, Takayasu disease, connective tissue disease)
- Peripheral atherosclerosis (systolic only with wide pulse pressure)

Renovascular hypertension
- Intrinsic renal artery disease
  - Intimal fibrosis (postinjury, idiopathic)
  - Medial (fibromuscular dysplasia, muscular hyperplasia)
  - Subadventitial (fibrosis or dysplasia)
  - Arteritis
  - Thrombotic
  - Embolic
  - Aneurysms, dissecting aneurysms
  - Fistulas
  - Neurofibromatosis
  - Associated with other congenital defects
    - Renal artery stenosis with coarctation
    - Uteropelvic junction obstruction
    - William syndrome
    - Atherosclerotic lesions
- Extrinsic compression
  - Renal parenchymal tumors
  - Paraaortic tumors
    - Neurofibroma
    - Pheochromocytoma
    - Ganglioneuroma
  - Paraaortic lymphatics
    - Lymphoma
    - Chronic granulomatous disease
  - Ectopic kidney position
  - Iatrogenic (ligature involving a normal or aberrant renal artery)

Renal parenchymal and structural disease
- Cystic disease
  - Infantile polycystic kidneys
  - Adult polycystic kidneys
  - Medullary sponge kidney (juvenile nephronophthisis) with Zellweger, Jeune, Goldenhar, trisomies D and E, and orofacial digital syndromes; short rib polydactyly; Ehlers-Danlos syndrome; various chromosome translocations
- Segmental hypoplasia (Ask-Upmark kidney)
- Hydronephrosis
- Pyelonephritis
- Glomerulonephritis
- Renal vein thrombosis (uncommon)
- Trauma
  - Page kidney (cellophane), resultant parenchymal compression
  - Transient hypertension after blunt abdominal trauma
- Nephrotic syndrome
- Hemolytic-uremic syndrome
- Sickle cell disease

Endocrine causes
- Congenital adrenal hyperplasia
  - 11-Hydroxylase deficiency
  - 17-Hydroxylase deficiency
- Cushing syndrome
  - Iatrogenic
- Hyperaldosteronism
  - Primary
  - Exogenous
  - Secondary
- Tumors
  - Pheochromocytoma, neuroblastoma, ganglioneuroblastoma, argentaffinoma, Wilms tumor, juxtaglomerular apparatus tumors
- Thyrotoxicosis
- Hyperparathyroidism
- Turner syndrome patients taking estrogens
- Oral contraceptives, syndrome of inappropriate antidiuretic hormone excess

Central nervous system hypertension
- Elevated intracranial pressure, ischemia
- Riley-Day syndrome (familial dysautonomia)
- Quadriplegia, polio, Guillain-Barré syndrome
- Absent corpus callosum, increased antidiuretic hormone–hypertension syndrome

Other causes
- Volume excess from polycythemia
- Stevens-Johnson syndrome
- Cyclic vomiting with dehydration
- Intussusception
- Femoral nerve traction

Modified from Inglefinger J. *Hypertension in childhood.* Philadelphia: Saunders, 1982.

The diagnosis of hypertensive encephalopathy should be viewed with some skepticism in the setting of hypertension that is chronic and not extremely severe and if a plausible alternative explanation of the encephalopathy exists. Lowering the systemic arterial blood pressure in many of the chronically hypertensive patients admitted to the intensive care unit (ICU) may be necessary, but it is not safe to do so as abruptly as one would with acutely hypertensive patients who are usually normotensive.

Children who recover from hypertensive encephalopathy can be expected to do well. In a 10-year study of 45 children with neurologic complications of hypertension, no neurologic or cognitive sequelae were noted on long-term follow-up.

Another neurologic problem associated with severe hypertension is the development of intracranial hemorrhage. Massive hemorrhage caused by hypertension may occur in a child with a berry aneurysm of the circle of Willis or after a recent neurosurgical procedure. Systemic hypertension in profoundly premature

TABLE 187-2. Conditions that may be Confused with Hypertensive Encephalopathy*

Illicit or therapeutic drugs
Uremic encephalopathy
Encephalitis or meningoencephalitis
Hypoglycemia
Hypocalcemia
Trauma
Low cerebral blood flow
Hepatic causes
Reye syndrome
Diabetic ketoacidosis
Seizure disorder
Hyperthyroidism or hypothyroidism
Psychosis
Cerebritis

*Hypertensive encephalopathy is defined as a hypertensive state with alternative (superimposed) explanation of encephalopathic features.

infants is thought to put them at risk for subependymal bleeding from the germinal matrix.

Cardiopulmonary Complications

Acute and severe hypertension can be associated with cardiac dilation, elevation of the left ventricular end-diastolic pressure, and symptomatic pulmonary edema. The normal myocardium handles the acute increase in left ventricular afterload relatively well. Children with acute glomerulonephritis do not typically have findings of a low cardiac output state as a result of increased afterload, and, typically, symptomatic pulmonary edema resolves rapidly without residual cardiac abnormality when the excessive intravascular blood volume associated with acute glomerulonephritis is lowered by diuretic therapy.

Some children have a limited cardiac reserve because of severe prematurity, congenital cardiac disease, or acquired cardiac disease. Under these circumstances, a hypertensive crisis may result in cardiovascular decompensation. Abruptly lowering the systemic arterial pressure is required in this setting. Cardiovascular decompensation with hypertensive crisis is more common in adults than in children because of the prevalence of overt or subclinical coronary artery atherosclerotic disease among adults with hypertension. Most children with hypertension have a hyperdynamic apex impulse, a dilated heart with an apex impulse displaced laterally, and a diastolic filling sound during a hypertensive crisis. Chronic hypertension is a risk factor for the development of atherosclerosis later in life. Chronic hypertension may be associated with left ventricular hypertrophy and arterial abnormalities. Acute aortic dissection has occurred in severely hypertensive children who did not have features of Marfan syndrome or other abnormalities of connective tissue. The degree of left ventricular hypertrophy ascertained by electrocardiography and echocardiography can give a clue as to the chronicity of hypertension. Left ventricular mass, as measured by echocardiography, is associated with long-term cardiovascular risk.

Complications in Other Organ Systems

Ophthalmic abnormalities may be related to severe hypertensive retinopathy. Nonneurologic manifestations of the effects of severe, acute hypertension in children are lower in frequency and severity compared with effects on the brain. Urgent therapy for hypertension might be considered in the child whose hypertension is associated with bleeding after cardiac surgery or whose hypertension might compromise the success of a renal transplant.

Renal Hypertension

An abnormal activation of the renin–angiotensin–aldosterone system is a significant cause of hypertension in children. Intrinsic renovascular hypertension (RVH), which arises from a disturbance of the circulation to one or both kidneys, is considered the prototypical lesion leading to renin-mediated hypertension. However, other renal diseases associated with the obliteration of blood vessels within the renal parenchyma are also associated with renin-mediated hypertension. The most common of these is the hypertension associated with renal scarring that results from reflux and recurrent pyelonephritis. Renin-mediated hypertension may also be seen as a complication of renal vein thrombosis, dysplastic kidneys, hypoplastic kidneys, polycystic kidneys, obstructive uropathy, and radiation nephritis. Rarely, juxtaglomerular cell tumors and nephroblastomas may produce renin directly and cause hypertension without affecting the renal circulation. Nephroblastomas, hamartomas, and arteriovenous malformations can also compress the renal artery, leading to ischemia and renin-mediated hypertension.

CLINICAL CHARACTERISTICS

Table 187-3 lists clinical clues that suggest RVH. RVH should be considered in any severe case of hypertension in a child whose condition is refractory to vasodilatory agents. An abdominal bruit, left ventricular hypertrophy (detected on echocardiogram), signs of secondary hyperaldosteronism (hypokalemia, mild alkalosis), and retinopathy suggest a chronic hypertensive disorder and should lead to a consideration of RVH. Finally, hypertension associated with a unilateral small kidney and an excellent response to ACE inhibitors is highly suggestive of RVH.

DIAGNOSTIC STUDIES

Renal arteriography remains the gold standard study for investigating RVH. The ultimate confirmation of RVH is the resolution of hypertension after surgical correction of the lesion. Considerable effort has been expended during the 1990s to evaluate the sensitivity and specificity of less invasive modes of investigation to spare the patient unnecessary surgical investigation. Although many of these tests are useful in screening for RVH in adults, their effectiveness has not been studied extensively in children. Furthermore, these tests have a low predictive value when used to screen the general population. Keeping in mind the limitations of these tests, viewing the results in light of the clinical picture, and using the tests judiciously in patients in whom the suspicion is high for RVH are all important.

Peripheral Renin Activity

The measurement of peripheral renin activity (PRA) has not been of value in screening or as a diagnostic test for RVH. PRA has a sensitivity and specificity of less than 75% and may be elevated or suppressed by many medications. In addition, many unrelated conditions including hyperthyroidism, congenial adrenal

TABLE 187-3. Clinical Clues that Suggest Renovascular Hypertension

Abrupt onset of severe hypertension
Epigastric, subcostal, or flank bruit
Progression to malignant-phase hypertension
Retinopathy
Hypokalemia
Plasma bicarbonate high-normal to elevated
Hypertension refractory to intensive antihypertensive regimen
Hypertension with unilateral small kidney
Excellent response to angiotensin-converting enzyme inhibitors
Transient impairment in renal function in response to angiotensin-converting enzyme inhibitor

insufficiency, pheochromocytoma, and salt-wasting renal diseases may elevate the PRA.

Renal Ultrasonography

Renal ultrasonography should be performed as a screening test in all children with hypertension. Ultrasonography provides accurate and meaningful information regarding kidney size, location, architecture, and contour. In newborns, it can detect vascular thrombosis secondary to umbilical artery catheters or dehydration. Many studies have been performed to evaluate the reliability of Doppler ultrasonographic imaging of renal arterial flow in diagnosing RVH. These studies have compared findings with angiography. Although the sensitivity is nearly 90% in adults, few studies have reproduced this degree of reliability in children. This difference may result from the differing etiologies of RVH in children and adults. In children, smaller vessels are more commonly involved and differences in renal blood flow cannot be resolved by Doppler imaging. In adults, RVH is often caused by atherosclerosis of larger vessels, which is more amenable to detection by Doppler imaging. Interestingly, one prospective study of children with renin-mediated hypertension showed that a negative Doppler imaging study was highly predictive for a cure with surgical or endovascular therapy. In any case, renal Doppler imaging should not be relied on to diagnose RVH at this time.

Radionuclide Evaluation

ACE inhibitors have been used in conjunction with radionuclide imaging to diagnose RVH. Renal function in a kidney that has a stenotic artery is dependent on the high renin levels produced by that kidney to maintain an elevated efferent arteriolar tone. This tone is depressed when an ACE inhibitor is given. When the kidney is visualized with radionuclide imaging after administration of an ACE inhibitor, a decreased uptake and clearance of the isotope from the affected kidney are present. This test has proved to be nearly 90% sensitive in diagnosing adults with suspected RVH. Studies in children have yielded conflicting results. Nevertheless, this study is helpful in identifying potential areas of disturbed renal circulation and is a valuable tool in the workup of suspected RVH. A negative test, however, should not preclude the diagnosis of RVH when the clinical picture is strongly suggestive of RVH.

Renal Arteriography

Renal arteriography with measurement of renal vein renin levels remains the gold standard in the diagnosis of RVH. These studies are usually performed simultaneously and provide both anatomic and functional information. The purpose of these studies is to visualize a functionally significant lesion. The presence of collateral vessels with a stenotic lesion is considered significant. Differential renal vein renin levels are obtained from effluent venous blood from each renal vein and from the inferior vena cava. In unilateral RVH, the affected kidney should have a renal vein renin activity of at least 1.5 times that of the vein of the unaffected kidney. In addition, a renal-to-systemic renin index is calculated with the level from the inferior vena cava. Differences in renin activity can be stimulated by sodium depletion or administration of an ACE inhibitor. The presence of a significant difference in renal vein activity is 90% predictive of a benefit from surgical intervention; however, many patients with a negative study also benefit from surgery.

CLINICAL MANAGEMENT OF RVH

The major objective of management of renin-mediated hypertension is to prevent the complications of hypertension by controlling blood pressure and preventing or slowing the loss of renal function. Control of moderate to severe hypertension is critical while the patient is undergoing evaluation. Long-term therapy may be medical using pharmacologic agents or surgical. Medical therapy has improved with the availability of ACE inhibitors since the 1980s. ACE inhibitors are the drugs of choice in children with renin-mediated hypertension. However, ACE inhibitors must be used with extreme caution in children with bilateral renal artery stenosis or evidence of a stenosis in a solitary kidney because they can cause renal failure in these circumstances. Thus, delaying initiation of ACE inhibitor therapy is prudent until these possibilities have been ruled out.

Surgical Options

Surgical options include nephrectomy, partial nephrectomy, revascularization by reconstructive vascular surgery, and autotransplantation. Another surgical therapeutic option is percutaneous transluminal renal angioplasty (PTRA). In this technique, a balloon catheter is used to dilate the constricted portion of the renal artery. This technique has a high degree of success in children with fibromuscular dysplasia. The lesions associated with neurofibromatosis, developmental anomalies of the aorta, and lesions secondary to arteritis are less amenable to treatment with PTRA. The restenosis rates vary from 10% to 30%. In many centers, PTRA is performed at the time of renal arteriography.

Artifacts in Blood Pressure Measurement

A common cause of artifactual hypertension is a cuff that is too small for the patient. The width of the cuff bladder should be approximately 40% to 50% of the circumference of the child's upper arm at its midpoint. This principle applies to both oscillometric and auscultatory methods of blood pressure determination.

Another type of artifact with auscultatory measurement of the systemic arterial pressure is the missed auscultatory gap. The auscultatory gap is a silent pressure interval between the onset of Korotkoff's sounds and their final disappearance or muffling. Failure to inflate the cuff to a sufficient pressure (i.e., 20 mm Hg above the point at which Korotkoff's sounds are heard on the first measurement confirmed by the disappearance of the radial pulse) or failure to listen for Korotkoff's sounds all the way down to zero can result in the appearance of a

TABLE 187-4. Drugs and Dosages for Use in the Treatment of Hypertensive Emergencies in Children

Drug	Dose	Comments
Diazoxide	1–10 mg/kg per dose IV	Should start at lower range; rapid infusion; watch for hypotension and hyperglycemia
Hydralazine	0.2–0.8 mg/kg per dose IV 1.05–5.00 mg/kg/d PO	Concerns about development of lupuslike phenomenon
Nitroprusside	0.5–8.0 μg/kg/min infusion	Cyanide and thiocyanate toxicity with prolonged high-dose therapy
Propranolol	0.1–2.0 mg/kg per dose	IV use with slow infusion and with capability to pace if bradycardia is excessive
Verapamil	0.1–0.2 mg/kg per dose	Should not be used if patient is younger than 6 months, is on beta blockers, or has congestive heart failure
Hydrochlorothiazide	0.5–2.0 mg/kg/d PO	More often for chronic therapy
Methyldopa	10–40 mg/kg/d	More often for chronic therapy
Esmolol	50–300 μg/kg/min infusion	Beta blocker with extremely rapid onset and termination of effect
Phentolamine	2.5–15.0 μg/kg/min infusion	Direct alpha blocker
Labetalol	0.5–3.0 mg/kg/hr infusion	Both alpha and beta blockade; little effect on cardiac output
Thorazine	0.5–1.0 mg/kg per dose IV	Sedative effects predominate; alpha-blockade side effect makes this agent useful after coarctation repair
Phenoxybenzamine	0.5–1.0 mg/kg IV	Investigational pediatric use as a vasodilator after heart surgery

sudden increase or decrease in blood pressure when it is measured accurately.

Treatment of Hypertensive Emergencies

Nitroprusside is an arteriolar dilator that lowers blood pressure by dropping the systemic vascular resistance. A nitroprusside infusion rapidly acts to lower the pressure and can be titrated to the arterial pressure desired. Blood pressure does not usually need to be decreased into the normal range to treat a hypertensive emergency. This is particularly true if chronic hypertension has been present before the hypertensive emergency. Nitroprusside must be used carefully because of the tendency of this drug to lower blood pressure below desired limits. Continuous blood pressure measurement with an indwelling arterial line is optimal during nitroprusside infusions. The usual dose ranges from 0.5 to 8.0 μg/kg/minute. High doses and prolonged infusions are associated with toxicity from cyanide and thiocyanate (Table 187-4).

A standard agent for lowering blood pressure in patients with hypertensive encephalopathy in the past has been diazoxide. An advantage is that this drug is less likely than nitroprusside to "bottom out" the blood pressure, but titration of effect is more difficult. The usual dose range is 3 to 5 mg/kg intravenously; however, a dose of 1 to 2 mg/kg has been found to be adequate in many cases, so an initial dose in the lower range is recommended. A dose of 10 mg/kg may be required in some cases. Diazoxide must be given in a rapid bolus because slow intravenous infusions result in binding of the drug by plasma proteins and loss of effect. Although diazoxide is unlikely to lower the blood pressure to an excessive degree, monitoring the pressure immediately after a bolus dose is wise. Appropriate management of excessive hypotension includes a volume infusion (e.g., 10 mL/kg of normal saline). Hyperglycemia is a side effect of diazoxide and is of particular concern when repeated doses are required.

Treating cerebral edema with an osmotic agent such as mannitol or glycerol and with hyperventilation sufficient to maintain the arterial P_{CO_2} in the low 30 mm Hg range may be necessary in some cases of hypertensive encephalopathy associated with profound brain swelling. Lowering blood pressure alone is sufficient in the vast majority of cases.

Use of nitroprusside to abruptly lower the blood pressure in the setting of a hypertensive crisis with congestive heart failure is reasonable. Volume reduction by diuretic therapy alone may ameliorate the findings of pulmonary edema in some of these cases. Diuretic therapy should be included for most patients with a hypertensive crisis that includes pulmonary edema. Patients in renal failure with a hypertensive crisis may not be responsive to diuretics. If substantial volume overload occurs, patients with renal impairment and cardiac dysfunction or cardiogenic pulmonary edema may need dialysis or plasmapheresis. Pericardial effusion is a common cause of radiographic cardiomegaly in the uremic patient. Cardiac tamponade in the uremic patient should be kept in mind as a possible cause of symptoms of heart failure. Abrupt volume reduction without treatment of cardiac tamponade in this setting is likely to result in further hemodynamic deterioration.

Abrupt onset of severe hypertension immediately after repair of coarctation of the aorta can result in neurologic and cardiovascular complications, increase the risk of postoperative bleeding, and lead to other findings of postcoarctectomy syndrome. Numerous antihypertensives have been used over the years. Our standard initial approach is a single dose of chlorpromazine (Thorazine, 0.5–1.0 mg/kg per dose intravenously), which lowers the blood pressure because of the side effect of alpha blockade, in addition to providing mild sedation. A single dose is often effective in lowering the blood pressure after coarctation surgery. Lowering pressure to the range of the preoperative pressure in the upper extremities is adequate.

Hydralazine is a common choice for the management of a hypertensive crisis after emergency treatment. Hydralazine can be given at a dose of 0.2 to 0.8 mg/kg intravenously or 1 to 5 mg/kg/day orally. A lupus-like syndrome occurs in some patients given hydralazine, but it is typically reversible when the drug is discontinued. Hydralazine is commonly used for patients who have hypertension associated with systemic lupus erythematosus including a hypertensive crisis.

Beta blockers may be useful adjuncts in the treatment of chronic hypertension. Intravenous beta-blocker therapy is rarely required for pediatric hypertension. If such therapy is needed, an agent with rapid onset and termination of action such as esmolol is the optimal choice. The emergency use of intravenous beta blockers in children is considered relatively hazardous, and the physician should be prepared to pace the rhythm if excess bradycardia occurs. The potential for negative inotropic effect is also a concern with the use of intravenous beta blockers. Labetalol has been useful for hypertensive emergencies in adults. Little experience exists in pediatric patients.

Alpha blockade with phentolamine is useful in treating hypertension occurring with hypercatecholamine states. Phentolamine treatment of pheochromocytoma cases and prophylaxis for pheochromocytoma at the time of surgery is standard. Phenoxybenzamine is an alpha blocker used in lowering systemic vascular resistance and systemic arterial pressure after infant heart surgery. Prazosin is an $alpha_1$ blocker used in chronic antihypertensive therapy but not in hypertensive emergencies.

Intravenous verapamil and other calcium channel blockers have been used to treat hypertension. They are also rarely used in the emergency treatment of hypertension. As with the beta blockers, the role of calcium channel blockers in hypertension is primarily as an adjunct in chronic therapy.

Angiotensin-converting enzyme inhibitors are valuable in the chronic treatment of hypertension, but they have little role in emergency management.

7 Gastrointestinal System

CHAPTER 188 Functional Constipation and Encopresis

Adapted from William J. Klish

Constipation is a common complaint in children and is one of the problems most frequently referred to the pediatric gastroenterologist. *Constipation* refers to both the frequency of defecation and the consistency of the stool. It is important to note that both of these parameters change normally with age and diet. The normal infant tends to pass a stool after each feeding, but this pattern varies considerably. Children older than 6 months tend to pass a stool at least once a day. Less frequent stools should be of concern if they are hard, dry, unusually large, or difficult to pass.

Encopresis denotes the syndrome of fecal soiling or incontinence secondary to constipation. Although psychological symptoms are often present in children with this problem.

Many general causes exist for constipation. Causes to be considered in the differential diagnosis of constipation are listed in Table 188-1.

TABLE 188-1. Causes of Constipation

Functional constipation and encopresis
Dietary causes
Protracted vomiting
Excessive intake of cow's milk
Lack of bulk in diet
Drugs that affect motility
Structural defects of the anus or rectum
Anterior displacement of the anus
Anal or rectal stenosis
Presacral teratoma
Rectal prolapse
Smooth muscle disease
Scleroderma
Dermatomyositis
Systemic lupus erythematosus
Primary chronic intestinal pseudoobstruction
Abnormal myenteric ganglion cells
Hirschsprung disease
Chagas disease
von Recklinghausen disease
Multiple endocrine neoplasia type IIB
Absence of abdominal musculature
Spinal cord defects
Spina bifida occulta
Myelomeningocele
Meningocele
Diastematomyelia
Paraplegia
Cauda equina tumor
Tethered cord syndrome
Metabolic and endocrine disorders
Hypothyroidism
Hypoparathyroidism
Renal tubular acidosis
Diabetes insipidus
Vitamin D intoxication
Idiopathic hypercalcemia
Hypokalemia
Neurologic and psychiatric conditions
Myotonic dystrophy
Amyotonia congenita
Mental retardation
Psychosis

PATHOPHYSIOLOGY

The rectum functions not as a storage area for fecal material but rather as a sensing organ that initiates the process of defecation. When stool moves into the rectum from the sigmoid colon, pressure is put on the wall and the rectal valves. This pressure initiates an impulse resulting in relaxation of the internal anal sphincter, which is experienced as the urgency felt just before defecation. If defecation is inconvenient, contraction of the external sphincter is initiated, first by reflex and then intentionally. The external sphincter is assisted by contraction of the puborectalis muscle, which helps constrict and angulate the anal canal. If the external sphincter is held contracted long enough, the reflex to the internal sphincter wanes and the urge to defecate disappears. When defecation is convenient, the external sphincter is consciously relaxed and stool is propelled by colonic peristalsis through the open anal canal. As stool enters the anal canal, a secondary reflex is initiated via the somatic nervous system that results in contraction of the abdominal musculature and assists in emptying the lower colon.

Constipation

Children who develop functional constipation associate discomfort with defecation. The most common reason for discomfort is an *anal fissure* resulting from either hard stool or the use of suppositories, enemas, or a rectal thermometer. Occasionally, the sense of discomfort results from a bad toilet-training experience. Whatever the cause, the result is the same. Whenever the child feels the sensation associated with relaxation of the internal anal sphincter, he or she aggressively contracts the external sphincter to prevent expulsion of stool and the pain it is expected to bring. Increased amounts of stool collect in the rectum, and over a period of months, the rectum gradually dilates. As it enlarges, it becomes less capable of propulsive peristaltic activity, which results in more stool retention. As the volume of the rectum increases, its sensory capacity diminishes, so that retention is easier. Eventually, the constipation becomes self-perpetuating.

Encopresis

Encopresis develops when the rectal vault enlarges sufficiently to exert pressure on the structures of the floor of the pelvis including the levator muscle. This muscle interdigitates with the anal sphincters. As it is pushed downward, the anal sphincters become distorted and the anal canal shortened. If the external anal sphincter is allowed to relax, it assumes a slightly open position. During activity, loose or mushy stool can then flow around firmer stool present in the rectum and leak out. Affected children instinctively know they have little control over the leakage at this point, so they often adopt a casual attitude that is frustrating to their parents. They constantly smell of fecal material, which may result in ridicule by their peers and secondary psychological problems.

CLINICAL FINDINGS AND DIAGNOSIS

The most common symptom associated with constipation is chronic recurrent abdominal pain. Enuresis is reported in approximately 30% of the children with encopresis. Urinary tract infection is a common complication in girls with chronic constipation.

Stools of very large caliber are another associated symptom. Parents must often break up stools mechanically to flush the toilet.

In children with encopresis, soiling is less common when the child is sedentary. Most children insist that they do not feel the stools coming and do not perceive the sensation of impending soiling until they actually feel stool in their underwear.

Poor appetite and poor growth are occasionally seen in association with constipation and may result from early satiety caused by the feeling of fullness of the colon.

The diagnosis of functional constipation or encopresis is made from the history and physical examination. Stool is often palpable in the abdomen, particularly in the left lower quadrant. Rectal examination reveals a short anal canal associated with a large, dilated rectum, full of stool. The external sphincter is intact.

A barium enema may show dilatation of the rectum to the anal verge. This is diagnostic of functional constipation and rules out Hirschsprung disease.

Rectal manometry can be helpful in distinguishing functional constipation from Hirschsprung disease and sacral nerve abnormalities. Functional constipation is associated with normal relaxation of the internal anal sphincter and no contraction of the external anal sphincter in response to considerable distention of the rectal ampulla. Normal contraction of the external anal sphincter should be elicited by stimulating the perianal skin to rule out abnormalities of sensory input.

TREATMENT

Simple constipation in the neonate is best treated with a nonabsorbable carbohydrate such as malt extract or lactulose. These can be titrated upward until the desired effect is achieved. In older children and adolescents with simple constipation, stool softeners such as docusate sodium (Colace) or bulking agents are suggested.

In children with long-standing functional constipation or encopresis associated with a megarectum, a laxative program is required. The rectal vault should first be emptied with a phosphosoda (Fleet) or soapsuds enema. No more than two enemas should be given in a single day. Once the rectum has been cleared of stool, a program of daily laxative administration should be initiated to allow the rectum to return to normal size. Laxatives such as flavored milk of magnesia should be given once per day. Adjustments are made daily until a dose is found that stimulates one or two normal bowel movements per day.

Patients should be reexamined at 1- to 2-month intervals, and a rectal examination should be performed to determine rectal vault size. Laxatives can be tapered when the rectal vault returns to normal size, which may take 6 months to 1 year. At that time, parents and children should be instructed about proper diet and the use of bulking agents to avoid hard stools. During laxative therapy, attempts should be made to establish a bowel habit. Once the parent determines when the laxative begins to stimulate, the child should be asked to sit on the toilet at that time each day. This behavior should continue after the laxative has been discontinued.

CHAPTER 189
Chronic Nonspecific Diarrhea of Childhood

Adapted from William J. Klish

Chronic nonspecific diarrhea is a common problem seen in children between 6 and 36 months of age. It consists of a pattern of two or more loose, voluminous stools per day (frequently containing undigested food particles) lasting for more than 4 weeks, unassociated with other symptoms such as pain or growth failure. Children with this syndrome are not usually bothered by the diarrhea.

ETIOLOGY

Malabsorption is not a factor. The etiology remains unknown with the cause of the diarrhea either being enhanced secretion of fluid in the bowel or interference with absorption of water and electrolytes from the colon. The classic symptoms may be preceded by an acute infection or by the child taking a course of a broad-spectrum antibiotic.

Some children drink large amounts of fruit juice. This intake plays some role in the perpetuation of the diarrhea, because enough poorly absorbed carbohydrate such as sorbitol or fructose can result in the stimulus for diarrhea. Lack of dietary fiber and other residue may help perpetuate the loose stools.

DIFFERENTIAL DIAGNOSIS

Disaccharide intolerance, infection, protein hypersensitivity, and, occasionally, inflammatory bowel disease can mimic chronic nonspecific diarrhea in presenting symptoms. Carbohydrate intolerance can be determined through the use of Clinitest tablets to screen for reducing sugars in the stool. A stool pH of less than 5.5 is suggestive of carbohydrate intolerance.

Most pathogenic bacteria don't produce diarrhea for several weeks. However, *Campylobacter jejuni* has been implicated in several cases of chronic diarrhea and must be ruled out with a stool culture. *Giardia lamblia* infection can have identical symptoms to chronic nonspecific diarrhea.

A complete blood count with differential, reticulocyte count, and stool guaiac test might give a clue to the presence of either protein hypersensitivity or inflammatory bowel disease. Eosinophilia is occasionally present in protein hypersensitivity.

TREATMENT

It should be stressed that diarrhea does not threaten the child's well-being. The syndrome improves with age, and most children have outgrown it by age 3 years. Furthermore, many therapies fail.

All children should be placed on a regular diet for age without excessive juices. If and when further therapies are needed, psyllium bulking agents are effective at minimizing the diarrhea. If no response is seen in 7 to 10 days, persisting with psyllium therapy is not necessary. Discontinuation of psyllium can be attempted after a few weeks and diarrhea may not recur.

Cholestyramine and metronidazole have also been used successfully to treat this syndrome.

TABLE 190-1. Causes of Gastrointestinal Bleeding

First 4 weeks
Swallowed maternal blood
Hemorrhagic disease of the newborn
Anal fissure
Hemorrhagic gastritis
Stress ulcers
Infective enterocolitis
Protein-sensitive enterocolitis
Necrotizing enterocolitis
Hirschsprung enterocolitis
Duplication cysts
Midgul volvulus
Vascular malformations
First 6 months
Nonspecific colitis
Anal fissure
Esophagitis
Infective enterocolitis
Protein-sensitive enterocolitis
Intussusception
Lymphonodular hyperplasia
Duplication cysts
Hirschsprung enterocolitis
Vascular malformations
6 months to 5 years
Epistaxis
Esophagitis
Esophageal varices
Gastritis
Infective enterocolitis
Clostridium difficile colitis
Lymphonodular hyperplasia
Intussusception
Meckel diverticulum
Vascular malformations
Henoch-Schönlein purpura
Hemolytic uremic syndrome
Neutropenic typhlitis
Polyps
Anal fissure
5 to 18 years
Same as for 6 months to 5 years plus
Tear in gastric mucosa (Mallory-Weiss syndrome)
Gastritis
Peptic ulcer
Chronic ulcerative colitis
Crohn's disease
Hemorrhoids

CHAPTER 190
Gastrointestinal Bleeding

Adapted from Marilyn R. Brown

Some types of gastrointestinal (GI) bleeding in children are common and relatively benign while others are less common and, occasionally, life threatening. Substances such as food dyes, beets (red appearance), iron and blueberries (black appearance) may give the appearance of blood in stool. Therefore, it is imperative that the physician first determines if the child has bled by use of a test for occult blood (Hemoccult or other). The diagnostic and treatment approach then hinges on differentiating bleeding from the upper (originating above the ligament of Treitz) or lower GI tract. Certain causes of GI bleeding are age dependent (Table 190-1) while others are age independent. A description of the color, location, and amount of blood is usually helpful. Proper terminology would include hemoptysis (coughing up blood), hematemesis (vomiting up blood), hematochezia (bright red blood per rectum) and melena (black or dark maroon stool).

AGE-INDEPENDENT ETIOLOGIES

At all ages, stress (burns, central nervous system trauma) and ingestion of nonsteroidal antiinflammatory drugs (NSAIDs) may lead to gastric stress erosions and ulcerations. Thrombocytopenia and coagulopathies should be considered a possibility in all ages. Although primary tumors of the GI tract are rare, they must be considered in the differential diagnosis at any age.

AGE-ASSOCIATED ETIOLOGIES

First 4 Weeks

In the first few days of life, hematemesis or the passage of bloody stools in a healthy newborn is most likely caused by swallowed maternal blood, which can be differentiated from fetal hemoglobin by the Apt alkali denaturation test. If the red blood denatures with alkali to a brown color, the hemoglobin is of adult origin. Hemorrhagic disease of the newborn with prolongation of the prothrombin time must be considered when vitamin K has not been administered. Breast-fed infants are particularly susceptible to this complication.

An anal fissure is a common cause of bleeding, usually initiated by the passage of a firm stool that makes a small tear along the anal canal. Stressed neonates may develop hemorrhagic gastritis or gastric stress ulcers. Necrotizing enterocolitis, Hirschsprung enterocolitis, midgut volvulus, and intestinal duplication cysts may also present with bleeding and must be kept in mind.

First 6 Months

Nonspecific colitis and protein-induced colitis are frequent causes of hematochezia in infants younger than 6 months. Gastroesophageal reflux is very common in infants and may cause reflux esophagitis with blood loss.

Among bacterial causes of bloody diarrhea, shigellosis, salmonellosis, *Campylobacter jejuni*, and enteroinvasive *Escherichia coli* may cause lower GI bleeding. Although *Clostridium difficile* organisms and toxin can be found in asymptomatic infants, antibiotic associated colitis can occur.

Allergic enterocolitis induced by milk, soy, or other proteins is a frequent cause of blood in the intestinal tract in the infant leading to protein-loss, hypoalbuminemia, and guaiac-positive stools. It may also occur in infants who are breast-fed; in these cases, the mother may be placed on a trial diet free of milk, soy, or other potential allergen. Allergic gastritis can lead to bloody vomitus.

6 Months to 5 Years

Epistaxis must always be considered as a cause of blood in vomitus. The blood loss from esophagitis associated with gastroesophageal reflux may be associated with "coffee ground" (dark brown) emesis, but it is often occult and may cause chronic anemia.

Intussusception (the telescoping of a proximal portion of the intestine into the distal portion) occurs most commonly during the first 2 years of life and usually presents with severe, colicky abdominal pain. The process may progress to vomiting, lethargy, "currant jelly" stools, with complete intestinal obstruction (see Chapter 192).

Meckel diverticulum, a remnant of the omphalomesenteric duct located in the ileum approximately 30 cm from the ileocecal valve, is often asymptomatic; however, when it contains gastric mucosa, acid secretion can cause ulceration in either the diverticulum or the adjacent ileum with subsequent painless bleeding presenting as black or maroon stools and anemia. The diagnosis is made by technetium Tc 99m pertechnetate radionuclide scan. Surgery is indicated for bleeding. A Meckel diverticulum may also act as a lead point for intussusception.

Henoch–Schönlein purpura (HSP) is a systemic vasculitis in which abdominal cramps and intestinal bleeding may precede the purpuric skin manifestations. Ileoileal intussusception may occur in HSP.

Juvenile colonic polyps (inflammatory hamartomas) are a common cause of intermittent painless hematochezia in children 2 to 5 years of age. The diagnosis is made by digital rectal examination, barium enema, sigmoidoscopy, or colonoscopy. Cauterization or polypectomy are the typical treatments.

5 to 18 Years

Repeated episodes of forceful vomiting may cause a small linear tear (Mallory–Weiss syndrome) at the gastroesophageal junction with minimal or moderate blood loss.

The spiral gram-negative organism *Helicobacter pylori* may inhabit the surface of mucosal epithelial cells of the stomach and, occasionally, the duodenum. Its presence is associated with local inflammation (chronic gastritis) (see Chapter 79).

The chronic inflammatory bowel diseases, Crohn's disease and ulcerative colitis, are of unknown etiology and characterized by a remitting–relapsing symptom pattern. These disorders are covered in separate chapters in this book.

Peutz–Jeghers syndrome consists of diffuse GI hamartomas associated with melanotic areas on the buccal mucosa and lips. Other chronic polyposes include juvenile polyposis coli, familial adenomatous polyposis, and Gardner syndrome (familial adenomatous polyposis associated with bony lesions, subcutaneous tumors, and cysts).

Vascular lesions take a variety of forms. Telangiectasias may be associated with Turner syndrome. Small angiodysplasias, hemangiomas, or arteriovenous malformations may occur, and arteriography may be helpful in diagnosis.

DIAGNOSIS AND THERAPY

A careful history and physical examination are helpful in most cases. The condition of the child determines the rapidity of the approach to diagnosis. If the child is unstable, the history, physical examination, diagnosis, and therapy must be performed rapidly.

Important elements of the history include age of the child; amount and character of the bleeding in vomitus or stool; presence of associated abdominal or rectal pain, diarrhea, drug ingestion, fever, and systemic symptoms such as joint pain or aphthous ulcerations; growth pattern; recent illnesses; foreign travel; and family history of GI or bleeding disorders.

Important components of the physical examination are evaluation of general appearance and vital signs; examination of skin for telangiectasias or purpura or melanotic spots on lips; examination for evidence of epistaxis, abdominal organomegaly, or tenderness or masses; and anorectal examination to verify the presence of blood in the stool and to identify fissures, fistulae, and distal polyps.

If upper GI bleeding is suspected, gastric aspiration should be performed. If necessary, upper endoscopy is attempted when the gastric aspirate after lavage is almost clear. If upper GI bleeding has stopped or has been minimal, an upper GI radiologic examination or upper endoscopy may be performed.

Regardless of the etiology, when lower GI bleeding is massive and ongoing, visualization through the colonoscope may be hindered by the blood. In these situations, a red blood cell scan or angiography with technetium Tc 99m sulfur colloid labeling may be helpful in identifying a site of bleeding. If these procedures do not identify a lesion, colonoscopy can be attempted after a large-volume cleansing electrolyte lavage. If diarrhea is present, a sigmoidoscopy is helpful in visualizing possible pseudomembranes associated with *C. difficile* infection. Biopsies may reveal amebae or distinguish between chronic and acute inflammatory changes. Stool cultures for *Shigella, Salmonella, C. jejuni, and Yersinia* should be obtained; tests should also be performed for *C. difficile* toxin and *E. coli* O157:H7.

Colonoscopy is most helpful in the diagnosis of inflammatory bowel disease, arteriovenous malformations that are visible through the mucosal surface, lymphonodular hyperplasia, and polyps. Barium enemas are valuable for the detection of polyps, inflammatory bowel disease, lymphonodular hyperplasia, Hirschsprung disease, and colonic duplication and for the diagnosis and treatment of intussusception.

Therapy for a massive GI hemorrhage deals with first resuscitating the patient by infusing normal saline or colloid. To determine the site of bleeding, a nasogastric tube may be placed into the stomach, and gastric contents are aspirated. An aspirate of red blood or "coffee ground" material indicates bleeding above the ligament of Treitz, although absence of blood does not rule out bleeding just distal to the pylorus. If fresh blood is present, saline lavage may be carried out until bleeding ceases. Further therapy for severe upper GI bleeding consists of possible blood replacement and neutralization of gastric acid. An intravenous infusion of a histamine$_2$ (H_2) receptor antagonist such as ranitidine or famotidine is used to decrease gastric acidity.

In addition to therapy with medications, endoscopy may be therapeutic for certain causes of GI bleeding. Sclerotherapy or rubber banding for varices, endoscopic heater probe (or laser) coagulation of bleeding sites, vasoconstrictive injections next to bleeding ulcers are possible.

CHAPTER 191

Peptic Ulcer Disease

Adapted from Kathleen J. Motil

Peptic ulcer disease (PUD) is an ulcerative condition of the stomach or duodenum that may be acute or chronic. PUD is classified as primary (idiopathic) when it occurs in otherwise healthy individuals and as secondary (stress) when underlying disorders associated with injury, illness, or drug therapy exist. Most primary peptic ulcers are chronic and more often duodenal in origin; most stress ulcers are acute and more often gastric in location.

PATHOGENESIS

The pathogenesis of PUD is thought to relate to an imbalance between destructive and defensive factors in the gastrointestinal (GI) tract. The destructive factors of the gastric mucosa include hydrochloric acid, pepsin, bile salts, ethanol, smoking, drugs, and stress, whereas the defensive factors include the unstirred mucus layer, bicarbonate secretion, mucosal blood flow, prostaglandins, and epithelial cell renewal. Acid is essential in the development of primary PUD. Any disruption of the gastric mucosal barrier can allow back-diffusion of secreted hydrogen ions from the gastric lumen back into the mucosal cells damaging the gastric tissue.

EPIDEMIOLOGY

The prevalence is estimated to be 1.7% in general pediatric practices and 3.4 per 10,000 pediatric hospital admissions. The male–to–female ratio is 2 to 3:1 with the exception of very young patients. Primary PUD occurs at any age, but its frequency is higher in older children and adolescents. Secondary stress ulcers are more common in infants younger than 6 months and are equal in frequency to primary peptic ulcers in children aged 6 months to 6 years.

PREDISPOSING FACTORS

Several entities have been implicated as predisposing factors for PUD in children. A family history of ulcers can be elicited in at least 50% of children with primary peptic disease. The role of emotional stress in the development of primary PUD is controversial. Emotional disturbances can be identified in nearly 40% of the children with PUD.

Exogenous factors such as alcohol and caffeine damage gastric mucosa and increase acid secretion, but there is no conclusive evidence that these factors are causal in the pathogenesis of ulcers. Cigarette smoking not only leads to duodenal ulcer formation but also slows healing and increases recurrence rates. Corticosteroid therapy is often complicated by the appearance of gastric ulcers. Similarly, aspirin and nonsteroidal antiinflammatory agents inhibit prostaglandin synthesis, thereby increasing the risk of gastric mucosal damage and ulcer formation. Stress ulcers in children can occur in conjunction with systemic illnesses such as sepsis, hypotension, respiratory distress, extensive burns, and brain injury.

H. pylori, a spiral, urease-producing bacterium, is associated with primary antral gastritis and peptic ulcerations in children. The prevalence of *H. pylori* colonization increases with age. Children from lower-income families are more likely to be infected than children from higher-income families. The eradication of *H. pylori* is associated with a pronounced reduction in the relapse rate of duodenal ulcers. Ulcer relapse is associated with either reinfection or recrudescence of *H. pylori* infection in medically noncompliant patients.

CLINICAL FEATURES

The clinical picture of PUD in children is variable and depends on the type of the ulcer and the age of presentation. Abdominal pain, generally localized to the epigastric or periumbilical area, is the most common presenting symptom of duodenal ulcers (Table 191-1). Typical duodenal ulcer pain that worsens with fasting, is relieved with meals, and wakens the patient at night is uncommon in children. Abdominal pain that is exacerbated by food, nausea, vomiting, and weight loss is a more common feature of gastric ulcers. Nausea, vomiting, and anorexia occur in 25% or less of the children with ulcer disease, and hematemesis and melena in less than 20%. Frontal headaches are present in approximately 10% of children. Failure to thrive can be associated with PUD.

Abdominal tenderness and overt GI bleeding are found on physical examination in at least one-half of the children with

TABLE 191-1. Presenting Features of Peptic Ulcer Disease in Children

Clinical feature	Frequency (%)
Symptom	
Abdominal pain	71
Epigastric	57
Periumbilical	32
"Typical"	9
Nausea	25
Vomiting	18
Hematemesis	18
Melena	13
Anorexia	17
Headache	11
Failure to thrive	3
Sign	
Abdominal tenderness	58
Gastrointestinal bleeding	53
Acute abdomen	22
Perforation	18
Obstruction	7
Anemia	11

TABLE 191-2. Differential Diagnosis of Peptic Ulcer Disease

Gastroduodenitis
Cholelithiasis
Zollinger-Ellison syndrome
Appendicitis
Chronic recurrent abdominal pain
Meckel diverticulum
Gastroesophageal reflux
Intussusception
Esophagitis
Infectious diarrhea
Pancreatitis
Inflammatory bowel disease

PUD. An acute abdomen with features of abdominal distention, decreased bowel sounds, and peritoneal irritation, consistent with the diagnosis of intestinal perforation or obstruction, occurs in nearly one-fourth of children at presentation.

LABORATORY, RADIOLOGIC, AND ENDOSCOPIC STUDIES

Approximately 10% of children with PUD have iron-deficiency anemia. In the presence of antral gastritis and PUD, *H. pylori* may be detected by an *H. pylori*–specific antibody serologic test or a carbon 13 urea breath test. A stool assay for *H. pylori* antigen is also available.

On upper Gi series, signs of PUD in the duodenum are characterized by a filling defect or a deformity of the duodenal bulb. Ulcer craters may also be found in the pyloric region leading to outlet obstruction. Overall, upper GI series detect PUD in 70% of the children who are studied with better performance demonstrating duodenal ulcers than gastric ulcers.

Endoscopy is the procedure of choice for the detection of PUD in children. Gastroesophagoduodenoscopy is indicated to make the initial diagnosis of PUD. Endoscopy confirms the diagnosis of PUD in 97% of the patients. A nodular appearance of the gastric antrum may be evident in a proportion of children with *H. pylori* infection. Confirmation of *H. pylori* requires cultures, measurement of urease activity [CLO (*Campylobacter*-like organism) test, Delta West, Australia], or Warthin–Starry silver stains of antral or duodenal biopsy tissue specimens.

DIFFERENTIAL DIAGNOSIS

The diagnosis of PUD in children may be difficult to make because the symptoms often mimic those of other diseases. Some common considerations in the differential diagnosis are listed in Table 191-2. The symptoms of abdominal pain, vomiting, and rectal bleeding may be common to many of these entities and lead to a significant diagnostic dilemma.

Nonspecific gastroduodenitis may present with the classic manifestations of PUD. Poorly localized, periodic abdominal pain, nausea, vomiting, bloating, flatus, and anorexia may occur. The condition is clinically indistinguishable from PUD, and the diagnosis must be confirmed by endoscopy and biopsies.

Zollinger–Ellison syndrome, an uncommon diagnosis in children, is characterized by hypersecretion of gastric acid, intractable ulcer disease, and intestinal malabsorption caused by a gastrin-secreting tumor (gastrinoma) of the pancreas.

Chronic recurrent abdominal pain occurs in approximately 10% of school-aged children and may be difficult to distinguish from PUD. The diagnosis of functional abdominal pain is usually made by a careful history and excluding organic illness through selected appropriate diagnostic studies including endoscopy if necessary.

Gastroesophageal reflux, esophagitis, pancreatitis, cholecystitis, and appendicitis may be confused with primary PUD because these illnesses have similar clinical features.

TREATMENT

The goal of medical therapy in PUD is to promote healing of the ulcer, relieve pain, and prevent complications. The control of gastric acid production by drugs and diet and the avoidance of factors that stimulate acid secretion are essential. The eradication of *H. pylori* from infected patients is imperative to prevent ulcer recurrence.

The medical management for PUD includes antacids and histamine$_2$ (H_2) receptor antagonists (e.g., ranitidine, famotidine). Antacids promote the healing of ulcers and provide relief of symptoms by neutralizing gastric acid. H_2 receptor antagonists are potent inhibitors of basal and food-stimulated acid production. Their use is associated with a healing rate of 90% in children with PUD. Maintenance therapy with H_2 receptor antagonists does not protect entirely against a recurrence of primary PUD.

Proton-pump inhibitors (e.g., omeprazole, lansoprazole) inhibit the hydrogen ion pump in the parietal cell, thereby blocking the final common pathway for acid formation. These drugs are indicated for the treatment of recalcitrant ulcers unresponsive to H_2 blocker therapy, hypersecretory states such as Zollinger-Ellison syndrome, and *H. pylori* antritis and duodenal disease.

Other medications such as sucralfate may be added to a therapeutic regimen. Sucralfate binds to the erosive surface of the ulcer and protects the mucosa from further damage. Other cytoprotective drugs (e.g., misoprostol) have not been sufficiently studied in children to warrant their use.

The most effective treatment regimen of *H. pylori*–associated PUD is combination drug therapy, which results in the successful eradication of *H. pylori* in 90% of compliant patients. Many regimens exist. The reader is directed to the Centers for Disease Control and Prevention (CDC) web site http://www.cdc.gov/ulcer/md.htm for updated recommendations.

Dietary intervention may also promote healing of the ulcer. Milk feedings have been found to increase the gastric pH and to prevent GI bleeding in hospitalized children. Food may ameliorate symptoms, although gastric ulcer pain can be exacerbated by acidic foods or beverages such as soft drinks, juices, pickles, tomatoes, and spices. Alcoholic beverages, cigarette smoking, aspirin, and other drugs that damage the gastric mucosal barrier are contraindicated.

The surgical management of PUD is reserved for patients with complications of ulcers including intractable pain, perforation, hemorrhage, and obstruction. Truncal or selective vagotomy with pyloroplasty, or in some instances antrectomy, is the most common procedure performed in children with PUD.

CHAPTER 192

Intussusception

Adapted from Mary L. Brandt

Intussusception is the most common cause of intestinal obstruction in infants aged 3 months to 3 years. Intussusception is rare in the first month of life and has a peak occurrence between the ages of 5 and 9 months.

PATHOPHYSIOLOGY

Intussusception is the result of invagination or telescoping of a portion of the bowel into the more distal bowel (Fig. 192-1). The *intussusceptum* is pulled along with its mesentery by peristaltic waves into the lumen of the *intussuscipiens*. When this occurs, the mesentery is compressed resulting in lymphatic obstruction and, subsequently, in venous obstruction. The intussuscepted mass quickly obstructs the intestinal lumen resulting in distention and peristaltic rushes proximal to the obstructing mass. With each peristaltic rush, the patient experiences colicky pain.

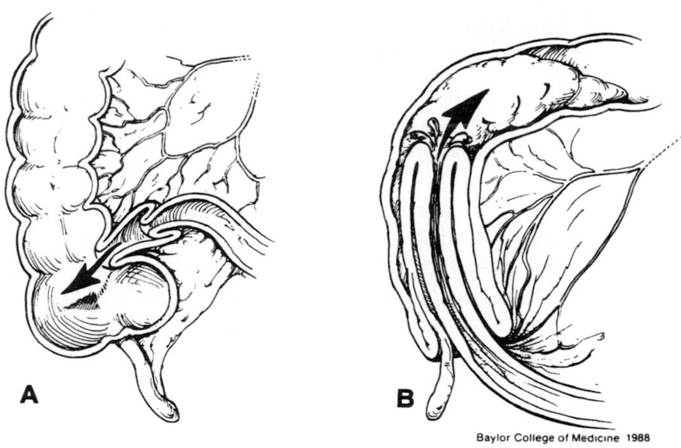

Figure 192-1. The development of an ileocolic intussusception. **A:** The invagination typically begins several centimeters proximal to the ileocecal valve. As the ileum is drawn into the more distal bowel, the lumen is obstructed and the mesenteric vessels become compressed. **B:** Edema and venous engorgement develop with accumulation of blood and mucus ("currant jelly") in the lumen of the colon. If not reduced, infarction of the intussusceptum occurs.

Eventually the hydrostatic pressure within the intussusception increases until it equals the arterial pressure, at which time arterial inflow ceases. The intestinal mucosa becomes ischemic with an outpouring of mucus into the intestinal lumen. Venous engorgement results in leakage of blood into the intestinal lumen, and the blood and mucus form the classic "currant jelly" stools. Although currant jelly stools are relatively diagnostic, they occur in only a small percentage of patients and are a late finding in intussusception.

ETIOLOGY

Most infants who develop intussusception are healthy and well nourished. Approximately 10% of patients have a previous history of diarrhea, and many have signs and symptoms of respiratory tract infections. In most cases, no clear cause of the intussusception can be identified. Hypertrophic lymphoid tissue of the bowel is usually found in patients with intussusception. This enlarged lymphoid tissue probably acts as the lead point for the intussusception. The association of intussusception with viral syndromes and the presence of this enlarged lymphoid tissue supports a viral etiology for the majority of the "idiopathic" intussusceptions. Adenovirus and rotavirus, in particular, have been implicated in the pathophysiology of intussusception.

Approximately 2% to 3% of older children with intussusception have, as the lead point, a recognizable lesion including polyps, Meckel diverticulum, nodular or ectopic pancreas, lymphomas, and benign tumors of the ileal wall. Localized edema or hemorrhage such as that seen in patients with Henoch-Schönlein purpura, abdominal trauma, hemophilia, and leukemia may also act as a lead point. Patients with cystic fibrosis may develop intussusception as a result of mucus-laden hypertrophied mucosal glands, which act as lead points, and as a result of the thick, tenacious fecal material associated with enzymatic insufficiency.

CLINICAL PRESENTATION

Nearly all affected infants present with vomiting and colicky pain. As few as 10% of children diagnosed with an intussusception have the classic triad of colicky abdominal pain, vomiting, and bloody stool. Early in the course of illness, the infant evacuates the distal colon and passes several partially formed stools. This can occasionally give the impression of diarrhea, and children are often misdiagnosed with gastroenteritis. It should be noted, however, that the pain of intussusception is more consistently episodic than that of gastroenteritis. As the intestinal obstruction progresses, vomiting becomes bile stained and eventually fecaloid. Waves of peristaltic rushes and colicky pain continue. During the intervals between peristaltic rushes, the infant appears to be in no discomfort, and the abdomen is soft and scaphoid. Children with intussusception may develop a profound lethargy mimicking a true coma, and this may be the presenting symptom.

At the time of presentation, a mass is usually palpable. Because 95% of the cases of intussusception are ileocolic with the invaginating bowel beginning just proximal to the ileocecal valve, the sausage-shaped mass can be found in the distribution of the colon, commonly in the area of the hepatic flexure but occasionally more distally. In 3% of the cases, the intussuscepting intestine prolapses through the rectum.

If complete intestinal obstruction ensues, the child may develop abdominal distention, fluid loss from vomiting and sequestration of intraluminal fluid, and continuous abdominal pain. If further delay in diagnosis and treatment occurs, infarction of the intussusceptum occurs. Clinical shock is also apparent in these children. In most cases, infarction of the intussusceptum is associated with generalized peritonitis; if untreated, the patient dies within 2 to 5 days.

DIAGNOSIS

The diagnosis of intussusception can be made with a careful history and high index of suspicion. On physical examination, a palpable sausage-shaped mass may be palpable in the abdomen.

Plain radiography of the abdomen may show small bowel obstruction, reduced gas in the jejunum, lateralization of the ileum, absence of stool in the rectum, and ability to visualize the intussusceptum as it is outlined by air in the lumen. Some centers use ultrasound with good accuracy to diagnose intussusception.

The gold standard for the diagnosis of intussusception in most institutions remains the contrast enema. Any infant or young child with signs and symptoms of distal small bowel or colonic obstruction, intermittent colicky pain, currant jelly or guaiac-positive stools, a sausage-shaped mass in the distribution of the colon, or profound lethargy with a negative central nervous system evaluation should undergo a diagnostic contrast examination.

TREATMENT

The treatment of suspected intussusception begins with a diagnostic, and often therapeutic, contrast enema. To be prepared, the child should be fluid resuscitated, and plans for surgery should be made in case the reduction attempt is unsuccessful or results in a perforation. Gastric aspiration through a nasogastric tube prevents further vomiting.

Once the diagnosis is confirmed by contrast enema, a decision must be made whether to attempt hydrostatic reduction (Fig. 192-2). The only absolute contraindications to hydrostatic reduction are free intraperitoneal air, physical signs of peritonitis, or systemic signs of compromised intestine. At present, contrast materials for reduction include air, water-soluble contrast, and barium. If the risk of perforation is high, air or water-soluble contrast is a better choice than barium. Treatment guidelines for the barium contrast enema are described in Table 192-1. Many institutions are very aggressive with contrast enemas to decrease the laparotomy rate.

Hydrostatic and pneumatic reduction is successful in 30% to 80% of the patients with intussusception. To be sure that complete reduction has occurred, contrast or air must be seen in the terminal ileum. For those children who come to surgery, successful operative reduction is possible in most patients; however, nearly 25% of infants require resection of bowel because reduction is impossible or the intestine is nonviable.

The recurrence rate after both hydrostatic reduction and surgical reduction is close to 5%; recurrences usually occur in the first 24 hours after the successful reduction.

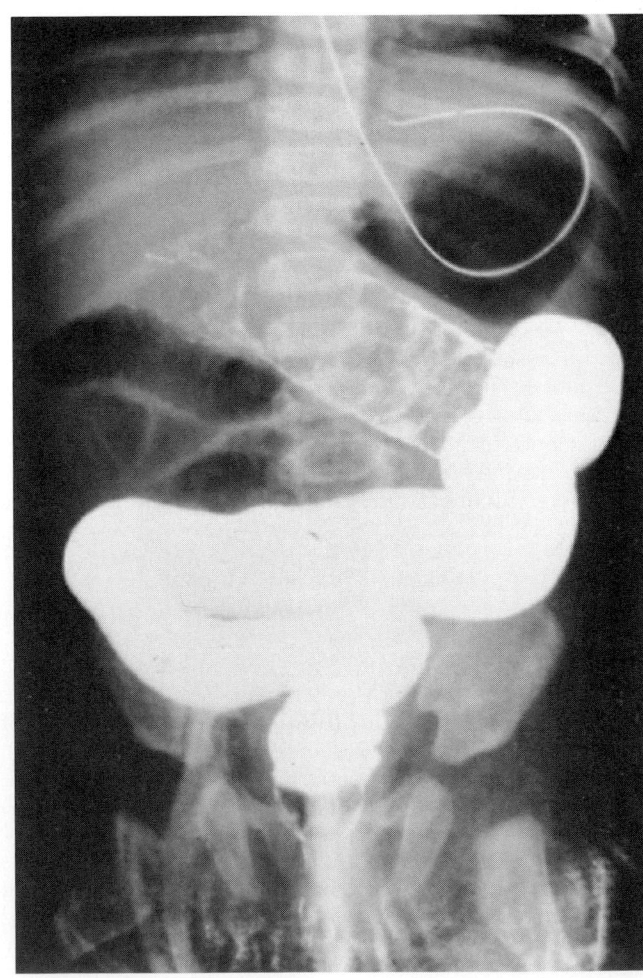

Figure 192-2. Barium enema study showing the coiled-spring pattern of barium around the intussusceptum in the transverse colon.

TABLE 192-1. Principles of Barium Enema Reduction of Intussusception

1. Notify operating room to prepare for emergency operation it barium reduction is not successful.
2. Initiate resuscitation with intravenous fluids and nasogastric suction.
3. Insert ungreased Foley catheter in rectum, distend balloon, and pull down against levators. Tape catheter in place and hold buttocks tightly together. Wrap legs.
4. Let barium run from a height of 3 feet, 6 inches above the table while intermittently fluoroscoping the patient.
5. Abandon procedure if barium column is stationary and its outline is unchanged for 10 minutes.
6. Reduction is marked by: free flow of barium well into the ileum, expulsion of feces and flatus with the barium, disappearance of the mass on physical examination, and clinical improvement of the child.
7. Failure to reduce the intussusception requires prompt operative intervention.

Adapted from Ravitch MM. Intussusception. In: Welch KJ, Randolph JG, Ravitch MM, et al., eds. *Pediatric surgery.* Chicago: Year Book, 1987:868.

CHAPTER 193

Oral Rehydration Therapy

Adapted from Mathuram Santosham, Katherine L. O' Brien, and Julius G. K. Goepp

Dehydration resulting from acute gastroenteritis (AGE) is a leading cause of child morbidity and mortality in the world. In the developing nations, over 3 million children younger than 5 years die annually from dehydration. Among children in the United States, dehydration accounts for approximately 300 deaths per year. In the United States, however, dehydration from AGE leads to some 200,000 hospitalizations, 1.5 million physician visits, and accounts for approximately $1 billion in direct medical costs.

Over the past 30 years, improved understanding of fluid and electrolyte transport in the gut has led to the development of physiologically appropriate solutions for oral fluid therapy. Such therapy, in combination with appropriate dietary management of the child with AGE, has come to be known as *oral rehydration therapy* (ORT). Although many practicing pediatricians viewed ORT with skepticism during the past 40 to 50 years, ORT is now viewed as a powerful, simple, and inexpensive approach that is credited with saving approximately 1 million lives annually. Paradoxically, ORT is used least in the industrialized countries where much of the original scientific research was done.

PATHOPHYSIOLOGY

A patient with AGE typically has sustained volume depletion reflecting losses not only of water but also of sodium and other electrolytes as well. Regardless of the measured serum sodium or potassium concentration, total body sodium and potassium content is invariably diminished during dehydration from AGE.

Oral Rehydration Solutions

ORT is based on sodium cotransport in the intestine. In this system, sodium absorption from the small intestine is promoted by the passive cotransport of small organic molecules such as glucose. Water absorption follows that of sodium so that osmotic equilibrium is maintained.

The composition of oral rehydration solutions (ORSs) has evolved since the 1970s. Today a single standard solution is recommended by the World Health Organization (WHO) and is used in most countries of the developing world. Solutions commercially available in the United States have lower sodium concentrations and lower osmolarity than the WHO solution, but studies have shown that these solutions are equally effective at fluid repletion.

GLUCOSE

When glucose concentrations in ORS exceed 3% (30 g/L), the osmotic pressure exerted by glucose in the intestinal lumen produces passive fluid loss greater than absorption, and diarrhea may be exacerbated. Table 193-1 shows the concentrations of glucose in the physiologically appropriate oral solutions, as well as that of other fluids still commonly used during diarrhea. It should be noted that soft drinks and juices all contain glucose in excess of 3%.

SODIUM

Early ORSs had comparatively high sodium concentrations of 100 to 120 mEq/L to address the hyponatremic dehydration seen in many patients with cholera. Current WHO solution has a sodium concentration of 90 mEq/L.

POTASSIUM

In children with AGE, potassium losses in stool and urine (under the influence of elevated aldosterone) lead to total body potassium depletion. Potassium losses sufficient to produce hypokalemia may result in ileus, which, in turn, may reduce intestinal fluid absorption. Partial repletion of potassium is an

TABLE 193-1. Composition of Fluids Frequently Used in Oral Rehydration[a]

Solution	Glucose/ CHO (g/L)	Sodium (mEq/L)	HCO_3 (mEq/L)	Potassium (mEq/L)	Osmolality (mmol/L)
Pedialyte	25	45	30	20	250
Infalyte	30[b]	50	30	25	200
Rehydralyte	25	75	30	20	310
WHO packet	20	90	30	20	330
Cola	700	2	13	0.1	750
Apple juice	690	3	—	32	730
Gatorade	255	20	3	3	330

CHO, carbohydrate; WHO, World Health Organization.
[a]Cola, juice, and Gatorade are shown for comparison only; they are not recommended for use.
[b]Rice syrup solids.

important aspect of fluid therapy in AGE. Approximately 20 mmol/L of potassium is provided in most ORSs. This potassium concentration is usually insufficient to fully replace most children's potassium losses. Early restoration of normal dietary intake provides a needed additional source of potassium.

BASE

Bicarbonate at 30 mEq/L has been a component of WHO-recommended ORS since 1975. Trisodium citrate provides three bicarbonate ions per molecule, is stabler than sodium bicarbonate, and is currently the source of base in these solutions.

OSMOLALITY

The osmotic burden presented by oral solutions to the gut is of great importance. Most full-strength fruit juices, punches, and soft drinks have high osmolality predominantly resulting from their sugar content and are unacceptable as the sole source of fluid replacement in diarrhea (Table 193-1). Fluids whose osmolality significantly exceeds that of serum (which is approximately 290 mOsm/L) can result in free water retained in the intestinal lumen. This effect not only reduces absorption of water but may also result in free water losses from the intravascular space contributing to or exacerbating hypernatremia.

Because of concerns that the WHO solution provided excessive amounts of sodium for children with noncholera diarrhea, various solutions with lower sodium concentrations and osmolarity have been evaluated for safety and efficacy. The current recommendations of the AAP state that all commercially available ORT solutions in the United States (with sodium concentrations between 50 mEq/L–90 mEq/L) can be used for both the rehydration and maintenance phases of fluid management.

Complex Carbohydrate Solutions

Although standard glucose based ORSs are effective at repletion of fluids and electrolytes, they have minimal effect on the volume and duration of stool output. In theory, by increasing the quantity of substrate available to the cotransport system, absorption of fluid could be promoted to the point of reversing water loss and actually reducing stool volume. In practice, because of the osmotic limitation alluded to previously, the concentration of free glucose that can be safely delivered in ORS is limited and should not exceed 3%. By contrast, solutions that contain complex carbohydrates (starches) are able to supply a much large number of glucose molecules in the intestinal lumen while imposing a relatively low osmotic load. Starch molecules are broken down into their constituent glucose residues by intestinal amylase enzymes. The free glucose molecules then function as organic substrate to cotransport sodium ions. The glucose molecules liberated by amylase at the intestinal brush border are rapidly absorbed so that high glucose concentrations do not develop in the lumen. By providing large amounts of substrate without imposing an *osmotic penalty*, starch-containing solutions may be capable of producing net fluid absorption in excess of losses.

Rice has been most thoroughly studied as a carbohydrate source. Among patients with noncholera diarrhea, minimal differences in output or duration of illness have been shown between rice based ORS and G-ORS.

DIETARY CONSIDERATIONS

For years, pediatricians have recommended delayed feeding until improvement or cessation of the diarrhea. This thinking has changed, and the current AAP practice parameter for management of children with diarrhea and dehydration recommends early feeding of appropriate foods to children with diarrhea once the dehydration has been sufficiently reversed. The nutritional consequences of fasting are profound. Children in the developing world may experience two to ten episodes of diarrhea annually, each of 3 to 5 days' duration. Serious caloric deprivation and ultimately growth retardation may ensue. Fasting has also been demonstrated to inhibit enterocyte renewal. Enteral feeding, on the other hand, has been shown to increase cell renewal in the gut and to diminish intestinal permeability.

Diminished absorption of lactose during diarrheal illness can occur. Although most children can safely tolerate lactose-containing feedings during diarrhea, their stool output should be monitored carefully. Those who develop significantly increased rates of stooling or abdominal distention should have lactose reduced or eliminated until they have recovered.

While human breast milk contains more lactose than cow's milk or milk-based formulas, studies have demonstrated reduced stool output among children who received continued breast-milk feedings compared with those whose feedings were interrupted.

DELIVERY OF ORAL REHYDRATION THERAPY

Like any other form of treatment, ORT must be delivered in a controlled and reliable fashion to be effective. When delivered in this manner, failure rates (i.e., the need for intravenous fluid therapy) should be less than 5%. Because of its simplicity, many health care providers tend to offer ORS to patients without properly instructing them in its use. When the families are properly educated, therapy is most likely successful.

In patients with uncomplicated AGE, the physical examination should be directed at the assessment of dehydration. Table 193-2 shows the clinical classification of dehydration. The management of the dehydrated child is divided into two phases: rehydration and maintenance. Replacement of ongoing fluid losses, as well as maintenance fluids and diet, should also be provided.

Rehydration Phase

In the rehydration phase, the total fluid deficit is intended to be replaced over a 4-hour period.

Children with mild or moderate dehydration should be given 60 to 80 mL/kg of ORS over 4 hours. Patients with severe dehydration (frank or impending shock) should receive an initial bolus of normal saline or Ringer's lactate by the intravenous or intraosseous routes at 40 mL/kg/hour until signs of shock resolve. The degree of dehydration should then be recalculated, and the ORS should be continued as outlined previously. While parenteral access is being sought, nasogastric infusion of fluid using a small (5–7 Fr.) soft catheter may be initiated at a rate of 30 mL/kg/hour, as long as the patient's airway protective reflexes remain intact.

At the end of each hour of rehydration, ongoing losses (stool and emesis) should be calculated and replaced. This fluid should consist of ORS (or isotonic intravenous fluid in children receiving initial parenteral therapy). Alternatively, parents may be instructed to provide 10 mL/kg (i.e., approximately 4 oz for a 12-kg child) of ORS for each diarrheal stool.

As soon as rehydration is complete, clinical assessment should be repeated. If signs of dehydration persist, the rehydration phase should be repeated until fluid repletion has occurred. When rehydration is complete, the maintenance phase is begun.

TABLE 193-2. Fluid Therapy Chart

Degree of dehydration	Signs[a]	Rehydration phase[b] (first 4 hr, repeat until no signs of dehydration remain)	Maintenance phase (until illness resolves)
Mild	Slightly dry mucous membranes, increased thirst	ORS 50–60 mL/kg	Breast-feeding, undiluted lactose-free formula, one-half strength cow's milk or lactose-containing formula
Moderate	Sunken eyes, sunken fontanelle, loss of skin turgor, dry mucous membranes	ORS 80–100 mL/kg	Same as above
Severe	Signs of moderate dehydration plus one or more of the following: rapid, thready pulse; cyanosis; rapid breathing; delayed capillary refill; lethargy; coma	IV or IO isotonic fluids (0.9% saline or Ringer's lactate), 40 mL/kg/hr until pulse and state of consciousness return to normal, then 50–100 mL/kg of ORS based on remaining degree of dehydration[c]	Same as above

ORS, oral rehydration solution.
[a]If no signs of dehydration are present, the rehydration phase may be omitted. Proceed with maintenance therapy and replacement of ongoing losses.
[b]Replace ongoing stool losses and vomitus with ORS, 10 mL/kg for each diarrheal stool and 5 mL/kg for each episode of vomitus.
[c]While parenteral access is being sought, nasogastric infusion of ORS may be begun at 30 mL/kg/hr, provided airway protective reflexes remain intact.

Maintenance Phase

The goals during the maintenance phase are twofold: to replace ongoing losses and to meet baseline metabolic fluid and nutritional needs. Ongoing stool losses should be replaced with ORS on a 1:1 basis. Ten mL/kg or approximately 4 oz of ORS should be given for each watery stool. Care providers should be instructed about the gastrocolic reflex that often results in a bowel movement immediately after a feeding and may result in poor compliance with ORT. Reassurance should be given that the fluid given by mouth is absorbed and is likely to exceed in quantity, the amount lost in stool.

Once the rehydration phase has been completed and vomiting has diminished, infants and children should be started back on regular feedings. For infants, this is typically breast feeding or infant formula (lactose free formulas may be used). For toddlers and children, foods high in complex carbohydrates and low in fats and simple sugars are optimal. Rice, bread, cereal, potatoes, vegetables, yogurt, lean meat, and fruit are good choices. Prescribing the standard BRAT (*b*anana, *r*ice, *a*pplesauce, *t*oast) diet is less acceptable to families than a careful description of preferred foods as above.

Use in ORT in Industrialized Nations

Health care providers in the industrialized world have been slow to take advantage of the benefits of ORT. Many physicians state lack of convenience, reluctance of support staff, insufficient training of support staff, and lack of reimbursement from third-party payors. For certain myths and misperceptions, the responses below may be used.

- *Myth: Parental involvement in the medical care of children is impractical.* Parents who have successfully provided ORS to their child and watched the child improve in their own hands often prefer the use of ORT to intravenous therapy.
- *Myth: ORT takes too long.* Several studies have favorably compared the timeliness of ORT with intravenous solutions. When 5 mL (1 tsp) of ORS is taken per minute, 300 mL (10 oz) is delivered hourly representing a rate of fluid administration sufficient to meet the needs of most children during the rehydration phase without inducing gastric distention.
- *Myth: ORT can only be used in mild dehydration.* Providers are often concerned that moderately or severely ill children will not tolerate ORS or that electrolyte abnormalities or acidosis mandate intravenous therapy. In fact, standard ORSs contain more base and potassium than standard intravenous solutions and are rapidly absorbed. As indicated previously, ORS can be rapidly delivered to the infant. Finally, a nasogastric tube may be used to deliver ORS to a child who is unable to drink (provided airway protective reflexes remain intact).
- *Myth: ORT cannot be used if a child is vomiting.* Although children with truly intractable vomiting require parenteral fluids for a time, most can be rehydrated enterally when small volumes are presented to the stomach. The use of a 5-mL syringe or medicine cup can facilitate fluid delivery. The volume of emesis is usually overestimated by parents and staff. More than 90% of infants who present with vomiting can be adequately hydrated with ORS when it is properly administered.

Real Obstacles to Implementation of Oral Rehydration Therapy

Although ORT is cheaper than intravenous therapy, the cost of the former is often borne by the parent because many third-party insurers do not pay for ORT in hospitals or clinics. Currently, commercially available solutions cost from $3 to $7 per liter, a prohibitive expense for many families. Public assistance programs such as WIC may provide solutions, but this is not universal in all states. One approach to the cost issue is to use packaged dry salts as is done by WHO. These packets (Oral Rehydration Salts, Jianis Bros., Kansas City, MO) provide salts for 1 L of ORS at less than $0.75 per packet. Mixing errors can occur and this risk must be weighed against the benefits. The AAP recommends the use of dry ORT packets when provided with an appropriately sized container for mixing to reduce the potential for misuse.

CHAPTER 194

Anorectal Malformations

Adapted from Nitsana A. Spigland
and David E. Wesson

Major anorectal malformations occur in 1 per 1,500 live births. Table 194-1 lists types of anorectal malformations according to gender, the level of rectal descent, and the presence or absence of a fistula. Through physical exam and imaging (X-ray, CT, MRI), one can identify the level of the rectum in relation to a line drawn between the pubis and the coccyx (pubococcygeal line) and the lowest quarter of the ossified ischium (I point). High lesions do not traverse the levator muscles and are located above the pubococcygeal line. Intermediate lesions partially traverse the levator muscle and end below the pubococcygeal line but above the I point. A low imperforate anus is below the level of the levator muscle and the I point.

Lesions close to the anus are more common than high and intermediate lesions in girls; high lesions are more common in boys. Nearly 80% of the boys with a high lesion have a fistula to the urinary tract, and nearly all girls with a high lesion have a fistula to the vagina or a cloacal anomaly (Figs. 194-1–194-2).

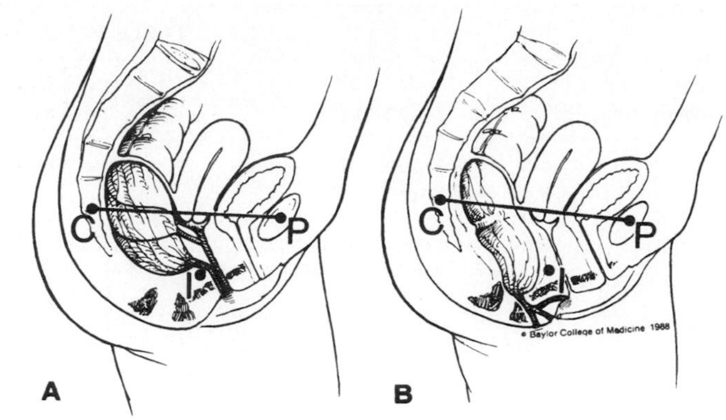

Figure 194-1. Anorectal anomalies in the female infant. **A:** High lesions usually have a fistula to the vagina, whereas intermediate lesions may have a fistula to the vagina or outside the hymen at the vestibule. **B:** Low lesions may also have a fistula to the vestibule or to the fourchette or perineum.

DIAGNOSIS

Several findings on physical examination suggest the level of an imperforate anus. A flat bottom with no crease or anal dimple and no evidence of an external sphincter predicts a high imperforate anus (Fig. 194-3). A well-developed raphe, anal dimple, and bucket-handle deformity usually suggest a low lesion.

Low lesions are more frequent in girls (Fig. 194-4). Nearly all girls with a low lesion have a fistula to the perineum in the form of an anterior ectopic anus (Fig. 194-5), a fistula to the fourchette, or a fistula to the vestibule, which is between the posterior fourchette and the hymenal ring. In patients with a single perineal opening, a cloacal anomaly must be considered.

Associated abnormalities should also be considered (see below).

ASSOCIATED MALFORMATIONS

Associated anomalies (reported in 40%–50% of the patients with imperforate anus) should be sought in infants with all forms of anorectal malformations. In addition to imperforate anus, esophageal atresia, vertebral anomalies, and radial and renal anomalies make up the VATER association. This association has been expanded to VACTERL, in which *C* represents cardiac lesions and *L* represents limb deformities. When any one of these anomalies is seen, the others should be sought with the appropriate studies.

Nearly 40% of the infants with imperforate anus have genitourinary anomalies. Unilateral renal agenesis is the most common defect occurring in 8% to 25% of the patients with imperforate anus.

Gastrointestinal anomalies occur in 10% to 15% of the children with imperforate anus. Esophageal atresia is the most common and is often associated with maternal polyhydramnios.

Cardiovascular anomalies are reported in 7% to 12% of the patients with imperforate anus. Ventricular septal defect and tetralogy of Fallot are two of the more common anomalies.

Skeletal anomalies are found in 6% to 20% of the patients with anorectal malformations. Vertebral anomalies, usually sacral, are the most common defect. As many as 50% of the patients with high lesions have sacral vertebral anomalies. Other abnormalities, referred to as *spinal dysraphism*, include intraspinal masses, lipomyelomeningoceles, tethered cord, and occult meningocele.

TABLE 194-1. Classification of Anorectal Malformations

Female	Male
High	**High**
Anorectal agenesis	Anorectal agenesis
With rectovaginal fistula	With rectourethral fistula
Without fistula	Without fistula
Rectal atresia	Rectal atresia
Intermediate	**Intermediate**
Rectovaginal fistula	Anorectal agenesis
Rectovestibular fistula	Rectourethral fistula
Anal agenesis without a fistula	Anal agenesis without a fistula
Low	**Low**
Anovestibular fistula	Anocutaneous fistula
Anocutaneous fistula	Anal stenosis
Anal stenosis	**Rare malformations**
Cloacal malformations	
Rare malformations	

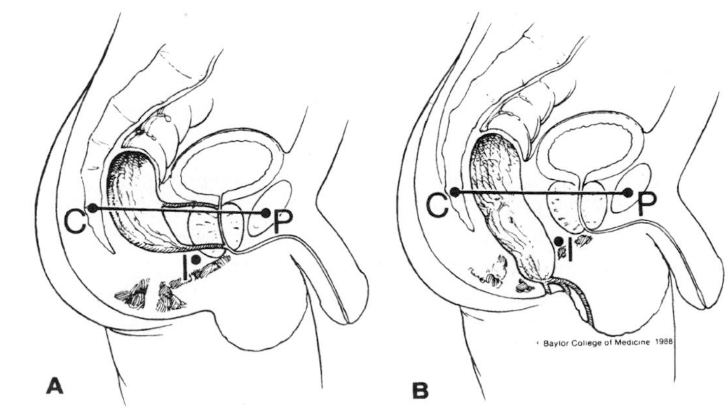

Figure 194-2. Anorectal anomalies in the male infant. **A:** Eighty percent of high and intermediate lesions have fistulas to the bulbar or membranous urethra. **B:** Ninety percent of male infants with low lesions have a fistula to the perineum or median raphe.

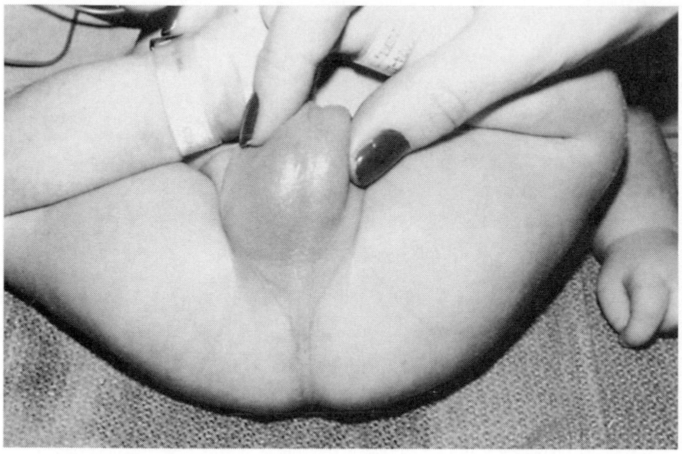

Figure 194-3. Perineum of a male infant with a high lesion and a rectourethral fistula. After 24 hours, there is no evidence of a fistula to the perineum or raphe. A colostomy was done on the second day of life and reconstruction of the anus and rectum at 1 year.

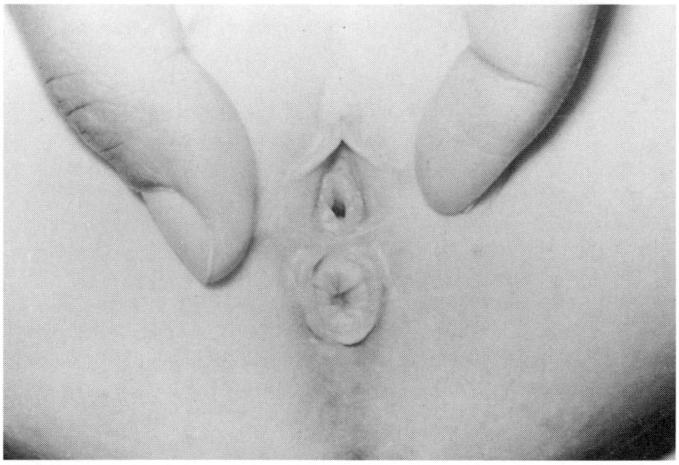

Figure 194-5. Ectopic perineal anus located posterior to the fourchette but anterior to the external sphincter. The patient did well with dilations until 6 months of age when the anus was moved to the normal location.

TREATMENT

The treatment of imperforate anus is directed by the pediatric surgeon and depends on the level of descent of the rectum and on the presence or absence of a fistula to the urinary tract, vagina, or perineum. Infants with low lesions and perineal fistulas may only require dilation of the tract to allow defecation. Children with high and intermediate lesions should undergo diverting colostomies as soon as the diagnosis is confirmed. This procedure is particularly important in patients with fistulas to the urinary tract. Failure to completely divert the feces from the fistula may result in recurrent urinary tract infections.

PROGNOSIS

Nearly all patients with low malformations have normal rectal function. The outcome of patients with high and intermediate malformations varies: A good outcome depends on operative technique, anatomic development or maldevelopment, and patient cooperation. In the early postoperative period, attention must be given to regular evacuations to prevent impactions. In some instances, daily laxatives or enemas are required. A significant number (up to 50%) of the patients with high anomalies have sacral vertebral defects. Patients with anomalies of S3 have varying degrees of neurologic deficit to the perineum including the rectal and bladder sphincters. Patients with absence of S2 to S5 have a complete neurologic loss to the perineum. These patients usually develop fecal or urinary incontinence. Finally, rarely does a child with a high anomaly have perfect rectal function. Toilet training may be difficult until the child is older, often 5 or 6 years of age. The rectal function and fecal continence continue to improve into early adolescence. If the patient and his or her family can be supported through the early postoperative years, rectal function nearly always improves to an acceptable level.

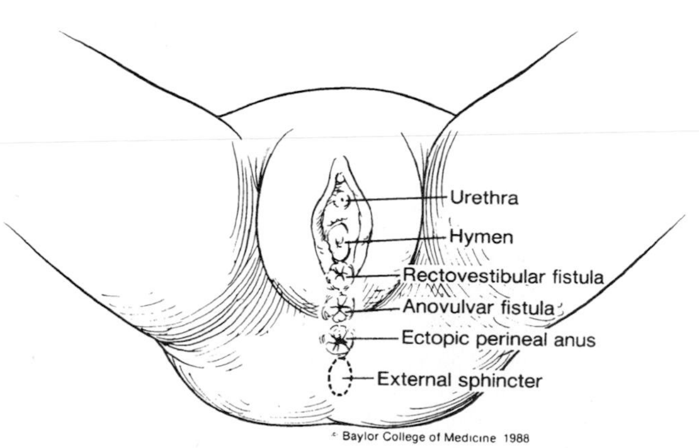

Figure 194-4. Appearance of fistulas on the female perineum.

CHAPTER 195
Ulcerative Colitis

Ulcerative colitis (UC) is a chronic relapsing inflammatory disease of the colon and rectum of unknown etiology. The inflammation in UC is limited to the colon and rectum. Table 195-1 contrasts the patterns of pathologic involvement in UC and Crohn's disease.

In UC, the distal colon is affected most severely. Inflammation is primarily limited to the mucosa and consists of *continuous* involvement with varying degrees of ulceration, hemorrhage, edema, and regenerating epithelium. Fistulas and perianal disease do not occur. The histology of UC lesions demonstrates continuous acute and chronic inflammation with mucosal and submucosal infiltration by polymorphonuclear leukocytes and mononuclear cells rarely extending beyond the muscularis. Cryptitis and crypt abscesses characterize acute inflammation.

ETIOLOGY

The cause of UC is unknown but involves a dysregulated immune response that injures colonic epithelial elements. Although no specific heritable patterns exist, 15% to 40% of the patients

TABLE 195-1. Comparative Features of Ulcerative Colitis and Crohn's Disease

	Ulcerative colitis	Crohn's disease
Site of disease		
Upper gastrointestinal tract	0%	20%
Ileum alone	0%	19%
Ileum and colon	Backwash ileitis	52%
Colon alone	85–90% (distal colon predominant)	9% (proximal colon predominant)
Rectum	Approximately 100%	Relative sparing
Rectum alone	10–15%	Rare
Perianal disease	Rare	25% (tags, fissures, abscesses)
Fistulas	0%	14% (enteroenteral, enterovesical, enterovaginal, enterocutaneous)
Gross pathology/radiology	Hemorrhagic mucosa, diffuse continuous inflammation, pseudopolyps, loss of haustra, no perianal disease	Segmental involvement, skip regions, focal aphthae, thickened bowel wall, serosal fat, narrow separate bowel loops, anal tags, fistulas
Histology	Mucosal and submucosal inflammation, cryptitis, crypt abscess and distortion, depletion of goblet cells	Transmural inflammation, noncaseating granulomas, prominent lymphoid tissue, preserved goblet cells, fibrosis

have other family members with inflammatory bowel disease with an incidence approximately ten times greater when a positive family history exists. However, concordance between monozygotic twins is only 20%, and HLA markers (e.g., DR2) and linkages to other genetic syndromes (e.g., Hirschsprung, Down, and Turner) indicate that other factors, environmental and genetic, may determine susceptibility given a familial predisposition. An autoantibody, perinuclear staining antineutrophil cytoplasmic antibody (pANCA), has been the most specific marker found in 70% of patients with UC and rarely in Crohn's disease. Rodent models of colitis, especially the interleukin-2 knockout mouse, support a hypothesized derangement of T-lymphocyte immunoregulation. The association of UC with a high familial prevalence of atopic diseases and extraintestinal manifestations of erythema nodosum, arthritis, uveitis, and vasculitis supports the presence of genetic immunologic factors in the pathogenesis. Early gastroenteritis and lack of breastfeeding have been proposed as risk factors. No data support a psychosomatic etiology in terms of stress, personality type, or psychiatric illness, although emotional and other psychosocial factors may affect the presentation and course of the disease.

EPIDEMIOLOGY

The incidence in the general population ranges from 3.9 to 7.3 cases per 100,000 with a prevalence ranging from 41.1 to 79.9 cases per 100,000 population. The disease is more prevalent in whites, particularly among those of Jewish backgrounds. Female patients outnumber male patients. The distribution of age at onset is bimodal with the major peak in the second and third decades and a second peak in the fifth and sixth decades. The disease is rare in children younger than 2 years, although cases in infants have been reported.

CLINICAL PRESENTATION

UC presents in at least four patterns that differ in the extent of mucosal inflammation and systemic disturbance (Table 195-2). The most common presentation is the insidious onset of diarrhea and hematochezia (overt rectal bleeding), usually without systemic signs. Disease is often confined to the distal colon and rectum; the physical examination is normal without abdominal tenderness; and the course remains mild with intermittent exacerbations.

Approximately 30% of patients have moderate signs of systemic disturbance and present with bloody diarrhea, cramps, urgency, anorexia, and weight loss. Physical examination may reveal abdominal tenderness, and stool shows varying amounts of blood and leukocytes.

Ten percent of cases are characterized as severe colitis. Features include bloody stools (greater than 6 per day), anemia, hypoalbuminemia, fever, and weight loss. A subgroup of these patients may not respond to medical therapy and may require early colectomy.

Extraintestinal manifestations of disease may be presenting features and may precede the manifestations of overt colitis. The first sign of disease may be growth disturbance characterized by decreased linear growth velocity. Thyroid abnormalities and arthritis involving peripheral large joints may precede and may not correlate with intestinal symptoms. Erythema nodosum may be seen on the extensor surfaces of the arms and legs before recognition of colitis.

COMPLICATIONS

The most serious complication of UC, toxic megacolon, occurs in fewer than 5% of the patients and is a medical and

TABLE 195-2. Patterns of Presentation of Ulcerative Colitis

Extraintestinal (<5%)
Growth failure, arthropathy, erythema nodosum, occult fecal blood, elevated sedimentation rate, nonspecific abdominal pain, altered bowel pattern, cholangitis
Mild disease (50–60%)
Diarrhea, mild rectal bleeding, abdominal pain
No systemic disturbance
Moderate disease (30%)
Bloody diarrhea, cramps, urgency, abdominal tenderness
Systemic disturbance: anorexia, weight loss, mild fever, mild anemia
Severe disease (10%)
More than six bloody stools per day, abdominal tenderness with or without distention, tachycardia, fever, weight loss, significant anemia, leukocytosis, hypoalbuminemia

surgical emergency. Dilitation of the diseased colon accompanied by fever, tachycardia, electrolyte disturbance, and dehydration occur. Some of these signs, particularly fever and tenderness, may be masked in patients taking high-dose corticosteroids. Colonic perforation, gram-negative sepsis, and massive hemorrhage can occur. Management should include stool bacterial culture, assay for *Clostridium difficile* toxins, broad-spectrum antibiotics, and high-dose corticosteroids. Patients who fail to respond promptly to these aggressive medical measures require colectomy.

With long-standing disease, a colonic stricture may occur. In adults, it may be caused by carcinoma; in children, benign postinflammatory fibrotic stricture is more likely.

DIAGNOSIS

A complete history should be obtained with attention to family history, exposure to infectious agents or antibiotic treatment, retardation in growth or sexual development, and extraintestinal manifestations. The physical examination should include assessment of hydration, nutritional status, and systemic and extraintestinal signs of chronic disease.

Leukocytosis or anemia may be present. The erythrocyte sedimentation rate is elevated in 70% to 90% of the patients. Serum protein and albumin levels may be low, as can levels of serum iron, zinc, and magnesium. Stool should be examined for blood, leukocytes, ova and parasites, and bacterial pathogens such as *Salmonella, Shigella, Campylobacter,* toxigenic or hemorrhagic *Escherichia coli, Aeromonas hydrophila,* and *Yersinia.* The colitis caused by the toxins of *C. difficile* may resemble the lesions in UC or Crohn's disease or may complicate underlying inflammatory bowel disease. An assay for *C. difficile* toxins should be obtained on all patients regardless of prior antibiotic treatment. Finding a pathogen does not exclude underlying inflammatory bowel disease in which the prevalence of secondary infections is increased.

Radiology

An abdominal radiograph can demonstrate colonic dilatation while a barium enema (BE) examination can be used to assess the character and extent of colonic disease. A BE should never be performed in patients with severe active colitis due to risk of perforation or provoking toxic megacolon. A BE may reveal the chronic changes of foreshortening, loss of haustrations, continuous involvement, and strictures, as well as spasm. An upper gastrointestinal barium series and small bowel follow-through with fluoroscopic study of the terminal ileum are often necessary to define small bowel involvement. Backwash ileitis may occur in UC, but no other signs of small bowel involvement should be present.

Flexible sigmoidoscopy or colonoscopy of the colon and ileum is the most sensitive and specific means of evaluating intestinal inflammation. Focal, segmental, or right-sided colonic inflammation with rectal sparing suggests Crohn's disease, and small bowel involvement should be excluded.

DIFFERENTIAL DIAGNOSIS

Other causes of rectal bleeding may be Meckel diverticulum, hemolytic–uremic syndrome, polyposis, hemorrhoids, or anal fissures. Colitis, characterized by fecal leukocytes with evidence of inflammation, may be caused by infection or allergy. Infection with *Salmonella, Shigella, Campylobacter, Yersinia, Aeromonas,* certain strains of *E. coli,* and *E. histolytica* may resemble UC and should be excluded. *C. difficile* pseudomembranous colitis may be present even in the absence of a history of antibiotic treatment. Food proteins, usually cow's milk or soy protein in infancy, may produce an allergic colitis difficult to distinguish from UC unless histology reveals a predominant eosinophilic infiltration of the mucosa.

THERAPY

Because UC is confined to the colon, total proctocolectomy is curative. However, because of the potential complications of surgery and the difficulties in adapting to an ileostomy and life without a colon, medical management is attempted initially. Surgery is reserved for failure to respond to medical management, severe hemorrhage or complications, chronic corticosteroid dependence, or excessive risk of carcinoma in long-standing disease.

Medical Therapy

Mild cases of colitis unaccompanied by systemic signs can be managed on an outpatient basis with rest, a low-residue diet, and the gradual introduction of sulfasalazine or a nonsulfa aminosalicylate (ASA) alternative. Response to treatment is expected within 2 weeks.

Moderate disease requires hospitalization for proper evaluation, observation for complications, and management. In addition to bed rest and a low-residue diet, corticosteroids are given. Sulfasalazine or a nonsulfa aminosalicylate alternative may be used as an adjunct. Failure to respond to this regimen warrants a trial of bowel rest with nutritional support by nasogastric elemental formula or parenteral nutrition. The immunosuppressant azathioprine or its active metabolite 6-mercaptopurine are useful in approximately 75% of cases of refractory disease.

Severe disease should be treated as an emergency with hospitalization and surgical consultation. Some of these patients eventually require colectomy for failure to respond to medical therapy or because of the emergence of life-threatening complications such as toxic megacolon. Parenteral nutritional support is necessary when complete bowel rest is needed. After blood and stool cultures (including toxin assays for *C. difficile*), broad-spectrum intravenous antibiotic coverage should be instituted with metronidazole, the drug of choice. High-dose corticosteroid treatment is often essential. Patients who fail to respond to a maximal medical regimen within 2 weeks ultimately require colectomy.

New options for immunosuppressive management are constantly being developed. Cyclosporine A or tacrolimus (FK-506) are immunosuppressive agents effective in controlling severe colitis until the slow-acting chronic immunosuppressive agents (azathioprine or 6-mercaptopurine) can exert their corticosteroid-sparing effects.

Nutritional Therapy

The provision of adequate nutrients is essential for optimal healing. Malabsorption is unlikely in UC, and increased metabolic requirements are small. Undernutrition is typically caused, however, by a reduced voluntary intake of calories and protein. Guidelines for supplementation are to provide at least 140% of the recommended daily allowance for height and age for both energy and protein. Continuous nocturnal nasogastric infusions of enteral formula through a soft Silastic catheter may be necessary for patients who cannot voluntarily increase their intake.

For severe disease, when bowel rest is desired as an adjunct to medical treatment, nasogastric feeding of an elemental formula or parenteral nutrition through a central venous catheter or elemental diet is necessary to achieve nutritional goals.

Surgery

Although, in most cases, medical management is successful in controlling UC and prolonged remissions are possible, a cure can be obtained only by surgical excision.

Indications for colectomy in acute UC include uncontrolled hemorrhage, severe colitis that fails to respond within 2 weeks to intensive treatment (including corticosteroids, antibiotics, bowel rest, and nutritional support), and complications of toxic megacolon, stricture, or perforation. Elective colectomy is indicated in patients with prolonged corticosteroid dependence or corticosteroid-induced complications, and long-standing disease or epithelial dysplasia of rectal or colonic mucosa, which increases the risk of carcinoma.

A partial or subtotal colectomy is usually performed leaving a rectal stump as a blind or Hartmann's pouch and creating a terminal ileostomy. If the rectal disease cannot be controlled or if ileostomy is preferred, proctectomy should be performed. The risks of extraintestinal complications and carcinoma remain, as long as residual diseased mucosa is present. If the disease in the rectal segment can be controlled with a combination of topical and systemic corticosteroids, performing a careful and complete rectal mucosectomy is possible with preservation of the pelvic nerves and the rectal musculature and sphincters through which the ileum may be pulled and anastomosed to the anus. Inflammation of the neorectum or ileal pouch, termed *pouchitis*, suggests stasis, possible Crohn's disease (which must be excluded by biopsy), or failure of complete dissection of the rectal mucosa before ileal pull-through. Metronidazole has been the most effective agent in treating pouchitis.

PROSPECTIVE MANAGEMENT AND PROGNOSIS

UC is a chronic disease requiring careful surveillance, patient education, and expert management by a team consisting of a pediatrician, gastroenterologist, nutritionist, psychiatrist or psychologist, social worker, and nurse. Most children have the potential for a full, active life with good general health. Ten percent of the patients experience only the presenting episode of colitis but must be followed long term because of the risk of cancer in later life. Approximately 20% of the patients have intermittent symptoms, 50% have chronic disease, and the remaining 20% have chronic, active, incapacitating disease.

The risk of colonic carcinoma in pediatric-onset UC increases by an estimated 10% to 20% per decade after the first 10 years of disease depending on the extent of involvement. Because the risk is cumulative, patients with persistent symptoms and pancolitis of early onset in youth are at greatest risk. Sigmoidoscopy and rectal biopsy, in conjunction with an annual colonoscopy, to detect dysplasia or polyps every 6 months have been recommended for patients with disease of more than 10 years' duration. However, such surveillance is costly, fallible, and not without morbidity, and the efficacy of surveillance in preventing lethal cancer is unproved. These considerations have led some physicians to advocate prophylactic colectomy in patients with long-standing disease that began in childhood or adolescence.

CHAPTER 196
Crohn's Disease

Adapted from W. Daniel Jackson and Richard J. Grand

Crohn's disease is a transmural inflammatory process that may affect any segment of the gastrointestinal (GI) tract from mouth to anus in a discontinuous fashion. The small bowel is involved in 90% of cases (generally the terminal ileum) and is responsible for many of the nutritional complications of Crohn's disease. When the colon is involved, the challenge exists for differentiation from other infectious and inflammatory bowel diseases. A table comparing the clinical features of Crohn's disease and ulcerative colitis is found in Chapter 195.

PATHOLOGY

The inflammation in Crohn's disease often appears as discrete focal ulcerations (i.e., aphthae) with relatively intact intervening mucosa. The rectum is relatively spared, but anal involvement is common with skin tags, anal fissures, and abscesses occurring in approximately 25% of patients. The inflammation of Crohn's disease is usually transmural resulting in stiffening of the small bowel loops caused by fibrosis; and adhesions, stricture formation, and fistulas to other loops of bowel, bladder, vagina, or skin.

Mucosal changes may resemble those of ulcerative or infectious colitis. Noncaseating granulomas may be found in as many as 50% of the patients.

ETIOLOGY

The cause of Crohn's disease is not specifically known, but factors such as genetics, luminal agents, altered mucosal integrity, and immunologic response likely play a role. A 67% concordance of disease in monozygotic twins exists. The pathogenesis of the chronic inflammation may involve dysregulation of the immune response to infectious, toxic, or dietary antigens or an appropriate immune response to an unusual antigen or infectious agent. While no specific organism is responsible for the pathogenesis, altered colonic flora or bacterial products may play a role given the attenuation of disease in sterile animal models and the therapeutic usefulness of antibiotics. An epidemiologic association of tobacco smoke exposure with Crohn's disease exists. Inappropriately regulated immune or cytokine responses have been implicated on the basis of the favorable response to corticosteroids, other immunosuppressive agents, and cytokine antagonists.

EPIDEMIOLOGY

Crohn's disease is more common than ulcerative colitis with an estimate of 3.5 new cases per 100,000 population per year. There is increased prevalence among whites, approximately equal male and female representation, and a bimodal age at onset, with peaks in the second and third and again in the sixth decades of life. No specific heritable pattern has been established.

CLINICAL PRESENTATION

The onset of Crohn's disease is insidious with nonspecific features of GI involvement or extraintestinal manifestations often

TABLE 196-1. Crohn's Disease: Patterns of Involvement

Extraintestinal signs and growth retardation
Anorexia, malaise, fatigue
Perianal disease, stomatitis
Erythema nodosum, pyoderma gangrenosum
Anemia, hepatitis, renolithiasis, arthritis, clubbing
Small bowel involvement
Diarrhea
Abdominal mass, postprandial cramps, nausea
Malabsorption
Mineral and vitamin deficiencies (iron, zinc, magnesium, folate, vitamin B_{12})
Colonic features
Diarrhea, urgency
Rectal bleeding, fecal leukocytes
Perianal fistula, abscess

leading to delayed or incorrect diagnosis. Diarrhea, abdominal pain, fever, and weight loss are the most common presenting features. Rectal bleeding, seen in 30% of Crohn's disease cases, is much less common than in ulcerative colitis.

Based on anatomic involvement, patients can present in one of three general patterns (considerable overlap may exist). Patients with the first pattern present with nonspecific extraintestinal manifestations and growth retardation (Table 196-1). Overt clinical signs of GI involvement may not appear for years, although this inflammation may be extensive enough to cause early satiety, nausea, anorexia, and distention as signs of malabsorption or impaired transit. Certain extraintestinal features that may be clues indicating the presence of Crohn's disease include perianal disease, oral aphthae, erythema nodosum, arthritis, uveitis, and digital clubbing. A microcytic anemia and an elevated erythrocyte sedimentation rate may be present.

Another pattern of presentation is produced by upper GI inflammation, which probably accounts for much of the postprandial cramping, early satiety, nausea, and anorexia that patients report. This can mimic acid peptic disease. Diarrhea and malabsorption can occur.

Colonic involvement may present as diarrhea associated with cramps and urgency to defecate. These signs, as well as overt rectal bleeding, may be difficult to distinguish from ulcerative colitis. Perianal disease (skin tags and fistulae) and relative sparing of the rectum are more frequent in Crohn's colitis than ulcerative colitis and may be the only differentiating features.

Extraintestinal Signs

Arthritis and arthralgias may occur in as many as 11% of cases and usually present as a seronegative monoarticular arthritis of large joints such as a knee or ankle or as a migratory polyarthritis. Arthritis may precede overt GI signs.

Less than 5% of patients develop cutaneous lesions of erythema nodosum or pyoderma gangrenosum. The latter condition is a severe deep ulceration of the skin, often preceded by minor trauma or associated with surgical incisions or stoma sites.

Liver involvement is seen in less than 10% of patients and correlates with bowel disease activity but rarely progresses to cirrhosis or chronic active hepatitis. Cholelithiasis can occur due to ileal dysfunction or resection that interrupts the enterohepatic circulation of bile acids leading to the decreased cholesterol solubility characteristic of lithogenic bile.

Calcium oxalate renal calculi can be caused by increased intestinal oxalate absorption accompanying steatorrhea and subsequent increased renal excretion. Recurrent urinary tract infections and pneumaturia may herald enterovesical fistulas.

Other signs include uveitis, aphthous stomatitis, osteoporosis; anemias of chronic disease and zinc deficiency with acrodermatitis.

Weight loss occurs in many children with Crohn's disease and may be as much as 12.5 kg. Impaired linear growth, retarded bone development, and delayed sexual maturation can be the result. These changes may be initially subtle and often precede overt bowel disease.

Inadequate energy intake may be the result of anorexia from altered taste, early satiety, or meal-related cramps or diarrhea. Some cases are complicated by excessive energy losses such as steatorrhea (29%) and increased enteric protein excretion (70%). Growth failure may occur with or without corticosteroid therapy. Although corticosteroids may suppress linear growth, their use in controlling the inflammation of Crohn's disease often permits growth to resume at normal rates.

COMPLICATIONS

The major intestinal complications of Crohn's disease are related to the transmural nature of the inflammation. Contiguous loops of bowel or other organs may become enveloped in inflammation. Adhesions, strictures, fistulas, and abscesses may develop with a risk of obstruction, bacterial overgrowth, and nutritional depletion. Massive hemorrhage and toxic megacolon, which are potential complications of ulcerative colitis, occur only rarely in Crohn's disease.

Although increased as high as 20 fold, the incidence of small bowel carcinoma is still low in patients with Crohn's disease, and the rates of colonic adenocarcinoma are lower than those in patients with ulcerative colitis. However, rates of colorectal cancer approach those of ulcerative colitis when adjusted for the extent of colonic involvement in Crohn's colitis.

DIAGNOSIS

The diagnosis of Crohn's disease is based on clinical presentation, radiologic findings, and mucosal appearance and histology after exclusion of alternative causes. A complete history should be obtained with attention to family history, exposure to infectious agents or antibiotic treatment, extraintestinal manifestations, and retardation in growth rate or in sexual development. Physical examination should include assessment of hydration, nutritional status, signs of peritoneal inflammation, and signs of systemic chronic disease. Features suggesting Crohn's disease are stomatitis; perianal skin tags, fissures, fistulas or inflammation; and digital clubbing. Fever, orthostasis, tachycardia, and abdominal tenderness, distention, or mass should be considered indications for admission to the hospital.

Laboratory Evaluation

The erythrocyte sedimentation rate is elevated in 90% of patients and may be useful as a marker of inflammatory activity. Total protein and albumin levels are typically low as are serum magnesium, iron, and plasma zinc levels. Ileal dysfunction may be revealed by low vitamin B_{12} and fat-soluble vitamin levels. Fresh stool should be obtained for visual inspection and laboratory examination for blood, leukocytes, and parasites; cultured for infectious pathogens including pathogenic *Escherichia coli* and *Yersinia enterocolitica;* and assayed for *Clostridium difficile* toxins.

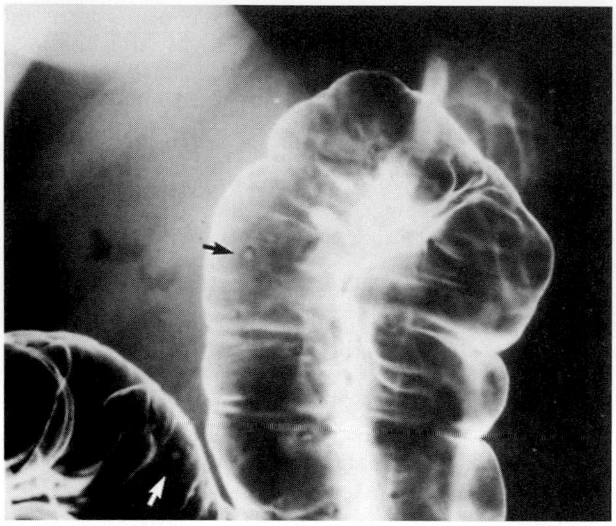

Figure 196-1. Air contrast barium enema in a patient with Crohn's disease demonstrating aphthae (*arrows*) in the splenic flexure.

Radiology

Although contraindicated in severe colitis, if mild to moderate clinical colitis is present and colonoscopy is unavailable, a barium enema study with air contrast may demonstrate characteristic aphthous lesions and show cecal or segmental involvement (Fig. 196-1). An upper GI series with small bowel follow-through or the more definitive enteroclysis study, combined with careful fluoroscopic study of the terminal ileum, is essential to define the small bowel involvement, which affects up to 90% of patients with Crohn's disease (Fig. 196-2). The small bowel enteroclysis study provides the best definition of small bowel lesions, stenosis, and fistulas.

An abdominal mass, persistent focal tenderness, fever, or obstruction should be evaluated by ultrasound or computed tomography to exclude abscess. Computed tomography can often demonstrate the bowel wall thickening, fat wrapping, or abscesses.

Endoscopy

Colonoscopy with biopsy of the colon and terminal ileum is the definitive test for evaluating Crohn's disease. As reflected in its pathology, the lesions of Crohn's disease may appear as discrete ulcerations or aphthae of the mucosa, often with a central exudate and corona of erythema. Severe or chronic disease may present with a cobblestone mucosal pattern caused by linear ulcerations and nodularity or with strictures or stenosis. Intervening areas may be normal in appearance and histologic characteristics and, hence, biopsies must be obtained from multiple sites.

DIFFERENTIAL DIAGNOSIS

Signs of inflammation (e.g., fever, abdominal cramps, tenderness), extraintestinal lesions, or an elevated sedimentation rate can often differentiate inflammatory causes of growth failure from endocrine or psychogenic syndromes such as growth hormone deficiency or anorexia nervosa.

Often the pediatrician is faced with a child with recurrent abdominal pain (RAP) as discussed in Chapter 197. The periumbilical nature of the pain in RAP is nonspecific but not pathognomonic for functional abdominal pain because it can also be characteristic of many children presenting with inflammatory bowel disease. If signs of inflammation are present, the child should be evaluated for Crohn's disease.

Pathogens such as *C. difficile, Y. enterocolitica,* enteropathogenic *E. coli, Aeromonas hydrophila, Giardia lamblia,* and *E. histolytica* must be excluded, along with the customary *Salmonella, Shigella,* and *Campylobacter* cultured in the setting of enterocolitis. These agents are often overlooked in the initial evaluation and may produce a chronic inflammatory picture resembling Crohn's ileocolitis.

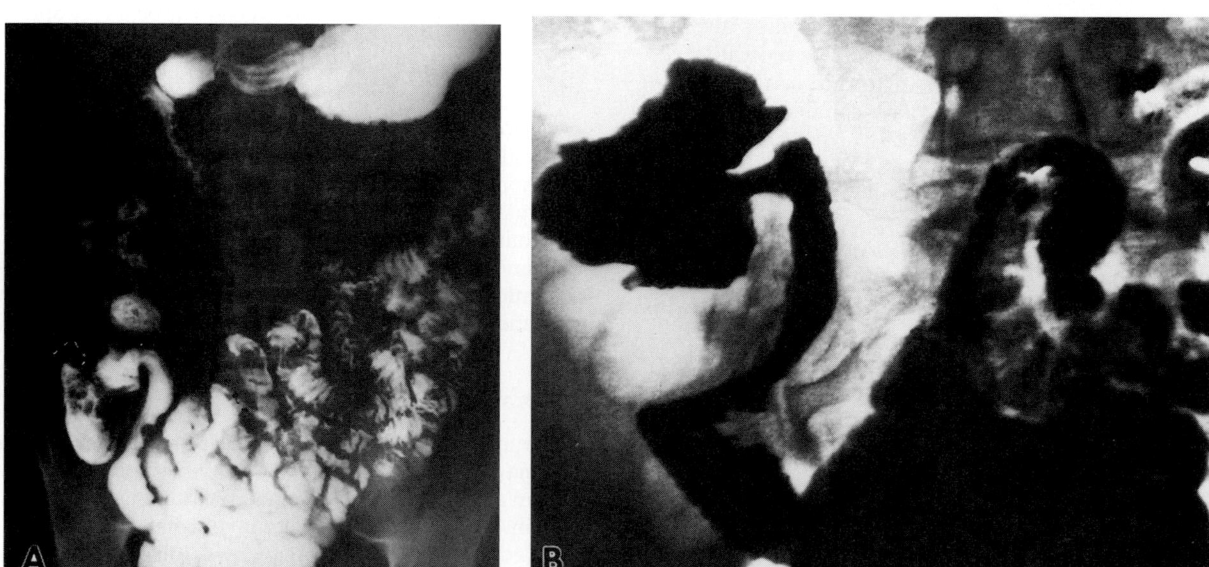

Figure 196-2. A: Enteroclysis small bowel study of a 15-year-old girl shows some distortion but no obstruction of the distal ileum and irregular cecal mucosa. **B:** Spot film of the terminal ileum reveals a long, constricted, and rigid segment with marked distortion at the ileocecal valve. The separation of loops indicates markedly thickened bowel walls.

THERAPY

Because no pharmacologic regimen has been shown to alter the long-term outcome of Crohn's disease, the goals of treatment are to minimize the morbidity of disease exacerbations without introducing iatrogenic morbidity. Optimal management mandates consultation with a pediatric gastroenterologist and may require the perspective of a pediatric surgeon.

Pharmacologic Therapy

Corticosteroid therapy is indicated for symptoms refractory to other agents, extensive small bowel disease, severe or persistent systemic and extraintestinal complications, and postoperative recurrences. Many differing dosage regimens may be used. Corticosteroids can effect short-term remissions of active small bowel disease in 70% of patients. Unfortunately, symptoms may recur with reduction of the dosage and many of these patients suffer relapse. Potential morbidity of high-dose corticosteroid therapy includes adrenal suppression, hypertension, osteoporosis, glaucoma, cataracts, pseudotumor cerebri, and altered body composition. An alternate-day dosing regimen may minimize these effects. A general principle is to use the least amount of corticosteroid necessary to control disease activity and allow growth and full function.

In as many as 75% of the patients who cannot be managed without high-dose or prolonged corticosteroids or who are at risk for complications of corticosteroid therapy, immunosuppressive agents (e.g., azathioprine, 6-mercaptopurine) are useful in establishing or maintaining remission and allowing reduction in corticosteroid dosage. Complications of bone marrow suppression and opportunistic infection are rare and can be weighed against the known morbidity of chronic corticosteroid treatment. Cyclosporine has been shown to have benefits that are short term with significant adverse effects. It may, however, have particular value in closing fistulas. Newer therapies such as human antiTNF-a antibodies (Infliximab) has been approved for patients with steroid-dependent or refractory disease, especially if complicated by fistula. Although costly, a 75% response rate in achieving sustained remission and healing of fistulas has been reported.

Sulfasalazine is useful in the management of Crohn's colitis. Sulfasalazine has side effects of headache, nausea, vomiting, and bloody diarrhea. Neutropenia and oligospermia are reversible side effects. Because the side effects of sulfasalazine are primarily caused by the sulfapyridine moiety and the antiinflammatory effects are caused by the topical activity of the relatively poorly absorbed 5-aminosalicylate moiety, alternative oral nonsulfa preparations of 5-aminosalicylic acid (5-ASA; Asacol, Pentasa, Dipentum) have been created to prevent proximal GI absorption. Evidence that all these agents are effective in the colitis of Crohn's disease, as well as ulcerative colitis exists.

Antimicrobial agents may have a role in reducing any bacterial antigen-stimulated inflammatory response. Metronidazole is the most effective antimicrobial agent and is indicated in patients with Crohn's colitis unresponsive to sulfasalazine or with complications of perianal disease or small intestinal bacterial overgrowth. Clinical series support its role in healing perineal fistulas with up to a 70% response rate for children with perianal disease. Ciprofloxacin has also proved efficacious in treating perianal disease including fistulas and abscesses with minimal toxicity in adults with Crohn's disease. Although quinolone antibiotics are not approved for use in children, more experience suggests their safety in courses of limited duration.

Nutritional Therapy

The goals of nutritional therapy in Crohn's disease must include recovery of metabolic homeostasis by correcting specific nutrient deficits and replacing ongoing losses, provision of sufficient energy and protein for positive nitrogen balance (i.e., protein synthesis) and healing, and promotion of catch-up growth toward premorbid percentiles.

Provision of at least 140% of the recommended daily allowance for total energy and protein is optimal. Nighttime nasogastric infusions may be necessary in patients who cannot voluntarily increase their intake. A gastrostomy tube is an option for those who cannot tolerate a nasogastric tube yet need chronic supplementation. In severe or complicated Crohn's disease, when enteral feeding is not possible, parenteral nutrition is necessary to achieve nutritional goals. Short-term remissions can be achieved by aggressive enteral or parenteral nutritional support alone.

Deficiencies in iron, folate, magnesium, or vitamin B_{12} should be corrected with appropriate supplements. Low plasma zinc levels, low cholesterol, or low alkaline phosphatase suggests a zinc deficit caused by low dietary intake or depletion caused by active mucosal inflammation and enteric losses. Treatment consists of supplements of zinc sulfate.

Surgery

Unlike ulcerative colitis, no definitive surgical cure for Crohn's disease exists. Surgery is reserved for the failed medical therapy and the acute and chronic complications of Crohn's disease such as intestinal obstruction or stricture, abscess or perforation, fistula, uncontrolled hemorrhage, or rare toxic megacolon. Local resection is more successful for isolated small bowel and ileocecal disease than for colitis. Intractable colitis is managed by total proctocolectomy with ileostomy or segmental colectomy with anastomosis. The endorectal pull-through operation used for intractable ulcerative colitis should never be used for Crohn's disease because of the risk of perirectal or pelvic abscess or perianal disease.

PROSPECTIVE MANAGEMENT AND PROGNOSIS

Crohn's disease is a chronic incurable disease requiring careful surveillance, patient education, and expert management by a team consisting of a pediatrician, gastroenterologist, nutritionist, psychiatrist or psychologist, social worker, and nurse. An alliance with a pediatric surgeon familiar with inflammatory bowel disease is essential for management of potential complications. The management of Crohn's disease in children requires adaptation of the patient to the lifelong unpredictable nature of this disease, the morbidity of chronic medication and hospital visits, and the demands of adolescent development.

Nutritional status, growth, sexual maturation, psychosocial adjustment to disease, and compliance with therapy should be monitored as carefully as one monitors the clinical signs and symptoms of disease activity. Most children with Crohn's disease can expect to live full, productive lives with good general health. Mortality is low, but morbidity is high, especially in patients with colonic involvement. Fertility is unaffected in Crohn's disease unless malnutrition or inflammatory damage to reproductive organs occurs.

CHAPTER 197

Chronic Recurrent Abdominal Pain

Adapted from William J. Klish

Chronic recurrent abdominal pain is a common problem in pediatrics. The symptom of abdominal pain is frightening to the average parent. Children often grip their stomachs, become pale and listless and, not surprisingly, parents worry about significant abdominal pathology such as appendicitis or malignancies. If the physician casually writes off the symptom as *functional or psychological*, he or she will lose the confidence of the parents, who observe their child in pain and know that the symptom is not "in the child's head." Physicians themselves frequently worry about missing a diagnosis in these cases, and this self-doubt may be subtly conveyed to the parents.

The physician should discuss the differential diagnosis with the parents at the beginning and rule out potential diagnoses in a logical manner. If the diagnosis of functional pain is made, the pediatrician should discuss it at length emphasizing that the pain is real and not life-threatening. These measures usually allay the fears of the parents sufficiently that they can deal with the symptom effectively.

DIFFERENTIAL DIAGNOSIS

Most children who have chronic recurrent abdominal pain unassociated with other significant symptoms have functional pain. However, because no specific diagnostic test is available, this diagnosis is one of exclusion.

The common entities that cause chronic recurrent abdominal pain of childhood, listed in their approximate order of frequency, are functional abdominal pain, lactose intolerance, simple constipation, musculoskeletal pain, parasitic infection, reflux esophagitis, *Helicobacter pylori* gastritis, peptic ulcer disease, and inflammatory bowel disease. Most of these diagnoses can be screened without a multitude of laboratory and radiographic examinations.

Lactose intolerance is probably the second most common cause of abdominal pain in childhood. If a child is programmed genetically to become lactase deficient, the activity of this enzyme gradually begins to decrease at approximately 4 to 6 years of age. If milk drinking continues at a constant rate, eventually the enzyme activity will not be sufficient to hydrolyze the entire amount of lactose ingested; as a result, some lactose spills into the distal small bowel and colon, where it is fermented by bacteria, and gases such as hydrogen and carbon dioxide are produced. This gas production, if great enough, may cause intestinal dilatation and pain. Early in the development of lactose intolerance, pain may be the sole symptom.

Dietary restriction may be the easiest way to establish lactose intolerance as a cause of abdominal pain. The child should be given a lactose-free diet for approximately 2 weeks. If the abdominal pain disappears, the diagnosis can be suspected. However, it should be confirmed by giving the child lactose again and observing for exacerbation of symptoms. Many recommend that this cycle be completed twice to ensure that lactose intolerance is present. After the diagnosis is established, the parents can be counseled on the avoidance of lactose containing foods and the use of occasional lactase supplementation. Because lactose intolerance is a dose-related phenomenon, most children can tolerate some lactose-containing foods.

Musculoskeletal pain arising from the abdominal muscles is a diagnosis that can be overlooked easily. School-aged children are frequently engaged in exercises that result in strained muscles. The pain is usually described as sharp and may be triggered by various activities or body positions. It is usually located at or near the insertion of the rectus or oblique muscles into the costal margin or iliac crest. Palpating along these insertions can establish the diagnosis.

Occasionally, intestinal parasites (e.g., *Giardia,* pinworms) may cause only abdominal pain. Stool should be examined for ova and parasites as part of the evaluation of all children with this problem.

Inflammatory bowel disease, *H. pylori* gastritis, and peptic ulcers usually cause enough symptoms that their diagnosis is apparent. However, an occasional patient may initially complain of nonspecific abdominal pain and nothing else. A complete blood count, reticulocyte count, sedimentation rate, *H. pylori* antibody test, and stool guaiac test are helpful to screen for these diagnoses.

If the child complains only of nonspecific abdominal pain and results of all of the prudent screening tests are negative, the physician should feel comfortable in making the diagnosis of functional abdominal pain.

TREATMENT

If the diagnosis of functional abdominal pain is made, discussing this diagnosis with the parents in the same manner as organic disease is helpful. The physician must convey the message that the pain is real but is not caused by a process that will become progressively worse and threaten the life of the child. The analogy of a headache in an adult is useful. The pain of a headache is real, but it is treated only as pain and, under normal circumstances, it is not allowed to interfere with daily responsibilities. A child's responsibility is to go to school, and pain should not prevent this from happening. If the pain is severe, it could be treated with medications such as acetaminophen. Antimotility agents are usually ineffective. Using a hot pad or hot water bottle as a counter-irritant is sometimes helpful. Above all, the physician should instill confidence in parents that the pain is not threatening to their child's well-being and will disappear as the child matures.

CHAPTER 198
Celiac Disease

Adapted from Carlos H. Lifschitz

The fraction of gluten called *gliadin* is the agent responsible for celiac disease. Prevalence figures vary from 1/2000 with some studies reporting prevalence of 1/100 (by serologic screening) in certain populations. The disease is more prevalent among persons who carry the HLA-DQ2 and HLA-DQ-8 antigens. It is also more likely in children with insulin dependent diabetes mellitus and trisomy 21.

As more is learned about celiac disease, it is clear that clinical manifestations are quite variable. The classic presentation of frothy, liquid, foul-smelling stools and a wasting syndrome beginning at 10 and 18 months of age (a time at which a sufficient amount of gluten is typically in the diet) may occur, but recent investigations have shown that celiac may present with, among other symptoms, constipation, recurrent abdominal pain, or growth retardation leading to short stature.

Laboratory analyses are nonspecific, and serum abnormalities such as low hemoglobin, iron, albumin, cholesterol, calcium, vitamin A, or carotene levels can be seen in any malabsprotion syndrome. Fat malabsorption may be quantified by means of a 72-hour stool collection (i.e., normal absorption, 95% of ingested fat). The gold standard for the diagnosis of celiac disease remains the small bowel biopsy demonstrating villous atrophy and a chronic inflammatory infiltrate of the lamina propria. As this test is invasive, however, many clinicians will first screen a suspected child with serologic tests. Validity of tests for autoantibodies against tissue transglutaminase and antiendomysial antibodies is superb with sensitivity and specificity of 90% to 95%. In cases of immunoglobulin A deficiency, which is associated with celiac disease, the test could provide a false-negative result.

Once the diagnosis is made, patients should be placed on a gluten-free diet. As many common dietary products contain gluten, the patient and family should meet with a qualified nutritionist. Another useful resource for families is the Celiac Disease Foundation (http://www.celiac.org/). Previous diagnostic algorithms required rechallenge with gluten and then repeat biopsy. Whether such diagnostic criteria currently need to be met depend on patient and clinician. Most experts recommend that affected patients remain on a gluten-free diet for life.

CHAPTER 199
Appendicitis

Adapted from Walter Pegoli, Jr.

Appendicitis is the most common condition leading to emergency abdominal operations in children and adolescents. An individual's risk for appendicitis is lowest during infancy and greatest during adolescence. Approximately 1% of all children at age 15 years or younger will develop appendicitis with a peak incidence between 10 and 12 years. In most published series, the incidence of perforation found at the time of surgery ranges between 10% and 50%.

PATHOPHYSIOLOGY

Luminal obstruction is the most common cause of acute appendicitis. Most often, obstruction results from inspissated fecal material (appendicolith). However, appendicoliths are present in only 30% to 50% of patients at the time of appendectomy.

Bacterial or viral infections can lead to periappendiceal lymphoid hyperplasia that can result in extrinsic compression and subsequent luminal obstruction. Obstruction is then followed by an increase in intraluminal pressure secondary to increased mucus production and venous engorgement. Unabated, this process leads to thrombosis of the microvasculature within the wall of the appendix. Vascular thrombosis with subsequent ischemia leads to necrosis and ultimate perforation of the appendiceal wall.

DIAGNOSIS

An understanding of the embryologic development of the appendix can aid clinicians in diagnosis. The appendix arises from the cecum during the eighth week of fetal development. It rotates from its initial position along the lateral aspect of the cecum to a more medial position near the ileocecal valve. Rotational arrest can occur at any point resulting in variations in the final position of the appendix within the abdominal cavity. This variability in position can lead to alterations in the location of maximal tenderness on physical examination when the appendix is inflamed.

Usually, patients present with the triad of nausea (with or without vomiting), fever, and abdominal pain. The pain associated with appendicitis exhibits a classic pattern of localization to the periumbilical region. As the inflammatory process continues and involves the entirety of the appendiceal wall, the parietal peritoneum becomes inflamed, and pain localizes in the right lower quadrant (RLQ) in the region of McBurney's point (located approximately two-thirds of the way between the umbilicus and the anterior superior iliac spine).

The differential diagnosis of RLQ pain is extensive (Table 199-1). Studies have shown that the most predictive finding in patients with appendicitis is abdominal pain that progresses to

TABLE 199-1. Differential Diagnosis of Right Lower Quadrant Pain

Medical conditions
Constipation
Diabetic ketoacidosis
Gastroenteritis
Hemolytic-uremic syndrome
Henoch-Schönlein purpura
Inflammatory bowel disease
Pneumonia
Primary peritonitis
Sickle cell crisis
Urinary tract infection
Gynecologic conditions
Ectopic pregnancy
Mittelschmerz
Ovarian torsion
Pelvic inflammatory disease
Surgical conditions
Intussusception
Meckel diverticulitis

point tenderness in the RLQ of the abdomen. The point of maximal tenderness, however, varies with the location of the appendix. For example, the tip of the appendix may lie across the psoas muscle or in the depths of the pelvis. In such situations, pain is not perceived in the classic position but rather as vague lower abdominal discomfort. However, one may elicit tenderness by extending the hip (psoas sign) or flexing and internally rotating the thigh (obturator sign). On rectal exam, focal tenderness in the right hemipelvis can be suggestive of acute appendicitis.

Although many different laboratory studies have been used to help to discriminate appendicitis from other causes of abdominal pain in children, none has been consistently reliable. An elevated leukocyte count with a predominance of polymorphonuclear cells in a patient with abdominal pain is consistent with a intraabdominal inflammatory process. This finding, however, is hardly specific for appendicitis. A urinary beta–human chorionic gonadotropin should be obtained to rule out pregnancy. On urinalysis, pyuria and/or hematuria should raise the question of genitourinary tract pathology but does not rule out the diagnosis of appendicitis. An inflamed appendix can lie over the ureter or bladder resulting in the irritation of its wall causing these findings on urinalysis.

On plain-film abdominal radiography, an appendicolith can be visualized in the RLQ in 10% to 20% of cases. In some centers, ultrasound is used to determine the thickness of the layers of the bowel wall and appendiceal compressibility. An edematous, distended (greater than 6 mm), or noncompressible appendix is suggestive of acute appendicitis. Sonography has the added advantage of diagnosing other processes, particularly female gynecological problems such as ovarian torsion and ectopic pregnancy.

Computed axial tomography (CAT) scanning continues to gain popularity for the diagnosis of appendicitis, in part, due to well done clinical studies and, in part, due to the wide availability of this modality. Studies have suggested that helical CT scan with rectal contrast can accurately diagnose appendicitis greater than 90% of the time.

MANAGEMENT

Appendectomy is the definitive treatment. Careful attention should be made to the patient's hydration status, particularly in cases of ruptured appendicitis where third-space fluid losses can be significant. Preoperative antibiotic therapy is empiric and is based on the extent of perceived intraabdominal contamination. An antibiotic should be chosen that is bactericidal to *Escherichia coli* and other enteric organisms. In patients with presumed nonperforated appendicitis, a broad-spectrum second-generation cephalosporin such as cefoxitin or cefotetan is usually adequate. Patients with a perforated appendix may require triple therapy with ampicillin, gentamicin, and metronidazole or clindamycin.

Patients with uncomplicated acute appendicitis require minimal postoperative care. Maintenance intravenous fluids should be maintained until the patient exhibits return of gastrointestinal function. Usually, this process occurs within the first 24 to 48 hours after surgery. A 24-hour course of perioperative antibiotics has been shown to be sufficient in uncomplicated cases. However, in patients with appendicitis complicated by perforation and defuse peritonitis or abscess formation, a nasogastric tube should be inserted while they are in the operating room and should be maintained postoperatively until gastrointestinal function returns. In the majority of cases, bowel function will not return for at least 5 days. Broad-spectrum antibiotics should generally continue until such patients are afebrile with normalizing laboratory parameters.

The most common complications in patients with appendicitis are wound infections and intraabdominal abscesses. Abdominal ultrasonography or computed tomographic scanning (or both) may identify an intraabdominal or pelvic abscess. Depending on location and size, abscess may be drained percutaneously or surgically.

CHAPTER 200
Pancreatitis

Adapted from Steven L. Werlin

ACUTE PANCREATITIS

Blunt abdominal trauma, viral infections, medications and multisystem disease account for the majority of pancreatitis of known etiology in children. Other causes are much less common (Table 200-1).

The healthy pancreas is protected by three factors: (a) pancreatic proteases synthesized as inactive proenzymes, (b) digestive enzymes in secretory granules, and (c) the presence of protease inhibitors. Acute pancreatitis is believed to occur after activation of proteolytic pancreatic proenzymes. This process then leads to autodigestion and further activation and release of active proteases. These activated enzymes then spill into the cytoplasm and interstitium initiating the inflammatory process.

Clinical Manifestations

Clinically, children with acute pancreatitis have midepigastric and periumbilical abdominal pain, often radiating to the back; vomiting; and, frequently, fever. The pain increases in severity for 24 to 48 hours. During this interval, vomiting may increase, and affected patients may require hospitalization for fluid and electrolyte therapy. Usually, acute cases are self-limited, and the prognosis is excellent.

Acute hemorrhagic pancreatitis, the most severe form of acute pancreatitis, is rare in children. In this life-threatening condition, affected children are severely ill and the pancreas may become necrotic and may be transformed into an infected, inflammatory, hemorrhagic mass or phlegmon. Shock, renal failure, infection, massive gastrointestinal bleeding may ensue.

Laboratory Findings

Serum amylase level is elevated for 4 to 5 days, whereas the lipase is increased for 8 to 14 days. Hyperamylasemia is nonspecific and may occur in diabetic ketoacidosis, burn patients,

TABLE 200-1. Etiology of Acute Pancreatitis in Children

Drugs and toxins
Alcohol
L-Asparaginase
Azathioprine
Cimetidine
Corticosteroids
Dideoxycytidine
Didanosine
Enalapril
Erythromycin
Estrogen
Furosemide
6-Mercaptopurine
Mesalamine
Methyldopa
Pentamidine
Scorpion bites
Sulfonamides
Sulindac
Tetracycline
Thiazides
Valproic acid
Hereditary pancreatitis
Infections
Coxsackie B virus
Epstein-Barr virus
Hepatitis A, B
Influenza A, B
Leptospirosis
Malaria
Measles
Mumps
Mycoplasma
Reye syndrome (varicella, influenza B)
Rubella
Rubeola
Obstructive causes
Ampullary disease
Ascariasis
Biliary tract malformations
Cholelithiasis and choledocholithiasis
Clonorchis
Duplication cyst
Endoscopic retrograde cholangiopancreatography complication
Pancreas divisum
Pancreatic ductal abnormalities
Postoperative conditions
Sphincter of Oddi dysfunction
Tumor
Systemic disease
Brain tumor
Collagen-vascular diseases
Cystic fibrosis
Diabetes mellitus
Head trauma
Hemochromatosis
Hemolytic uremic syndrome
Hyperlipidemia types I, IV, V
Hyperparathyroidism
Kawasaki disease
Malnutrition
Organic acidemia
Peptic ulcer
Periarteritis nodosa
Renal failure
Systemic lupus erythematosus
Transplantation (bone marrow, heart, liver, kidney, pancreas)
Trauma
Blunt injury
Child abuse
Surgical trauma
Total body cast

and in the presence of an elevation of salivary amylase, as may occur in parotitis. Fractionation of serum amylase into the salivary and pancreatic components can be performed readily in most clinical laboratories. Serum lipase is more specific for acture pancreatitis.

On abdominal X-ray, a sentinel loop of small bowel or a segmental ileus may be seen. Ultrasonography (US) and computed tomography (CT) are the most commonly used imaging modalities, but their use is rarely warranted in uncomplicated cases. They can be helpful to evaluate for complications such as peripancreatic abscesses.

Treatment

Treatment is typically supportive and aimed at balancing fluid and electrolyte needs and controlling pain. Opiates are typically necessary for pain control. Usually, improvement occurs in 2 to 4 days. Patients with acute pancreatitis may be fed when clinical symptoms have resolved and the serum amylase has returned to near normal. A low-fat diet is typically recommended for several weeks.

PANCREATIC PSEUDOCYST

Pancreatic pseudocyst formation is an uncommon sequela of pancreatitis. Pseudocysts are delineated by a fibrous wall in the lesser peritoneal sac, which may enlarge or extend in almost any direction. A pseudocyst is suggested when an episode of pancreatitis fails to resolve, when an abdominal mass develops after an episode of pancreatitis, or when pancreatitis relapses shortly after resolution. Clinical features may include pain, nausea, vomiting, and jaundice. The most useful diagnostic techniques are ultrasound (Fig. 200-1), CT scanning and endoscopic retrograde cholangiopancreatography (ERCP).

Most pseudocysts smaller than 4 cm resolve spontaneously. Treatment of nonresolving pseudocysts involves drainage (percutaneously or endoscopically) or surgery. If surgery is required, the pseudocyst must be allowed to mature for 4 to 6 weeks before surgical drainage is performed.

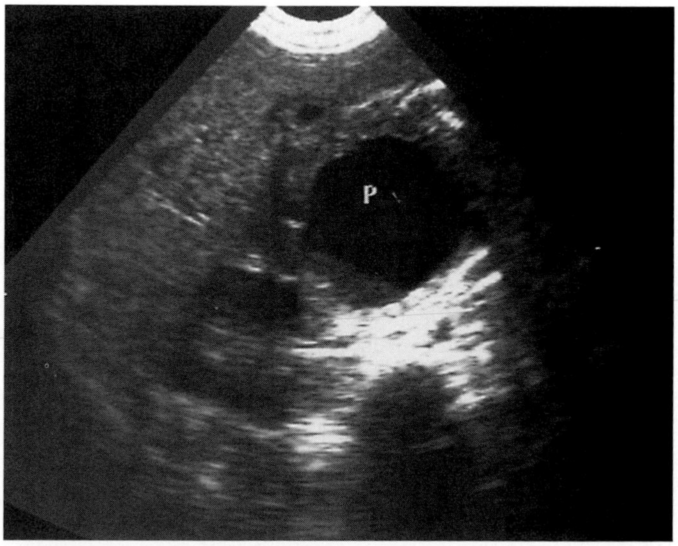

Figure 200-1. Pancreatic pseudocyst (*P*). This pseudocyst, 5 cm in diameter, developed in a 16-year-old boy 2 weeks after recovery from an episode of acute pancreatitis. (Courtesy of Dr. John Sty.)

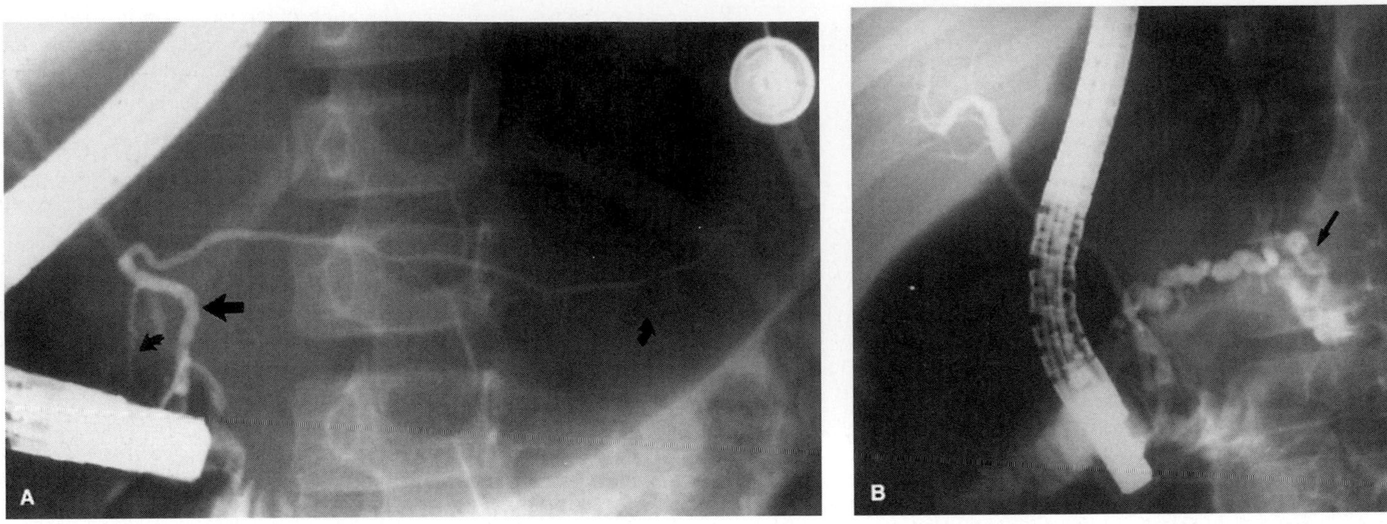

Figure 200-2. A: Normal pancreatogram. Note the excellent visualization of the side branches. Main pancreatic duct (*large arrow*); side branches (*small arrows*). (Courtesy of Dr. Anthony Bohorfoush.) **B:** Chronic pancreatitis. Note dilatation and tortuosity of the main pancreatic duct. Filling defects represent intraductal stones (*arrow*).

CHRONIC PANCREATITIS

The definition of acute pancreatitis and its differentiation from chronic pancreatitis have been the subject of much dispute. The definition accepted most widely holds that acute pancreatitis is an isolated episode with complete morphologic and histologic resolution. Acute pancreatitis may recur but, unless structural damage occurs, it rarely becomes chronic.

Usually, chronic or recurrent pancreatitis in children is due to hereditary pancreatitis, traumatic damage, cystic fibrosis, or anomalies of the pancreatic or biliary ductal systems. Frequently, symptoms begin in the first decade but are usually mild at onset. Although spontaneous recovery from each attack occurs in 4 to 7 days, episodes become progressively more severe.

Hereditary pancreatitis is diagnosed when the disease is present in successive generations of a family. The gene for hereditary pancreatitis has been localized to the short arm of chromosome 7 and has been cloned. Two different mutations on the cationic trypsinogen gene that have been identified allow autoactivation of trypsinogen to trypsin.

All children who have experienced more than one episode of pancreatitis must be evaluated thoroughly. Serum lipid, calcium, and phosphorus levels are determined. In the appropriate clinical setting, stools are evaluated for ascaris. A sweat test is performed. Plain-film abdominal radiographs are evaluated for the presence of pancreatic calcifications. US or CT is performed to detect the presence of a pseudocyst or biliary lithiasis.

ERCP, which defines the anatomy of the gland, should be considered in the evaluation of children with nonresolving pancreatitis, recurrent acute pancreatitis, or chronic pancreatitis and before operation in patients with pseudocyst (Fig. 200-2). In such cases, ERCP may detect unsuspected anatomic defects amenable to surgical therapy.

CHAPTER 201

Cholecystitis

Adapted from Kathleen J. Motil

Cholecystitis is an inflammatory disease of the gallbladder that may be acute or chronic, with further classification as calculous or acalculous, and based on the presence or absence of gallstones. Gallstones are present in 80% to 85% of children who have this disorder. Chronic cholecystitis with cholelithiasis is the most common pattern occurring in almost two-thirds of children with this diagnosis.

ETIOLOGY AND PATHOGENESIS

Acute cholecystitis may result from any of three primary events in the gallbladder: bile stasis, an inflammatory response, or ischemia (Table 201-1). Stasis usually results from obstruction of the cystic duct due to gallstones, starvation, dehydration, and immobilization. Inflammatory responses are usually incited by

TABLE 201-1. Pathophysiology of Cholecystitis

Acute cholecystitis
Bile stasis
Obstruction (gallstones, lymph nodes, tumor)
Starvation
Immobilization
Inflammation
Bile salts
Lysolecithin
Pancreatic juice
Bacteria
Ischemia
Torsion
Systemic vascular disease
Chronic cholecystitis
Recurrent obstruction and inflammation

bile salts, lysolecithin, pancreatic juice, and bacteria. Torsion of the gallbladder or systemic vascular disease may lead to ischemic changes of the biliary tract.

EPIDEMIOLOGY

The incidence of cholecystitis in children ranges from less than 1% to 4%. Girls are affected more commonly than boys after adolescence, and whites are almost twice that number in the African-American population. Acalculous cholecystitis more commonly affects younger children, and calculous cholecystitis occurs more frequently in adolescents.

PREDISPOSING FACTORS

Several entities have been implicated as predisposing factors for cholecystitis in children (Table 201-2). Hemolytic disease (congenital spherocytosis, sickle cell anemia, and thalassemia), total parenteral nutrition of prolonged duration, and ileal abnormalities such as ileal resection or Crohn's disease are some of the more common causes. Infections such as parasitic infestations (e.g., with *Giardia, Ascaris*), infectious hepatitis (e.g., type A), urinary tract infections, scarlet fever, endocarditis, and pneumonia have been implicated as infectious causes of cholecystitis in 12% of patients. Congenital or acquired malformations of the biliary tract (e.g., choledochal cyst) have been implicated in the development of cholecystitis. Cystic fibrosis and cirrhosis have also been associated with gallbladder disease.

CLINICAL FEATURES

Clinical presentation can be variable with very few symptoms or florid illness. Episodic right upper quadrant abdominal pain (with abdominal tenderness on exam) radiating to the back or shoulder is the most common complaint. Vomiting occurs in nearly half the patients. Jaundice and fever may also be present.

TABLE 201-2. Factors Associated with Cholecystitis in Childhood

Factors	Frequency (% of cases)
Hemolytic disease	37
Ileal abnormalities	37
Pregnancy	31
Obesity	27
Total parenteral nutrition	19
Infection	12
Family history of biliary disease	12
Previous abdominal surgery	9
Cystic fibrosis	7
Biliary tract anomalies	6
Cirrhosis	4
Trauma	1
Other (congenital anomalies, drugs, ventilatory support)	<1

Infrequently, a mass may be palpated and may be associated with acute acalculous cholecystitis.

LABORATORY AND RADIOGRAPHIC STUDIES

Laboratory studies including liver function tests are of limited diagnostic value but, typical screening labs include liver function tests, serum amylase, bilirubin, and alkaline phosphatase. A complete blood cell count and hemoglobin electrophoresis may be indicated to determine the presence of an underlying hemolytic disorder.

Significant abnormalities such as gallbladder dilatation or thickened walls can be demonstrated in at least 90% of the children who undergo abdominal ultrasound. Hepatobiliary imaging with a technetium Tc 99m–labeled iminodiacetic acid derivative may be useful to demonstrate a nonfunctioning gallbladder. Endoscopic retrograde cholangiopancreatography (ERCP), a radiologic technique used to diagnose diseases of the biliary tract and pancreas, may suggest cystic or common bile duct obstruction in the absence of visualization of the gallbladder. The major indications for diagnostic ERCP in this setting are obstructive jaundice and recurrent pancreatitis, both of which may be found in the presence of cholelithiasis.

An abdominal flat plate may serendipitously show asymptomatic calcified gallstones. Because gallstones are not calcified in at least 50% of children, they are not seen on a plain radiograph of the abdomen. Moreover, calcifications constitute a nonspecific finding that is consistent with other diagnoses including tuberculosis, bacterial or amebic abscesses, intrahepatic calculi, hemangioma, echinococcal cysts, neuroblastoma, and hepatic neoplasms.

DIFFERENTIAL DIAGNOSIS

Cholecystitis should be considered early in the differential diagnosis of abdominal pain, especially in high-risk children who have a family history of gallbladder or sickle cell disease. The principal conditions to consider in the differential diagnosis of cholecystitis are appendicitis, pancreatitis, gastroesophageal reflux, esophagitis, peptic ulcer disease, hepatitis, hepatic abscess or tumor, intussusception, pyelonephritis or nephrolithiasis, and pneumonitis.

Cholecystitis may be difficult to differentiate from acute pancreatitis and the processes may simultaneously occur. Cholelithiasis may cause acute pancreatitis as stones traverse the common bile duct and ampulla of Vater.

TREATMENT

The treatment of acute cholecystitis includes discontinuation of oral feedings, hydration, and correction of electrolyte abnormalities. Opiates can be used for pain relief. Antibiotics such as ampicillin and gentamicin or a second generation cephalosporin are used to treat acute cholecystitis because they are excreted in bile or provide adequate coverage for enteric organisms.

Laparoscopic cholecystectomy is the treatment of choice for the management of uncomplicated acute cholecystitis. The current recommendation is to proceed with surgery 3 to 7 days after bowel rest and antibiotics have been initiated. If the child has not responded to bowel rest and antibiotics, or complications of cholecystitis are apparent, surgery must be performed immediately.

Surgery is also the preferred treatment for chronic cholecystitis, particularly in the case of cholelithiasis. Controversy exists about the treatment of asymptomatic cholelithiasis in children. Because spontaneous disappearance of gallstones in infancy has been reported, a 2- to 3-month period of observation may be warranted for an asymptomatic patient who has sludge or noncalcified stones in the gallbladder. However, elective cholecystectomy is advised for all symptomatic patients, patients with calcified stones, and asymptomatic patients in whom sludge or noncalcified stones do not resolve after 2 to 3 months. Laparoscopic cholecystectomy is considered the procedure of choice in the treatment of symptomatic cholelithiasis.

COMPLICATIONS

A serious complication of acute cholecystitis is perforation causing pericholecystic abscess with possible generalized peritonitis or fistula formation into the bowel. Surgical intervention is indicated for these complications. Less frequently, ascending cholangitis, liver abscess, or sepsis may complicate the clinical course of acute cholecystitis.

The complications of chronic cholecystitis in the absence of cholelithiasis are minimal. Patients with gallstones are at risk for recurrent bouts of acute cholecystitis, pancreatitis, perforation, bile peritonitis, biliary obstruction, biliary cirrhosis, and cancer of the gallbladder.

8
Endocrine System

CHAPTER 202
Parathyroid Glands

Adapted from John L. Kirkland

HYPOPARATHYROIDISM

Hypoparathyroidism in children is rare, excluding transient hypoparathyroidism in neonates. Hypoparathyroidism is recognized biochemically by hypocalcemia usually associated with hyperphosphatemia. The clinical manifestations of hypocalcemia are secondary to neuromuscular instability. The most common presentation is a seizure. Numbness and tingling sensations in the extremities may precede the seizure. Chvostek sign (stimulation of the ipsilateral facial muscle by tapping the facial nerve in front of the ear), Trousseau sign (carpopedal spasm produced by inflation of the blood pressure cuff to greater than the systolic blood pressure for 2 minutes), laryngospasm, bronchospasm, and prolonged QT intervals on electrocardiography can occur. The etiology of hypoparathyroidism and treatment of hypocalcemia are discussed in the following sections.

Autoimmune Hypoparathyroidism

Hypoparathyroidism may occur alone or as part of an autoimmune complex. Addison disease and mucocutaneous candidiasis are most frequently associated with hypoparathyroidism. Hypoparathyroidism also occurs as part of the autoimmune polyendocrinopathy–candidiasis–ectodermal dystrophy syndrome. A consistent component is immunologic destruction of the hormone-producing cells. Approximately 30% to 40% of patients have antibodies against the parathyroid gland, but the role of antibodies as causative is uncertain.

Hypocalcemia clinically presents with tetany, seizures, and neuromuscular irritability in children with hypoparathyroidism. Mucocutaneous candidiasis may precede the hypoparathyroidism. Other endocrinopathies include hypoadrenalism, hypogonadism, hypothyroidism, and diabetes mellitus. Lymphocytic infiltration of the parathyroid glands is a common pathologic finding.

A child with hypoparathyroidism should be examined frequently for other endocrinopathies. Many cases are secondary to an autosomal recessive gene, and genetic counseling may be warranted.

NEONATAL HYPOCALCEMIA

Neonatal hypocalcemia occurring within the first 24 hours of age is defined as early, whereas hypocalcemia occurring after the second or third day of life is defined as late. Early neonatal hypocalcemia may develop from agenesis or hypoplasia of the parathyroid gland, either as an isolated finding or as part of a recognizable group of clinical findings. DiGeorge syndrome was originally described in infants with congenital absence of the thymus and the parathyroid glands, as well as deficient cell-mediated immunity. Later descriptions included cardiovascular malformations involving the aortic arch. These included truncus arteriosus and aortic arch syndromes. Additional findings include dysmorphic features of the face such as low-set ears, short philtrum, micrognathia, and a small "fish-like" mouth. Velocardiofacial syndrome includes facial dysmorphisms, palatal abnormalities, congenital heart disease, and other clinical findings consistent with DiGeorge syndrome. Genetic analysis of both conditions reveals chromosome 22q11 deletions suggesting a common origin with clinical overlap that should be designated as the chromosomal 22q11 deletion syndrome. An autosomal dominant trait has been documented in some cases. The natural history is quite variable with the hypoparathyroidism resolving in some affected children during the first year.

Other causes of early neonatal hypocalcemia include preterm delivery with low birth weight, birth asphyxia, and presence of diabetes in the mother. The etiologies of these disorders are poorly understood. Possible reasons for the hypocalcemia include increased calcitonin levels, target-organ resistance to 1alpha, 25-dihydroxyvitamin D, delayed feeding, decreased PTH excretion, and diminished biological effects of PTH.

Late neonatal hypocalcemia developing on the second or third day of life may occur secondary to hypoparathyroidism of any etiology, either as an isolated entity or as part of a syndrome. Examples of the latter include Kearns–Sayre syndrome and Kenny–Caffey syndrome. Maternal hyperparathyroidism may produce neonatal hypocalcemia caused by suppression of neonatal PTH. Increased phosphorus intake of any cause including cow's milk–based formulas may lower serum calcium.

Why only a small percentage of neonates fed a high phosphate-containing milk develop hypocalcemia is unclear. The increased phosphorus levels may antagonize PTH actions or secretion of PTH or produce increased calcium and phosphorus deposition in bones leading to hypocalcemia.

Illnesses

Acute illnesses in children including gram-negative sepsis, toxic shock syndrome, and acquired immunodeficiency syndrome are often associated with hypocalcemia secondary to hypoparathyroidism. The etiology of the hypoparathyroidism in ill children is unknown, but it may be related to macrophage-generated interleukins that mimic calcium ionophores. A critically ill child admitted to an intensive care unit is a prime candidate for hypocalcemia. Recognition of hypocalcemia may be delayed because of concurrent resuscitation or diagnostic procedures. However, correction of the hypocalcemia is mandatory because many cardiovascular agents require normal concentrations of calcium for biological effects. Ionized calcium levels, as opposed to total serum calcium levels, reflect the child's true calcium status, because disturbances in total serum calcium determination from hypoalbuminemia, fluctuations in the pH, and the presence of radiographic contrast media may influence total serum calcium measurements.

ISOLATED HYPOPARATHYROIDISM

Isolated hypoparathyroidism not associated with other endocrine diseases, or as a result of thyroid surgery, can occur. The etiology of isolated hypoparathyroidism is usually unknown, but its clinical and laboratory findings, as well as its treatment, are identical to those of other forms of hypoparathyroidism. The familial forms may be caused by gene mutations near the PTH gene located on the short arm of chromosome 2. Hypoparathyroidism also occurs as a consequence of iron deposition in the parathyroid gland from frequent transfusions such as in thalassemia major or as a result of copper deposition such as in Wilson disease.

HYPOMAGNESEMIA

Chronic magnesium deficiency, either congenital or acquired, produces hypocalcemia secondary to diminished production and effectiveness of PTH. Interestingly, acute-onset hypomagnesemia increases production of PTH. Chronic hypomagnesemia caused by urinary or gastrointestinal losses develops from unknown cellular defects. Affected individuals have other metabolic disturbances such as hypokalemia. Acquired hypomagnesemia is usually secondary to another disease such as intestinal malabsorption. Clinical manifestations usually consist of tetany, carpopedal spasms, or seizures. Laboratory findings include serum levels of magnesium less than 1.5 mEq/L. Treatment consists of magnesium administered intravenously, intramuscularly, or orally. Magnesium levels should be frequently measured. Diarrhea may result from oral administration of magnesium. If diarrhea develops, the oral replacement dosage should be decreased accordingly, then slowly increased.

Laboratory Findings

The characteristic laboratory findings of hypoparathyroidism include hypocalcemia and hyperphosphatemia. PTH levels are low in most situations discussed previously. Radiographs of bones usually do not show any diagnostic features. The differential diagnosis includes hypocalcemia for other reasons such as phosphate-induced hypocalcemia; renal failure; and hypocalcemic rickets, although reduced levels of serum phosphorus usually distinguish it. Clinical history, laboratory assessment, and radiographs can facilitate the evaluation. Children with pseudohypoparathyroidism (end-organ resistance to PTH action) present with hypocalcemia and hyperphosphatemia, but PTH levels are elevated.

Treatment of Hypocalcemic Disorders

The acute treatment of symptomatic hypocalcemia in the previously mentioned disorders can be generalized if modifications are made for each etiology. Intravenous calcium is usually required. Pediatricians frequently use 10% calcium gluconate initially as an intravenous solution. Infants with seizures and laryngospasm may require an initial dose of 1 to 2 mL/kg. The infusion of calcium should be slow, 1 mL or less per minute, paying strict attention to the heart rate or an electrocardiographic monitor. Bradycardia is an indication to decrease the rate of calcium infusion. Subsequent intravenous calcium is administered at a rate of 25 to 100 mg of elemental calcium per kilogram of body weight per day depending on the severity of the hypocalcemia and the serum calcium levels. Extravasation of intravenous calcium may result in tissue necrosis. This complication may develop despite the continuous monitoring of intravenous sites prompting some physicians to administer intravenous calcium only as an intermittent bolus. However, intermittent dosages of intravenous calcium may decrease serum pH, rapidly increase tonicity, and produce an intermittent "overshoot" hypercalcemia. A 10% calcium chloride solution can also be used for intravenous treatment, but it is more irritating to the veins than calcium gluconate. Ten milliliters of 10% calcium chloride can be diluted with 50 mL of 5% glucose solution to administer intravenously. Oral treatment with calcium supplementation may be initiated immediately. Calcium glubionate (Neo-Calglucon) contains 23 mg of elemental calcium per milliliter, whereas calcium lactate powder is 13% elemental calcium (i.e., 100 mg of calcium lactate has 13 mg of elemental calcium). Other commercial preparations have varying amounts of elemental calcium. The amount of calcium supplementation administered should be monitored monthly by serum calcium determinations. The amount of elemental calcium administered to maintain eucalcemia varies from 50 to 150 mg/kg/day. Because calcium administered through the gastrointestinal system is dependent on the presence of 1alpha, 25-dihydroxyvitamin D or its analogues, it is not surprising that treatment of hypoparathyroidism with calcium alone is rarely successful.

Treatment with vitamin D or its analogues is the only method available now to treat chronic hypocalcemic states such as hypoparathyroidism. Most vitamin D supplementation is undertaken with dihydrotachysterol, 25-hydroxyvitamin D, or 1alpha, 25-dihydroxyvitamin D. Vitamin D was previously used in large amounts, but its long half-life made adjustments in dosage difficult. Dihydrotachysterol is administered in a dose of 0.05 to 0.50 mg/day. A liquid solution facilitates small changes in the dosage required to maintain eucalcemia. Begin 25-Hydroxyvitamin D at 20 μg a day or on an every-other-day basis, and then increase the dosage slowly. Experience in infants and children is limited. A 1alpha, 25-dihydroxyvitamin D is initiated with a dose of 0.25 μg/day and is increased to several micrograms per day depending on the response of the serum calcium level. This preparation has a more rapid onset of action than dihydrotachysterol, and therapeutic manipulation is easier.

Another preparation of 1alpha, 25-dihydroxyvitamin D may be administered intravenously, but its use in children is limited.

The goal of long-term management is to maintain eucalcemia and eucalciuria. Children should obtain monthly tests for calcium levels and take 24-hour urine collections twice yearly for calcium content. The optimal serum calcium level is in the low range of normal. For children older than 8 years, the urinary calcium level should be less than 0.3 mg of calcium per milligram of creatinine. For children younger than 8 years, urinary calcium levels should be less than 0.8 mg of calcium per milligram of creatinine depending on the child's age. Older patients may require serum calcium levels slightly below the normal range to avoid hypercalciuria.

HYPERPARATHYROIDISM

Hyperparathyroidism is uncommon in pediatric patients, but it is extremely important because an aggressive therapeutic approach may prevent chronic renal diseases from developing as a consequence of nephrocalcinosis. The clinical manifestations of hypercalcemia from any cause are similar. Initially affected are the neuromuscular and gastrointestinal systems. Muscle weakness, paralysis, or hyporeflexia may be observed in the former, whereas constipation, anorexia, and nausea may be observed in the latter. Antidiuretic hormone action on the kidney may be affected adversely with resulting polyuria and polydipsia suggesting diabetes insipidus. Nephrocalcinosis may occur later. The cardiovascular symptoms may reveal bradycardia and a reduced QT interval. The etiologies of hyperparathyroidism are discussed in the following sections. Nonparathyroid gland hypercalcemia in children is mentioned briefly.

Neonatal Severe Hyperparathyroidism

A rare form of hypercalcemia in neonates is neonatal severe hyperparathyroidism. Pathologic examination reveals hyperplasia of the parathyroid glands. Inactivating mutations of the calcium-sensing receptor disable the normal negative feedback mechanisms that control the secretion and production of PTH. The mutations cause the parathyroid gland cells to sense incorrectly hypocalcemic serum levels resulting in the stimulation of PTH production and secretion. Genetic analysis suggests that neonatal severe hyperparathyroidism is a homozygous form of familial hypocalciuric hypercalcemia. Thus, the neonates inherit mutated calcium-sensing receptor genes from both parents and, as a result, have severe hypercalcemia. However, de novo mutations in the calcium-sensing receptor are reported. The increased PTH levels promote resorption of bones producing hypercalcemia, as well as increased renal tubular loss of phosphate. Attempts to control hypercalcemia with dietary restrictions of calcium may result in rickets. Failure to thrive occurs frequently. Medical treatment, as outlined, is usually inadequate to manage the hypercalcemia, and total parathyroidectomy is required. Parathyroid gland autoimplants are successful in some cases in which ectopically transplanted parathyroid tissue can be selectively removed as required to maintain eucalcemia. Subtotal parathyroidectomy has a significant risk for the continuation or recurrence of hypercalcemia in neonates.

PARATHYROID ADENOMA AND PARATHYROID GLAND HYPERPLASIA

Hypercalcemia in older children may be secondary to hyperparathyroidism from parathyroid adenoma and chief cell hyperplasia. Presenting clinical signs may include paralytic ileus, osseous deformities, and personality changes, or the child may be asymptomatic. Unfortunately, many cases are undiagnosed until hypercalcemic complications develop. The diagnosis is confirmed biochemically by hypercalcemia, hypophosphatemia, and elevated PTH levels. Hypercalciuria may be present. Radiographic findings include osteitis fibrosa cystica and genu valgum. Advances in sonographic techniques and the use of technetium 99m sestamibi scans may assist in presurgical localization and differentiate between parathyroid gland hyperplasia and adenoma. Hypocalcemia may occur after surgery as remaining parathyroid tissues recover from suppression and calcium deficits in bone are replaced.

Multiple Endocrine Neoplasia Type I

Multiple endocrine neoplasia type I, or Wermer syndrome, is characterized by neoplasia of the pancreas, anterior pituitary gland, and parathyroid gland. Multiple endocrine neoplasia type I is an autosomal dominant inherited disease with high penetrance and variable expression. Hyperparathyroidism occurs in 90% of patients. Pancreatic tumors and pituitary adenomas occur less frequently. Almost all patients with hyperparathyroidism have enlargement and hyperplasia of parathyroid tissue. Genetic analysis reveals a loss of heterozygosity at chromosome 11q13 loci producing inactivation of a tumor-suppressor gene. Some cases have an onset in neonates. Hypercalcemia, elevated levels of PTH, and the familial occurrence confirm the diagnosis. Treatment consists of subtotal parathyroidectomy (three and one-half glands) with implants of a small amount of parathyroid tissue to the muscles of one extremity.

FAMILIAL HYPOCALCIURIC HYPERCALCEMIA

Familial hypercalcemic hypocalciuria is an autosomal dominant form of hypercalcemia previously known as familial benign hypercalcemia. The diagnosis is unsuspected in most children unless other family members have hypercalcemia. The cardinal findings are mild to moderate hypercalcemia and relative hypocalciuria. Serum calcium levels are rarely greater than 14 mg/dL. Urinary calcium expressed in terms of milligram of calcium per milligram of creatinine for age is normal or slightly elevated, but it is less than would be expected from the degree of hypercalcemia. Nephrocalcinosis does not occur. PTH levels are normal, but they are elevated for the degree of hypercalcemia. Phosphorus levels are variable. Serum magnesium levels are elevated in some children. Other biochemical studies related to calcium and vitamin D metabolism such as 1alpha, 25-dihydroxyvitamin D, calcitonin, urinary cAMP levels, and radiographic examination of the skeleton do not reveal consistent abnormalities or have normal results. The asymptomatic nature of this disorder, as opposed to the signs and symptoms of hypercalcemia secondary to hyperparathyroidism, can corroborate the diagnosis.

The etiology is secondary to an inactivating mutation of the calcium-sensing receptor. The defective gene has been localized in some families to the long arm of chromosome 3. The inactivation of the calcium-sensing receptor results in mild to moderate resistance to the inhibitory effects of hypercalcemia on PTH secretion. Surgical removal of all parathyroid tissue results in hypoparathyroidism. Removal of only parts of the parathyroid gland does not improve the hypercalcemia. No treatment is currently recommended.

Nonparathyroid Gland Hypercalcemic Disorders

WILLIAMS SYNDROME

Individuals with Williams syndrome are usually small for gestational age with facial abnormalities, hypotonia, motor retardation, supravalvular aortic stenosis, and a gregarious and friendly character ("cocktail party" personality). The hypercalcemia usually resolves by the end of the first year of life. The gene responsible for this disorder has been localized to the long arm of chromosome 7. Deletions of the entire elastin gene result in Williams syndrome, whereas partial deletions result in isolated supravalvular aortic stenosis.

IDIOPATHIC INFANTILE HYPERCALCEMIA

Excessive maternal supplementation of vitamin D during pregnancy results in birth defects similar to Williams syndrome. The infants may have supravalvular aortic stenosis and musculoskeletal abnormalities as observed in Williams syndrome. The hypercalcemia persists for longer than 1 year. Elevated levels of PTHrP may occur with hypercalcemia.

IMMOBILIZATION HYPERCALCEMIA

Fractures in weight-bearing limbs frequently require immobilization. Immobilization may infrequently produce hypercalcemia and hypercalciuria. The etiology is unknown, but it may be related to the normally fast turnover of calcium in the skeletal system of children. The best treatment is ambulation, but calcitonin administration may lower serum calcium levels.

HYPOPHOSPHATASIA

Severe infantile hypophosphatasia is an autosomal recessive disorder resulting from a deficiency of the isoenzyme alkaline phosphatase. The lack of this bone enzyme results in deficient mineralization and rickets. Hypercalcemia results from an imbalance in absorption of calcium and deposition of calcium in bones. Urinary phosphoethanolamine levels may be elevated, but the test is not pathognomonic. No effective treatment exists for this disorder, but hypercalcemia may improve with calcitonin.

HYPERCALCEMIC GRANULOMATOUS DISORDERS

Numerous granulomatous diseases (including sarcoidosis, tuberculosis, and neonatal subcutaneous fat necrosis) have been associated with hypercalcemia. The macrophages involved in the granuloma produce increased amounts of 1alpha, 25-dihydroxyvitamin D. Treatment with glucocorticoids has been effective in producing eucalcemia.

Laboratory Findings

Elevated levels of PTH concomitant with hypercalcemia and hypophosphatemia usually distinguish hyperparathyroidism from other etiologies. The negative feedback system between calcium and PTH permits differentiation from other causes of hypercalcemia. For example, low levels of PTH accompany the hypercalcemia of hypervitaminosis D. Ultrasound and radiopharmaceutical evaluation of parathyroid gland size permit differentiation of hyperplasia and adenomas. The diagnosis of familial hypercalcemic hypocalciuria is usually based on a normal level of PTH, relative hypocalciuria, modest hypercalcemia, and the same biochemical findings in other family members.

Treatment of Hypercalcemic Disorders

Treatment of hypercalcemia secondary to hyperparathyroidism must include treatment of the underlying disorder. The acute treatment requires hydration, which can be performed orally in cooperative children, or by intravenous methods in uncooperative ones. Twice the maintenance fluid rates or more are used. Dehydration secondary to nausea, vomiting, and polyuria can occur with hypercalcemia. The total fluid replacement volume should include deficits, as well as the increased maintenance amounts. The administration of intravenous saline after rehydration offers an added benefit because calcium excretion is enhanced by sodium excretion. Furosemide, 2 mg/kg/day, or other loop diuretics may be used, because they increase sodium excretion, as well as calcium excretion. Glucocorticoids such as prednisone, 2 mg/kg/day, are useful because they decrease intestinal absorption of calcium. Sunlight, any form of vitamin D, and dairy products should be avoided during hypercalcemia. The previously mentioned treatments usually suffice in children, but further treatment can be undertaken with calcitonin, 2 U/kg every 6 hours; phosphorus; mithramycin; peritoneal dialysis; and pamidronate, 20 to 60 mg intravenously in a single dose. The latter forms of treatment have been used in adults, and their experience in children is limited.

CHAPTER 203
Thyroid Disorders

Adapted from Patricia A. Donohoue

HYPOTHYROIDISM

Hypothyroidism is defined as a state in which the thyroid gland fails to secrete sufficient quantities of thyroid hormone (see Chapter 276 for a listing of normal thyroid function test values). Primary hypothyroidism results from a problem inherent to the gland itself, and secondary or central hypothyroidism results from the failure of pituitary stimulation of the thyroid gland. Primary and central hypothyroidism can be either congenital or acquired.

Congenital Hypothyroidism

Congenital hypothyroidism is a disease with an overall prevalence of approximately 1 in 4,000 live births including 1 of 2,000 persons of Far Eastern or Hispanic descent, 1 of 5,500 persons of European descent, and 1 of 32,000 persons of African descent. Ninety-five percent of all cases are sporadic, and 5% are genetic, most often reflecting a dyshormonogenesis. It has a 2:1 female–to–male predominance, and associations with specific HLA types have been reported in certain populations. Newborn screening for congenital hypothyroidism is performed in all 50 states in the United States, but the methods of screening vary. Healthy, premature infants have lower T_4 concentrations than term infants of the same chronologic age, which must be considered when evaluating the results of the newborn screen. If the newborn screen blood sample is obtained within the first day of life, the TSH level may be falsely elevated because of the peripartum TSH surge.

ETIOLOGY

Permanent primary hypothyroidism denotes irreversible failure of the thyroid gland to produce sufficient thyroid hormone. The most common cause is an ectopic thyroid gland, which results from improper migration during fetal development. It accounts for more than two-thirds of all cases detected by newborn screening worldwide. The ectopic thyroid tissue can often be demonstrated by technetium Tc 99m scanning, and it is found most commonly at the base of the tongue (i.e., lingual thyroid). These aberrantly located glands do not function properly and do not produce an adequate amount of thyroid hormone.

The next most common cause of congenital primary hypothyroidism is hypoplasia, or aplasia of the gland, and this thyroid dysgenesis may result from the same pathophysiologic process, as does ectopy of the gland. In some cases, immunoglobulins have been implicated in the pathogenesis. A TSH-binding inhibitor immunoglobulin (TBII) has been described in sibling cases of nongoitrous neonatal hypothyroidism and in association with maternal chronic lymphocytic thyroiditis. TBII may be associated with a transient form of hypothyroidism in the newborn. TBII is detectable in both maternal and infant sera. Another antibody, known as *thyroid growth-blocking immunoglobulin*, has been associated with thyroid dysgenesis. It can block the growth of thyroid cells *in vitro*. Antithyroglobulin and antimicrosomal antibodies are not known to play direct roles in the pathogenesis of congenital hypothyroidism.

The third most common cause of congenital primary hypothyroidism is dyshormonogenesis, an inborn error of thyroid hormone synthesis, secretion, or metabolism. Dyshormonogenesis is responsible for most of the familial cases of congenital hypothyroidism. The most common form is a defect in the organification of iodide. Congenital hypothyroidism may result from maternal radioactive iodine treatment, if it has been given after the eighth week of gestation when fetal iodide trapping has begun.

Transient primary hypothyroidism is a self-limited process, and the cause is determined by a careful history. The causes include maternal iodine deficiency (e.g., endemic goiter), fetal or neonatal exposure to iodine (e.g., maternal medications, amniofetography, painting of the cervix, painting of the umbilical stump), maternal antithyroid drugs, maternal antibodies (e.g., TBII) and, rarely, association with the nephrotic syndrome (i.e., urinary loss of iodine). Transient hypothyroidism is more likely to occur in premature rather than full-term infants. Although transient, some of these conditions may require temporary treatment with thyroid hormone. Hypothyroxinemia of prematurity (low T_4 with normal TSH) is not clearly understood, but treatment with thyroxine is not generally recommended.

Permanent central hypothyroidism is generally associated with congenital hypopituitarism and may account for as many as 5% of cases of congenital hypothyroidism. Hypopituitarism may be associated with midline craniofacial defects (e.g., septooptic dysplasia, cleft lip, cleft palate), pituitary aplasia, idiopathic hypopituitarism, and malformations of the CNS.

TABLE 203-1. Signs and Symptoms of Congenital Hypothyroidism

Large fontanelles	Prolonged jaundice
Umbilical hernia	Constipation
Macroglossia	Lethargy
Mottled, dry skin	Difficulty feeding
Hypotonia	Cool skin (hypothermia)
Abdominal distention	Sleeps through the night (newborn period)
Hoarse cry	Goiter (rare)
Respiratory distress	

Low T_4 level without hypothyroidism is most commonly caused by TBG deficiency, an X-linked recessive disorder with a frequency similar to that of central hypothyroidism. TBG deficiency is easily differentiated from true hypothyroidism because the level of free T_4 is normal, the T_3RU level is high, and the TBG level is low. This condition does not require treatment. Low T_4 levels may occur in ill neonates as a manifestation of the euthyroid sick syndrome (i.e., nonthyroidal illness), which is discussed later.

DIAGNOSIS AND CLINICAL CHARACTERISTICS

Congenital hypothyroidism is diagnosed only rarely from clinical abnormalities. These children have normal birth weight and length and a slightly larger than average head circumference at birth, and one-third have longer than average gestation: Most cases are detected as a result of newborn screening tests, which must be confirmed by thyroid function tests using a venous blood sample. The dried blood filter-paper test is not a satisfactory confirmatory test.

Certain clinical features of hypothyroidism, listed in Table 203-1, may suggest the diagnosis before the results of the newborn screening tests are available. The hormonal patterns found in congenital hypothyroxinemia are summarized in Table 203-2. A variety of other neurologic and learning disorders including hearing loss, ataxia, attention deficit disorder, abnormalities of muscle tone, and speech defects have been associated with untreated congenital hypothyroidism. Somatic growth and skeletal development are also impaired. With severe hypothyroidism, cardiac failure may develop.

TREATMENT

The treatment of congenital hypothyroidism consists of replacement of thyroid hormone with oral levothyroxine in a single daily dose of 8 to 10 $\mu g/kg/day$. The total replacement dose may be used at the outset of therapy, unless evidence of cardiac disease is present, in which case, a stepwise increase in dosage

TABLE 203-2. Hormonal Patterns in Congenital Hypothyroxinemia

	First newborn screen		Follow-up confirmation			
Cause	*T_4*[a]	*TSH*	*T_4*	*T_3RU*	*TSH*	*Free T_4*
Primary hypothyroidism	Low	High	Low	Low/normal	High	Low
Central hypothyroidism	Low	Normal[b]	Low	Low/normal	Normal[b]	Low
Transient hypothyroidism	Low	High	Normal	Normal	Normal	Normal
Thyroid-binding globulin deficiency[c]	Low	Normal	Low	High	Normal	Normal

T_3RU, triiodothyronine resin uptake; T_4, thyroxine; TSH, thyroid-stimulating hormone.
[a]Many state newborn screening programs do not measure T_4, but only thyroid-stimulating hormone levels.
[b]The normal level of thyroid-stimulating hormone seen in central hypothyroidism is inappropriately low for the decreased level of free T_4.
[c]The diagnosis of thyroid-binding globulin deficiency is made most accurately by demonstration of a low thyroid-binding globulin level.

is recommended. Breast-feeding is not a substitute for replacement therapy because thyroid hormones, although measurable in breast milk, do not provide adequate serum levels in the hypothyroid infant. The goals of treatment include maintenance of the T_4 level in the upper half of the normal range for the age, being careful to avoid overtreatment because of the complications of neonatal hyperthyroidism. In primary hypothyroidism, several months of treatment may be necessary before the TSH level normalizes. Rarely, the pituitary set-point for TSH release may be elevated in these patients causing the TSH level to remain high, despite normal free T_4 and T_3 levels.

With prompt and adequate treatment, children with congenital hypothyroidism have the potential to have normal somatic and intellectual growth and development. If left untreated, severe mental retardation and neurologic dysfunction ensue and are more severe in children with primary than central hypothyroidism. Patients in whom treatment is begun before 6 weeks of age have an average IQ of 100. If treatment is begun at 6 weeks to 3 months, the average IQ decreases to 95; if begun at 3 to 6 months, the average IQ is 75. After 6 months, the average IQ is 55 or less.

The sequelae of untreated congenital hypothyroidism are devastating. If an infant has evidence of congenital hypothyroidism on the basis of the newborn screen result and a speedy diagnosis cannot be made after the confirmatory test results have been obtained, therapy should be initiated before establishing the diagnosis. In infants with a possible central hypothyroidism, adrenocorticotropic hormone deficiency must be ruled out before starting thyroid hormone replacement. Levothyroxine treatment is inexpensive and has a low risk if thyroid hormone levels are measured frequently. In uncertain cases, the child should be treated until 2.5 to 3.0 years of age when the medication can be temporarily discontinued for 1 to 2 months without risk, while a diagnosis is established.

Acquired Hypothyroidism

Acquired hypothyroidism appears after the newborn period in a child who did not have congenital hypothyroidism. The estimated prevalence is 1 in 500 to 1,000 school-aged children, with a female–to–male preponderance of 4:1. Certain types of acquired hypothyroidism are familial in origin.

ETIOLOGY

Primary acquired hypothyroidism in childhood is characterized by low T_4 levels, elevated TSH, and a variety of clinical manifestations (Table 203-3). The most common cause is chronic lymphocytic thyroiditis (CLT), also known as *Hashimoto thyroiditis*. A defect in cell-mediated immunity results in lymphocytic infiltration and enlargement of the thyroid gland. Titers of antithyroglobulin and antimicrosomal antibodies are elevated in more than 80% of patients. Patients with CLT present with nontender enlargement of the gland, which may be asymmetric or even nodular in appearance. The patients are often euthyroid, but some may present with transient hyperthyroidism or have signs and symptoms of hypothyroidism.

CLT may occur alone or in association with other autoimmune endocrine diseases known as the *autoimmune polyglandular syndromes types I and II* (Table 203-4). Because of this association, patients with CLT should be observed for signs of other autoimmune processes, some of which may result in severe illnesses such as Addison disease and diabetes mellitus. An increased incidence of CLT exists among patients with chromosomal abnormalities including Down syndrome, Turner syndrome, and Klinefelter syndrome. This factor is particularly important for patients with Down syndrome because many of the clinical manifestations of hypothyroidism are also seen in patients with Down syndrome and may cause a delay in diagnosing the hypothyroidism.

Several nonimmune-mediated causes of acquired hypothyroidism exist. Subacute thyroiditis may produce hypothyroidism in some patients. Environmental causes of primary hypothyroidism include goitrogen ingestion (e.g., iodides, antithyroid drugs, other medications; see Table 203-5), thyroidectomy, and radioactive iodine ablative therapy. Infiltrative diseases that can cause hypothyroidism include Langerhans histiocytosis and nephropathic cystinosis.

Central acquired hypothyroidism is caused by pituitary or hypothalamic dysfunction. This central process itself may be primary (i.e., idiopathic) or the result of another disease process. Idiopathic hypopituitarism is manifested by deficiencies of some or all of the anterior pituitary hormones including TSH, growth hormone, adrenocorticotropic hormone, luteinizing hormone, and follicle-stimulating hormone. Hypopituitarism can be secondary to infiltrative disease (e.g., histiocytosis), tumor (e.g., craniopharyngioma), head trauma, surgery, and radiation therapy. A greater chance of posterior pituitary

TABLE 203-3. Signs and Symptoms of Acquired Hypothyroidism

Short stature, decreased growth velocity
Obesity, myxedema
Goiter (primary hypothyroidism)
Delayed skeletal and dental age
Cold intolerance
Constipation
Dry, cool skin
Thinning of hair
Lethargy
Delayed reflex return
Bradycardia
Delayed puberty
Abnormal menses
Precocious puberty (rare)
Muscular pseudohypertrophy (rare)
Galactorrhea (rare)*

*Hypothalamic thyroid-releasing hormone stimulates prolactin release from the posterior pituitary. In primary hypothyroidism, increased thyroid-releasing hormone may produce hyperprolactinemia and galactorrhea.

TABLE 203-4. Clinical Features of Autoimmune Polyglandular Syndromes

Type I	Type II
Primary hypothyroidism	Primary hypothyroidism
Primary hypogonadism	Primary hypogonadism
Vitiligo	Vitiligo
Pernicious anemia	Pernicious anemia
Alopecia	Alopecia
Malabsorption	Malabsorption
Adrenal insufficiency	Adrenal insufficiency
Mucocutaneous candidiasis	Myasthenia gravis
Chronic active hepatitis	Type I diabetes mellitus
Hypoparathyroidism	Hyperthyroidism
Onset in infancy or childhood	Onset in adults
Probably autosomal recessive	Autosomal dominant
No HLA association	HLA-B8, -DR3 associated

TABLE 203-5. Drugs that Influence Thyroid Hormone Levels

Characteristic	Drug	Effect
Drugs that have a transient CNS effect to alter thyroid hormone levels	Octreotide, dopamine, L-dopa, glucocorticoids	Decreased TSH secretion
	Metoclopramide	Increased TSH
Drugs that directly decrease thyroid hormone synthesis, most often by decreasing iodide organification; exceptions are nitroprusside, which inhibits iodide trapping, and lithium, which inhibits release of T_4 and T_3 from thyroglobulin	*p*-Aminosalicylate, phenylbutazone, sulfonamides, aminoglutethimide, nitroprusside, lithium, inorganic iodide*	Decreased T_4 and free T_4; increased TSH
Compounds that decrease the gut absorption of orally administered thyroxine	Cholestyramine, soybean flour, aluminum hydroxide, ferrous sulfate, sucralfate	Decreased T_4 and free T_4 and thus increased TSH
Drugs that inhibit the binding of T_4 and T_3 to TBG; phenytoin also acts to increase cellular uptake of T_4, which decreases the free T_4 concentration	Salicylates, phenylbutazone	Decreased T_4; normal free T_4 and TSH
	Phenytoin	Decreased T_4 and free T_4; normal T_3 and TSH
Drugs that change uptake or metabolism of thyroid hormones, including decreased conversion of T_4 to T_3	Heparin	Normal T_4; increased free T_4; normal T_3 and TSH
	Phenytoin	Decreased T_4 and free T_4; normal T_3 and TSH
	Glucocorticoids	Decreased T_4, free T_4, and T_3; normal TSH
	Propanolol	Decreased T_3 (only in hyperthyroidism)
	Amiodarone	Complex effects may cause hypothyroidism or hyperthyroidism, but most patients are euthyroid with slightly high TSH levels early in treatment
	PTU, methimazole	Decreased T_4 and T_3; increased TSH; PTU: levels decreased peripheral T_4 to T_3 conversion
Drugs that induce hepatic mixed function oxidases and enhance clearance of thyroxine; effect may be accompanied by increased T_4 to T_3 conversion	Diphenylhydantoin, phenobarbital, carbamazepine, rifampin	Decreased T_4 and free T_4 with normal T_3 and TSH because of combined effects
Drugs that enhance T_4 to T_3 conversion	Exogenous growth hormone	Decreased T_4 and free T_4; normal T_3 and TSH
Drugs that induce autoimmune thyroiditis	Interferon-alpha	Induction of antithyroid antibodies with transient hypothyroidism or hyperthyroidism
	Interleukin-2	Transient painless thyroiditis

CNS, central nervous system; PTU, propylthiouracil; T_3, triiodothyronine; T_4, thyroxine; TBG, thyroxine-binding hormone; TSH, thyroid-stimulating hormone.

*Many commonly used compounds contain iodide, including expectorants, amiodarone, topical antiseptics, radiographic contrast dyes, and antiasthmatic drugs.

Adapted from Kaplan MM. Interactions between drugs and thyroid hormones. *Thyroid Today* 1981;4:5; Burger AG. Effects of certain pharmacologic agents on the peripheral metabolism of thyroxine. In: Ingbar SH, Braverman LE, ed. *Werner's the thyroid: a fundamental and clinical text.* Philadelphia: Lippincott–Raven, 1986:351; Surks MI, Sievert R. Drugs and thyroid function. *N Engl J Med* 1995;333:1688.

involvement occurs in secondary hypopituitarism than in idiopathic hypopituitarism. Posterior pituitary involvement is most often manifested by the presence of diabetes insipidus (i.e., vasopressin deficiency).

TSH deficiency is usually associated with generalized pituitary or hypothalamic dysfunction. Isolated TSH deficiency is rare and may be caused by a lack of TRH stimulation (e.g., receptor defects in the pituitary, tumor invasion of the critical hypothalamic nuclei), or it may be idiopathic.

DIAGNOSIS AND CLINICAL CHARACTERISTICS

The diagnosis of hypothyroidism is usually straightforward. The clinical features are listed in Table 203-3. The earliest sign of hypothyroidism in a child is often a slowing of the linear growth rate, as skeletal growth is sensitive to thyroid hormone levels, which is reflected in a delayed bone age and often in delayed puberty. In rare cases of primary hypothyroidism, precocious puberty occurs as a result of secretion of luteinizing hormone and follicle-stimulating hormone accompanying the increased TSH release. These children may have normal or relatively advanced bone ages caused by the effects of sex steroids, but they do not have the associated pubertal growth spurt. A severe loss of height potential may occur.

Except in the rare cases of peripheral resistance to thyroid hormone, circulating levels of T_4 and T_3 are low in hypothyroidism. Tests that assess concentrations of thyroid hormone-binding proteins (e.g., T_3RU, TBG level) or free T_4 levels must be performed before therapy is initiated. TSH levels help differentiate primary from secondary hypothyroidism. The cause of primary hypothyroidism can often be determined by careful history of goitrogen exposure, surgery, or radiation exposure or from assessment of antithyroid antibody levels. Determination of the cause of secondary hypothyroidism must involve an assessment of other aspects of the hypothalamic-pituitary system, and radiologic studies of the brain may be necessary to rule out tumor or infiltrative disease.

TREATMENT

The treatment of acquired hypothyroidism is thyroid hormone replacement with a single daily dose of oral levothyroxine

(3 to 5 μg/kg/day for children decreasing to 1 to 3 μg/kg/day for adults). In cases of hypothyroidism caused by exposure to goitrogen, treating the hypothyroidism by eliminating exposure to the goitrogen may be possible.

Monitoring the growth rate and T_4 levels in all patients and the TSH levels in patients with primary hypothyroidism is important. Many children who commence treatment after longstanding hypothyroidism may experience school and behavioral problems, which may be related to a decrease in attention span and an increase in energy level, as they become euthyroid.

The euthyroid sick syndrome, also known as the low T_3 syndrome, is a condition present in patients with nonthyroidal illness in whom the total T_3 level is lower than normal, the total T_4 level is often low, and the TSH level is in the normal range. The rT_3 levels may be elevated or normal. Impaired conversion of T_4 to T_3 results in low T_3 levels. The patient's illness may cause increased metabolic clearance of T_4 and a decreased ability of the pituitary to secrete TSH. As a result, total concentration of T_4 may decrease, but free T_4 may remain normal because of the presence of a circulating inhibitor of T_4 binding to TBG. In cases of a low level of free T_4, tissue hypothyroidism may exist in this syndrome, but it may be adaptive and even beneficial in severe illness. If the patient recovers from the underlying illness, serum TSH levels increase and may become elevated before the T_3 and T_4 levels return to normal. Replacement therapy with T_4 is not recommended.

HYPERTHYROIDISM

Hyperthyroidism occurs when excessive amounts of circulating thyroid hormone are present. The clinical manifestation is called thyrotoxicosis. Like hypothyroidism, hyperthyroidism may be congenital or acquired. Hyperthyroidism in childhood is rare and accounts for fewer than 5% of all cases of hyperthyroidism.

Congenital Hyperthyroidism

Congenital hyperthyroidism, more often called neonatal thyrotoxicosis, occurs almost exclusively in infants of mothers with Graves disease. Neonatal thyrotoxicosis may be transient, lasting up to several weeks, or prolonged, lasting more than 6 months. Neonatal thyrotoxicosis is a serious illness requiring prompt and aggressive management. This disease occurs in as many as 1 of 70 infants of mothers with Graves disease. It has an equal gender distribution, unlike the later-onset form of thyrotoxicosis, which has a female preponderance. If maternal TSI titers are more than five times the normal values, regardless of whether she has had ablative thyroid therapy, the risk of neonatal thyrotoxicosis is greatly increased. Neonatal thyrotoxicosis accounts for approximately 1% of all cases of pediatric thyrotoxicosis.

ETIOLOGY

The cause of the transient form of neonatal thyrotoxicosis is probably transplacental passage of TSI (i.e., maternal immunoglobulin G). The prolonged or persistent form of the disease may be caused by endogenously produced TSI from the infant's own lymphocytes or from transplacentally acquired maternal lymphocytes.

DIAGNOSIS AND CLINICAL CHARACTERISTICS

The diagnosis is made on the basis of clinical findings combined with elevated levels of T_4, free T_4, and T_3. Fetal tachycardia and intrauterine growth retardation may suggest the diagnosis.

Affected patients often have low birth weight and microcephaly. They also exhibit marked irritability and hyperactivity, tachycardia, tachypnea, prominent eyes, thyroid enlargement, and a failure to gain weight despite marked hyperphagia. The glandular enlargement may be so marked that it causes respiratory distress requiring endotracheal intubation. Other features include vomiting, severe diarrhea, hepatosplenomegaly, jaundice, thrombocytopenia, and cardiac failure. The mortality rate of untreated cases is 15% to 25%, and death is usually caused by cardiac failure. The severity of the disease does not correlate with the size of the goiter, but it may be related to maternal TSI levels.

Long-term complications of neonatal thyrotoxicosis can occur even in patients who receive prompt and adequate treatment. These complications include premature craniosynostosis and neurodevelopmental defects, particularly intellectual impairment; both may be caused by intrauterine thyrotoxicosis. The intellectual impairment usually correlates with premature craniosynostosis, but a direct effect of thyrotoxicosis on the developing brain cannot be ruled out.

TREATMENT

The treatment of neonatal thyrotoxicosis is directed toward immediate management of the symptoms and reduction in the amount of thyroid hormone produced. This treatment may need to be initiated in the intensive care nursery with adequate cardiopulmonary monitoring and venous access.

Therapy consists of a combination of Lugol solution (5% iodine and 10% potassium iodide), given as one drop every 8 hours; propylthiouracil, administered as 5 to 10 mg/kg/day; and propranolol, given at a dosage of 2 mg/kg/day. Treatment with dexamethasone is helpful in some cases. If no improvement occurs within 24 hours, the doses of Lugol solution and propylthiouracil should be increased by at least 50%. If evidence of cardiac failure arises, the infant should be given digitalis promptly. Adequate caloric intake is vital in these hypermetabolic infants. Serum levels of thyroid hormone must be carefully monitored to ensure adequate therapy and to avoid hypothyroidism. In milder cases, Lugol solution and propranolol may not be needed.

Acquired Hyperthyroidism

Acquired hyperthyroidism is most often caused by Graves disease (i.e., autoimmune thyrotoxicosis). The female–to–male ratio ranges from 3:1 to 5:1. It has a familial tendency and an association with HLA types B8 and DR3. It may occur in the autoimmune polyglandular syndrome. Emotional stress, as a precipitating factor of thyrotoxicosis, has been frequently described.

ETIOLOGY

The cause of Graves disease is autonomous hyperfunction of the thyroid gland stimulated by TSI. TSI levels are elevated in most patients. TSI binds to the TSH receptors on the thyroid cells producing the stimulatory effect. Graves disease is serologically related to CLT in that antithyroid antibodies may be elevated in patients with Graves disease and in their unaffected family members. The events that stimulate the production of TSI and their relation to antithyroid antibodies are unknown.

DIAGNOSIS AND CLINICAL CHARACTERISTICS

The diagnosis of Graves disease is based on the combination of clinical findings (Table 203-6) and the characteristic elevations of thyroid hormone levels. The thyroid gland is almost invariably enlarged, and tachycardia, nervousness, and widened pulse pressure occur in more than 80% of patients. Most patients

TABLE 203-6. Signs and Symptoms of Hyperthyroidism

Goiter
Anxiousness, nervousness
Tachycardia
Widened pulse pressure
Increased appetite
Weight loss or gain
Tremor
Proptosis
Heat intolerance
Increased growth velocity
Diarrhea
Sleep disturbances
Fatigue

experience weight loss, although weight gain may occur because of a significantly increased appetite. Proptosis or exophthalmos is a common finding, but the Graves ophthalmopathy in children is usually less severe than that in adults.

The thyroid hormone profile characteristically shows elevated total T_4, free T_4, and T_3 levels accompanied by very low or undetectable levels of TSH. In some cases, the T_3 level is elevated with a normal level of T_4 (i.e., T_3 toxicosis). The source of T_3 in patients with T_3 toxicosis is direct secretion by the gland. In these patients, the contribution of T_3 secreted by the gland may equal or exceed that of peripheral T_4 deiodination to the total circulating T_3.

In patients with hyperthyroidism without exophthalmos, differentiating among early CLT, subacute thyroiditis, and Graves disease may be difficult. If TSI levels are not elevated, a radioactive iodine uptake scan aids in the diagnosis. Characteristically, patients with Graves disease have elevated uptake that is not suppressed with administration of T_3. Patients with CLT or subacute thyroiditis generally have normal or decreased uptake of ^{123}I.

TREATMENT

The mainstay of medical management is antithyroid medication with methimazole (Tapazole) or propylthiouracil (PTU). Both are equally effective in decreasing the production of T_4 and T_3 by the thyroid gland, but PTU also blocks the peripheral deiodination of T_4 to T_3. PTU is not known to significantly decrease thyroid gland secretion of T_3 and, therefore, may not provide a significant advantage over methimazole in patients with T_3 toxicosis. The dosage of PTU is 5 to 10 mg/kg/day, divided into three equal doses. The daily dose of methimazole is approximately one-tenth that of PTU, and it has the advantage of a longer serum half-life allowing twice-daily or even once-daily doses. If the symptoms of thyrotoxicosis are particularly bothersome to the patient, they may be alleviated by treatment with propranolol concomitantly with antithyroid medication until the symptoms improve. With successful treatment, the patient should become euthyroid within 6 weeks.

The medical therapy of thyrotoxicosis is somewhat controversial. In some centers, the dosage of antithyroid medication is increased until the patient becomes hypothyroid, at which time, thyroid hormone replacement is added to the regimen. This increase gives the theoretical advantage of maximal suppression of the gland minimizing the likelihood of relapse. This theory has been supported by clinical trials. In other centers, the dose of antithyroid medication is titrated to maintain the patient in a euthyroid state. After the patient becomes euthyroid using either method, treatment is continued for usually not less than 1 year before the child is assessed for remission by a T_3 suppression test or by discontinuing antithyroid medication. If relapse occurs, the antithyroid medication can be restarted, or alternative treatment can be instituted.

Approximately 5% to 10% of patients treated with antithyroid medication experience side effects from the medication. Most of these side effects are minor and include erythematous skin rashes, urticaria, and arthralgias. Granulocytopenia is the most frequent serious side effect and is generally heralded by a fever or sore throat. Vasculitis, at times severe enough to cause pulmonary hemorrhage, is another serious side effect. If side effects occur, discontinuation of the drug generally reverses the problem. The patient may then be treated with a different antithyroid preparation; however, the same reaction may occur.

If medical treatment is not successful because of side effects, frequent relapses, or inability to comply with the treatment schedule, or if the patient or physician prefers an immediate cure, thyroid ablative therapy should be implemented. Iodine 131 ablation has been widely used to treat thyrotoxicosis in adults. Its use in children has been limited because of a theoretical risk of the later development of thyroid or other malignancies. However, the data currently available suggest that ^{131}I treatment in childhood or adolescence does not affect the risk of developing thyroidal or nonthyroidal cancers or leukemia and does not increase the risk of birth defects in the patients' offspring. Remission from thyrotoxicosis should occur within several weeks, and remission is most often followed by permanent hypothyroidism after several months.

Surgical subtotal thyroidectomy is effective and has low morbidity when performed by an experienced surgeon. The patient must be euthyroid for surgery, and preoperative treatment with iodides such as Lugol solution is often recommended to decrease vascularity of the gland. The risks include those associated with general anesthesia, as well as hypothyroidism (up to 50%); transient hypocalcemia (10%–20%) and, rarely, hypoparathyroidism; recurrent laryngeal nerve damage; or recurrence of thyrotoxicosis.

PROGNOSIS

The prognosis for children with Graves disease is generally good. Evidence suggests that with antithyroid medication alone, remission of Graves disease, defined as being euthyroid for 1 year after stopping medication, occurs at a rate of approximately 25% every 2 years. In some cases, relapse of hyperthyroidism or spontaneous hypothyroidism may occur after remission.

A rare but life-threatening complication of Graves disease is thyroid storm, also called thyrotoxic crisis, which is a clinical diagnosis based on the manifestations of exaggerated and uncontrolled hyperthyroidism. Patients generally present with marked hyperthermia and tachycardia and may develop cardiac failure, vomiting, diarrhea, and CNS abnormalities including confusion, apathy, and coma. Thyroid storm can be precipitated by many events but is most often associated with infection, surgery, or trauma. The therapy includes aggressive antithyroid treatment including PTU or methimazole, Lugol solution, or lithium carbonate; prevention of thyroid hormone action with beta-blockade; antipyretics; support of life-threatening conditions using intravenous hydration, oxygen, and digitalis; and treatment of any underlying infection.

THYROMEGALY

Thyromegaly, or enlargement of the thyroid gland or goiter, is uncommon in children. Causes include neoplasm, infiltration, inflammation, or stimulation of the gland. The enlargement may be diffuse or nodular (Table 203-7). Enlargement of certain nonthyroidal structures may mimic thyromegaly.

TABLE 203-7. Causes of Thyromegaly
Diffuse
Hashimoto thyroiditis
Thyrotoxicosis
Graves disease
Thyroiditis
Thyroid-stimulating hormone–secreting adenoma
Pituitary resistance to thyroid hormone
Goitrogen exposure
Dyshormonogenesis
Iodine deficiency (endemic)
Idiopathic (simple) goiter
Acute, subacute thyroiditis
Nodular
Hashimoto thyroiditis
Thyroid cyst
Thyroid adenoma
Hyperfunctional (hot)
Hypofunctional (cold)
Thyroid carcinoma
Papillary
Follicular
Mixed papillary or follicular
Anaplastic
Medullary
Nonthyroidal masses

CHAPTER 204
Adrenal Disorders

Adapted from Patricia A. Donohoue

ABNORMALITIES OF THE ADRENAL CORTEX

Congenital Adrenal Hyperplasia

Congenital adrenal hyperplasia (CAH) is a family of diseases caused by an inherited deficiency of any of the enzymes necessary for the biosynthesis of cortisol (Fig. 204-1). These enzymes, with the exception of 3-beta-hydroxysteroid dehydrogenase, are members of the cytochrome P-450 family. These cytochromes are microsomal or mitochondrial terminal oxidases involved in electron transport and require NAD and flavoproteins as cofactors. Deficiency of any one of these enzymes results in decreased production of cortisol and increased secretion of ACTH. With stimulation by ACTH, the adrenal cortex becomes hyperplastic and steroid precursors preceding the enzymatic block accumulate. These accumulated precursors are shunted, if possible, to a steroidogenic pathway that is unaffected by the enzymatic block. Each form of CAH is manifested by the clinical features produced by deficient end products (e.g., glucocorticoid, mineralocorticoid, androgen) and by accumulated or shunted precursors (e.g., mineralocorticoid or androgen excess). CAH is inherited as an autosomal recessive disorder and has an equal gender distribution. A summary of these diseases and their clinical features is given in Table 204-1. The severity of the clinical features varies among families representing very severe to mild or even asymptomatic forms.

The most common form of CAH is caused by 21-hydroxylase (21-OH) deficiency, which accounts for more than 90% of the cases. The most severe form, the salt-losing form, is caused by complete absence of 21-OH activity and results in cortisol and

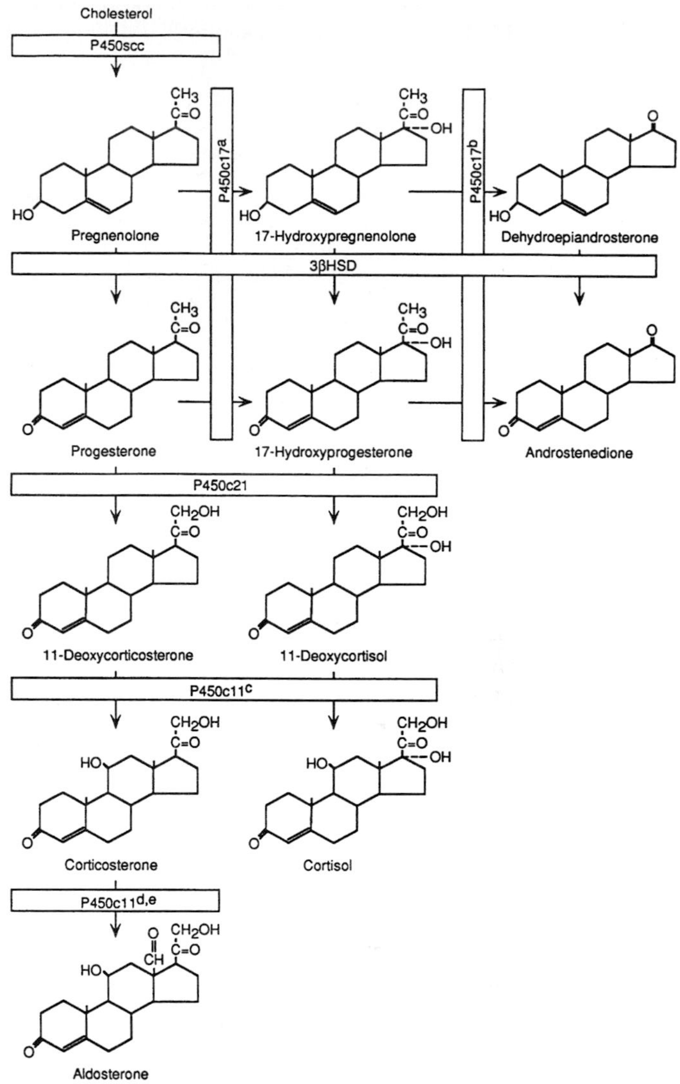

Figure 204-1. Adrenal steroid biosynthetic pathways. The 20-hydroxylase, 22-hydroxylase, and 20,22-desmolase are activities of the same P450scc enzyme. Both 17α-hydroxylase and 17,20-desmolase activities are properties of the same P450c17 enzyme. However, 11β-hydroxylase and CMO activities are properties of two different isozymes of P450c11, encoded by different genes. The single enzyme that has CMOI and CMOII activities is termed aldosterone synthase. In addition, several isoforms of 3β-HSD exist, some of which are expressed in extraadrenal sites. 3β-HSD, 3β-hydroxysteroid dehydrogenase, Δ^5,Δ^4-isomerase; CMO, corticosterone methyl oxidase; P450c11[c], 11β-hydroxylase; P450c11[d], 18-hydroxylase (CMOI); P450c11[e], 18-dehydrogenase (oxidase) (CMOII); P450c17[a], 17α-hydroxylase; P450c17[b], 17,20-desmolase (lyase); P45c21, 21-hydroxylase; P450scc, 20-hydroxylase, 22-hydroxylase, 20,22-desmolase.

mineralocorticoid deficiencies. Affected girls have ambiguous genitalia at birth caused by hypersecretion of adrenal androgens, which are converted to testosterone (Fig. 204-2). Usually, affected and untreated girls and boys present with symptoms of acute adrenal insufficiency, known as a *salt-losing crisis*, at ages 1 to 3 weeks.

The simple virilizing form is caused by a partial 21-OH deficiency. Patients with this disease produce adequate amounts of cortisol and aldosterone under the stimulation of excess ACTH and elevated plasma renin activity (PRA) levels but at the expense of excess androgen production. Girls may present with ambiguous genitalia or postnatal virilization, and boys may present with suspected isosexual precocious puberty, although the testes remain prepubertal in size. The combined frequency of the

TABLE 204-1. Clinical Features of the Different Forms of Congenital Adrenal Hyperplasia at Diagnosis

Deficient enzyme	Clinical form	Elevated levels	Abnormal sexual development
21-Hydroxylase			
Complete deficiency	Salt-losing	Urinary 17-ketosteroids, plasma 17-hydroxyprogesterone, plasma androstenedione, PRA, ACTH	Girls: ambiguous genitalia
Partial deficiency	Simple virilizing	Same as in complete deficiency	Girls: ambiguous genitalia Boys and girls: postnatal virilization
Mild deficiency	Attenuated, late-onset	Same as in complete deficiency, but milder elevations	Female adults or adolescents: hirsutism, menstrual irregularities
11β-Hydroxylase*	Hypertensive	Urinary 17-hydroxycorticosteroids, urinary 17-ketosteroids, plasma DOC, plasma 11-deoxycortisol, plasma androstenedione	Girls: ambiguous genitalia Boys and girls: postnatal virilization
17α-Hydroxylase	Hypertensive	Plasma DOC, plasma corticosterone	Boys: absent or incomplete virilization
3β-Hydroxysteroid dehydrogenase			
Complete deficiency	Salt-losing	Plasma DHEA, 17-hydroxypregnenolone, PRA, ACTH	Boys and girls: ambiguous genitalia
Partial deficiency	Mild	Plasma DHEA, 17-hydroxypregnenolone	Female adolescents: hirsutism, premature pubarche
Cholesterol side-chain cleavage	Salt-losing "lipoid"	No steroids produced	Boys: absent virilization

ACTH, adrenocorticotropic hormone; DHEA, dehydroepiandrosterone; DOC, 11-deoxycorticosterone; PRA, plasma renin activity.
*A late-onset form of 11β-hydroxylase deficiency has been reported.

salt-losing and simple virilizing forms approximate 1 in 10,000 to 13,000 births among whites. The incidence among populations of Asian and African descent is somewhat lower.

A mild degree of 21-OH deficiency, the attenuated, late-onset or nonclassic form, manifests as hirsutism or menstrual irregularities in adolescent or adult female patients. In the asymptomatic or cryptic form, biochemical abnormalities consistent with 21-OH deficiency are present, but no clinical features are evident.

Diagnosis

The diagnosis of CAH caused by 21-OH deficiency is made when elevated levels of hormones preceding the enzymatic block (Fig. 204-1) are demonstrated in a child with the typical clinical findings. A female infant with virilization of the external genitalia or a male infant with a salt-losing crisis (dehydration with hyponatremia, hyperkalemia, and acidosis) has elevated plasma 17-hydroxyprogesterone, progesterone, and androstenedione levels, increased urinary 17-ketosteroids, elevated PRA and ACTH levels, and normal or low serum cortisol concentration. Older children who present with inappropriate virilization (i.e., simple virilizing form) have normal cortisol and electrolyte levels but the same elevated hormone levels as those described for the younger group. Such children also have growth acceleration and advanced skeletal age caused by the effects of androgens.

In the salt-losing form, treatment is first directed at correcting the life-threatening metabolic abnormalities of adrenal crisis by correcting dehydration with intravenous saline and dextrose, correcting hyperkalemia with insulin and glucose, if necessary, and, after a blood sample is obtained for steroid hormone measurements, replacing glucocorticoid with the rapidly acting intravenous glucocorticoid, hydrocortisone (Solu-Cortef), at a "stress" dosage, which is three times the calculated dose for daily physiologic replacement. Because parenteral mineralocorticoid preparations are no longer available, prolonged treatment with high-dose glucocorticoids is necessary until oral mineralocorticoids can be tolerated. This treatment allows sufficient mineralocorticoid effect from the glucocorticoid preparation to achieve a lowered serum potassium concentration and adequate urinary sodium retention. In many cases, supplemental sodium chloride must be added for infants to maintain normal serum electrolyte levels.

Treatment

Treatment with glucocorticoids promptly decreases the ACTH level and the excess androgen production. Children with the salt-losing form of CAH have a lifelong requirement for

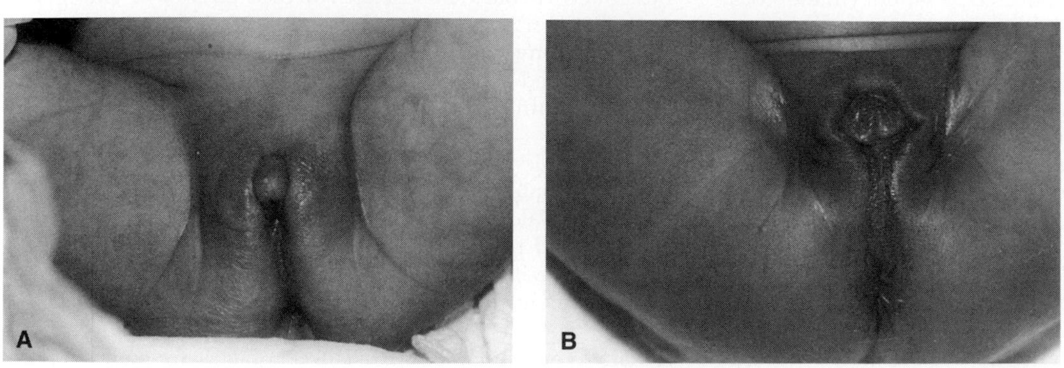

Figure 204-2. Ambiguous genitalia in female pseudohermaphrodites with congenital adrenal hyperplasia. Both cases exhibit enlargement of the clitoris, posterior fusion of the vaginal orifice, and development of rugae of the labia majora. **A:** Female infant with salt-losing 21-hydroxylase deficiency. **B:** Female infant with 11β-hydroxylase deficiency.

glucocorticoid replacement, but they may tolerate discontinuation of daily mineralocorticoid therapy when they reach adulthood. Careful titration of glucocorticoid therapy is necessary because the balance between undertreatment (i.e., androgen excess) and overtreatment (i.e., cushingoid features) may be within a narrow dosage range and varies significantly from patient to patient.

For the simple virilizing form of 21-OH deficiency, mineralocorticoid therapy is not generally needed. However, in some patients, mineralocorticoid supplementation has been used successfully to decrease the required glucocorticoid dose for adequate suppression of adrenal androgen levels. Glucocorticoid therapy must be titrated for optimal results, as in the salt-losing form. Treatment of the late-onset form of 21-OH deficiency is with glucocorticoid replacement as well.

In treating patients with all forms of this disease (as for all children receiving glucocorticoid therapy), the dosage must be increased during times of stress; parents must be trained to administer intramuscular hydrocortisone during times when children cannot take the medication orally.

Prognosis

The prognosis for children with 21-OH deficiency is good with careful follow-up and titration of hormonal replacement therapy. Some degree of morbidity is associated with surgical correction of the external genitalia in girls, and it may be significant if multiple surgical procedures are needed. Fertility is normal in males with the salt-losing form, but females with this form may have decreased fertility. In the simple virilizing form and late-onset forms, fertility is generally unaffected in males and females who receive adequate treatment.

Prenatal Diagnosis

The prenatal diagnosis of 21-OH deficiency is available for families at risk using one of several methods. The diagnosis can be made in the presence of elevated amniotic fluid levels of 17-hydroxyprogesterone and androstenedione. The genes for 21-OH lie within the HLA complex on chromosome 6 and are inherited with the HLA complex. If the HLA haplotypes of a previously affected sibling are known and no HLA recombination has occurred, the 21-OH status of the fetus can be determined by the HLA type of amniotic cells. Amniotic fluid cells and chorionic villus biopsy specimens can be analyzed directly for 21-OH gene mutations if the genotype of a previously affected sibling is known.

Prenatal Treatment

Prenatal treatment has proved effective in preventing or reducing the ambiguity of the genitalia in female infants, but only if it is instituted early in the first trimester. A mother at risk is treated with dexamethasone until chorionic villus sampling or amniocentesis can provide information about the genetic gender and 21-OH genotype or HLA type of a fetus. If the fetus has an XY karyotype or if it has a normal 21-OH genotype, the dexamethasone should be stopped. If the treatment must be continued until term, the dose of dexamethasone required for adequate suppression of amniotic fluid levels of 17-hydroxyprogesterone (and thus reduced risk of female virilization) may produce maternal cushingoid features.

Unaffected siblings can be tested for 21-OH deficiency carrier status to provide genetic counseling. In response to an intravenous ACTH stimulation test, heterozygotes have normal baseline levels with an exaggerated increase in levels of the steroid precursors progesterone and 17-hydroxyprogesterone. Determination of HLA types or 21-OH genotypes may be used to confirm the biochemical findings.

PRIMARY ADRENAL INSUFFICIENCY

Primary adrenal insufficiency or failure is usually caused by Addison disease. The most common cause of Addison disease is autoimmune destruction of the adrenal cortex, as occurs in the autoimmune polyglandular syndromes. Approximately 45% of patients with autoimmune Addison disease (i.e., caused by antiadrenal antibodies) develop one or more other autoimmune endocrinopathies, most often thyroid disease. Other, rarer causes of primary adrenal failure are congenital adrenal hypoplasia, bilateral adrenal hemorrhage (as in the Waterhouse–Friderichsen syndrome), trauma, thrombosis, infection (e.g., tuberculosis), destruction caused by tumor metastases, or degeneration (as seen in adrenoleukodystrophy).

In primary adrenal failure, decreased or absent production of all three groups of adrenal steroid hormones occurs. In most cases, the signs and symptoms of adrenal insufficiency, particularly the hyperpigmentation associated with increased ACTH, develop slowly. ACTH and other substances (beta–endorphin) stimulate melanocytes and result in hyperpigmentation. The clinical features of adrenal insufficiency are listed in Table 204-2.

Diagnosis

The diagnosis is based on demonstration of elevated ACTH levels combined with decreased or absent cortisol and mineralocorticoid production. The fasting 8 a.m. cortisol level is low and fails to rise with ACTH stimulation. The fasting glucose value may be low, and hyponatremia with hyperkalemia may be present. Usually, PRA is elevated. Adrenal androgen levels may be below normal in adolescent patients. Antiadrenal antibody levels should be measured, as should antibodies to other endocrine glands.

Treatment

Treatment includes physiologic replacement with glucocorticoid and mineralocorticoid. Glucocorticoid dosage must be increased during times of stress.

TABLE 204-2. Signs and Symptoms of Adrenal Insufficiency

Glucocorticoid deficiency
Fasting hypoglycemia
Increased insulin sensitivity
Decreased gastric acidity
Gastrointestinal symptoms (e.g., nausea, vomiting)
Fatigue
Headaches
Mineralocorticoid deficiency
Muscle weakness
Weight loss
Fatigue
Nausea, vomiting, anorexia
Salt craving
Hypotension
Hyperkalemia, hyponatremia, acidosis
Androgen deficiency (in older children and adults)
Decreased pubic and axillary hair
Decreased libido
Increased proopiomelanocortin cleavage products
Hyperpigmentation due to melanocyte stimulation

SECONDARY ADRENOCORTICAL INSUFFICIENCY

Secondary adrenocortical insufficiency is usually caused by ACTH deficiency. Rarely, resistance to ACTH may occur. ACTH deficiency may be caused by idiopathic hypopituitarism (congenital), congenital malformations of the pituitary or hypothalamus, destruction of the pituitary or hypothalamus (infection, hemorrhage, tumor, irradiation, infiltrative disease), or iatrogenic causes (prenatal glucocorticoid treatment of the mother or postnatal pharmacologic glucocorticoid treatment).

In the absence of primary adrenal disease, ACTH deficiency does not result in mineralocorticoid deficiency. Therefore, hyponatremia, hyperkalemia, and dehydration are not seen as manifestations of ACTH deficiency. In fact, cortisol deficiency may result in decreased renal clearance of free water resulting in fluid retention. Often, it is apparent in diabetes insipidus patients who may appear to have improvement of their disease if ACTH deficiency develops.

Diagnosis

The diagnosis of ACTH deficiency is based on absence of the 8 a.m. peak in serum cortisol and the lack of response to tests of ACTH secretion (insulin-induced hypoglycemia, glucagon stimulation, metyrapone). In cases of partial ACTH deficiency, affected patients may produce enough ACTH for normal daily physiologic needs (normal 8 a.m. cortisol, normal 24-hour urinary 17-hydroxycorticosteroids) but may be unable to respond to stress and will fail the tests of stimulated ACTH secretion. In any child with ACTH deficiency, the secretion of other anterior and posterior pituitary hormones must be assessed carefully.

Treatment

ACTH deficiency is treated with glucocorticoid at physiologic replacement doses. The dosage must be titrated carefully to prevent overtreatment, which seems to occur at lower doses in children with ACTH deficiency than in those with primary adrenal failure. Mineralocorticoid treatment is unnecessary.

ADRENOCORTICAL HYPERFUNCTION

Adrenocortical hyperfunction is manifested most often by the effects of glucocorticoid excess called Cushing syndrome.

Etiology

The most common cause of Cushing syndrome is iatrogenic administration of pharmacologic doses of a glucocorticoid as an antiinflammatory or immunosuppressive agent. Other causes of Cushing syndrome are rare in childhood (Table 204-3). These causes include ACTH-dependent hypercortisolism (Cushing disease) and primary adrenal hypercortisolism. Among children who have hypercortisolism and are not receiving exogenous glucocorticoids, those younger than 7 years are more likely to have a primary adrenal cause. Those older than age 7 are more likely to have ACTH-dependent hypercortisolism. The clinical features of hypercortisolism are listed in Table 204-4.

TABLE 204-3. Causes of Cushing Syndrome

ACTH-independent
Iatrogenic (e.g., glucocorticoid therapy)
Adrenocortical tumors (e.g., adenoma, carcinoma, micronodular disease)
ACTH-dependent
Hypothalamic CRH-producing tumor
Pituitary ACTH-producing tumor
Ectopic CRH-producing tumor (e.g., pancreas, lung)
Ectopic ACTH-producing tumor (e.g., lung, bronchus, gut)
Iatrogenic (e.g., ACTH therapy)
Increased serotonin levels (e.g., idiopathic)

ACTH, adrenocorticotropic hormone; CRH, corticotropin-releasing hormone.

Diagnosis

The diagnosis of Cushing syndrome is based on demonstration of hypercortisolism and the determination of its source in patients not receiving glucocorticoid treatment. Measurement of serum cortisol levels at 8 a.m. and in late afternoon may fail to show the normal diurnal variation. However, the diurnal pattern may not mature in normal children until after they are 3 years old. The value of serum ACTH levels is limited. Low levels do not rule out the possibility of an ACTH-producing tumor, but high levels usually rule out a primary adrenal cause. Usually, the 24-hour urinary 17-hydroxycorticosteroid levels and free cortisol levels are elevated, as are 17-ketosteroid levels in some cases.

In children with equivocal clinical features and baseline static test results, an overnight dexamethasone suppression test may be the most advantageous dynamic screening test. After a single dose of dexamethasone (20 μg/kg given orally at 11 p.m.), the 8 a.m. serum cortisol should be less than 5 μg/dL in a normal child. If the child fails the overnight test, a low-dose and then a high-dose dexamethasone suppression test should be performed (Table 204-5). Failure to respond to the low-dose test in conjunction with appropriate suppression on the high-dose test suggests an ACTH-producing pituitary adenoma. Failure to respond to the high-dose dexamethasone test suggests an ectopic ACTH-producing tumor or an adrenal tumor. If a pituitary, adrenal, or ectopic ACTH-producing tumor is suspected, radiologic imaging studies must be performed to visualize the tumor. Some ACTH-producing pituitary tumors are microadenomas, visible only at the time of transsphenoidal pituitary exploration.

Treatment

The treatment of Cushing syndrome is removal of the cause of hypercortisolism. In cases of iatrogenic disease, that procedure is not always possible because the nature of the disorder requires glucocorticoid treatment. In cases of ACTH-dependent disease, the source of ACTH production must usually be

TABLE 204-4. Clinical Features of Hypercortisolism

Obesity with violaceous striae (generalized in infants, truncal in older children with moon facies or buffalo hump)
Decreased height velocity (short stature, delayed bone age)
Plethora, increased hematocrit
Easy bruising
Hypertension
Osteoporosis
Glucose intolerance
Poor wound healing
Increased frequency of infections
Renal stones, hypercalciuria
Weakness, muscle wasting (unusual in infants)
Depression

TABLE 204-5. Normal Plasma and Urinary Steroid Hormone Levels with Static and Dynamic Tests

Test		Values	
Static tests			
Plasma cortisol[a]		*μg/dL*	
	Cord blood	5–17 (13.1)[b]	
	Premature infants (day 4)		
	26–28 wk	1–11 (6.0)	
	31–35 wk	2.5–9.1 (6.4)	
	Full-term infants		
	3 d	1.7–14 (6.2)	
	1–7 d	2–11 (4.4)	
	1–12 mo	2.8–23 (9.4)	
	Children 1–16 yr (8 a.m.)	3–21 (9.8)	
	Adults		
	8 a.m.	8–19 (11.0)	
	4 p.m.	4–11 (5.9)	
Urinary 17-hydroxycorticosteroids (17-OHCS)		*mg/g creatinine*	*mg/24 hr*
	Prepubertal children		
	1–5 yr	1.7–6.4 (4.1)	0.2–2.5 (0.8)
	5–10 yr	2.2–6.0 (3.5)	0.5–2.5 (1.2)
	Prepubertal children and adults		
	Male	2.4–4.3 (3.2)	3–10 (6.4)
	Female	1.6–3.6 (2.3)	2–6 (2.8)
Urinary free cortisol		*μg/g creatinine*	*μg/24 hr*
	Prepubertal children	7–25 (15)	3–9 (5.2)
	Adult men	7–45 (21)	11–84 (40)
	Adult women	9–32 (19)	10–34 (20)
	Pregnancy	14–59 (38)	16–60 (47)
Dynamic tests			
Adrenal capacity	Plasma cortisol at 1 hour is double baseline level and >18 μg/dL		
Rapid IV test: 0.25 mg Cortrosyn immediately			
Prolonged test: 20 U/m^2 Acthar gel IM every 12 hours for 3 days, or 0.25 mg Cortrosyn IV over 8–12 hours beginning at 8 a.m. for 3 days	Urinary 17-OHCS: three to fivefold increase over baseline		
ACTH capacity[c]			
Oral metyrapone: 15 mg/kg every 4 hours six times from 8 a.m. to 4 a.m.	Urinary 17-OHCS increase two- to fourfold or serum 11-deoxycortisol increase to >10 ng/dL		
Oral metyrapone: 30–40 mg/kg (up to 3.0 g) at midnight	8 a.m.: Increase in serum 11-deoxycortisol to >7 μg/dL, with a decrease in serum cortisol to <5 μg/dL		
Regular insulin 0.05–0.10 U/kg IV or glucagon 0.1 mg/kg IM	Rise in serum cortisol by 10 μg/dL or to >20 μg/dL		
Pituitary suppression test			
Single-dose dexamethasone: 20 μg/kg up to 2 mg orally at 11 p.m.	Serum cortisol <5 μg/dL at 8 a.m. (fasting)		
Prolonged dexamethasone: 5 μg/kg up to 0.5 mg orally every 6 hours for 2 days, then 40 μg/kg up to 2 mg every 6 hours for 2 days	Suppression or urinary 17-OHCS to <3 $mg/m^2/d$		

ACTH, adrenocorticotropic hormone; IM, intramuscularly; IV, intravenously.
[a]Stress or anxiety may cause elevation of cortisol levels for above the stated normal range.
[b]Normal ranges and means (in parentheses) are based on reference ranges from Endocrine Science Laboratories, Calabasas Hills, California, and are used with permission.
[c]In many centers, metyrapone no longer is available for diagnostic testing. Insulin-induced hypoglycemia or glucagon stimulation will be the tests of choice for ACTH capacity. The specific details of the glucagon stimulation test are detailed in Vanderschueren-Lodeweyckx M, Wolter R, Malvaux P, et al. The glucagon stimulation test effect on plasma growth hormone and on immunoreactive insulin, cortisol, and glucose in children. *J Pediatr* 1974;85:182.

removed surgically. In cases of pituitary Cushing disease, medications such as cyproheptadine and bromocriptine have been more effective in lowering ACTH levels in adults than in children. Bilateral adrenalectomy was once the only treatment for ACTH-dependent disease, but most patients then developed Nelson disease (i.e., pituitary enlargement due to hyperplasia of ACTH-producing cells). In primary adrenal disease, adrenalectomy (unilateral in the case of a tumor and bilateral in micronodular disease) is the treatment of choice. The side effect of these treatments most commonly encountered is adrenal insufficiency caused by ACTH deficiency or adrenalectomy. In the case of unilateral adrenalectomy, the contralateral adrenal gland will need time to recover from prolonged lack of ACTH stimulation. Patients who undergo pituitary exploration have a small risk of developing panhypopituitarism.

Prognosis

The prognosis for patients with Cushing syndrome is based on the underlying cause. Patients with adrenal or pituitary adenomas have a good prognosis after adequate surgical resection.

Those who have adrenal or ectopic ACTH-producing carcinomas have a poorer prognosis. Hypersecretion of adrenal androgens may be caused by CAH or by an adrenal tumor. In addition, feminizing adrenocortical tumors have been described. Adrenal tumors including adenomas and carcinomas are rare in childhood; they are treated by surgical resection and, in some cases, by adjunctive therapies.

Hypersecretion of mineralocorticoids may be caused by the hypertensive form of CAH (Table 204-1) or by primary hyperaldosteronism. In 11-OH or 17-OH deficiency, glucocorticoid replacement therapy results in lowering of mineralocorticoid levels. Hyperaldosteronism is exceedingly rare in childhood and treated with the aldosterone inhibitor spironolactone. Rare causes of apparent mineralocorticoid excess include an inherited defect in the conversion of cortisol to cortisone and licorice ingestion.

ABNORMALITIES OF THE ADRENAL MEDULLA

Pheochromocytoma

Pheochromocytoma is rare in childhood but must be considered in children with hypertension or other symptoms of catecholamine excess. This tumor may arise from any chromaffin tissue, but it is found most often in the adrenal medulla. Bilateral adrenal or extraadrenal tumors are a feature more common in pediatric than in adult pheochromocytomas, and they are often associated with the familial multiple endocrine neoplasia (MEN) syndromes. The neoplasias associated with the various MEN syndromes are listed in Table 204-6. Features consistent with these associated tumors (e.g., medullary carcinoma of the thyroid) should be sought in any patient with pheochromocytoma. The MEN syndromes are inherited in an autosomal dominant manner and are expressed variably. The MEN type I syndrome is due to germline mutations of a gene termed MEN1. The MEN type II syndromes (i.e., IIA and IIB) and familial medullary carcinoma of the thyroid are caused by germline activating mutations of the RET protooncogene. Tumor cells from sporadic pheochromocytomas may contain mutations of this gene as well. Pheochromocytomas are also associated with neuroectodermal dysplasias (e.g., neurofibromatosis). Pheochromocytoma is benign in more than 90% of pediatric patients. The disorder shows a male preponderance among children with this tumor, but the sex ratio is reversed in adults. The peak incidence occurs between 9 and 12 years in the pediatric group. The signs and symptoms of pheochromocytoma are those of catecholamine excess (Table 204-7). These features vary greatly and are likely to be paroxysmal, but the hypertension may be sustained. Hypertensive crisis may occur during anesthesia.

TABLE 204-6. The Multiple Endocrine Neoplasia Syndromes

Neoplasia	MEN type I[a]	MEN type IIa[b]	MEN type IIb
Pheochromocytoma		+	+
Medullary thyroid carcinoma		+	+
Multiple neural tumors			+
Parathyroid hyperplasia	+	+	
Pancreatic islet tumors	+		
Anterior pituitary tumors	+		

+, the tumor is associated with the syndrome.
[a]Also known as *Wermer syndrome.*
[b]Also known as *Sipple syndrome.*

TABLE 204-7. Signs and Symptoms of Pheochromocytoma

Hypertension
Sweating
Flushing
Palpitations and tachycardia
Emotional lability
Headache
Nausea and vomiting
Constipation
Polyuria and polydipsia

Diagnosis

The diagnosis of pheochromocytoma is based on demonstration of increased catecholamines and their metabolites in a 24-hour urine collection and in blood. These substances are urinary free epinephrine and norepinephrine, metanephrine, and VMA. Urinary VMA levels may be elevated falsely with certain drugs such as aspirin, penicillin, and sulfa preparations. If these test results are inconclusive, a clonidine suppression test may be useful.

Clonidine causes a decrease in blood catecholamine levels only if they are not elevated as a result of secretion from an autonomous source. If suspected from the biochemical tests, the tumor can usually be localized by ultrasonography, computed tomography, magnetic resonance imaging, or intravenous pyelography. Venography to demonstrate elevated levels of catecholamines should be performed only after administration of adequate alpha–blockade with phentolamine mesylate (Regitine) to prevent a hypertensive crisis. Scintigraphic imaging with ^{131}I-metaiodobenzylguanidine (MIBG scan) has been used to demonstrate the presence of a pheochromocytoma. MIBG is similar in structure to norepinephrine and is concentrated in tissues that are synthesizing catecholamines by means of norepinephrine in storage granules.

Treatment

The treatment of pheochromocytoma is surgical excision and requires extensive preoperative treatment with alpha- and beta–blockade and with alpha–methyltyrosine if needed. If bilateral adrenalectomy is necessary, treatment for primary adrenal insufficiency must be promptly instituted. Postoperative recordings of blood pressure and catecholamine levels are needed to monitor for tumor recurrence. Malignant tumors are diagnosed on the basis of functional tumor in nonchromaffin tissue areas. Benign tumors may cause blood vessel or capsular invasion, but they do not spread beyond chromaffin tissue areas. Malignant tumors grow slowly and are resistant to irradiation and chemotherapy. Symptoms are treated medically with various degrees of success.

NEUROBLASTOMA

Neuroblastoma is one of the most common solid tumors of childhood and may arise from the adrenal medulla. It can be sporadic or familial. The diagnosis is based on demonstration of elevated homovanillic acid or VMA levels in the urine and radiologic localization. The treatment and prognosis of neuroblastoma are discussed in Chapter 172.

Other Tumors

Other tumors of the adrenal medulla include ganglioneuroblastoma and ganglioneuroma. These tumors may manifest with chronic watery diarrhea as a result of tumor secretion of vasoactive intestinal peptide. The diarrhea resolves after excision of the tumor.

CHAPTER 205
Puberty and Gonadal Disorders

Adapted from Leslie P. Plotnick

In most girls, puberty begins between 8 and 13 years of age and is completed, on average, in 4.2 years (range, 1.5–6.0 years). A 1997 study by Herman-Giddens et al., showed that a substantial portion of girls have pubertal changes at age 7 years. The changes occurred earlier in black than in white girls. The time from the onset of breast buds to menarche is 2.3 ± 1.0 years. In 99% of boys, puberty begins between 9 and 14 years of age and is completed, on average, in 3.5 years (range, 2.0–4.5 years).

If a girl shows signs of pubertal maturation before 7 to 8 years of age or a boy shows signs before 9 years of age, the child should be evaluated for precocious puberty. If no signs of pubertal development occur by 13 years of age in girls or by 14 years of age in boys, the child should be evaluated for pubertal delay. The timing of progression of puberty is also important. Pubertal changes that progress too rapidly or arrest in progression require evaluation.

TABLE 205-1. Precocious or Inappropriate Sexual Development

True or central precocious puberty (central gonadotropin secretion)
Idiopathic
Central nervous system tumors: hamartomas, gliomas (with neurofibromatosis), and others
Other central nervous system disorders: trauma, postinfectious, hydrocephalus, radiation, surgery
Severe primary hypothyroidism
Precocious puberty independent of pituitary gonadotropins
Girls
Exogenous estrogen exposure
Estrogen-secreting tumors (adrenals or ovaries)
Ovarian cysts
McCune-Albright syndrome
Boys
Exogenous androgen exposure
Adrenal androgen secretion
Congenital adrenal hyperplasia
Adrenal tumors
Testicular androgen secretion
Tumors
Familial Leydig cell hyperplasia
Gonadotropin-secreting tumors
McCune-Albright syndrome
Heterosexual development
Virilization in girls
Congenital adrenal hyperplasia
Adrenal tumors
Ovarian tumors
Feminization in boys
Adrenal tumor
Testicular tumor
Increased peripheral conversion of androgens to estrogens
Variations of normal puberty
Premature thelarche
Premature adrenarche
Pubertal gynecomastia

PRECOCIOUS SEXUAL DEVELOPMENT

Causes of precocious or inappropriate sexual development are listed in Table 205-1. In evaluating a child for sexual precocity, a careful medical and family history is imperative. Does the child have any history of a central nervous system (CNS) disorder? What is the child's growth pattern? Is there evidence of linear growth acceleration? Previous growth measurements are valuable. When did the various pubertal changes begin? How fast have these changes progressed? Is the child outgrowing clothes and shoes rapidly? Has the child's appetite increased? When did the parents and siblings have pubertal changes? Is there a history of early sexual development in any relatives? Questions regarding exposure to any exogenous source of sex steroids must be asked. Creams and pills can contain sex steroids, especially estrogens, and oral contraceptives are readily found in many homes. Are any athletes in the home taking anabolic steroids?

The physical examination should include a careful examination of the fundi. The child's skin should be inspected for signs of oiliness, acne, and café au lait spots. The thyroid should be palpated. The presence of axillary hair and odor, the amount of breast tissue, and whether the nipples and areolae are enlarging and thinning should be evaluated. The abdomen should be carefully palpated for masses. The amount, location, and character of pubic hair should be noted.

In girls, the clitoris, labia, and vaginal orifice should be examined carefully. Is there evidence of maturation of the labia minora? Does the vaginal mucosa look red and shiny (prepubertal) or pink and dull (estrogenized)? Is the clitoris of normal size? Are vaginal secretions evident on the genitalia or on the child's underwear?

In boys, the stretched length and width of the penis should be evaluated. Careful palpation and measurement of the testes is key. Are the testes prepubertal in length (less than 2.5 cm), or are they enlarging? Is there a difference in size and consistency of the two testes suggesting a unilateral mass? Transillumination of the testes may be helpful, especially if size discrepancies exist. Is the scrotum thinning, or does it look thick and nonvascular (i.e., prepubertal)? Are the results of the neurologic examination normal?

TRUE OR CENTRAL PRECOCIOUS PUBERTY

True or central precocious puberty is caused by early maturation of hypothalamic GnRH secretion. This form of precocious puberty is much more common in girls than in boys. In many cases, no definable CNS abnormality can be found, and the problem falls into the idiopathic category, which occurs more frequently in girls than in boys. In idiopathic precocious puberty, although the onset is at an early age, the pattern and timing of progression of pubertal events are normal.

CNS tumors, especially hypothalamic hamartomas, are known causes of central precocious puberty and neuroimaging with computed tomography (CT) or magnetic resonance imaging (MRI) is recommended. Neurofibromas, gliomas, and other tumors have been found with some frequency. Other CNS lesions such as hydrocephalus, posttrauma, and postinfectious encephalitis or meningitis are associated with precocious puberty. Hypothalamic hamartomas contain GnRH neurons that function independently of CNS inhibition.

Children with central precocious puberty have accelerated linear growth, advanced bone ages, and pubertal levels of LH, FSH, and the sex steroids estradiol and testosterone. Because LH and FSH levels fluctuate, single samples may be inadequate to make this diagnosis. Multiple samples, which may be taken at 20-minute intervals for 1 or more hours, are helpful. A GnRH infusion with LH and FSH levels determined at regular intervals helps clarify this diagnosis. Newer, highly sensitive gonadotropin assays may allow the diagnosis of central precocious puberty by a single basal LH measurement or by a single LH measurement 40 minutes after a subcutaneous GnRH injection. In boys, the finding of bilateral pubertal-sized testes almost always indicates central precocious puberty. This is an extremely important point in the physical examination because it determines the diagnostic workup.

Early attempts to treat central precocious puberty with medroxyprogesterone (Provera) and the weak androgen danazol successfully reversed some secondary sex characteristics but did not prevent bone age acceleration and compromise of adult stature.

The discovery that the pulse frequency of endogenous GnRH is important for pituitary LH and FSH secretion has had a major effect on designing treatments for blocking LH and FSH release. GnRH agonists that provide consistent, not fluctuating, GnRH levels lower LH and FSH levels. Long-acting GnRH analogues have been successful in inhibiting pituitary LH and FSH release and in stopping the progression of puberty. In many cases, secondary sex characteristics have regressed. Treatment with GnRH analogues produces a prepubertal hormonal state, and growth acceleration, bone age advancement, and the progression of secondary sex characteristics cease.

The decision to treat should depend on several factors. First, the age of the child and his or her adjustment to the pubertal changes must be considered. A 2-year-old child is in need of treatment, but a 7-year-old child may psychologically handle the changes well. The rapidity of pubertal progression, as well as chronologic age, must be considered. In the older child with precocious puberty, the major issues in deciding whether to treat are the magnitude of bone age advancement and the rapidity of its progression, the degree of compromise of adult stature, and the decreases in predicted adult height.

In some patients with severe prolonged untreated primary hypothyroidism, precocious sexual development may be seen and is associated with pubertal levels of LH and FSH. These patients exhibit poor linear growth and usually delayed bone age. When the thyroid-stimulating hormone overproduction is suppressed by exogenous thyroxine, the LH and FSH concentrations decrease to prepubertal levels, and the pubertal changes regress.

PRECOCIOUS PUBERTY INDEPENDENT OF PITUITARY GONADOTROPINS

Girls

Girls with precocious puberty independent of pituitary gonadotropins have a nongonadotropin-stimulated or independent source of estrogens producing their pubertal changes. An exogenous source of estrogens must be sought. The use of skin creams and medications must be pursued and the labels read to see whether they contain estrogen. Birth control pills are widely used and, although they may not be in the child's home, grandparents, friends, and baby-sitters may keep them in unprotected locations. In some cases, ingestion of animal protein, especially poultry, has been reported to produce estrogenization in a child if the animal received estrogens.

Estrogen-producing tumors of the ovary and adrenal gland must be considered. Adrenal estrogen-producing tumors are rare and are associated with high estradiol levels and increased levels of other adrenal sex hormones. They should be visible with abdominal CT or MRI scans. Estrogen-producing ovarian tumors are more common and may be palpable during careful bimanual examination. As with adrenal tumors, estradiol levels are usually high. Ultrasound and CT scans usually demonstrate the ovarian mass. Ovarian cysts, associated with high levels of estradiol, are another cause of gonadotropin-independent precocious puberty and are demonstrable with imaging. Sometimes ovarian cysts are recurrent.

Treatment entails removal of the estrogen source if exogenous exposure is the cause. If an adrenal or ovarian tumor is found, surgical excision and, if the tumor is malignant, additional treatment is indicated. Ovarian cysts are difficult to treat because they may recur, and surgical excision may make no difference in the patient's long-term clinical course.

McCune–Albright syndrome is an unusual syndrome of irregular café au lait spots, polyostotic fibrous dysplasia, and precocious puberty. McCune–Albright syndrome is seen in both sexes. Excessive hormone production by other glands (e.g., thyroid) may be present. McCune–Albright syndrome is caused by a mutation in the gene that codes for the alpha subunit of Gs, the G protein that stimulates adenyl cyclase formation. This mutation produces constitutive activation. Treatments with ketoconazole (see following discussion) and testolactone (an aromatase inhibitor) have been tried with variable success.

Boys

Boys with gonadotropin-independent precocious puberty have a source of androgens independent of central gonadotropin secretion. Exogenous androgen exposure must be considered. With the widespread abuse of androgens (i.e., anabolic steroids) by athletes, young children are at risk for exposure.

An adrenal source of androgens including an adrenal tumor or an adrenal biosynthetic defect (e.g., 21-hydroxylase deficiency, 11-hydroxylase deficiency) causes precocious puberty in boys. Those with an adrenal or exogenous androgen source show clinical virilization including linear growth acceleration and bone age advancement but have prepubertal testes on examination.

Adrenal tumors are associated with high levels of adrenal androgens that are not suppressed with glucocorticoid administration. CT or MRI is important in establishing the diagnosis. Adrenal enzyme deficiencies show characteristic precursor and androgen patterns, and the elevated androgen levels are suppressible with exogenous glucocorticoids.

Testicular tumors may produce elevated androgens and cause precocious puberty. On examination, the testes show a size discrepancy; the testis with the tumor is larger and often has an irregular consistency.

The syndrome of premature Leydig cell maturation or familial testotoxicosis is gonadotropin-independent, but premature Leydig cell maturation with pubertal levels of testosterone occurs despite prepubertal LH patterns. Because maturation of spermatogenesis occurs, these patients are fertile.

Activating mutations in the LH receptor causes this disorder.

Treatment of gonadotropin-independent precocious puberty in boys entails removal of the androgen source in exogenous exposure. Excision of adrenal or testicular tumors is indicated with additional treatment if the lesions are malignant. Adrenal enzyme deficiencies require appropriate glucocorticoid replacement.

GnRH analogue treatment is not useful in familial Leydig cell hyperplasia. Some reports indicate that ketoconazole, which inhibits enzymes in the testosterone biosynthetic pathway, may be a useful treatment.

An additional cause of precocious puberty in boys is human chorionic gonadotropin (hCG)-producing tumors. These tumors may be in the CNS (i.e., germinoma) or elsewhere in the body (e.g., hepatoma, hepatoblastoma, teratoma, chorioepithelioma). Because some LH assay antibodies cross react with hCG, laboratory test results may show factitiously elevated LH and prepubertal FSH levels. Specific assays document that the gonadotropin is hCG. Because a gonadotropin is being secreted, the testes are enlarged, and boys with this problem clinically may resemble those with central precocious puberty.

Heterosexual Development

Heterosexual development is defined as virilization in girls and feminization in boys. When it occurs before the normal age of puberty, it can be called heterosexual precocity. But whether it occurs at a prepubertal age or later, the diagnostic causes, evaluation, and treatment are the same.

Adrenal and ovarian lesions can cause virilization in girls. Adrenal enzyme deficiencies (e.g., 21-hydroxylase, 11β-hydroxylase, and 3β-hydroxysteroid dehydrogenase deficiencies) produce virilization. Typically, girls with these enzyme deficiencies have genital ambiguity as neonates, but other manifestations may occur later, sometimes as subtle as hirsutism or acne in a teenager or adult. Adrenal or ovarian androgen-producing tumors must be sought in any female patient with virilization by measuring plasma levels of sex steroids and by diagnostic imaging with ultrasound, CT, or MRI.

Boys with signs of feminization may have an adrenal estrogen-producing tumor, a testicular tumor, or increased peripheral conversion of androgens to estrogens, as with a familial increase in aromatase activity or certain tumors such as hepatomas.

Measurement of sex hormone levels, diagnostic imaging, tests of suppression with glucocorticoids, and adrenocorticotropin (ACTH) stimulation tests are helpful in defining the cause.

VARIATIONS OF NORMAL PUBERTY

Premature Thelarche

Premature thelarche is a common entity with clinical evidence of mild estrogenization in girls, typically between 1 and 4 years of age. Breast enlargement, which may be unilateral, occurs, often without nipple and areolar development. No sexual hair develops, and no linear growth acceleration occurs. This is an isolated phenomenon, and lack of progression is the hallmark. Laboratory test results show incomplete estrogenization of the vaginal mucosa, a normal bone age, and prepubertal gonadotropin patterns. Estradiol levels are usually prepubertal, but they may be slightly increased.

Postulated causes include ovarian cysts and transient pituitary gonadotropin secretion. No treatment is necessary. Close follow-up is important because the early stages of precocious puberty may be clinically indistinguishable from those of premature thelarche.

Premature Adrenarche

Premature adrenarche is caused by early activation of adrenal androgens producing pubic and axillary hair development and axillary odor. In girls, the pubic hair often begins on the labia. No other signs of pubertal changes and no signs of abnormal virilization exist. If signs of gonadarche are observed, an evaluation for precocious puberty is indicated. If virilization occurs, a workup for virilizing lesions is necessary. Some children with premature adrenarche may have mild neurologic problems. Height and bone age are often slightly greater than the mean but fall within two standard deviations. Plasma adrenal androgens and urinary androgen metabolites (17-ketosteroids) are increased to the early pubertal range.

Typically, premature adrenarche occurs in 6- to 8-year-old children, but it may be seen in much younger children. The sexual hair gradually increases. Evidence suggests that a substantial percentage of children with this diagnosis may have mild 21-hydroxylase deficiency, and an ACTH stimulation test is useful for this diagnosis. In some girls, premature adrenarche may be a marker of polycystic ovarian syndrome.

Pubertal Gynecomastia

Pubertal gynecomastia is common in teenage boys, typically beginning in Tanner stage 2 or 3 and lasting for approximately 2 years. In some boys, the ratio of estradiol to testosterone may be elevated. Severely affected boys may require surgical reduction.

Tamoxifen and testolactone may be effective for treating gynecomastia in moderate cases. Pathologic causes of gynecomastia must be considered. Hypogonadism [e.g., Klinefelter syndrome (47XXY)]; partial androgen insensitivity; partial blocks in testosterone biosynthesis; hyperthyroidism; adrenal, testicular, or LH and hCG-producing tumors; liver tumors or disease; and chronic debilitating illness causing malnutrition have all been associated with gynecomastia. A variety of drugs can cause gynecomastia: androgens, estrogens, hCG, psychoactive drugs (e.g., phenothiazines), marijuana and other street drugs and alcohol, testosterone antagonists (e.g., ketoconazole, cimetidine, spironolactone), and antituberculosis and cytotoxic agents.

Obese teenage boys may present with large breasts that are only adipose tissue and of no pathologic consequence. However, determining whether glandular breast tissue exists in an extremely obese boy may be difficult.

DELAYED PUBERTY

The causes of delayed puberty are listed in Table 205-2. An evaluation for pubertal delay is indicated if no signs of puberty are observed in a girl by 13 years of age or in a boy by 14 years of age. Evaluation is also indicated if an arrest in pubertal maturation occurs.

The differential diagnosis of delayed or absent puberty rests on the initial gonadotropin levels. If LH and FSH levels are high, a primary gonadal abnormality exists. If LH and FSH levels are normal or low, a search for central hormonal abnormalities or chronic disease must be undertaken.

TABLE 205-2. Causes of Delayed Puberty

Elevated gonadotropin levels
Gonadal failure: autoimmune, chemotherapy or radiation, traumatic, infectious, postsurgical, torsion, "vanishing testes," pure gonadal dysgenesis, myotonic dystrophy
Complete androgen insensitivity syndrome
Complete 17α-hydroxylase deficiency
Chromosomal abnormalities
Turner syndrome
Klinefelter syndrome
Other sex chromosome abnormalities
Normal or low gonadotropin levels
Constitutional delay of growth and adolescence
Hypopituitarism
Isolated luteinizing hormone/follicle-stimulating hormone deficiency associated with hyposmia or anosmia (Kallmann syndrome)
Multiple hormone deficiencies
Chronic disease
Malnutrition; excessive exercise
Syndromes
Prader-Willi
Laurence-Moon-Biedl

Elevated Gonadotropin Level

Patients with elevated LH and FSH levels have evidence of bilateral gonadal failure and lack of appropriate sex steroid levels to feed back centrally. After LH and FSH levels are found to be elevated, a karyotype should be determined. Common causes of gonadal failure are chemotherapy, radiation therapy, and autoimmune glandular failure.

Girls with the XY karyotype who have complete androgen insensitivity develop breasts at the appropriate age, but no sexual hair develops, and no menses occur. Girls with the XY karyotype and complete 17α-hydroxylase deficiency (i.e., no sex steroids can be formed) have no secondary sex characteristics. If these syndromes are partial, enough androgen is present to cause genital ambiguity in the neonate or virilization during puberty.

Turner syndrome is a common cause of absent breast development and elevated gonadotropin levels. Turner syndrome is invariably associated with short stature and often with other anomalies including webbed neck, increased nevi, high-arched palate, shield chest, coarctation of the aorta, renal anomalies, an increased arm-carrying angle, and edema of the hands and feet. Most girls with this syndrome have a 45X karyotype, but many have a mosaic pattern (45X/46XX) or an X-chromosomal structural abnormality (e.g., ring or isochrome). Buccal smears are not adequate for this diagnosis. Sexual hair develops in girls with Turner syndrome because adrenal androgens are not affected.

Boys with Klinefelter syndrome (47XXY) usually come to attention because of gynecomastia and small testes (i.e., inadequate masculinization). They are usually clinically normal at birth, and throughout childhood they are tall with slim builds and long limbs. They may also have mosaic chromosome patterns (e.g., 46XY/47XXY) or multiple X chromosomes.

Treatment of patients with gonadal failure involves replacing sex steroids. Depending on the age of the patient and whether height is an issue, replacement can be done gradually over several years or more abruptly.

In young teenaged boys, injectable testosterone can be used. A typical regimen is testosterone enanthate administered intramuscularly in a dose of 50 mg/month initially and gradually increased to full adult doses of 300 mg every 3 weeks. Long-term replacement therapy with oral testosterone preparations is not recommended because of the hepatotoxicity of 17-alpha-alkylated steroids. Testosterone patches are now available and can be used to induce and maintain puberty.

In girls, conjugated estrogens can be started at 0.3 mg/day with doses increased gradually until satisfactory breast development is achieved. After 1 to 2 years of estrogen treatment or if vaginal spotting occurs, treatment with estrogens in cycles of approximately 25 days per month, with a progestational agent overlapping for approximately the last 10 to 14 days of each cycle, should be started. Estradiol can also be given in gradually increasing doses. Depot estrogen preparations given monthly have been used. New transdermal estrogen patches may be useful in long-term treatment. After adequate estrogenization has occurred, long-term treatment can be achieved with a combination oral contraceptive pill.

Normal or Low Gonadotropin Levels

The most common cause of pubertal delay is constitutional delay, which is discussed in Chapter 206. Usually, a careful physical examination in a mid-teenaged boy reveals signs of early puberty, which progresses on follow-up examinations. Reassurance may be all that is necessary. However, more severely affected boys may be psychologically disabled by this problem, and a short course of exogenous testosterone (e.g., testosterone enanthate given intramuscularly as 50–100 mg/month for 4–6 months) should be seriously considered. Short courses of modest doses do not appear to adversely affect ultimate stature. A bone age radiograph should be obtained as part of the evaluation for delayed puberty, and bone age should be monitored whenever androgens are used.

Isolated gonadotropin deficiency may or may not be associated with anosmia or hyposmia (i.e., Kallmann syndrome). Kallmann syndrome is caused by lack of fetal GnRH neuron migration caused by lack of adhesion molecule production (coded by the KAL gene). Hypogonadotropic hypogonadism may be difficult to differentiate from constitutional delay in certain cases, and overnight gonadotropin sampling or GnRH testing may be helpful. Baseline LH and FSH levels may not differentiate prepubertal or hypogonadotropic from early pubertal levels. Search for an organic cause requires CNS imaging. Prolactin-secreting pituitary adenomas may produce gonadotropin deficiency. LH and FSH deficiency is more commonly associated with other pituitary hormone deficiencies, especially growth hormone deficiency. The differential diagnosis of hypopituitarism is discussed in Chapter 207. Induction and maintenance of puberty in these patients must be coordinated with other hormonal replacement therapy. Traditionally, puberty has been induced and maintained with exogenous sex steroids, as discussed earlier in this chapter. Gonadotropin injections can be used to induce fertility in patients with central gonadotropin deficiency. GnRH has been given in pulsatile fashion to induce puberty and to produce fertility.

Some adolescent girls may develop normally, but because they lack normal central cyclic function, they do not have normal menses. Any chronic disease during childhood and adolescence may delay puberty and growth. Particular attention must be paid to the possibility of subtle gastrointestinal disease, especially inflammatory bowel disease, and to the patient's nutritional status. Inadequate caloric intake or excessive exercise can delay puberty and cause amenorrhea.

Certain syndromes are associated with central gonadotropin deficiency, particularly the Prader–Willi and Laurence–Moon–Biedl syndromes. Hypothyroidism can cause delayed puberty or precocious puberty.

Blind children may have pubertal delay, and associated pituitary-hypothalamic dysfunction must be considered in these children.

In virtually all patients with primary gonadal failure or central gonadotropin deficiency, treatment with sex steroids can induce and maintain satisfactory sexual maturation and satisfactory sexual functioning. Patients with central gonadotropin deficiency have hope for fertility with the use of gonadotropins or GnRH preparations.

CHAPTER 206
Growth Disorders

Adapted from Leslie P. Plotnick

SHORT STATURE OR POOR LINEAR GROWTH

A child with a height below the third percentile or whose growth curve has been crossing percentiles downward should be carefully examined for a pathologic cause of poor growth (Table 206-1). Probably the largest category of causes of poor growth is major organ system disease. Most patients in this category have a disorder that is not subtle, and the history and physical examination disclose the problem without extensive laboratory testing. However, some disorders may not be evident from history and physical examination and, therefore, require laboratory studies for diagnosis.

Genetic Short Stature and Constitutional Growth Delay

Familial or genetic short stature is a common cause of short stature in children. Usually the parents' heights are in the lower normal percentiles for adults. This is not a disorder: These children are entirely normal. Their heights are usually at or slightly below the third percentile but not at or more than 3 SD below the mean. They have normal growth velocities, and their height curves parallel the third percentile. Their bone ages are normal, and their pubertal growth spurts are normal in timing and magnitude.

One or both of the parents may be short for a pathologic reason such as familial growth hormone (GH) deficiency or mild chondrodysplasias, which the child may have inherited. If a parent's height is more than 2 SD below the mean (i.e., less than the third percentile) or if the parent is disproportionately short for his or her family, both parent and child may have a pathologic cause for their short stature.

Constitutional slow growth with delayed adolescence, called constitutional delay, is another common diagnostic category. This variant of normal growth is seen more frequently in boys than in girls. Typically, affected children lag 2 to 4 years behind average in height, bone age, and pubertal development. Often, the family history in parents, older siblings, or other family members is positive for this growth pattern.

If growth rate is normal, the height is at or slightly below the third percentile, a positive family history exists, and the bone age is delayed by 2 to 4 years, no additional evaluation is needed. However, if any concern about a subnormal growth velocity exists, further evaluation is indicated. Patients with early inflammatory bowel disease or with milder degrees of GH deficiency may initially resemble children with constitutional delay. Because growth velocity gradually drops with age and is at its lowest just before the pubertal growth spurt begins (Fig. 206-1), teenagers with constitutional delay may spend a prolonged time at this low rate. Growth velocity should be assessed in relation to both bone age and chronologic age. The combination of familial or genetic short stature and constitutional delay may occur producing significant growth retardation.

TABLE 206-1. Causes of Short Stature or Poor Linear Growth

Major organ system disease
Central nervous system
Cardiac
Pulmonary
Hematologic
Renal
Gastrointestinal or nutritional
Chromosomal disorders: Turner syndrome, others
Inborn errors of metabolism
Intrauterine growth retardation
Familial or genetic short stature
Constitutional delay of growth and adolescence
Endocrine disorders
Cortisol excess (exogenous or endogenous)
Hypothyroidism
Pseudohypoparathyroidism
Poorly controlled diabetes
Growth hormone deficiency (e.g., idiopathic, organic, familial, psychosocial)
Growth hormone insensitivity (resistance)
Shifting linear percentiles
Skeletal disorders
Nutritional
Deprivation or psychosocial dwarfism
Medications

Endocrine Causes of Short Stature

Endocrine abnormalities are another diagnostic category of short stature. Cortisol excess (i.e., cortisol in greater amounts than physiologic needs) produces short stature, whether the excess cortisol is exogenous (caused by oral, topical, or inhalant glucocorticoids) or endogenous (as in Cushing disease). Children with cortisol excess have a subnormal linear growth rate, delayed bone age, and typical cushingoid clinical features: round, plethoric "moon" face; centripetal obesity; increased dorsal fat pad ("buffalo hump"); and proximal muscle weakness. When the source of excess glucocorticoids is removed, the growth rate increases, but the ultimate height can be compromised by years of glucocorticoid excess.

Hypothyroidism is a distinct endocrine cause of short stature characterized by a subnormal linear growth rate, increased weight gain, and a delayed bone age. When the diagnosis is made and appropriate treatment given, children undergo catch-up growth, although their ultimate height can be compromised. The threshold for performing thyroid function tests should be low for a child with a question of poor growth rate because the diagnostic tests and treatment are of minimal risk, inexpensive, and effective. Treatment often has dramatic effects on clinical signs and symptoms and on growth. Patients with pseudohypoparathyroidism have a characteristic phenotype that includes short stature. Poorly controlled insulin-dependent diabetes mellitus may be associated with short stature and poor linear growth rate. The growth retardation in poorly controlled diabetes can be severe. Improving metabolic control usually normalizes the growth rate, and catch-up growth can occur.

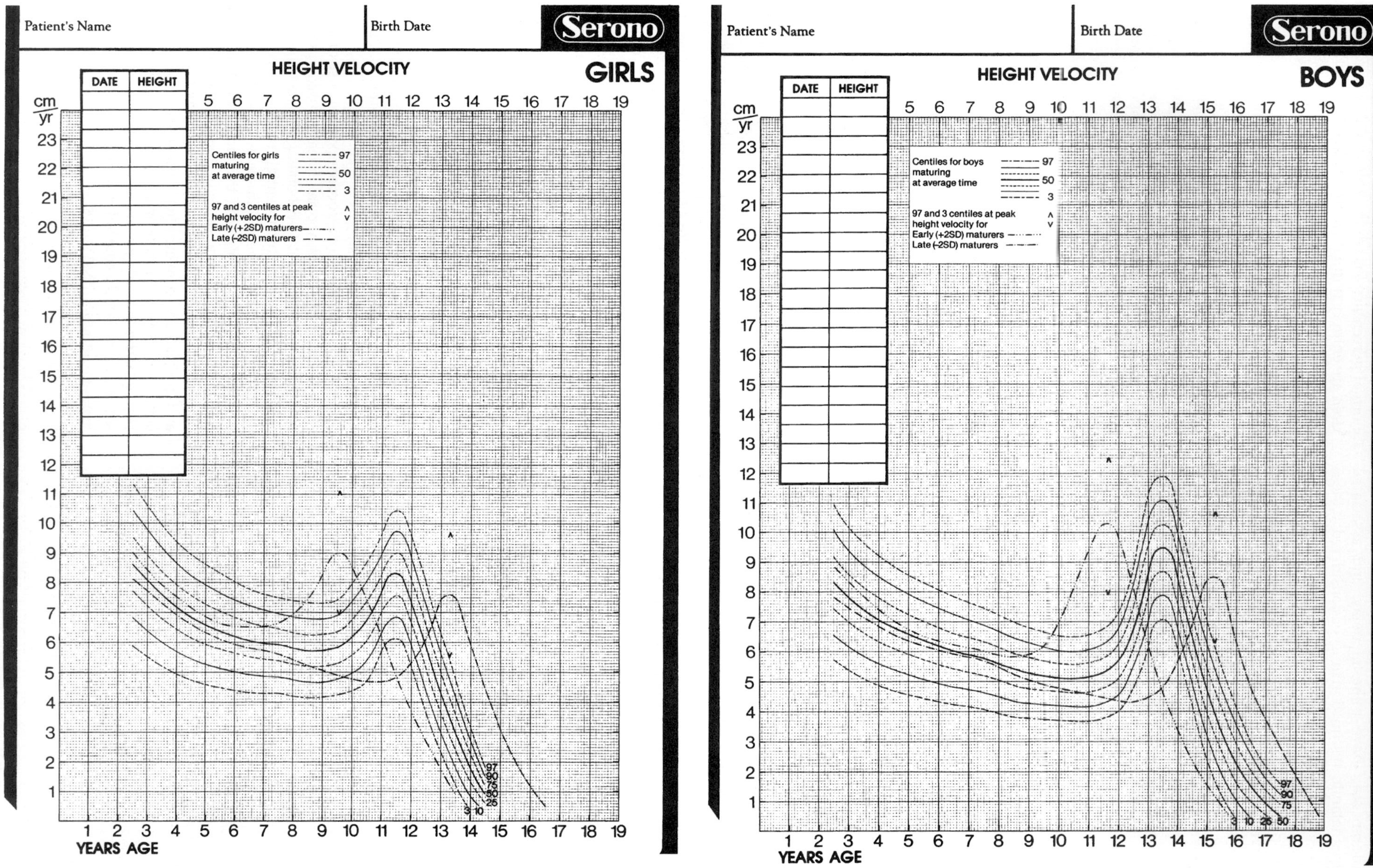

Figure 206-1. Growth velocity curves for girls and boys including early and late pubertal patterns. (Reprinted with permission from Tanner JM. North American growth and development longitudinal standards. Height: distance and velocity for girls and boys. *J Pediatr* 1985;107. Distributed by Serono Laboratories, Randolph, MA.)

Growth Hormone Deficiency

GH deficiency is a diagnostic category that has undergone considerable flux. GH deficiency may be idiopathic, organic, or familial; occasionally, it is psychosocial and reversible. It may occur alone or with other pituitary hormone deficiencies. Children with classic GH deficiency have short stature, poor linear growth rate, and delayed bone age, and they are usually chubby. They may have fasting hypoglycemia, and boys may have small penises. They fail to release normal amounts of GH in response to certain standard pharmacologic stimuli and levels of GH-dependent proteins such as insulin-like growth factor-1 (IGF-1; somatomedin-C) may be low. Various degrees of GH deficiency occur; there is a continuum from normal GH secretion to classic GH deficiency, and where a physician draws the line between normal and abnormal is arbitrary. Some patients respond normally to pharmacologic tests but have low physiologic 24-hour GH secretion, and some have borderline responses to pharmacologic tests; both groups of patients may have partial GH deficiency or neurosecretory defects. Rarely, some patients secrete normal amounts of immunologically active GH that is biologically subactive. Patients in these categories may have been previously classified as having constitutional delay. The level of IGF-1 in these patients may be borderline or low.

The diagnosis of classic GH deficiency remains clear-cut, but the standards of diagnosis of the lesser degrees of GH compromise or of biologically subactive GH are less clear. Because some or many of these patients may benefit from treatment with exogenous GH, this is an important concern for pediatric endocrinologists.

Specific causes of GH deficiency, isolated or associated with other pituitary hormone deficiencies, are congenital abnormalities including septooptic dysplasia, trauma, central nervous system (CNS) infections, vascular abnormalities, irradiation for malignancies, tumors (e.g., craniopharyngiomas), and infiltrative processes such as histiocytosis.

Miscellaneous Causes of Poor Growth and Short Stature

Renal disorders, particularly renal tubular acidosis, require evaluation by electrolytes, chemistries, and urinalysis. Particularly difficult to define are patients with gastrointestinal (GI) abnormalities. Patients with inflammatory bowel disease, especially Crohn's disease, may have growth failure for several years before GI symptoms become evident. A complete blood cell count with an erythrocyte sedimentation rate test may be helpful, but GI contrast studies and endoscopy are required to make the diagnosis. Patients with celiac disease may not have the classic history of malabsorption stools and hyperphagia. These children are often thin and have poor appetites. Certain laboratory tests (antigliadin antibodies and antiendomysial antibodies) may help with this diagnosis, but the only definitive diagnostic test is a small-bowel biopsy. The decision as to when to do the more extensive GI studies (e.g., radiologic, endoscopic) rests on the persistence of a poor growth rate over time with other laboratory tests remaining normal and no other diagnosis being made, especially if the child's weight is affected more than his or her height. Malnutrition of any cause including malabsorption or inadequate caloric intake is associated with poor growth.

Growth retardation is often seen as part of the clinical picture in children with a variety of inborn metabolic errors. Intrauterine growth retardation (IUGR) is another category associated with short stature. Children who are severely small for gestational age at birth often have poor postnatal growth. These children may have dysmorphic features indicating a specific syndrome associated with IUGR. They may be nondysmorphic but thin, especially with very thin extremities, minimal body fat, and thin, narrow faces. Bone ages may be delayed or normal. Chromosomal disorders are often associated with poor growth. They are usually evident from characteristic dysmorphic features and developmental delay. Turner syndrome and its variants (i.e., absence or structural abnormalities of one X chromosome or a mosaic pattern) may manifest with classic phenotypic features or may have only minor clinical features. Girls with non45X karyotypes (i.e., mosaics, rings, isochromes, or partial X deletions) are more likely to lack the classic phenotypic features. All short girls with subnormal growth rates should have banded karyotyping as part of the laboratory evaluation. Buccal smears are not adequate because they do not reveal structural abnormalities or mosaic patterns. Banded karyotyping is expensive and adds considerably to the cost of the evaluation. However, Turner syndrome may be as common as GH deficiency and should be considered in all short girls. Growth curves for girls with Turner syndrome are available.

Craniopharyngiomas are the most common tumors associated with pituitary and hypothalamic deficiencies. They are tumors of the Rathke pouch and are usually suprasellar, but they may be entirely intrasellar. Patients with craniopharyngiomas usually present with headache, visual abnormalities, and neurologic symptoms. They may also have symptoms of diabetes insipidus and growth failure. On physical examination, they may have visual defects (e.g., field cuts, optic atrophy, papilledema) and signs of pituitary hormone deficiencies. CNS imaging identifies the tumors. Treatment is surgical excision, often followed by radiation therapy, and appropriate hormonal replacement therapy.

Syndromes of primary GH insensitivity or resistance occur because of defects in the GH receptor or its signal transduction or IGF-1 synthesis. Secondary causes of GH insensitivity include inhibiting GH antibodies, malnutrition, liver disease, and renal failure.

Some children who are born smaller or larger than their genetic growth potential gradually shift percentiles, up or down, for height and weight. A typical example is a child who, at birth, is in the 90th percentile for length and weight but whose parents are in the tenth percentile for height. During the first 1 to 2 years of life, this child gradually decelerates to approximately the tenth percentile. Sometimes differentiating this pattern from pathologic growth is difficult. The key points are a gradual deceleration of height and weight proportionally, deceleration not below the genetically anticipated percentile, and, once the percentile is reached, velocities normalizing, and height and weight remaining at that percentile. If the deceleration is abrupt and falls to less than the fifth percentile or to a percentile below the parents' percentile, further evaluation is needed.

Skeletal dysplasias are obvious causes of poor growth. The skeletal abnormalities are usually evident on physical examination, as are abnormal arm spans and upper and lower segment ratios. Radiologic studies can help identify the specific abnormalities.

Nutritional deficiencies are an important cause of growth retardation throughout the world. In the developed countries, they may be caused by GI pathology, familial psychosocial problems, or self-imposed caloric deprivation. The last is an important problem in the United States.

Psychological factors have also been associated with poor growth. Growth abnormalities can be caused by severe caloric deprivation. Children in disturbed families may have psychosocial dwarfism with disturbed eating and sleeping behaviors and transient pituitary hormone deficiencies, especially of GH and adrenocorticotropic hormone. When the child is removed from the adverse home environment, catch-up growth occurs and the hormonal levels normalize.

Various medications may produce poor growth. Glucocorticoids were discussed earlier in this chapter. Stimulants such as amphetamines and methylphenidate, especially in high doses, have been associated with impairment of weight and height.

Evaluation of Short Stature or Poor Linear Growth Velocity

The evaluation of a child with poor growth begins with a careful history. Height and growth patterns and the timing of puberty in parents, siblings, and other relatives should be obtained. Gestational age and length and weight at birth are important. Anything in the history to suggest major organ system pathology should be heeded, remembering that renal and GI disorders can be quite subtle. The child's psychological adjustment to his or her stature should be investigated, as should the overall family functioning. Nutritional issues should be discussed.

The child's growth curve should be evaluated carefully. If no previous growth data are available, questions about changes in shoe and clothing sizes and about how the child's growth compares with that of siblings and peers can be helpful. For example, "He used to be a head taller than his sister, who's 3 years younger, but now they're the same height," is revealing information. Every effort should be made to obtain previous height and weight data. The entire complete physical examination is important. Any features of chronic disease should be elicited. Accurate height and weight measurements are mandatory. Careful fundoscopic examination looking for evidence of optic nerve abnormalities and confrontation visual fields should be performed. Because dentition reflects bone age, the age appropriateness of primary and secondary teeth should be assessed. Are there any dysmorphic features of the face or body habitus or extremities? The thyroid should be carefully palpated. Are there signs of sexual maturation? If the patient is a boy, is the penis abnormally small? Are there any clinical features of cortisol excess or of Turner syndrome? Is the child's appearance proportionate or disproportionate for arm span and for upper and lower segment ratios? If there are clues to a specific diagnosis, a complete laboratory workup is unnecessary. For example, if the child appears normal on examination and the history and growth curve strongly suggest familial short stature, no workup is necessary. Perhaps only a bone age evaluation to assess predicted height should be performed. If the child is clearly cushingoid, the specific cause should be pursued.

In the many children in whom no clear cause is evident after history and physical examination, we recommend the following initial laboratory workup: complete blood count with erythrocyte sedimentation rate, chemistry panel including electrolytes, urinalysis with specific gravity and pH (urine culture if any signs of infection are present), bone age, thyroid hormone levels (i.e., T_4, T_3RU, TSH), IGF-1, banded karyotyping for girls, possibly an insulin growth factor binding protein (IGF-BP3), and anti-endomysial antibodies.

Any specific abnormalities should be investigated further, but if nothing abnormal is seen other than perhaps a significant bone age delay, the next step depends on the clinical impression and on the child's growth curve and current growth rate. Growth is an ongoing dynamic process, and evaluation over time is useful. If a child's growth rate is persistently subnormal such that he or she gradually or abruptly falls away from a normal curve, formal GH testing is indicated.

Tests for GH deficiency are summarized in Table 206-2. An inadequate response to a screening test indicates the need for definitive testing. For classic GH deficiency to be diagnosed, a patient must fail two definitive pharmacologic tests. Most laboratories use a level of 7 to 10 ng/mL peak value as the cut-off point between normal and subnormal. Different assays have different normal ranges. Low levels of IGF-1 and of an IGF-binding protein, IGF-BP3, also indicate GH deficiency. The best method for diagnosis is unclear. Some cases of GH deficiency may be caused by mutations in genes coding for GH, the GH-releasing hormone receptor, or transcription factors (e.g., Pit-1). Patients with other disorders of the GH–IGF-1 axis have been described. A biologically subactive GH molecule or an abnormality in the GH receptor (i.e., Laron dwarfism) causes an inability to generate normal amounts of IGF-1. Administration of exogenous GH can help differentiate patients with biologically subactive GH from those with GH insensitivity, because a response of an increase in IGF-1 and an increase in growth rate occurs only in patients with biologically subactive GH and not in those with GH insensitivity. IGF-1 synthetic defects and resistance to IGF-1 have been described.

TABLE 206-2. Tests for Growth Hormone Deficiency

Screening tests
Exercise: before and after 20 minutes of jogging on a level surface or up and down stairs
Sleep: useful for inpatients; measure growth hormone approximately 45 minutes after onset of nightime sleep
Definitive pharmacologic tests (arginine through glucagon in the following list measure ability of the hypothalamic-pituitary unit to secrete growth hormone)
Arginine
L-Dopa
Insulin hypoglycemia
Clonidine
Glucagon
Growth hormone–releasing factor (i.e., measures only pituitary growth hormone function)
Physiologic tests: sampling every 20 to 30 minutes, intermittently or with a continuous blood withdrawal pump

Partial GH deficiency can be difficult to diagnose. A subnormal growth rate, delayed bone age, and low or low-normal IGF-1 levels are clues. Twenty-four-hour physiologic GH monitoring may help with this diagnosis. Ultimately, a trial of GH therapy may be useful.

Newer methods include the measurement of GH-binding proteins. GH-binding protein is the circulating extracellular part of the GH receptor. The levels of IGF-binding proteins, mainly IGF-BP3, correlate with GH production and may be a screening tool for GH deficiency. Synthetic small (six–seven amino acids) GH-releasing peptides and nonpeptide GH secret-agogues produce GH release but not through GH-releasing hormone. Some of these compounds are undergoing clinical trials.

Despite the sophisticated diagnostic testing available, some children have clearly negative workup results, do not fit the diagnosis of constitutional delay, and are left with a diagnosis of idiopathic short stature. Children in this category need careful follow-up because a specific cause may become evident with time.

TREATMENT OF SHORT STATURE

If a specific diagnosis is made, the condition is treated appropriately. For example, if primary hypothyroidism is found, thyroid replacement therapy is indicated. This section primarily discusses treatment with exogenous GH for children with GH disorders, IUGR, Turner syndrome, familial short stature, constitutional delay, and idiopathic short stature.

Until the spring of 1985, GH in the United States and elsewhere was obtained exclusively from cadaver pituitaries. In the United States, it was distributed by the National Hormone and Pituitary Program for patients in research protocols and, starting in the mid-1970s, through several commercial companies by prescription. The supply was limited. Most children treated were GH deficient. In 1985, pituitary GH was withdrawn because a few young men treated with pituitary GH in the 1960s and 1970s died of Creutzfeldt–Jakob disease, a slow virus disease similar to kuru and scrapie. It seemed likely that the slow virus particles had contaminated some pituitary GH preparations in the past, and because it was impossible to ensure that this could not occur with later preparations, the hormone was withdrawn from use. Fortunately, studies with recombinant DNA-produced biosynthetic GH were already under way. In October 1985, the first of these was approved for use in GH-deficient children, and in May 1987, a second preparation became available. Several other preparations have also been approved.

Pituitary GH and biosynthetic GH have identical effects. Patients taking biosynthetic GH may have measurable antibodies to GH in low titers. This finding is not clinically significant; no effect on growth rate has been noted.

A GH-deficient child usually grows 3 to 4 inches in the first year of treatment and 2 to 3 inches in each successive year. Catch-up growth to the normal range may be gradual. Recommended doses are different for different preparations. Daily treatment using approximately 0.20 to 0.30 mg/kg/week divided into six or seven subcutaneous injections has supplanted thrice-weekly therapy for many patients because of data documenting better growth rates on daily treatment regimens.

GH has also been approved for use in growth failure associated with chronic renal insufficiency and in Turner syndrome. Use for other diagnostic categories is investigational. It may be modestly effective in helping some children with IUGR grow faster.

Boys with constitutional delay may clearly benefit from treatment with androgens during their teenage years. Low-dose testosterone given by monthly injection for 4 to 6 months can gently accelerate growth, bone age, and spontaneous puberty. Anabolic steroids may be helpful for younger children with constitutional delay, although these are not routinely used.

Some children with mild deficiencies in GH secretion may clinically resemble patients with constitutional delay. Because these patients may benefit from GH treatment, a trial of GH may be considered for patients with subnormal growth velocities and low-normal IGF-1 levels. Children with familial short stature grow at normal velocities and do not need any treatment to help them achieve a genetically appropriate height. Often, parents exert tremendous pressure to intervene in some way and put the child on GH treatment. In some families, the focus on being taller as a cure for all ills suggests the need for psychiatric intervention. Whether GH treatment can increase the adult height of nonGH-deficient short children has not been definitely demonstrated, and this issue remains controversial.

Idiopathic short stature is a leftover diagnostic label for short children who do not fall into any specific diagnostic category. A child who is inappropriately small for the family; who has a negative history, physical examination, and laboratory evaluation; and who does not fit the category of constitutional delay is considered to have idiopathic short stature.

The use of GH treatment in children with constitutional delay, familial short stature, and idiopathic short stature has been studied by several investigators. A national study is under way. In some published studies, as many as 50% of treated children had significant increases in their growth rates. After GH treatment is stopped, the growth rate in many patients decelerates, sometimes to or below the pretreatment growth rate. Data are variable about whether ultimate adult stature is affected. However, for a child who is very short (i.e., height more than 2.5–3.0 SD below normal) and especially one with a subnormal growth rate, a trial of GH treatment may be considered, although, again, this is controversial.

The side effects of biosynthetic GH treatment include development of various degrees of insulin resistance (although hyperglycemia is rare), mild sodium and water retention that is not clinically significant, development of antiGH antibodies that is not clinically significant, and transient lowering of thyroxine levels. Occasionally, slipped capital femoral epiphyses, worsening of scoliosis, and gynecomastia have been reported, but whether these are related to GH treatment remains unclear.

The most concerning issue about GH therapy is the possibility that it could increase the development of malignancies, especially leukemia. Studies in GH recipients do not show an increase in leukemia in those without risk factors (i.e., prior tumors), but a less than twofold overall increase in risk may exist. GH therapy does not increase the risk of recurrence of CNS tumors.

GH-releasing factor, through pulsatile infusion pump or bolus injections, has been shown to stimulate linear growth velocity in GH-deficient children with hypothalamic defects. This approach has not been better than GH treatment in effect and ease of administration. Trials with IGF-1 are ongoing in patients with GH-receptor defects.

Tall Stature and Excessive Linear Growth

Most children with tall stature (i.e., height more than 2 SD above the mean) have familial or genetic tall stature; their parents or other family members are tall. This, like familial short stature, is not pathologic. These children grow above the 95th percentile, but their growth curves are parallel to it. Their linear growth velocities are normal, and their bone ages are normal. Their pubertal growth spurt is normal in timing and magnitude, although they tend to grow in the upper normal velocity percentiles.

Certain syndromes are associated with tall stature and should be sought on examination. Marfan syndrome, cerebral gigantism, homocystinuria, Klinefelter syndrome (XXY), and XYY karyotypes are associated with tall stature.

Nutritional obesity is often associated with tall stature. Obese children typically show linear growth in the upper normal percentiles and may also have bone ages at the upper limits of normal (i.e., approximately 1 to 2 SD above the mean). This growth is in contrast to the weight gain associated with endocrine abnormalities such as hypothyroidism, Cushing disease, and GH deficiency in which linear growth rate is subnormal and bone age is delayed. Endocrine abnormalities can also cause tall stature. Children with hyperthyroidism may have an excessive linear growth rate during the hyperthyroid period, but this finding is not usually a presenting complaint.

GH excess (i.e., pituitary gigantism) causes excessive linear growth rates. GH excess is rare in childhood and adolescence and is usually caused by a pituitary GH-producing tumor or sometimes by excess GH-releasing factor production from a hypothalamic or peripheral tumor such as a pancreatic tumor. Some children with tall stature and excessive linear growth rates have precocious sex hormone secretion caused by central precocious puberty or a variety of gonadal or adrenal abnormalities (see Chapter 205). Children with precocious sex hormone secretion initially have excessive linear growth rates. However, the hormones also cause rapid bone age advancement and early epiphyseal fusion, which compromise adult stature.

High doses of sex steroids can be used to treat tall stature if the predicted adult height is excessive. Patients have been reported with aromatase deficiency that cannot convert androgen to estrogen, and one patient was reported to have an estrogen receptor defect. All have tall stature, lack of epiphyseal fusion, and osteopenia, despite normal or elevated androgen levels. These patients indicate the crucial role of estrogen in stopping linear growth by causing epiphyseal fusion.

CHAPTER 207
Pituitary Disorders

Adapted from Leslie P. Plotnick

DISORDERS OF ANTIDIURETIC HORMONE

Antidiuretic hormone (ADH, vasopressin) is released from the posterior pituitary by neurons originating in the hypothalamic supraoptic and periventricular nuclei. ADH release is mediated through osmoreceptors and baroreceptors, and secretion increases in response to hypovolemia and hyperosmolality. ADH acts by means of the kidney to reabsorb water, which decreases urine volume and increases urine osmolality.

Diabetes Insipidus

Diabetes insipidus is a disorder of subnormal ADH secretion or reduced kidney responsiveness to ADH. Renal responsiveness can be established by monitoring the response to exogenous vasopressin. ADH deficiency may be genetic, but it is more often caused by lesions in the hypothalamic area, commonly tumors and infiltrative disorders such as histiocytosis. Trauma, inflammatory processes, and vascular abnormalities are also causes of ADH deficiency.

ADH deficiency manifests with symptoms of polyuria and polydipsia with large volumes of dilute urine. Symptoms are often dramatic and may be abrupt in onset. The search for an organic cause requires head computed tomographic scans or magnetic resonance imaging, a search for histiocytosis, and an evaluation for dysfunctions of other areas of the hypothalamic-pituitary axis.

The best diagnostic test is water deprivation. This test should be performed under careful observation in a well-hydrated child. Body weight, urine and serum sodium and osmolality, and urine volumes should be measured at baseline, frequently during the test, and at the end of the test. ADH levels can be measured at the onset and conclusion of the test, but the ADH level is not essential for the diagnosis. If serum osmolality and serum sodium values increase above normal in the context of poor urine concentration, the diagnosis of diabetes insipidus is made. A weight loss of a maximum of 5% is allowed. At the end of the water deprivation test, exogenous ADH [injection of aqueous vasopressin or deamino-8-D-arginine vasopressin (DDAVP) or intranasal DDAVP] is given to assess renal responsiveness.

Children with psychogenic or neurogenic polydipsia as the primary problem must be differentiated from those with diabetes insipidus. These children usually have low serum sodium and osmolality. Diabetes insipidus caused by ADH deficiency is treated with exogenous ADH. The best mode of treatment is with intranasal DDAVP, a long-acting analogue of arginine vasopressin. To eliminate nighttime awakening to urinate and drink, treatment begins with low doses that are gradually increased. DDAVP can also be given parenterally. In many patients, DDAVP can be given every 12 hours. An oral DDAVP preparation is now available, but higher doses are needed. Because infant diets have a low solute load, their urine should remain dilute, and long-acting ADH preparations may more readily produce hyponatremia. A shorter-acting spray (e.g., lysine vasopressin; duration, 4–6 hours) can be given before bedtime to produce short-lasting antidiuresis during the night.

An intact thirst mechanism allows patients on ADH preparations to easily regulate their fluid balance on their own, as long as they have free access to water. In the unusual patient with abnormal thirst, regulation becomes difficult, and strict prescriptions of fluid intake must be given.

Syndrome of Inappropriate Antidiuretic Hormone Secretion

Excess endogenous or exogenous ADH without fluid restriction leads to water intoxication: water retention and weight gain, hyponatremia, and production of small amounts of concentrated urine. The typical symptoms are lethargy, weakness, nausea, vomiting, headaches, and seizures.

In children, the most likely causes of the syndrome of inappropriate antidiuretic hormone secretion are intracranial disease (e.g., meningitis), neurosurgery, head trauma, and pulmonary disease. Malignancies producing excess ADH are uncommon in children.

The treatment is fluid restriction. In severe cases, use of hypertonic saline with diuretic therapy (e.g., furosemide) may be indicated. Slow and steady correction is required.

Excess Prolactin Secretion

Prolactin is the one pituitary hormone whose major physiologic control is an inhibiting factor, dopamine. Pathologic processes occur when prolactin is secreted in excess amounts because of a prolactin-secreting pituitary adenoma or when loss of hypothalamic dopamine inhibition occurs because of interruption of normal pathways, especially by trauma, tumors, or infiltrative processes in the hypothalamus. Certain drugs (e.g., phenothiazines, cimetidine, opiates) can cause hyperprolactinemia. Excess prolactin suppresses pituitary LH and FSH secretion and is associated with galactorrhea. The decrease in LH and FSH leads to impotence, oligomenorrhea, amenorrhea, infertility, and delayed puberty.

The diagnosis of excess prolactin secretion is made by finding an elevated prolactin level in a euthyroid, nonpregnant patient. CNS imaging with computed tomographic scans or magnetic resonance imaging and a workup for evidence of other dysfunction of the hypothalamic-pituitary unit is necessary. Very high prolactin levels are usually associated with large tumors.

Treatment options include careful observation, medical therapy with dopamine agonists, and surgery. Dopamine agonists (bromocriptine or cabergoline) are the major therapeutic options, and the response to treatment is rapid. In some cases, bromocriptine therapy has been associated with regression in tumor size. Surgery, especially transsphenoidal for microadenomas, is not uniformly successful, and recurrences are frequent. For patients who do not respond well to bromocriptine or surgery, radiation therapy may be indicated.

CHAPTER 208

Type 1 (Insulin-Dependent) Diabetes Mellitus

Adapted from Leslie P. Plotnick

DEFINITION AND DIAGNOSTIC CRITERIA

Type 1 diabetes is the type most frequently found in children and adolescents. Patients with type 1 diabetes are insulinopenic and need exogenous insulin to prevent ketosis and to preserve life. Type 2 diabetes is most commonly found in adults and obese persons. Primarily, insulin resistance without adequate compensatory insulin secretion causes this type of diabetes. Thus, a relative, not absolute, insulin deficiency occurs. Affected patients are not dependent on insulin for survival or ketosis-prone, but they may need exogenous insulin for metabolic control, and they can develop ketosis in certain situations. Sometimes distinguishing between type 1 and type 2 is difficult at presentation. Other specific types of diabetes occur due to causes including genetic defects in beta-cell function [maturity-onset diabetes in youth (MODY)] and insulin action or are caused by diseases of the exocrine pancreas.

To be diagnosed with diabetes, a child or adolescent must have classic symptoms with a random plasma glucose level at or above 200 mg/dL (11.1 mmol/L). If the patient is asymptomatic, fasting plasma glucose must be at or above 126 mg/dL (7.0 mmol/L) or the 2-hour plasma glucose levels on an oral glucose tolerance test must be at or above 200 mg/dL. The asymptomatic criteria require confirmation by repeat testing (on another day). The diagnosis of diabetes in a child is rarely subtle. Most children present with the classic symptoms of polyuria, polydipsia, polyphagia, weight loss, and lethargy. Glucose tolerance testing is rarely necessary for diagnosis.

Epidemiology

The prevalence of type 1 diabetes in the United States in children and adolescents varies somewhat according to different sources with most studies reporting a rate of 1.2 to 1.9 cases per 1,000 members of the population of this age group. Incidence increases with age and peaks in early to middle puberty. A seasonal distribution of newly diagnosed cases exists: For unknown reasons, more cases are diagnosed in the cooler months. Male and female subjects are approximately equally affected.

Etiology

Beta-cell destruction occurs in genetically susceptible people. At least 80% of the functional beta-cell mass must be destroyed before overt glucose intolerance occurs. The process of beta-cell destruction in most cases is immune-mediated, probably takes months or years, and may be initiated by external, environmental factors. One hypothesis is that the exposure to the environmental factors may be recurrent and intermittent or continuous (e.g., viral infections, dietary factors, environmental toxins, stress) rather than a single triggering event. Viruses or other environmental factors may precipitate beta-cell destruction by direct damage (exposing antigens for future immunologic attack) or by molecular mimicry caused by similar protein sequences in beta-cell antigens and the offending agent (e.g., virus, bovine serum albumin). The damaged beta cell presents antigens recognized as nonself to the immune system. The autoimmune processes release cytokines that are destructive in the beta cells directly or that destroy tissue by generating free radicals because beta cells have low levels of antioxidants.

Most patients with newly diagnosed type 1 diabetes have measurable immunologic markers: islet cell antibodies (ICAs) and insulin autoantibodies (IAAs). ICAs may be cytoplasmic or surface antibodies. High-titer ICAs confer a greater risk of subsequently developing type 1 diabetes than low titers. ICAs are probably more predictive in children, as is the persistence of positivity. Another important immunologic marker is insulin autoantibodies. Insulin autoantibodies in combination with ICA and high-titer insulin autoantibodies are associated with an increased risk of developing type 1 diabetes. Other beta-cell autoantigens including glutamic acid decarboxylase (GAD) have been identified.

Pathophysiology

Insulin is the body's major anabolic hormone. In the fed state, it stimulates energy storage in the forms of glycogen, protein, and adipose tissue. When insulin levels are low or deficient, mobilization of stored substrate occurs (i.e., glycogenolysis, proteolysis, lipolysis) and tissue uptake of glucose is inhibited. Because insulin is a potent antilipolytic hormone, a greater degree of insulin deficiency is required for lipolysis than for glucose intolerance to occur. In the early stages of insulin deficiency, hyperglycemia predominates, and a more severe degree of insulin deficiency is necessary for ketonuria, ketonemia, and acidosis to develop.

In addition to insulin deficiency, a relative excess of counterregulatory hormones (e.g., growth hormone, cortisol, glucagon, catecholamines) must exist to produce the picture of diabetic ketoacidosis (DKA). Hyperglycemia produces an osmotic diuresis causing the symptoms of polyuria and polydipsia. Passive electrolyte loss occurs, along with the osmotic diuresis. Weight loss is caused by the general catabolic state and the osmotic diuresis. Eventually, dehydration results and is especially severe if the child cannot drink enough fluid to compensate for the diuresis, as in the case of vomiting or a decreased level of consciousness. Lipolysis results in ketone production causing metabolic acidosis.

Clinical Presentation

Most children with type 1 diabetes present with the classic symptoms of polyuria, polydipsia, polyphagia, and weight loss; many also complain of lethargy. If the diagnosis is not made and treatment is not begun, further metabolic decompensation occurs with worsening DKA. In young children and infants, the diagnosis is more likely to be missed in its early stages because of difficulty in recognizing early symptoms, and children of these ages are more likely to present with severe ketoacidosis. If pediatricians specifically inquire about the classic symptoms in patients with nonspecific signs of illness and weight loss, this diagnosis is more likely to be made quickly. Early diagnosis avoids further metabolic decompensation and the risks of DKA.

Most children with new-onset type 1 diabetes have symptoms of less than 1 month's duration, but some have had mild to moderate symptoms for several months. Questions about bedwetting, nocturia, number of diapers used, or leaving class to use the bathroom may help uncover polyuria.

Type 1 diabetes must be considered in any child with clinical dehydration who continues to urinate regularly. Too often, frequent urination leads the parent or physician to incorrectly conclude that the child is not dehydrated. Routine dipstick testing for urine glucose and ketones in patients with nonspecific symptoms such as lethargy, weight loss, nausea, and vomiting and in those with specific type-1 diabetes symptoms could greatly enhance the early diagnosis of this disease before severe metabolic decompensation has occurred.

New-onset type 1 diabetes may be managed in an inpatient or outpatient setting depending on the severity of the patient's metabolic abnormalities and the health care resources available.

Management

INSULIN

Regular insulin is rapid acting and is the standard insulin used to rapidly treat hyperglycemia, ketosis, and DKA. A new, faster-acting insulin was approved for use in August 1996. Insulin lispro (Humalog, Eli Lilly) is a biosynthetic analogue of regular insulin and is absorbed and cleared more rapidly than regular insulin and, therefore, more closely mimics pancreatic insulin secretion. It can even be used effectively after a meal in children with unpredictable eating habits. Semilente is another short-acting insulin. Neutral protamine Hagedorn (NPH) or Lente is intermediate in peak and duration of action. Ultralente is a long-acting insulin with duration of more than 24 to 36 hours. However, human Ultralente may have a much shorter duration of action (Table 208-1).

Most children and adolescents require at least two injections per day of short- and intermediate-acting insulin to achieve satisfactory metabolic control; the injections are administered shortly before breakfast and dinner. During the honeymoon period, when insulin requirements are at a minimum, one injection per day may be satisfactory for control (see clinical course). Except for this period, achieving control with a single daily injection is nearly impossible. Absorption may vary from different injection sites and is more rapid in exercised sites and at higher temperatures. Injection into hypertrophied sites may slow absorption.

Frequent blood glucose monitoring is necessary so that patients can respond to the levels by adjusting their insulin doses. For example, if an occasional fasting blood glucose level falls above the target range, the morning short-acting insulin dose should be increased. If the fasting blood glucose level is increased for several consecutive days, the evening NPH dose should be increased.

During the honeymoon period, dose requirements may drop to less than 0.5 U/kg/day. Except during this period, most preadolescent children need approximately 0.75 to 1.00 U/kg/day. Teenagers usually require approximately 1.0 to 1.2 U/kg/day after the first few years of the disease.

TABLE 208-1. Timing of Action of Available Insulins

Insulin	Onset (hr)	Peak (hr)	Usual duration (hr)
Lispro	0.25	0.5–1.0	3
Regular			
Human	0.5–1.0	2–3	3–6
Pork	0.5–2.0	3–4	4–6
NPH/Lente			
Human	2–4	4–10	10–16
Pork	4–6	8–14	16–20
Ultralente			
Human	6–10	Minimal (?)	18–20
Animal	8–14	Minimal	24–36
Mixed (70% NPH, 30% regular)			
Human	0.5	2–12	24

NPH, neutral protamine Hagedorn.

Patients on a twice-daily dosage regimen typically need approximately two-thirds of the total dose in the morning and one-third before dinner. The doses are usually split between one-third short-acting (regular or lispro) and two-thirds NPH to one-half short-acting and one-half NPH. More short-acting insulin is usually required in the morning because of an early morning glucose rise. This early morning glucose increase (i.e., dawn phenomenon) may be caused by normal nocturnal increases in some counterregulatory hormones.

Other insulin regimens may be needed to achieve adequate control. Often, the evening dose must be separated with short-acting insulin given before dinner and NPH at bedtime to maintain adequate insulin levels throughout the entire night and to avoid hypoglycemia during the hours between 1:00 and 4:00 a.m. Sometimes additional short-acting insulin is needed before lunch, although this may be difficult to arrange in a school-aged child (without interfering with his or her school schedule), or before a midafternoon snack.

Ultralente can be used to provide a continuous, fairly steady insulin level with a once- or twice-daily dose with short-acting insulin given before each meal. The use of continuous subcutaneous insulin infusion pumps can be considered in highly motivated and conscientious patients. Short-acting insulin is used for continuous subcutaneous infusion to achieve a continuous basal rate with bolus doses given before meals.

When insulin doses are more than 1.5 U/kg/day and especially when they are at or more than 2 U/kg/day, overtreatment must be considered. Excess insulin doses can worsen control and produce a clinical picture of widely variable blood glucose values. The Somogyi phenomenon is rebound hyperglycemia after hypoglycemia, which may be asymptomatic. This is caused by release of counterregulatory hormones (e.g., catecholamines, cortisol, glucagon, growth hormone) in response to hypoglycemia.

MEDICAL NUTRITION MANAGEMENT

Diet is a cornerstone of diabetes management. Children and adolescents with type 1 diabetes require a nutritionally balanced diet with adequate calories and nutrients for normal growth. The recommended diet usually contains 50% to 55% carbohydrate calories, 20% protein, and approximately 30% fat. Most carbohydrate calories are complex carbohydrates, and the fat portion should emphasize low levels of cholesterol and saturated fats. Timing of meals and snacks should minimize blood glucose variability. In addition to the usual three meals, mid-afternoon snacks are necessary, particularly because they are timed to coincide with the typical peak of the morning NPH insulin dose and with most after-school sports activities.

Bedtime snacks are important for most children receiving evening NPH doses. Mid-morning snacks are useful in preschool-aged children, but most school-aged children find them disruptive to their school routine. This snack is not usually recommended after a child begins elementary school. Occasional treats should be allowed by the diet plan, and patients and families should learn how to adjust insulin doses for times of increased caloric intake such as holidays and birthdays. Calorie control with avoidance of obesity is necessary for certain patients. A sense of satiety and a diet that fits with the family's food preferences are necessary for maximum and realistic adherence to dietary recommendations. The diet should be individualized for each child and family. Nutritional management is complex, especially in sophisticated regimens when carbohydrate counting and insulin-to-carbohydrate ratios are used to determine insulin doses. This regimen is best prescribed by a nutritionist with expertise in diabetes management.

EXERCISE

Physical fitness and regular exercise are important for all patients with type 1 diabetes. Insulin requirements may be lower, metabolic control improved, and self-esteem and body image better in the physically fit child. During periods of exercise, extra calories or lower insulin doses may be needed to prevent hypoglycemia. Blood glucose monitoring to assess the effects of exercise on blood glucose and the response to these therapeutic maneuvers should be performed to arrive at an effective regimen for the individual patient. Regular exercise should be encouraged at any age because it can then become part of the child's health care regimen.

When metabolic control is poor (e.g., the child has hyperglycemia, especially with ketosis), the stress of exercise may worsen metabolic control. Some patients have a delayed hypoglycemic response to exercise and, if this response occurs, adjustments in insulin dose and calories become necessary.

MONITORING

One of the major advances since the late 1970s has been the technique of self-monitoring blood glucose. Numerous reagent strips, glucose meters, and finger-lancing devices are available. Glucose meters are small, portable, and accurate.

Blood glucose is traditionally monitored before meals, before snacks (e.g., mid-morning, mid-afternoon, bedtime), and in the middle of the night at approximately 3:00 a.m., the anticipated lowest nighttime point, if evening NPH is used. Approximately four recorded readings a day usually provide enough information to assess and achieve control. During a period of metabolic instability, more frequent monitoring is necessary. Fasting and preprandial blood glucose readings in the 70 to 150 mg/dL range, postprandial levels of less than 180 to 200 mg/dL, and 3:00 a.m. values greater than 65 to 80 mg/dL indicate good control.

A specified insulin dose is appropriate when the blood glucose values are in this target range. Doses of short-acting insulin can be changed using a sliding scale (Table 208-2) when a specific blood glucose level is outside the target range. For example, if the fasting blood glucose is 50 mg/dL one day, less regular insulin is needed that morning. When patterns outside the target range occur, NPH doses can be adjusted to achieve blood glucose levels in the target range. For example, if fasting values are approximately 50 mg/dL for several consecutive days, the evening NPH dose should be reduced. Most physicians increase the target ranges for infants and small children and aim for blood glucose values less than 200 mg/dL. Blood glucose determinations before lunch and bedtime snacks are necessary to fine-tune short-acting insulin doses.

TABLE 208-2. Example of an Insulin Regimen for a 30-kg Child

	Sliding scale regular dose	
Blood glucose	***Morning (before breakfast) 12 NPH***	***Evening (before dinner) 6 NPH***
<50	3	2
50–100	4	3
100–150	5	4
150–200	6	5
200–250	7	6
250–300	8	7
>300	9	8

NPH, neutral protamine Hagedorn.

The measurement of glycosylated hemoglobin (HbA1c) levels is another major advance in diabetes management. This is an objective level that measures an average blood glucose reading over approximately the previous 2 months. Various methods are available, and normal ranges vary. The method used in the Diabetes Control and Complications Trial (DCCT) had a normal HbA1c range of less than 6.05%. Some patients can achieve values in the normal or near-normal range with relative ease. These children may have some residual endogenous insulin secretion. Diabetes management teams can be successful in helping patients achieve improved HbA1c levels, but some patients may not achieve levels in the goal range.

Urinary ketones should also be monitored. Even patients who monitor blood glucose accurately and regularly need to check urinary ketones, particularly when the blood glucose levels are above 250 mg/dL, when they have a fever, when they feel nauseous or are vomiting, or when they are just not feeling well. This monitoring is important in achieving the goal of aborting DKA episodes by treating early ketosis.

Blood lipids should be monitored periodically. Because type 1 diabetes is associated with other autoimmune diseases, especially thyroid disease, periodic monitoring should be performed (e.g., thyroid antibodies, thyroid-stimulating hormone, thyroxine). Patients should be seen by the health care team approximately every 3 months. Regular monitoring for ophthalmologic complications and for nephropathy are discussed later in this chapter.

EDUCATION

Education is fundamental to diabetes management and control. Patients and families need to understand all aspects of diabetes including acute and long-term complications. They must understand details of insulin action including duration and timing, injection techniques, dietary information, blood glucose monitoring, and urinary ketone checks.

Education must be appropriate to the child's age and the family's educational background, and it must be ongoing. Shifting responsibility from parent to child for diabetes self-care skills (e.g., insulin injections) should be done gradually and when the child shows interest and readiness to do so. Premature shifting of responsibility may be a cause of deterioration in metabolic control. Diabetes management teaching is best handled by a diabetes management team including a physician, nurse educator, dietitian, and psychologist or psychiatric social worker.

CLINICAL COURSE

After the initial presentation, most children with newly diagnosed type 1 diabetes undergo a honeymoon period or remission phase. During this period, the remaining functional beta cells regain the ability to produce insulin, possibly as a result of elimination of hyperglycemia. Measurement of C-peptide levels has demonstrated that improved insulin secretion occurs during this phase. Because endogenous insulin secretion increases, requirements for exogenous insulin decrease, usually dropping to less than 0.5 U/kg/day. Hypoglycemia becomes a potential problem. This phase usually begins within 1 to 3 months after diagnosis and lasts for several months, sometimes as long as 12 to 24 months. The honeymoon period is a period of relative well-being with metabolic normality, as indicated by normal glycosylated hemoglobin levels. Information about the honeymoon period must be included in the education of the newly diagnosed patient, because denial of disease and subsequent failure to monitor are likely to occur, unless patients and families learn about this phase and expect its occurrence and its end. As this phase ends, the remaining beta cells lose their capacity to secrete insulin, and requirements increase for exogenous insulin. This phase usually occurs gradually, but, as in cases of acute infection, it may be abrupt. Careful monitoring and frequent dose adjustments are extremely important during the end of the remission phase, and close contact between the patient and physician is necessary.

COMPLICATIONS

Acute Effects

HYPOGLYCEMIA

Hypoglycemia (i.e., blood glucose less than 50–60 mg/dL) occurs in patients on insulin whether or not they are in tight metabolic control, but it occurs more frequently when blood glucose levels are kept close to normal. Hypoglycemic symptoms may be mild (i.e., adrenergic symptoms of tremors, sweating, hunger, palpitations), moderate (i.e., adrenergic plus neuroglycopenic symptoms of headache, irritability or other mood change, sleepiness, confusion, inattentiveness, impaired judgment, weakness), or severe (i.e., unresponsiveness, coma, convulsions). Mild and moderate reactions can be treated by ingesting simple sugars (i.e., 10–15 g of glucose). Moderate reactions may require assistance by another person and additional carbohydrates. Severe reactions require treatment with intravenous glucose or parenteral glucagon (0.1 mg/kg to a maximum of 1.0 mg intramuscularly or subcutaneously). All patients' families, day-care providers, teachers, coaches, and others should learn the signs and symptoms of hypoglycemia, have a readily available source of glucose to treat it (e.g., a tube of cake frosting), and ideally have and know how to use glucagon injections to treat severe reactions. Evidence suggests that a longer duration of disease and tight metabolic control and more hypoglycemic episodes are associated with a diminished counter-regulatory hormone response to hypoglycemia, and some patients develop hypoglycemic unawareness. These factors increase the risk of severe hypoglycemia. Young children often cannot notify their parents of hypoglycemic symptoms, and goals for metabolic control may need to be loosened. Some concern exists that hypoglycemia may have deleterious effects on learning. Fear of hypoglycemia, particularly after a severe reaction, may cause long-lasting acceptance by patients and families of unacceptably high blood glucose levels (greater than 200 mg/dL).

HYPERGLYCEMIA AND KETOSIS

Patients with type 1 diabetes and their families must learn how to adjust insulin doses to treat the inevitable hyperglycemia that occurs with type 1 diabetes or when to call their health care provider for assistance. Ketosis may occur occasionally or more frequently, and patients must know how to respond.

DIABETIC KETOACIDOSIS

DKA is a common and potentially life-threatening acute complication of type 1 diabetes. DKA is the most common cause of death in patients with type 1 diabetes younger than their mid-20s. Mortality may be as high as 6% to 10%. See Chapter 69 for a complete review of DKA.

SICK DAY MANAGEMENT

Deterioration of metabolic control during infections in children is caused, in part, by the increase in stress or counter-regulatory hormones, which have hyperglycemic and lipolytic effects and produce relative insulin deficiency and requirements for increased insulin. Alternatively, because decreases in caloric intake occur with illness in children, especially with nausea and vomiting, insulin requirements may drop, and hypoglycemia may occur. The goals of sick day management are the prevention and treatment of hypoglycemia and significant hyperglycemia and the prevention of DKA. The physician's advice is essential, as is parental supervision. Sick day management should not be left to a child or teenager. The underlying illness (e.g., infection) needs to be diagnosed and treated. The basis of management includes frequent blood glucose and urinary ketone checks (at least every 4 hours for blood glucose and every void for urinary ketones); insulin adjustment (using short-acting insulin) based on blood glucose levels and urinary ketones; and substitution of equivalent calories of sugar-containing fluids (e.g., soda, fruit juice, jello, popsicles) if the child cannot or will not eat solids. Depending on the type of illness, the insulin dose may be the usual NPH or Lente dose with short-acting insulin doses adjusted up or down for blood glucose levels; a decrease in the NPH or Lente dose with short-acting insulin adjusted for blood glucose levels; or only short-acting insulin given approximately every 4 hours. Persistent vomiting (i.e., several times in a row so that no calories are retained) or refusal to take fluids or food orally requires an emergency department or clinic visit. Glucagon must be available in the home. Supplemental short-acting insulin at doses of 10% to 20% of the 24-hour requirement given every 4 to 6 hours are often effective in preventing significant hyperglycemia and in clearing or preventing ketosis.

Chronic Effects

AUTOIMMUNE DISEASE

Associated autoimmune disease, particularly thyroid dysfunction, occurs with greater frequency with type 1 diabetes. Thyroid function should be monitored periodically (every few years at a minimum) in patients with type 1 diabetes.

JOINT DYSFUNCTION

Limited joint mobility, perhaps caused by glycosylation of tissue proteins, is a marker for long-term poor control and is associated with other complications (e.g., retinopathy, nephropathy, and neuropathy). The hands and other joints should be examined.

GROWTH DISTURBANCE

Linear growth is negatively affected by poor diabetic control. Decreased growth velocity crossing percentiles downward for height and weight, eventual short stature, and delayed skeletal and sexual maturation are associated with chronic under treatment with insulin. An extreme form of this—the Mauriac syndrome, or diabetic dwarfism—rarely occurs and is usually associated with hepatomegaly. Careful height and weight measurements should be obtained at every appointment and plotted on growth curves, so that deviations from normal velocities can be detected early. Alternatively, treatment with excessive insulin doses often leads to excessive weight gain causing the weight curve to cross percentiles upward. The maintenance of normal growth curves for height and weight is an important goal of diabetes management.

RETINOPATHY

Most patients with type 1 diabetes develop background retinopathy after 15 to 20 years of the disease. The percentage of patients developing proliferative retinopathy is less with studies reporting incidences of 20% to 50%. Approximately 5% to 10% of patients with type 1 diabetes become blind. Early treatment with laser photocoagulation can significantly reduce the rate of progression to blindness. All patients with type 1 diabetes should be evaluated annually by an ophthalmologist with regular-interval eye examinations performed by the child's pediatrician and diabetes physician. These yearly examinations should begin within 5 years of the onset of the disease.

NEPHROPATHY

Approximately 30% to 40% of patients with type 1 diabetes eventually develop end-stage renal disease and need dialysis or transplantation. End-stage renal disease is an important cause of morbidity and mortality. Diabetic nephropathy is characterized by proteinuria, which may be severe, producing a nephrotic syndrome, hypertension, initial hyperfiltration (i.e., increased glomerular filtrate rate), and progressive renal insufficiency (i.e., increasing serum creatinine and urea nitrogen, decreasing glomerular filtrate rate). Glomerular damage, especially mesangial expansion and basement membrane thickening, is the most characteristic histologic finding. A genetic predisposition may be an important underlying factor. All patients with type 1 diabetes should be monitored by urine microalbumin, at least, annually after the first few years of the disease but perhaps starting in the first year after the diagnosis. Blood pressure should be monitored accurately several times a year. After hypertension, overt proteinuria, or elevation in serum creatinine or urea nitrogen is found, monitoring of renal function several times each year and consultation with a nephrologist is warranted. Microalbuminuria (less than 200–250 mg/day) is a marker for the early stages of nephropathy. Low-protein diets have been successful in slowing or preventing progression of renal insufficiency in type 1 diabetes, but concerns exist about their use in growing children.

Hypertension is an extremely important factor known to accelerate the progression of nephropathy. It should be aggressively treated. Angiotensin-converting enzyme inhibitors are recommended. Whether using angiotensin-converting enzyme inhibitors to lower blood pressures, already in the normal range, is useful in preventing or retarding nephropathy is not known. Patients should avoid other risk factors such as smoking.

NEUROPATHY

Symptomatic diabetic neuropathy, peripheral or autonomic, is uncommon in children and adolescents with type 1 diabetes, although changes in nerve conduction may be measured after 4 to 5 years of the disease. Overall, neuropathy is a common type 1 diabetes complication, and its frequency increases with the duration of disease and degree of hyperglycemia. Improvements in glycemic control may help neuropathic symptoms. Clinical trials of aldose reductase inhibitors have reported serious side effects.

MACROVASCULAR COMPLICATIONS

Patients with type 1 diabetes tend to have coronary artery, cerebrovascular, and peripheral vascular disease more often, at an earlier age, and more extensively than the nondiabetic population. Hypertension, elevated blood lipid levels, and cigarette smoking are other risk factors for developing macrovascular complications. Risk factor assessment including lipid panels, blood pressure measurements, and determining if the patient smokes should be done, and treatment should be instituted as indicated.

CHAPTER 209
Childhood Obesity

Adapted from William H. Dietz

Childhood obesity has now become the most prevalent nutritional disease of children and adolescents in the United States. Estimates from the third National Health and Nutrition Examination Survey (NHANES III) indicate that more than 20% of children in the United States are overweight. Furthermore, comparison of the prevalence of obesity in NHANES III (completed in 1994) with data from earlier NHANES surveys indicates that the prevalence has increased by more than 30% since 1980. The prevalence of obesity and its association with a variety of morbidities in childhood and adolescence indicate that the prevention of obesity in the nonobese and the treatment of obesity among those who are already overweight must become high priorities for pediatricians.

IDENTIFICATION

A consensus conference has suggested that childhood and adolescent obesity should be identified through the use of the body mass index (BMI; weight in kilograms/height in meters^2) (Fig. 209-1). The BMI appears to be a reasonable index of adiposity because it correlates reasonably well with the percentage of body weight attributable to fat and does not covary with height as much as the weight-for-height index. Furthermore, the National Center for Health Statistics will soon release new BMI tables. The appropriate cut-off points for the identification of obesity will probably remain the 85th and 95th percentiles. The 95th percentile is identified by a BMI of 30 in young adults, which corresponds to grade 2 obesity in adults. Therefore, this approach will make the identification of childhood and adolescent obesity parallel to the criteria used to identify adult obesity.

Because of the concern about spuriously labeling a child as overweight who may have an increased BMI because of an increase in muscle or bone mass, the approach indicated in Fig. 209-1 should be followed in the assessment of a child with an increased BMI. One approach to distinguish children with an increased BMI attributable to fat from those whose BMI reflects an increase in fat-free mass or bone is the measurement of the triceps skinfold thickness. The triceps skinfold thickness provides a relative but direct measure of body fat. If a child has an increased BMI but normal triceps skinfold thickness, the child is likely overweight but not overfat. Both the child and the family should be reassured that the child's increased BMI represents a growth variant, but that continued monitoring is essential. If the child has an increased triceps skinfold thickness, the additional screening tests noted in Fig. 209-1 should be performed to assess whether an associated morbidity exists. Children whose BMI is at the 85th percentile, or children who have had rapid weight gain of more than two BMI units annually, should be considered at risk and followed carefully.

PERIODS OF RISK

Identification of the periods of risk for the development of childhood and adolescent obesity helps identify the times and populations that represent reasonable targets for counseling efforts. Young children at greatest risk for the development of adult

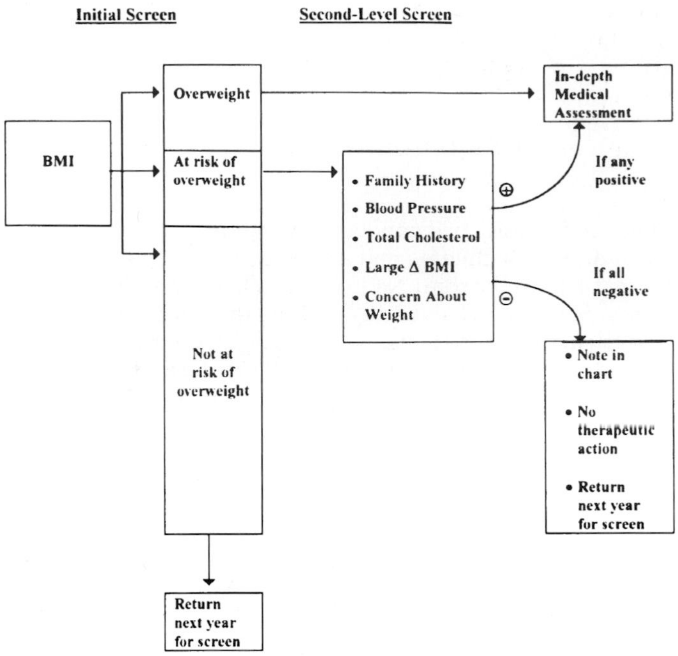

Figure 209-1. Algorithm for the assessment of children with an increased body mass index (BMI). Children with a BMI greater than the 95th percentile should receive in-depth assessment including measurement of the triceps skinfold thickness (TSF) to confirm that the increase in BMI is attributable to an increase in fat. If both the BMI and TSF are increased, a complete history and physical examination are required to exclude the syndromes and complications associated with obesity. Biochemical measures should include a fasting lipoprotein profile, fasting insulin, and urinalysis. Children whose BMI is between the 85th and 95th percentiles require a more detailed history and a close follow-up to ensure that their weight gain does not progress. Children with a BMI between the 85th and 95th percentile who have a family history of obesity, elevated blood pressure or cholesterol, a large change in BMI, or who are concerned about their weight should have an in-depth assessment like that for children or adolescents whose weight exceeds the 95th percentile. (Reprinted with permission from Himes JH, Dietz WH. Guidelines for overweight in adolescent preventive services: recommendations from an expert committee. The Expert Committee on Clinical Guidelines for Overweight in Adolescent Preventive Services. Am J Clin Nutr 1994; 59:307.)

obesity are children of two obese parents, regardless of the weight status of the child. Therefore, counseling with respect to diet and activity for children of two obese parents should begin early. The first important period of risk for persistent obesity independent of the risk of parental obesity is the period of adiposity rebound, which occurs at ages 4 to 6 years in at-risk individuals. After an initial increase in the BMI in the first year of life, the BMI begins to decline and reaches a nadir at 6 to 8 years under normal circumstances. Thereafter, the BMI begins to increase again during what is known as the period of adiposity rebound. Children in whom adiposity rebound begins early are at increased risk for persistent obesity, independent of parental obesity. The factors that begin to operate during the period of adiposity rebound remain uncertain. Factors in early childhood that affect food preference or that alter the regulation of food intake may begin to affect adiposity at this time. Alternatively, because this period often represents the first exposure of the child to environments that affect food or activity outside the home, environmental influences may alter energy balance to promote gains in body fat.

The second period of risk for the development of obesity or its complications is adolescence. Body fat increases in girls during adolescence, whereas body fat decreases in boys. In girls, however, body fat is deposited gluteally, whereas body fat in boys is deposited centrally. Visceral fat deposition increases the risk of a variety of cardiovascular morbidities such as hyperlipidemia, glucose intolerance, and hypertension. The risk of persistent obesity in adolescent girls is, therefore, greater than in boys, but the risk of subsequent mortality associated with obesity in boys is greater than in girls. Morbidity in adulthood associated with adolescent obesity is greater in both genders than in adults who were not obese during adolescence.

ASSOCIATED SYNDROMES AND COMPLICATIONS

The history and physical examination must exclude the causes and associated complications of obesity. The quartet of signs or symptoms that suggest an associated syndrome include dysmorphic features, short stature, impaired vision, and hypogonadism or gonadal dysfunction. Their presence should initiate additional tests to exclude the more common syndromes listed in Table 209-1. At any age, obesity in children or adolescents is associated with an increased frequency of cardiovascular risk factors. Hypertension must be excluded by blood pressure determinations with an appropriately sized cuff. Elevated low-density lipoprotein cholesterol, decreased high-density lipoprotein cholesterol, and hypertriglyceridemia should be sought by a fasting lipoprotein profile. A fasting insulin determination helps exclude glucose intolerance. Children or adolescents with acanthosis nigricans (i.e., hyperpigmentation in specific locations such as the nape of the neck, the axillae, and the groin) are at particular risk for glucose intolerance.

The most urgent complications of obesity include sleep apnea, pseudotumor cerebri, Blount disease (tibia vara), and imminent slipped capital femoral epiphysis. Sleep apnea is characteristically associated with snoring and daytime somnolence. Tonsillar enlargement may contribute to sleep apnea, and a tonsillectomy may be curative. However, obese children should receive careful postoperative monitoring after a tonsillectomy, because postoperative peripharyngeal edema may cause a fatal respiratory obstruction. Headaches and papilledema require a careful workup to confirm pseudotumor and exclude malignancies. Blount disease or bowing of the lower extremities associated with overgrowth of the medial aspect of the proximal metaphysis requires weight reduction to halt the progression of the disease or to prevent recurrence after surgical correction. Slipped capital femoral epiphysis usually presents with hip pain and a limp. The morbidities associated with these complications merit aggressive weight reduction therapy.

Causality

Obesity can only result from an energy intake in excess of energy expenditure. However, whether energy intake is a more important factor than energy expenditure remains unclear.

TABLE 209-1. Syndromes Associated with Childhood Obesity

Alström-Hallgren syndrome
Carpenter syndrome
Cohen syndrome
Laurence-Moon-Biedl syndrome
Polycystic ovary disease
Prader-Labhart-Willi syndrome
Pseudohypoparathyroidism
Turner syndrome

Limitations in the measurement of energy intake and energy expenditure, and the lack of longitudinal measures of each, contribute to our lack of knowledge about these critical features of obesity. Therefore, although the discussion that follows considers logical causal factors, only a limited number of studies link these behaviors to the onset or persistence of obesity.

Studies of dietary intake have focused on the role of dietary fat in the genesis of obesity. Dietary fat is calorically denser than carbohydrate, and in contrast to carbohydrate, increased fat intake is not associated with increased fat oxidation. Therefore, excessive fat intake may predispose to fat deposition. However, the recent increases in the prevalence of obesity in the U.S. population have occurred despite a reduction in the proportion of dietary energy derived from fat. Furthermore, restriction of dietary fat alone in children whose caloric intake was not limited produced no differences in the change in BMI over a 1-year period. Nonetheless, the conclusion that fat plays no role in the genesis or persistence of obesity must be tempered by several limitations of the dietary methodologies. Approximately one-third of an average family's income spent on food is spent on food consumed outside the home. Furthermore, almost 70% of children consume lunch away from home, and almost 20% of children consume breakfast or dinner outside the home. The foods consumed on these occasions, especially if they are fast food or take-out foods, tend to be higher in fat and calories and are often consumed in larger portions than comparable foods that are prepared and consumed at home. A second area that deserves increased attention is the pattern of food intake. Although children who consume a greater quantity of fruit and vegetables should be less likely to become overweight, no data yet link increased fruit and vegetable intake to a reduced risk for the development of obesity. Likewise, no data yet link snack frequency or snack choice to the development of obesity. Family interactions around food constitute a final area of interest and concern. Parental control of the quantity of food intake may impair the ability of the child to regulate energy balance. No population-based studies have examined this variable to determine whether the prevalence of obesity is increased in families in which parents attempt to regulate food intake.

Energy expenditure constitutes the second variable in the energy balance equation. Few definitive studies have examined the link between resting metabolic rate, the energy spent on activity, or total daily energy expenditure and the development of obesity. The few short-term studies that have examined this problem have failed to demonstrate that reductions in any one of these components of energy expenditure place children or adolescents at increased risk for the development of increased adiposity. At the outset of high school, 50% of boys but less than 30% of girls participate in regular vigorous activity. By the end of high school, participation among boys declines slightly, whereas among girls, the rates decline to approximately 15%. Although no data yet link the decline in vigorous activity in girls to the development of obesity during adolescence, the coincidence of the decline in vigorous activity with the period at which the prevalence of obesity increases in girls should not be dismissed.

Inactivity or sedentary behavior appears to represent a domain that is independent of activity. Television viewing represents the most important form of inactivity for children and adolescents in the United States. The average child spends approximately 3 to 4 hours per day watching television. Furthermore, several cross-sectional population studies and one prospective study have linked the amount of time spent viewing television with the development of obesity in children and adolescents. Although children who are watching television are sedentary, the effects of television viewing on obesity may not be attributable to the effects of television on activity. Television viewing also affects food consumption. Advertisements for food constitute the most frequent commercials on children's television programs. Consumption of the foods advertised on television and food consumption while watching television are directly related to the prevalence of obesity. Therefore, the effects of television viewing on the prevalence of obesity may reflect both inactivity and increased food consumption.

The effects of television viewing on obesity suggest that the covariance of behaviors may play an important role in the development of obesity. Several additional studies suggest that this may be the case. In one study, for example, inactivity covaried with a high fat diet and tobacco use. Although adolescent girls may use cigarettes to control their weight, cigarette smoking may also increase the deposition of intraabdominal fat. Whether the effects of cigarette use on abdominal fat can be used to discourage cigarette smoking or whether increases in activity decrease gains in body fat and discourage cigarette smoking has not yet been examined.

PREVENTION AND TREATMENT

The natural history of obesity suggests that several periods in childhood and adolescence should be targeted for prevention. These include infancy, the period of adiposity rebound, and adolescence, particularly in girls. In infancy and early childhood, as previously indicated, the highest risk of obesity occurs in the child whose parents are both overweight, regardless of the weight status of the child. Therefore, families with two obese parents should be targeted for preventive efforts. Although the focus of prevention has not been clearly determined, several logical targets exist. Infants who are breast-fed accept the introduction of new foods more readily than infants who are fed formula. Although not carefully studied, acceptance of a variety of foods by infants may enhance the likelihood that when they are older, children will accept foods such as fruits and vegetables that are likely to reduce the caloric density of the diet. In addition, mothers who are restrained eaters or who try to control the quantity of food that their child consumes have children who are less capable of controlling their own caloric intake. This observation suggests that parents should be in charge of what their children are offered and when, and children can decide whether to eat what is offered or not. Implicit in this division of responsibility is that if children do not decide to eat what is offered, parents are not obligated to offer alternative choices. After children learn that they will be hungry if they do not eat what is offered, it is much more likely that they will consume that food when it is next offered. However, negotiations about food must be conducted in a neutral manner, and failure to accept what is offered should not be met with a punitive response. Otherwise, attitudes about food will likely develop an emotional overlay. Finally, children should not be encouraged to eat, because encouragement may make it less likely that the child will consume the food he or she is encouraged to eat. In each of these areas, parents may need assistance in building the skills necessary to negotiate these developmental steps successfully.

After early childhood, the obesity of the child or adolescent has a greater effect than parental obesity status on the risk of persistence. The two groups at greatest risk for persistent obesity are children with onset of obesity during the period of adiposity rebound and girls during adolescence. At any age, the more severely overweight have an increased risk of persistent obesity.

The first goal of therapy should be weight maintenance. In children whose weight is 20% to 30% in excess of ideal, weight maintenance may be the only therapy required for the child to return to the normal weight range. The goal of weight maintenance may be easiest for the male preadolescent, in whom adolescence is accompanied by a loss of fat and an increase in fat-free mass.

Because the child's dietary choices and exercise patterns occur in a family context, the family must be included in decisions about what modifications are necessary and how they should be implemented. How primary care providers approach families of overweight children is critical. Questions to the family such as "How concerned are you about your child's weight?" help establish whether the family views the child's weight as a serious problem and may help establish their readiness for change. A family that does not view their child's weight as a serious problem should be counseled regarding the potential adverse physical and psychosocial effects of obesity and told that the primary-care provider will be happy to help them if they become more concerned. A question such as "What do you think has made your child overweight?" addresses what the family views as the cause of their child's obesity and moves the discussion toward therapy. A question such as "What changes do you have to make to control your child's weight?" allows the family to begin to define the changes necessary to achieve weight maintenance and, subsequently, weight loss. In families in which adolescents are in conflict with their parents about what and when they should eat, the neutrality of the primary-care provider often provides the successful arbitration that allows an alliance with the adolescent and support for the adolescent's role in self-care.

The same rules that govern the division of responsibility previously outlined apply to the overweight child and adolescent. Careful dietary histories to establish caloric intake are not helpful, because they underestimate food intake. However, dietary histories that focus on the pattern of food intake or the consumption of high-caloric-density snacks may offer specific targets for reduction or elimination. Consumption of foods outside the home at day-care, school, or after-school programs may represent an important source of excess calories in families that carefully control the foods offered at home.

Activity also plays a crucial role in weight maintenance and reduction. Increased activity increases energy expenditure. Although several studies suggest that increases in activity play a modest role in weight reduction, at least one study of adults demonstrated a significant effect of increased activity on weight maintenance. Furthermore, increased activity, particularly resistance training, may reduce the losses of fat-free mass that may accompany weight loss.

As Epstein has clearly demonstrated, reductions in inactivity may be a more effective approach to weight loss in children than efforts to increase activity. In the context of a program that included parents and children and comparable control of caloric intake by the elimination or reduction of specific high-caloric-density foods, a program that reinforced children for the reduction of inactivity produced greater short-term and 1-year weight losses than one that reinforced children for increased activity. In most cases, the reduction in inactivity was achieved by a reduction in television viewing. Furthermore, the attitudes of children toward vigorous activity were more positive among children reinforced for reductions in inactivity than among children reinforced for increased activity. The lack of improvement in attitudes among children reinforced for increased activity may reflect a forced choice. Children who were reinforced for increased activity may have felt pressured to increase their activity and were, therefore, less positive about their choices than children who were reinforced to decrease their inactivity and who chose freely what to do in place of inactivity.

How to achieve increases in activity by advice given in primary-care settings has not been carefully investigated. Parents should be encouraged to limit television time, not only because of the positive effect such limitations have on obesity but also on a wide variety of other behaviors. Furthermore, children must be given opportunities to play. Time with parents walking or playing outdoors is valued by both participants. One important hazard is the guilt that working parents feel when their schedules offer few opportunities for their children to play. In many neighborhoods, safe environments for children do not exist. In these cases, alliances with other groups committed to neighborhood safety and community improvement may help to make schools or other facilities available for children to play after school or on weekends.

Children or adolescents with morbid complications of their obesity such as sleep apnea, Blount disease, slipped femoral capital epiphysis, or pseudotumor cerebri are candidates for rapid weight loss. A consensus on the treatment of the morbidly obese child or adolescent, defined as a body weight 200% of ideal, does not yet exist. In cases where either a morbid complication of obesity or morbid obesity exists, however, referral to a specialist in the treatment of obese children and adolescents is warranted. In such cases, aggressive family therapy used in conjunction with a low-calorie diet such as the protein-modified fast may be warranted.

At present, drug therapy must be reserved for those adolescents with either a morbid complication of obesity or those who have failed more conservative approaches to weight reduction. The experience with cardiac complications associated with the combination of phentermine and D-fenfluramine suggests that if pharmacotherapy is used to treat obesity, a study protocol and informed consent should be required. However, our limited experience with phentermine and D-fenfluramine, and the preliminary data in adults with the pancreatic lipase inhibitor and the serotonin reuptake inhibitor, which are about to be marketed, suggest that only modest weight losses can be expected from these medications. As with more restrictive dietary therapy, the use of medications to treat obesity should be deferred to an obesity treatment specialist.

9 Inborn Errors of Metabolism

CHAPTER 210 Introduction to Inborn Errors of Metabolism

Adapted from Rebecca S. Wappner and Bryan E. Hainline

DEFINITION

Inborn errors of metabolism are genetically determined abnormalities in the biochemical processes of the body. Most often, a single defective protein disrupts a metabolic pathway at a specific step leading to excessive accumulation of immediate or precursor substrates and deficiency of immediate and subsequent products of the reaction.

Individual disorders result from point mutations, deletions, or other alterations of DNA or RNA processing. Defects may

TABLE 210-1. Clinical Manifestations of Inborn Errors of Metabolism

	General type of disorder								
Clinical manifestation	*AA*	*OA*	*UREA*	*FAO*	*MIT*	*CARB*	*PER*	*MPS*	*SL*
Episodic nature	++	++	++	++	+	+	−	−	−
Poor feeding	+	+	++	+	+	+	+	−	−
Abnormal odor	+	+	−	+	−	−	−	−	−
Lethargy, coma	+	++	++	++	+	+	−	−	−
ALTE	+	+	+	+	+	+	−	−	−
Seizures	+	+	+	−	+	+	+	+	+
Developmental regression	+	+	+	−	+	−	+	++	+
Hepatomegaly	+	+	+	+	+	+	+	+	+
Hepatosplenomegaly	−	−	−	−	−	−	−	+	+
Splenomegaly	−	−	−	−	−	−	−	−	+
Hypotonia	+	+	+	+	+	+	+	+	+
Cardiomyopathy	−	+	−	+	+	+	+	+	+
Coarse facies	−	−	−	−	−	−	−	++	+
Birth defects	−	+	−	+	+	−	+	−	−
Hypoglycemia	+	+	−	+	+	+	−	−	−
Acidosis	+	++	−	+	+	+	−	−	−
Hyperammonemia	+	+	++	+	+	−	−	−	−
Ketosis	+	+	−	+	−	+	−	−	−
Hypoketosis	−	−	−	+	−	−	−	−	−

++, usually present; +, may be present; −, usually not present; AA, amino acidopathies; ALTE, acute life-threatening event; CARB, disorders of carbohydrate; FAO, mitochondrial fatty acid oxidation defects; MIT, mitochondrial disorders of oxidative phosphorylation; MPS, mucopolysaccharidoses; OA, organic acidopathies; PER, peroxisomal disorders; SL, sphingolipidoses; UREA, disorders of the urea cycle.
Adapted from Wappner RS. Biochemical diagnosis of genetic diseases. *Pediatr Ann* 1993;22:283.

occur in nuclear-encoded genes located on the autosomes or X chromosome or in mitochondrial DNA. Most disorders produce abnormalities in a single enzyme protein, but a regulatory, protective, or activator protein for the enzyme can be involved. Other inborn errors may be due to faulty transport of molecules. Occasionally, several enzymes may be affected giving a composite clinical picture incorporating features of several enzyme deficiencies. Conversely, identical clinical phenotypes may be seen with mutations in different proteins.

Most of the disorders are inherited as autosomal recessive traits. Some are inherited as X-linked conditions, whereas others show maternal, or mitochondrial, inheritance.

CLINICAL PRESENTATION

Clinical presentation varies widely. The disorders affecting essential pathways often present with early, severe disease (i.e., urea cycle defects or organic acidemias). Others disorders are indolent and associated with the gradual onset of organomegaly (i.e., Gaucher disease) or neurologic impairment (i.e., phenylketonuria). Still others are benign and result in no significant clinical problems (i.e., iminoglycinuria or pentosuria). Inborn errors of metabolism may present at any age with mild variants of all forms reported in adolescents and adults.

Often, the pattern of clinical findings suggests the pathway affected. Acidosis and hyperammonemia (with clinical features of encephalopathy, coma, or death) occur in disorders involving amino acid or organic acid metabolism. Disorders of fatty acid oxidation and carbohydrate metabolism present with lethargy, encephalopathy, and hypoglycemia at times of decreased carbohydrate intake or fasting. Hepatomegaly and hypotonia are frequently noted. Lactic acidosis, cardiomyopathies, myopathies, and other neurologic symptoms are commonly seen with mitochondrial disorders. Lysosomal storage disorders are characterized by progressive hepatomegaly, splenomegaly, neurologic regression, short stature, and coarse facies. Frequently, patients with peroxisomal disorders have dysmorphic features and neurologic problems. Other inborn errors present with only psychomotor handicaps.

A history of cyclic vomiting and lethargy, especially if related to intake of protein or specific carbohydrates, should arouse suspicions, as should repeated episodes of apparent life-threatening events. A family history may possibly reveal similarly affected individuals or unexplained early infant deaths.

Table 210-1 lists patterns of clinical findings associated with certain groups of the disorders.

ACUTE METABOLIC DISEASE

In addition to life support measures, metabolic derangements of acidosis and hypoglycemia should be corrected. This may require hemodialysis or hemofiltration. All sources of protein should be stopped, and the patient should be given only glucose as the carbohydrate source. Vitamins or cofactors for the suspected disorder may be given after diagnostic specimens are obtained. Consultation with a specialist in metabolic disorders should be requested at this time.

Samples for diagnostic testing are most helpful when obtained during the symptomatic period. Urine organic acid analysis, plasma amino acid analysis, and other specialized tests are now widely available through reference labs. Further molecular genetics testing such as mutational analysis or linkage studies are often warranted.

If the patient is gravely ill and time does not allow consultation with a metabolic specialist, samples of frozen plasma or serum (2 mL or more) and frozen urine (10 mL or more), along with dried blood filter-paper dots (as used for newborn screening) should be collected. If the affected patient dies, quick-frozen samples of muscle and liver should also be obtained, preferably within 1 hour of death, and should be stored without preservative at −70°C. In addition, a skin biopsy for cultured fibroblasts should be performed, and the sample should be placed in a sterile container without preservative or in tissue culture media. Then the samples may be used for diagnostic testing after consultation with the metabolic specialist.

CHAPTER 211

Disorders of Amino Acid and Organic Acid Metabolism

Adapted from Rebecca S. Wappner

DISORDERS OF PHENYLALANINE AND TYROSINE METABOLISM

Phenylalanine and tyrosine are precursor amino acids for important compounds such as thyroid hormone, neurotransmitters, and melanin. Phenylalanine is an essential amino acid (it cannot be synthesized in the body). Tyrosine may be synthesized from phenylalanine. Both phenylalanine and tyrosine are present in natural foods. The metabolism of phenylalanine and tyrosine is shown in Fig. 211-1.

Phenylketonuria

Phenylketonuria (PKU) results from deficient activity of phenylalanine hydroxylase (PAH). It occurs in 1 in 12,000 births and is seen most frequently among persons of white and Asian backgrounds. Affected patients appear normal at birth. Untreated, they gradually develop severe mental retardation, microcephaly, hyperreflexia, seizures, autistic-appearing behaviors, eczematoid-appearing rashes, and pigment dilution over the first few years of life.

Untreated patients have markedly elevated blood and urine levels of phenylalanine, which interfere with brain growth and myelination. Phenylalanine metabolites such as phenylacetic acid and phenylpyruvic acid (known also as phenylketones) are also elevated. Increased levels of phenylacetic acid will result in a "mousy" body and urine odor.

Presently, newborn screening for PKU occurs throughout the United States. Neonates with positive screening should be promptly referred to a program that specializes in PKU care for confirmation and treatment of their disorder. Control of blood phenylalanine levels before age 1 month leads to the most favorable prognosis. Once it has occurred, loss of intellectual potential is not regained on treatment. Foods low in or devoid of phenylalanine, yet containing tyrosine, are used. Small amounts of phenylalanine are given, as it is necessary for growth. Keeping the phenylalanine level within the recommended range requires measurement of blood phenylalanine and frequent dietary adjustments.

As a group, treated PKU patients have a mean IQ approximately one-half of a standard deviation lower than that of their peers. A significant number of older treated children are also affected with learning disabilities and behavioral problems.

Dietary control of blood phenylalanine levels including the use of special medical foods is needed indefinitely for optimal function. Children and adolescents who discontinue the special diet have increasing problems with "executive" planning skills, school performance, and behavior.

PKU is inherited as an autosomal recessive trait. Multiple mutations have been found at the PAH gene site on chromosome 12q22–q24.1. Many individuals with PKU are, in fact, compound heterozygotes for two different mutations. Carrier detection and prenatal diagnosis are available by using molecular genetic techniques in families in whom the exact mutation or polymorphisms at the PAH locus are known.

Certain mild variants of PKU allow a nearly normal dietary phenylalanine intake and do not require the use of special medical foods. Blood phenylalanine levels are elevated persistently (greater than 2 mg/dL) but are lower than the levels seen with classic PKU.

The offspring of women with uncontrolled PKU during pregnancy have a significantly increased risk for cardiac malformations, microcephaly, psychomotor retardation, poor prenatal and postnatal growth, and an unusual facies similar to that seen with fetal alcohol exposure. The psychomotor development of the offspring has been shown to be inversely related to the mother's blood phenylalanine level during pregnancy. All offspring of

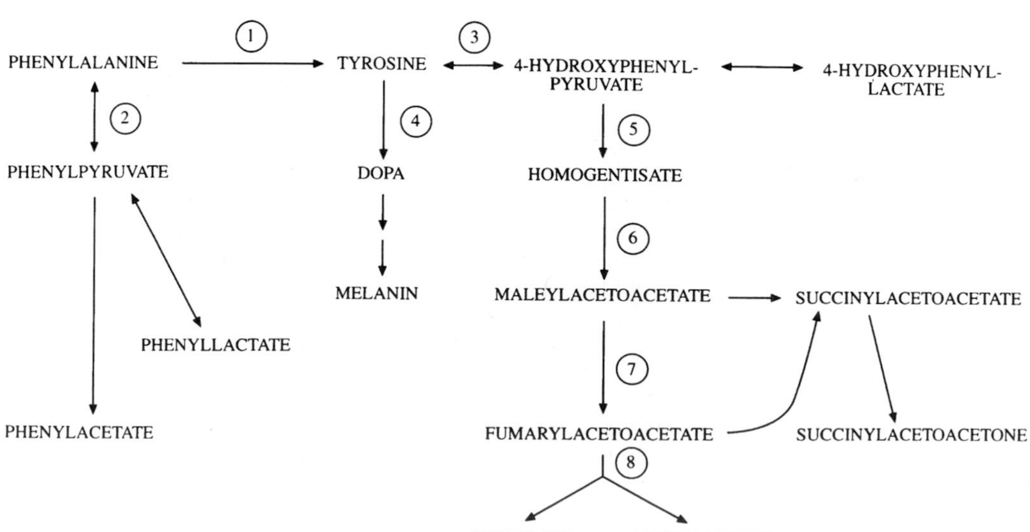

Figure 211-1. Metabolism of phenylalanine and tyrosine. 1, phenylalanine hydroxylase; 2, phenylalanine aminotransferase; 3, tyrosine aminotransferase; 4, tyrosine hydroxylase; 5, 4-hydroxyphenylpyruvate dioxygenase; 6, homogentisic acid oxidase; 7, maleylacetoacetate isomerase; 8, fumarylacetoacetate hydrolase. DOPA, 3,4-dihydroxyphenylalanine.

PKU mothers will be carriers for PKU; approximately 1 in 150 offspring will also have PKU depending on the carrier status of the father.

Tyrosinemia

TYROSINEMIA TYPE I

Hepatorenal tyrosinemia, also known as hereditary tyrosinemia or tyrosinemia type I, results from deficient activity of fumarylacetoacetate hydrolase (FAH). The disorder is inherited as an autosomal recessive trait. In the general population, it occurs in 1 in 100,000 to 120,000 births. Clinical manifestations of tyrosinemia result from elevated levels of succinylacetone and succinylacetoacetone, which accumulate as a result of the deficient FAH activity.

Progressive hepatic synthetic dysfunction starts in infancy. Elevated transaminase levels and jaundice may be seen with some patients developing hepatic failure by 1 year of age. Others may have acute hepatic crises with rising liver enzymes, jaundice, ascites, and possible gastrointestinal bleeding. Although acute hepatic crises are most likely to occur during infancy, they can happen at any age. Affected patients who survive early infancy develop progressive macronodular cirrhosis. Developing hepatic nodules may transform into hepatocellular carcinoma, which occurs in approximately 18% of patients older than age 2 years. Liver transplant may be necessary.

Most affected children with tyrosinemia are developmentally normal. Psychomotor regression is rare unless acute hepatic encephalopathy develops from hepatic failure. Patients can, however, develop acute episodes of neurologic crisis that begin as painful paresthesias with autonomic symptoms sometimes occurring. Repeated neurologic crises may lead to chronic weakness.

Varying degrees of renal tubular dysfunction can occur. Nephromegaly is noted in 80% of patients with nephrocalcinosis in 33%.

Special dietary therapy devoid of or low in phenylalanine, tyrosine, and methionine, along with limited amounts of natural protein, results in improved tyrosine levels. However, diet therapy alone will not stop the production of succinylacetone, prevent the progression of liver and kidney disease, or reduce the risk for neurologic crises or hepatocellular carcinoma. Treatment with 2-(2-nitro-4-trifluoromethylbenzoyl)-1,3-cyclohexanedione (NTBC), an inhibitor of 4-hydroxyphenylpyruvate dioxygenase, reduces succinylacetone production and should be started, along with dietary therapy, once the disorder is confirmed. Even with NTBC therapy, affected patients may still go on to develop hepatocellular carcinoma and might require liver transplantation.

Newborn screening for tyrosinemia type I is done by measurement of tyrosine or succinylacetone levels in dried blood filter-paper cards. For confirmation, elevated levels of urinary succinylacetone and succinylacetoacetone may be demonstrated with special gas chromatography–mass spectroscopy techniques. Deficient activity of FAH may be documented in erythrocytes, peripheral blood lymphocytes, or liver biopsy samples. Mutations in the FAH genetic locus on chromosome 15 have been shown in affected patients.

TYPE II TYROSINEMIA

Oculocutaneous tyrosinemia, also known as type II tyrosinemia or the Richner–Hanhart syndrome, is associated with deficient activity of tyrosine aminotransferase and inherited as an autosomal recessive trait. Although symptoms usually start during the first year of life, late presentations may be seen. Affected patients develop a corneal dystrophy with erosions, ulcerations, opacities, and plaques. Painful, hyperkeratotic plaques develop on the palms and soles and are occasionally seen at the elbows, knees, and ankles. Approximately one-half of affected patients have psychomotor handicaps. Levels of tyrosine and tyrosine metabolites are elevated in body fluids. Treatment with a lowered tyrosine and phenylalanine diet typically results in clinical improvement. Deficient activity of tyrosine aminotransferase may be shown in liver biopsy samples. Usually, affected patients will be detected by newborn tyrosinemia screening that uses measurement of tyrosine levels.

DISORDERS OF TRANSSULFURATION

The transsulfuration pathway is shown in Fig. 211-2. Methionine, an essential amino acid, is converted to homocystine and is subsequently metabolized through cystathionine and cystine to inorganic sulfur, which is excreted from the body. Homocystine may also be remethylated to methionine by two pathways, which use either 5-methyltetrahydrofolate or betaine as methyl donors for the reaction. Because the demand for methyl groups is often greater than the amount that dietary methionine can supply, at least one-half of the homocystine produced from methionine is remethylated to methionine.

Homocystinuria

Homocystinuria may occur as a result of cystathionine synthase deficiency. It may also be the result of defects in the remethylation pathway catalyzed by methionine synthase, which converts homocystine to methionine.

Cystathionine Synthase Deficiency

Classic homocystinuria is associated with deficient activity of cystathionine synthase. The disorder is inherited as an autosomal recessive trait and has an incidence of approximately 1 in 344,000 births. Elevated levels of methionine and homocystine with low cysteine levels are found in affected patients. These patients appear normal at birth, then, because of elevated homocystine levels, slowly develop features of the disease during early childhood. Interference in the cross-linkage of collagen leads to dislocated lens, osteoporosis, scoliosis, and a marfanoid body habitus. Most patients are tall with long, thin extremities. In contrast to Marfan syndrome, they often have decreased range of motion at the elbows and knees (Fig. 211-3). Elevated homocystine levels disrupt the vascular endothelium and thrombus formation leading to pulmonary emboli, myocardial infarctions, and cerebrovascular accidents can occur at any age. The average intelligence quotient is 64 and patients may have unusual personalities, behavioral problems, and other neuropsychiatric problems.

Plasma and urine amino acid determinations will show elevated levels of methionine and homocystine and lowered levels of cystine. Deficient activity of cystathionine synthase may be shown in lymphocytes or in skin fibroblasts.

Treatment is aimed at reducing homocystine levels and normalizing cystine levels. Methionine-free medical foods with added cystine help to accomplish this. Betaine as a methyl donor for remethylation of homocystine can also be used. Treatment is indicated for life.

Approximately 50% of patients with homocystinuria have residual cystathionine synthase activity and, thus, less severe clinical manifestations of the disorder. Many of these patients have normal intelligence. Some of these patients are responsive to high dose pyridoxine.

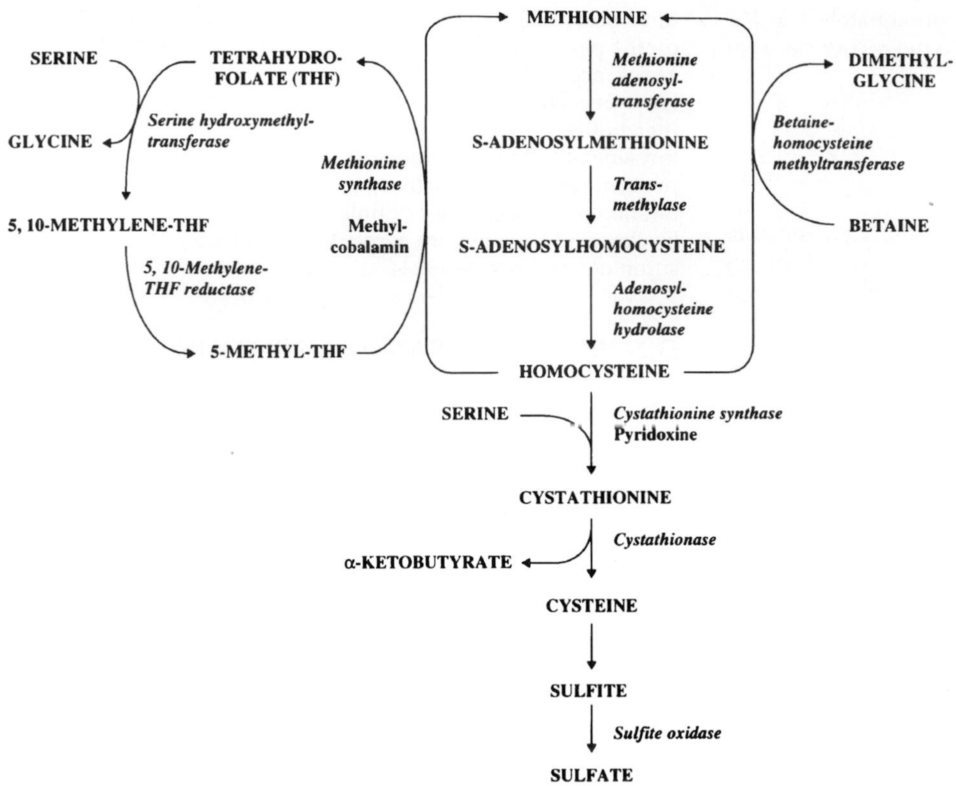

Figure 211-2. The transsulfuration pathway.

The gene that encodes for cystathionine synthase (CBS) is located at chromosome 21q22.3. At least 17 mutations in the CBS gene have been reported. Some of the mutations are associated with pyridoxine responsiveness. Carrier detection may be performed if the mutation or polymorphisms at the CBS locus are known. Prenatal diagnosis is available.

Newborn screening for homocystinuria is performed in some states and in Europe by testing blood methionine levels in dried blood filter-paper samples. Due to slow rise in methionine, the levels in a particular patient at the first newborn screen may not be high enough. A second newborn screen may be necessary. Affected infants started on dietary therapy in early infancy may have complications such as psychomotor handicaps and dislocated lenses prevented or delayed in onset. It is not clear if early dietary treatment prevents thrombotic risks as patients age.

HOMOCYSTINURIA DUE TO REMETHYLATION DEFECTS

Patients with homocystinuria may have deficient activity of methionine synthase or inherited disorders in folate or cobalamin metabolism that affect methionine synthase activity. Homocystine levels are elevated but, to a degree, less than that seen with cystathionine synthase deficiency. Methionine levels are low or normal. Cystathionine levels may be elevated. Usually, progressive central nervous system disorders are seen, in addition to features of classic homocystinuria. All the disorders are inherited as autosomal recessive traits. Prenatal diagnosis is available. Carrier detection may be performed if the mutation or polymorphisms at the genetic loci involved are known. Nutritional deficiencies of folate or cobalamin may result in similar biochemical and clinical abnormalities.

DISORDERS OF AMMONIA METABOLISM

Excess dietary or waste nitrogen is typically converted to urea by a series of reactions known as the urea cycle (Fig. 211-3). Disorders of the urea cycle are associated with the accumulation of ammonia and its precursors, which can lead to cytotoxic

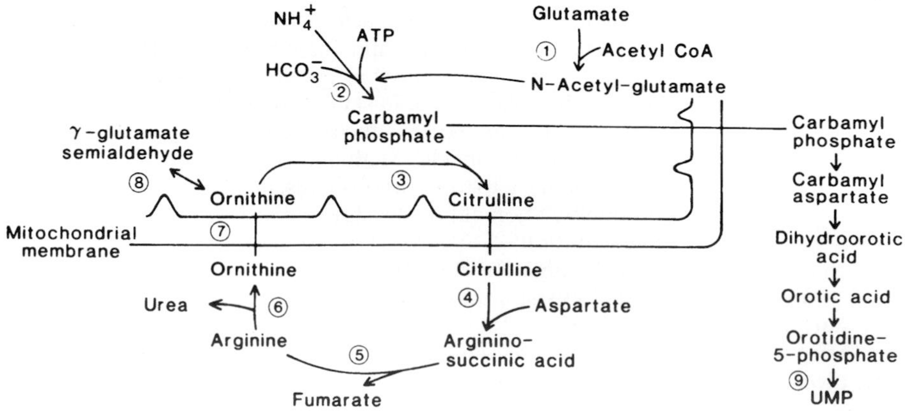

Figure 211-3. Urea cycle. 1, N-acetylglutamate synthetase; 2, carbamyl phosphate synthetase I; 3, ornithine transcarbamylase; 4, argininosuccinate synthetase; 5, argininosuccinate lyase; 6, arginase; 7, mitochondrial ornithine transport defect (hyperammonemia-hyperornithinemia-homocitrullinuria); 8, ornithine aminotransferase; 9, decarboxylase, site of allopurinol block in pyrimidine pathway; ATP, adenosine triphosphate; CoA, coenzyme A; UMP, uridine monophosphate.

changes in the brain and liver. As ammonia rises, patients develop poor feeding, anorexia, behavioral changes, irritability, vomiting, lethargy, ataxia, and seizures. Eventually, coma, apnea, circulatory collapse, and cerebral edema ensue. A classic case of hyperammonemia is a neonate who appears asymptomatic for 24 to 48 hours and then develops progressive neurologic deterioration. Milder forms of urea cycle defects may present later in life with either an acute decompensation or as the underlying etiology of neurologic and psychomotor findings in older children and adults.

As a group, the disorders are estimated to occur in approximately 1 in 30,000 live births. All the disorders of ammonia metabolism are inherited as autosomal recessive traits, except for ornithine transcarbamylase (OTC) deficiency, which is inherited as an X-linked trait, and transient hyperammonemia of the newborn, which is not thought to be entirely genetic.

The diagnosis of a specific urea cycle disorder is made on the basis of the pattern of plasma and urine amino acid abnormalities and the presence or absence of orotic aciduria. Confirmation of specific enzymatic deficiencies requires erythrocytes, cultured skin fibroblasts, or liver biopsy. Molecular genetic studies can confirm the diagnosis and aid in carrier detection.

Treatment of acute hyperammonemia is a medical emergency. During the first episode, blood and urine samples should be collected for testing, but treatment should not be delayed. All exogenous protein sources should be stopped and intravenous glucose should be given to prevent protein catabolism. Hemodialysis or hemofiltration is often needed to quickly reduce ammonia levels. The duration of time in coma is inversely related to outcome. Therefore, prompt referral to a tertiary medical center is indicated for all of these patients.

Drugs that use alternate pathways for waste nitrogen excretion such as sodium benzoate and sodium phenylacetate may be used intravenously to control acute mild to moderate hyperammonemia (less than 350 μmol). These drugs can also be used enterally to maintain plasma ammonia levels within the normal range. Sodium benzoate combines with glycine to form hippurate. Sodium phenylacetate combines with glutamine to form phenylacetylglutamine. Both products are rapidly excreted by the kidneys.

Once hyperammonemia is resolving (less than 100 μmol), medical foods, free of protein or with protein content composed of only essential amino acids, are given to meet basic caloric and other nutrient needs. Specific amino acids with L-citrulline or L-arginine are given for relative insufficiencies of these amino acids and to "prime" the urea cycle.

Even with aggressive medical therapy, only 30% to 50% of neonates who develop hyperammonemic coma survive the neonatal period. Most of those who do survive have neurologic deficits. Later acute episodes, usually precipitated by intercurrent infections or excessive protein intake, can also lead to further neurologic sequelae or death. Liver transplantation, done before significant neurologic impairment has occurred, has been shown to correct the biochemical abnormalities in children affected with severe forms of carbamyl phosphate synthetase I and ornithine transcarbamylase deficiencies.

Carbamyl Phosphate Synthetase I Deficiency

Carbamyl phosphate synthetase I (CPS I) is a mitochondrial enzyme that catalyzes the formation of carbamyl phosphate from ammonia, adenosine triphosphate, and bicarbonate in the presence of N-acetylglutamate. N-acetylglutamate, a critical cofactor for this reaction, is formed from acetyl CoA and glutamate in the presence of N-acetylglutamate synthetase. Inhibition of N-acetylglutamate synthetase by organic acids, especially propionic acid, is thought to be the reason for the secondary hyperammonemia seen with organic acidurias.

Most patients with CPS I deficiency (less than 10% of normal CPS I activity) present with neonatal hyperammonemic coma. Partial deficiencies with 10% to 25% of normal enzyme activity have been reported with later onset of symptoms. Treatment includes a fairly restrictive daily protein intake, medical foods with only essential amino acids, L-citrulline, and either combined sodium benzoate and sodium phenylacetate or high-dose phenylbutyrate. The disorder is inherited as an autosomal recessive trait. The gene that encodes for CPS I, located at chromosome 2q35, has been cloned and sequenced.

Ornithine Transcarbamylase Deficiency

OTC deficiency, the most common of the urea cycle disorders, is inherited as an X-linked trait. Usually, affected male individuals present as neonates with severe hyperammonemia. Less severely affected male patients with 10% to 25% of normal enzymatic activity have a disorder of later onset. Many patients die, despite aggressive management. For those who survive, therapy includes restricted protein intake, medical foods with only essential amino acids, L-citrulline, and either combined sodium benzoate and sodium phenylacetate or high-dose phenylbutyrate. The enzymatic deficiency may be confirmed with liver biopsy or by molecular genetic studies.

Female individuals who are heterozygous for OTC deficiency have a wide clinical spectrum ranging from being affected as severely as hemizygous affected male individuals to being asymptomatic. The degree of relative lyonization (random X chromosome inactivation) in hepatocytes of normal and abnormal OTC genes in female individuals determines the clinical severity of their disease.

Female relatives of affected patients should be evaluated to determine whether they are carriers for OTC deficiency. At least 50 mutations at the OTC locus at chromosome Xp21.1 have been identified. Molecular genetic techniques are also available for both carrier detection and prenatal diagnosis in families with known mutations or polymorphisms at the OTC locus.

Transient Hyperammonemia of the Newborn

Patients with transient hyperammonemia of the newborn present with symptomatic hyperammonemia during the first 2 days of life. Often, they are premature infants who rapidly develop respiratory distress, lethargy, and coma. Frequently, plasma ammonia levels are massively elevated (2,000–4,000 μmol). For individuals who survive, recurrent hyperammonemia is rare, even with a normal protein intake. The etiology for the disorder is unknown but may be related to a transient immaturity of the urea cycle.

DISORDERS OF BRANCHED-CHAIN AMINO ACID METABOLISM

The branched-chain amino acids (BCAA) leucine, isoleucine, and valine are essential amino acids needed for protein synthesis and growth. The metabolism of the BCAA is illustrated in Fig. 211-4. Most disorders of BCAA cause metabolic acidosis from accumulation of organic acids. Secondary inhibition of the urea cycle with hyperammonemia may occur. Bone marrow depression may result in neutropenia, thrombocytopenia, or pancytopenia. The severe forms of the disorders present early with life-threatening illness. Less severe forms present at later

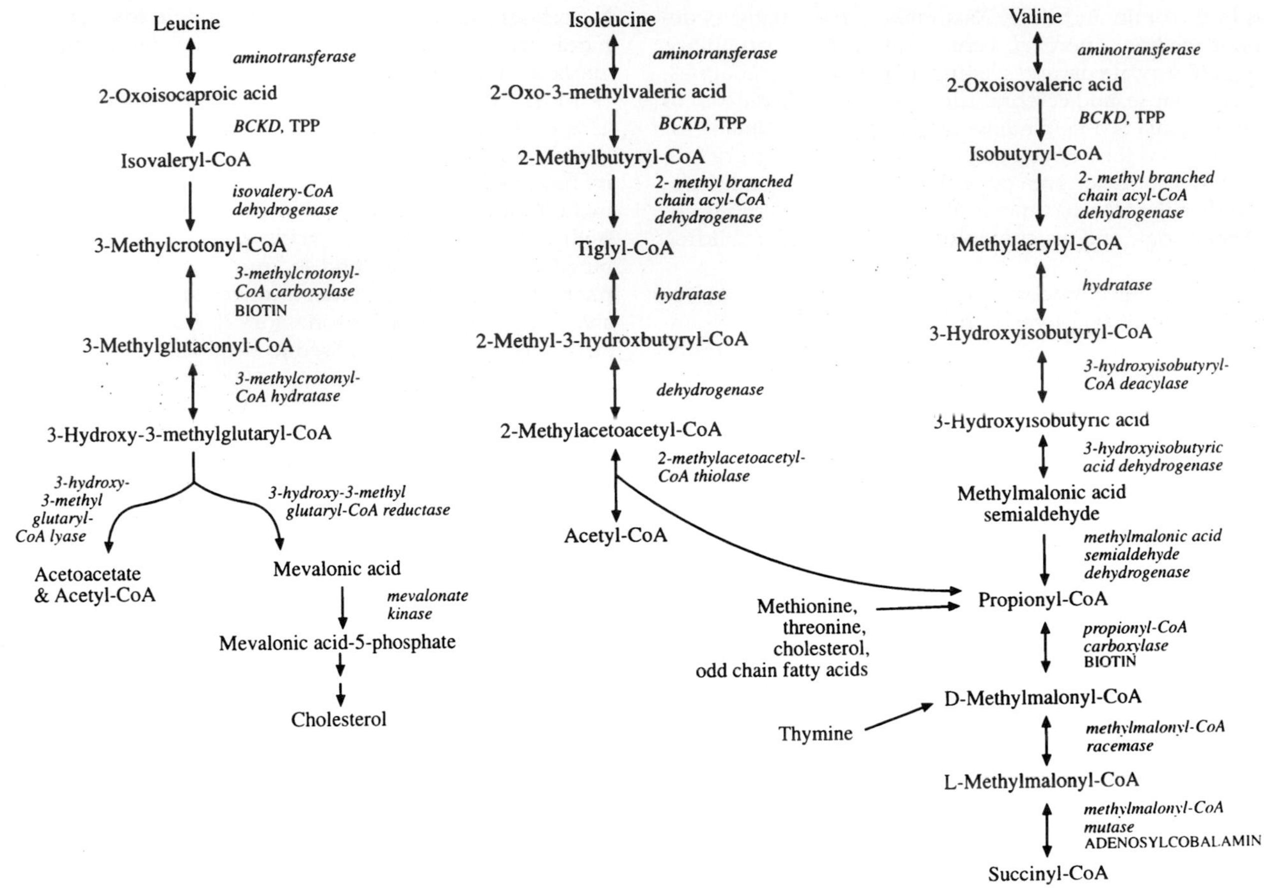

Figure 211-4. Metabolism of the branched-chain amino acids. BCKD, branched-chain alpha-ketoacid (2-oxoacid) dehydrogenase complex; CoA, coenzyme A; TPP, thiamine pyrophosphate.

ages with psychomotor handicaps, seizures, episodic lethargy or vomiting, or acute metabolic decompensation with intercurrent illness. Maple Syrup Urine Disease is discussed below.

Maple Syrup Urine Disease

MSUD occurs in approximately 1 in 200,000 births. It is most common among the Mennonites of eastern Pennsylvania, in whom it has an incidence of 1 in 176. MSUD results from deficient activity of the branched-chain amino acid alpha-ketoacid dehydrogenase (BCKD) complex.

Patients with MSUD have elevated levels of the BCAA leucine, isoleucine, and valine and their corresponding alpha-ketoacids (BCKA), 2-oxoisocaproic acid, 2-oxo-3-methylvaleric acid, and 2-oxoisovaleric acid, respectively. The disorder derives its name from the 2-oxo-3-methylvaleric acid, which has an odor similar to maple syrup or burnt sugar.

MSUD exists in five forms. The most common, classic form presents early in life with poor feeding, irritability, lethargy, alternating hypotonia and hypertonia, abnormal movements, and seizures, which progress to cerebral edema and coma. Severe metabolic acidosis and ketosis occur, often with hyperammonemia and hypoglycemia. Even with aggressive therapy, many infants affected with the disorder do not survive the neonatal period. Those who do are at risk for subsequent acute episodes of metabolic decompensation with intercurrent illnesses or other times of decreased caloric intake.

Milder forms of MSUD occur in patients with some residual enzymatic activity of the BCKD complex. An intermediate form presents most often after the newborn period with failure to thrive, vomiting, ataxia, and psychomotor handicaps. Biochemical findings will be milder but similar to those seen with classic MSUD. Treatment of acute episodes and long-term management are similar to those for classic MSUD. For crises, this consists of glucose, electrolytes, and bicarbonate (if indicated) to correct acidosis. Hemofiltration or hemodialysis may be required to correct the acidosis or hyperammonemia. Enteral feedings with special medical foods or intravenous hyperalimentation with special amino mixtures devoid of the BCAA are then used. Maintenance therapy includes the use of special medical foods devoid of the BCAA. Limited amounts of natural protein to supply leucine requirements, along with small amounts of valine, and, occasionally, isoleucine are given to maintain plasma BCAA within the recommended measured treatment range.

Newborn screening for MSUD is available in some areas of the United States. Most programs test for leucine levels in dried blood filter-paper samples. Mutations in genes that encode for the three major components of the BCKD complex have been demonstrated in patients with MSUD. Carrier detection is available for those families in whom the genetic mutation or polymorphisms are known.

CHAPTER 212
Disorders of Mitochondrial Fatty Acid Oxidation

Adapted from Bryan E. Hainline
and Rebecca S. Wappner

FATTY ACID METABOLISM

During normal fasting, mitochondrial beta-oxidation of fatty acids is an important source of energy. After long-chain fatty acids are mobilized from adipose tissue, they are transported, bound to albumin, the liver and other tissues, where plasma membrane uptake is mediated by fatty acid–binding proteins. The fatty acids are "activated" to their coenzyme A (CoA) esters by long-chain acyl-CoA synthase, transported across the mitochondrial membrane by a carnitine-mediated system, and oxidized to ketone bodies in the mitochondrial matrix. Disorders involving mitochondrial beta-oxidation of fatty acids are characterized by faulty ketone body formation, impaired energy production, and the accumulation of partially oxidized fatty acid metabolites during periods of stress and fasting. The disorders have widely varying clinical manifestations. All are inherited as autosomal recessive traits.

As shown in Fig. 212-1, long-chain (C10–C25) fatty acids are activated by long-chain acyl-CoA synthase (located in the outer

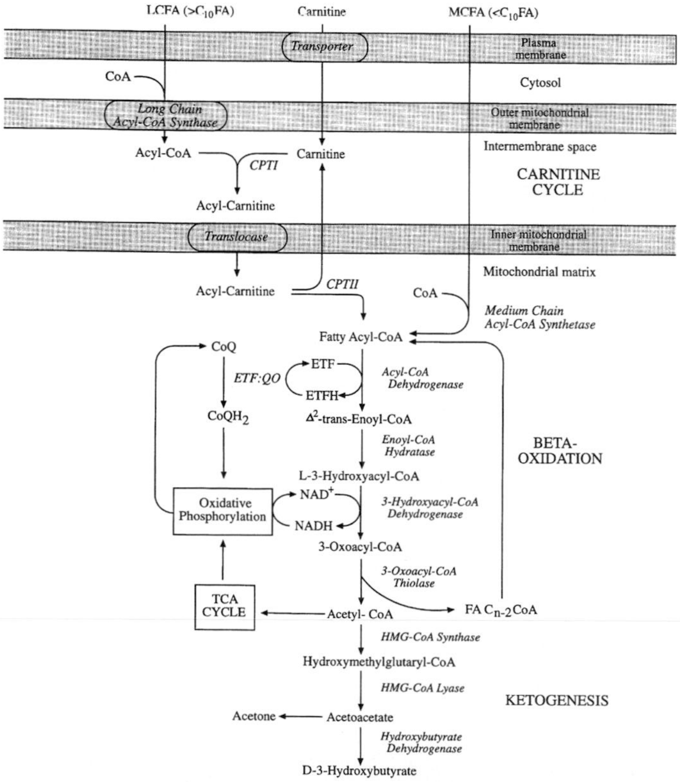

Figure 212-1. Mitochondrial metabolism of fatty acids. C, carbon length; CoA, coenzyme A; CoQ, coenzyme Q; $CoQH_2$, reduced coenzyme Q; CPT, carnitine palmitoyl transferase; ETF, electron transport flavoprotein; ETF:QO, ETF:ubiquinone oxidoreductase; FA, fatty acid; LCFA, long-chain fatty acids; MCFA, medium-chain fatty acids; NAD^+, oxidized form of nicotinamide adenine dinucleotide; NADH, reduced form of nicotinamide adenine dinucleotide; TCA, tricarboxylic acid (citric acid).

mitochondrial membrane) to form long-chain acyl-CoA esters. Then the esters are transesterified with carnitine by carnitine palmitoyl transferase (CPT) I, which resides on the inner aspect of the outer mitochondrial membrane. The long-chain acylcarnitines (and nonesterified carnitine) cross the inner mitochondrial membrane by a process mediated by carnitine-acylcarnitine translocase. On the matrix side of the inner mitochondrial membrane, the long-chain acylcarnitines are reesterified to long-chain acyl-CoA esters by a separate transferase, CPT II. Medium-chain (C6–C12) and short-chain (C4 and C6) fatty acids do not need carnitine-mediated transport to transverse the membranes. They are "activated" to their respective acyl-CoA esters by medium- or short-chain acyl-CoA synthases (synthetases) located in the mitochondrial matrix before entering the beta-oxidation pathway. With each cycle through the pathway, the fatty acid–CoA ester is reduced in length by two carbons to form an acetyl-CoA group that can be metabolized further to ketone bodies in the liver and kidneys or can enter the tricarboxylic acid cycle in heart and skeletal muscle. The beta-oxidation pathway includes a series of chain length-specific acyl-CoA dehydrogenases: enoyl-CoA hydratases, 3-hydroxyacyl-CoA dehydrogenases, and 3-oxoacyl-CoA thiolases. The four acyl-CoA dehydrogenases are flavoproteins that transfer electrons from acyl-CoA esters to electron transfer flavoprotein (ETF) and, subsequently, to the mitochondrial electron transport chain to form adenosine triphosphate. Very long-chain acyl-CoA dehydrogenase (VLCAD) is a membrane-bound protein that catalyzes the oxidation of fatty acids with chain lengths of 16 to 24 carbons; long-chain acyl-CoA dehydrogenase (LCAD) catalyzes the reaction for 12- to 18-carbon fatty acid esters; medium-chain acyl-CoA dehydrogenase (MCAD) catalyzes the reaction for chain lengths of 4 to 14 carbons; and short-chain acyl-CoA dehydrogenase (SCAD) catalyzes the reaction for chain lengths of 4 or 6 carbons. Fatty acid acyl-CoA esters with odd chain lengths are similarly oxidized until a three-carbon propionyl-CoA is formed. Unsaturated fatty acids require additional enzymes, long- and short-chain 3-cis, 2-trans-enoyl-CoA isomerase and 2,4-dienoyl-CoA reductase, for complete beta-oxidation of these compounds. An enzyme related to SCAD may be responsible for oxidation of branched-chain substrates. The long-chain activities for enoyl-CoA hydratase, 3-hydroxyacyl-CoA dehydrogenase, and 3-oxoacyl-CoA thiolase exist as a "trifunctional" protein complex. Individual soluble enzymes with short-chain enoyl-CoA hydratase, short-chain 3-hydroxyacyl-CoA dehydrogenase, and 3-oxoacyl-CoA thiolase activities have been found in the mitochondrial matrix.

The acetyl-CoA and acyl-CoA esters formed as a result of beta-oxidation that exit the mitochondrial matrix by carnitine-mediated transport similar to that for the entrance of long-chain acyl-CoA esters. Acetyl-carnitine is formed by carnitine acetyltransferase and is transported by the translocase to the cytosol.

ETF and ETF:ubiquinone oxidoreductase (ETF:QO) are proteins that mediate the transfer of electrons from flavin-containing acyl-CoA dehydrogenases (i.e., VLCAD, LCAD, MCAD, SCAD, and others) to the main respiratory chain at the level of ubiquinone (coenzyme Q). The energy of these electrons is used for the formation of adenosine triphosphate and the ultimate reduction of molecular oxygen to form water.

L-Carnitine (gamma-trimethyl-beta-hydroxy-butyrobetaine) is needed for transport of long-chain fatty acid acyl-CoA esters into the mitochondrial matrix and for the return of acyl-CoA intermediates to the cytosol. L-Carnitine also functions to remove the metabolites of faulty beta-oxidation and certain other abnormal organic acids from the mitochondrial matrix by forming carnitine esters with these compounds. The abnormal acylcarnitine compounds are then transported to the cytosol, from which they exit the cell, enter the circulation, and are excreted in the urine. Usually, plasma carnitine measurements are reported as total, free, and esterified in micromolar concentrations. In some patients with disorders of beta-oxidation or organic acidemias, both the total and free carnitine levels are low. In other patients, the total plasma carnitine level is normal, but the esterified fraction is abnormally high (greater than 40% of total carnitine). This condition results in a relative deficiency of free carnitine, which is needed for appropriate fatty acid transport.

Dietary sources of carnitine include meats and dairy products. Endogenous carnitine may be synthesized from methylated lysine, which can be derived from muscle proteins such as myosin. Usually, secondary carnitine deficiency states are associated with organic acidemias or faulty beta-oxidation. Deficiencies may also be seen in patients with renal tubular disorders, vitamin C and pyridoxine deficiencies, strict vegetarian diets, total parenteral nutrition, hemodialysis, and valproate anticonvulsant therapy.

Systemic carnitine deficiency, regardless of its etiology, results in faulty fatty acid oxidation and has been associated with poor tolerance of fasting, hypoketotic hypoglycemia, liver dysfunction, hypotonia, myopathies, cardiomyopathies, and recurrent myoglobinuria and myalgias.

DISORDERS OF FATTY ACID OXIDATION

Medium-Chain Acyl-CoA Dehydrogenase Deficiency

MCAD deficiency, the most common of the disorders of fatty acid oxidation, occurs in approximately 1 in 13,000 births. This disorder is seen almost exclusively in whites. Most patients present between ages 5 and 24 months with vomiting, lethargy, and hypotonia that occur after a decreased carbohydrate intake associated with an intercurrent illness or fasting. Hypoglycemia, mildly elevated blood ammonia, and increased liver enzyme levels are usually noted. Any acidosis is usually mild. Urine and plasma ketones may be either absent or inappropriately low (but detectable) for the degree of hypoglycemia and elevation of free fatty acids.

Some patients are identified by screening or clinical presentation in the newborn period, while others may remain asymptomatic for long periods of time. Metabolic crises are characterized by a deteriorating course that progresses from encephalopathy to coma and death from cardiorespiratory collapse or cerebral edema. Approximately 25% of patients die with their first episode. This disorder may be misdiagnosed as Reye Syndrome, sepsis, or sudden (unexplained) infant death syndrome. Autopsy findings include fatty infiltration of the liver and abnormal appearance of mitochondria on electron microscopy.

With episodes, affected individuals accumulate metabolites of medium-chain length (C6–C12), especially octanoic acid and 4-decanoic acid. As a result of the excessive accumulation of fatty acyl-CoA intermediates of medium-chain length in the mitochondria, alternative pathways of microsomal (omega and $omega_1$) oxidation and peroxisomal beta-oxidation become involved and lead to excessive production of $omega_1$-hydroxy acids and medium-chain dicarboxylic acids such as adipic, suberic, and sebacic acids. Organic acid analysis may detect these metabolites in the blood or urine of patients during episodes. Acyl-CoA compounds may be conjugated with glycine and carnitine. Abnormal metabolites of medium-chain length may be detected by urinary acylglycine conjugates (stable isotope dilution gas chromatography–mass spectrometry) or by plasma or dried blood filter-paper sample acylcarnitine profiles.

Between episodes, asymptomatic affected patients may have normal routine organic acid studies. However, urine acylglycine or dried blood filter-paper or plasma acylcarnitine profiles are usually abnormal. Frequently, affected patients have abnormal plasma and urinary carnitine levels with lowered total and elevated esterified fractions. Such patients should not be subjected to a provocative fast because of the possibility of inducing a fatal acute episode. The use of acylcarnitine profiles from dried blood filter-paper samples has not only allowed identification of asymptomatic affected children but has also led to retrospective diagnosis in children who have died including several affected newborns. Deficient activity of MCAD in cultured skin fibroblasts may be shown by finding disease-specific labeled metabolites by tandem or electrospray mass spectrometry assay after feeding with carbon 14- or deuterium-labeled palmitate or linoleate.

Molecular genetic analysis of the MCAD gene has led to localization of the gene on chromosome 1p31 and elucidation of the underlying mutations. A common point mutation at position 985 of the MCAD cDNA (K304E) is present in approximately 90% of patients with the disorder. Twenty-one less common mutations account for the remaining alleles. Confirmation of the disease and determination of carrier status for the common mutation may be performed using DNA extracted from dried blood filter-paper samples. Prenatal diagnosis may be done by molecular genetic techniques or by using the labeled-metabolite assay.

The basis for treatment is the avoidance of fasting and lipolysis. Frequent meals or feedings with a high carbohydrate and relatively lowered fat intake is recommended. Medium-chain triglyceride (MCT) oil in any form should be avoided. Treatment should be started as soon as the diagnosis is considered, even if test results are not yet available. The prescription form of L-carnitine supplementation is indicated in symptomatic patients. Once the disorder is recognized and treated, many patients do well. However, residual neurologic dysfunction from severe episodes will persist.

Long-Chain Hydroxyacyl-CoA Dehydrogenase and Trifunctional Protein Deficiency

In isolated LCHAD deficiency, symptoms of nonketotic hypoglycemia, carnitine deficiency, cardiomyopathy, liver dysfunction, pigmentary retinopathy, muscle weakness, and peripheral neuropathy may be seen. Affected patients may present with sudden and rapid circulatory collapse. Other patients experience a later onset of symptoms including muscle weakness, rhabdomyolysis, progressive hypotonia, and fatty infiltration of the liver.

During pregnancy, mothers carrying children affected with LCHAD may develop acute fatty liver of pregnancy (AFLP) syndrome or HELLP (*h*ypertension, *e*levated *l*iver enzymes, *l*ow *p*latelets) syndrome. All children born of mothers with either AFLP or HELLP syndrome during pregnancy should be evaluated for LCHAD.

With episodes, affected patients excrete 3-hydroxydicarboxylic acids and 3-hydroxymonocarboxylic acids. Plasma or dried blood filter-paper acylcarnitine profiles are abnormal. Plasma carnitine levels reveal elevated esterified fractions. The defective enzyme activity and abnormal metabolites can be demonstrated in cultured skin fibroblasts in a manner similar to those discussed for the foregoing disorders. Treatment includes avoidance of fasting and prompt treatment of episodes. Treatment with L-carnitine and MCT supplementation is also indicated.

CHAPTER 213
Disorders of Carbohydrate Metabolism

Adapted from Rebecca S. Wappner

CARBOHYDRATE METABOLISM

Dietary carbohydrate polymers and disaccharides are hydrolyzed to monosaccharides by enzymes in the brush border of intestinal villi. The free monosaccharides—glucose, galactose, and fructose—are then absorbed and transported to the liver, where they are used rapidly. Glucose may be formed by the metabolism of dietary carbohydrates, from degradation of glycogen, or by gluconeogenesis from amino acids, glycerol, and lactate. All sources for free glucose must be converted to glucose-6-phosphate except for that resulting from the action of debrancher enzyme on glycogen. In addition to being used for free glucose, glucose-6-phosphate may also be used for glycogen synthesis; for glycolysis and the production of lactate and CO_2 by the Embden–Meyerhof pathway; for the production of the reduced form of nicotinamide adenine dinucleotide and CO_2 by entering the pentose cycle; and for glucuronate formation. The major disorders of carbohydrate metabolism involve the intermediary metabolism of glycogen, galactose, and fructose.

DISORDERS OF GLYCOGEN SYNTHESIS AND DEGRADATION

Glycogen Metabolism

Glycogen, the principal storage form of carbohydrate in humans, is found primarily in liver and muscle. Glycogen is synthesized from glucose-1-phosphate by the actions of three enzymes (Fig. 213-1). Uridine diphosphate (UDP)-glucose pyrophosphorylase combination converts glucose-1-phosphate to UDP-glucose. Glycogen synthetase catalyzes the transfer of glucosyl residues from the UDP-glucose to a glycogenin protein molecule to form a glycogen primer. Glycogen synthetase also catalyzes the attachment of additional glucosyl residues in alpha-1,4-linkage to lengthen the chains. The brancher enzyme, amylo-1,4-1,6-transglucosylase, creates the branch points by attaching glucosyl residues in alpha-1,6-linkage to the linear chains.

Glycogen degradation involves sequential removal of nonreducing terminal glucosyl residues by a phosphorylase system and the debrancher enzyme. Phosphorylase exists in both inactive (b) and active (a) forms. Conversion of the phosphorylase

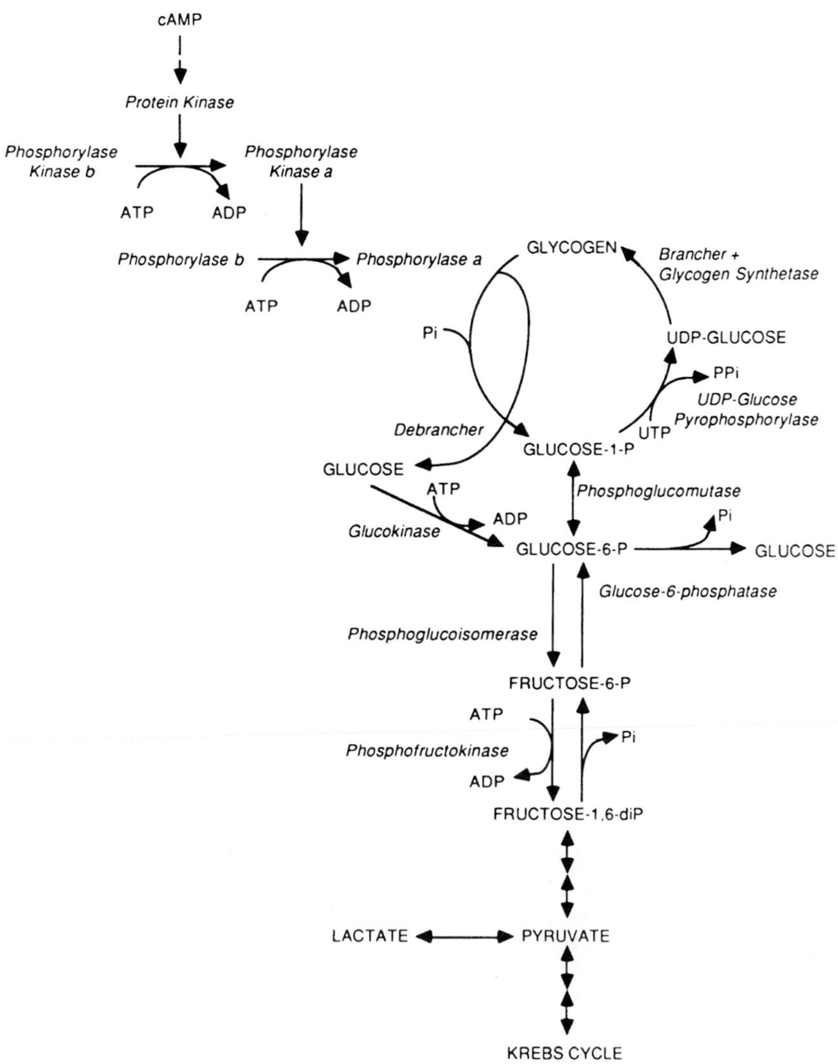

Figure 213-1. Glycogen synthesis and degradation. ADP, adenosine diphosphate; ATP, adenosine triphosphate; cAMP, cyclic adenosine monophosphate; diP, diphosphatase; P, phosphatase; Pi, inorganic phosphate; PPi, inorganic pyrophosphate; UDP, uridine diphosphate; UTP, uridine triphosphate.

to the active form requires the presence of adenosine triphosphate (ATP) and active phosphorylase kinase. Phosphorylase kinase also exists in inactive (b) and active (a) forms and is activated in the presence of ATP by a protein kinase generated in response to increased cyclic adenosine monophosphate (cAMP) formation from hormonal and chemical influences on the hepatic parenchymal cell plasma membrane. The activated phosphorylase a cleaves the alpha-1,4-linkages of the outer chains to within four glucosyl residues of the branch points and liberates glucose-1-phosphate. Then debrancher enzyme is needed for further degradation to proceed. Debrancher functions both as a transferase, which moves the three outermost glucosyl residues to another linear chain, and as an amylo-1,6-glucosidase, which then removes the final glucosyl residue in branched alpha-1,6-linkage with liberation of free glucose. In this manner, approximately 10% free glucose and 90% glucose-1-phosphate is released. The glucose-1-phosphate is converted to glucose-6-phosphate by phosphoglucomutase. Then, glucose-6-phosphate is converted to free glucose and inorganic phosphate by the glucose-6-phosphatase system.

The active site of microsomal glucose-6-phosphatase is located within the lumen of the endoplasmic reticulum. Substrates and products of its activity, thus, must cross the endoplasmic reticulum membrane. Six different proteins are now recognized to be necessary for normal hepatic glucose-6-phosphatase activity. The catalytic subunit of glucose-6-phosphatase hydrolyzes glucose-6-phosphate. A "stabilizing protein" for the catalytic subunit is also needed for enzymatic activity; the stabilizing protein is a regulatory calcium-binding protein. At least four microsomal transport proteins are also involved. The microsomal transport protein T1 transports glucose-6-phosphate, the substrate for the reaction, into the lumen of the endoplasmic reticulum. Transport proteins T2-alpha and T2-beta transport inorganic phosphate and inorganic phosphate, pyrophosphate, and carbamyl phosphate, respectively, across the microsomal membrane and out of the lumen, where they would inhibit glucose-6-phosphatase activity. Further, transport protein GLUT7 (formerly termed T3), one of a family of proteins that transport glucose across plasma membranes, transports free glucose from the lumen to the cytosol.

The synthesis and degradation of hepatic glycogen are regulated primarily by cAMP, glucose, and glycogen. An increased demand for blood glucose results in increased activation of phosphorylase and suppression of glycogen synthetase activity. Hepatic glycogen functions as a reserve for blood glucose. In contrast, muscle glycogen functions mainly as a fuel reserve for ATP generation, which is needed during exercise and usually does not contribute to blood glucose levels. Under anaerobic conditions, muscle glycogen can also be degraded to lactate by glycolysis.

Glycogen storage disorders may have primarily hepatic or muscle involvement.

Hepatic Glycogen Storage Disorders

The hepatic glycogen storage disorders are estimated to occur in at least 1 in 60,000 births. All of these disorders cause some degree of hepatomegaly and (usually) hypoglycemia. The presence of fasting hypoglycemia, the response to glucagon in the fasting and fed state, the response of blood glucose to the administration of other carbohydrates such as galactose, and the type of glucose response noted with a glucose tolerance test may be used to help differentiate between the disorders. All fasting and tolerance testing should be done with caution and close observation of the patient. For the severe disorders, the presence of lactic acidosis and hypoglycemia may be considered a relative contraindication to proceeding with fasting, glucagon stimulation, and other tests in the classic fashion. Liver and muscle biopsies may be performed to assess the total content of glycogen and the type of glycogen structure present and to document deficient activity of specific enzymes. Most important is that an experienced laboratory be contacted before obtaining the samples to ensure appropriate handling. Because many of the disorders may be documented by enzymatic analysis or by molecular genetic techniques in leukocytes, erythrocytes, or cultured skin fibroblasts, these less invasive procedures should be performed first, if possible.

All the disorders are inherited as autosomal recessive traits except for three forms of type IX glycogen storage disease (GSD), which are inherited as X-linked traits. Carrier detection and prenatal diagnosis vary, depending on the tissue distribution of the enzyme involved and whether molecular genetic testing is available for the specific disorder.

Type Ia (von Gierke Disease)

Type Ia GSD, also known as hepatorenal GSD, is associated with deficient activity of glucose-6-phosphatase in liver, kidney, and intestine. Patients have a defective catalytic subunit of the enzyme. Affected individuals experience marked hepatomegaly, lactic acidosis, and hypoglycemia. The disorder is diagnosed most often between ages 3 and 4 months but may be recognized in the neonatal period. Milder forms may present at later ages with hepatomegaly and short stature. Other clinical features include a doll-like appearance, decreased muscle mass, renal enlargement, vomiting, diarrhea, and failure of maturation in puberty. Many affected infants are obese, as a result of demanding frequent feedings, including nocturnal feedings beyond the time this behavior usually disappears.

Fasting hypoglycemia may be profound and often demonstrates clinical symptoms in the untreated patient. This tolerance of hypoglycemia is thought to be the result of the ability of these patients to use alternative substrates for glucose in the brain. Glucose-6-phosphatase is essential for the normal release of hepatic free-glucose, whether it is the product of glycogenolysis or gluconeogenesis. Dietary carbohydrates other than glucose also cannot be converted to glucose because the conversion involves glucose-6-phosphatase as the final step. The fasting hypoglycemia results in activation of phosphorylase and hepatic glycogenolysis, which leads to the formation of glucose-6-phosphate. The glucose-6-phosphate is then metabolized to lactate by glycolysis. Gluconeogenesis is also stimulated, and a recycling between lactate and glycogen occurs resulting in a net increase in lactate. Stimulation of the glycolytic and gluconeogenic pathways also results in elevated triglyceride, cholesterol, very low-density lipoprotein, free fatty acid, and uric acid levels. Xanthomas, lipemia retinalis, gout, and uric acid nephropathy may occur.

Liver transaminases are normal or only slightly elevated. Within the liver parenchyma, adenomatous nodules may develop, which, before current dietary therapy, were occasionally reported to transform into hepatic carcinoma. Abnormal bleeding tendencies that occur are thought to result from decreased platelet adhesiveness associated with the hypoglycemia. Hypercalcuria and, occasionally, renal tubular dysfunction may be present during childhood. Frequently, adults develop progressive renal disease including focal segmental glomerulosclerosis and interstitial fibrosis.

Because patients with type I GSD frequently become hypoglycemic after 2 to 3 hours of fasting, any tolerance or stimulation test should be done cautiously and with intravenous glucose at hand. Glucose tolerance testing gives a diabetic-type early response. Fasting insulin levels are low. No glycemic response to galactose occurs (1–2 g/kg of 20% solution, orally or intravenously). Glucagon stimulation (20–30 μg/kg intramuscularly or intravenously; maximum dose, 1 mg) will, occasionally, produce a response, which is defined as a rise in blood glucose of 50% more than baseline. Lactic acid levels will rise with fasting and with glucagon or galactose administration. Glycogen content is elevated in liver, kidney, and intestine. Glycogen structure is normal. On liver biopsy, the hepatocytes are noted to have glycogen in the nuclei and lipid droplets of varying size in the cytoplasm. Cirrhosis is not evident. The diagnosis may be confirmed by demonstrating a recognized mutation at the glucose-6-phosphatase gene locus in peripheral leukocytes or by measurement of glucose-6-phosphatase in liver or intestinal biopsy samples. Prenatal diagnosis and carrier detection are readily available only in families in whom the molecular defects are known.

Treatment is directed at supplying continuous exogenous glucose. Infants are given a formula with glucose or glucose polymers as the only carbohydrate source. Older children are given similar enteral supplements and are restricted in their intake of natural sources of galactose and fructose. Frequent daily feedings every 2 to 3 hours are supplemented with nocturnal nasogastric or gastrostomy drip feeding. Uncooked cornstarch slurries may be used with older children and adults. Clinical and laboratory improvement is remarkable with dietary therapy. Usually, hepatic adenomas regress. Long-term survival is possible. However, affected patients continue to be at risk for significant acidosis and hypoglycemia with intercurrent illnesses or if enteral feedings are interrupted. Renal transplantation has been performed for renal failure. Liver transplantation has been shown to correct attendant biochemical abnormalities and should be considered if malignant transformation of adenomas occurs.

Muscle Glycogen Storage Disorders

TYPE V GLYCOGEN STORAGE DISEASE (McARDLE DISEASE)

Types V GSD affects only muscle. It is associated with deficient activity of muscle phosphorylase. Elevated muscle glycogen content and the enzymatic defect may be demonstrated on muscle biopsy. With exercise, the increased requirement for ATP requires glycogenolysis. As the enzymatic defect occurs in the glycolytic pathway, affected patients are noted to have increased fatigability. Between ages 20 and 40 years, severe muscle cramps, myoglobinuria, and elevated blood levels of lactate dehydrogenase, aldolase, and creatine kinase are noted with exercise. After age 40, the cramps and myoglobinuria are less evident, but muscle wasting and weakness appear with increasing severity. Skeletal muscle biopsy reveals increased glycogen deposits in the cytoplasm beneath the sarcolemma. Treatment involves avoidance of strenuous exercise, which may result in myoglobinuria and acute renal failure.

DISORDERS OF GALACTOSE METABOLISM

Galactose Metabolism

Galactose, the major dietary carbohydrate in infants, must be converted to glucose to be used as an energy source. This conversion occurs primarily in hepatocytes by the Leloir pathway. Galactose is first phosphorylated to galactose-1-phosphate by a specific galactokinase. The galactose-1-phosphate then reacts with UDP-glucose to form UDP-galactose and glucose-1-phosphate in the presence of galactose-1-phosphate uridyl transferase. UDP-galactose is converted to UDP-glucose by UDP-galactose-4-epimerase. The UDP-glucose formed may reenter the Leloir pathway at the transferase step and react with pyrophosphate to form glucose-1-phosphate, or it may be used to form glycogen in the presence of glycogen synthetase.

Galactose may also be reduced by a nonspecific aldose reductase in the presence of the reduced form of nicotinamide adenine dinucleotide to form galactitol. In patients with kinase and transferase deficiencies, elevated galactitol levels lead to osmotic swelling and disruption of lenticular fibers resulting in cataract formation.

UPD-galactose may also be synthesized in the body from glucose-1-phosphate by reversing the Leloir pathway. In this manner, UDP-galactosyl residues needed for biosynthesis of macromolecules such as gangliosides may be generated even in the absence of dietary galactose. The UDP-galactose may also be converted to galactose-1-phosphate by pyrophosphorylase, which is thought to be the source of the galactose-1-phosphate seen in patients with well-controlled transferase deficiency.

Galactose-1-Phosphate Uridyl Transferase Deficiency (Classic Galactosemia)

Galactose-1-phosphate uridyl transferase deficiency is the most common disorder of galactose metabolism. It is inherited as an autosomal recessive trait and, in its classic form, occurs in approximately 1 in 62,000 births. Affected infants appear normal at birth. With the ingestion of dietary galactose, symptoms of failure to thrive, vomiting, diarrhea, and lethargy are usually evident by age 1 week. Prolonged physiologic jaundice or the appearance of hepatotoxic jaundice may be evident after age 1 week with increased direct bilirubin. Exchange transfusion and phototherapy may be indicated. Hepatomegaly and abnormal liver function tests are common. Nuclear cataracts (on slit-lamp examination) appear within days or weeks and may become irreversible. Renal tubular dysfunction with generalized aminoaciduria, proteinuria, and galactosuria develops. Marasmus and an encephalopathy follow. The symptoms are rapidly progressive, and most untreated infants do not survive past age 6 weeks. Deaths are due most commonly to liver failure and septicemia, especially with Escherichia coli. The cataracts are thought to be the result of lenticular accumulation of galactitol, as with the kinase deficiency. Galactose-1-phosphate levels are elevated markedly in the tissues and are thought to be responsible for the hepatic, renal, and central nervous system manifestations of the disorder.

The presence of nonglucose-reducing substances in the urine may be demonstrated, as in galactokinase deficiency. Assuming the child has not been transfused, the disorder can be confirmed by demonstrating deficient activity of galactose-1-phosphate uridyl transferase in erythrocytes.

Newborn screening programs test for elevated blood galactose (Paigen test) or galactose-1-phosphate (Paigen test) or screen for the transferase by spot enzyme assay (Beutler test). All screening tests should be confirmed with more definitive testing. Any suspicion of the disorder should prompt the clinician to put the patient on a galactose-free diet while awaiting confirmatory testing. Carrier testing and prenatal diagnosis are available.

Treatment includes strict dietary restriction of all galactose and lactose sources. Affected children improve gradually and dramatically when placed on the diet. Markedly elevated galactose-1-phosphate intracellular levels decrease slowly and may remain elevated for 10 to 15 days. Some persistent mild elevation of erythrocyte galactose-1-phosphate may be seen in patients compliant with galactose restriction and is thought to occur as a result of *in vivo* formation from UDP-galactose. The hepatic and renal manifestations improve slowly and may be entirely reversed. The cataracts improve significantly, but residua may remain. Effects on the central nervous system and ovaries, however, are not reversible. Approximately 60% of patients who are treated early have later psychomotor difficulties and learning disabilities, especially in expressive language, mathematics, and spatial relationships. Behavioral problems with attention deficits and other psychological problems may occur. At least 70% of women have hyper-gonadotropic hypogonadism with ovarian atrophy. Amenorrhea can be primary or secondary. Men have normal gonadal function. Dietary restriction should continue indefinitely.

DISORDERS OF FRUCTOSE METABOLISM

Fructose Metabolism

Sucrose and small amounts of fructose and sorbitol are widely distributed in fruits, vegetables, and other natural and sweetened foods and comprise a major portion of the daily dietary carbohydrate consumption in Western societies. After hydrolysis of sucrose, a large portion of ingested fructose is absorbed unchanged in the small intestine and is transported to the liver, the main site of fructose metabolism. Some of the fructose is converted to glucose in the small intestine, and some is metabolized in muscle, adipose tissue, and the kidneys. Ingested sorbitol is converted to fructose by sorbitol dehydrogenase.

Fructose is converted to intermediates of the gluconeogenic and glycolytic pathways and is metabolized primarily to glucose and lactate (Fig. 213-2). Fructokinase catalyzes the phosphorylation of fructose to fructose-1-phosphate. In normal individuals, this process is associated with a decrease in intracellular inorganic phosphate and ATP concentration and with secondary transient mild hyperuricemia, hypermagnesemia, hyperkalemia, hypophosphatemia, and hypoglycemia. An exaggeration of this response is thought to be the basis for the clinical symptoms seen in hereditary fructose intolerance. Fructose-1-phosphate is cleaved to D-glyceraldehyde and dihydroxyacetone

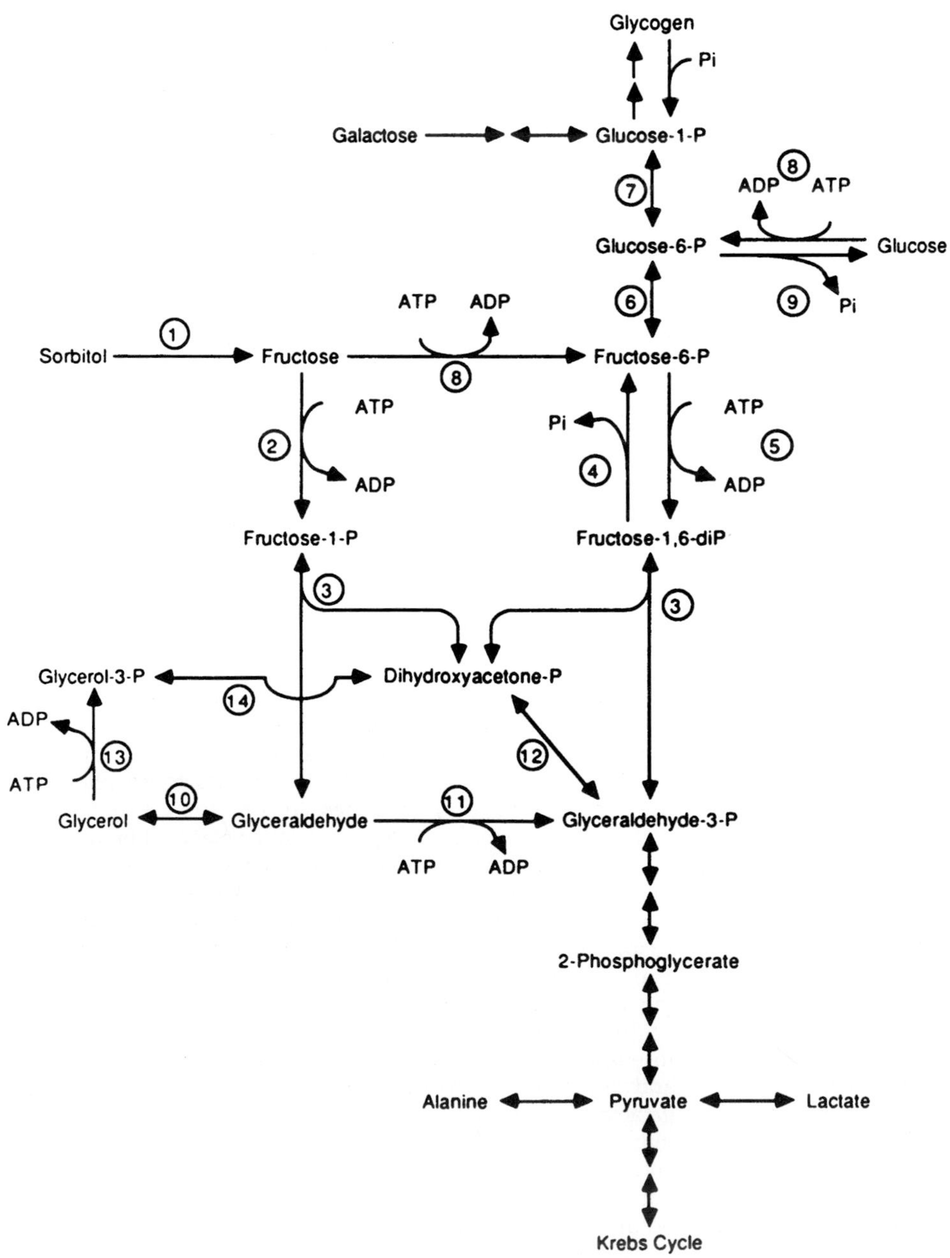

Figure 213-2. Pathways of fructose metabolism. 1, sorbitol dehydrogenase; 2, fructokinase; 3, fructoaldolase; 4, fructose-1,6-diphosphatase; 5, phosphofructokinase; 6, phosphohexose isomerase; 7, phosphoglucomutase; 8, hexokinase; 9, glucose-6-phosphatase; 10, alcohol dehydrogenase; 11, triokinase; 12, triose phosphate isomerase; 13, glycerol kinase; 14, glycerophosphate dehydrogenase; ADP, adenosine diphosphate; ATP, adenosine triphosphate; P, phosphate; Pi, inorganic phosphate.

phosphate in the presence of aldolase. Aldolase also catalyzes the cleaving of fructose-1,6-diphosphate to D-glyceraldehyde-3-phosphate and dihydroxyacetone phosphate. Three forms of aldolase exhibit different tissue distributions: Aldolase B is the major form in liver, aldolase A is the major form in muscle, and aldolase C is the major form in brain.

Fructose-1-Phosphate Aldolase B Deficiency (Hereditary Fructose Intolerance)

Fructose-1-phosphate aldolase B deficiency, an autosomal recessive disorder, is associated with reduced activity of aldolase B in the liver, renal cortex, and small intestine. Considerable heterogeneity is seen in residual activity among affected patients who usually have less than 15% of normal hepatic aldolase B activity. The true incidence of the disorder is unknown; it is estimated to occur in 1 in 20,000 individuals in Switzerland.

The symptoms of this disorder, which occur only after the ingestion of dietary fructose, are related to acute hypoglycemia and chronic hepatic and renal dysfunction. In young infants, usually the symptoms do not start until weaning or the introduction of fruits, vegetables, and juices. Symptoms may occur before this time if the infant is taking a formula with fructose or sucrose as the carbohydrate source. The symptoms of an acute ingestion, which are more severe in young infants than in older children and adults, are associated with hypoglycemia and include sweating, trembling, emesis, lethargy, coma, seizures, and even shock and death. Acute fructose ingestion results in depletion of intracellular inorganic phosphate and ATP and in secondary inhibition of gluconeogenesis and glycolysis. More chronic symptoms include poor feeding, failure to thrive, vomiting, diarrhea, irritability, tremors, hepatomegaly, hepatic dysfunction leading to cirrhosis and hepatic failure, and proximal renal tubular dysfunction of the Fanconi type. The accumulation of fructose-1-phosphate in the liver, kidney, and small intestine is thought to be responsible for these manifestations. The pattern of these chronic symptoms with intermittent acute episodes associated with the ingestion of fructose-containing foods, points to the disorder clinically. Older children and adults will have a nutritional history of avoidance of fructose and may be referred for bizarre eating patterns.

Laboratory findings associated with acute episodes will include hypoglycemia, hypophosphatemia, hypermagnesemia, hyperuricemia, hyperkalemia, lactic acidosis, and fructosemia and fructosuria. The presence of a nonglucose-reducing substance in the urine should be confirmed as fructose by sugar chromatography. Fructosuria will not be present in those patients with intake of foods or fluids with other carbohydrate sources and may not be seen in patients with poor intake or patients without recent exposure to fructose. Laboratory findings from chronic exposure are associated with hepatic dysfunction and proximal renal tubular dysfunction. Liver biopsy samples reveal diffuse steatosis, scattered hepatic necrosis, periportal and intralobular fibrosis, and cirrhosis in later stages. Renal biopsy reveals granulation and vacuolization of epithelial cells with dilated proximal tubules. Small intestinal biopsy samples may exhibit submucosal or serosal hemorrhages.

Treatment with avoidance of all dietary sources of sucrose and fructose including that in foods and medications should be instituted once the disorder is suspected. Sorbitol is metabolized to fructose and, thus, must also be avoided. Acute episodes respond to intravenous glucose infusion. Once a fructose-restricted diet is started, clinical improvement is usually evident within days. After several weeks of treatment, an intravenous fructose tolerance test with a maximum dose of 200 mg/kg may be administered with caution. The disorder can also be documented by demonstrating a known mutation at the aldolase B gene locus in peripheral leukocytes or by enzymatic assay of aldolase B in biopsy samples from the liver or small intestine. Because aldolase B is not expressed in cultured skin fibroblasts or amniocytes, carrier and prenatal testing is only available for families in whom the molecular genetic defect is known.

CHAPTER 214
Peroxisomal Disorders

Adapted from Rebecca S. Wappner

PEROXISOMAL FUNCTION

Peroxisomes are small, subcellular organelles associated with a number of recognized biochemical functions and disorders. The name peroxisomes was coined when catalase, which reduces hydrogen peroxide to water, and a series of oxidases were found to be localized to this organelle.

At least 40 enzymatic reactions are known to happen in peroxisomes. Abnormalities noted in patients with peroxisomal disorders have included catalase deficiency and reduced beta-oxidation of very long-chain fatty acids (VLCFA; carbon chain length greater than 22). Faulty beta-oxidation of VLCFA can lead to elevated plasma levels and tissue storage of VLCFA.

CLASSIFICATION OF PEROXISOMAL DISORDERS

The peroxisomal disorders are classified into two groups: those disorders of peroxisomal biogenesis and those disorders associated with deficient activity of a single peroxisomal enzyme. The first group includes, among others, Zellweger syndrome and classic and severe neonatal adrenoleukodystrophy (ALD). Among other diseases, the second group comprises disorders such as "Zellweger-like" conditions termed pseudo-Zellweger syndrome and X-linked adrenoleukodystrophy (ALD).

DISORDERS ASSOCIATED WITH DEFECTS IN PEROXISOMAL BIOGENESIS

Zellweger Syndrome

Zellweger syndrome (cerebrohepatorenal syndrome) is characterized by major dysmorphic features including a flat midfacial area with shallow orbital ridges and epicanthal folds, large fontanelle, flat occiput, high prominent forehead, dolichocephaly, Brushfield spots, mild micrognathia, external ear anomalies, and transverse palmar creases. Patients may be affected with retinitis pigmentosa and impaired vision, hearing problems, hepatomegaly with impaired function, and cirrhosis. Impaired cortisol response to adrenocorticotropic hormone or adrenal atrophy can also occur. Marked generalized hypotonia, present from birth, is often associated with feeding and respiratory problems. Some patients also have congenital cataracts, glaucoma, cardiac defects, and elevated serum iron levels. Abnormal fetal brain development with macrogyria and polymicrogyria, and failure of myelination and white matter development lead to progressive psychomotor retardation and seizures. Most children have pronounced failure to thrive and do not live past 6 months of age (Fig. 214-1).

Zellweger syndrome is associated with generalized peroxisomal dysfunction. Current therapy is only symptomatic and

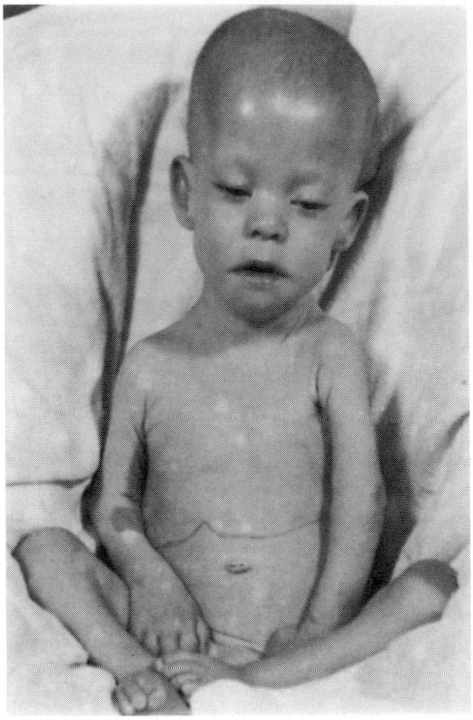

Figure 214-1. Child with Zellweger syndrome at age 8.5 months. (The spots are from film processing and are not caused by hypopigmentation.)

supportive. This includes correction of coagulopathies with vitamin K and adrenal corticosteroid hormone replacement therapy if indicated. The disorder is inherited as an autosomal recessive trait. The molecular basis for the disorder has been shown for some of the patients. Most commonly, a molecular defect occurs in PEX1. Prenatal diagnosis is available. Carrier detection is only available in families where the molecular defect is known.

DISORDERS ASSOCIATED WITH DEFICIENT ACTIVITY OF A SINGLE PEROXISOMAL ENZYME

X-Linked or Childhood Adrenoleukodystrophy (ALD) and Adrenomyeloneuropathy (AMN)

X-linked or childhood ALD is characterized by the onset between 4 and 8 years of age, changes in behavior or school performance, disturbances in vision or hearing, abnormalities in gait and coordination, dysarthrias, and dysphagia. A progressive central and peripheral nervous system demyelination develops with gradual loss of vision, hearing, mental and motor abilities, and the development of seizures. Most boys die within 3 to 5 years after the onset of symptoms. Adrenocortical atrophy or insufficiency and a suppressed response to adrenocorticotropic hormone may be noted. Occasionally, a patient will exhibit Addison disease before the neurologic symptoms are noted. Some affected male subjects, ascertained through family studies, do not develop progressive neurologic disease.

AMN, an adult variant of ALD that usually occurs in men in their 20s, is characterized by progressive spastic paraparesis, sensory deficits, and polyneuropathy. Often, a history of adrenal insufficiency exists. Primary hypogonadism with low testosterone and elevated follicle-stimulating hormone levels usually occurs. Because both ALD and AMN are inherited as X-linked traits and have occurred in the same sibship, AMN is considered to be a milder phenotypic variant of ALD. Some female carriers for ALD/AMN also develop progressive neurologic disorders with spastic paraparesis.

ALD and AMN result from defective degradation of VLCFA. Reduced activity of peroxisomal very long-chain acyl-CoA synthetase (also known as lignoceroyl-CoA synthetase), the first step in beta-oxidation of VLCFA, has been shown in cultured fibroblasts from affected patients. Patients with ALD and AMN, as well as most female carriers of these disorders, have elevated plasma levels of VLCFA. Affected male subjects accumulate saturated VLCFA in the ganglioside of cerebral white matter and in the cholesteryl ester fraction of the adrenal cortex and cerebral white matter (Fig. 214-2).

Treatment with hormone replacement therapy is indicated for adrenal and testosterone insufficiency. Investigational studies have shown that dietary restriction of C26:0, along with glycerol trierucate (C22:1) and glycerol trioleate (C18:1) supplementation, results in lowered plasma levels of VLCFA. Some affected male patients with ALD appear to respond to this therapy if it is started before the onset of neurologic symptoms. Whether the therapy prevented neurologic progression in these patients or whether these patients were the fortunate ones destined not to have progressive neurologic disease was unclear. The therapy is not effective in patients with AMN. Agents that modify inflammatory responses are also being investigated. Bone marrow transplantation can be considered for male patients with ALD

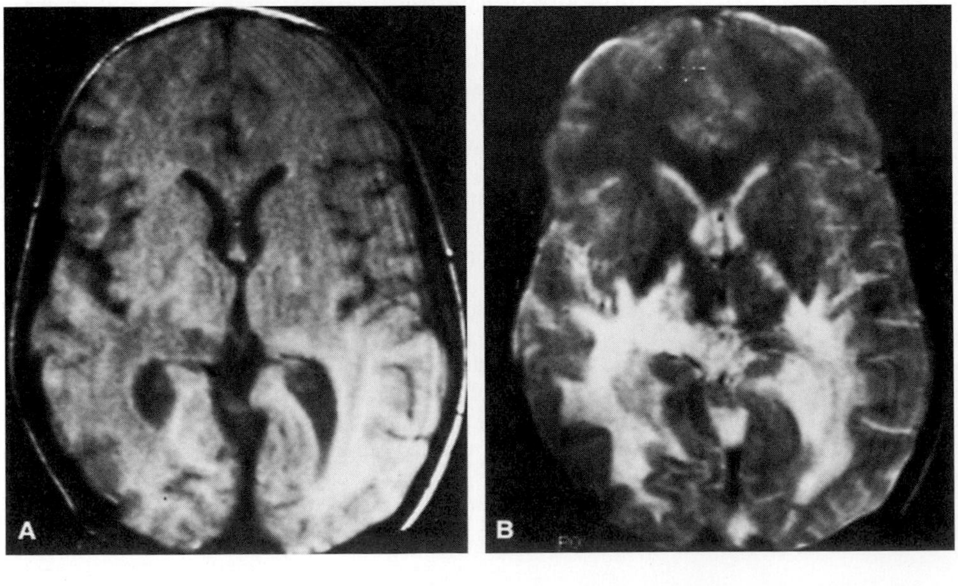

Figure 214-2. Adrenoleukodystrophy. T1-weighted magnetic resonance image (**A**); T2-weighted magnetic resonance image (**B**). Note the increased periventricular signal in the posterior areas.

early in their disease and before significant neurologic involvement develops.

The gene ALDP, located at chromosomal location Xq28, is associated with ALD/AMN. ALDP encodes the ALD protein, which is thought to be a peroxisomal transport protein involved with the import or anchoring of very long-chain acyl-CoA synthetase at the peroxisomal membrane. Multiple different mutations at the ALDP locus have been reported in affected male patients. Because approximately 10% to 15% of obligate female carriers for ALD/AMN have false-negative results when tested by plasma VLCFA levels alone, molecular genetic techniques using mutational analysis must be used for true accuracy in carrier detection. This testing is especially important if a sister is being considered as a bone marrow transplant donor.

CHAPTER 215
Heritable Disorders of Connective Tissue

Adapted from Michael J. Wright and Harry C. Dietz III

MARFAN SYNDROME AND RELATED PHENOTYPES

Marfan syndrome is a dominantly inherited disorder with a birth incidence estimated to be approximately 1 in 10,000. This is likely an underestimation, however, as many of those affected have few signs. The genetic defect in Marfan syndrome was discovered in the early 1990s. Diagnosis, however, still depends on the identification of specific clinical features (Table 215-1).

The increased total height, part of the distinctive appearance of Marfan syndrome, is largely explained by the lower segment measured from the symphysis pubis to the floor in an individual standing in bare feet. Consequently, the upper segment–lower segment ratio is decreased as compared to controls. Usually, the ratio is more than 2 SD below the mean for age and, in general terms, less than 1.0 at 0 to 5 years; less than 0.95 at 6 to 7 years; less than 0.90 at 8 to 9 years; and less than 0.85 in those older than 10 years. Upper extremity involvement is reflected in an increased span-height ratio with greatest diagnostic significance given to values greater than 1.05.

Arachnodactyly is a subjective finding that can be assessed by eliciting the "thumb sign" (positive if the proximal phalanx projects beyond the ulnar border of the palm when the thumb is opposed maximally) and the "wrist sign" (positive if the distal phalanges of the thumb and little finger overlap when the wrist is encircled by the contralateral hand). Joint laxity may give rise to recurrent dislocation. Instability of the ankle and pes planus can cause difficulties with ambulation. Later in life, arthritis may develop in previously hypermobile joints.

The axial skeleton is also involved: Scoliosis with or without kyphosis of the thoracic spine occurs in approximately 10% of cases. Spondylolisthesis may be found in the lumbosacral spine. Physiologic thoracic kyphosis can be replaced by a "straight back" or even by thoracic lordosis; in association with the pectus excavatum, this condition may give rise to significant reduction in anteroposterior diameter of the chest. Pectus excavatum and carinatum arise as a result of rib overgrowth, which may also cause chest asymmetry.

Abnormalities of the bones of the skull and face manifest as dolichocephaly, a long thin face, a high arched palate giving rise to dental crowding and malocclusion, and retrognathia or prognathia.

The increased mortality associated with Marfan syndrome at all ages is explained almost exclusively by cardiovascular complications. The most common cardiovascular complications are mitral valve prolapse and aortic root dilation. The aortic root dilation predisposes an affected individual not only to aortic regurgitation but also to the most feared of all complications of Marfan syndrome: aortic dissection and rupture. Usually, dilation is limited to the ascending aorta, but it may extend to the abdominal aorta and to the pulmonary vasculature.

Subluxation or complete dislocation of the lens is the classic ocular sign in Marfan syndrome. This condition may be present at birth but can present or progress throughout childhood. Formal slit-lamp examination is essential to confirm this feature, but the presence of iridodonesis (a shimmering of the iris as accommodation occurs) is indicative. In addition to myopia and retinal detachment secondary to increased length of the eyeball, glaucoma and cataracts occur at greater than expected frequency and earlier in life than in the general population.

Dural ectasia has become recognized as a feature of both diagnostic and clinical importance. In this defect, the neural canal is enlarged with erosion of sacral bone. Usually, this condition remains asymptomatic but should be considered in the differential diagnosis of back or leg pain in individuals with Marfan syndrome. Rarely, dural ectasia produces a meningocele presenting as a pelvic mass.

Often, spontaneous pneumothorax is perceived as a common complication of Marfan syndrome; in reality, it is relatively rare. Pulmonary function may be compromised by severe scoliosis and chest wall deformity.

Diagnosis

The current diagnostic criteria for Marfan syndrome are shown in Table 215-1. The discovery of the molecular basis of Marfan syndrome has not allowed for the creation of a definitive and universally applicable diagnostic test, due to the large number of causative mutations and the fact that related, but separate, conditions can be caused by mutations in the same gene.

Specialized investigations required are slit-lamp examination, echocardiography, and plasma amino acid analysis (to exclude the diagnosis of homocystinuria). To make a diagnosis of Marfan syndrome in an individual with no family history, major criteria are required in two organ systems with involvement of a third. If a major criterion is already established by reason of family history, major criteria must be met in one organ system and another must be involved.

Management

Management of cardiac complications can have beneficial effects on morbidity and mortality. Yearly echocardiograms are recommended in those patients without symptoms (more often in patients with significant cardiac involvement). Surgical intervention should be considered when the aortic root diameter approaches twice the upper limit of normal for an individual's body surface area or the absolute measurement exceeds 5.0 to 5.5 cm. Severe left ventricle enlargement or dysfunction is an indication for surgical repair or replacement of the aortic or mitral valves.

Beta-blockade has been shown to slow the rate of aortic root dilation and to reduce the incidence of aortic regurgitation and dissection. Contact sports, competitive sports, exercise to the point of exhaustion, and exertion against a fixed resistance (e.g., weight lifting) should be avoided because of the increased risk

TABLE 215-1. Diagnostic Criteria for Marfan Syndrome*

	Major criteria	Minor criteria	Involvement
Family history	First-degree relative who meets diagnostic criteria Marfan-causing *FBN1* mutation Haplotype around *FBN1* associated with confirmed Marfan inherited by descent	None	Major criterion must be met or family history is noncontributory
Skeletal	Presence of any four of the following: Pectus carinatum Pectus excavatum requiring surgery Reduced upper segment–lower segment ratio or span/height >1.05 Positive wrist and thumb signs Scoliosis >20 degrees or spondylolisthesis Extension <170 degrees at elbow Medial displacement of the medial malleolus causing pes planus Protrusio acetabulae	Pectus excavatum Joint hypermobility High arched palate with dental crowding Facial appearance	Two of the components of the major criteria or one of the components of the major criteria and two minor criteria
Ocular	Ectopia lentis	Flat cornea (by keratometry) Increased globe length (by ultrasound) Hypoplastic iris or hypoplastic ciliary muscle causing decreased miosis	Two minor criteria
Cardiovascular	Dilation of the ascending aorta with or without aortic regurgitation involving at least the sinuses of Valsalva Dissection of the ascending aorta	Mitral valve prolapse with or without mitral regurgitation Dilation of main pulmonary artery without other cause at age 40 years or younger Calcification of the mitral annulus at age 40 years or younger Dilation or dissection of the descending thoracic or abdominal aorta at age 50 years or younger	One major or one minor criterion
Pulmonary	None	Spontaneous pneumothorax Apical blebs (radiographically)	One minor criterion
Skin and central nervous system	Lumbosacral dural ectasia	Striae atrophicae not associated with marked weight changes, pregnancy, or repetitive stress Recurrent or incisional herniae	One major or one minor criterion

*To make a diagnosis of Marfan syndrome in an individual with no family history requires major criteria in two organ systems and involvement of a third. If there is a family history, major criteria must be met in one organ system and another must be involved.

of aortic dilation, rupture, or dissection. Antibiotic prophylaxis should be prescribed to prevent bacterial endocarditis.

The development and progression of scoliosis should be monitored by clinical and radiographic assessment. Management of hypermobile joints may require physical therapy to increase strength of surrounding muscle groups and may call for splinting to allow for adequate function. Correction of chest deformity should be delayed as long as possible, unless pulmonary function is compromised severely. Often, repair in childhood is unsuccessful, as a result of recurrence with continued growth. In adolescence and adulthood, the development of arthritis and back pain can become a major and difficult management issue.

Management of ectopia lentis in individuals with Marfan syndrome requires the expertise of an experienced ophthalmologist. Otherwise, patients should be evaluated yearly for the complications mentioned above.

Often, individuals with Marfan syndrome display significant problems with psychosocial adjustment. Contact with other affected families and individuals of similar age through organizations such as the National Marfan Foundation can be very helpful in this regard.

To date, mutations causing Marfan syndrome have been found only in the gene FBN1. Fibrillin-1, the gene product, is the major component of the extracellular microfibril. Fibrillin monomers combine to form multimeric fibers and aggregate with other structural proteins to form microfibrils. A large number of different mutations have been found in FBN1 precluding effective population screening.

Ehlers–Danlos Syndromes

The Ehlers–Danlos syndromes (EDS) comprise a heterogeneous group of disorders with cardinal features such as hyperextensible skin with a velvety texture, dystrophic scarring, easy bruising, joint hypermobility, and connective tissue fragility. Two classification systems for EDS are compared in Table 215-2. Types I, II, and III are described below.

TYPE I

The cardinal features of EDS are present to a severe extent in EDS type I with particularly prominent skin elasticity and joint hypermobility giving rise to early degenerative arthritis. Pes planus and scoliosis are common and thought to be due to ligamentous laxity, which is also responsible for delayed motor development. Dystrophic scarring is marked with the formation of cigarette-paper scars and characteristic scars on the forehead and under the chin when affected children begin to walk. Mitral valve prolapse has been described in as many as 50% of cases.

TABLE 215-2. Classification of Ehlers-Danlos Syndromes

Berlin nosology (Beighton et al., 1988)	Villefranche nosology (Beighton et al., 1998)
Type I	Classic
Type II	Classic
Type III	Hypermobility
Type IV	Vascular
Type V	Other forms
Type VI	Kyphoscoliosis
Type VII A and B	Arthrochalasia
Type VII C	Dermatopraxis
Types VIII, X, and XI Progeroid Ehlers-Danlos syndromes and unspecified forms	Other forms

TYPE II

The phenotype in EDS type II is similar to the phenotype in EDS type I but is less severe. In particular, scarring and bruising are less severe, and motor development is normal. Mitral valve prolapse may be present.

Both EDS type I and type II are inherited in an autosomal dominant manner and, in some families who have been described, individuals with features of both phenotypes are found. Molecular genetic studies have shown that both EDS type I and type II can be caused by mutations in type V collagen. However, not all families show linkage to this locus, but linked and unlinked families appear clinically indistinguishable.

TYPE III

The dominantly inherited EDS type III has been mistakenly called the benign hypermobility syndrome. The skin manifestations are, at worst, mild, but joint hypermobility giving rise to recurrent dislocation, joint pain in adolescence and adulthood, and early arthritis are common and often severely disabling symptoms. A mutation in type III collagen has been found in a family with what could be classified as either EDS type III or what was known as EDS type XI, now called *familial joint instability syndrome*.

CHAPTER 216

Lysosomal Storage Disorders

Adapted from Rebecca S. Wappner

Lysosomes are cytoplasmic organelles that contain hydrolytic enzymes responsible for the degradation of a variety of compounds including mucopolysaccharides, sphingolipids, and glycoproteins. Deficient activity of a specific lysosomal acid hydrolase leads to progressive accumulation of partially degraded material, which distends the cells and disrupts cellular function. The reduced activity of an acid hydrolase may be the result of a genetic mutation at the enzyme locus that results in lowered specific activity or reduced stability of the enzyme, failure of formation of a protective protein or activator for the enzyme, or failure of formation of a recognition marker on the enzyme, which targets it for lysosomal location. Lysosomal storage of material may also result from failure of active transport of small molecules from the lysosome.

The clinical findings are related to the type of compound stored and its natural distribution in the body. All the disorders are inherited as either autosomal recessive or X-linked traits. For many of the disorders, the associated genes have been mapped and cloned. Heterogeneity has been noted in the molecular basis for many of the disorders and often correlates with the varying clinical presentations.

Current therapy consists of symptomatic and supportive therapy for the patient and family. Enzyme replacement therapy is only available for type I Gaucher disease and may become available for other lysosomal storage disorders in the future. Bone marrow transplantation may be considered, especially for those disorders that do not have central nervous system involvement.

MUCOPOLYSACCHARIDOSES

The mucopolysaccharidoses are associated with lysosomal accumulation of partially degraded acid mucopolysaccharides (MPS). MPS, also termed glycosaminoglycans, are large molecules composed of linear repeating sulfated hexuronate or hexosamine disaccharide units attached to a protein core. MPS are normally degraded by a series of acid hydrolases but deficiency results in partial degradation of the molecules and lysosomal storage of the residual fragments.

The degradation of heparan sulfate, dermatan sulfate, keratan sulfate, or chondroitin sulfate, alone or in combination, may be involved depending on the specific hydrolase affected. Disorders associated with heparan sulfate storage usually have central nervous system involvement and progressive mental retardation, those disorders associated with dermatan sulfate storage are usually associated with visceral and bone involvement, and those disorders associated with keratan sulfate storage have bone involvement as their major clinical feature.

Radiography shows a distinct pattern of abnormalities termed *dysostosis multiplex*. The skull is enlarged and elongated (dolichocephaly) and the calvarium thickened. The sella may be J-, wooden shoe-, or boot-shaped. The vertebral bodies in the lower thoracic and upper lumbar areas have a beaking of the anterior inferior surface caused by hypoplasia of their anterosuperior areas (Fig. 216-1). A dorsal kyphosis, or gibbus deformity, develops. The ribs are thickened, except where they join the spine, and they have an oar-shaped appearance (Fig. 216-2). The metacarpals have a proximal narrowing with distal widening giving them a baby-bottle appearance. The pelvis shows flaring of the iliac bones, shallow acetabular areas, and progressive coxa valga. The long bones become shortened, thickened, and may have signs of expansion of the medullary cavity. Hypoplasia of the odontoid process may occur.

The age of onset, severity, and pattern of clinical and radiographic findings help to distinguish between the various types of mucopolysaccharidoses. Although urinary MPS testing may be helpful in some cases, the diagnosis is made on the basis of enzymatic testing. Demonstration of deficient activity of a specific lysosomal hydrolase may be done with serum or peripheral leukocytes for most of the disorders. Cultured skin fibroblasts may be required for others.

Hurler Syndrome (Mucopolysaccharides I-H)

Hurler syndrome is associated with deficient activity of alpha-L-iduronidase and excessive storage of heparan and dermatan sulfate. Hurler syndrome is inherited as an autosomal recessive trait and occurs in approximately 1 in 100,000 births.

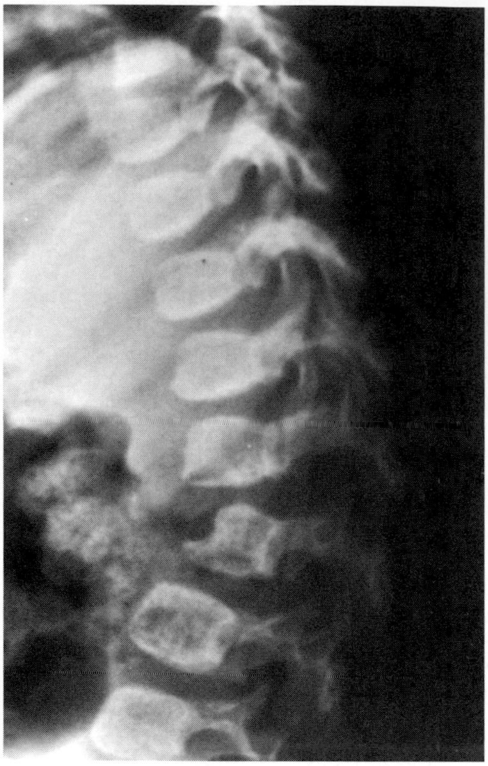

Figure 216-1. Lateral spine radiogram in Hurler syndrome.

Hurler syndrome is considered to be the most severe of the mucopolysaccharidoses and is the prototype for the group of disorders.

Children with Hurler syndrome appear normal at birth. Between 6 and 12 months of age, they have the onset of gradual coarsening and prominence of facial features with flattening of the midfacial areas and widening of the nasal bridge. Clouding of the corneas, gingival hyperplasia, and thickening of the alveolar ridge develop. Dental eruption is delayed. Deafness may occur. Respiratory involvement results from thickening of the soft tissues in the nasal and pharyngeal areas. Initially, the child may have persistent rhinorrhea or noisy breathing. Gradual upper airway obstruction may result in sleep apnea and cor pulmonale. Cardiac involvement usually develops between 2 and 5 years of age and may result in thickened valve leaflets, pseudoatheromatosis of the coronary arteries, cardiomyopathy, and congestive heart failure. Hepatosplenomegaly develops during the first year. Usually, no physiologic problems are associated with the disorder, except for occasional hypersplenism with thrombocytopenia or pancytopenia. Umbilical and inguinal hernias often require surgical correction (Fig. 216-3).

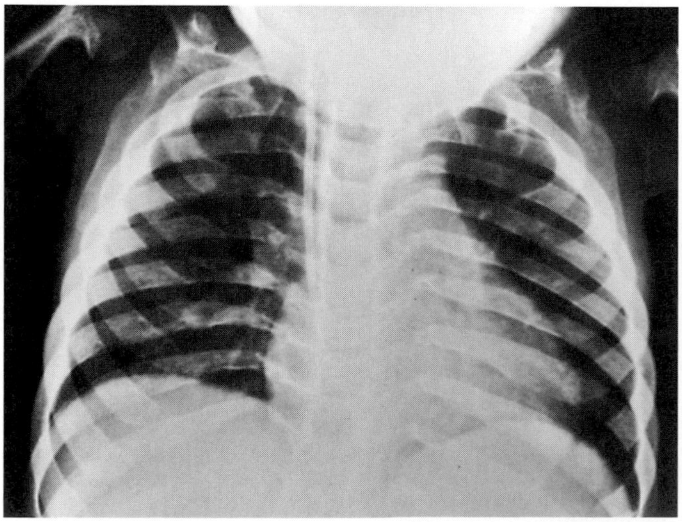

Figure 216-2. Anteroposterior chest radiogram in Hurler syndrome.

Bone growth is delayed, and there is usually minimal linear growth after 2 to 3 years of age. The gibbus deformity, a dorsolumbar kyphosis, develops during the first year and may progress. The head becomes enlarged and dolichocephalic with prominence of the frontal areas and suture lines. Radiography shows a progression of the dysostosis multiplex as described previously. Overproduction of collagen and elastin may accompany the MPS storage and result in joint stiffness, carpal tunnel syndrome, thickening of the meninges with hydrocephalus, and decreased compliance of the thoracic cage.

Psychomotor development appears normal for the first year, remains on a plateau for 1 to 2 years, then gradually regresses. Physical limitations are noted as a result of the joint stiffness and bone involvement. Contractures in the lower extremities lead to a "jockey stance," and the hands become stiff and claw-like in appearance with limited manual dexterity. Physical therapy may be prescribed with the restriction that flexion and extension of the neck should not be done because of possible hypoplasia of the odontoid process. Adaptive equipment may be of benefit. Most children eventually become wheelchair-bound and do not live past their early teenage years. Death may occur earlier from cardiopulmonary involvement.

Hurler syndrome may be confirmed by demonstrating deficient activity of alpha-L-iduronidase in peripheral leukocytes or cultured skin fibroblasts. At least 46 mutations have been identified at the alpha-L-iduronidase locus (*IDUA*) that are associated with Hurler syndrome. Carrier detection is available, but considerable overlap exists between carriers and noncarriers with enzymatic testing. More accurate carrier detection may be done in families of patients in whom the exact genetic mutation is known. Prenatal diagnosis is available with both chorionic villi sampling and cultured amniotic fluid cells.

Hunter Syndrome (Mucopolysaccharides II)

Hunter syndrome is an X-linked disorder associated with deficient activity of iduronate sulfatase and storage of heparan and dermatan sulfate. Both severe (type A) and mild (type B) forms exist. The clinical features of the severe form are similar to those of Hurler syndrome, except that the onset is between 1 and 2 years of age, the course of the disease is somewhat slower, and no corneal clouding occurs (Fig. 216-4). Deafness is common. Skin lesions consisting of ivory raised papules are often noted on the upper back and lateral upper arms and thighs. Patients commonly survive until the second or third decades. The milder type of this disorder usually has normal intelligence and survival into the sixth or seventh decade.

SPHINGOLIPIDOSES

The sphingolipidoses are associated with lysosomal accumulation of glycosphingolipids, gangliosides, and sphingomyelin. Faulty degradation of the molecules results from deficient activity of a lysosomal acid hydrolase or a missing sphingolipid

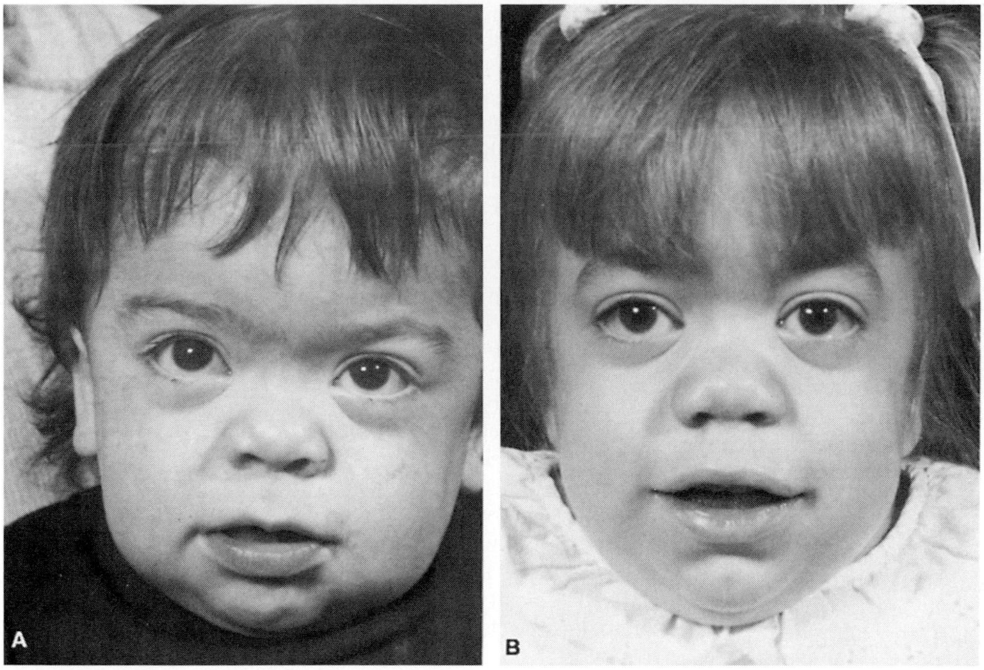

Figure 216-3. Face in Hurler syndrome. Aged 27 months (**A**); aged 37 months (**B**).

activator protein needed for enzyme-lipid stabilization and interaction.

Ceramide, the basic structure for these molecules, is composed of sphingosine, to which a long-chain fatty acid, usually C16, has been attached at the amino group. Attachment of neutral carbohydrate groups in an oligosaccharide chain occurs at the hydroxyl group of the sphingosine. The attachment of a glucosyl residue in beta linkage as the first neutral sugar leads to a glucosylceramide (glucocerebroside) series of glycosphingolipids. Attachment of a galactosyl residue leads to a galactosylceramide (galactocerebroside) series. The neutral sugars of the oligosaccharide side chain may be in alpha or beta linkage and are derived from glucose, galactose, *N*-acetyl-galactosamine, or *N*-acetyl-glucosamine. If the first neutral sugar is a sulfated galactosyl, the compound is called a *sulfatide*. If sialic acid, or *N*-acetyl-neuraminic acid, is attached to the neutral sugars, the structure is termed a *ganglioside*.

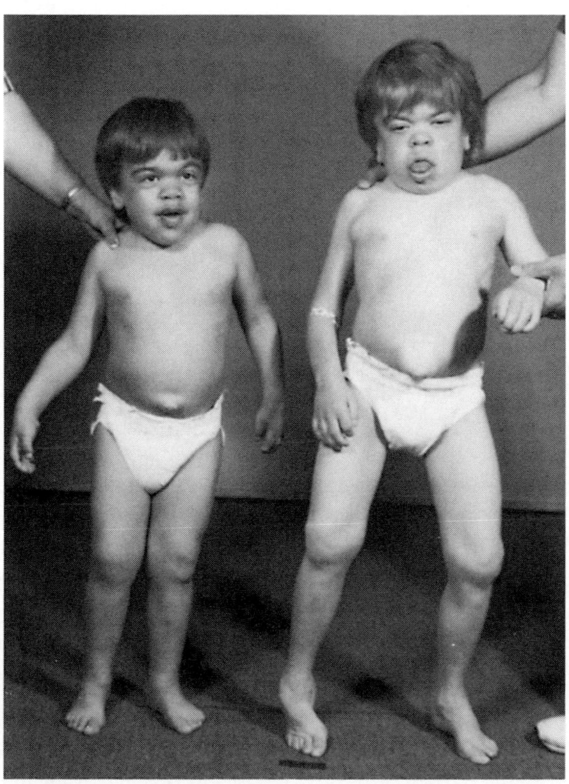

Figure 216-4. Brothers, ages 5 and 15 years, with Hunter syndrome.

Current nomenclature of the gangliosides, according to the Svennerholm classification, is determined by the number of sialic acid residues that are attached to the oligosaccharide chain (M = mono, D = di, T = tri) and by the number (5 minus n) of neutral sugars in the chain. For example, GM_1 ganglioside would have one sialic acid residue and four (5 minus 1) neutral sugars in the oligosaccharide chain attached to the ceramide. Degradation of glycosphingolipids involves stepwise removal of the neutral sugars, sulfate, and sialic acid by a series of lysosomal hydrolases.

GM_2 Gangliosidoses

The GM_2 gangliosidoses are a group of autosomal recessive disorders associated with cerebral degeneration secondary to lysosomal storage of GM_2 ganglioside and related glycosphingolipids. The disorders are associated with deficient activity of the beta-hexoaminidases or the GM_2 activator protein.

Beta-hexosaminidase has two subunits, alpha and beta, which are the products of two separate genetic loci, *HEXA* and *HEXB*, located on chromosomes 15 and 5, respectively. The isoenzymes of beta-hexosaminidase are comprised of different combinations of these subunits. Hexosaminidase A is composed of an alpha and a beta subunit, whereas hexosaminidase B contains two beta subunits. Hexosaminidase A usually accounts for 55% to 70% of the total hexosaminidase-specific activity, whereas hexosaminidase B accounts for 30% to 45%. Genetic mutations at the alpha subunit gene locus lead to hexosaminidase A deficiency and Tay–Sachs disease. Mutations at the beta subunit gene locus lead to deficiency of both hexosaminidase A and B and result in Sandhoff disease. A GM_2 activator protein, encoded by the

GM2A locus on chromosome 5, is needed for stabilization of the GM_2 ganglioside-hexosaminidase A complex. At least 54 mutations at the *HEXA* locus, 12 at the *HEXB* locus, and 2 at the *GM2A* locus have been characterized to date.

Tay–Sachs Disease (GM_2 Gangliosidosis, Type 1)

Tay–Sachs disease is associated with the storage of GM_2 ganglioside and progressive central nervous system degeneration. Affected children are usually normal at birth. Between 6 and 12 months of age, hypotonia and psychomotor retardation become evident and an exaggerated startle response to stimuli, hyperacusis, may be noted. Starting at approximately 1 year of age, spasticity, loss of vision, seizures, and macrocephaly develop. Cherry red spots in the macular area may be seen as early as 3 months of age and represent a normal red macular area surrounded by a white area of storage. Affected children usually require nasogastric or gastrostomy feedings and have problems with oral secretions after 18 to 24 months of age. Intercurrent respiratory problems frequently occur. Most affected children die between 3 and 4 years of age. The diagnosis is confirmed by measurement of hexosaminidase A in serum, plasma, peripheral leukocytes, or cultured skin fibroblasts. Severe deficiency of hexosaminidase A exists, which may be expressed in specific activity units or as a percentage of the total enzyme. Because hexosaminidase B is not affected and may be increased, the total amount of beta-hexosaminidase is normal.

The disorder is most common in individuals of Eastern European Jewish ancestry among whom the carrier rate is 1 in 27. Since the 1970s, community education and carrier testing programs have identified at-risk couples, in which both individuals are carriers for Tay–Sachs disease, before the birth of an affected child. The current recommendation is that all couples of Eastern European Jewish ancestry have carrier testing performed before conception so that timely and appropriate genetic counseling can be given. Because the carrier rate among individuals of other backgrounds is approximately 1 in 200, the possibility of Tay–Sachs disease should not be excluded in nonJewish children if the disorder is suspected on clinical grounds. Prenatal diagnosis is available using chorionic villi sampling or amniocentesis.

Fabry Disease (alpha-Galactosyl-Lactosyl Ceramidosis)

Fabry disease is an X-linked disorder associated with deficient activity of alpha-galactosidase (formerly termed *alpha-galactosidase A*). Storage of glycosphingolipids with terminal galactosyl residues in alpha linkage such as globotriaosylceramide, galabiosylceramide, and blood group B substances occurs in the eyes, kidneys, skeletal and cardiac muscle, the central and autonomic nervous systems, and the vascular endothelium and smooth muscle throughout the body.

Clinical symptoms are usually evident by 10 years of age. Acroparesthesia is often the presenting symptom. Intermittent painful crises lasting minutes to days may involve the extremities or the abdomen. Because episodes are often accompanied by a low-grade fever and an elevated erythrocyte sedimentation rate, they may be mistaken for other causes of an acute abdominal crisis. A characteristic whorl-like corneal dystrophy with spoke-like or propeller-like cataracts may be seen. Angiokeratoma corporis diffusum consisting of punctate, flat to slightly raised, dark red to blue-black papules usually appear in clusters in areas between the umbilicus and knees (bathing suit area). Angiokeratoma may also be found on the conjunctiva or mucosal surfaces. Hypohidrosis is common.

With advancing age, affected patients complain of fatigue, weakness, and poor vision. Cardiac involvement may lead to myocardial infarction, cardiomyopathies, or conduction defects. Vascular involvement of the central nervous system may lead to aneurysms, vascular occlusion, or hemorrhage. Patients frequently become hypertensive. Renal dysfunction, initially evident as proteinuria, usually progresses to renal failure by 30 to 40 years of age. Renal dialysis or transplantation may be indicated.

Deficient activity of alpha-galactosidase may be shown in peripheral leukocytes or cultured skin fibroblasts. Low-dose diphenylhydantoin or carbamazepine may improve the acroparesthesia and painful crises. Enzyme replacement therapy to replace the missing alpha-galactosidase enzyme activity was approved in the United States in April 2003 (Fabrazyme®, Genzyme Corp., Cambridge, MA.). Accurate carrier detection may be done with molecular genetic techniques. Prenatal diagnosis is available.

Female carriers for Fabry disease often have milder, but similar, clinical findings. The most frequent of these is corneal dystrophy. With advancing age, many become symptomatic, and deaths may occur from vascular, renal, or cardiac involvement, as in male subjects.

Gaucher Disease (Glucocerebrosidosis)

Gaucher disease is an autosomal recessive disorder associated with deficient activity of beta-glucocerebrosidase (beta-glucosidase). Storage of glucocerebroside (glucosylceramide) occurs in the reticuloendothelial system. Three forms of the disorder vary in clinical severity.

Type 1, the chronic, nonneuronopathic form of Gaucher disease, is the most common sphingolipid storage disorder. Affected patients may present at any age with asymptomatic splenomegaly. More severely affected patients present during childhood with massive splenomegaly and pancytopenia. Hepatomegaly with mildly elevated liver function test results also occurs. Cirrhosis and liver failure occasionally develop. Infiltration of the bone marrow interferes with bone growth and mineralization and compounds the pancytopenia. Pulmonary storage may lead to abnormal pulmonary function and cor pulmonale. Bone marrow and other tissues from the reticuloendothelial system have large, lipid-laden, fusiform histiocytes with dense eccentric nuclei that resemble wrinkled tissue paper or crumpled silk (Gaucher cells). Radiography shows an expanded cortex of the distal femur termed an *Erlenmeyer-flask deformity;* bone erosion with cyst-like changes of varying sizes are noted. Painful avascular crises in long bones and vertebral bodies, pseudoosteomyelitis, and avascular necrosis of the femoral or humeral heads may occur. Serum acid phosphatase levels are elevated from bone involvement. Older patients may have yellow or brown discoloration of the exposed skin or pingueculae on the conjunctiva. Primary central nervous system disease does not occur. The disorder is slowly progressive, and many patients who present in childhood live well into adult life. Other patients have a relatively mild disease and are identified by splenomegaly when they are adults.

Enzyme replacement therapy with infusions recombinant DNA derived glucocerebrosidase (Cerezyme®, Genzyme Corp., Cambridge, MA.) results in significant clinical improvement in symptomatic patients. Responses in hematologic parameters and reduction in the size of the liver and spleen occur more rapidly than skeletal changes. Although extremely expensive, enzyme replacement therapy should be considered for any symptomatic patient with type 1 Gaucher disease. Bone marrow transplantation may also be considered, but it is associated with considerable risks when compared with enzyme replacement therapy. Gene transfer therapy is being investigated.

Before enzyme replacement therapy was available, many patients required splenectomy for persistent thrombocytopenia and bleeding diatheses. Postsplenectomy management should include prophylactic antibiotics and immunization, as for other asplenic individuals. Orthopedic problems are often difficult to treat and should be referred to specialists who are experienced with Gaucher patients.

Type 2, the acute neuronopathic form of Gaucher disease, has its onset between birth and 18 months of age. Massive hepatosplenomegaly is accompanied by rapidly progressing central nervous system deterioration. Trismus, strabismus, and retroflexion of the head are pathognomonic. Spasticity, hyperreflexia, and seizures occur. Feeding and respiratory problems are common. Death usually occurs by 2 years of age. Treatment is symptomatic and supportive. Enzyme replacement therapy has been shown to improve organomegaly and hematologic status but does not prevent central nervous system deterioration.

Type 3, the subacute neuronopathic form of Gaucher disease, has features of both types 1 and 2. Most cases occur in individuals with northern Swedish (Norrbottnian) ancestry. The onset of hepatosplenomegaly in childhood usually precedes the progressive neurologic symptoms. Behavioral changes, oculomotor apraxia, extrapyramidal and cerebellar signs, seizures, and developmental regression occur. Many patients live into early adulthood. Enzyme replacement therapy improves organomegaly and hematologic status and appears to stabilize and, in some cases, has improved central nervous system involvement.

The diagnosis for all three types of Gaucher disease is established by the demonstration of deficient activity of beta-glucosidase in peripheral leukocytes or cultured skin fibroblasts in experienced laboratories. Molecular genetic studies help differentiate between type 1 and type 3 disease in young patients. Atypical juvenile cases have been associated with deficiency of sphingolipid activator protein 2 (saposin C). Carrier detection and prenatal diagnosis are available.

10
Nervous System

CHAPTER 217
Cerebral Palsy

Adapted from Bruce K. Shapiro and Arnold J. Capute

DEFINITION AND EPIDEMIOLOGY

Cerebral palsy is a disorder of movement and posture that results from an insult to, or anomaly of, the immature central nervous system (CNS). This definition recognizes the central origin of the dysfunction and differentiates cerebral palsy from neuropathies and myopathies. The definition implies that the cause is static and excludes progressive neurologic disorders. The simplicity of the definition belies the diversity of the dysfunctions that result from diffuse neurologic damage.

Cerebral palsy is the most common movement disorder of childhood. Estimates of its frequency vary from 1 to 6 per 1,000, but more recent studies report a prevalence of 1 to 2 per 1,000. The lower rate should be regarded as a minimum estimate because milder cases are not included; more severe cases may be obscured by other developmental disabilities such as seizure disorders or mental retardation, and the most severe cases may die.

Traditionally, spastic cerebral palsy has been the most frequent type accounting for approximately 50% of cases. It is followed by athetosis (approximately 20% of cases), rigidity, ataxia tremor, and mixed forms (approximately 25% of cases). Most cerebral palsy is found in children who do not possess identifiable risk factors. Traditional risk factors associated with cerebral palsy are birth asphyxia, prematurity, and intrauterine growth retardation. When risk factors are analyzed in a multivariate fashion, the strongest determinants of cerebral palsy are not related to events of labor or delivery.

The impact of prematurity on the incidence of cerebral palsy is not clear. As neonatal care has improved, the incidence of cerebral palsy in heavier-birth-weight groups has decreased. Very low-birth-weight (VLBW) infants (less than 1,500 g) may have a higher incidence of cerebral palsy, but the lower number of children at this birth weight should modify the contribution that these children make to the total pool of cerebral palsy cases.

Some studies have reaffirmed the relationship between maternal infection and cerebral palsy. Multiple gestations markedly increase the incidence of cerebral palsy. Some researchers have suggested that cytokines are the mediators that tie together infection, asphyxia, multiple births, and prematurity.

DIAGNOSIS

Neonatal Period

In the neonatal period, cerebral palsy cannot be diagnosed by clinical methods. The relative immaturity of the full-term newborn limits the prognostic ability of the neonatal examination. Although a normal neurologic examination may be reassuring, abnormal findings in the neonatal period do not usually prognosticate cerebral palsy.

Advances in noninvasive techniques of neuroimaging, particularly in ultrasonography, have provided an alternative means of assessment that may better predict cerebral palsy than the clinical examination. Periventricular cysts, although uncommon, are specific for cerebral palsy. As the natural history of ultrasonic lesions is better appreciated and as techniques for assessing metabolism and blood flows (e.g., emission tomography) are increasingly applied to neonates, the chance of diagnosing cerebral palsy in the neonatal period improves.

Birth to 6 Months

The earliest presentations of cerebral palsy are subtle because the infant has not yet developed a wide range of volitional movement. Feeding difficulties related to hypotonia or uncoordinated sucking and swallowing, difficulty with diapering because of adductor tightness, and behavioral disturbance such as impaired periodicity, excessive colic, or cerebral irritability are common manifestations of cerebral palsy.

The motor examination of the young infant is made difficult by the differential maturation of the underlying precursors of volitional movement. Flexor hypertonus occurs in full-term newborns and normalizes during the first half-year. Primitive reflexes appear during the last trimester of pregnancy, are displayed at birth, and are suppressed during the first 6 months of life. Movement is undifferentiated and reciprocating initially, but it becomes more specific as the infant ages. Although rolling is usually considered the first motor milestone, predictable motor sequences that may assist early diagnosis occur before rolling.

Observing spontaneous movement is the most important aspect of the motor examination. Decreased amounts of the movement may be generalized or confined to specific limbs. The baby may not kick equally, may exhibit fisting in one hand but not the other, may transfer in only one direction, or may show hand preference at too early an age. Such asymmetries are not normal.

Eliciting movements may yield information about axial abilities. In the prone position, the baby may clear the face at birth, lift the head by 1 month, lift the chest by 2 months, get up on the forearms by 3 months, and push up on the wrists by 4 months. By 5 months, the infant should be able to shift weight in a prone position while attempting to obtain a toy. In prone suspension, many infants are able to move their faces perpendicularly to the plane of their bodies with vertebral extension (i.e., Landau reflex) by 3 months. The full-term baby has only minimal overshoot when being pulled into the sitting position, and the 2-month-old infant can maintain the head in line with the body if gently displaced laterally from supported sitting. The 4-month-old infant flexes the neck from a supine position. The newborn can step and momentarily support his or her weight when held in vertical suspension (i.e., neonatal positive support). By 2 to 3 months, the infant loses this stepping response and is able to support his or her weight (i.e., mature positive support response). Neuromotor signs indicating increased lower extremity tone such as "scissoring" or assumption of an equinus position are not normal.

The components of early movement may assist in delineating the nature of the dysfunction, but they are distant from the motor action and are not directly related. Passive tone assessment or measurement of deep tendon reflex activity yields little in infants of this age. Primitive reflexes are difficult to interpret except when they are abnormally absent or in obligatory forms or when the most immature of the primitive reflexes exist (e.g., a Moro reflex beyond 6 months or stepping beyond 2 months).

If the pediatrician sees generalized decreases in movement, notices asymmetric findings, or elicits a neurodevelopmental examination that approximates that of an infant of one-half the child's chronologic age, the examination is abnormal. The examination has limited prognostic value because the situation is likely to change with maturation. However, early identification permits early intervention and monitoring. An abnormal motor examination requires delineation of other areas of neural functioning because dysfunction is usually diffuse.

6 to 18 Months

Motor delay is the basis for the diagnosis of cerebral palsy. However, lesser motor delays may not be significant and resolve with maturation. One technique for qualifying the amount of motor delay is to compare the child's motor age with the chronologic age to develop a motor quotient. Motor quotients of less than 50% are associated with significant motor dysfunction and should be investigated further.

The examination of the infant who is motor delayed consists of assessing the degree and duration of primitive reflexes, evaluating the child for postural responses that should be developing, noticing reactions that are never normal (e.g., asymmetry), and searching for neurologic dysfunction in other areas such as language.

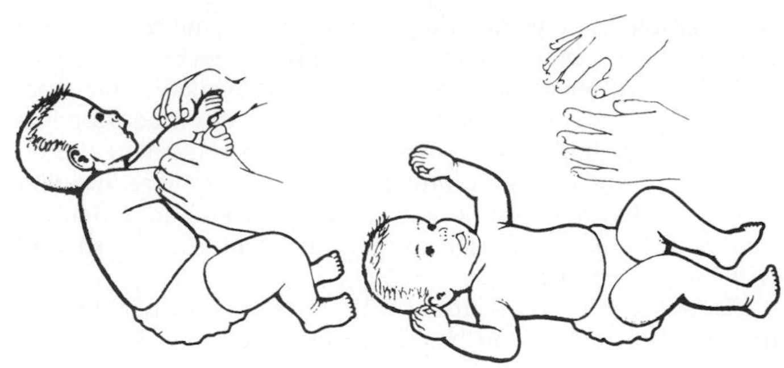

Figure 217-1. The Moro, or embrace, reflex is elicited by sudden neck extension or by slapping the side of the baby's pillow. The reflex is present at birth and disappears at 3 to 6 months.

As is true of the younger infant, direct observation of spontaneous movement is a sensitive method for detecting movement disorders. Watching the child's sitting; locomotion in prone posture, standing, and walking, as well as transitions between postures, reveals important information about gross movement. Assessment of transferring, reaching, raking, finger isolation (e.g., pincer use), and voluntary release reveals the status of the upper extremities.

The interweaving of the suppression of the primitive reflexes and the onset of postural responses serves as the basis for volitional movement. Persistence of significant primitive reflex activity beyond the first half-year is abnormal. The Moro reflex (Fig. 217-1), or embrace response, is elicited by sudden neck extension or by slapping the side of the pillow; extension, adduction, and abduction of the upper extremities occur, followed by semiflexion of fingers, wrists, and elbows. The asymmetric tonic neck reflex (Fig. 217-2), or "fencer" response, is elicited by turning the child's head laterally with relative extension of the limbs on the chin side and relative flexion on the occiput side. The tonic labyrinthine reflex (Fig. 217-3) is elicited by extending or flexing the neck. This maneuver alters the relation of the labyrinths and is associated with shoulder retraction and hip extension or shoulder protraction and hip flexion. If present to a substantial

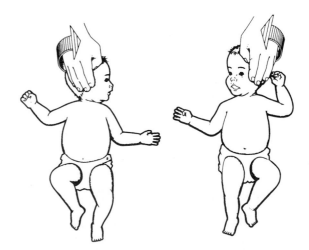

Figure 217-2. In the asymmetric tonic neck reflex, or "fencer" response, limbs extend on the side to which the chin is turned, and limbs on the opposite side are flexed. The reflex is present at birth and disappears at 3 to 6 months.

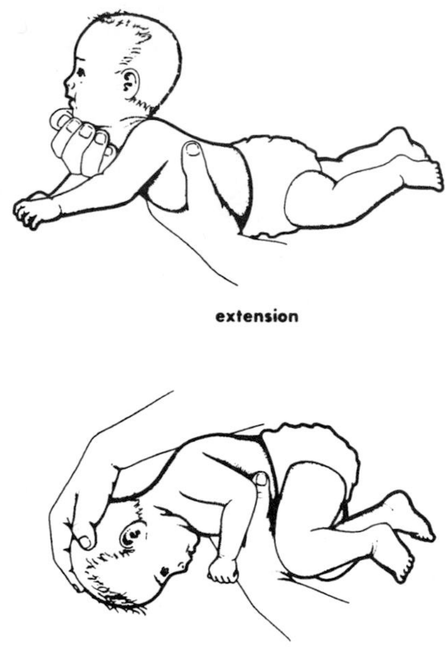

Figure 217-3. The tonic labyrinthine reflex is elicited by extending or flexing the neck. The reflex is present at birth and disappears at 3 to 6 months.

degree, these three reflexes interfere with midline activities, inhibit rolling, and preclude sitting.

A fourth reflex is the positive support reflex of the neonatal type (Fig. 217-4), which gives some indication of neurologic integrity of the lower extremities. It is elicited by stimulating (i.e., bouncing) the hallucal areas on a firm surface; the result is momentary lower extremity extension followed by flexion caused by cocontractions of the hip flexors and extensors. This neonatal or immature response is followed at 2 to 3 months of age by the more mature one in which the extremities support the body weight for a longer period.

Just as important as the delineation of movement-inhibiting primitive reflexes is the evaluation of postural responses (e.g., righting, equilibrium). Postural responses appear in the second half of the first year of life and coincide with volitional movement. Postural responses keep the head and neck in vertical alignment with the body. The 5-month derotative responses are defined as the body following the turning of the head in a derotative fashion or the head following the axial displacement of the body. Resistance to anterior displacement by extension of the arms (i.e., anterior propping) occurs at 5 months, lateral propping is seen at 7 months, and posterior propping is noted at 9 months. Anterior propping is associated with the ability to sit in a tripod fashion; lateral propping correlates with independent sitting; and posterior propping permits pivoting in sitting. Propping responses without primitive reflex activity portend a good prognosis in the motor-delayed child.

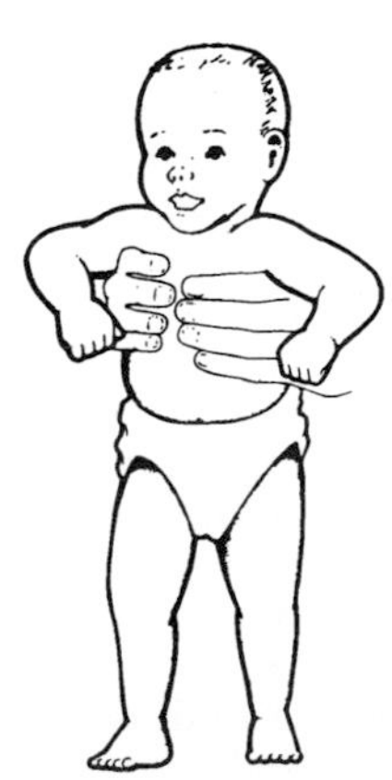

Figure 217-4. The positive support reflex is elicited by bouncing the hallucal areas on a firm surface. It is present at birth and disappears at 2 to 3 months.

Physiologic Classification

Cerebral palsy can be divided into two major groups, the pyramidal (spastic) and the extrapyramidal (nonspastic) types. Extrapyramidal cerebral palsy can be subdivided into choreoathetoid, ataxic, dystonic, and rigid forms. These groups are clinically useful but are not well correlated with neuropathologic findings.

The signs used to differentiate spastic from nonspastic types are listed in Table 217-1. The neurologic findings of the pyramidal type are consistent and persistent varying little with movement, tension, emotion, or sleep. Variability is the main feature of extrapyramidal types; findings are increased with activity, tension, and emotions and decreased with sleep or relaxation.

The characteristic type of hypertonus seen in spasticity is clasp knife, similar to the opening and closing of a penknife with a consistent hitch. The tone in extrapyramidal types varies from hypotonic to hypertonic. Extrapyramidal hypertonus is of the lead pipe or candle-wax type, but it is variable and can be diminished by repetitive movement (i.e., "shaking it out"). The persistence of spastic hypertonus may be a factor in the development of contractures. The variability of extrapyramidal tone may protect against contractures.

Pathologic reflexes such as Babinski or Chaddock are readily elicited in spastic forms. A true Babinski reflex must be differentiated from the extensor plantar response that is seen as part of athetotic posturing. Primitive reflexes are more evident in the extrapyramidal forms.

Topographic Classification

The topographic classification is limited to the spastic types. Generally, it is not used with extrapyramidal types because these types show four-limb involvement and are classified by the nature of the movement disorder. The topographic axis includes hemiplegia, diplegia, quadriplegia, and bilateral hemiplegia.

Hemiplegia (i.e., hemiparesis) describes involvement of either lateral side of the body. The upper extremities are more impaired than lower ones, and upper extremity dysfunction usually brings the child to attention.

Diplegia refers to four-limb involvement with the upper limbs only minimally involved, although significant lower extremity impairment is present. The good upper extremity function seen in diplegia is of major assistance to habilitative efforts. The designation *paraplegia* is reserved for spinal and lower motor neuron dysfunctions such as myelodysplasia.

Spastic quadriplegia is four-limb involvement with significant impairment of all extremities. Upper limbs may be less impaired than lower ones, but substantial functional limitations exist. Some researchers consider quadriplegia a furtherance of diplegia.

Bilateral hemiplegia designates significant spasticity of both sides of the body with upper extremities more significantly impaired. Monoplegia and triplegia are combinations of hemiplegia and quadriplegia.

TABLE 217-1. Distinguishing Signs of Spastic and Nonspastic Types

Sign	Pyramidal (spastic) type	Extrapyramidal (nonspastic) type
Movement	Decreased	Disordered, but may be decreased in rigidity
Oral motor	Suprabulbar type (flat facies)	Athetotic (grimacing) or suprabulbar type; common oral reflexes are root, palmomental, increased gag
Tone changes	Consistent and persistent; remain relatively constant when infant is asleep or challenged	Variable, changes with tension, challenge, or sleep (usually hypotonic when asleep or quiet)
Tone quality	Clasp-knife spasticity; sudden give followed by resistance or vice versa (similar to the opening or closing of a penknife); more exaggerated with sudden increase in tendon stretching	Lead pipe or candle-wax rigidity; sustained resistance throughout extension or flexion of a limb, brought out by slow movement
Primitive reflexes	Present (not noticeable as with choreoathetoid cerebral palsy)	Present; most evident in this type of cerebral palsy
Deep tendon reflexes	Hyperreflexia predominates, 3 or 4+ (frequently accompanied by overflow movement)	Normal or mildly increased, 1 to 3+
Babinski, Chaddock, Oppenheim, or Gordon	Present	Absent, not to be confused with the athetotic positioning of the toes and foot (extensor plantar response) due to the posturing seen with choreoathetoid movement
Ankle clonus	Sustained ankle clonus evident	Unsustained ankle clonus; possible to have some ankle clonus present
Contractures	Nonpositional contractures	Positional contractures such as hip and knee flexion contractures when child has been in a wheelchair for months or years

From Shapiro BK, Palmer FB, Capute AJ. Cerebral palsy: history and state of the art. In: Gottlieb M, Wilhams J, eds. *Textbook of developmental pediatrics.* New York: Plenum Publishing, 1987.

TREATMENT

The treatment of cerebral palsy is directed toward maximizing function and preventing secondary handicaps. Normality is rarely achieved, although functional outcomes are not uncommon. Treatment objectives change as the child ages.

In the preschool years, enhancing communication becomes increasingly important. Communicative abilities are more closely related to long-term outcome than is motor function. The most efficient means of communication is oral. However, oral communication may not be possible for some children, and alternative methods may be used to circumvent oral motor dysfunction. Children whose motor dysfunction is sufficiently severe to make intelligible speech unlikely, but who possess the necessary cognition, may be treated with augmentative methods of communication that circumvent oral communication. These methods may range from boards that require looking at the proper answer, to scanning systems, to pointing, to computer-synthesized speech.

As the child ages, concerns about communication evolve into concerns about school performance. Cognitive deficits, peer acceptance, and environmental issues are areas that commonly require intervention. Management of motor deficits focuses on the prevention of postural deformity and seeks to maintain gross motor function.

Motor Therapy

The motor deficit in cerebral palsy results from the combination of abnormal tone and abnormal control of movement. Normalizing tone may permit the expression of more functional abilities. Most techniques are designed to decrease hypertonus and its effects. Low tone in extreme forms is treated by positioning and support. Shifting tone is the most difficult to treat. No techniques have been consistently effective in achieving control of disordered movement.

Specific techniques of handling are the mainstay of physical therapy. In young infants and in children with severe motor deficits, handling techniques are supplemented by positioning. Positioning seeks to diminish asymmetries and tonic influences of primitive reflexes and to normalize tone. Proper positioning enhances the child's opportunity to interact with the environment. Benefits for oral motor function may be seen in improved feeding abilities and less difficulty in handling secretions. Modified seating devices ensure that most children can be in an upright position, in addition to prone and side-lying positions.

Drugs may be used to decrease hypertonus. Diazepam is the agent most commonly used, although baclofen and dantrolene sodium are effective. Tizanidine hydrochloride has also been recommended for spasticity. For extrapyramidal dysfunction, L-dopa/carbidopa or trihexyphenidyl hydrochloride has been used. Most of the experience with these agents is not derived from their use in children with cerebral palsy, and only limited data exist regarding their effects in motor and nonmotor areas (e.g., effects on learning with long-term use). Pharmacologic approaches must be coupled with targeted, measurable goals.

Nerve blocks with agents such as alcohol or phenol have been used to treat localized motor dysfunction caused by spasticity (e.g., heel cord tightness or adductor overactivity). Botulinum toxin has been used as well. These agents are more specific than other forms of pharmacotherapy, but the effects are not permanent.

Bracing may be used to assist function, prevent deformity, or normalize tone. For example, in children who have spastic diplegia and obligatory positive supporting responses such as marked equinus, bracing of the ankle and foot may be used to stretch tight muscles and prevent contracture or provide a more stable base for walking.

Surgical goals are similar to those of other motor therapies: improvement of function and prevention of deformity. Surgical approaches have moved away from consideration of static, single-joint function to more dynamic approaches. This move has been facilitated by techniques such as gait analysis that objectively quantify movement in great detail and permit the delineation of individual muscle action during the course of a movement. As a result, lower extremity surgery is becoming more specific to the physiologic disturbance.

Hand function is essential to the ultimate outcome in cerebral palsy. Good hand function may permit the person with cerebral palsy to circumvent other motor deficits. Surgical approaches to aid upper extremity function have traditionally been deferred until late adolescence to allow for full growth and maximal patient cooperation.

Neurosurgical approaches to cerebral palsy primarily seek to alter the abnormal control of movement. Some techniques also normalize tone. Selective posterior rhizotomy is the most commonly applied neurosurgical technique. Ventrolateral thalamotomy, cerebellar pacing, and electronic stimulation have also been used.

CHAPTER 218
Developmental Defects

Adapted from Marvin A. Fishman

HYDROCEPHALY

Hydrocephaly is a congenital or acquired disorder in which an excessive amount of cerebrospinal fluid (CSF) is present within the cerebral ventricles. More CSF is produced than can be reabsorbed. Increased pressure within the ventricular system may be transitory or persistent. *Noncommunicating hydrocephaly* refers to conditions in which the ventricular fluid does not communicate with the fluid in the basal cisterns or spinal subarachnoid spaces. It implies a block of the CSF flow within the ventricular system. In communicating hydrocephaly, the block is outside the ventricular system or its exit foramina.

CSF is formed within the ventricular system, mainly by the choroid plexus, through the processes of active secretion and diffusion. The fluid exits the ventricular system by way of foramina in the fourth ventricle and circulates into the lumbar and subarachnoid spaces. Most CSF absorption takes place at the arachnoid villi leading to venous channels of the sagittal sinus. In adults, the total CSF volume is approximately 150 mL, and only 25% is within the ventricular system. The rate of formation is approximately 20 mL/hour, and the CSF turns over three to four times per day.

Etiology

Congenital hydrocephalus may result from congenital malformations of the nervous system including isolated aqueductal stenosis or may be associated with other malformations including the Dandy–Walker malformation. The latter consists of a large cyst in the posterior fossa continuous with the fourth ventricle and partial or complete absence of the cerebellar vermis. A common associated malformation syndrome is that of meningomyelocele with Chiari malformation. Other syndromes include a sex-linked form of aqueductal stenosis and chromosomal anomalies resulting in syndromes with additional multiple congenital malformations. Arachnoid cysts or congenital tumors may obstruct the ventricular system. Congenital hydrocephalus may be caused by intrauterine infections, which cause inflammation of the ependymal lining of the ventricular system or the meninges in the subarachnoid space, subsequently occluding the CSF pathways. Among the more common infections causing congenital hydrocephalus are rubella, cytomegalovirus infection, toxoplasmosis, and syphilis.

Hydrocephalus may be acquired postnatally secondary to infections of the nervous system (e.g., bacterial meningitis), brain tumors, and arachnoiditis due to bleeding into the subarachnoid space from a ruptured arteriovenous malformation, aneurysm, or trauma. Premature infants may develop hydrocephalus secondary to intraventricular hemorrhage.

Clinical Characteristics

The primary process (e.g., tumor, infection, bleeding) and the symptoms and signs caused by increased ICP secondary to the hydrocephalus may contribute to the clinical picture. The severity of the findings is influenced by the rate at which the hydrocephalus develops and the development of alternate pathways of CSF absorption. Nonspecific symptoms include headaches that are variable in location and intensity; these occasionally occur early in the morning and are associated with vomiting. Personality and behavior changes including irritability or indifference sometimes occur. Lethargy and drowsiness are relatively late symptoms. Nausea and vomiting are secondary to increased ICP, particularly with posterior fossa lesions. Nonspecific signs include third and sixth cranial nerve deficits, which result in paresis of extraocular muscles and may lead to diplopia. Papilledema may be a late finding if the ICP is not markedly elevated and the process is a slow, chronic one. Changes in vital signs occur relatively late and indicate distortion of the brainstem. In young children, the anterior fontanelle may become full or distended; this condition is accompanied by excessive head growth and dilatation of scalp veins. The setting-sun sign is produced by paralysis of upward gaze so that the sclera is visible above the iris. Spasticity develops first in the lower extremities and then in the arms and results from stretching of motor fibers around the bodies of the lateral ventricles. Dilatation of the third ventricle may cause pressure on the hypothalamus resulting in disturbances in sexual development and in fluid and electrolyte imbalance. Specific deficits produced by focal lesions include hemiparesis, ataxia, tremor, speech and language disorders, gaze disorders, facial weakness, and difficulty in swallowing. Seizures are unusual, isolated presenting symptoms of childhood brain tumors.

Diagnosis and Therapy

Neuroimaging techniques such as computed tomographic (CT) or magnetic resonance imaging (MRI) have made the diagnosis of hydrocephalus relatively straightforward. The pattern of ventricular dilatation, the presence of interstitial edema (i.e., CSF in the white matter surrounding the ventricles), and an underlying cause for obstruction of CSF flow are usually readily apparent (Fig. 218-1). The CSF should be examined if a relatively recent infection is suspected, or if subarachnoid bleeding is suspected, but no evidence of such is found on neuroimaging studies. In infancy, chronic subdural hematomas may present in a similar fashion and can be detected by neuroimaging procedures.

Treatment includes specific therapy for any underlying condition associated with the hydrocephalus such as brain tumor, abscess, and chronic meningitis. Surgery is the most effective means of treating progressive hydrocephalus; a shunt system placed between the cerebral ventricles and the peritoneal cavity is the most commonly used technique. The shunt allows diversion of the CSF into the peritoneal cavity, where it is absorbed. Shunt placement is a palliative measure and not a cure. The complication rate is relatively high. Problems encountered include

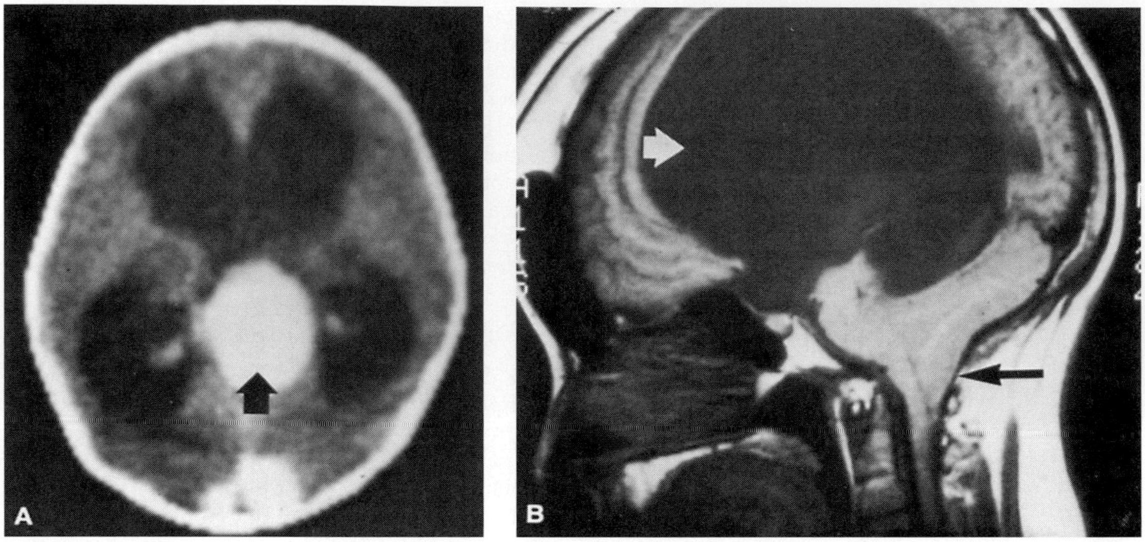

Figure 218-1. **A:** Computed tomographic (CT) scan with contrast enhancement demonstrates hydrocephalus secondary to an aneurysm of the vein of Galen (arrow). **B:** A magnetic resonance image (MRI) in the sagittal plane demonstrates hydrocephalus (white arrow) and a Chiari type II malformation (black arrow) with downward displacement of the brainstem into the cervical canal. (Courtesy of Dr. Clark Carrol, Texas Children's Hospital, Houston, TX.)

mechanical obstruction of the shunt system and infections within it, which may produce meningitis or ventriculitis. Shunt infections may be indolent and are often caused by organisms that are not usually considered pathogens such as *Staphylococcus epidermidis*. Medical therapy designed to decrease CSF production may be used when the hydrocephalus is slowly progressive and perhaps transitory. Such conditions include the ventricular enlargement, sometimes seen after subarachnoid hemorrhage or meningitis. The therapeutic agents used include acetazolamide, furosemide, and glycerol. These agents may also be used in the interim between the removal of an infected shunt system and insertion of a new system.

CHIARI MALFORMATION

The Chiari malformation involves the brainstem and lower portion of the cerebellum. These structures are displaced downward into the cervical canal. Various degrees of the malformation occur. In type I, caudal cerebellar tonsillar ectopia is present, and the cerebellar tonsils extend into the foramen magnum for more than 5 mm. In type II, the medulla and fourth ventricle are elongated and extend into the spinal canal. The downward displacement may be such that the cervical cord is kinked on itself, and the foramen magnum and upper cervical canal may be packed tightly with the displaced tissue. Almost always, an associated meningomyelocele is present. In the rare type III malformation, an associated cervical spina bifida with herniation of brain tissue through the defect is present. As a result of the distal displacement, lower cranial nerves and cervical spinal nerve roots may be stretched. Associated nervous system abnormalities are often present. Children with meningomyeloceles and hydrocephalus usually have an associated Chiari malformation. It may also be associated with hydromyelia and syringomyelia. Other minor malformations include beaking of the tectal plate and large massa intermedia.

Type II Chiari malformations usually occur in children with spina bifida and hydrocephalus. The symptoms and signs are caused by the malformations. With significant downward displacement of the hindbrain, stretching of the lower cranial nerves may occur, which can produce facial paralysis, hoarseness or stridor, or difficulty swallowing. If the upper segments of the spinal cord are involved, motor deficits in the arms may be seen. Cerebellar ataxia and vertical nystagmus have also been described in patients with Chiari malformation.

The symptoms related to Chiari malformation type I include neck pain, back pain, scoliosis, torticollis, motor dysfunction, and apnea. The ages of the patients range from 1 month to 14 years. Some children have associated syringomyelia. The downward displacement of the hindbrain can be detected by neuroimaging procedures (Fig. 218-1). In addition to MRI of the posterior fossa, MRI of the spinal cord may be necessary to detect the associated malformations.

Shunting of an associated hydrocephalus and repair of the meningomyelocele are the first procedures attempted in treating these patients. If these do not improve the symptoms attributable to hindbrain or cervical cord dysfunction, occipital decompression and cervical laminectomy should be considered.

SYRINGOMYELIA AND HYDROMYELIA

Syringomyelia is a rare condition in children. It is a cavity within the spinal cord lined by glial elements and is paracentral in location. The cavity may extend over many segments or be isolated to just a few. The cervical area is often involved. If the syrinx extends into the brainstem, the condition is known as *syringobulbia*. Syringomyelia may be associated with abnormalities of the cervicomedullary junction including Chiari malformation, intramedullary spinal cord tumors, spinal cord trauma, and arterial insufficiency to the cord. The signs and symptoms depend on the location of the syrinx and any associated condition. Often, wasting of the small muscles of the hands and sensory deficits involving the arms are present. Deep tendon reflexes may be absent. Involvement of the descending tracts may cause spasticity in the lower extremities. A dissociated sensory disturbance with loss of pain and temperature sensation but preservation of touch may occur; it may show a segmental distribution and is due to destruction of the commissural fibers of the spinal cord by the cavity. The diagnosis may be made by

MRI of the spinal cord. Treatment consists of therapy for the primary lesion such as associated tumor or cervical medullary junction abnormality, and decompression of the syrinx itself in some patients.

Hydromyelia involves symmetric dilatation of the central canal of the spinal cord. The enlarged canal is lined by ependyma and often communicates with the fourth ventricle. The enlargement may extend over many segments and may include the entire length of the spinal cord. It is often associated with other malformations including communicating hydrocephaly, Chiari malformation, and aqueductal stenosis. The signs and symptoms are often related to the associated malformations, and therapy is directed toward them. Whether any findings are related to the dilatation of the central canal itself is unclear.

MACROCEPHALY

Macrocephaly refers to a head size 2 SD above the mean. The condition can have many causes. Table 218-1 lists the more common conditions associated with large head size. In some children, a large brain (i.e., megalencephaly) may be the underlying condition. It may be familial and may not be accompanied by any additional symptoms and signs or may include an associated mental deficiency and other neurologic abnormalities such as hypotonia.

Infants who are macrocephalic and whose head growth parallels a normal growth pattern, but is above the 95th percentile, have been described. Imaging demonstrates slight ventricular dilatation and increased width of the subarachnoid space over the convexities of the hemispheres. The development of most of these children is normal or only slightly delayed. If head growth continues parallel to the 95th percentile, no intervention is necessary. The exact cause of this condition is uncertain. It has been called *extraventricular obstructive hydrocephalus, benign communicating hydrocephalus,* and *external hydrocephalus*. Another possibility is that the fluid over the convexities represents small subdural hematomas with secondary hydrocephalus. The diagnosis can be established by CT or MRI, and the children can be followed with serial head circumference measurements. Any deviation from the anticipated growth pattern warrants repeat neuroimaging studies. Usually, by the preschool years, the head size deviates less from the 95th percentile, and the fluid collections remain stable or decrease.

MICROCEPHALY

Microcephaly indicates a head size smaller than 2 SD below the mean. The condition is due to a small brain (i.e., microencephaly), the causes of which are many. In primary microcephaly, no identifiable insult occurs to the developing brain that, subsequently, inhibits its growth. The primary microcephalies include familial forms and cases that seem to occur in isolation. Newborn infants with primary microcephaly do not often exhibit striking deficits, unlike the infants who have sustained a major insult *in utero*. Eventually, intellectual impairment becomes apparent, and some children develop motor deficits and epilepsy. Other anomalies sometimes associated with microcephaly include agyria, lissencephaly, micropolygyria, schizencephaly, macrogyria, and heterotopia. These infants usually have severe deficits that are apparent in the neonatal period. Microcephaly can result from a variety of disorders due to chromosomal anomalies—from intrauterine infections secondary to inherited metabolic disorders, from intrauterine anoxia or vascular events, and from insults in the perinatal period.

TABLE 218-1. Large Head Syndromes

Hydrocephaly
Congenital
Aqueductal stenosis: with or without meningomyelocele and Chiari malformation
Communicating: with or without meningomyelocele and Chiari malformation
Dandy-Walker syndrome
Hydranencephaly
Porencephaly
Holoprosencephaly
Genetic
Chromosomal malformation
Sex-linked
Cysts
Infectious
Postinflammatory disease (meningitis)
Viral (cytomegalovirus, mumps, other)
Parasitic (toxoplasmosis)
Vascular
Postsubarachnoid hemorrhage
Arteriovenous malformation
Vein of Galen aneurysm
Tumor
Choroid plexus papilloma
Posterior fossa neoplasm
Other
Subdural
Effusion
Hematoma
Hygroma
Empyema
Neurocutaneous disorders
Neurofibromatosis
Tuberous sclerosis
Multiple hemangiomatosis
Incontinentia pigmenti
Basal cell nevus syndrome
Neurocutaneous melanosis
Toxic-metabolic causes
Benign increased intracranial hypertension associated with antibiotics, vitamins, endocrine disorders, catch-up growth after malnutrition, galactosemia, anemias
Cranioskeletal dysplasias
Anemias
Achondroplasia
Osteogenesis imperfecta
Osteopetrosis
Metaphyseal dysplasia
Platybasia
Fibrous dysplasia (Albright syndrome)
Storage and degenerative diseases
Leukodystrophies
Canavan spongy degenerative disease
Alexander disease
Lysosomal disease
Tay-Sachs disease
Generalized gangliosidosis
Mucopolysaccharidosis
Metachromatic leukodystrophy
Peroxisomal disorders
Neonatal adrenoleukodystrophy
Amino acid disorders
Maple syrup urine disease
Unknown causes
Cerebral gigantism
Megalencephaly
Familial
Dominant
Beckwith-Wiedemann syndrome

CHAPTER 219
Epilepsy

Adapted from Daniel G. Glaze

Epilepsy is the symptomatic expression of underlying brain pathology or disordered brain function, not a disease in the usual sense. The incidence of epilepsy has been reported to range from 0.8% to 1.1%. Epilepsy is the most common neurologic disorder seen in children, and approximately 50% of all cases of epilepsy start in childhood. Epilepsy is defined as a randomly recurring symptom complex resulting from an episodic disturbance of central nervous system function associated with an excessive, self-limited, neuronal discharge. Variation in clinical manifestations results from variation in the portion of the brain involved.

CLASSIFICATION AND DESCRIPTION OF SEIZURE TYPES

The classification system for epileptic seizures currently in use (Table 219-1) is based on both clinical and electroencephalograph (EEG) features. It divides seizures into two major categories, generalized and partial. Generalized seizures are those in which the clinical features indicate the involvement of both cerebral hemispheres from the start. Consciousness is usually impaired and, when motor involvement is present, it is bilateral and relatively symmetric from the beginning. Conversely, clinical features suggesting that only a limited or functional area of one cerebral hemisphere is involved characterize partial seizures. They begin focally, although they may become generalized. Partial seizures are divided further into those with elementary or simple symptomatology and those with complex symptomatology. In children, elementary partial seizures are most commonly focal motor or focal sensory phenomena, and consciousness is preserved unless secondary generalization occurs. Complex partial seizures usually have their origin in temporal or frontal lobe structures, and the clinical features encompass a spectrum of complex phenomena including behavioral automatisms, alterations of perception, hallucinations, changes in affect and memory, and ideational distortions.

TABLE 219-1. Classification of Epileptic Seizures

Generalized seizures
Tonic-clonic
Clonic
Tonic
Atonic
Myoclonic
Absence
Partial seizures
Elementary symptomatology
With motor symptoms
With sensory symptoms
Complex symptomatology
With impairment of consciousness only
With cognitive symptomatology
With affective symptomatology
With psychosensory symptomatology
Compound forms
Secondarily generalized

Reprinted with permission from Commission on Classification and Terminology of the International League Against Epilepsy. Proposal for revised clinical and electroencephalographic classification of epileptic seizures. *Epilepsia* 1981;22:489.

Generalized Seizures

TONIC-CLONIC TYPE

Generalized tonic-clonic seizures are clinically characterized by an abrupt arrest of activity and an immediate loss of consciousness. The tonic phase, consisting of sustained, generalized contraction of flexor or extensor muscles, usually lasts only a few seconds. The clonic phase that follows is characterized by symmetric, rhythmic, clonic activity consisting of alternating contraction and relaxation of major appendicular or axial muscle groups. The clonic phase is longer in duration than the tonic phase, but it often terminates spontaneously in less than 5 minutes. Respiration may be irregular and stridulous, and sphincter incontinence may or may not be present. The clonic phase is usually followed by a variable period of confusion and lethargy, which may persist from minutes to hours, and sleep is common.

CLONIC TYPE

Clonic seizures are identical to the clonic phase of tonic-clonic seizures. Generalized tonic seizures are characterized by sustained contraction of flexor or extensor muscle groups giving the child a stiff or rigid appearance. A coarse tremor may be superimposed, but it should not be confused with the rhythmic, alternating muscle contraction and relaxation of clonic activity. A distinction can often be made by asking the parents to supplement their verbal description with a demonstration of what they observed. Postictal signs and symptoms similar to those seen following generalized tonic-clonic seizures are also associated with both clonic and tonic seizures.

ATONIC TYPE

Atonic seizures are characterized by the abrupt loss of postural tone and limpness. In contrast to akinetic seizures, the loss of consciousness lasts for several minutes, and usually postictal confusion and lethargy or sleepiness result.

MYOCLONIC TYPE

Myoclonic seizures are characterized by brief, random contractions of a muscle or group of muscles occurring unilaterally or bilaterally, either singly or in clusters. Consciousness is usually preserved. Myoclonic seizures are most often seen with progressive or degenerative types of encephalopathy accompanied by intellectual deficits, as well as other overt abnormalities, on neurologic examination. Akinetic or "drop" attacks are a subclass of myoclonic seizures and are characterized by a precipitous loss of postural tone. The child abruptly becomes limp and drops to the floor. With nonambulatory infants, precipitous loss of tone resulting in head nodding or slumping forward may occur. The duration of myoclonic seizures is only a few seconds, and immediate resumption of normal activity with no postictal lethargy or confusion occurs.

ABSENCE TYPE

Absence seizures are clinically characterized by brief episodes of altered awareness during which transient arrest of activity occurs and the child appears to stare blankly. The duration of these episodes is seldom longer than 5 to 10 seconds, but they can recur many times a day. They are rarely seen in children younger than 3 years, and most have their onset before 10 years of age. Commonly, the child is not aware that a seizure has occurred and is frequently assumed to be daydreaming. A child who is daydreaming, however, is aware of doing so and usually responds when his or her name is called or he or she is touched. In contrast, a child with absence seizures usually denies awareness of any lapse and does not respond to verbal or physical stimuli. Subtle motor activity such as rhythmic eye blinking, drooping of the head, or slight movements of the arms may accompany the staring episodes. The seizure is terminated by the immediate return of environmental awareness, and the child may resume an activity at the point where it was interrupted. A generalized, symmetric three-per-second spike and wave pattern is the EEG hallmark of absence seizures.

Partial Seizures

The initial features of a partial seizure are especially important. Tonic deviation of the head and eyes to one side, or some other localized motor or sensory feature preceding a secondarily generalized tonic-clonic seizure, may be a clue to focal cortical origin of the attack. In children, elementary partial seizures are usually focal motor or sensory. The initial feature may be focal twitching involving the distal portion of an extremity, which may remain localized or spread to become a hemiconvulsion. Similarly, focal sensory seizures may be initiated by the appearance of a sensation of numbness or tingling in an extremity, which may remain confined to that area or spread to involve the entire side of the body. Consciousness is often preserved, but lost if secondary generalization occurs.

COMPLEX PARTIAL SEIZURES

Complex partial seizures have a variety of clinical expressions and are subclassified on this basis. One form that has impairment of consciousness only is characterized by transient, blank staring or confusion. These episodes can be mistaken for absence seizures, but the attacks usually last 30 seconds or longer, whereas absence episodes commonly last less than 10 seconds. An EEG can be helpful in distinguishing between the two forms because a three-per-second generalized spike and wave pattern is the hallmark of absence seizures, whereas focal discharge from temporal or frontal areas is seen in complex partial seizures.

PARTIAL SEIZURES WITH COGNITIVE CHANGES

Another form of partial complex seizure involves *cognitive symptomatology*. This form is clinically characterized by an abrupt alteration in mental state that involves disruption of time relationships and memory. Older children sometimes describe feelings of unreality, remoteness, detachment, or depersonalization. Forced thinking, a deluge of thoughts, or perseveration of a thought have also been described. *Déjà vu* or *jamais vu*, the impression of an inappropriate familiarity or unfamiliarity with a place or situation, may occasionally be reported. Attacks characterized by *affective symptomatology* may be described as inexplicable feelings of fear or dread or other emotional experiences that abruptly intrude on the patient's prevailing affective state. Attacks characterized by *somatosensory disturbances* are notable for distortions of perception or hallucinations. Some children report transient distortions of perception concerning the size of objects (micropsia or macropsia), and others describe hallucinations involving taste or smell, as well as formed visual hallucinations.

PARTIAL SEIZURES WITH AUTOMATISM

Probably the most familiar complex partial seizure is the psychomotor attack that is characterized by semipurposeful motor automatisms. The stereotyped automatisms may be persistent in nature, and the child exhibits continuing repetition of the activity in which he or she was engaged before the onset of the seizure. For example, if the child was walking, he or she may continue to walk, but without purposeful direction. If the child was writing, he or she may continue to move the pencil across the page without producing decipherable script. The simplest types of automatisms are masticatory, sucking, and lip-pursing movements. Patting, scratching, or picking at clothing may also be seen. More complex behaviors such as fumbling with clothing, as if to undress, or turning about, as if searching for something, are less common. Finally, *compound forms* that incorporate various elements of the several varieties just described may be seen. In an individual child, the form taken is usually stereotyped from one attack to another.

EPILEPTIC SYNDROMES

Infantile Spasms

Infantile spasms or infantile massive spasms are peculiar to infancy and early childhood with a peak incidence of onset between 2 and 7 months of age. They have been described as occurring in three clinical forms. Flexor spasms consist of sudden flexion of the neck, trunk, and extremities, which may be so violent that the torso will jackknife at the waist. Extensor spasms consist of abrupt extension of the neck and trunk with adduction or abduction of the extremities. The predominant form is a mixed flexor-extensor spasm most commonly consisting of flexion of the neck, trunk, and arms with extension of the legs and, less commonly, flexion of the legs and extension of the arms. Infantile spasms tend to occur in clusters with each cluster consisting of two to 125 individual spasms. Each individual spasm lasts only for a few seconds, although a cluster may extend over several minutes. Spasms rarely occur during actual sleep but frequently occur on arousal. In most instances, the EEG shows the distinctive pattern of hypsarrhythmia.

Infantile spasms must be distinguished from benign myoclonus of early infancy and benign neonatal sleep myoclonus, which are characterized by normal EEG results, normal development, and occurrence during sleep. Massive spasms are frequently misinterpreted as startle responses or attacks of colic. A careful history usually elicits the absence of a preceding startle stimulus or the information that the episodes are too precipitous in onset and offset and too short in duration to fit the usual clinical picture of colic. Although crying may follow an infantile spasm, it is not the inconsolable crying encountered in infants with cramping abdominal pain.

Infantile spasms have been divided into two broad groups. In the idiopathic or cryptogenic group, no demonstrable cause is present, the child's development has usually been normal until the onset of spasms, and the results of computed tomographic (CT) scans of the brain are normal. In the symptomatic group, a specific etiologic factor can be identified, developmental or neurologic abnormalities have preceded the onset of spasms, and the results of computed tomographic (CT) scans of the brain are often abnormal. The cryptogenic group represents no more than 10% to 15% of the total, and it has a better prognosis than the symptomatic group.

Causes associated with the symptomatic group of infantile spasms include cerebral dysgenesis, intrauterine infections, and genetic disorders. Two syndromes of cerebral dysgenesis that have been associated with infantile spasms are the Miller–Dieker syndrome (lissencephaly with or without a chromosome 17 abnormality) and Aicardi syndrome (girls with agenesis of the corpus callosum, distinctive chorioretinopathy, and mental retardation).

The relationship of pertussis immunization to the onset of infantile spasms has generated interest and concern for many years. Well-designed, controlled epidemiologic studies have failed to prove an association between DTP immunization and infantile spasms. Children receive their initial DTP immunizations at an age when infantile spasms have their onset. The administration of pertussis vaccine is associated with a short-term increase in the risk of seizures (mostly febrile seizures), and complete recovery is expected. Children whose neurologic problems begin soon after immunization warrant a full diagnostic workup.

LENNOX–GASTAUT SYNDROME

The Lennox–Gastaut syndrome is one type of symptomatic generalized epilepsy, and it is age-dependent. The Lennox–Gastaut syndrome is characterized in early childhood by the onset of mixed seizures (including tonic, tonic-clonic, atonic, akinetic or myoclonic, and absence), refractoriness to common antiepileptic drugs (AEDs), an abnormal EEG pattern (generalized, slow spike and slow wave activity), and a high incidence of developmental and mental retardation. This syndrome is frequently preceded by infantile spasms. Etiologic factors are similar to those outlined with infantile spasms. In 30% of the cases, the Lennox–Gastaut syndrome appears in children who have no antecedents, previous epilepsy, or clinical or neurologic evidence of brain damage and who have had previously normal development.

BENIGN EPILEPSY OF CHILDHOOD (ROLANDIC SEIZURES)

Benign focal epilepsy of childhood (also called *benign epilepsy of childhood with rolandic or centrotemporal spikes*) is a form of partial epilepsy characterized by an onset between the ages of 4 and 10 years. The seizures typically occur during sleep, although daytime seizures may also be seen. The seizures begin most frequently with clonic twitching of one side of the face. Involvement of the tongue or an upper extremity, and secondary generalization may occur. If the child is awake, he or she may experience paresthesias involving the mouth and throat. The child usually appears well immediately after the seizure. The occurrence of seizures during sleep may cause uncertainty as to whether the child has had a nightmare or a seizure. The children are otherwise well and have a history of normal development. Neuroimaging studies in these children have been unremarkable. The EEG is characterized by independent spike discharges occurring focally in one or both central (rolandic) regions. Focal spike activity is enhanced during sleep and may only occur at this time. EEG background activity is otherwise normal. Both the seizures and the spike focus typically have a short natural history and are usually resolved by puberty or soon after. This natural history, in addition to normal development of the child and normal results of neuroimaging studies, suggests the terminology of benign focal epilepsy. The EEG trait (the central spike with a normal background) may be inherited as an autosomal dominant gene with a particular age penetrance. The inheritance pattern of the seizures is familial, but appears to be multifactorial. Similar varieties of benign focal epilepsy have been identified in association with temporal, parietal, and occipital spike foci.

ANCILLARY LABORATORY STUDIES

Electroencephalography

A routine EEG should always be recorded during wakefulness and sleep and, in older children, during hyperventilation and photic stimulation. Because normal organizational and frequency characteristics change rapidly with advancing age and cerebral maturation, it is of particular importance that the interpretation of EEGs in infants and young children be done by an electroencephalographer who has had specific training and experience with this age group.

The duration of a routine EEG recording in most laboratories is approximately 1 hour. This 1-hour sample is taken to be representative of the patient's cerebral electrical activity during any average 24-hour period. An obvious potential exists for sampling to take place at a time when no epileptiform activity is present. A sleep-deprived EEG or a routine EEG obtained at a subsequent date may demonstrate abnormalities that were not evident in the initial sample. The yield of useful information is enhanced when the EEG can be scheduled in particular relationship to a clinical seizure. The EEG should be recorded as soon as possible after any seizures that occur in neonates and infants up to 6 months of age. If an EEG is recorded in children with febrile seizures who are 6 to 36 months of age, it should be delayed until 5 to 10 days after the seizure because the child's postictal brain wave activity may be transiently and diffusely slow for several days and its significance misinterpreted. For patients with nonfebrile seizures, the EEG should be recorded as soon as possible after the event.

Normal EEG results should not necessarily dissuade a physician from making a diagnosis of epilepsy in the face of a convincing clinical description. Similarly, abnormal EEG results do not necessarily confirm a clinical suspicion of epilepsy. The type and location of an abnormality is expected to correlate with the clinical data. When the available clinical and EEG data do not provide a basis for confident classification regarding seizure type, or in cases in which pseudoseizures are suspected, video-EEG monitoring may be justified.

Neuroimaging

Routine skull radiography is seldom indicated or helpful, except when overt bony pathology is detected by physical examination. Neuroimaging studies may be indicated in cases of partial seizures, or if the history and physical examination suggest structural lesions, degenerative diseases, or a congenital structural abnormality. High-resolution ultrasound is a useful technique in the investigation of premature infants and term neonates with seizures. Magnetic resonance imaging (MRI) has virtually replaced CT in the evaluation of patients with epilepsy. MRI allows for the clear imaging of intraparenchymal structures without bony artifacts and exposure to ionizing radiation; allows acquisition of multiplanar anatomic data and the ability to reconfigure the data for enhanced visualization; and visualizes important substrates of epilepsy such as malformations of cortical development, abnormal neuronal and glial proliferation, abnormal neuronal migration, tumors, vascular malformations, encephalomalacia, and mesial temporal sclerosis.

MEDICAL TREATMENT

Population studies suggest that approximately 70% of patients in whom epilepsy is diagnosed ultimately become free of seizures and that the majority can expect to discontinue anticonvulsant medication. A higher likelihood of remission has been reported in children than in adults. Children with epilepsy in association with mental retardation or cerebral palsy, however, have low rates of remission. The literature does not reflect universal agreement on the optimal duration of anticonvulsant therapy. In most instances, a seizure-free period of at least 2 to 3 consecutive years is a conservative objective before the gradual withdrawal of medication should be considered. Monitoring serum drug levels at reasonable intervals can provide a guideline for adjusting drug dosages as the child grows. Complete seizure control is not possible in some children and, in those instances; the occurrence of an occasional seizure is preferable to an increase in the dosage of anticonvulsants to levels that produce sedation and dysequilibrium, which compromises both cognitive function and social interaction.

Treatment after the Nonfebrile First Seizure

The initiation of AED therapy, after an initial, nonfebrile seizure in otherwise well children, continues to be controversial. The decision to treat should be individualized and take into consideration the risk of seizure recurrence, consequences of having another seizure, and the risks of AED therapy. The observation that many children, possibly as many as one-half, who present with a single unprovoked seizure that do not experience a second seizure has resulted in many clinicians electing not to begin AED therapy after the first seizure. Some children may have a benign developmental disorder of seizure threshold that they outgrow. These include children whose generalized tonic-clonic seizures begin between 1 and 10 years of age, have normal neurologic examinations, and normal or nonspecific abnormal EEG results and children with benign epilepsy with rolandic spikes.

The importance of identifying epileptic syndromes has been recognized. For example, children with West syndrome (infantile spasms), childhood absence epilepsy, and juvenile myoclonic epilepsy have high recurrence risks, whereas children with benign epilepsy with rolandic spikes appear to have good outcomes without AED therapy. Some physicians believe that the stigma attached to the diagnosis of epilepsy and the potential adverse side effects of AEDs, especially on behavior and cognitive function, outweigh the risk of recurrent seizures.

The risk for recurrence in children with a first, nonfebrile seizure has been addressed in only a few studies and has been reported to vary from 52% to 61%. Past studies indicated that recurrence rates are much higher after a second seizure (79%–90%), and most seizures recur within 6 months of the first (70%–74%). Recurrence rates are highest in patients with abnormal results on neurologic examination, focal spikes in the EEG, and complex partial seizures. Recurrence rates in otherwise normal children, who have normal EEG results after the first, nonfebrile, generalized tonic-clonic seizure, range from 10% to 30%. The diagnosis of epilepsy is conventionally made after two unprovoked seizures.

Antiepileptic Drugs

Optimal response to drug therapy and control of seizures can be obtained in approximately 70% of children if a few general principles are observed carefully:

- Initiate therapy with a drug that is known to be effective for the specific type of seizure disorder being treated. If several drugs are equally effective, start with the one that is least toxic and least expensive and requires the least amount of laboratory monitoring.
- Always initiate therapy with a single drug. The introduction of more than one variable complicates the assessment of side effects and therapeutic efficacy.
- Start with a dosage that falls near the lower end of the known therapeutic range (Table 219-2).
- Dosage intervals should be based on the half-life of the drug being used. It may be necessary to administer drugs with relatively short half-lives, two to three times a day. Even though drugs with long half-lives such as phenobarbital can be delivered in a single daily dose, transient sedation may be noted at peak levels, or sluggishness may be seen during the early morning hours when the total dose is delivered at bedtime.
- Maintain the initial dosage for an interval that is sufficient to achieve a steady state before assessing therapeutic efficacy or checking blood levels. Drug metabolism and excretion begin almost immediately after absorption, and the drug continues to accumulate in the body until the elimination rate is in equilibrium with the daily intake. As a general rule, long-term oral administration for approximately five times the half-life of the drug is required to achieve a steady state.
- If the initial dosage does not produce satisfactory seizure control, advance it incrementally until seizure control is obtained or the patient exhibits dose-related side effects (sedation, ataxia, etc.). Serum concentrations of anticonvulsants can be measured as a guideline for adjusting the administered dosage.

TABLE 219-2. Commonly Used Antiepileptic Drugs: Dosage and Side Effects

Drug	Oral dosage (mg/kg/d)	How supplied	Side effects
Carbamazepine (Tegretol)	10–30	100-, 200-mg tablets; 100-mg/5-mL suspension; 100-, 200-, 400-mg extended-release tablets	Diplopia, vertigo, ataxia, sedation, nausea and vomiting, thrombocytopenia, leukopenia, and agranulocytosis
Ethosuximide (Zarontin)	20–40	250-mg capsules; 250-mg/5-mL syrup	Abdominal pain, anorexia, nausea and vomiting, headache, dizziness, photophobia, aplastic anemia, leukopenia, agranulocytosis
Phenobarbital	3–8	8-, 15-, 16-, 30-, 32-, 65-, 100-mg tablets; 20-mg/5-mL elixir	Sedation, hyperkinesis, ataxia, nystagmus
Phenytoin (Dilantin)	3–8	50-mg tablets; 30-, 100-mg capsules; 30-mg/5-mL suspension; 125-mg/5-mL suspension	Nystagmus, ataxia, sedation, hypertrichosis, gum hyperplasia, leukopenia, agranulocytosis
Primidone (Mysoline)	5–30	50-, 250-mg tablets; 250-mg/5-mL suspension	Sedation, hyperkinesis, ataxia, nystagmus
Valproic acid (Depakene, Depakote)	10–40	250-mg/5-mL syrup; 250-, 500-mg capsules; 125-, 250-, 500-mg tablets; 125-mg "sprinkles"; 100-mg/mL IV solution	Nausea and vomiting, increased appetite with weight gain, anorexia with weight loss, transient alopecia, hepatic failure, anemia, leukopenia, thrombocytopenia, acute pancreatitis

- If the addition of a second drug becomes necessary, add only one drug at a time. If little or no improvement was seen with the initial drug, consider withdrawing it gradually after the second drug has reached therapeutic blood levels and seizures are significantly improved or controlled.
- No logic supports the simultaneous administration of two drugs in the same chemical group.
- Periodic laboratory monitoring is indicated when drugs that are known to have a significant incidence of hematologic or hepatic side effects are being used.
- The withdrawal of AEDs should always be gradual to avoid the precipitation of status epilepticus.

Blood Level Monitoring

The blood levels of AEDs that define a therapeutic range are intended to be used as general guidelines, always in the context of the clinical state of the child. The lower limit of the range identifies the minimal level that is required to produce seizure control in the average patient. The upper limit identifies the level at which the average patient exhibits clinical symptoms of dose-related toxicity. Seizures can be controlled in a few children with blood levels somewhat lower than the minimum range, but others require and tolerate levels somewhat above the maximum. The circumstances in which blood levels can be useful in clinical decision making are as follows: 5 to 14 days (five times the drug half-life) after treatment has been initiated at a given dosage, or after a change is made in the dosage (levels drawn before a steady state is achieved will not accurately reflect the optimal concentrations that can be achieved with the dose being used); when previously controlled seizures begin to recur (the most common explanation for this circumstance is noncompliance, but occasionally a child will have been allowed to outgrow a dosage); when clinical symptoms of toxicity become evident or when suspected drug interactions need assessment; and every 6 to 8 months in a rapidly growing child, especially one whose seizures have been easily controlled at low therapeutic levels.

COMMONLY USED DRUGS

Currently, of AEDs approved by the U.S. Food and Drug Administration for the treatment of seizures, six, either alone or in some combination, are used for seizure control in the majority of children who are responsive to medical therapy. These six drugs are phenobarbital, phenytoin, carbamazepine, ethosuximide, valproic acid (VPA), and primidone (Table 219-2). Evidence indicates that therapy with a single agent suffices for the majority of children, but a significant number require more than one drug. Phenobarbital, phenytoin, carbamazepine, and VPA have been used successfully in the control of generalized tonic-clonic, clonic, and tonic seizures. Ethosuximide is the usual drug of choice in the treatment of absence seizures, and VPA appears to be equally effective. VPA, ethosuximide, and clonazepam have been useful in patients with myoclonic and akinetic seizures. Adrenocorticotropic hormone and prednisone are the only agents proven to be effective in infantile spasms. Some studies have suggested that VPA may have efficacy in the treatment of infantile spasms; however, these observations have not been verified in a controlled trial. Clonazepam has limited usefulness because of sedative side effects and the development of drug tolerance. Elementary partial seizures have responded to carbamazepine, phenytoin, and phenobarbital. Carbamazepine is the drug of choice in the treatment of complex partial seizures; phenytoin, primidone, and phenobarbital are effective second choices.

Drug Interactions

Chlorpromazine, prochlorperazine, chlordiazepoxide, anticoagulants, estrogens, chloramphenicol, cimetidine, and isoniazid may elevate blood levels of phenytoin by impairing its metabolism. Antacids taken in proximity to a dose can almost completely impair the absorption of phenytoin. Carbamazepine levels are increased by troleandomycin, erythromycin, cimetidine, and isoniazid. Carbamazepine accelerates theophylline metabolism.

Newer Antiepileptic Drugs and the Ketogenic Diet

Of children with epilepsy, 20% to 25% do not achieve adequate seizure control with standard AEDs and 5% to 10% are truly intractable. These observations have supported the development of newer AEDs, renewed interest in the ketogenic diet, and use of surgical approaches for the management of childhood epilepsy. Although a discussion of epilepsy surgery is beyond the scope of this chapter, an awareness of the newer AEDs and the ketogenic diet is important for physicians who provide general care for children with epilepsy, and a brief overview of these topics is presented.

Lamotrigine

Lamotrigine (LTG) comes in tablets of 25, 100, 150, and 200 mg, and serum therapeutic levels are 2 to 20 mg/L. In addition to effectiveness for partial seizures, LTG appears especially effective in the treatment of generalized epilepsies in children including generalized absence seizures and Lennox–Gastaut syndrome, although it is less effective for treatment of myoclonic seizures. Side effects include increase in seizure frequency and rash. A higher incidence (in comparison with adults) of rash, typically maculopapular, but including Stevens–Johnson syndrome, has been reported in children. Rash typically occurs within 2 to 8 weeks, but it has been reported on the first day and as late as the fifth month after LTG initiation. The occurrence of rash, in some reports, has been related to rapid escalation of the dose of LTG and to concurrent use of VPA. After discontinuance of VPA, LTG has been reintroduced without recurrence of rash. As monotherapy, its half-life is 24 hours; used with VPA, 59 hours; and used with enzyme-inducing AEDs (carbamazepine, phenytoin, phenobarbital), 15 hours. Twice-a-day dosing is possible. Therefore, when added to VPA, the starting dose is 0.5 mg/kg/day with 0.5 to 1.0 mg/kg/day increases every 1 to 2 weeks; with enzyme-inducing AEDs, the starting dose is 2 mg/kg/day with increases every week of 1 to 2 mg/kg/day to a suggested maximum dose of 10 mg/kg/day, although higher doses have been used without significant side effects.

Gabapentin

Gabapentin (100-, 300-, 400-mg capsules; therapeutic serum level, 4–10 mg/L) has no significant interactions with other drugs and is not metabolized in the liver. Side effects can include weight gain and involuntary movements. Drawbacks include a short half-life (5–7 hours) necessitating multiple daily doses, and that it is renal-function dependent, has a limited spectrum of effectiveness, is ineffective against primary generalized seizures such as absence and myoclonic seizures, and has limited effectiveness as monotherapy in children. The suggested pediatric daily dose is 30 to 60 mg/kg/day.

Topiramate

Topiramate (TPM) is available as 25-, 100-, and 200-mg tablets and 15- and 25-mg sprinkle capsules, and it has a therapeutic serum level of 2 to 25 mg/L. Clinical evidence is emerging that TPM may be effective in pediatric epilepsies. In addition to effectiveness against partial seizures, TPM may also have efficacy for generalized seizures and may be useful in the treatment of Lennox–Gastaut syndrome. Increases in the phenytoin serum levels reportedly occur occasionally with the addition of TPM. Side effects include confusion, psychomotor slowing, and difficulty with concentration. Rarely (1.5%), renal stones have been reported. Therefore, attention to hydration is emphasized, as TPM is a weak carbonic anhydrase. In children, starting doses of 1 to 3 mg/kg/day or 25 mg/day have been suggested; the half-life is 21 to 22 hours, so twice a day dosing is possible.

Tiagabine

Tiagabine (TGB) (4-, 12-, 16-, and 20-mg tablets) appears to be an effective AED for partial seizures, but it may be contraindicated in patients with primary generalized seizures. Short half-life (8 hours monotherapy; 2–3 hours when used with carbamazepine or phenytoin), decreased rate of absorption with food, and diurnal variation (lower levels in evening than morning) may complicate the use of TGB. Side effects include generalized weakness (dose dependent), abnormal thinking, and depression. The possibility of long-term ophthalmologic effects has been suggested because of potential binding of melanin to the retina and uvea.

Ketogenic Diet

Interest in the ketogenic diet has had a resurgence. However, the diet has a long history as an effective and safe method for treatment of intractable childhood epilepsy. Its use predates almost all AEDs, except phenobarbital and bromides. Many clinical reports indicate that at least one-third to two-thirds of patients benefit from the use of the diet. Whether the effect of the diet is caused by the direct anticonvulsant effect of high levels of ketones or to a ketone-induced secondary change in cerebral metabolism is unclear. Current practice has been to initiate the diet in children intractable to medical therapy. The diet appears to be most effective for patients with symptomatic forms of epilepsy that are hard to control, especially epileptic encephalopathies associated with atypical absence seizures, myoclonic seizures, and atonic seizures. The diet, to a lesser degree, may have efficacy for partial seizures. Although the diet is most successful in children aged 2 to 5 years, it has been used in infants and older children. Infants must have adequate nutrition to support growth and development. The ketogenic diet produces a state of chronic ketosis by manipulation of protein, fat, and carbohydrates. To achieve the required amount of daily calories for daily activity, fat is added to achieve a fat-to-carbohydrate ratio of 4:1 or 3:1 and, thereby, leads to the accumulation of ketone bodies. A daily intake of protein of 0.75 g per 1.2 kg is maintained to meet requirements for growth. A highly motivated family and an experienced dietitian are key to the successful use of the diet. The diet should be given at least a 4- to 6-week trial with ketosis well maintained. If the frequency of seizures has not significantly changed, a return to standard therapy should be considered. If a significant decrease in the number of seizures occurs, the diet should be maintained for 2 years, an attempt to reduce and stop AEDs should be made and, at the end of 2 years, the diet should be discontinued gradually. Potential side effects include reduction in bone mass, renal calculi, thinning of hair and, rarely, alopecia. The long-term cardiovascular effects need further study. Sugar-free supplements of multivitamins and calcium need to be provided. The use of medium-chain triglyceride oil is an alternative to the traditional diet. Evidence suggests that medium-chain triglycerides can reduce the likelihood of hypoglycemia and high cholesterol levels, which have been reported with the 4:1 diet. Control of sugar intake while on the diet is strict, and commonly used medications such as antibiotics, as well as daily used substances such as toothpaste, must be closely monitored for their carbohydrate intake.

Discontinuing Antiepileptic Drugs

The use of AEDs in children involves at least three major decisions. Two of these, whether to start AEDs and which AED to use, have been discussed. The third concerns when to discontinue AED therapy. To reduce further exposure to AEDs, a growing tendency is to remove children from AED therapy after shorter seizure-free periods. The decision to discontinue AEDs should take into consideration the likelihood of when remission may occur for an individual patient, the benefits versus potential adverse effects of continuing AED therapy, and the risks associated with discontinuing medication. The risks of seizure relapse after discontinuing AED in children have varied between 6% and 40% depending on the population studied, the types of epilepsy and their causes, and the follow-up period.

The American Academy of Neurology, recognizing that withdrawal of AEDs is a common problem in the management of patients with epilepsy and that the decision is often made in the absence of data, has developed practice parameters to serve as a guideline for making this decision. It suggests that children or adults meeting the following profile have the greatest chance for successful drug withdrawal:

- Seizure-free for 2 to 5 years while taking AEDs
- Single type of partial or generalized seizure
- Normal neurologic examination and normal IQ
- EEG normalized with treatment

The recommendation is that drug withdrawal be offered to patients who meet this profile and who have complied with treatment. Children meeting this profile are expected to have at least a 69% chance for successful withdrawal. However, discontinuation of AEDs may be appropriate in patients not meeting this profile, even though the risk of recurrence may be higher than 31% for these children.

COUNSELING PATIENTS AND PARENTS

Diagnosing the condition and initiating appropriate drug therapy are only the initial steps in caring for a child with a seizure disorder. Parents and children often have many questions, misconceptions, and fears. They always want to know if the child will outgrow seizures, what to do during a seizure, and how seizures may influence participation in school and sports. Dispelling misconceptions and providing guidance are just as important as dispensing medication.

Frequently, parents are concerned that their child might die during a seizure. One should emphasize that the objective of maintenance drug therapy is to prevent seizure recurrence and that a period of observation is required to optimize the medication dosage. If further seizures occur, they will most likely be brief. Most seizures terminate spontaneously within 5 minutes, and death, as a result of seizures, is exceedingly rare. Indeed, fatalities are usually the consequence of the patient being engaged in a potentially hazardous activity when a seizure occurs (swimming unattended, operating a motorized vehicle, or climbing to some high place).

Parents should be reassured that the brevity of most seizures obviates the necessity of rushing to the emergency department. If a seizure persists beyond 10 to 15 minutes, seeking medical assistance is appropriate. Teachers and school nurses should also be advised that sending a child home after a brief, uncomplicated seizure is not necessary. Excessive zeal in this regard can only diminish self-esteem, raise anxiety levels, and alter social interaction with classmates. The family should be fully informed of the rationale for drug choice and use and of the potential dose-related and nondose-related side effects. Compliance can be enhanced by advising the patient to use an inexpensive, compartmentalized pillbox to hold daily medications for 1 week.

Precautions

In general, the child with epilepsy should be treated as a normal child with a few notable precautions. As with all children, swimming should always be supervised. Until seizures are well controlled, bicycle riding should be restricted to low-traffic residential areas, and climbing onto rooftops should be discouraged. Sports and athletic activities are often extremely important to young people, and decisions regarding participation should involve the parents, patient, and physician in an open discussion. In most instances, epilepsy should not exclude a child from participation in sports activities. Situations in which a seizure could cause a dangerous fall such as rope climbing, activities on parallel bars, and high diving should be avoided, as should competitive underwater swimming. Participation in contact collision sports should be given individual consideration. Common sense suggests, however, that contact or collision sports might pose significant risks to a patient who is continuing to have several seizures per month.

Immunizations

Current recommendations state that pertussis immunization may adversely affect seizure risk and should be deferred in children with a personal history of seizures and in those with certain neurologic conditions such as tuberous sclerosis, certain inherited metabolic disorders, or other conditions predisposing them to seizures. The pertussis component of DTP vaccine should be eliminated from subsequent immunizations in the child who has had a seizure within 48 hours of a prior DTP immunization.

Puberty

Puberty has traditionally been considered to have an adverse effect on the course of epilepsy, especially in girls. An increase, a decrease, and no change in seizure frequency during puberty have been reported. Physicians have been cautioned against withdrawing AEDs during this period, even when the patient has met currently accepted criteria for discontinuing therapy. This attitude is not supported by the evidence, however.

Teratogenesis

Physicians have a special obligation to adolescents and potentially sexually active girls and their parents in making them aware of the potential teratogenic effects of AEDs. No woman should receive AEDs unnecessarily and, in the girl who has been free of seizures for several years, consideration should be given to gradual withdrawal of medication before a pregnancy is planned. The discontinuation of AEDs in pregnant women who have required medication to control seizures is not recommended because prolonged seizures could cause serious harm to both the woman and the fetus.

Most AEDs in current use have been reported to produce congenital malformations ranging from minimal defects such as cleft lip (amenable to satisfactory cosmetic repair) to major cardiac defects and spinal dysraphism. In general, however, the pregnant woman with epilepsy who requires drugs for seizure control has approximately a 90% chance of delivering a normal child. Daily folate supplementation (suggested dose 4–6 mg/day) for women of childbearing age that are receiving AEDs is recommended, especially for those receiving VPA.

Driver's Licensure

The restriction imposed by epilepsy on eligibility for a driver's license is a major concern for adolescents and teenagers. In some instances, the aspiration for licensure can be a potent motivation for compliance with medication regimens. Legal requirements and the duration of restrictions vary from state to state, and physicians must be acquainted with the regulations of the state in which they practice. In general, the recommendation is that patients be free of seizures for at least 9 to 12 consecutive months before being licensed to drive. The physician may be required to attest to the seizure-free interval and to the patient's compliance with the prescribed drug regimen. For medicolegal purposes, it may be useful for the physician to document by an entry in the clinical record that the patient and the parents have been advised of the relevant regulations.

CHAPTER 220

Febrile Seizures

Adapted from Marvin A. Fishman

Febrile seizures are a worldwide problem and occur in 2% to 4% of children younger than 5 years. A febrile seizure is defined as a convulsion associated with an elevated temperature greater than 38°C occurring in a child who is younger than 6 years. Exclusions to the diagnosis include a history of a previous afebrile seizure, central nervous system infection or inflammation, or acute systemic metabolic abnormalities that may produce convulsions. Febrile seizures are classified into two groups based on their clinical features. Simple (benign) febrile seizures are those that last less than 15 minutes, do not have focal features and, if they occur in a series, have a total duration of less than 30 minutes. Complex febrile seizures last more than 15 minutes, have focal features or postictal paresis, and occur in series with a total duration greater than 30 minutes.

PATHOGENESIS

Febrile seizures are an age-related phenomenon and occur in children between the ages of 6 months and 6 years. The reason that febrile seizures occur only in infants and young children is unclear, as is the mechanism whereby fever induces the seizure.

Febrile seizures occur during both bacterial and viral infections and may occur more frequently in patients with illnesses that are accompanied by severe constitutional symptoms. One study found that infection with human herpesvirus 6 accounted for approximately one-third of the first-time febrile seizures in children 2 years old or younger. The convulsion often takes place as the temperature is rapidly increasing but may occur as it is declining. Genetic factors appear to be important in the expression of the condition. An increased incidence of febrile seizures exists among first-degree relatives—10% to 20% of parents and siblings—of children with febrile seizures. The concordance rate for febrile seizures in monozygotic twins is much higher than that in dizygotic twins in whom the rate is similar to that of other siblings. Siblings and parents of patients with febrile seizures have a 4% to 10% incidence of epilepsy. Also, siblings of patients with epilepsy are at increased risk for febrile seizures.

CLINICAL CHARACTERISTICS

The vast majority of febrile seizures are simple. Prolonged convulsions occur in fewer than 10% of children with febrile seizures, and focal features are seen in fewer than 5%. Generalized seizures are mainly clonic, but both atonic and tonic episodes have been noted. Involvement of the facial and respiratory muscles is frequently noted. Complex febrile seizures occur as the initial convulsion in the majority of children who experience them. An initial simple febrile seizure can be followed by a subsequent complex febrile seizure, however, and vice versa. Children usually have significantly elevated body temperatures, but approximately 25% of febrile convulsions occur in children whose temperatures are between 38°C and 39°C. Children who have repeated febrile seizures do not always experience them with the same degree of fever. Also, they do not occur every time the child has a temperature elevation similar to the one associated with the preceding febrile seizure. The majority of febrile seizures are seen on the first day of illness and, in some children, they are the first sign of the accompanying infection.

DIFFERENTIAL DIAGNOSIS

The main concern in evaluating an infant or child with a febrile convulsion is the possibility of underlying meningitis or encephalitis. A thorough evaluation by an experienced clinician almost always detects the child with meningitis. If the only indication for performing a lumbar puncture is a febrile seizure, meningitis is found in less than 1% of patients. Less than one-half of these patients have bacterial meningitis. In children who have meningitis presenting with seizures, as many as 40% (particularly younger infants) may not have meningeal signs. They may have other symptoms and findings, however, which strongly suggest the presence of meningitis. Thus, a diagnosis of bacterial meningitis based solely on a routine evaluation of CSF after a febrile seizure is exceedingly rare.

Seizures are usually distinguished easily from other types of involuntary movements occurring in sick infants. Chills usually consist of fine rhythmic oscillatory movements about a joint and are not clonic in nature. They rarely involve facial or respiratory muscles. Also, chills are not accompanied by a loss of consciousness, which occurs during a generalized seizure.

The detection of an underlying metabolic disorder presenting as a seizure in a febrile child is rare. A careful review of the history usually provides other clues suggesting the likelihood of an underlying problem.

DIAGNOSTIC TESTS

The routine performance of lumbar punctures in all children with febrile seizures does not seem warranted. Children who might be considered candidates for examination of the CSF include young infants, children whose febrile seizure occurs after the second day of illness, cases in which the clinician is unsure of his or her judgment regarding the presence or absence of meningitis, and situations in which it is not possible to observe the patient. The American Academy of Pediatrics recommends that after the first seizure with fever in infants younger than 12 months, performance of a lumbar puncture should be strongly considered. The routine performance of skull radiography in children with febrile seizures is not generally helpful. If imaging of the brain is indicated [by abnormal head size, an abnormal neurologic examination (especially with focal features), or signs or symptoms of increased intracranial pressure], computed tomography (CT) or magnetic resonance imaging (MRI) should be performed. Measurement of serum electrolytes, blood sugar, calcium, and urea nitrogen concentrations are of very low yield and need not be routinely performed. They should be done when the results of the history or physical examination indicate a need for them. Patients with significant vomiting, diarrhea, and abnormal fluid intake may be suspected of having acute metabolic disturbances, and routine serum chemistries should be performed in these children. The routine use of electroencephalography (EEG) in all children with febrile seizures is not warranted. A tracing obtained within 1 week or less of the seizure is abnormal in at least one-third of these children. Febrile convulsions of long duration or with focal features increase the likelihood that abnormalities will be found. Abnormal EEG results do not identify children in whom epilepsy will subsequently develop and should not be used as the basis for deciding which children need anticonvulsant therapy.

TREATMENT

Short-Term Treatment

A child who is actively convulsing needs to be treated urgently, especially if the seizure has been present for 5 minutes or longer and shows no signs of abating. Immediate attention should be directed toward ensuring that the patient has an adequate airway, is breathing well, and has satisfactory perfusion and circulatory status. Blood should be obtained for the determination of electrolyte and glucose levels, if indicated. At this point, antiepileptic drugs should be administered, intravenously if possible. One strategy is to give a short-acting anticonvulsant such as lorazepam (0.05–0.10 mg/kg). If seizures persist, an additional dose can be repeated. The clinician should be ready to intubate the child if respirations become inadequate. Rarely, additional treatment with phenytoin (15–20 mg/kg) may need to be given if seizures persist. It should be administered slowly to avoid the development of cardiac dysrhythmias and hypotension. For persistent status epilepticus, phenobarbital may need to be administered (20 mg/kg).

Rectally administered diazepam, at a dosage of 0.5 mg/kg (maximum, 5 mg), has been used for the control of febrile seizures. Rectally administered diazepam is effective in approximately 80% of patients. After the seizures are under control, the fever should be treated with antipyretic agents such as acetaminophen or ibuprofen.

Prophylactic Treatment

Controversy exists regarding which children should be treated with antiepileptic drug therapy to prevent recurrent febrile seizures. Continuous administration of phenobarbital and maintenance of a serum level of at least 15 μg/mL reduce the risk of recurrence to approximately one-third of what might be expected with no treatment (approximately 10%–15% versus 30%–40%). An alternative for the prevention of recurrent febrile seizures is the intermittent administration of diazepam during febrile illnesses. A dose of 0.33 mg/kg every 8 hours during the first few days of the febrile illness is as effective as the continuous administration of phenobarbital in reducing repeated episodes. Although the incidence of recurrent febrile seizures can be reduced, no data prove that treatment decreases the incidence of sequelae associated with prolonged seizures or the development of epilepsy, which occurs at greater frequency in children who have febrile seizures than in the general population. Because febrile seizures have so few sequelae and such a good prognosis in the vast majority of children, the benefits of therapy must be considered carefully and compared with the side effects of the medication. Changes in behavior and sleep patterns are noted in approximately 30% to 40% of children who are given phenobarbital, and these changes are severe enough to require discontinuation of the drug in 20%. Phenobarbital does not appear to have a significant negative effect on intellectual development and cognitive function in children.

Of the three aspects of the natural history—recurrence rate, development of sequelae, and development of epilepsy—only the recurrence rate can be modified with antiepileptic drug therapy. The prophylactic use of additional anticonvulsant agents (Table 220-1) such as primidone and valproic acid has been shown to be effective in reducing the incidence of recurrent febrile seizures. However, the continuous use of anticonvulsants to prevent the recurrence of febrile seizures is rarely indicated. In children who have a high likelihood of developing epilepsy, the decision must be made whether to institute anticonvulsant therapy at the time of the febrile seizures or to wait until the epilepsy actually develops.

Because fever is the precipitating event in febrile seizures, attempts at reducing elevated temperature are a logical approach. Attempts at parent education including detailed written and oral instructions regarding the use of antipyretics have been made. The recurrence rate among patients whose parents were so instructed was 25%, which is similar to that of an untreated population.

TABLE 220-1. Antiepileptic Drug Treatment and Seizure Recurrence

	Percentage of patients with recurrent febrile seizures	
	Treated	***Control or inadequate treatment***
Carbamazepine	18.5	25
	81.3[a]	—
Diazepam	12[b]	42
Phenobarbital	13	34
Phenytoin	32	34
Primidone	10	57
Valproate	13	47

[a]Phenobarbital failures.
[b]Intermittent treatment.

PROGNOSIS

The prognosis for children with febrile seizures can be divided into three categories: recurrence rate for febrile seizures, development of neurologic sequelae, and development of epilepsy. The major factor influencing the recurrence of febrile seizures is the age of the infant at the time of the first seizure. The younger the child, the more likely that febrile convulsions will recur. If the first seizure occurs when the child is younger than 1 year, the recurrence rate is approximately 50% to 65%, in contrast to a rate of 28% if the first seizure occurs after that point. If the first seizure does not occur until at least 2.5 years of age, the recurrence rate is reduced to approximately 20%. Other factors that have been shown in some studies to influence the recurrence rate have been abnormal development before the first febrile seizure, a history of afebrile seizures in parents and siblings, and the number of subsequent febrile illnesses. Approximately 50% to 75% of recurrences take place within 1 year of the initial seizure, and approximately 90% occur within 2.5 years. This recurrence rate can be influenced by the intermittent use of rapidly acting antiepileptic drugs or continuous prophylactic treatment.

Neurologic sequelae reported as a result of febrile seizures include death, status epilepticus, motor coordination deficits, mental retardation, and learning and behavioral problems. The exact incidence of these complications is uncertain, but it appears to be exceedingly low. They occur only in children who have experienced complex febrile seizures. Many of the reports documenting these complications have been anecdotal and derived from biased populations consisting of children who were evaluated at hospitals or clinics. In population-based studies, the incidence of these complications is very low. In the National Collaborative Perinatal Project, approximately 5% of children who had febrile seizures had episodes lasting longer than 30 minutes. No children in that study sustained permanent motor deficits, and none of the patients had impaired mental development unless afebrile seizures subsequently developed. Another study has also confirmed that status epilepticus as a result of febrile seizures does not cause new neurologic deficits. Children with prior neurologic abnormalities have a higher risk of subsequent febrile, as well as afebrile seizures, than normal children after an episode of status epilepticus.

Children who have febrile seizures are at increased risk for the development of epilepsy. In a normal child who has a simple febrile seizure, this risk may be twice that of the general population, or 1.0% versus 0.5%. Abnormal neurologic development in the presence of complex febrile seizures, particularly focal seizures, greatly increases the risk by as much as 30- to 50-fold. In the National Collaborative Perinatal Project, children who were neurologically abnormal and had a focal seizure had a 15.4% incidence of afebrile seizures by 7 years of age. In a population-based study in Rochester, Minnesota in which patients were observed into adulthood, the risk ranged from 2.4% among children with simple febrile convulsions to as high as 49% among children with focal, prolonged, and repeated episodes within 24 hours. In the National Collaborative Perinatal Project, one-half of the children who had nonfebrile seizures never had recurrent febrile seizures. Thus, recurrence does not appear to be a prerequisite for the development of epilepsy.

CHAPTER 221
Headache

Adapted from Arthur L. Prensky

CHRONIC HEADACHE SYNDROMES

Migraine Headaches

In 1988, the Classification Committee of the International Society for Headache redefined migraine headaches. The diagnosis of common migraine would require at least five attacks of headaches, each lasting over 4 hours and accompanied by nausea and vomiting or photophobia and phonophobia, as well as two of the following: unilateral location, pulsating quality, an intensity that inhibits daily activities, or aggravation by routine physical activity. Common migraine is defined as "migraine without aura." The diagnosis presumes that neither the history nor the physical examination suggests other diseases that would produce repeated headaches. The Committee then defined migraine with aura. The aura can be brief, as in classic migraine, or prolonged, as in complicated migraine. The Committee separated ophthalmoplegic migraine, a rare disorder most common in infants, in which repeated attacks of headaches are associated with paresis of one or more ocular cranial nerves in the absence of demonstrable intracranial lesion, from retinal migraine, in which repeated attacks of headaches occur that are associated with scotoma or blindness in one eye.

The suitability of these criteria for the diagnosis of migraine headaches in children has been questioned repeatedly because making the diagnosis of migraine by these criteria is extremely difficult if no gastrointestinal symptoms are present. Another generally accepted group of criteria for the diagnosis of migraine in children is one that includes repeated episodes of headaches accompanied by at least three of the following symptoms: (a) recurrent abdominal pain (with or without headaches) or nausea or vomiting; (b) an aura, which is usually visual but may be sensory, motor, or vertiginous; (c) throbbing or pounding pain; (d) pain restricted to one side of the head (although it may shift sides from one headache to the next); (e) relief of pain by brief periods of sleep; and (f) family history of migraines in one or more immediate relatives.

CLINICAL CHARACTERISTICS

Children with common migraines usually have nausea or some type of abdominal distress, are helped by sleep, and have a family history of migraines. Localized, throbbing pain and an aura are seen more frequently during and after puberty. These criteria have been criticized for placing excessive emphasis on a family history of similar headaches. Migraines in children differ from those in adults in that approximately 60% of patients affected before age 12 are male compared with approximately 33% in the adult population; unilateral headaches are less common in prepubertal children; and a visual aura is much less frequent. The incidence of epilepsy with migraines ranges from 5.4% to 12.3% in children in various series, but in adults, it is less than 3%. Nausea and vomiting occur in approximately the same percentage of cases for both adults and children, and approximately 70% of children and adults have a strong family history of migraines. Childhood migraines are more likely to vary in frequency than in severity. Children who otherwise fit the criteria for the diagnosis of migraines may have one headache a month and then gradually, or sometimes abruptly, begin to have three to five headaches a week. Occasionally, the exacerbations can be related to changes in mood, particularly depression, or to stress. However, frequently, no predisposing factor can be found to explain the variation in headache frequency or severity.

DIAGNOSIS

The diagnosis of migraines is made by history. The physical examination is generally normal. Laboratory studies are not usually needed for confirmation unless physical signs or a doubtful history is present. Aspects of the clinical history that should alert the physician to study the child further include (a) a strong family history of occlusive cerebrovascular disease early in life or of intracranial hemorrhage, (b) persistent localization of headaches to one side of the cranium with never a shift to the other hemisphere, (c) onset of motor or sensory symptoms well after the headache has started rather than before the headache, (d) failure of motor or sensory symptoms to clear within 24 hours after the headache has ceased, and (e) association of focal headaches with partial seizures involving the same hemisphere. Focal physical findings or evidence of increased intracranial pressure on examination also indicate the need for further evaluation or even hospitalization. Neuroimaging usually clarifies whether these symptoms or signs are associated with an underlying structural disorder of the brain. At the present time, magnetic resonance imaging (MRI) scans of the brain and the arterial system are the most satisfactory studies to rule out an underlying disorder. Unless seizures are suspected, the electroencephalogram (EEG) has little place in the evaluation of a child suspected of having migraines.

Many children have symptoms that are said to be "migraine variants." Children who have migraine variants may not have a headache with each attack. The syndrome is related to migraines on the basis of one or two pieces of information: (a) a strong family history of migraines or (b) the known tendency of children with these disorders to develop more typical forms of migraines later in life. Patients who have or later develop migraines may have isolated attacks of confusion or loss of memory. They may have recurrent attacks of delirium. These patients may not complain of headaches, although a strong family history may suggest migraines. Motion sickness is a very common symptom in patients who have or will develop migraines. Recurrent attacks of paroxysmal vertigo in younger children (benign paroxysmal vertigo) are considered a migraine variant, although not all of these children later develop migraines. Children with benign paroxysmal vertigo have a normal neurologic examination and a normal EEG. Infants who have attacks of hemiplegia that alternately affect the left and right sides of the body have been considered to have a migraine variant, often because a strong family history of migraines is seen and many of these children later go on to complain of migraines. However, these children often have other paroxysmal phenomena such as tonic spells and movement disorders and many do not develop normal physical or mental function as they grow older. Although some investigators have claimed success in modifying this disorder by treating the infants or children with calcium channel blockers, the relationship between migraines and alternating infantile hemiplegia is still not clear.

Some children with recurrent episodes of abdominal pain develop typical migraine headaches later in life. Paroxysmal abdominal pain is more likely to be a migrainous than an epileptic syndrome, although paroxysmal EEGs are common with the disorder. Most children with recurrent abdominal pain do not have either migraines or epilepsy when they are followed into adult life.

TREATMENT

The treatment of migraines can be divided into two parts: (a) the treatment of the acute attack and (b) prevention of numerous future attacks.

Several principles guide the treatment of an acute migraine headache:

- Drug therapy is more likely to be effective if it is used before the headache becomes severe, which may necessitate taking medication to school. Oral medication does not work once the patient has started to vomit.
- Unless they are specifically contraindicated, over-the-counter preparations should be used initially.
- The more frequent the headache, the more reluctant the physician should be to prescribe powerful but addicting analgesics. These drugs should not be given to patients who experience more than six headaches per month. When patients have frequent headaches that occur three or four times per week, the use of even simple analgesics (e.g., ibuprofen or acetaminophen) can potentiate the recurrence of headaches as patients strive to withdraw from the drug.
- If headaches are relatively infrequent but the pain is severe and disabling and interrupts activities, the initial dose of an analgesic should be a large one if it does not have a sedative added to it. Aspirin is not generally used for the treatment of headaches in children at the present time because of its association with Reye syndrome. The current recommendation is to give acetaminophen, 20 mg/kg, at the onset of the headache and to give 10 to 20 mg/kg in 2 or more hours if needed, up to four times per day. Ibuprofen should be given initially in a dose of 20 mg/kg, up to 800 mg/kg in one dose to be repeated in 2 to 4 hours, but no more than three doses should be given in 24 hours. Furthermore, the drug should not be used if the patient begins to complain of abdominal pain, dizziness, or tinnitus. Naproxen sodium can be given to children older than 12 years. One tablet should be taken at the onset of the headache, and the dose may be repeated up to three times a day at 8- to 12-hour intervals. Again, nausea that worsens or epigastric pain is a contraindication to continued use of the drug. If these mild analgesics fail, commercial preparations such as Fioricet (acetaminophen/caffeine/butalbital) or Midrin (isometheptene/Apap/dichloralphenazone) may be used in older children. One to two tablets can be taken at the onset of the headache and the dose can be repeated in 30 to 60 minutes. Adolescents should take two tablets at the onset of the headache, a third tablet at 60 minutes from onset, and a fourth tablet at 90 minutes from onset, if indicated. Stronger, addicting medications such as oxycodone or butorphanol should be reserved for extremely severe, infrequent headaches. The latter drug can be given by nasal spray and, thus, can relieve pain, even in the presence of vomiting.

Ergotamine preparations still have a place in the treatment of infrequent migraine attacks, although they potentiate nausea and vomiting. Children aged 6 to 12 should take 1 mg at the onset of a headache and 0.5 mg every 30 to 60 minutes thereafter, until a total of 4 mg is ingested or the vomiting or headache subsides. Children aged 12 to 18 may take 1 to 2 mg at the onset of a headache and 1 mg every 30 minutes thereafter, until a total of 6 mg is reached. Some of these preparations come as suppositories. If these are being used, 2 mg should be taken at the onset of the headache; the drug can be given again in 1 hour if needed. The same dosage is used for sublingual preparations. Intramuscular injections of dihydroergotamine mesylate can be given as well. One milligram is injected at the onset of the headache; the dose can be repeated twice at 1-hour intervals, but no more than 3 mg should be given to a patient in a 24-hour period. Use in children is restricted to those older than age 12.

Sumatriptan has not been approved for use in children, but it is widely used, nevertheless. It can be given orally, by subcutaneous injection, or by nasal spray. The injectable form reaches much higher blood levels more rapidly than the oral or nasal forms and should be reserved primarily for adolescents. Regardless of the patient's age, the first dose should be given in an emergency department under the direction and immediate supervision of a physician. The injectable form is prepared for adults and comes in a 6-mg stat dose. Patients younger than 18 years should not receive more than 0.1 mg/kg. Twenty-five to 50 mg of sumatriptan can be given orally at the onset of the headache and repeated in 1 hour if needed. If that program is ineffective, no further treatment with this drug is indicated. The total dosage orally should not exceed 100 mg/day.

Migraines may also be treated prophylactically when the headaches occur more frequently than four times per month and, thus, could require excessive pain medication for relief. Prophylactic medications include propranolol (1–2 mg/kg/day in three divided doses), cyproheptadine hydrochloride (0.3 mg/kg/day in three divided doses), amitriptyline hydrochloride (1–2 mg/kg/day), phenobarbital or phenytoin (3–5 mg/kg/day), and calcium channel blockers.

In the past decade, the most common forms of headaches in children have begun to be treated by biofeedback and relaxation therapy. Initial studies were poorly controlled, but increasing evidence indicates that pediatric, as well as adult, patients with common migraines and tension headaches respond to this type of treatment.

The use of special diets to treat headaches is not generally successful, nor is desensitization to common allergens. No substantial evidence has established that migraines are an allergic disorder. However, some children do get headaches after eating specific foods that contain amines such as tyramine. Chocolate, cheese and other milk products, and wine are major offenders. Some children also seem to have an increased number of headaches if they drink a great deal of soda containing caffeine or diet soda containing aspartame. Most of these children ingest one to two cans of soda a day, or more. If the relationship of a headache to a specific food is well established, withdrawal of the particular food from the diet can be helpful.

Adolescent women who have migraines with aura have a somewhat higher incidence of stroke. This risk is increased if they take birth-control pills, and, hence, this form of birth control should be avoided by such patients.

Other Types and Causes of Headaches

TENSION HEADACHES

Differentiating common migraines from tension headaches solely by the description of the headache is often difficult. No single factor in the history separates them, and people who have either type of headache tend to have a normal physical examination. The Classification Committee of the International Headache Society indicates that tension headaches may last from 30 minutes to 7 days. The pain is a pressing or tightening type of pain that is mild to moderate in intensity, is bilateral, and does not worsen with routine physical activity. Nausea and vomiting are absent, but either phonophobia or photophobia may be present. These criteria are used to differentiate tension headaches from migraine headaches. However, in children at least, the differentiation using these criteria is not sharp. Children who appear to have tension and not migraine headaches by other criteria have nausea and vomiting when the headache is extremely severe. Many children with migraines do not have both photophobia and phonophobia, but only one or the other. Some children with migraines do not have gastrointestinal symptoms. Other factors in the history help the physician make a diagnosis. Tension headaches tend to occur and to be more severe during periods of obvious stress. This association is seen with migraines, but it is not as clear-cut. Migraine headaches tend to involve the frontal and, to a lesser degree, the temporal regions of the head or to be localized to one side of the head; tension headaches tend to involve the occipital or temporal regions bilaterally and often extend to the neck. They also tend to be diffuse. Tension headaches tend to be continuous; they fluctuate throughout the day, but they often never disappear. Patients who have tension headaches are less likely to have immediate family members who have typical migraine headaches.

The pain resulting from tension headaches can usually be treated by analgesics such as those recommended for the treatment of pain in children with migraines. When tension headaches occur frequently, biofeedback and relaxation therapy are useful. Antidepressants may occasionally help patients who have chronic tension headaches. However, the population of children whose headaches are related to depression, an anxiety neurosis, or a conversion reaction requires a psychiatric referral.

Many adolescents and a few children younger than age 12 years have chronic daily headaches. These patients have tight-pressing, generally nonthrobbing, headaches lasting part or all of the day, virtually every day. The headaches are diffuse or bilateral, unassociated with gastrointestinal symptoms, and frequently do not inhibit daily activities. However, many children with this type of headache are unable to go to school. Yet a careful search fails to reveal that they are stressed at school in any way. In our experience, the majority of children with chronic daily headaches have had headaches in the past that meet the criteria for the diagnosis of migraines and have headaches that are migrainous in quality when their chronic headaches are severe (i.e., they frequently vomit, their headaches become worse with activity, and they have photophobia or phonophobia or both). Children who have these headaches often have a family history of migraines. However, their headaches are not unilateral, they do not throb, they have no aura, and they are not relieved by sleep. Chronic daily headaches are the most difficult form of cephalgia to treat. Fortunately, they tend to disappear over several years, even if therapy is unsuccessful. This is the type of headache for which the excessive use of analgesic agents may compound the recurrence of pain when drug use is decreased. The use of increasingly powerful analgesics leads to addiction. The headaches sometimes respond to tricyclics or other types of antidepressants, even if no history of frank depression exists. However, the response is not as gratifying as that seen with simple migraine. Biofeedback and relaxation therapy may also be of help, but again, the results are not as satisfactory as those with simple migraine or episodic tension headaches.

SINUS HEADACHES

Chronic or recurrent headaches occur in approximately 15% of children with chronic sinusitis. Sinus disease may also exacerbate the symptoms of migraines in children who are subject to that disorder. Frequently, no increase in temperature occurs. The most common accompanying symptoms are rhinorrhea, postnasal drip, coughing, sneezing, wheezing, and headache. However, none of these symptoms predicts sinus infection. Pain or pressure over the frontal or maxillary sinuses may be present, and these cavities can fail to transilluminate. (The frontal sinuses form later in childhood and are not fully developed in most children until the end of puberty.) Most sinus headaches in children result from infection of the sphenoid or ethmoid sinuses, which cannot be palpated or visualized by transillumination in the office. Pain from these sinuses is usually referred to the frontotemporal region but can occur over any part of the cranial vault. Sinus headaches often occur at the same time each day, build slowly, are often throbbing, and vary quite markedly with change in position because positional change may promote sinus drainage. Although simple analgesics may help decrease the pain of sinus headaches, sustained relief usually depends on long-term therapy for the underlying disease with appropriate antibiotics and nasal decongestants. In less tractable disorders, the sinuses may have to be drained surgically and passages opened to prevent them from becoming infected once again.

OCULAR HEADACHES

Pain in or around the eye is usually caused by local diseases of the eye. The sclera is often red. Light, movement of the eye, or pressure on the eyeball may make the pain worse. Severe eye pain caused by glaucoma, uveitis, inflammation of tissues of the orbit, or masses within the orbit are rarely confused with headaches from other sources. Errors of refraction and strabismus are not associated with an increased incidence of headaches, other than perhaps in hypermetropia or astigmatism; the latter usually produces a dull, aching sensation in and about the eye or, at worst, a mild frontal headache when the eyes are used for close work such as reading for a long period.

TEMPOROMANDIBULAR JOINT DISEASE

The most common symptoms of temporomandibular joint disease are pain in the face and jaws, stiffness of the jaws in the morning, sounds of clicking or movement of the joint when chewing, and fatigue when chewing. Patients with temporomandibular joint disease often clench their jaws and have bruxism. Patients who have these symptoms including older children and adolescents often complain of chronic headaches. The pain is predominantly in the temporal or frontotemporal region and may be unilateral or bilateral. At other times, throat, occipital, neck, and back pain are complaints. The physical examination is helpful if limited movement of the temporomandibular joint occurs or a click is palpated when the patient makes chewing movements. Pain may also occur when the lateral mandibular muscles are pressed. Evaluations of children who have malocclusion and require orthodontic treatment do not indicate that they have more symptoms related to temporomandibular joint disease than other children of the same age. Whether temporomandibular joint disease contributes to chronic headache in children remains uncertain. Many children exhibit bruxism but have little else in the way of symptoms or signs to suggest joint disease. If sufficient findings exist to suspect that the joint is the cause of chronic cephalgia, the patient should be referred to a dental surgeon for occlusal splint therapy.

EPILEPSY

Lateralized or generalized headaches frequently follow epileptic seizures and occasionally precede partial seizures as an aura. No consensus exists as to whether headaches can be the sole manifestation of an epileptic seizure. Headaches, often diagnosed as migraines, occur more frequently in children who have epilepsy than in the general pediatric population. Children who have complex-partial seizures tend to have headaches of brief duration and abrupt onset and termination at times when they are not having an epileptic seizure. These headaches are usually relieved by anticonvulsant therapy; however, this does not mean that the headaches represent a seizure, because anticonvulsants are effective in relieving migraine in children who have no history or signs of epilepsy.

TRAUMA

A traumatic injury to the head may produce intracranial lesions that are associated with headaches. Some patients with acute traumatic lesions, particularly intracerebral hemorrhage or acute subdural bleeding, may be alert enough to complain of headaches. If so, the pain is usually severe and nonthrobbing. It is often localized on the same side as the site of the lesion, but it is sometimes diffuse. Intracranial injuries can also be associated with more chronic, increasingly severe headaches, which, again, may be localized or diffuse and may have no other special characteristics. This type of headache is seen with enlarging subdural hematomas. Regardless of the severity or location of the headache, severe or persistent cephalgia that follows cranial trauma should be investigated by neuroimaging, even if the patient does not have neurologic signs.

Chronic or recurrent headaches may follow head trauma when no focal lesion is revealed by cerebral imaging. As noted, trauma can be a triggering stimulus for the onset or worsening of migraines. Headaches are also an integral part of the postconcussive syndrome, which also includes dizziness and personality changes. Fortunately, the syndrome is less common in children than in adults. When the headaches occur, they can persist for months. Standard criteria for the diagnosis of a postconcussive headache require that the concussion be severe enough to have caused a transient loss of consciousness or posttraumatic amnesia lasting longer than 10 minutes. The headaches should occur within 14 days of regaining consciousness. The postconcussion syndrome is often accompanied by anxiety, irritability, and, at times, frank depression. These emotional changes may help to prolong the headache and make it more intense.

Traumatic injury to the soft tissue of the neck may be a cause of chronic cervicogenic headaches, which are usually referred to the occipital area of the head. On examination, the paraspinal muscles of the neck are frequently tender, and the head may be restricted in this range of motion.

The treatment of posttraumatic headaches depends on their causes. The therapy for posttraumatic migraines does not differ from that of migraines in children who have not been traumatized. Analgesics are used to treat postconcussive headaches; however, as in other syndromes with chronic daily headaches, these agents may be abused and may be difficult to withdraw, so they become a part of the continuing problem. If these headaches persist for months and no associated structural lesion is discovered, the child may need a psychiatric evaluation.

Subacute Headache Syndromes

Children with subacute headache syndromes but have had no headaches or rare headaches until 2 to 3 months before evaluation are brought to a physician because, during this brief period, their headaches have become increasingly frequent and severe. Distinguishing intracranial causes from extracranial causes of such headaches by history alone may not be possible. However, certain features of the headache suggest the possibility that the cause is more likely an intracranial lesion. These features include (a) severe occipital headaches; (b) headaches made worse by straining, sneezing, or coughing; (c) headaches that awaken the patient from a deep sleep; (d) headaches that are exacerbated or improved markedly by a change in position; (e) headaches associated with projectile vomiting or vomiting without nausea; and (f) headaches with a history of focal seizures. Headaches that occur day after day in the same area with increasing intensity are also worrisome. Even if one or more of these symptoms are present, statistically, the majority of children do not have an intracranial lesion. Patients who have had headaches caused by intracranial mass lesions almost always have physical findings if the headaches have been present for several months. These findings include papilledema, unilateral or bilateral sixth nerve palsies, ataxia, and spasticity (particularly in the lower extremities), as well as more localized indications of brain dysfunction involving movement, vision, or language, depending on the site of the lesion. Although physical findings are much more suggestive of an intracranial lesion, all children with a history of subacute headaches whose pain is becoming progressively worse or more frequent should be investigated by neuroimaging.

INTRACRANIAL LESIONS

Headaches result from intracranial lesions for one of two reasons: (a) A localized or generalized increased pressure occurs within the skull, which stretches and distorts vessels at the surface of the brain or distorts the meninges, which also contain pain-sensitive fibers, or (b) the pain-sensitive fibers in these brain coverings become irritated by infection or bleeding. Tumors or other masses such as an abscess or hemorrhage are usually responsible for local distortion of brain vessels or meninges. However, nearly 80% of tumors in children occur either in the posterior fossa or near the midline. Thus, they can frequently obstruct the circulation of cerebrospinal fluid resulting in hydrocephalus. When this occurs, the elevation of intracranial pressure is more diffuse, and the headache is frequently bifrontal or generalized rather than localized over one part of the hemicranium.

PSEUDOTUMOR CEREBRI

Pseudotumor cerebri produces the same type of headache that is found when intracranial pressure is elevated from other causes such as a mass lesion or hydrocephalus. Frequently, vomiting or blurred vision are accompanying complaints, and papilledema, sixth nerve palsies, ataxia and, less frequently, spasticity may be found on physical examination. As the name implies, no mass is found on neuroimaging. Now that visualizing the dural sinuses by MRI techniques is possible, an increasingly large proportion of patients with pseudotumor are found to have occlusion of one of the dural sinuses. However, in the majority of cases, the cause is still unknown. Pseudotumor cerebri is more frequent in obese females and has been associated with both high and low levels of serum vitamin A, use of drugs such as lithium or antibiotics, and disorders of endocrine function.

TREATMENT

The treatment of headaches resulting from tumor or hemorrhage is not within the scope of this chapter. If the diagnosis of pseudotumor cerebri is made, the patient may often be relieved by a single lumbar puncture performed for diagnostic reasons. If, as is often the case, symptoms recur and intracranial pressure returns to high levels within 3 to 4 days, dexamethasone (2–4 mg every 6 hours) may be used for 3 to 5 days and then withdrawn rapidly. Alternatively, acetazolamide (20 mg/kg/day) can be given in three divided doses. If this treatment fails to relieve the patient's symptoms, repeated lumbar punctures may be needed whenever the symptoms recur. Oral glycerol is still infrequently used as an osmotic agent to lower intracranial pressure. The dosage is increased gradually from 0.5 to 2.0 mg/kg/day in three divided doses as tolerated. Obesity and chronic diarrhea are complications of this form of therapy. The major danger of chronic elevation of intracranial pressure due to pseudotumor is damage to the visual system, and vision should be followed on a regular basis by an ophthalmologist. In intractable pseudotumor that cannot be treated by drugs or repeated lumbar puncture, the optic nerve must be protected. This protection can be accomplished in one of two ways: fenestration of the optic nerve sheath, which protects the nerve against high pressures or, alternatively, placement of a lumbar peritoneal shunt that reduces intracerebral pressure.

Acute Headache Syndromes

Common intracranial causes of acute, severe headaches are a mass lesion, infection, and intracranial hemorrhage. Extracranial causes include migraines, tension headaches, and, rarely, sinusitis. The most decisive factor in the child's history is whether this is the first such headache the child has experienced or another headache in an already established pattern that has been evaluated in the past. Determining whether this particular headache has been associated with an unusual antecedent event such as head injury, seizure, fever, or changes in sensory or motor function is also important. Critical physical findings include meningismus, focal neurologic signs, papilledema or split sutures, evidence of cranial trauma including blood in or behind the ear, and a depressed level of consciousness.

If this is the first attack of severe cephalgia without a significant prior headache history, immediate neuroimaging is recommended if any of the following is present: history of recent trauma, recent onset of seizures, unusual behaviors predating the headache, fever, meningismus, papilledema, focal neurologic signs, or a depressed level of consciousness. Early neuroimaging is indicated if the physician feels the need to use drugs that significantly depress consciousness to relieve the child's pain. Meningeal irritation usually results in an acute, diffuse, rapidly progressive headache that becomes so intense, it may be unbearable. If the cause of the irritation is bleeding, the onset may be explosive (a "thunderclap" headache) and the headache may become excruciating within a matter of a minute or two. Many of these patients do not have focal neurologic signs, but, frequently, a disturbance of orientation or of consciousness occurs. The physical examination may show nuchal rigidity resulting from meningeal irritation, but if the insult is relatively recent, it may not yet be pronounced. Occasionally, the examiner can see perivenous or subhyaloid hemorrhages in the eye resulting from high intracranial pressure and the extravasation of subarachnoid blood.

A lumbar puncture should be considered if a fever without a cause accompanying the headache is present, or if meningismus and new neurologic signs or abnormal behaviors are present, although neuroimaging results are normal. If a child is febrile with meningismus without evidence of focal signs or elevated intracranial pressure, proceeding with a lumbar puncture before obtaining a computed tomographic (CT) or MRI scan may be appropriate.

The presence of abnormal findings on lumbar puncture or an acute or subacute abnormality on neuroimaging dictates that the child be hospitalized. If these tests are normal, the child may still need to be hospitalized if clinical evidence of elevated intracranial pressure or new neurologic signs are present. In the face of pernicious vomiting, a child may have to be hospitalized for rehydration. Children may also require hospitalization for the treatment of intractable pain or, rarely, for acute psychiatric care.

If the child has no evidence of an intracranial lesion and has a prior headache history that indicates migraines, tension headaches, or recurrent sinusitis, pain can be relieved by the intramuscular administration of 1 to 2 mg/kg of meperidine and 1 mg/kg of hydroxyzine. The use of morphine or morphine derivatives to relieve pain is rarely necessary. If the child is agitated, sedation with pentobarbital or chloral hydrate may be necessary. This therapy usually requires hospital admission for observation. If the child has acute sinusitis, that infection must be treated appropriately.

Most children who present to the emergency department with severe headaches have already been diagnosed as having migraines. If this diagnosis is substantiated by history, physical examination, and necessary laboratory tests, other methods of treating the acute pain and vomiting are available including the intravenous administration of 0.1 to 0.2 mg/kg of chlorpromazine or 0.2 mg/kg of prochlorperazine, up to a maximum of 10 mg. Dyskinetic and dystonic movements may occur, and sedation is frequent. However, the vomiting and headache often stop. Adolescents may respond to a 10-mg intravenous dose of ketorolac tromethamine (Toradol) to relieve pain. Older children may also be given up to 6 mg of sumatriptan subcutaneously (approximately 0.1 mg/kg). If the headache cannot be broken by these means, the child may require dihydroergotamine administered intravenously at 0.02 mg/kg up to 1.0 mg. Patients are usually pretreated with metoclopramide administered intravenously at 0.2 mg/kg up to 10 mg. An initial test dose of 20% of the final calculated dose should be given first to test the patient's tolerance to the drug. The child may need to be admitted to the hospital. Dihydroergotamine can be given intravenously every 8 hours for up to 3 days. Often, 48 to 72 hours is required for a patient with a difficult, severe migraine to respond. In the interim, the patient may need to be sedated or treated with narcotics.

CHAPTER 222
Disorders of the Anterior Horn Cell

Adapted from Julie Thorne Parke

Damage to the anterior horn cells is clinically characterized by weakness, atrophy, and hyporeflexia. Fasciculations are common. Because the dorsal sensory root is not involved in these disorders, sensory abnormalities are not present. Motor nuclei in the brainstem are commonly involved, so bulbar involvement is frequently seen.

ACUTE INFANTILE SPINAL MUSCULAR ATROPHY (ACUTE WERDNIG–HOFFMANN DISEASE, SPINAL MUSCULAR ATROPHY TYPE I)

Patients with the most severe form of SMA present a stereotypic picture with the onset of symptoms occurring within the first 6 months of life. In one-third of cases, the onset occurs *in utero* with a notable decrease in fetal movements during the last months of pregnancy. These children are hypotonic and weak in the neonatal period, and they have significant feeding difficulties and respiratory distress. Other children may appear normal for the first few weeks of life while generalized weakness of the extremities, trunk, and bulbar muscles gradually develops. A typical *frog-leg* posture characterized by abduction of the arms with flexion at the elbows and abduction of the legs with flexion at the knees is seen in the early stages of the disease.

Clinical Characteristics

Physical examination reveals marked hypotonia and generalized and symmetric weakness. Movements may be limited to flickering of the fingers and toes. The tendon reflexes are almost invariably absent. The child is unable to support the head and cannot straighten the trunk when held in ventral suspension. Respirations are shallow, and chest movements may be paradoxic. Feeding difficulties occur early, and secretions pool in the mouth as swallowing becomes further impaired. Visible atrophy and fasciculations of the tongue may be present. The extraocular muscles are not affected. The child appears alert and attentive, and development is normal with the exception of motor skills. Contractures are not common in the early stages of the disease, although a small percentage of patients have congenital contractures or dislocation of the hip. The natural course is one of gradually increasing weakness with feeding difficulties and respiratory compromise. In most cases, death occurs from a pulmonary infection with respiratory failure before the patient reaches 3 years of age.

Diagnosis

Electromyographic examination plays an important role in the investigation of patients with suspected SMA-I. Typically, fibrillations occur at rest suggesting active denervation, and a marked reduction of motor unit potentials on voluntary effort is also seen. Regular, repetitive involuntary firing of single motor units appears to be unique to the acute form of SMA. The large, complex, polyphasic motor unit potentials that are characteristic of chronic denervation are not seen in young infants with this disorder. Histologically, striking differences in the muscle occur between SMA-I and other neurogenic atrophies. Large groups of small, round or oval fibers with well-preserved architecture are present suggesting an arrest in maturation rather than atrophy of mature muscle fibers (Fig. 222-1).

Treatment

The treatment of acute infantile SMA is limited to supportive care. Respiratory insufficiency frequently becomes a problem before 1 year of age, and survival beyond 2 years is rare. Because of the poor prognosis of these children, artificial ventilation rarely, if ever, is justifiable. Appropriate genetic counseling is mandatory.

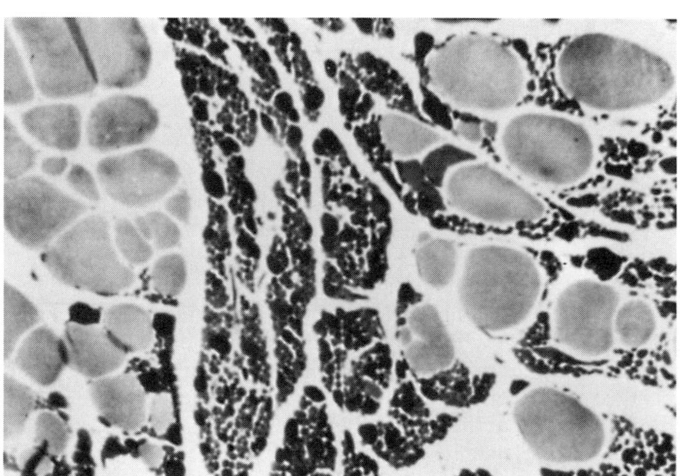

Figure 222-1. Muscle biopsy sample of a patient with Werdnig–Hoffman disease showing characteristic groups of rounded, atrophic type II (dark) muscle fibers adjacent to groups of normal sized or hypertrophic type I (light) muscle fibers.

INTERMEDIATE SPINAL MUSCULAR ATROPHY (CHRONIC WERDNIG–HOFFMANN DISEASE, SPINAL MUSCULAR ATROPHY TYPE II)

Intermediate SMA usually presents in the middle of the first year of life. Development is appropriate until approximately 6 months of age when motor milestones become delayed. The child may learn to sit independently and to stand, but independent walking is not usually achieved.

Clinical Characteristics

Weakness is symmetric, and proximal muscles tend to be involved more severely than distal muscles. Involvement of the truncal muscles is often prominent leading to kyphoscoliosis. Usually, a fine tremor of the hands is present. Tongue fasciculations and atrophy are noted in approximately one-half of the patients, but chewing and swallowing difficulties are rare. The deep tendon reflexes are absent or diminished. As in patients with the acute form of the disease, intelligence is normal. The course of the illness varies, and long periods in which the disease appears to be static may occur. Many patients have a stable course after the initial months of progressive weakness and may survive until adult life.

Diagnosis

Results of the electromyographic examination differ somewhat from those found in patients with the acute form of intermediate SMA in that fibrillation potentials are not prominent and motor unit action potentials tend to be polyphasic and large in amplitude. Examination of muscle biopsy samples reveals features similar to those found in acute infantile SMA, although large sheets of atrophic fibers are not usually seen. The muscle biopsy is helpful in making the diagnosis, but it is not a reliable indicator of the prognosis.

Treatment

No specific treatment is available for this disorder. Therapy should be directed toward preventing contractures by a combination of physiotherapy, bracing, and orthopedic procedures. Attention should be paid to maintaining correct posture of the spine because scoliosis may be rapidly progressive and can cause severe thoracic distortion adding to the respiratory impairment.

JUVENILE SPINAL MUSCULAR ATROPHY (KUGELBERG–WELANDER DISEASE, JUVENILE PROXIMAL HEREDITARY MUSCULAR ATROPHY)

Typically, juvenile SMA begins between 5 and 15 years of age, although earlier and later times of onset have been described. Weakness frequently starts in the hip girdle causing difficulty in walking, climbing stairs, and rising from a seated position.

Clinical Characteristics

As pelvic girdle weakness progresses, the child may use the hands to push off the knee when rising from the floor (Gowers maneuver). The calf muscles may appear hypertrophied in comparison with the atrophic thigh muscles leading to the erroneous diagnosis of Duchenne or Becker muscular dystrophy. Involvement of the shoulder and arm muscles becomes apparent in the later stages of the illness. Facial weakness and bulbar symptoms are rare. Most patients remain ambulatory until their third or fourth decade, at which time, severe hip weakness necessitates the use of a wheelchair. Skeletal deformities are not common early in the disease, but kyphoscoliosis and contractures may occur when the patient becomes wheelchair bound.

Diagnosis

Laboratory studies are important in this disorder, as it may be clinically indistinguishable from a number of other types of myopathy. The serum creatine phosphokinase level is elevated in approximately one-half of the patients, but it is rarely as high as that seen in individuals with Duchenne dystrophy. Electromyography reveals evidence of denervation and reinnervation with fibrillations, fasciculations, and large-amplitude polyphasic potentials. Muscle biopsy samples show signs of denervation with angular, atrophic fibers and fiber-type grouping. In the early stages of the disease, juvenile SMA may resemble Duchenne muscular dystrophy, particularly if significant calf hypertrophy is present. The absence of toe walking and heel-cord tightening may help differentiate SMA from Duchenne dystrophy. Facioscapulohumeral muscular dystrophy, limb-girdle dystrophy, and inflammatory myopathies are also included in the differential diagnosis.

INFECTIOUS DISEASES INVOLVING THE ANTERIOR HORN CELL

Poliomyelitis is an acute viral disease that exhibits a specific predilection for the anterior horn cells. The illness begins with fever, malaise, and, frequently, gastrointestinal symptoms. These symptoms are followed by a meningitic illness with stiffness and pain in the neck and pain in the back muscles. In a small percentage of infections, paralysis develops during the acute meningeal illness. Occasionally, paralysis may be delayed for 1 to 2 weeks after the meningeal symptoms. The legs are usually more involved than the arms, but weakness may occur in any muscle group. The muscular weakness may be associated with fasciculations and pain initially and then progress to a flaccid paralysis. Muscular involvement may be asymmetric and restricted to muscles in one extremity, or it may involve the trunk and all the extremities. Bulbar involvement occurs in 10% to 30% of children with paralytic poliomyelitis causing difficulty in swallowing or breathing. Examination of the cerebrospinal fluid reveals lymphocytosis with a normal glucose level and a normal or slightly elevated protein level. The virus cannot be isolated from the cerebrospinal fluid, but it may be recovered from stool suspensions or throat washings. Electromyography reveals evidence of denervation (fibrillation potentials) after a period of approximately 3 weeks. As recovery progresses, polyphasic motor unit action potentials of increasingly large amplitude are recorded indicating reinnervation.

The prognosis of patients with paralytic poliomyelitis varies depending on the site and severity of the paralysis. The mortality in bulbar disease is approximately 10% with death usually resulting from respiratory failure. The mortality associated with spinal poliomyelitis is approximately 1%. Gradual improvement occurs in most cases, but many patients are left with residual weakness. Poliomyelitis has become a rare disease since the advent of widespread immunization, but sporadic cases still occur.

Coxsackievirus infections occasionally show an affinity for anterior horn cells causing a paralytic illness similar to poliomyelitis. Numerous other viruses and immunizations have been associated with the development of transverse myelitis with anterior horn cell involvement. Transverse myelitis begins abruptly 1 to 3 weeks after a viral illness. Severe back or root pain is usually the initial symptom and may be accompanied by fever, malaise, neck stiffness, and diffuse muscular aching. Disruption of the anterior horn cells in the cervical or lumbar enlargements causes a flaccid paralysis of the extremities. Because involvement of the cord is not limited to the anterior horn cells but involves corticospinal tracts as well, the flaccidity may change gradually to spasticity. A sensory loss extending to the level of cord impairment is detectable, and bowel and bladder dysfunctions occur in almost all patients.

CHAPTER 223

Basal Ganglia and Neurotransmitter Disorders

Adapted from Joseph Jankovic

Biochemical or structural pathology in the basal ganglia may be manifested by movement disorders, groups of neurologic diseases, or syndromes that are characterized either by slowness, paucity, and "freezing" of voluntary movement (bradykinesia, akinesia) or by excess abnormal involuntary movement (hyperkinesia, dyskinesia). The diagnosis of a particular movement disorder primarily depends on careful observation of the clinical phenomena. Often, the bradykinetic movement disorders are accompanied by rigidity, postural instability, and loss of automatic associated movements. The hyperkinetic involuntary movements are differentiated phenomenologically according to their characteristic clinical features: rapidity and duration of contractions, rhythmicity, pattern, and suppressibility (Table 223-1). In general, abnormal involuntary movements are exaggerated with stress and disappear during sleep; however, certain forms of myoclonus and tics may persist during all stages of sleep. In a clinic devoted to movement disorders, tics are the hyperkinetic movements most commonly observed in children, followed in lessening frequency by dystonia, stereotypies, choreoathetosis, tremors, and myoclonus.

COMMON DISEASES

Parkinson Disease

Usually, Parkinson disease (PD) is a condition of middle and late life, but the incidence of early-onset parkinsonism (before age 40) and juvenile parkinsonism (before age 20) seems to be increasing. Although the rigid, akinetic form of parkinsonism appears to be more common in the juvenile cases, the typical resting tremor is present in many affected patients. Dystonia (often involving the legs), levodopa-induced dyskinesias, and clinical fluctuations seem to be particularly common in the juvenile cases. Some patients with familial juvenile parkinsonism belong to the group with the "hereditary dystonia-parkinsonism syndrome." Rare patients with juvenile parkinsonism who were examined at autopsy have been noted to have depigmentation of the substantia nigra, but Lewy bodies have not been detected. The absence of Lewy bodies does not indicate that these patients did not have PD but probably reflects an age-related susceptibility of the neuronal

TABLE 223-1. Differential Diagnosis of Hyperkinetic Movement Disorders

	Tremor			
Clinical features	***At rest***	***Postural***	***Kinetic***	**Chorea**
Characteristics	3- to 7-Hz supination-pronation oscillatory ("pill rolling"): hands, legs, lips, jaw (alternating contractions of antagonists)	4- to 12-Hz flexion-extension oscillatory movement with arms outstretched: hands, arms, head, voice, legs (simultaneous contractions of antagonists)	3- to 5-Hz intention tremor on finger-to-nose and heel-to-shin test	Rapid, abrupt, flowing, unsustained, random, semipurposeful, nonpatterned; athetosis is a slow chorea (writhing movement)
Associated features	Bradykinesia, rigidity (cog-wheel), shuffling gait, postural instability, hypomimia, micrographia	Dystonia, parkinsonism, and hereditary peripheral neuropathy, torticollis, parkinsonism	Ataxia, titubation, dysdiadochokinesia, loss of check and other cerebellar or brainstem signs	"Milkmaid's grip," darting tongue, orofacial dyskinesia, hypotonia, pendular or "hung-up" reflexes, dementia in Huntington disease, carditis in Sydenham chorea
Etiology	Parkinson disease, secondary parkinsonism, heterogeneous disorders with parkinsonian features	Physiologic, accentuated physiologic, essential cerebellar outflow (midbrain rubral, wing beating)	Cerebellar disorders and tumors, multiple sclerosis, brainstem and cerebellar strokes	Huntington disease, rheumatic fever (Sydenham), drug-induced hyperthyroidism, static encephalopathy, pregnancy, vasculitis, electrolyte metabolic imbalance
Treatment	Anticholinergics, amantadine, levodopa or carbidopa, dopamine agonists	Propranolol and other beta-blockers, benzodiazepines, phenobarbital, pyrimidine, clonazepam, amantadine, alcohol	No effective treatment, wrist-arm weights, thalamotomy	Treat underlying disorder, dopamine-blocking or depleting agents, cholinergic agents

cytoskeleton to develop the cytoplasmic inclusions. The neurotoxin 1-methyl-4-phenyl-1,2,3,6-tetrahydropyridine produces inclusions similar to Lewy bodies but only in aged animals. Although many cases of juvenile parkinsonism are sporadic, genetic predisposition in juvenile parkinsonism is frequent. One form of autosomal recessive juvenile PD has been linked to a locus on chromosome 6q25.2–27. Many other types of parkinsonism, some of which have their onset in childhood (Table 223-2), have been identified.

Wilson Disease

Wilson disease (WD) is one of the most important causes of juvenile parkinsonism and other movement disorders. Failure to diagnose this condition may have tragic consequences including death as a result of irreversible liver cirrhosis and profound neurologic deficit. The gene for this autosomal recessive hepatolenticular degenerative disease has been linked to the esterase D locus on the long arm of chromosome 13. Numerous mutations have been identified in the WD gene, which encodes copper-transporting P-type adenosine triphosphatease (ATPase) and has been termed *ATP7B*. The prevalence of the gene in the overall population is approximately 1%, although symptomatic WD is relatively rare (estimated prevalence, 30 per 1 million). The hepatic and neurologic dysfunction associated with WD is caused by a defect in copper metabolism resulting from a reduction in the rate at which copper is incorporated into ceruloplasmin and a decrease in the rate at which it is excreted from the liver. Usually, low ceruloplasmin levels are found in patients with WD, but they do not seem to be the primary defect because some patients with the disease and some heterozygotes have normal levels. Furthermore, the ceruloplasmin gene has been mapped to chromosome 3, not to chromosome 13. The excess copper not only accumulates in the liver and brain but can also cause renal tubule damage, osteoporosis, and arthropathy. Kayser–Fleischer rings, the best-recognized ophthalmologic sign of WD, are caused by the deposition of copper in the cornea.

Usually, the onset of WD is between adolescence and age 40, and its presentation seems to be age-dependent with hepatic failure being more common in children and neurologic or psychiatric symptoms more frequent in adults. In a nonselected population of 31 patients with WD, the mean age at onset was 21 ± 5 years. Sixty-one percent had neurologic symptoms, 13% had liver symptoms, and 10% had a combination of neurologic and liver problems. Approximately one-third of patients had psychiatric symptoms at disease onset including depression, emotional lability, personality change, and slow mentation. Another one-third had neurologic symptoms, particularly parkinsonism, pseudobulbar palsy, tremor, and dystonia; 14% had symptoms of liver disease; and 17% had their condition diagnosed by family screening. The most common neurologic findings at first evaluation were dysarthria (97%), dystonia (65%), dysdiadochokinesia (58%), rigidity (52%), gait and postural abnormalities (42%), tremor (32%), abnormal eye movements (32%), hyperreflexia (29%), drooling (23%), and bradykinesia (19%).

Because of its variable clinical expression, often the diagnosis of WD is delayed. Almost all patients with neurologic disease have Kayser–Fleischer rings, but this yellow-brown deposit at

TABLE 223-1. *(Continued)*

Stereotypy	Dystonia	Ballism	Myoclonus: *Generalized*	Myoclonus: *Segmental*	Tics
Repetitive, purposeless movements resembling normal voluntary movements	Sustained, twisting, usually low but may be rapid and may progress to fixed contractures (dystonic postures)	Abrupt, random, forceful, violent, flinging, usually proximal and unilateral, often spontaneously remits	Abrupt, irregular, brief, jerklike contractions of one or more muscles occurring synchronously or asynchronously, may be stimulus-sensitive	Rhythmic contraction of agonists, not stimulus-sensitive, may persist during sleep	Rapid, sudden, unpredictable, coordinated jerks preceded by inner urge, waxing and waning, temporarily suppressible
Often associated with akathisia (sensory and motor restlessness)	Torticollis, writer's cramp, blepharospasm, spasmodic dysphonia, essential tremor, hypertrophy of contracted muscles	Initial hemiparesis, later choreoathetosis	Encephalopathy, seizures, dementia, periodic electroencephalogram, enhanced somatosensory evoked potentials	Palatal myoclonus may be associated with bulbar palsy; spinal myoclonus may be associated with myelopathy	Vocalizations, coprolatia, echolalia, copropraxia, echopraxia, obsessive-compulsive behavior, attention deficit disorder, sleep disturbance
Usually drug-induced (tardive dyskinesia) schizophrenia, autism, mental retardation, Rett syndrome	Dystonia musculorum deformans, adult-onset torsion dystonia, drug-induced	Lesion of contralateral subthalamic nucleus (hemorrhage, infarction, rarely tumor)	Postanoxic, uremic, and other encephalopathies, Creutzfeldt-Jakob disease, subacute sclerosing panencephalitis, myoclonic epilepsy, Ramsay Hunt syndrome	Brainstem or spinal cord infarction, hemorrhage, myelitis, demyelinating disease	Gilles de la Tourette syndrome, transient tic of childhood
May improve with dopamine blockers or depleters, beta-blockers, opioid agonists or antagonists	Muscle relaxants, anticholinergics, tetrabenazine, baclofen, dopamine agonists, levodopa for diurnal dystonia, C botulinum toxin injections, thalamotomy	Dopamine-blocking or depleting agents, thalamotomy	Clonazepam, 5-hydroxytryptophan, sodium valproate, piracetam, lisuride	Tetrabenzine, 5-hydroxytryptophan, clonazepam, anticholinergics	Dopamine-blocking or depleting agents

the limbus of the cornea may also be noted in patients with primary biliary cirrhosis and active hepatitis with cirrhosis. Occasionally, a "sunflower cataract" may be seen as a result of copper deposition in the lens.

Usually, the diagnosis of WD is confirmed by the demonstration of low serum copper and ceruloplasmin levels, increased urine copper concentrations after a dose of penicillamine, and a rise in the level of copper in the liver (Table 223-3). The ratio of radioactivity in the plasma at 24 hours to that at 2 hours after the administration of an oral or intravenous dose of copper 64 is less than 0.5 in patients with WD (the equivalent value being greater than 0.8 in normal individuals). Other laboratory abnormalities often detected in patients with WD include aminoaciduria, hypercalciuria, glycosuria, leukopenia, hemolytic anemia, thrombocytopenia, and renal tubal deficit. In approximately one-half of affected patients, computed tomographic (CT) scanning of the brain reveals characteristic hypodense areas in the region of the basal ganglia, and often magnetic resonance imaging (MRI) reveals on T2-weighted images hypointensity that extends from the globus pallidum into the putamen. Extensive degeneration of the corpus striatum, particularly the putamen, is seen at autopsy. Also, the cerebellum, brainstem, and subcortical white matter may be involved.

The goals of treating WD patients are to reduce copper intake and to create a negative copper balance by increasing copper output in the urine. D-penicillamine has been used successfully to chelate copper at dosages of 0.5 to 2.0 g/day. However, penicillamine often produces considerable toxicity including fever, urticaria, leukopenia, nephritis, thrombocytopenia, systemic lupus erythematosus, hemolytic anemia, Goodpasture syndrome, pyridoxine deficiency, and a syndrome resembling myasthenia gravis. Hydrochloride (Syprine) in dosages of 400 to 800 mg three times daily before meals has been approved for the treatment of penicillamine-sensitive patients with WD. In addition to the chelating agents, zinc sulfate at a dosage of 300 to 1,200 mg/day between meals may reduce copper absorption. When early diagnosis is made and dietary and chelating therapies are instituted, the progression of liver and neurologic dysfunction can be halted and even reversed. At least 2,000 μg of copper should be excreted during the first 24 hours of penicillamine therapy. Approximately one-third of patients with WD experience deterioration despite penicillamine therapy, but most improve, sometimes after a latent period lasting several weeks or months. In patients with parkinsonian symptoms, levodopa and anticholinergic therapy may provide symptomatic relief.

Besides the treatment of patients with symptomatic WD, of paramount importance is screening all their relatives and instituting therapy immediately if the disease is diagnosed in any of them. Patients who fail to improve with chelating or other pharmacologic therapy may experience marked relief of neurologic symptoms several months after liver transplantation.

Huntington Disease

The usual onset of Huntington disease (HD) occurs in the fourth and fifth decades of life, but it is seen in approximately 10% of affected patients during childhood or adolescence. Both

TABLE 223-2. Classification of Parkinsonism

Primary Parkinson disease
Idiopathic, dominated by:
- Tremor
- Postural instability, gait difficulty
- Akinesia (freezing)
- Dementia
- Depression
- Sensory disturbance
- Autonomic dysfunction

Inherited, associated with essential tremor, dystonia, or peripheral neuropathy
Young-onset, associated with dystonia or essential tremor

Secondary parkinsonism
Drugs (dopamine-blocking and -depleting drugs, alpha-methyldopa, lithium, diazoxide, flunarizine, cinnarizine)
Toxins (manganese, mercury, carbon monoxide, cyanide, carbon disulfide, methanol, ethanol, MPTP)
Metabolic (parathyroid, acquired hepatocerebral degeneration, GM, gangliosidosis, Gaucher disease)
Encephalitis and postencephalitic syndrome
Slow virus (Creutzfeldt-Jakob disease)
Vascular (multiinfarct, Binswanger disease)
Brain tumor
Trauma and pugilistic encephalopathy
Hydrocephalus (normal and high-pressure)
Syringomesencephalia

Multiple system degenerations (parkinsonism plus)
Sporadic
- Progressive supranuclear palsy (ophthalmoparesis)
- Shy-Drager syndrome (dysautonomia)
- Olivopontocerebellar atrophy (ataxia)
- Parkinsonism–dementia–amyotrophic lateral sclerosis complex
- Striatonigral degeneration
- Corticodentonigra degeneration with neuronal achromasia
- Alzheimer disease

Inherited
- Huntington disease
- Wilson disease
- Hallervorden-Spatz disease
- Familial parkinsonism-dementia syndrome
- Familial basal ganglia calcification
- Neuroacanthocytosis
- Spinocerebellar-nigral degeneration and Joseph disease
- Glutamate dehydrogenase deficiency

MPTP, 1-methyl-4-phenyl-1,2,3,6-tetrahydropyridine.
Modified from Jankovic J. Parkinson's disease and related disorders of movements. In: Calne DB, ed. *Handbook of experimental pharmacology.* Berlin: Springer-Verlag, 1989:227.

juvenile and adult-onset HD are autosomal dominant traits with a defective gene mapped to a terminal band of the short arm of chromosome 4. The gene mutation was found to consist of an unstable enlargement of the CAG repeat sequence at 4p16.3. The majority of patients with juvenile HD have the akinetic-rigid syndrome termed the Westphal variant. Other features of juvenile HD include dementia, seizures, and ataxia. In addition, patients with juvenile HD are more likely to have inherited the abnormal gene from their father than their mother, and they tend to segregate within families. Although the medium-sized spiny neurons (type I cells) are usually affected first in the adult form of HD, the large spiny cells have been suggested to degenerate first in the juvenile form. In contrast to the caudate nucleus, which is typically involved in the adult form of HD, the putamen seems to be most damaged in the juvenile form of the disease.

The diagnosis of HD can be established with 100% accuracy with the demonstration of the presence of more than 30 CAG repeats in one of the alleles in the HD gene. The psychological and social impact of such testing, however, must be carefully considered before presymptomatic individuals are tested.

The most remarkable biochemical change observed in the brains of adults with HD is a reduction in the activity of glutamic acid decarboxylase, particularly in the corpus striatum, substantia nigra, and other basal ganglia. In contrast, thyrotropin-releasing hormone, neurotensin, somatostatin, and neuropeptide Y are increased in the corpus striatum. The depletion of gamma-aminobutyric acid in the corpus striatum may result in disinhibition of the nigral-striatal pathway. Coupled with the accumulation of somatostatin, the net result may be the release of striatal dopamine, which results in chorea. Dopamine-blocking drugs such as haloperidol, and dopamine-depleting agents including tetrabenazine, are often useful in controlling chorea. In patients with childhood HD, which is usually manifested by parkinsonian features, levodopa may provide symptomatic relief.

TABLE 223-3. Laboratory Tests in Wilson Disease

Laboratory tests (units)	Normal	Wilson disease
Serum copper (μg/dL)	90–140	<60 (10–100)
Serum ceruloplasmin (mg/dL)	24–45	<15 (0–30)
Urine copper (μg/24 hr)	<40	>200 (100–1,000)
Urine copper after penicillamine (μg/6 hr)	<400	>800
Liver copper (μg/g wet weight)	<10	>30
Liver uptake (^{64}Cu at 24 hr)	>60%	<50%
Plasma (^{64}Cu 24:2 hr ratio)	>0.8	<0.5

HYPERKINETIC MOVEMENT DISORDERS

Tremor

Essential tremor (ET) is the most common cause of an oscillatory involuntary movement during childhood (Table 223-4). ET may start at any age including infancy. One form of infantile ET is the hereditary chin tremor, which consists of rhythmic, three-per-second contractions of the chin that are often associated with deafness and are inherited in an autosomal dominant pattern. Another form of ET that begins during infancy or early childhood is so-called shuddering attacks. Affected children may have more than 100 attacks a day, but symptom-free intervals may last as long as 2 weeks. The attacks are characterized by bursts of rapid trembling of the entire body occasionally associated with head turning, involuntary sniffing, and throat clearing. During the attacks, affected children usually sink to the floor; the attacks may persist during sleep.

In addition to these forms of ET, the characteristic action-postural tremor may also be seen in children. Often, the slower tremor (approximately 6.5 Hz) involves the head and neck, whereas the more rapid tremor (8 to 12 Hz) tends to involve the hands. Many other variants of ET have been recognized, however. Although ET is usually "benign," it can occasionally progress to a very disabling movement disorder interfering with writing, feeding, speaking, and other activities of daily living.

Usually, ET is inherited in an autosomal dominant manner, and a locus has been found on chromosome 2p22–p25. Although neurotransmitter abnormalities in the basal ganglia are suspected to underlie ET, no pathologic changes have been documented in the few brains that have been examined at autopsy. Besides the beta-blockers, primidone, lorazepam, alprazolam,

TABLE 223-4. Classification of Tremors

- **Rest tremors**
- *Parkinson tremor*
- Parkinson disease
- Secondary parkinsonism
  - Postencephalic
  - Toxic disorder (phenothiazines, butyrophenones, metoclopramide, reserpine, tetrabenazine, carbon monoxide, manganese, MPTP, carbon disulfide)
  - Tumor
  - Trauma
  - Vascular disorder
  - Metabolic tremor: hypoparathyroidism, chronic hepatocerebral degeneration
- Parkinsonism plus (heterogeneous system degenerations)
- Olivopontocerebellar atrophy
- Progressive supranuclear palsy
- Wilson disease
- Huntington disease
- *Spasmus nutans*
- *Hereditary chin quivering*
- *Other*
- Midbrain (rubral) tremor
- Severe essential tremor
- Roussy-Lévy syndrome
- **Action tremors**
- *Postural tremors*
- Physiologic tremor
  - Normal physiologic tremor
  - Accentuated physiologic tremor
    - Stress-induced (anxiety, fight, fatigue, fever)
    - Endocrine (thyrotoxicosis, hypoglycemia, pheochromocytoma)
    - Drugs, toxins (epinephrine, isoproterenol, caffeine, theophylline and other sympathomimetic agents, levodopa, amphetamines, lithium, tricyclic antidepressant, phenothiazines, butyrophenones, thyroxine, hypoglycemic agents, adrenocorticosteroids, alcohol withdrawal, mercury, lead, arsenic, bismuth, carbon monoxide, methylbromide, monosodium glutamate, sodium valproate, metrizamide, meperidine)
- Essential tremor
  - Autosomal dominant
  - With peripheral neuropathy: Charcot-Marie-Tooth disease (Roussy-Lévy syndrome)
  - With other movement disorders (parkinsonism, torsion dystonia, spasmodic torticollis, myoclonus)
  - Factors that accentuate physiologic tremor and also enhance or unmask essential tremor
  - Vitamin E deficiency
- Action tremor of parkinsonism
- Neuropathic tremor
  - Peripheral neuropathies
  - Motor neuron disease
- Cerebellar postural hypotonic tremor (titubation)
- Midbrain ("rubral") tremor
- Dystonic (axial) tremor
- *Kinetic (intention) tremor*
- Cerebellar outflow tremor (superior cerebellar peduncle lesion)
  - Multiple sclerosis
  - Posterior circulation strokes
  - Cerebellar degenerations
  - Wilson disease
  - Drugs, toxins (phenytoin, barbiturates, lithium, meperidine, alcohol, mercury, 5-fluorouracil, vidarabine, amiodarone, cimetidine, tocainide)
- Midbrain ("rubral") tremor
- Primary handwriting tremor
- Dystonic (distal) tremor
- Familial benign chorea and tremor
- *Miscellaneous tremors and other rhythmic movements*
- Idiopathic
- Hysterical
- Involuntary rhythmic movements not classified as tremors
  - Cardiac and respiratory movements
  - Convulsions
  - Nystagmus
  - Segmental myoclonus
  - Oscillatory myoclonus
  - Asterixis
  - Fasciculations
  - Clonus
  - Minipolymyoclonus
  - Shivering
  - Shuddering
  - Head flopping or nodding movements

MPTP, 1-methyl-4-phenyl-1,2,3,6-tetrahydropyridine.
Modified from Jankovic J. *Neurologic consultant.* New York: Lawrence Della Corte, 1984:1.

clonazepam, amantadine, clonidine, and ethanol may improve ET.

Other oscillatory involuntary movements occasionally seen in infants and children are "head nodding," which is often associated with congenital nystagmus including spasmus nutans, and the "bobble-headed doll's syndrome," which is seen with diencephalic lesions including third-ventricle cysts or tumors, craniopharyngioma, hydrocephalus, and hypothalamic lesions.

Chorea, Athetosis, and Ballism

Chorea consists of continuous, unsustained, rapid, abrupt, and random contractions, whereas athetosis consists of nonpatterned, writhing movements that represent a form of "slow chorea." In contrast, ballism is a form of severe, coarse chorea; usually, it is unilateral (hemiballism) and is often the result of a lesion in the contralateral subthalamic nucleus and adjacent structures. Many acquired and hereditary types of chorea can become manifest during childhood (Table 223-5). Almost all normal infants make movements that resemble chorea, but usually this physiologic chorea resolves by age 8 months. Children with attention deficit disorder and hyperactivity have distal chorea called *chorea minima*.

HEREDITARY CHOREA

Although the majority of children with HD have a parkinsonian syndrome, approximately one-fourth have chorea. Another form of hereditary chorea is benign hereditary chorea, an autosomal dominant disorder that may present during infancy, childhood, or adolescence. Although it is benign, it may persist as a lifelong condition and may rarely be associated with intellectual impairment. Usually, caudate atrophy is not seen, but ^{18}F-2-fluorodeoxyglucose positron emission tomography may indicate decreased cerebral glucose metabolism in the caudate nucleus.

Another cause of genetic childhood chorea is the Lesch–Nyhan syndrome. This complex motor-behavioral syndrome is inherited as an X-linked recessive trait and is a result of defective activity of the enzyme hypoxanthine-guanine phosphoribosyltransferase. The diagnosis is suspected when a young boy with delayed developmental milestones, spasticity, and choreoathetosis develops self-mutilating behavior and is found to have

TABLE 223-5. Classification of Choreas

Developmental choreas
Physiologic chorea of infancy
Kernicterus, cerebral palsy, "minimal cerebral dysfunction" (the choreiform syndrome)
Hereditary choreas
Amino acid disorders
Glutaric acidemia, cystinuria, homocystinuria, phenylketonuria, Hartnup disease, argininosuccinicaciduria
Carbohydrate disorders
Mucopolysaccharidoses, mucolipidoses, galactosemia, pyruvate dehydrogenase deficiency
Lipid disorders
Sphingolipidosis (Krabbe), globoid cell leukodystrophy, metachromatic leukodystrophy, Gaucher, GM_1 and GM_2 gangliosidosis, ceroid lipofuscinosis
Other metabolic disorders
Lesch-Nyhan syndrome, Leigh disease, sulfite-oxidase deficiency, porphyria
Heredodegenerative disorders
Hallervorden-Spatz, ataxia-telangiectasia, tuberous sclerosis, Sturge-Weber, Wilson disease, myoclonus epilepsy, familial inverted choreoathetosis, hemoglobin SC disease, xeroderma pigmentosum, Pelizaeus-Merzbacher, familial striatal necrosis, Huntington disease, benign familial chorea (hereditary chorea without dementia), choreoacanthocytosis (amyotrophic chorea), paroxysmal kinesigenic choreoathetosis, paroxysmal dystonic choreoathetosis (Mount-Reback), familial calcification of the basal ganglia, Joseph disease, olivopontocerebellar atrophies (hereditary ataxia)
Drug-induced and toxic choreas
Antipsychotic neuroleptics
Tardive dyskinesia
Antiparkinsonian drugs
Dopaminergic (levodopa, bromocriptine, pergolide, lisuride), amantadine, anticholinergics
Anticonvulsants
Phenytoin, carbamazepine
Noradrenergic stimulants
Amphetamines, methylphenidate, aminophylline, theophylline, caffeine, pemoline
Steroids
Oral contraceptives, anabolic steroids
Opiates
Methadone
Miscellaneous drugs
Amoxapine, antihistamines, cimetidine, cyclizine, diazoxide, digoxin, isoniazid, lithium, methyldopa, metoclopramide, reserpine, triazolam, tricyclic antidepressants
Toxins
Alcohol intoxication and withdrawal, carbon monoxide, manganese, mercury, thallium, toluene, glue sniffing
Metabolic disorders
Hyponatremia and hypernatremia, hypocalcemia, hypoglycemia and hyperglycemia, hypomagnesemia, hepatic encephalopathy (acquired hepatocerebral degeneration), renal encephalopathy
Endocrine disorders
Hyperthyroidism, hypoparathyroidism, pseudohypoparathyroidism, hyperparathyroidism, chorea gravidarum (pregnancy), Addison disease
Nutritional disorders
Beriberi, pellagra, vitamin B_{12} deficiency in infants
Infectious disorders
Sydenham chorea (poststreptococcal), scarlet fever (streptococcal erythrogenic toxin), diphtheria, pertussis, typhoid fever, viral encephalitis (mumps, measles, varicella, echovirus, influenza), postvaccinal, neurosyphilis, mononucleosis, legionnaires' disease, bacterial endocarditis, sarcoidosis, mycobacterium tuberculosis, bacterial meningitis
Immunologically mediated chorea
Systemic lupus erythematosus, periarteritis nodosa, Behçet syndrome, Henoch-Schönlein purpura, multiple sclerosis
Cerebrovascular choreas
Basal ganglia infarction, basal ganglia hemorrhage, arteriovenous malformation, polycythemia vera, migraine, transient cerebral ischemia
Miscellaneous choreas
Posttraumatic, epidural hematoma, subdural hematoma, electrical injury to the nervous system, brain tumor, degeneration of nucleus centrum medianum of thalamus, hydrocephalus

Modified from Kurlan R, Shoulson I. Facial choreas. In: Jankovic J, Tolosa E, eds. *Advanced neurology*, vol 49, New York: Raven, 1988.

sand-like deposits in his urine. Often, affected patients have complications of hyperuricemia including gouty arthritis, tophus formation, and obstructive nephropathy. Cerebrospinal fluid studies of monoamine metabolites and postmortem biochemical assays have provided evidence for reduced dopamine and norepinephrine turnover in patients with this disorder.

SYDENHAM CHOREA

The high frequency of complications of chronic rheumatic heart disease in patients with Sydenham chorea (SC) suggests an association between rheumatic fever and this neurologic disorder. Unlike arthritis and carditis, which occur soon after such infection, chorea and various neurobehavioral symptoms may be delayed for 6 months or longer and may be the sole manifestation of rheumatic fever. Coincident with a dramatic decline in cases of acute rheumatic fever, the incidence of SC is also decreasing rapidly. Of 240 patients admitted with the diagnosis of SC to the University of Chicago Hospital between 1951 and 1976, only 8% were seen after 1968. Irritability, emotional lability, and other behavioral problems usually accompany the involuntary movements of this disorder. In approximately 20% of cases, the chorea is strictly unilateral (hemichorea). Besides chorea, other clinical features of SC include the "milkmaid's grip," "spooning," and "hung-up" reflexes. In most cases, the chorea subsides within 5 to 15 weeks, but it may recur in as many as 30% of patients within 2 years. Recurrence is particularly likely during pregnancy (chorea gravidarum). Usually, although the motor symptoms resolve completely, mental changes (particularly emotional lability) and cardiac problems may persist indefinitely. Persistent dopaminergic supersensitivity in affected individuals has been suggested by the high frequency of adverse reactions to central stimulants and to neuroleptics, together with psychotic features.

In addition to elevated titers of antistreptolysin, IgG antibodies reacting with neurons in the caudate and subthalamic nuclei have been found in the majority of patients. Because a latency period of approximately 1 to 6 months may occur after the streptococcal infection before the onset of chorea, patients with SC may have normal erythrocyte sedimentation rates and normal antistreptolysin and antistreptococcic antibody levels. The pathology of SC has not been studied well, but some brains have had vasculitis, chiefly involving the basal ganglia, cortex, and cerebellum. Besides SC, many other infectious causes of chorea including meningitis exist.

Although cephalosporins are equally effective, penicillin G, 500 to 1,000 mg four times per day, or one intramuscular injection of 600,000 to 1.2 million units of benzathine penicillin, is considered the drug of choice for pharyngitis caused by beta-hemolytic streptococcal infection. Despite an adequate (10-day) course, the bacteriologic failure rate is as high as 15%, and some patients

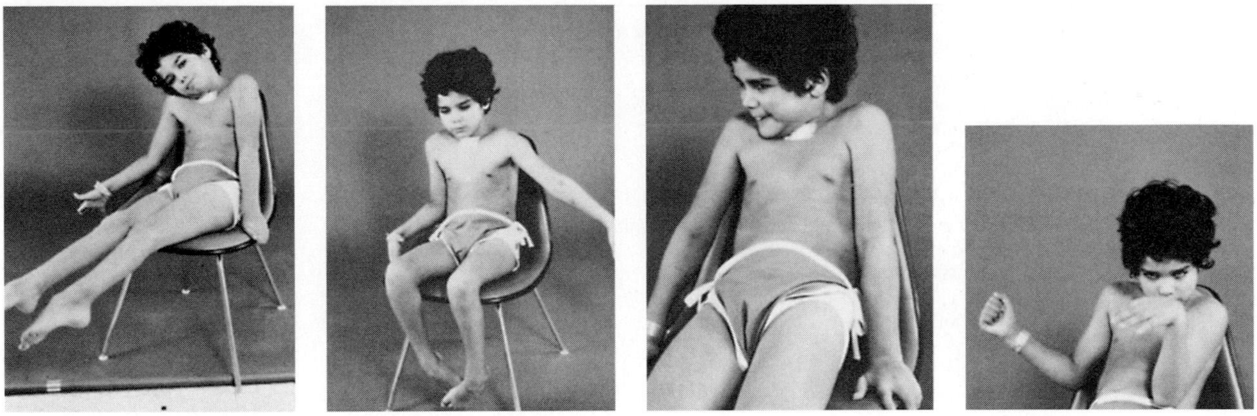

Figure 223-1. An 8-year-old boy with autosomal dominant, generalized torsion dystonia. As a result of severe dystonic contractions, he had muscle breakdown, myoglobinuria, and renal failure requiring a temporary curarization and tracheostomy. (Reproduced with permission from Jankovic J, Fahn S. Dystonic disorders. In: Jankovic J, Tolosa E, eds. *Parkinson's disease and movement disorders,* 3rd ed. Baltimore: Williams & Wilkins, 1998:513.)

develop rheumatic fever. Therefore, oral rifampin, 20 mg/kg every 24 hours in four doses, is recommended during the last 4 days of the 10-day course of penicillin therapy. Alternately, oral rifampin, 10 mg/kg, can be given every 12 hours for 8 doses with one dose of intramuscular benzathine penicillin G. Another alternative is oral clindamycin, 20 mg/kg/day in three doses for 10 days. The best ways to prevent rheumatic fever are accurate diagnosis and adequate treatment of the initial acute pharyngitis. Penicillin prophylaxis is advisable in all patients for at least 10 years. In addition to an initial course of penicillin followed by the administration of prophylactic oral penicillin until the patient reaches 20 years of age, a trial of corticosteroids, haloperidol, pimozide, reserpine, or tetrabenazine may be needed in severe cases.

Dystonia

Dystonia consists of repetitive, patterned, twisting, and sustained movements that may be either slow or rapid. The distribution of dystonia seems to be age-dependent; in children, often the disorder starts distally, whereas in adults, a cranial-cervical distribution is more common. Approximately 30% of all patients with dystonia have onset of the involuntary movements before they reach age 20. Childhood dystonia tends to progress to generalized dystonia, but usually adult dystonia remains focal or segmental (Fig. 223-1). Hemidystonia (unilateral dystonia) involving one-half of the body seems to be particularly common among children and young adults (Fig. 223-2). Approximately three-fourths of patients with hemidystonia have evidence of a structural lesion in the contralateral basal ganglia, particularly the putamen. The causes include infarction or hemorrhage in one-third and perinatal trauma in one-fifth of cases. In many patients with secondary dystonia, particularly children, a delay of several years after the acute event may often occur before the contralateral hemidystonia becomes manifest.

Dystonic states may be classified (according to cause) into primary dystonia, secondary dystonia, or psychogenic dystonia (Table 223-6). The term *primary dystonia* has replaced the old terminology of *dystonia musculorum deformans* and *idiopathic torsion dystonia*. By definition, primary dystonia, whether sporadic or inherited, is not associated with any other neurologic impairment such as intellectual, pyramidal, cerebellar, or sensory deficits. Approximately 20% of patients with primary dystonia, however, have associated tremor that is phenomenologically identical to ET; in some families, dystonia and ET can coexist. Cerebral palsy is probably the most common cause of secondary dystonia seen in children, but many other causes of secondary dystonia exist (Table 223-6).

Accurate diagnosis is the first step in treating patients with torsion dystonia. Usually, more extensive diagnostic investigation is prompted by the presence of atypical features such as impaired intellect, seizures, neuroophthalmologic abnormalities, ataxia, corticospinal tract signs, sensory deficits, severe speech disturbance, and unilateral distribution of the dystonia (Table 223-7). WD is one of the most important causes of dystonia because it is curable. Another treatable, and possibly preventable, type of childhood dystonia is the drug-induced form. Dystonic

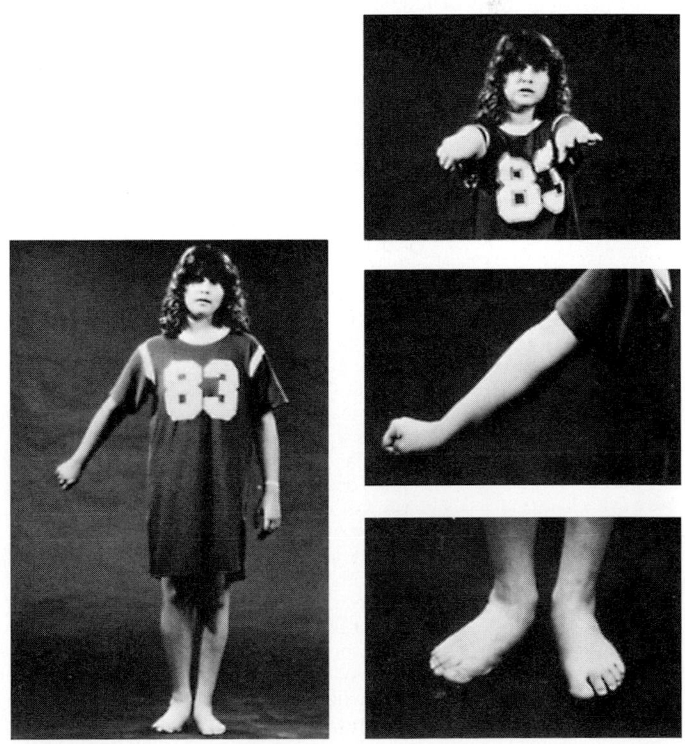

Figure 223-2. A 14-year-old girl with right hemidystonia as a result of left striatal injury at age 2. (Reproduced with permission from Jankovic J, Fahn S. Dystonic disorders. In: Jankovic J, Tolosa E, eds. *Parkinson's disease and movement disorders,* 3rd ed. Baltimore: Williams & Wilkins, 1998:513.)

TABLE 223-6. Classification of Dystonic States

Primary idiopathic dystonia
Inherited (hereditary torsion dystonia, dystonia musculorum deformans)
Autosomal dominant
Autosomal recessive (pseudodominant)
X-linked recessive
Dystonia with marked diurnal variation*
Paroxysmal kinesigenic and nonkinesigenic dystonia*
Parkinsonism-dystonia*
Sporadic (idiopathic torsion dystonia)
Generalized
Segmental (usually secondary dystonias)
Hemidystonia
Multifocal
Focal (torticollis, occupational cramps, oromandibular dystonia, blepharospasm, spasmodic dysphonia)
Secondary dystonia
Associated with other neurodegenerative disorders
Wilson disease
Huntington disease
Parkinsonism
Progressive supranuclear palsy
Progressive pallidal degeneration
Hallervorden-Spatz disease
Joseph disease
Ataxia-telangiectasia
Multiple sclerosis
Neuroacanthocytosis
Rett syndrome
Intraneuronal inclusion disease
Infantile bilateral striatal necrosis
Familial basal ganglia calcifications
Associated with metabolic disorders
Amino acid disorders
- Glutaric aciduria type I
- Methylmalonic acidemia
- Homocystinuria
- Hartnup disease
- Tyrosinosis

Lipid disorders
- Metachromatic leukodystrophy
- Ceroid lipofuscinosis
- Juvenile dystonic lipidosis ("sea-blue" histiocytosis; GM_1- and GM_2-variant gangliosidoses: neurovisceral storage disease with supranuclear ophthalmoplegia)

Miscellaneous metabolic disorders
- Leigh disease
- Leber disease and mitochondrial encephalopathies
- Lesch-Nyhan syndrome
- Triosephosphate isomerase deficiency
- Vitamin E deficiency

Result of known specific cause
Perinatal cerebral injury and kernicterus (possibly be delayed in onset)
Infection: viral encephalitis, encephalitis lethargica, tuberculosis, Reye syndrome, subacute sclerosing panencephalitis, Creutzfeldt-Jakob disease, acquired immunodeficiency syndrome; syphilis; acute infectious torticollis
Paraneoplastic brainstem encephalitis
Head trauma
Peripheral trauma
Atlantoaxial dislocation, subluxation, plagiocephaly
Gastroesophageal reflux (Sandifer syndrome)
Cerebrovascular injury
Brain tumor
Arteriovenous malformation
Central pontine myelinolysis
Cerebral ectopia and syringomyelia
Tortiocular tilt
Toxins (manganese, carbon monoxide, carbon disulfide, methane, wasp sting)
Drugs (levodopa, bromocriptine, antipsychotics, metoclopramide, fenfluramine, ergots, anticonvulsants)
Psychogenic dystonia

*Also may occur sporadically.
Modified from Jankovic J, Fahn S. Dystonic syndromes. In: Jankovic J, Tolosa E, eds. *Parkinson's disease and movement disorders.* Baltimore: Urban and Schwarzenberg, 1988:283.

TABLE 223-7. Investigation of Patients with Atypical Dystonia

Blood studies
Ceruloplasmin, copper, creatine phosphokinase, myoglobin, glucose, lactate, pyruvate, uric acid, creatinine, workup for autoimmune disease
Examination of red blood cells for acanthocytosis or sickle cell disease; lymphocytes for vacuolation (light microscopy) or inclusions (electron microscopy)
Leukocytes (lysosomal enzymes, hypoxanthine guanine phosphoribosyltransferase)
Urine studies
Screening tests (amino acids, 24-hour copper, column chromatography for oligosaccharides and mucopolysaccharides)
Cerebrospinal fluid studies
Lactate, pyruvate
Biopsies
Liver (morphology, copper)
Bone marrow ("sea-blue" histiocytes, vacuolation)
Skin (fibroblasts for lysosomal enzymes)
Conjunctivae (neuronal inclusions)
Rectal mucosa (neuronal inclusions)
Muscle (mitochondrial abnormalities)
Brain (neuronal inclusions or deposits)
Other studies
Slit-lamp examination for Kayser-Fleischer ring, cataracts, etc.
CT or MRI (basal ganglia calcifications or necrosis and other abnormalities)
PET scan (glucose metabolism, blood flow, ^{18}F-L-dopa, receptor ligand studies)
Spine radiographs or myelogram (atlantoaxial subluxation, Klippel-Feil deformity)
Upper gastrointestinal study (hiatal hernia in Sandifer-Kinsbourne syndrome)
Videotape (quantitative rating scale and polyelectromyograph for documentation)
Electrophysiologic studies (electroencephalogram; electroetinogram; visual-brainstem, somatosensory, and cortical evoked responses; polysomnography; electromyography; nerve conduction tests) (particularly useful in evaluation of paroxysmal and posttraumatic dystonia)

CT, computed tomography; MRI, magnetic resonance imaging; PET, positron emission tomography.
Modified from Jankovic J, Fahn S. Dystonic syndromes. In: Jankovic J, Tolosa Ed, eds. *Parkinson's disease and movement disorders.* Baltimore: Urban and Schwarzenberg, 1988:283.

movements may be caused by levodopa, bromocriptine, anticonvulsants, and ergots, but only the dopamine receptor blocking drugs such as the antipsychotics and antiemetics produce persistent tardive dystonia. Although acute transient dystonic reaction is a well-recognized complication of therapy with these drugs, a small percentage of patients treated with the neuroleptics have persistent and often disabling dystonia. In such cases of tardive dystonia, the offending drug should be stopped and, if no spontaneous improvement occurs, the patient should be given trials of muscle relaxants, anticholinergic drugs, and tetrabenazine. Approximately two-thirds of children with idiopathic torsion dystonia obtain some benefit from high-dose anticholinergic therapy (30–60 mg/day of trihexyphenidyl). When trihexyphenidyl is used, it must be introduced in small doses and increased gradually over a period of several weeks or months until symptomatic improvement is noted or side effects such as mental dullness, blurring of vision, and other anticholinergic adverse reactions prevent further increase in the dosage. In addition to anticholinergic drugs, we find that tetrabenazine, a monoamine-depleting agent, is effective in some patients with dystonia; occasionally, we combine it with pimozide, a postsynaptic dopamine receptor–blocking drug. Other drugs that occasionally prove useful in the treatment of dystonia include oral and intrathecal baclofen, carbamazepine, valproate, primidone, and lithium. All patients with childhood-onset dystonia, particularly when the disorder is combined with parkinsonism, should be treated with levodopa because they may have DRD. When pharmacologic therapy fails, *Clostridium botulinum* toxin injections may be tried, particularly for patients with focal dystonia. Usually, stereotactic thalamotomy, cervical rhizotomy, and other surgical therapies are reserved for patients who have disabling dystonia and whose disease does not respond to pharmacologic therapy or chemodenervation with botulinum toxin.

Tics

Approximately 25% of normal children have transient tics rendering this the childhood-onset involuntary movement most frequently seen in a movement disorders clinic. One of the most common causes of pathologic tics in childhood is the Gilles de la Tourette syndrome (TS). This motor-behavioral disorder is the expression of a genetic disturbance affecting the central nervous system. Usually, the onset is between ages 2 and 15, although in some cases, the initial manifestation may not be appreciated until the age of 21. The clinical expression of TS is gender-influenced: In boys, motor and vocal manifestations seem to dominate, whereas in girls, behavioral problems such as obsessive-compulsive disorder (OCD) seem more common. In addition to OCD, other comorbidities, particularly attention deficit disorder with or without hyperactivity, occur sometime during the course of the illness in a majority of patients with TS.

In addition to such simple tics as blinking, facial grimacing, shoulder shrugging, and head jerking, many patients with TS have complex sequences of coordinated movements including bizarre gait, kicking, jumping, body gyrations, scratching, and seductive or obscene gestures. The waxing and waning nature of tics, the irresistible urge before a tic and relief after a tic, the temporary suppressibility of the tics, and the recurrence of tics during sleep often result in the misdiagnosis of the disorder as having a psychogenic origin. The psychogenic nature of the condition is also erroneously suggested by the involuntary vocalizations that occur, which range from simple noises to coprolalia (obscene words), echolalia (repetition of words), and palilalia (repetition of a phrase or word with increasing rapidity). Coprolalia, although it is one of the most recognizable symptoms of TS, has been seen in only 40% of our patients, thus far. Many patients also experience copropraxia, echopraxia, bizarre thoughts and ideas, thought fixation, compulsive ruminations, and perverse sexual fantasies. Sleep complaints including restlessness, insomnia, enuresis, somnambulism, nightmares, and bruxism have been noted in approximately one-half of our patients, and approximately two-thirds had evidence of motor tics recorded by polysomnography. If a broad spectrum of behavioral problems is included, approximately 1% of all individuals manifest one or more aspects of the TS gene.

Disturbance in the mesencephalic-mesolimbic system, which results in disinhibition of the limbic system, has been suggested as the pathogenetic mechanism underlying TS. Neither imaging nor postmortem studies of brains of patients with TS have shown any abnormalities consistently.

Although haloperidol is recommended most frequently for TS, we find fluphenazine, pimozide, and tetrabenazine to be more effective and better tolerated. Patients with predominant behavioral symptoms, particularly impulse control problems and rage attacks, may benefit from clonidine and the selective serotonin uptake inhibitors. The selective serotonin uptake inhibitors are also fairly effective in treating associated OCD. When TS is associated with attention deficit disorder with or without hyperactivity, central nervous system stimulants such as methylphenidate, dextroamphetamine (Dexedrine), and guanfacine may be needed. These agents, however, should be used cautiously because they may precipitate or exacerbate tics.

Myoclonus

In contrast to tics, myoclonus is a simple, jerk-like movement that is not coordinated or suppressible and is often activated by volitional movement. Benign neonatal sleep myoclonus, which occurs in the first month of life, is usually stimulus-sensitive and occurs in the early stages of sleep. It should be differentiated from neonatal seizures and infantile spasms. Usually, essential myoclonus begins before age 20, is inherited in an autosomal dominant pattern, and may be associated with ET.

Cortical myoclonus may be manifested as a continuous, repetitive, focal jerking. It can be triggered by external stimuli or evoked by muscle stretch reflex or by quick, passive, movement of distal phalanx (cortical reflex myoclonus) or by movement (cortical action myoclonus). Cortical reflex myoclonus is characterized by a time-locked electroencephalographic (EEG) event preceding the myoclonic movement and by enhanced amplitude of the somatosensory evoked potential. The most common causes of epilepsia partialis continua include cortical stroke and Rasmussen encephalitis, a disorder of childhood or adolescence caused by focal cortical lesion or inflammation, possibly caused by viral infection. In contrast to the hyperexcitable sensorimotor cortex that underlies cortical myoclonus, presumably reticular reflex myoclonus is the result of hyperexcitable brainstem reticular formation, particularly the nucleus reticularis gigantocellularis.

Progressive myoclonus epilepsy consists of myoclonus, seizures, and a progressive clinical course. One form of progressive myoclonus epilepsy, Unverricht–Lundborg disease (also known as *Baltic myoclonus*), is characterized by stimulus-sensitive myoclonus that usually begins when affected patients are between ages 6 and 15. Such patients also have dysarthria, ataxia, intention tremor, and mild intellectual decline, and most become bedridden within 5 years after onset of the disease. Epileptiform EEG findings may be seen as long as 3 years before the onset of clinical symptoms. The disease is inherited in an autosomal recessive pattern, and at least some cases may be associated with mitochondrial myopathy and encephalopathy. Another form of progressive myoclonus, Lafora body disease, usually begins in patients between ages 11 and 18 and is characterized by progressive dementia, apraxia, and cortical blindness with total disability resulting within 5 to 8 years after onset. Biopsy of the skin (particularly the axillary skin), liver, muscle, or brain reveals typical inclusions (Lafora bodies) that are positive on periodic acid–Schiff staining.

Ramsay Hunt syndrome is a group of heterogeneous disorders dominated by a combination of progressive myoclonus and cerebellar ataxia. Myoclonus may also be a manifestation of viral encephalitis and is typically seen in patients with subacute sclerosing panencephalitis. In this subacute disorder, progressive dementia and "slow" myoclonus, which occur approximately every second, are associated with periodic complexes on the EEG. Another form of myoclonic encephalopathy that occurs in young children is the opsoclonus–myoclonus syndrome or the "dancing eyes–dancing feet" syndrome. Usually, it is seen after a febrile illness or in association with a neuroblastoma, and marked improvement may be achieved with steroid therapy. Stimulus-sensitive myoclonus resembles another jerk-like movement disorder called *the startle disease* or *hyperexplexia*. Hereditary hyperexplexia, an autosomal dominant disorder of childhood, has been found to be caused by a point mutation in the gene coding for the alpha-1 subunit of the glycine receptor on chromosome 5, but not all forms of hereditary hyperexplexia are caused by the same genetic and physiologic abnormality. Small myoclonic jerks (minipolymyoclonus) have also been reported in children with chronic spinal muscular atrophy. The idiopathic, generalized, or segmental forms of myoclonus may improve with treatment using clonazepam, sodium valproate, 5-hydroxytryptophan, tetrabenazine, reserpine, levodopa, trihexyphenidyl, lisuride, and piracetam.

Stereotypies

Stereotypies are repetitive, purposeless, and seemingly voluntary movements such as chewing, rocking, and twirling or touching. These movements are usually seen in the setting of infantile autism or mental retardation. Attention has been increasingly directed toward another disorder characterized by marked stereotypy: Rett syndrome. This condition occurs only in girls who have normal prenatal and perinatal growth and development. At the age of 6 to 18 months, they regress in their verbal and motor skills, lose purposeful use of their hands, and have jerky ataxia and typical stereotyped movements of the hands resembling hand washing and kneading. In addition to the motor manifestations, girls with Rett syndrome often have breath-holding spells, hyperventilation, loss of facial expression, poor eye contact, bruxism, dystonia, occasional seizures, apparent insensitivity to pain, and a variety of self-injurious and aggressive behaviors. The pathogenesis of Rett syndrome is unknown, and the vast majority of the cases occur sporadically, although some are familial.

CHAPTER 224
Leukodystrophies

Adapted from Alan K. Percy

METACHROMATIC LEUKODYSTROPHY (SULFATIDE LIPIDOSIS)

Metachromatic leukodystrophy is an autosomal recessive disorder with an incidence of 1 per 40,000 people. The biochemical basis is the inability to degrade the sphingolipid, sulfatide, or galactosyl-3 sulfate ceramide. Sulfatide, along with galactosylceramide, is an important constituent of myelin. Metachromatic leukodystrophy exhibits deficiency of sulfatide sulfatase (arylsulfatase A), the lysosomal enzyme responsible for the degradation of sulfatide. This deficiency results in the accumulation of sulfatide in both neural and nonneural (especially kidney and gallbladder) tissues, where it can be detected as metachromatic granules. Both central and peripheral myelin are abnormal. Neuropathology consists of widespread loss of myelin and oligodendroglia in the brain and segmental demyelination of the peripheral nerves.

Forms of the Disease

Metachromatic leukodystrophy occurs in three principal forms: late infantile (the most common), juvenile, and adult (Table 224-1). The distinction of separate phenotypes is arbitrary because the variability reflects more a continuum of phenotypes than separate entities. As specific mutations are identified, the genotype-phenotype correlations become clearer, and the continuum of clinical involvement becomes more evident.

TABLE 224-1. Characteristics of Sulfatide Lipidoses

Characteristic	Late infantile	Juvenile	Adult	Multiple sulfase deficiency
Age at onset	6–24 mo	4–8 yr	15 yr or older	6–18 mo
Prognosis	Death in 5–6 yr	Death in 10–15 yr	Slow progression	Death by age 10–12 yr
Mode of inheritance	AR	AR	AR	AR
Neurologic signs	Gait difficulty, hypotonia, ataxia, rapid deterioration	Gait difficulty, ataxia, intellectual decline	Dementia, depression, psychosis, motor difficulty	Gait difficulty, hypotonia, ataxia, rapid deterioration
Systemic signs	—	—	—	Coarse features, hepatosplenomegaly, skeletal deformity, ichthyosis
Stored material	Sulfatide	Sulfatide	Sulfatide	Sulfatide, cholesterol sulfate, mucopolysaccharide sulfate
Enzyme defect	Sulfatide sulfatase (arylsulfatase A)	Sulfatide sulfatase (arylsulfatase A)	Sulfatide sulfatase (arylsulfatase A)	Multiple sulfatases
Feasibility of prenatal diagnosis	Yes	Yes	Yes	Yes

AR, autosomal recessive.

Diagnosis and Treatment

The diagnosis of metachromatic leukodystrophy is accomplished by careful clinical assessment and performance of appropriate laboratory studies. The diagnosis is suggested by a history of regression and progressive deterioration of motor function and signs of gait difficulties with weakness, hypotonia, hyporeflexia, and extensor plantar responses in the early forms or behavioral and motor disability in older children or adolescents. Nerve conduction velocities are reduced as a reflection of peripheral nerve involvement. The cerebrospinal fluid (CSF) protein level is increased. Computed tomography (CT) or magnetic resonance imaging (MRI) reveals symmetric white matter lesions in the early forms of the disease and may demonstrate cortical atrophy in the later forms. Definitive diagnosis is made by establishing decreased activity of the enzyme arylsulfatase A, preferably in leukocytes or skin fibroblast cultures. The availability of biochemical analysis has greatly diminished the role of peripheral nerve biopsy, which typically reveals metachromatic granules.

No effective treatment is available for metachromatic leukodystrophy. Enzyme replacement by bone marrow transplantation has possible benefit in terms of improved arylsulfatase A activity and slowed disease progression, but convincing evidence of long-term efficacy within the central nervous system is lacking. Careful consideration should be given to therapies that may modify the natural history in a way that would produce greater chronicity without affecting resolution. Supportive therapy is indicated to ensure proper nutrition and to treat medical problems including seizures, as they occur.

GLOBOID CELL LEUKODYSTROPHY (GALACTOCYLCERAMIDE LIPIDOSIS, KRABBE DISEASE)

Globoid cell leukodystrophy is an autosomal recessive disorder that has an incidence in Sweden of approximately 1 per 50,000 people but is apparently less common outside Scandinavia. The biochemical abnormality involves the inability to degrade the sphingolipid galactosylceramide, also called *galactocerebroside.* Galactocerebroside is an important component of myelin. Hence, both the central and peripheral nervous systems are affected in this disorder. Globoid cell leukodystrophy represents a fundamental failure in myelinogenesis. The small amount of myelin that is formed (less than 1% of normal) has a normal composition. Also, unlike metachromatic leukodystrophy, with its marked storage of sulfatide, an actual deficiency of galactocerebroside occurs in this disorder.

Forms of the Disease

Globoid cell leukodystrophy occurs in two principal forms: infantile (the more common) and late-onset (Table 224-2).

TABLE 224-2. Globoid Cell Leukodystrophy

Characteristic	Infantile	Late infantile
Age at onset	Infancy	1–5 yr
Prognosis	Death by age 2 yr	Death by age 10–12 yr
Mode of inheritance	Autosomal recessive	Autosomal recessive
Neurologic signs	Irritability, extensor rigidity, optic atrophy, cortical blindness, rapid deterioration	Ataxia, gait difficulty, vision loss, psychomotor decline
Stored material	Galactosylceramide, galactosylsphingosine (psychosine)	Galactosylceramide, galactosylsphingosine (psychosine)
Enzyme defect	Galactosylceramide beta-galactosidase	Galactosylceramide beta-galactosidase
Feasibility of prenatal diagnosis	Yes	Yes

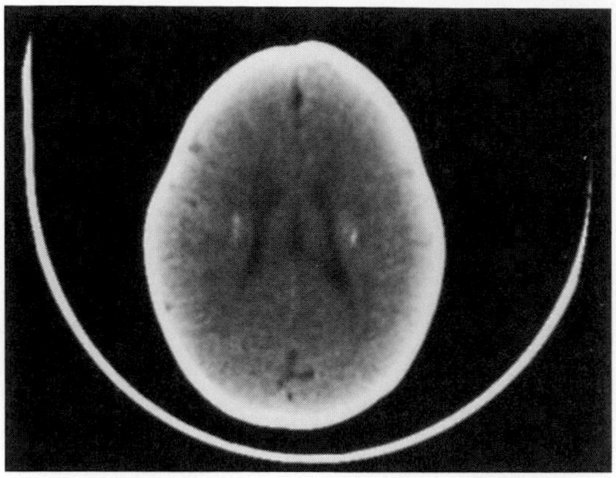

Figure 224-1. Nonenhanced brain computed tomographic (CT) scan of an infant with galactosylceramide lipidosis (Krabbe disease) demonstrating lesions of increased density adjacent to the lateral ventricles.

Diagnosis and Treatment

The definitive diagnosis of globoid cell leukodystrophy can be made by enzymatic assay. Galactocerebroside beta-galactosidase activity, mapped to chromosome 14, is deficient and can be assayed in leukocytes and fibroblast cultures. As in metachromatic leukodystrophy, numerous mutant alleles have been identified in this disorder providing phenotype-genotype correlations for the variant forms. The need for enzyme analysis will be suggested by a careful history and physical assessment and by the demonstration of reduced nerve conduction velocities and marked elevation of the CSF protein level (usually in excess of 3 g/L). CT will show decreased white matter and increased density of the internal capsule, thalamus, and basal ganglia (Fig. 224-1). MRI will reflect the failure of myelination by demonstrating reversal of the usual gray-white appearance.

Effective therapy for globoid cell leukodystrophy is lacking. Nevertheless, supportive care is important to assist the family during this difficult period.

ADRENOLEUKODYSTROPHY

Adrenoleukodystrophy, first described as an X-linked disorder, is now recognized as a multifaceted complex that includes adrenoleukodystrophy and adrenomyeloneuropathy, both of which are X-linked, and an autosomal recessive form that appears in infancy (Table 224-3).

Forms of the Disease

Adrenoleukodystrophy, the most common of the three disease forms, is a progressive disorder of young boys aged 3 to 16 (mean age, 8 years) that generally begins with personality changes or altered school performance and motor deficit. Seizures occur in 20% of children and occasionally signal the onset of the disorder. Motor involvement may be unilateral at first. Although expression of disease is highly variable, progression is generally relentless and results in profound psychomotor retardation, spasticity, and extensor posturing. Death occurs within 10 years of diagnosis. Adrenal insufficiency is clinically important in approximately 40% of children, although an equal number may have inadequate cortisol response to adrenocorticotropic hormone challenge. An "Addison disease only" phenotype of adrenoleukodystrophy is now recognized and may account for 40% of cases of Addison disease in men.

Diagnosis and Treatment

The clinical diagnosis of adrenoleukodystrophy is based on careful history and physical examination, characteristic changes seen on CT (confluent hypodensities in parietooccipital white matter with contrast enhancement at the margins suggesting active demyelination; Fig. 224-2) or MRI (symmetric periventricular signal increase) examination, normal nerve conduction velocities, abnormal brainstem auditory-evoked responses (prolonged interpeak latency between waves I and V), and elevated CSF protein levels. In contrast, adrenomyeloneuropathy is characterized by normal CSF protein levels and normal results on CT scans of the brain (with mild atrophy, a possible late finding) but abnormal nerve conduction velocities and brainstem auditory-evoked responses. In addition

TABLE 224-3. Adrenoleukodystrophy Complex

Characteristic	Adrenoleukodystrophy	Adrenomyeloneuropathy	Neonatal adrenoleukodystrophy
Age at onset	3–16 yr (mean, 8 yr)	20–40 yr	Infancy
Prognosis	Death in 1–10 yr	Prolonged survival	Death in 1–4 yr
Mode of inheritance	XLR	XLR	AR
Neurologic signs	Behavior problems, poor school performance, quadriparesis, blindness	Spastic paraparesis, distal neuropathy, urinary retention, impotence	Hypotonia, seizures, rapid deterioration, mild dysmorphism, hepatomegaly
Systemic signs	Hypoadrenalism in 50%, diminished response to ACTH, skin hyperpigmentation	Hypoadrenalism, hypogonadism	Normal adrenal function, hypoplastic adrenal glands
Stored material	Very long-chain fatty acids	Very long-chain fatty acids	Very long-chain fatty acids, phytanic acid, bile acid precursors, reduced plasmalogens
Enzyme defect	Peroxisomal fatty acyl-CoA synthetase import	Peroxisomal fatty acyl-CoA synthetase	Absent or deficient peroxisomes
Feasibility of prenatal diagnosis	Yes	Yes	Yes

ACTH, adrenocorticotropic hormone; AR, autosomal recessive; XLR, X-linked recessive.

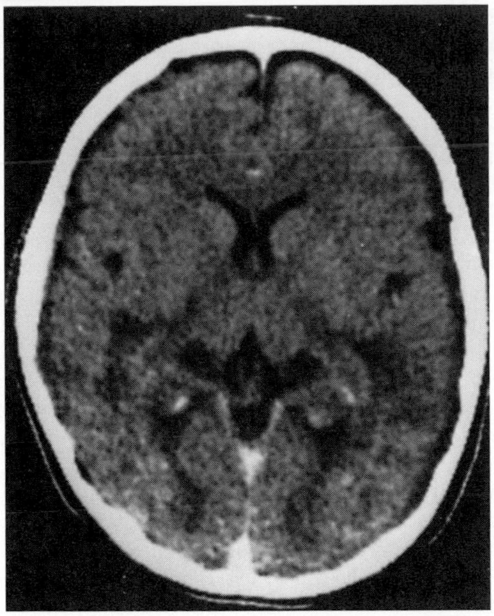

Figure 224-2. Enhanced brain computed tomographic (CT) scan of a child with adrenoleukodystrophy indicating symmetric low-density lesions located posteriorly in the parietooccipital regions with areas of contrast enhancement.

to having elevated very long-chain fatty acid levels and altered peroxisomes, children with neonatal adrenoleukodystrophy demonstrate reduced plasmalogens and elevated phytanic acid and pipecolic acid levels in plasma. Marked abnormalities of brainstem auditory-evoked responses, visual-evoked responses, and electroretinography (EEG) may also assist in the clinical diagnosis.

Heterozygote detection may be accomplished reliably for adrenoleukodystrophy by combining the measurement of very long-chain fatty acid levels and ratios with brainstem auditory-evoked responses. As many as 15% of possible heterozygotes for adrenoleukodystrophy may still escape detection, however. With regard to the neonatal form, heterozygote detection is not possible. Nevertheless, prenatal diagnosis is feasible for each disorder in families known to be at risk.

Fifteen percent or more of female heterozygotes for adrenoleukodystrophy may have a generally mild form of the disease. Such cases are characterized by a progressive spastic paraparesis, mild peripheral neuropathy, normal adrenal function, and elevated very long-chain fatty acid levels in plasma or fibroblasts.

Effective therapy for the various forms of adrenoleukodystrophy is actively being sought. Bone marrow transplantation for enzyme replacement has not been helpful in neurologically impaired children with the disorder, but it may retard disease onset in normal or mildly affected patients. Dietary therapy aimed at restricting the intake of long-chain fatty acids and at modifying their endogenous formation seems to function similarly by restricting disease onset in presymptomatic individuals. Nevertheless, the treatment of progressive disease is ineffective.

CHAPTER 225

Hereditary and Acquired Types of Myopathy

Adapted from Darryl C. De Vivo
and Salvatore DiMauro

HEREDITARY TYPES OF DYSTROPHY

X-Linked Diseases

DUCHENNE-TYPE MUSCULAR DYSTROPHY (DMD)

DMD is the most severe form of progressive primary muscular degeneration and is associated with a genetic abnormality in band 1 of region 2 of the short (p) arm of the X chromosome. This genetic locus is designated Xp2.1. Approximately 1 in 3,000 live-born male infants have this condition with one-third of all cases representing new mutations. The dystrophy is manifest at birth, becomes clinically evident between ages 3 and 5, and progresses inexorably over the next two decades before culminating in the death of affected patients. Most patients become wheelchair-dependent between ages 10 and 12. Complications result from cardiac involvement, nervous system involvement, musculoskeletal deformities, and failing respiratory function. Levels of serum enzymes that originate from skeletal muscle are elevated, most notably creatine kinase (CK). The CK value is very high after birth and remains remarkably elevated during the presymptomatic phase permitting early diagnosis of siblings at risk. Rarely, affected infants are clinically involved. Infant macroglossia has been noted on occasion, and motor milestones may be delayed. One-third of patients with DMD are late walkers (i.e., they do not walk independently until between ages 15 and 18 months). Parents retrospectively report developmental clumsiness and motor sluggishness in running, climbing stairs, rising from the ground after falling, and pedaling a tricycle. Abnormalities of gait and posture appear in middle childhood with the emergence of increasing lumbar lordosis, pelvic waddling, frequent falling, and Gowers sign. Although it is distinctive in DMD, Gowers sign may be seen in patients with any condition that causes pelvic girdle weakness. Enlargement of the musculature becomes evident with characteristic involvement of calf, gluteal, lateral vastus, deltoid, and infraspinatus groups. Weakness is more evident in the proximal muscles, and tendon reflexes are diminished at the knees, biceps, and triceps. Only in the preterminal phase are the distal tendon reflexes noticeably affected. Contractures of the iliotibial bands, hip flexors, and heel cords develop before ambulation is lost. After ambulation is lost, the muscles decrease in size, contractures progress with loss of joint mobility, and kyphoscoliosis develops with further compromise of respiratory function.

Cardiac involvement is evident in all patients with DMD but is rarely the cause of death. Similarly, cardiac abnormalities may be noted in female carriers of DMD, even when the serum CK values are normal. Degenerating muscle fibers and small foci of fibrosis are scattered throughout the myocardium and conduction systems. The posterobasal region and adjacent lateral wall of the left ventricle are commonly and prominently involved. The electrocardiographic (ECG) changes are distinctive: tall right precordial R waves and deep Q waves in the left precordial and limb leads.

Nervous system involvement has been recognized since the earliest descriptions of DMD. It is a nonprogressive process and may be associated with "atrophy" of the brain seen on computed tomography (CT). Some patients also have macrocephaly. The mean IQ is approximately 80, and individual IQ values correspond to a gaussian, bell-shaped distribution curve.

The electromyogram (EMG) is distinctively myopathic with decreases in the amplitude and duration of the compound action potential and enrichment of the interference pattern. A large number of the motor units are polyphasic, and occasional sparse fibrillation potentials are consistently observed. Sensory and motor conduction velocities are normal.

Etiology and Treatment

The etiology of DMD is genetic, but the pathophysiology remains obscure. This obscurity will not be the case much longer, however, because antibodies are now available for the gene product. The protein, termed dystrophin, has a molecular weight of 440 kd, and its structure and function are expected to be elucidated in the near future. Then DMD and its allelic variants will be definable by immunochemical methods, and more rational therapeutic interventions including gene therapy can be contemplated. The traditional methods of care will remain applicable until the disease can be prevented from appearing or progressing. Family counseling, physical therapy, proper use of orthotic devices, selective surgical interventions to treat joint contractures and spinal deformities, and dietary management are important interventions that improve the quality and length of life for patients with DMD. Clinical trials of promising therapeutic regimens have been conducted during the last several years by the Collaborative Investigation of Duchenne Dystrophy (CIDD) group sponsored by the Muscular Dystrophy Association. The CIDD group has documented the clinical course of DMD carefully and has developed rigorous protocols to assess the efficacy of various drugs and hormones in its treatment. Treatment with prednisone, 0.75 mg/day, has been shown in double-blind, placebo-controlled trials to slow the decline of muscle strength and to increase muscle mass.

Differential Diagnosis

The differential diagnosis of DMD includes autosomal recessive limb-girdle dystrophy presenting in early life (Tunisian form), BMD, Emery–Dreifuss dystrophy, congenital muscular dystrophy, muscle carnitine deficiency, the childhood form of acid maltase deficiency, and juvenile spinal muscular atrophy (Kugelberg–Welander syndrome). Female patients with clinical features of DMD must undergo genetic and cardiologic examination. Such patients may represent sporadic cases of autosomal recessive limb-girdle dystrophy manifesting carriers of DMD or genuine examples of DMD resulting from selective chromosomal aberrations. These aberrations include Turner syndrome (XO karyotype), mosaic states (X/XX or X/XX/XXX), a structurally abnormal X chromosome, an X autosomal translocation, and, perhaps more important, a skewed inactivation of the X chromosome favoring the one carrying the mutant gene.

BECKER MUSCULAR DYSTROPHY (BMD)

BMD represents a more benign version of DMD. BMD is similar to DMD, but the age of onset is later, and the progression is slower. Pseudohypertrophy is striking, and frequently pes cavus deformities are present in patients with BMD. Unlike in DMD, cardiac and nervous system involvement is unusual, but "pure" dilated cardiomyopathy can occur in patients with BMD in the absence of muscle weakness. Patients with BMD may have children, although infertility is higher in this population. All female progeny are obligate carriers, and all sons are unaffected. Loss of ambulation is the single best discriminator between DMD and BMD. The treatment approaches and genetic counseling are similar to those for DMD.

Autosomal Types of Dystrophy

MYOTONIC DYSTROPHY

Myotonic dystrophy follows a pattern of autosomal dominant inheritance. Gene mapping studies have localized the defect to the long arm of chromosome 19. The unstable gene mutation is an expanding trinucleotide sequence. This amplification correlates with the clinical phenomenon of anticipation. In general, patients with myotonic dystrophy do not complain of their myotonia, and infants with congenital myotonic dystrophy have no clinical or electrical evidence of the disorder. In contrast, patients with the nonprogressive forms of myotonia are aware of their disease and are bothered by this symptom, and myotonia can be demonstrated in infancy. Virtually all systems are involved in this condition. Severe brain involvement may occur in the congenital form, and adults have mental deterioration. Smooth, striated, and cardiac muscle tissues are affected. Myotonia involves striated muscle and anal sphincter; smooth-muscle involvement has been seen in the gastrointestinal tract, gallbladder, uterus, ureter, and ciliary body of the eye. Endocrine disturbances include testicular tubular atrophy, pituitary dysfunction, and diabetes mellitus associated with peripheral insulin resistance. Baldness and cataracts are common, as is hypogammaglobulinemia. Cataracts are represented as multicolored subcapsular opacities best visualized by slit-lamp examination.

Virtually all affected infants with congenital myotonic dystrophy demonstrate that the mother is the affected parent, despite the fact that the gene is transmitted as an autosomal dominant trait. Numerous complications of pregnancy have been recognized including an increased rate of spontaneous abortion, reduced fetal movements, polyhydramnios, uterine inertia during labor, and postpartum hemorrhage (often associated with retained placental fragments). Neonatal mortality is increased, and affected infants display numerous abnormal features. Neonatal respiratory distress, paralyzed diaphragm, hypotonia, bilateral facial weakness, talipes, and delayed motor and mental retardation are common clinical features. Myotonia is conspicuously absent and is not clinically evident until later in the first decade of life. Congenital hip dislocation and hernias are the result of muscular laxity. Mild mental retardation is evident in most, if not all, affected children, and hydrocephalus has been reported in some instances. The correlation between maternal myotonic dystrophy and the congenital form of the disease is overwhelming but unexplained. An expansion of the CTG triplet repeat at the 3′ end of the gene located on chromosome 19q13.3 is the molecular basis for this disease. Clinical anticipation in successive generations is associated with an increasing number of nucleotide triplet repeats.

Treatment of the various types of myotonia is specifically directed toward their symptoms and the debilitating features of myotonic dystrophy. The myotonia may be relieved with quinine sulfate, procainamide, or phenytoin. Additionally, patients with myotonic muscular dystrophy seldom complain of the myotonia, and treatment of the condition is indicated less frequently. Quinine sulfate and procainamide may be hazardous when given to patients with cardiac conduction disturbances. Patients with the nonprogressive types of myotonia do not have cardiac involvement but are very troubled and disabled by the myotonia.

Patients with myotonic dystrophy need general medical supervision and support. Cardiac conduction disturbances and sensitivity to various anesthetics may be life-threatening.

Medical and rehabilitative intervention, insertion of cardiac pacemakers, treatment of respiratory problems, and the use of various orthotic devices are helpful.

THE PERIODIC PARALYSES

Numerous conditions of diverse etiology may result in periodic paralysis. Often, high or low serum potassium values are associated with this syndrome. The primary periodic paralyses are inherited as an autosomal dominant trait, whereas the secondary disorders result from acquired conditions that perturb body water and electrolyte status or thyroid function. The genetically determined conditions are associated with modest disturbances of potassium homeostasis, in contrast to the nongenetic conditions. Thyrotoxic periodic paralysis resembles hypokalemic periodic paralysis. It is remarkably more common in men (6:1) and Asians (3:1). The condition is sporadic and resolves with effective treatment of the hyperthyroidism.

The primary periodic paralyses are hypokalemic, hyperkalemic, and normokalemic. A fourth (rarer) form of periodic paralysis is associated with a bidirectional ventricular tachycardic dysrhythmia.

The hypokalemic form presents in middle to late childhood. Attacks are accompanied by a modest fall in the serum potassium level and in urinary retention of sodium, potassium, chloride, and water. These electrolyte changes can produce a characteristic ECG change. The attacks may be provoked by the ingestion of carbohydrate or sodium or by excitement. Initially, the attacks are infrequent, but daily attacks may occur during early adulthood. The episodes decrease in frequency in late adulthood, but older patients may have a fixed limb weakness. Glucose-insulin infusion may provoke an attack, and oral potassium salts attenuate the episode. These findings are diagnostic of the condition. Mutations in the calcium channel gene have been associated with hypokalemic periodic paralysis.

The hyperkalemic form is also inherited as an autosomal dominant trait with initial presentation during the first or second decade of life. The serum potassium value rises modestly during the attack, accompanied by a kaliuresis. Some patients have myotonia involving facial, lingual, thenar, or finger extensor muscles; others do not. The presence of myotonia in a subset of patients with hyperkalemic periodic paralysis suggests genetic linkage with paramyotonia congenita. This apparent association will be resolved when the genetic basis of these clinically diverse conditions is understood. Primary hyperkalemic periodic paralysis can be provoked by the oral administration of potassium chloride. Mutations in the sodium channel gene (SCN4A) have been identified in patients with hyperkalemic periodic paralysis.

The normokalemic form is more debatable as a distinct nosologic entity. Again, as with the other primary forms, it is transmitted as an autosomal dominant trait with onset in childhood. It is provoked by potassium loading (in some families but not others), exposure to cold, alcohol, and rest after physical activity. Glucose administration has no effect, but sodium loading may reduce the weakness.

The periodic paralysis associated with cardiac tachycardic dysrhythmias also has some heterogenous elements. It is inherited, possibly as a dominant trait, but the total number of reported cases is only six. Three cases were thought to be hyperkalemic, one normokalemic, and one hypokalemic. Dysmorphic features that have been described include short stature, clinodactyly, microcephaly, midfacial hypoplasia, low-set ears, and cryptorchidism. The cardiac dysrhythmia is potentially fatal. Two affected patients have died suddenly.

The muscle biopsy sample often reveals few or absence of abnormalities in patients with the periodic paralyses during the early symptomatic years, even during a paralytic episode. Later, a distinctive vacuolar myopathy develops. Often, these biopsy changes correlate with fixed limb weakness.

Lack of electrical excitability of muscle fiber surface membranes is common to the various forms of primary periodic paralysis, and an abnormality of the sodium channel characterizes the electrophysiologic study results in patients with paramyotonia congenita and those with hyperkalemic periodic paralysis (in agreement with molecular genetic data). The resting membrane potential, studied *in vitro*, is reduced in patients with primary hypokalemic periodic paralysis and in those with the acquired form associated with thyrotoxicosis. Both insulin and thyroid hormone are known to increase the activity of the sodium-potassium pump, but this information does not facilitate an understanding of the clinical symptomatology associated with modest decreases in serum potassium values.

Treatment begins with accurate diagnosis of the syndrome. Aggravating environmental factors must be avoided to minimize the frequency and intensity of the attacks. Acetazolamide is the preferred drug for both the hypokalemic and hyperkalemic forms of primary periodic paralysis; it may also be useful in the paralysis associated with cardiac dysrhythmias. Treatment of the paralysis, however, may worsen the cardiac disturbance. Imipramine has been useful in one patient in controlling the dysrhythmia. Acetazolamide is ineffective in treating the paralysis associated with hyperthyroidism. Propranolol is helpful, but control of the thyroid disease is more important.

Hereditary Types of Myopathy

MITOCHONDRIAL DISEASES

Defects of mitochondrial metabolism are being recognized with increasing frequency. Morphologic abnormalities of mitochondria have been observed in some patients. Mitochondria were overly abundant, very large, or misshapen. A distinctive abnormality of mitochondria was evident at the light-microscopical level with the modified Gomori trichrome stain, and fibers containing this abnormality were labeled ragged-red. Ragged-red fibers (RRFs) are distinctive and usually represent the morphologic counterpart of suspected or proven biochemical defects that affect the inner mitochondrial membrane. Current information suggests that RRFs are seen in those mitochondrial diseases associated with a defect involving intramitochondrial protein synthesis. The muscle morphology may be normal in patients with other mitochondrial diseases, however, such as carnitine palmitoyl transferase (CPT) deficiency. This fact emphasizes the need for a classification scheme predicated on biochemical and molecular genetic criteria.

The mitochondrial diseases of muscle or brain can be subdivided into five major groups according to the site of the biochemical lesion: defects of mitochondrial transport, defects of substrate use, defects of the Krebs cycle, defects of oxidation-phosphorylation, and defects of the respiratory chain (Table 225-1). A discussion of all of these defects is beyond the scope of this text book (see Oski's Pediatrics, 3rd edition for a complete discussion of each defect).

Primary mitochondrial DNA defects occur sporadically or are inherited as maternal, nonmendelian traits. Maternal inheritance resembles X-linked and autosomal dominant inheritance patterns in that the maternally transmitted trait is passed from affected mothers to their children and the disease appears in consecutive generations. The maternally inherited trait differs from the X-linked inherited trait because both male and female progeny inherit the condition from their mothers. Similarly, the maternally inherited trait differs from the autosomal dominant

TABLE 225-1. Classification of Mitochondrial Diseases

Defects of mitochondrial transport
Adenine nucleotide translocator deficiency
Carnitine deficiency
Carnitine-acylcarnitine translocase defect
Carnitine palmitoyl transferase deficiency
Defects of substrate use
Pyruvate carboxylase deficiency
Biotinidase deficiency
Pyruvate dehydrogenase complex deficiency
Long-chain acyl-CoA dehydrogenase deficiency
Medium-chain acyl-CoA dehydrogenase deficiency
Short-chain acyl-CoA dehydrogenase deficiency
Glutaric aciduria type I
Glutaric aciduria type II (multiple acyl-CoA dehydrogenase deficiency)
Isovaleric acidemia
Defects of the Krebs cycle
Dihydrolipoyl dehydrogenase defect
Fumarase deficiency
Succinate dehydrogenase defect
Alpha-ketoglutarate dehydrogenase complex defect
Defects of oxidation-phosphorylation coupling
Defects of the respiratory chain

trait because a higher percentage (theoretically, 100%) of the progeny are affected. The phenotypic expression of a maternally inherited trait is modulated by replicative segregation and the threshold effect. These two concepts are predicated on the facts that multiple mitochondrial DNA copies are found in each mitochondrion and that hundreds or thousands of mitochondria are found in each cell. As a result, the distribution of wild-type mitochondrial DNA and mutated mitochondrial DNA drifts randomly in each successive cell division. As the percentage of mutated mitochondrial DNA copies approaches a theoretic threshold, the cellular phenotype reflects the genotype and displays energy failure.

Kearns–Sayre syndrome is characterized by three fundamental criteria: pigmentary degeneration of the retina, ophthalmoplegia, and clinical onset before age 20. Often, other signs occur including heart block, cerebellar syndrome, and an elevated cerebrospinal fluid (CSF) protein concentration in excess of 100 mg/dL. RRFs are present in skeletal muscle obtained at biopsy, and sensorineural hearing loss is frequent. Endocrine disturbances are associated with this syndrome, and short stature is a common problem. Diabetes mellitus and hypoparathyroidism may develop and may contribute to fatal episodes of coma or to seizures, respectively. A spongy degeneration is seen without exception in the brain of all patients examined at autopsy. Basal ganglia calcification is observed in all patients with hypoparathyroidism. Folic acid levels are reduced in the CSF, and coenzyme Q10 concentrations in serum and muscle are decreased. Replacement therapy has been proposed on the basis of these observations. A cardiac pacemaker is necessary as therapy for heart block.

Virtually all reported cases of Kearns–Sayre syndrome have been sporadic, and approximately 98% of affected patients have major, single deletions of the mitochondrial genome. Sporadic cases of progressive external ophthalmoplegia have also been associated with these deletions suggesting that this abnormality of ocular motility is the minimal clinical expression of Kearns–Sayre syndrome. Large mitochondrial DNA deletions have also been observed in infants with Pearson syndrome, a frequently fatal sporadic disease of infancy manifested by pancytopenia and pancreatic exocrine dysfunction. In addition, large mitochondrial DNA deletions were recently described in a family with maternally inherited diabetes mellitus and deafness, but later this family was also found to have harbored an mtDNA duplication, which can explain both the origin of the deletion and the maternal inheritance.

Myoclonus epilepsy and RRFs (MERRF) are otherwise known as the *Fukuhara syndrome*. The clinical expression of this disease is dominated by myoclonus, ataxia, limb weakness, and generalized seizures. Most patients have symptoms in childhood or early adolescence. Associated signs often include dementia, optic atrophy, short stature, hearing loss, and proprioceptive sensory loss in the legs.

Although spongy degeneration of the brain is common, neuronal loss is also frequently seen in MERRF, and it preferentially affects the cerebellum, brainstem, and spinal cord. CT scans and magnetic resonance imaging (MRI) reveal brain atrophy. Characteristically, electroencephalography shows paroxysmal epileptiform discharges that are either focal or generalized. Often, the blood and CSF lactate values are increased, but usually the CSF protein level is normal. Endocrine disturbances have been limited to one case of "hypothalamic disorder" and one case of isolated adrenocorticotropic hormone deficiency. Positron emission tomography revealed cerebral and cerebellar hypometabolism in one case.

MERRF is inherited as a maternal trait. Muscle biopsy shows RRFs, which are cytochrome oxidase negative. The mutation associated most commonly with MERRF is in the $tRNA^{Lys}$ gene (A83344G). No effective treatment is available for patients with MERRF, aside from seizure control.

MELAS (mitochondrial myopathy, encephalopathy, lactic acidosis, and stroke-like episodes) has been described in numerous patients. The original criteria included normal early development, short stature, seizures, and sudden onset of hemiparesis, hemianopsia, or cortical blindness. Dementia was prominent in several cases, as was episodic vomiting, headache, and hearing loss. CT scan revealed focal lucencies in several cases and basal ganglia calcifications in some cases. Diffuse spongy degeneration of the brain and focal encephalomalacia were seen at autopsy. Muscle biopsy shows RRFs but, unlike those found in other mtDNA-related disorders, most RRFs in MELAS are cytochrome oxidase–positive; another morphologic peculiarity of MELAS is the mitochondrial proliferation in the walls of blood vessels. Marked deficiency of the reduced form of nicotinamide-adenine dinucleotide (NADH)–cytochrome *c* reductase (complex I) has been reported in approximately 35% of affected individuals. MELAS is inherited as a maternal trait, and approximately 80% of patients fulfilling the clinical criteria for this condition have a mutation in the $tRNA^{Leu(UUR)}$ gene of mtDNA (*A3243G*). Several other mutations, both in tRNA genes and in protein-encoding genes, have been associated with MELAS. Coenzyme Q10 is beneficial in treatment, and vigorous attempts should be made to control seizure activity.

Several other conditions with mitochondrial DNA point mutations have been described. Leber hereditary optic neuropathy, a maternally inherited condition, is associated with three "primary" mutations, all of them in genes encoding complex I subunits: G3460A in ND1; G11778A in ND4; and T14484C in ND6. Approximately ten additional point mutations in complex I genes ("secondary mutations") put affected patients at increased risk of developing Leber hereditary optic neuropathy. A maternally inherited condition associated with NARP (neuropathy, ataxia, and retinitis pigmentosa) and with developmental delay has been linked with a mtDNA point mutation—T8993G—affecting subunit 6 of adenosine triphosphate synthase (ATPase, complex V). Patients with an abundance of this point mutation are seen in early infancy with maternally inherited Leigh syndrome. Other mutations in the ATPase 6 have been associated with Leigh syndrome or bilateral striatal necrosis. By 1998, more than 50 point pathogenic mutations in mtDNA had been reported reflecting the explosive pace of discoveries in this area.

CHAPTER 226

Phakomatoses and Other Neurocutaneous Syndromes

Adapted from Sharon E. Plon
and Vincent M. Riccardi

NEUROFIBROMATOSIS TYPE 1 (VON RECKLINGHAUSEN DISEASE)

NF-1 occurs with a frequency of approximately 1 in 2,500 to 4,000 persons. It is passed on as an autosomal dominant trait; however, approximately one-half of the index cases represent new mutations, so that a negative family history is common in the pediatric setting. The disorder is essentially the same whether it is inherited or results from a new mutation. NF-1 is highly variable in its expression from one family to another, from one person to another within a given family, and from one body part to another within a given person. Its penetrance (i.e., the likelihood that the mutant gene will express itself if it is present) is close to 100%. The gene mutated in NF-1 resides on the proximal long arm of chromosome 17, specifically in band 17q11.2, and has been isolated. Molecular testing for mutations associated with NF-1 is currently available and can aid in genetic counseling of families.

Features

Café au lait spots are the hallmark of NF-1. They are almost always present in patients with segmental NF and do not cross the body's midline. They are variably seen in patients with NF-2. In patients with NF-1, the hyperpigmented macules are usually larger than 15 mm in diameter and have sharply defined edges and a uniform intensity of coloration (Fig. 226-1). Café au lait spots often develop during the first year of life and increase in number during the first few years of life. The pattern of café au lait spots then stabilizes. Café au lait spots are different from freckling, which in NF-1 is most likely to occur in regions of skin apposition, particularly the axilla.

Neurofibromas are of four types: cutaneous, subcutaneous, nodular plexiform, and diffuse plexiform. Cutaneous neurofibromas are the most common variety, eventually occurring in virtually all patients with NF-1. Often, they do not appear until just before puberty or coincident with it. They are present in highest density over the trunk (Fig. 226-2). Subcutaneous neurofibromas usually become apparent toward the end of the first decade of life or in early adulthood, and they may be painful or tender. Nodular plexiform neurofibromas are complex clusters of subcutaneous-like neurofibromas along proximal nerve roots and major nerves. With continued growth along the spinal column, they often lead to spinal erosion and, eventually, spinal cord compression. Diffuse plexiform neurofibromas with or without overlying hyperpigmentation are congenital lesions that tend to enlarge steadily with age, at times perniciously (Fig. 226-3). Both diffuse and nodular plexiform lesions can result in significant morbidity.

Lisch nodules are relatively specific for NF-1. These lesions of the iris are found in less than 10% of patients with NF-1 who are younger than 6 years, but various investigators report their frequency to range from 90% to 100% in patients who are older than 10 years. If large in size or number, they may be easy to see with an ordinary ophthalmoscope, but ruling out their presence

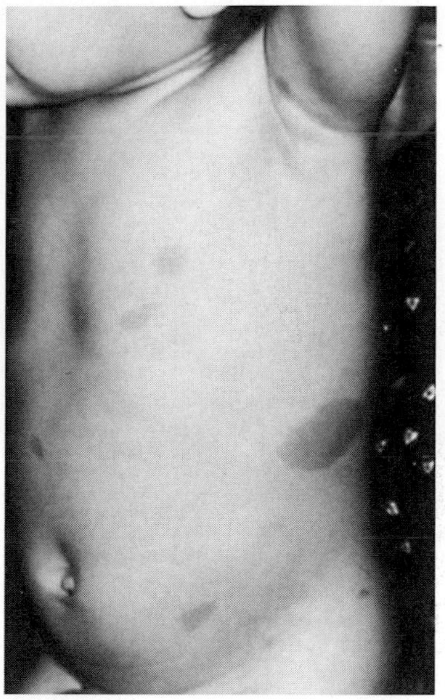

Figure 226-1. In patients with neurofibromatosis type 1, café au lait spots are usually larger than 15 mm in diameter, the edges are usually sharply defined, and the intensity of the coloration is uniform.

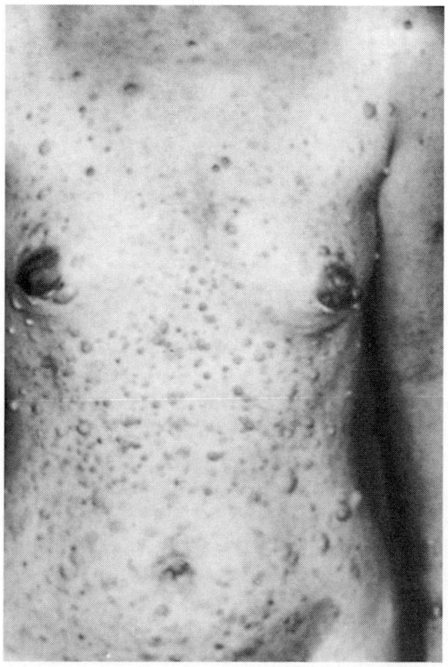

Figure 226-2. Cutaneous neurofibromas are not often apparent until puberty and are present in highest density over the trunk.

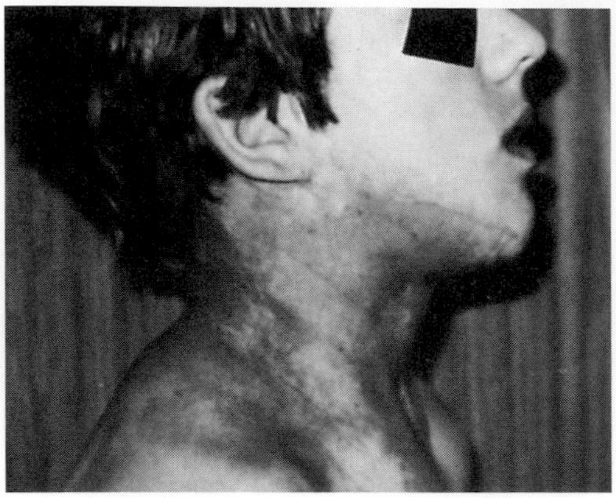

Figure 226-3. Plexiform neurofibromas with or without overlying hyperpigmentation are congenital lesions that tend to enlarge steadily with age.

requires careful slit-lamp examination by an ophthalmologist who is familiar with these lesions. Examination of parents for the presence of Lisch nodules can be very useful in determining whether an affected child carries a new mutation or inherited it from an affected parent.

Optic pathway gliomas are characteristic of NF-1 occurring in 15% of patients with this disorder. In approximately 5% of children with NF, these lesions result in morbidity including blindness. However, given the variable natural history of these lesions and the controversy concerning appropriate treatment, no consensus with regard to recommendations for routine neuroimaging to detect these lesions presymptomatically has been established. In addition to optic gliomas, children with NF-1 are at increased risk for other central nervous system (CNS) neoplasms.

Learning disabilities, distinct from mental retardation, are present in 40% to 60% of children with NF-1. These disabilities may be foreshadowed by infantile muscular hypotonia or a delay in attaining developmental milestones but, in any event, they are usually apparent by the time the child begins the first grade of school. Mental retardation occurs in approximately 8% of patients with NF-1, but its presence should not be presumed to be the result of NF-1 until an investigation for other causes has been completed and found to be negative or unrevealing. Mental retardation and dysmorphic features are found with children who have a large deletion encompassing the whole NF-1 gene. Speech impediments may involve articulation or language elements and are usually obvious by 3 years of age.

Pseudarthrosis, or bowing of the tibia, may occur as an independent lesion, but it is often one of the characteristic congenital lesions of NF-1. The congenital nature of the pseudarthrosis may be masked by a delay in diagnosis until weight bearing or walking is attempted. Any child with tibial pseudarthrosis should be presumed to have NF-1 until proven otherwise. The scoliosis that is typical of NF-1 usually involves the cervical and upper thoracic spine and has an anterior angulation (kyphosis). It frequently becomes apparent between 6 and 10 years of age. Renovascular hypertension is one of the clinical problems of NF-1 that can be anticipated and treated effectively. All individuals who have NF-1 are at risk for the disorder and must receive regular blood pressure monitoring, regardless of their age, although adolescents and pregnant women are most likely to be affected. Pheochromocytoma is another source of systemic hypertension, both intermittent and sustained, that is important because it is one of the preventable causes of untimely death among patients with NF-1.

Neurofibrosarcoma probably has an overall frequency of less than 5% among patients with NF-1. Although the magnitude of this risk may be small, the relative risk is at least two orders of magnitude above that of the general population. Thus, a neurofibrosarcoma must be ruled out in a child with a history suggestive of such a lesion (i.e., pain, a rapidly enlarging tumor, or an otherwise unexplained neurologic deficit).

Several other common medical conditions show an increased frequency in NF-1. One of these is puberty disturbance. More important, premature or delayed puberty may indicate the presence of a chiasmal or hypothalamic glioma, which may be amenable to treatment. Short stature is seen in at least 16% of patients with NF-1. Macrocephaly is also present in 16% or more of affected patients. This finding is not always apparent in infancy and is not correlated with any known functional compromise. Although pruritus occurs in only approximately 10% of patients with NF-1, pruritus associated with an actively growing neurofibroma may indicate that the lesion warrants close observation.

Diagnosis

The diagnostic criteria for NF-1 are met in an individual if two or more of the following are found: six or more café au lait spots larger than 5 mm in greatest diameter in prepubertal individuals and larger than 15 mm in greatest diameter in postpubertal individuals; two or more neurofibromas of any type, or one plexiform neurofibroma; freckling in the axillary or inguinal regions; optic pathway glioma; two or more iris Lisch nodules; a distinctive osseous lesion such as sphenoid wing dysplasia or thinning of long-bone cortex with or without pseudarthrosis; and a first-degree relative (parent, sibling, or offspring) with NF-1 diagnosed by the above criteria.

Screening and Follow-Up

The current recommendation is that children suspected of having NF-1 be evaluated in a multidisciplinary NF clinic. Such a clinic normally includes specialists from the following disciplines: genetics, neurology, dermatology, neurosurgery, and plastic surgery. The first purpose of a screening evaluation is to confirm the diagnosis of NF-1 by identifying features of the disease that are not apparent from the history and general physical examination. The second goal of clinic care is to detect potentially compromising lesions before they become symptomatic, thereby minimizing the ultimate severity of the symptoms (e.g., identifying an optic pathway glioma before it causes irreversible blindness). At the initial visit, a full family history is taken and the genetics of NF including potential recurrence risk in other offspring is explained to the parents.

In addition to a full physical, dermatologic, and neurologic examination, additional evaluation includes a slit-lamp ocular examination to identify Lisch nodules, choroidal hamartomas, hypertrophied corneal nerves, and, perhaps, signs of an optic pathway glioma. As previously mentioned, the use of neuroimaging for asymptomatic children with NF-1 is controversial. However, many clinicians who follow children with NF-1 continue to perform neuroimaging on patients younger than 3 years to look for optic pathway tumors. Intelligence quotient determination and psychologic evaluation are useful to identify learning disabilities so that special efforts can be initiated on behalf of the youngster in school. If the results of a detailed history, physical examination, and presymptomatic screening fail to reveal any potentially serious problems, annual routine follow-up visits are recommended.

Treatment

Medical therapy for problems arising from NF-1 is similar to that used for the same conditions when they occur in the absence of NF-1. Problems associated with NF-1 that are most likely to require medical treatment include seizures, headaches, hyperactivity and learning disabilities, anxiety, and renovascular hypertension. The use of oral contraceptives is not absolutely contraindicated in patients with NF-1, although evaluation on an individual basis is obviously appropriate. Antineoplastic chemotherapy has no role in the treatment of neurofibromas. Its role in the treatment of optic pathway gliomas is still investigational, and its use in the treatment of neurofibrosarcomas is problematic. Radiotherapy for neurofibromas has no proven effect. It appears to be useful in the treatment of at least some optic pathway gliomas, although this therapy is controversial.

Surgery is the mainstay of therapy for patients with NF-1, particularly for removing or debulking tumors (e.g., neurofibromas, neurofibrosarcomas, pheochromocytomas), for treating skeletal dysplasia (e.g., tibial pseudarthrosis, sphenoid wing dysplasia), for correcting scoliosis or kyphoscoliosis, and for treating at least some individuals with renovascular or other types of vascular compromise. In general, the surgical removal of neurofibromas is associated with suboptimal results; the tumors tend to recur, and the possibility of a consequent neuropathy is significant. Surgical removal of a neurofibroma should be undertaken only if a specific major goal can be established beforehand.

NEUROFIBROMATOSIS TYPE 2 (BILATERAL ACOUSTIC NEUROFIBROMATOSIS)

Features

The definitive feature of NF-2 is the presence of bilateral acoustic neuromas, which are actually vestibular schwannomas. Intracranial and spinal cord meningiomas also frequently occur, as do spinal cord astrocytomas. Paraspinal schwannomas and neurofibromas are common at all levels, but particularly in the cervical and lumbar regions. Cutaneous and subcutaneous neurofibromas are generally few in number and infrequently present. Cutaneous schwannomas are relatively common, even in early childhood; they may have the same coloration as the skin or be slightly hyperpigmented with or without associated hypertrichosis. Their size ranges from 3 to 8 mm. Café au lait spots are few in number and relatively pale in color, and they tend to be somewhat less clearly demarcated and larger in size than those that are typical of NF-1. Posterior subcapsular cataracts are consistently present, even at a young age. Retinal hamartomas are another feature of NF-2. Both the cataracts and the retinal hamartomas may be particularly useful features for delineating the diagnosis of NF-2 in a child. This disease is distinct from NF-1; in particular, optic pathway gliomas, Lisch nodules, and plexiform neurofibromas are not features of NF-2.

Diagnosis

In contrast to the diagnosis of NF-1, the diagnosis of NF-2 may be difficult to establish in children. The inclusive diagnostic criteria for NF-2 are the following: bilateral eighth cranial nerve masses seen with neuroimaging studies [computed tomography (CT) or, preferably, magnetic resonance imaging (MRI)]; or a first-degree relative with NF-2 and either a unilateral eighth cranial nerve mass or two of the following: neurofibroma, meningioma, spinal astrocytoma, schwannoma, and posterior subcapsular cataracts. Often, the condition is asymptomatic through the first 15 years of life, although the cutaneous schwannomas, cataracts, and retinal hamartomas may be detectable during this period. The most frequent symptoms include headaches, hearing loss, and tinnitus, which are most often unilateral in the earliest stages of the disease. Once symptoms appear, however, progression is generally constant and relatively gradual, although rapid deterioration occasionally occurs. The progression of symptoms results from the appearance and growth of the various CNS tumors. Pregnancy or, in some cases, the use of oral contraceptives leads to the onset of symptoms from meningiomas, acoustic neuromas, or both. Recognition of the disorder usually results from the development of symptoms from a CNS tumor or the presence of an affected first-degree relative. Occasionally, the detection of a paraspinal neurofibroma or schwannoma may lead to the correct diagnosis.

Treatment

Surgery for the removal or debulking of intracranial, spinal, or paraspinal tumors is the mainstay of therapy for patients with NF-2. The consequences of surgical removal of an acoustic neuroma may include further hearing loss and ipsilateral facial nerve palsy, although efforts are being made to use operative strategies that preserve hearing and facial nerve function. In addition, stereotactic radiation has been used with arguable success. Brainstem implants to restore some degree of hearing have been helpful for some patients. Because some acoustic neuromas have few or minor associated symptoms, even when they are quite large, the size of the tumor alone should not be used to time surgery. Women with NF-2 should be advised that pregnancy would almost certainly make the condition worse. Unlike in patients with NF-1, oral contraceptive use is generally contraindicated in individuals with NF-2 because it may seriously aggravate the growth and symptoms of the intracranial tumors. Severe disorientation may occur when patients are diving or swimming underwater, and drowning may result. All individuals who have or are at risk for NF-2 should be advised of this risk and should be cautioned never to swim alone.

TUBEROUS SCLEROSIS

Tuberous sclerosis (TS) is characterized by depigmented lesions of the skin, tumors of the CNS, and ocular hamartomas; it shows an autosomal dominant pattern of inheritance. Because it combines developmental abnormalities of the skin, nervous system, and eyes, this disorder has traditionally been grouped with the neurofibromatoses and von Hippel–Lindau disease (VHL) in the category known as the *phakomatoses*.

Diagnosis

When multiple features of TS are present, the diagnosis is relatively easy to make. When only one feature is present, the diagnosis is likely to be considered only tentatively, if not overlooked entirely. Establishing the diagnosis of TS depends on detecting the presence of two or more of the following features:

- *Skin:* hypopigmented macules usually elliptic in shape (ash-leaf spots); fibroadenomas (adenoma sebaceum, shown in Fig. 226-4), typically involving the malar regions of the face; periungual fibromas; shagreen patches, most commonly seen over the lower trunk; and a distinctive brown patch on the forehead. The latter lesion is especially important, as it may be the first and most readily recognizable feature of TS to be

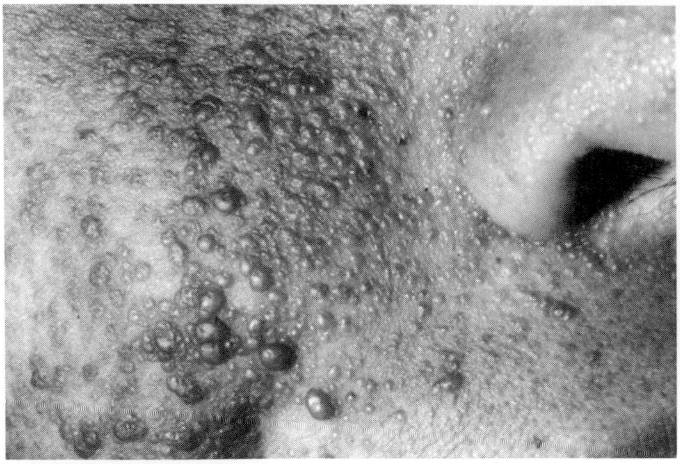

Figure 226-4. Fibroadenomas (adenoma sebaceum) in a child with tuberous sclerosis at age 7.

appreciated on physical examination of neonates and infants with the disorder.

- *Teeth:* characteristic pits of the enamel.
- *Eyes:* choroidal hamartomas; hypopigmented defects of the iris.
- *CNS:* periventricular tubers; cerebral astrocytomas; sacrococcygeal chordomas; nonspecific electroencephalographic (EEG) abnormalities including hypsarrhythmia.
- Cardiovascular system: cardiac rhabdomyomas; aortic and major artery constrictions.
- *Kidneys:* renal angiomyolipomas.
- *Lungs:* diffuse interstitial fibrosis.

Seizures of all types, but particularly myoclonic jerks, associated with hypsarrhythmia, and mental retardation are the most common symptoms leading to the consideration of the diagnosis of TS. MRI scans of the brain in patients with TS are virtually diagnostic and should be obtained for all individuals suspected of having the disorder. Heart failure or a cardiac murmur may indicate the presence of a cardiac rhabdomyoma, and deficient circulation or decreased pulses may indicate the presence of arterial tree involvement. Renal failure or an abdominal mass may lead to the recognition of hamartomatous kidney involvement. Dyspnea may indicate the presence of pulmonary involvement, but this anatomic feature of TS is often found coincidentally.

Treatment

No medical treatment is available for TS itself. The medical treatment used for seizures and other complications (e.g., heart failure, renal failure) is the same as if TS were not present, unless surgery on the primary lesions is indicated. For example, surgical removal of a cardiac rhabdomyoma may be warranted, and some clinicians encourage an aggressive surgical approach to the renal angiomyolipomas, at least in advanced cases.

VON HIPPEL–LINDAU DISEASE

VHL is traditionally grouped with the neurofibromatoses and TS as a phakomatosis because of the direct involvement of the CNS, vascular abnormalities, diffuse cystic changes in multiple organs, and malignant tumors of the kidney that characterize the disease. It, too, is an autosomal dominant, heritable condition and is due to mutations in the VHL gene on chromosome 3.

Diagnosis

The diagnostically distinctive feature of VHL is retinal vascular hamartoma. When retinal vascular hamartomas are found, the presence of other features of the disorder add credence to the diagnosis. In the absence of retinal vascular hamartomas, establishing the diagnosis requires detecting a combination of the other features or detecting one of the other features plus identifying an affected first-degree relative.

Retinal vascular hamartomas may be associated with visual disturbances and glaucoma; they can often be appreciated by direct ophthalmoscopy. Usually, but not always, they are unilateral. CNS vascular hamartomas (cerebellar hemangioblastomas) similar to those seen in the eye are another key feature of the disorder. Other characteristic tumors include renal cell carcinoma, pheochromocytoma, epididymal cystadenoma, and pancreatic cysts. Diffuse cystic lesions throughout the kidneys may accompany the renal cell carcinomas. Other tumors may include oat cell carcinoma of the lung, pancreatic carcinoma, and hepatocellular carcinoma. Each of these features may be seen independently of VHL.

Treatment

The hallmark of treatment is careful surveillance by imaging of brain and abdomen, as well as yearly ophthalmologic examination. All patients with VHL should be carefully followed in a center familiar with the multiple complications of this disorder. Medical treatment of VHL is the same as that generally recommended for pheochromocytomas, renal cell carcinomas, or other tumors. The knowledge that the patient is at increased risk for recurrent or ipsilateral renal cell carcinoma influences the surgeon toward kidney-sparing surgery. The treatment approach to the vascular hamartomas is complex and must be tailored to the individual lesions.

Surgical removal of renal cell carcinomas and pheochromocytomas is the preferred treatment. Unlike in TS, a surgically conservative approach to the treatment of renal cysts is usually advised. The use of laser technology to treat the ocular angiomatosis has some merit and should be considered as one therapeutic approach.

STURGE–WEBER DISEASE

Sturge–Weber disease (SWD) is also called *encephalofacial angiomatosis* and is traditionally known as the "fourth phakomatosis." It differs from the neurofibromatoses, TS, and VHL by virtue of the absence of three features: cutaneous pigmentation defects, a clear excess of tumors, and heritability. In addition, the relatively large number of variant or atypical cases renders accurate comparisons difficult.

Features

In addition to a facial port wine stain and intracranial angiomatosis, primary involvement of the anterior chamber of the eye, specifically the trabecular network, and Schlemm canal may lead to glaucoma (in either eye) in as many as 30% of patients with SWD. Macrocephaly and cutaneous xanthogranulomas may also be seen. No one feature is uniformly associated with any other, and histopathologic features cannot establish a diagnosis beyond confirming the type of lesion.

Diagnosis

The diagnosis of SWD depends on the presence of a port wine stain (nevus flammeus) on the face, primarily in the first division of the trigeminal nerve; leptomeningeal angiomatosis (including angiomatous involvement of the choroid plexus or choroid of the eye); or both.

Treatment

No medical treatment is available for SWD, and the role of surgical treatment has yet to be defined. The use of lasers to treat the facial and ocular angioma lesions has been, at least, partially successful.

ALBRIGHT SYNDROME

Albright syndrome (AS) is also known as Albright–McCune–Sternberg syndrome or polyostotic fibrous dysplasia. The cardinal features of the disorder are fibrous dysplasia of one or more bones, precocious puberty, and café au lait spots. Although some features of AS overlap with those of one or more of the neurofibromatoses (e.g., café au lait spots), the diseases rarely present a diagnostic dilemma. AS is due to mutations in specific G protein subunits that regulate signal transduction from membrane receptors.

Features

The fibrous dysplasia of AS may involve any bone, but the most frequent sites are the femur, tibia, pelvis, phalanges, ribs, and humerus. Radiography reveals a combination of radiolucent and radiopaque elements, except at the base of the skull, where diffuse sclerosis is usually seen. Precocious puberty or sexual precocity, as it relates to this disorder more accurately, is termed pseudoprecocious puberty; that is, blood levels of sex steroids are elevated, but levels of gonadotrophic hormones are normal. Early spermatogenesis and fertility can accompany these endocrine changes. Café au lait spots, when they are present, are usually fewer in number and larger in size than those seen in patients with NF (particularly NF-1). Hyperthyroidism may be seen in 30% or so of patients with AS. Other features including acromegaly and elevated levels of growth hormone in the blood, intramuscular myxomas, hyperplastic reticuloendothelial tissues, and lymphoid or myeloid metaplasia have also been reported, although much less frequently.

Treatment

Treatment of the premature puberty is best carried out under the auspices of a specialized pediatric endocrinology center. Bone grafting and subsequent surgical procedures to correct deformities may be indicated depending on the extent and complications of the lesions. Close observation of the fibrous dysplasia lesions for malignant degeneration is warranted.

CHAPTER 227

Diseases of the Neuromuscular Junction

Adapted from Julie Thorne Parke

Numerous different conditions may interfere with the transmission of the electrical impulse across neuromuscular junctions, which consist of the terminal portion of a motor nerve, the synaptic cleft, and the end-plate region of a muscle. Neuromuscular transmission can fail if insufficient acetylcholine is released (presynaptic process) or if the number of acetylcholine receptors is insufficient to interact with the acetylcholine (postsynaptic disorder). Neuromuscular transmission failure may also occur when inhibition of or a deficiency in acetylcholinesterase occurs causing a depolarization block (Table 227-1).

JUVENILE MYASTHENIA GRAVIS

Clinical Characteristics

The juvenile and adult forms of myasthenia gravis are autoimmune disorders characterized by an autoimmune attack on the acetylcholine receptor. Circulating antibodies to the acetylcholine receptor bind to the receptor on the muscle end plate blocking its function. Usually, the onset of juvenile myasthenia gravis occurs after age 10, although it can appear much earlier. Girls are affected more commonly than boys. The cardinal feature of the disease is easy fatigability. Usually, the onset is gradual with symptoms most apparent in the afternoon or evening when the patient is tired. Occasionally, the onset is fairly sudden and may appear to have been precipitated by an infectious illness. Characteristically, the weakness abates with rest and worsens with sustained effort. In approximately one-half of patients, weakness first appears in the ocular muscles causing ptosis or diplopia (Fig. 227-1). Frequently, ptosis is asymmetric and may be unilateral. It tends to fluctuate during the day and to vary from day to day. Involvement of the ocular muscles is variable, but it may be severe causing a total ophthalmoplegia. Approximately one-fourth of affected patients have weakness of the

TABLE 227-1. Disorders of Neuromuscular Transmission

Presynaptic
Botulism
Eaton-Lambert syndrome
Hypermagnesemia
Hypocalcemia
Snake bite
Antibiotics
Congenital myasthenia gravis
? Tick paralysis
Inhibition or deficiency of acetylcholinesterase
Organophosphates
Congenital myasthenia gravis
Postsynaptic
Autoimmune myasthenia gravis
Curare (D-tubocurarine)
alpha-Bungarotoxin
Congenital myasthenia gravis

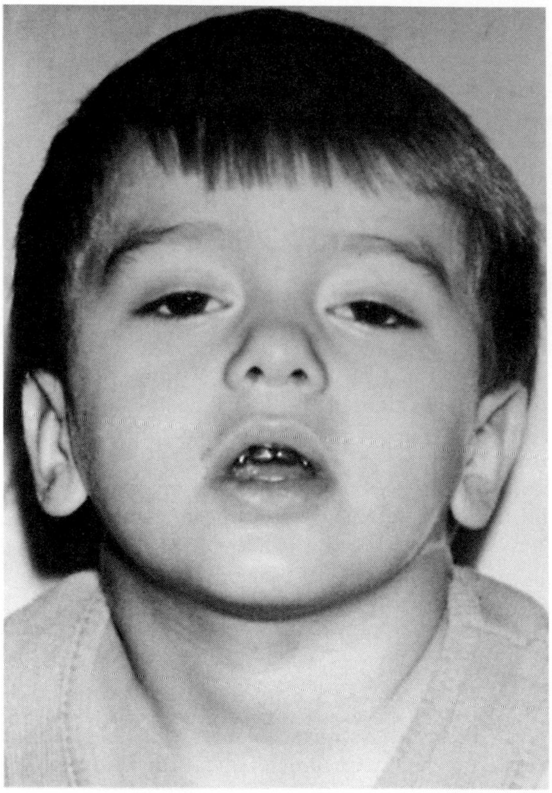

Figure 227-1. Four-year-old child with juvenile myasthenia gravis exhibiting fluctuating ptosis and bilateral facial weakness.

bulbar musculature resulting in difficulties in speaking, swallowing, or chewing. The facial muscles are involved in most affected patients. Weakness of the palate and tongue may render speech unintelligible. Affected children's voices may be strong initially becoming softer and less distinct during continued conversation. Difficulty chewing food is a common problem, and many patients support their jaw in one hand to assist with chewing. Swallowing difficulties and choking spells may occur. Weakness of the muscles of the neck, particularly the neck extensors, causes the head to fall forward. Patients with predominantly bulbar symptoms are at risk of developing respiratory failure, particularly during an intercurrent infection.

A smaller number of children (approximately 20%) have generalized weakness of the extremities. Fatigability may be demonstrated in younger children by having them climb stairs or hold their arms outstretched for an interval. In older children, repetitive testing of deltoid strength or performance of multiple deep knee bends may help to disclose the weakness. Regardless of the distribution of weakness, the principal features are a fluctuating quality in the weakness and a susceptibility to fatigue. These features differ from those of other neuromuscular disorders, which produce relatively constant symptoms.

Diagnostic Studies

Usually, the diagnosis of myasthenia gravis can be made on the basis of the history and physical examination, and it may be confirmed by pharmacologic tests. A small dose of an anticholinesterase drug produces a dramatic improvement in strength. Edrophonium chloride (Tensilon) is preferred because of its rapid onset and short duration of action. The availability of acetylcholine is increased by inhibiting the enzyme cholinesterase, thereby improving neuromuscular transmission. A placebo injection of normal saline should be given before the edrophonium. A test dose of one-tenth of the total dose is given initially. If no complications occur with the test dose, the remainder of the full dosage of 0.2 mg/kg (maximum dosage, 10 mg) is given intravenously. Affected patients' heart rate and blood pressure must be monitored throughout the test, and atropine sulfate should be immediately available because a cholinergic crisis occasionally occurs manifest by extreme bradycardia or transient respiratory weakness requiring ventilatory support. Usually, a marked but short-lived improvement in weakness is seen in patients with myasthenia. Neostigmine may be used if a longer effect is necessary to evaluate limb strength.

Electrophysiologic studies are helpful in documenting transmission failure at neuromuscular junctions. Antibodies to the human muscle acetylcholine receptor are found in the serum of as many as 90% of patients. However, the patients with negative antibody test results are typically those with purely ocular weakness or mild generalized weakness in whom the diagnosis is uncertain. A negative test result does not exclude the diagnosis.

Treatment and Prognosis

Numerous different therapeutic modalities are available for treating myasthenia gravis. The selected approach should consider the age of affected patients, the severity of the disease, and the potential benefits and risks of each form of therapy. Cholinesterase inhibitors improve neuromuscular transmission by inhibiting the enzymatic degradation of acetylcholine prolonging its effect on muscle end plates. These agents result in symptomatic improvement in strength in most patients with myasthenia gravis and may be sufficient to produce normal or near-normal strength in some. Pyridostigmine bromide (Mestinon) and neostigmine bromide (Prostigmin) are the agents most commonly used (Table 227-2). The dosage of cholinesterase inhibitor used and the dosing interval must be carefully adjusted on the basis of close clinical observation. The dosage required by given individuals may vary during the day and from one day to the next. A cholinergic crisis may result from excessive anticholinesterase dosing as a result of the accumulation of acetylcholine at neuromuscular junctions (Table 227-3).

TABLE 227-2. Cholinesterase Inhibitors in the Treatment of Myasthenia Gravis

	Equivalent doses			Starting oral doses		
Drug	***Oral***	***IM***	***IV***	***Infant***	***Older child***	***Adult***
Pyridostigmine bromide (Mestinon)	60	2	0.7	4–10 mg every 4 hr	30 mg every 4 hr	60 mg every 4 hr
Neostigmine bromide (Prostigmin)	15	—	—	1–2 mg every 4 hr	7.5–10.0 mg every 4 hr	15 mg every 4 hr
Neostigmine methylsulfate	—	0.5	0.5	—	—	—

TABLE 227-3. Side Effects of Cholinesterase Inhibitors

Muscarinic
Abdominal cramps
Diarrhea
Nausea
Vomiting
Increased salivation
Increased bronchial secretions
Irritability
Anxiety
Sleep disturbances
Coma
Seizures
Nicotinic
Muscle fasciculations
Muscle weakness

Clinicians may have difficulty in distinguishing between an overdose of anticholinesterase medications (producing weakness in respiratory muscles) and respiratory distress from myasthenic crisis (causing respiratory insufficiency). Close monitoring of affected patients' muscle strength, pulmonary function, and ability to adequately cough is critical during these periods. Elective intubation and ventilatory support should be instituted before respiratory insufficiency occurs.

Other treatment modalities including thymectomy, corticosteroid therapy, and immunosuppressive agents are aimed more directly at the basic immunologic mechanism of the disease. Corticosteroid therapy given on an alternate-day schedule is effective in many patients who have an incomplete response to anticholinesterase drugs. However, the complications of corticosteroid therapy in young children may make its long-term use unsatisfactory. The importance of the thymus gland in myasthenia gravis has long been recognized, and thymectomy has been accepted as a successful method of treatment. The beneficial effects of thymectomy are not fully understood, but likely the thymus sensitizes lymphocytes to form antibodies directed at the acetylcholine receptors in the postsynaptic membrane. Total removal of the thymus gland is essential for maximal benefit. Often, the postoperative care of affected children is complex, and careful monitoring and observation in an intensive care setting are required. The efficacy of thymectomy appears to be greatest in patients with primarily bulbar symptoms. It is less effective and not generally recommended for patients with solely ocular symptoms. Plasmapheresis has been used as an intensive, short-term intervention in patients with myasthenia. It is helpful in patients who have had a short-term exacerbation of weakness during myasthenic crisis or after a thymectomy. It is also used to produce rapid improvement in strength in preparation for thymectomy.

The prognosis for patients with juvenile myasthenia gravis is relatively good, in that complete or partial remissions occur in 25% within 2 years of disease onset. Often, however, the disease is characterized by a fluctuating course of remissions and exacerbations. The severity of symptoms varies, and some children have severe disease necessitating frequent hospitalizations and mechanical ventilatory support. Approximately 80% of children improve after thymectomy.

TRANSIENT NEONATAL MYASTHENIA GRAVIS

The syndrome of transient neonatal myasthenia gravis is found in infants born of mothers with myasthenia gravis. The disease is caused by the transplacental passage of the IgG acetylcholine receptor antibodies and occurs in approximately 15% of the newborn children of affected mothers. Usually, symptoms appear in the first few hours after birth, although the onset may be delayed for several days. Initial symptoms include hypotonia, diffuse muscle weakness, respiratory distress, and feeding difficulties. Ptosis or ocular motility problems may occur. Usually, symptoms last for several weeks, but they may persist for several months. The affected children fully recover and have an incidence of the later onset of myasthenia gravis no greater than that in the general population. The severity of an affected mother's illness is not correlated with the occurrence or severity of her infant's myasthenia. The diagnosis of neonatal myasthenia can be made by performing repetitive nerve stimulation studies, documenting the presence of circulating antibody to acetylcholine receptors, and evaluating the response to short-acting anticholinesterase medication. Supportive care and anticholinesterase agents are necessary in approximately 80% of patients.

CONGENITAL MYASTHENIA GRAVIS

Several rare varieties of congenital myasthenia gravis exist exhibiting onset at birth or in early childhood and persistent symptoms. Usually, the disorders are familial, and most are inherited through an autosomal recessive mechanism, with the exception of the dominantly inherited slow-channel syndrome. Congenital myasthenia gravis differs from acquired myasthenia gravis by lack of evidence of an autoimmune etiology. Detailed physiologic and morphologic studies have identified specific abnormalities in neuromuscular junctions in patients with several of the syndromes (Table 227-4). Similar to other disorders of neuromuscular transmission, the syndromes are characterized by fluctuating

TABLE 227-4. Distinguishing Features of Congenital Myasthenic Syndromes

Features	Defect in ACh synthesis or mobilization	End-plate AChE deficiency	Slow-channel syndrome	End-plate AChR deficiency
Inheritance	Recessive	Recessive	Dominant	Recessive
Abnormal fatigability	+	+	+	+
Reduced muscle bulk	−	+	+	Occasionally +
Hyporeflexia	−	+	±	−
Age at onset of symptoms	At birth	At birth	Variable	At birth
Response to anticholinesterase drugs	+	−	±	+
Circulating AChR antibodies	−	−	−	−

ACh, acetylcholine; AChE, acetylcholinesterase; AChR, acetylcholine receptor.
Adapted from Engel A. Myasthenia gravis and myasthenic syndromes. *Ann Neurol* 1984;16:519.

weakness. Because of their heterogenous pathophysiology, the clinical manifestations of these syndromes vary. Recurrent episodes of apnea may occur. Severe ocular muscle weakness is characteristic of several of the syndromes. Bulbar or respiratory involvement may be accentuated by crying or prolonged activity. Motor milestones may be delayed. Progression of symptoms may occur during adolescence; in some cases, presentation may not occur until adolescence or early adult life. Patients with these disorders do not respond to immunosuppressive therapy or to thymectomy. The response to acetylcholinesterase inhibitors varies. The slow-channel syndrome and acetylcholinesterase deficiency syndrome may be worsened by acetylcholinesterase inhibitors.

BOTULISM

Pathophysiology

The exotoxin of *Clostridium botulinum* is one of the most potent neurotoxins known. It is absorbed from the intestine or an infected wound and is distributed in a hematogenous manner to peripheral cholinergic nerve synapses such as neuromuscular junctions. The toxin irreversibly blocks acetylcholine release from the presynaptic nerve terminals. Recovery occurs by sprouting of terminal motor neurons and the formation of new motor end plates.

In children and adults, poisoning may occur after ingestion of the toxin in inadequately cooked or improperly canned food. The anaerobic bacillus and the exotoxin it produces are destroyed by heat, so proper cooking of food should eliminate outbreaks. At high altitudes, where water boils at a lower temperature, the exotoxin is not destroyed during boiling accounting for the greater frequency of botulism in mountain locales. The majority of outbreaks of botulism can be traced to home-canned foods, particularly vegetables, fruits, fish, and condiments. Wound botulism results from infection of traumatized tissue by the organism with subsequent toxin production. Most cases occur subsequent to wounds sustained in open fields or on farms, particularly compound extremity fractures.

A third type of botulism, infant botulism, differs from food-borne and wound botulism because it is caused by ingestion of the spores of *C. botulinum* rather than by the exotoxin. It occurs almost exclusively in children in the first year of life, usually in those between ages 5 and 12 weeks. The ingested spores colonize the intestinal tract and produce the *C. botulinum* toxin. Frequently, the source of the spores is not found. Honey has been implicated as the source in approximately 20% of patients, and environmental sources such as yard soil have been implicated in other cases.

Seven antigenically distinct types of *C. botulinum* toxin have been identified. Disease in humans is primarily caused by toxin types A, B, E, and F. Almost always, type E botulism can be traced to fish and fish products. Almost all cases of infant botulism have been caused by toxin types A or B.

Clinical Characteristics

Clinical symptoms appear within 1 to 2 days after the consumption of contaminated food or within 1 to 2 weeks after wound inoculation. The initial symptoms of food-borne infection may resemble those of food poisoning: vomiting, diarrhea, and abdominal pain. Commonly, similar symptoms develop in several members of a family. Weakness of the extraocular muscles occurs causing blurred vision and diplopia. Failure of convergence may be the first symptom. Often, vision problems are accompanied by other bulbar symptoms including dizziness, dysarthria, and dysphagia. Some patients have only bulbar symptoms; others have varying degrees of extremity weakness. Weakness may occur fairly rapidly after the ingestion of large amounts of toxin causing a flaccid paralysis and respiratory failure. In wound botulism, the toxin is released slowly into the circulation so that the onset of symptoms and the progression of weakness are slower. Examination reveals involvement of the extraocular muscles. Pupillary responses may or may not be affected. Typically, tendon reflexes are absent, but they may be present. Sensory abnormalities are not seen. In patients with milder disease, fatigability is not as prominent as in patients with myasthenia gravis.

The clinical appearance of infant botulism is different from that of food-borne or wound botulism. Constipation is the first sign of illness, although frequently this symptom may be overlooked. Infants gradually become listless and weak over a period of days to weeks. As the bulbar muscles become involved, difficulty in feeding occurs, and the cry becomes weaker. Drooling and pooling of food and secretions in the posterior pharynx may occur. Ptosis, ophthalmoplegia, and diminished facial expression are present. Most often, hypotonia and generalized muscle weakness are initially manifest as a loss of head control. Respiratory arrest may abruptly occur in patients with severe disease. Botulism may be responsible for some cases of unexpected sudden death in infancy.

Diagnostic Studies

Electrophysiologic studies are helpful in demonstrating a disturbance in neuromuscular transmission in patients with botulism. The compound muscle action potential elicited by a single stimulus to the nerve is small, and the amplitude declines with repetitive stimulation at a slow rate. Repetitive stimulation at fast rates produces an increase in the amplitude of muscle action potentials. Needle examination demonstrates a distinctive pattern of brief, small, abundant motor unit potentials that may be diagnostic of botulism in the context of the clinical syndrome. Confirmation of the diagnosis of botulism depends on detecting the toxin or the organism in affected patients or in the implicated food. In infant botulism, the organism may be isolated from stool culture.

Differential Diagnosis

Botulism in children must be distinguished from myasthenia gravis, Guillain–Barré syndrome, tick paralysis, and chemical intoxications. Typically, myasthenia gravis patients have preserved pupillary reactions and, usually, do not have areflexia. Fatigability is much more prominent in myasthenia gravis, and the edrophonium chloride (Tensilon) test result is dramatically positive. Clinical differentiation from Guillain–Barré syndrome may be difficult. Usually, Guillain–Barré syndrome patients have ascending weakness with a later onset of cranial nerve involvement. Frequent paresthesias and elevated cerebrospinal fluid protein content also help to distinguish this disorder. Electromyography is helpful in differentiating both Guillain–Barré syndrome and myasthenia gravis from botulism.

In addition to these disorders, the differential diagnosis of infant botulism includes Werdnig–Hoffmann disease, poliomyelitis, and diphtheria. The early extraocular muscle and pupillary involvement, the symmetry of weakness, and the absence of fever or pharyngitis, in addition to the characteristic electrophysiologic findings, should increase the suspicion of botulism.

Treatment and Prognosis

The treatment of all forms of botulism is directed toward aggressive supportive care with particular attention paid to respiratory support. Generally, the prognosis is good if the patient is adequately supported, although recovery may be very slow taking weeks to many months in severely affected individuals. In cases of food-borne botulism, if affected patients are seen early, emetics and gastric lavage should be used to reduce the amount of unabsorbed toxin. Antitoxin may be given, although evidence of its efficacy once neurologic manifestations have occurred is lacking. If food-borne botulism is suspected, state and federal health officials should be notified immediately. The treatment of wound botulism includes exploration and débridement of the site, in conjunction with antitoxin and antibiotic therapy. Guanidine may be of some value in improving muscle strength in mild or moderately severe cases of food-borne or wound botulism. Infant botulism is a self-limiting disease generally lasting 2 to 6 weeks. The use of antitoxin and antibiotics has not been shown to influence its course. Antibiotics may exacerbate symptoms because bacterial death may liberate *C. botulinum* toxin increasing the amount of toxin in the gastrointestinal tract. Aggressive supportive care is required throughout the period of hypotonia and weakness, and many infants require prolonged ventilator support. Constipation may persist for months and may improve with the use of stool softeners and adequate hydration. The mortality with botulism is 20% to 25% in cases of food-borne or wound botulism. The mortality of recognized cases of infant botulism is approximately 3%. Relapse of infant botulism after apparent resolution of clinical symptoms may occur making close follow-up necessary.

TICK PARALYSIS

Pathophysiology

A progressive, ascending flaccid paralysis may be caused by the attachment of certain species of ticks. In North America, the disease is most commonly caused by *Dermacentor andersoni* (wood tick) or *Dermacentor variabilis* (dog tick). *Ixodes holocyclus* (scrub tick) is the cause of the disease in Australia. Most cases of tick paralysis occur in the spring or summer and involve young children, especially girls with long hair. Frequently, the tick attaches near the hairline, where it remains unnoticed. Clinical symptoms begin within several days after the tick attaches. Tick paralysis is thought to be caused by a toxin released by the ticks, but the exact mechanism and site of the toxin's action are not known. The toxin may prevent depolarization in the terminal portions of the motor neurons.

Clinical Characteristics

Tick paralysis may begin with general symptoms such as irritability and diarrhea. Initial neurologic signs include gait ataxia and areflexia. Weakness of the legs then becomes apparent and advances in an ascending, symmetric pattern to involve the trunk and upper extremities. If the tick remains attached, the weakness may progress to involve the bulbar musculature producing dysarthria, dysphagia, blurred vision, and facial weakness. Respiratory compromise may occur. Patients may complain of numbness and tingling of the extremities, but objective sensory abnormalities are rare.

Diagnostic Studies

Routine laboratory studies are not helpful in establishing the diagnosis of tick paralysis. The cerebrospinal fluid protein level is normal, which helps to distinguish tick paralysis from Guillain–Barré syndrome. Usually, electrophysiologic studies reveal a reduced amplitude of the compound muscle action potential with no significant incremental or decremental response with repetitive stimulation. Motor and sensory nerve conduction velocities are slightly decreased in the distal segments.

Treatment and Prognosis

Recovery occurs within 1 to 5 days after removal of the tick. Intensive supportive care with assisted ventilation for respiratory failure may be required during this period. The tick must be removed for recovery to occur. Removal is achieved best by covering the tick with petrolatum to cause it to withdraw before removing it with forceps. Care should be taken to remove the entire tick so that secondary infection does not occur.

NEUROMUSCULAR TOXINS

Numerous pharmacologic and environmental agents may interfere with neuromuscular transmission (Table 227-5). Organophosphates such as parathion cause irreversible inhibition of acetylcholinesterase resulting in an accumulation of acetylcholine in the synaptic cleft. These insecticides cause muscle paralysis with prominent autonomic symptoms. Common neuromuscular-blocking agents used in anesthesia such as succinylcholine may cause prolonged paralysis in patients with clinical or subclinical myasthenia gravis. Numerous antibiotics such as neomycin, streptomycin, kanamycin, colistin, and tetracycline interfere with the release of acetylcholine aggravating preexisting neuromuscular transmission problems. Several other drugs including propranolol, phenytoin, and corticosteroids may have a similar effect on neuromuscular transmission. The treatment of drug-induced neuromuscular blockade consists of supportive care and the substitution of a different drug.

TABLE 227-5. Drugs Affecting Neuromuscular Transmission

Antibiotics (tetracyclines, trimethoprim, polymyxins, aminoglycosides, lincomycin, clindamycin)
beta-Adrenergic blockers (propranolol)
Phenytoin
Procainamide
Quinidine
Chloroquine
Lithium
Phenothiazines
Succinylcholine
Pancuronium bromide
Anticholinesterases
Adrenocorticotropic hormone
Corticosteroids

CHAPTER 228

Peripheral Neuropathy

Adapted from Julie Thorne Parke

Involvement of the peripheral nerves may occur in a variety of different disorders including systemic diseases, infections, and poisonings. In addition, degeneration of the peripheral nerves is a major feature in numerous diseases. Diseases of the peripheral nerve have been classified in several ways. They may be categorized according to type of functional impairment (motor, sensory, autonomic, or mixed), site of pathologic involvement (primary involvement of axon or myelin), clinical course and tempo (acute, subacute, or chronic), or presumed etiology. None of these systems of classification are entirely satisfactory, and combinations of clinical, electrophysiologic, and pathologic features are usually used to determine the etiology. Despite a thorough diagnostic search, the cause of polyneuropathy remains obscure in more than one-half of all cases.

INFLAMMATORY POLYRADICULONEUROPATHY (GUILLAIN–BARRÉ SYNDROME)

The most common cause of acute weakness from peripheral nerve involvement is GBS. This syndrome is characterized by the acute or subacute development of a polyradiculoneuropathy, usually after an upper respiratory tract infection or an episode of gastroenteritis. Numerous infectious agents including Epstein–Barr virus, coxsackievirus, influenza viruses, echoviruses, cytomegalovirus, and Mycoplasma pneumoniae have been associated with the illness. *Campylobacter jejuni* infection has been associated with GBS, particularly the axonal form. GBS may follow immunization against rabies. Pathologically, the disorder is characterized by the presence of inflammatory lesions with segmental demyelination scattered throughout the peripheral nervous system. The most severely involved segments are the rootlets and the proximal portions of the peripheral nerves.

Much evidence supports an immunologic basis for this disease. The neuropathologic and clinical features are similar to those of an experimental condition known as experimental allergic neuritis, which is induced in animals by the injection of peripheral nerve tissue with Freund adjuvant. Experimental allergic neuritis can be passively transferred between animals by sensitized lymphocytes but not by serum suggesting that experimental allergic neuritis is mediated by a delayed hypersensitivity mechanism. The prevailing opinion is that demyelination in GBS is secondary to a cell-mediated immune response that is directed against a component of peripheral myelin. Humoral immunity has also been found to be altered in patients with GBS, and it may contribute to the pathogenesis of the disorder.

Clinical Characteristics

Clinical symptoms typically follow an antecedent infection after a latent period that varies in length from several days to several weeks. The most common initial symptoms are numbness and paresthesias of the hands and feet, followed by progressive weakness involving all four extremities. Motor impairment usually begins in the lower extremities and progresses in an ascending pattern to involve the upper extremities, trunk, and cranial nerves. A descending pattern of weakness has also been observed. Occasionally, the onset is abrupt with simultaneous involvement of all extremities. The weakness is usually symmetric, although minor differences between the sides may occur.

A spectrum of motor involvement varying from mild weakness to a complete flaccid quadriplegia occurs. Muscle stretch reflexes are markedly reduced or absent. Involvement of the cranial nerves is common with facial diplegia occurring in 50% of patients. Lower cranial nerve dysfunction may give rise to dysarthria and difficulty in swallowing and coughing. Significant respiratory muscle weakness occurs in 20% of patients and may necessitate artificial ventilation. Sensory symptoms are much less prominent than weakness, but a distal sensory loss, particularly involving proprioception and vibratory sensation, may be present.

The autonomic nervous system is frequently involved with episodes of paroxysmal hypertension or hypotension, tachycardia or bradycardia, facial flushing, and sweating abnormalities. Bowel and bladder functions may be impaired early in the course of the disease, but sphincter dysfunction is usually short-lived. The neurologic symptoms evolve fairly rapidly over the first few days with maximum disability reached within 1 week in most cases. A stable period of 1 to 3 weeks occurs, after which recovery begins. The recovery may be rapid taking place in 6 to 8 weeks, or it may be slow lasting many months.

Many patients with GBS have some variation in clinical presentation or laboratory test results. The currently accepted criteria for the diagnosis of this syndrome are listed in Table 228-1. Several variants of GBS are recognized; the most common one occurring in childhood is a syndrome of acute external

TABLE 228-1. Criteria for Diagnosis of Guillain-Barré Syndrome

Required
Progressive motor weakness in more than one extremity
Areflexia (or distal areflexia with hyporeflexia of biceps and knee jerks)
Strongly supportive
Clinical features (in order of importance):
Progression up to 4 weeks into illness
Relative symmetry
Mild sensory symptoms or signs
Cranial nerve involvement (facial weakness in 50%)
Recovery beginning 2–4 weeks after progression ceases
Autonomic dysfunction
Absence of fever at onset of symptoms
Cerebrospinal fluid features:
Protein level elevated after first week of symptoms
Ten or fewer mononuclear leukocytes per microliter
Electrodiagnostic features:
Nerve conduction slowing or block (80%)
Prolongation of F wave latencies
Casting doubt
Marked, persistent asymmetry of weakness
Persistent bowel or bladder dysfunction
Bowel or bladder dysfunction at onset
More than 50 mononuclear leukocytes per microliter in cerebrospinal fluid
Presence of polymorphonuclear leukocytes in cerebrospinal fluid
Sharp sensory level
Rule out the diagnosis
Current history of hexacarbon abuse
Abnormal porphyrin metabolism
Recent diphtheritic infection
Evidence of lead neuropathy or intoxication
Purely sensory syndrome
Definite diagnosis of poliomyelitis, botulism, hysterical paralysis, or toxic neuropathy

Adapted from Asbury AK. Diagnostic considerations in Guillain-Barré syndrome. *Ann Neurol* 1981;9(suppl):1.

ophthalmoplegia, ataxia, and areflexia known as the Miller–Fisher syndrome. The ophthalmoplegia is often bilateral and may be complete with pupillary involvement. The course is usually benign with recovery taking place within 3 to 6 months.

Differential Diagnosis

Numerous entities may produce a clinical picture similar to that of GBS. The ascending form of acute transverse myelitis and early cord compression may initially be difficult to distinguish from GBS. The presence of pyramidal tract signs, a clear sensory level, and persistent sphincter disturbances support involvement of the spinal cord rather than the root and peripheral nerve. Acute paralytic poliomyelitis may present with weakness simulating GBS, but generally more systemic symptoms, more marked meningeal signs, and a cellular response in the CSF are present. Uncommon conditions that may cause acute symmetric weakness include porphyria, diphtheritic polyneuropathy, heavy metal intoxication, systemic lupus erythematosus, periodic paralysis, tick paralysis, rabies, and botulism.

Laboratory Findings

The most important laboratory finding in patients with GBS is an elevated cerebrospinal fluid (CSF) protein content without a pleocytosis (albuminocytologic disproportion). The total CSF protein level may be normal in the early stages of the illness, but it is elevated in almost all patients after an interval of several days. The protein content continues to increase after the disease stabilizes reaching a peak 2 to 4 weeks after the onset of the disease and ranging from 45 to 800 mg/dL.

Electrophysiologic studies are helpful in diagnosing GBS with abnormalities of motor and sensory conduction occurring in 90% of patients. Characteristic electrodiagnostic features include marked slowing of conduction velocities, prolonged distal latencies, and dispersion of the evoked responses. Proximal nerve conduction, which is characteristically slow and can be measured by studying the latency of the F response, may be the only abnormal electrophysiologic finding in the early stages of the disease. In later stages of the disease, electromyographic studies may show denervation potentials indicating axonal damage, which is associated with a poor prognosis for complete recovery.

Treatment

The treatment of GBS is largely supportive. Careful monitoring of respiratory function is important during the early stages of the illness to prevent death as a result of respiratory failure. Elective intubation and mechanical ventilation should be used aggressively in patients with any evidence of respiratory compromise because respiratory failure may abruptly occur if they become fatigued. Good nursing care and physiotherapy are important in severely affected patients. Most children with GBS recover completely, although the convalescence may be prolonged. The value of corticosteroids in the treatment of GBS has been debated, but no convincing evidence exists to support their use. Plasmapheresis and intravenous immunoglobulin have been shown to be beneficial both in shortening the length of the illness and in lessening the associated long-term disability.

OTHER NEUROPATHIES

Postinfectious Neuropathies

Bell palsy, an acute paralysis of the face, is the most common postinfectious neuropathy. It frequently occurs after mild upper respiratory tract infections or episodes of otitis media. It may also occur in conjunction with Lyme disease. Patients often complain of pain localized in the ear, which is followed by the rapid development of weakness of the entire side of the face. The nasolabial fold on the affected side is flattened, and the child may be unable to close the eye. Taste sensation may be altered, and hyperacusis may occur as a result of involvement of the nerve to the stapedius muscle.

The prognosis for recovery is good, particularly if the paralysis is not complete. Convalescence begins within a few days to several weeks. Some evidence suggests that treatment with corticosteroids may be beneficial if started within 2 to 3 days of the onset of weakness. Therapy should include measures to protect the exposed cornea of the affected eye by taping and using artificial tears. The differential diagnosis of an acute facial palsy includes demyelinating disease, brainstem tumor, otitis media, and mastoiditis.

A painless abducens nerve paralysis may occur after a nonspecific viral illness. The prognosis for this type of cranial nerve VI palsy is excellent with improvement beginning in 3 to 6 weeks and total recovery seen in most children by 3 months. Isolated oculomotor, glossopharyngeal, and hypoglossal nerve palsies occur much less commonly.

Brachial Plexopathy

An acute brachial plexopathy may occur in children after acute febrile illnesses or immunizations. The disorder is characterized by the sudden onset of pain in the shoulder and upper arm, followed by the rapid development of flaccid weakness primarily involving the muscles that are innervated by the upper roots of the brachial plexus. The paralysis may be severe, and atrophy of the affected muscles occurs. Sensory loss is minimal or absent. Electrophysiologic studies reveal slowing of nerve conduction velocities, low-amplitude evoked responses, and evidence of denervation. Physiotherapy is required to prevent contractures because recovery tends to be very slow occurring over many months.

Genetically Determined Neuropathies

The genetically determined neuropathies tend to be slowly progressive, symmetric disorders that may be inherited as either an autosomal dominant or a recessive trait (Table 228-2). These forms of neuropathy are predominantly motor and are usually associated with deformities of the feet such as pes cavus and hammer toe. The foot deformities may precede the development of weakness by many years and, in some cases, may be the only manifestation of the disease. The hereditary neuropathies are classified on the basis of clinical, electrophysiologic, genetic, and pathologic features. The specific metabolic defects are known in only a minority of the disorders (Table 228-3).

Hereditary Sensory Autonomic Neuropathies

Hereditary sensory neuropathies occur much less frequently than sensorimotor neuropathies. The major feature of type I and type II forms of these conditions is distal sensory loss with painless ulceration of the feet. The severity varies widely. Type I is inherited dominantly; type II is a recessive trait. Type II sensory neuropathy usually presents in infancy or early childhood with severe sensory loss and may affect the hands and trunk, as well as the feet. Progressive and nonprogressive types occur. Autonomic disorders are frequently seen. Pathologically, either the number of myelinated fibers is decreased or the fibers are totally absent.

TABLE 228-2. Hereditary Motor and Sensory Neuropathies

Disorder	Inheritance	Age of onset	Clinical features
HMSN-I (hypertrophic peroneal muscular atrophy)	Autosomal dominant	Childhood	Awkward gait, weakness and atrophy of anterior tibial and peroneal muscles; later hand involvement; sensory loss minimal; slow nerve conduction velocities
HMSN-II (neuronal form of peroneal muscular atrophy)	Autosomal dominant	Late childhood	Normal or near normal nerve conductions with low-amplitude response
HMSN-III (Déjérine-Sottas disease)	Autosomal recessive	Infancy	Delayed motor development; marked sensory loss; small stature with skeletal deformities; cranial nerve involvement; deafness; nerve conductions markedly reduced; elevated cerebrospinal fluid protein level
HMSN-IV (Refsum disease)	Autosomal recessive	Early childhood to second decade	Abnormal gait, sensory deficits, exacerbations and remissions of weakness; ataxia; retinitis pigmentosa, progressive deafness; cardiomyopathy; ichthyosis; elevated cerebrospinal fluid protein level; abnormal electro-retinogram; slow nerve conduction velocities; accumulation of phytanic acid

HMSN, hereditary motor and sensory neuropathy.

Familial dysautonomia (Riley–Day syndrome) is a sensory neuropathy notable for its involvement of the autonomic nervous system. Familial dysautonomia is a rare familial disorder that is inherited in an autosomal recessive manner, primarily in individuals of Jewish ancestry with onset in infancy. It has been localized to chromosome 9 at 9q31–q33. Familial dysautonomia is characterized by poor feeding, vomiting, irritability, and pulmonary infections. Signs of autonomic dysfunction include abnormal temperature regulation, decreased or absent tearing, blotching of the skin, and hypotension. The tongue is smooth and lacks fungiform papillae. Generalized insensitivity to pain involving the cornea, as well as the skin, is present. Muscle stretch reflexes are decreased or absent. Mental retardation has been reported. Death usually occurs in early childhood. Motor nerve conduction velocities are slightly slow. Several metabolic abnormalities including increased amounts of homovanillic acid and decreased amounts of vanillylmandelic acid in the urine, as well as reduced levels of plasma dopamine beta–hydroxylase, the enzyme that converts dopamine to norepinephrine, have been reported.

Toxic Neuropathies

Many pharmaceutical agents and toxic chemicals have been implicated as causes of peripheral neuropathy. The onset of these polyneuropathies is usually insidious after prolonged exposure to the toxin. A careful history of drug use and environmental exposure to toxins is of utmost importance in making a diagnosis.

TABLE 228-3. Hereditary Neuropathies with Known Biochemical Abnormality

Disorder	Inheritance	Biochemical defect	Associated clinical features
Acute intermittent porphyria	Autosomal dominant	Uroporphyrinogen 1 synthetase deficiency	Abdominal pain: acute psychosis; progressive weakness; tachycardia; hypertension.
Krabbe disease	Autosomal recessive	Galactocerebroside beta-galactosidase deficiency	Irritability; spasticity; loss of milestones in early infancy; elevated cerebrospinal fluid protein level. Death within 1–2 years.
Metachromatic leukodystrophy	Autosomal recessive	Arylsulfatase A deficiency	Ataxia; spasticity; intellectual regression; loss of reflexes at age 2–3 years; elevated cerebrospinal fluid protein level. Slower juvenile form.
Adrenoleukodystrophy	X-linked recessive	Peroxisomal defect in fatty acid oxidation (very long-chain fatty acid accumulation)	Behavior changes; gait disturbance; vision loss; adrenal insufficiency between ages 5 and 10 years. Later onset forms occur.
Refsum disease	Autosomal recessive	Peroxisomal defect (alpha-oxidation of long-chain fatty acids, phytanic acid accumulation)	Ataxia; ichthyosis; deafness; retinitis pigmentosa; progressive sensorimotor neuropathy.
Fabry disease	X-linked recessive	alpha-Galactosidase A deficiency	Painful sensory neuropathy (burning feet); angiokeratomas in bathing-suit distribution; renal failure; stroke.
Bassen-Kornzweig disease (abetalipoproteinemia)	Autosomal recessive	beta-Lipoprotein deficiency	Fat malabsorption; vitamin A, E, and K deficiencies; progressive ataxia; retinitis pigmentosa; developmental retardation; acanthocytosis; low cholesterol level.
Tangier disease	Autosomal recessive	alpha-Lipoprotein deficiency	Yellow tonsils; hepatosplenomegaly; sensory neuropathy.

TABLE 228-4. Toxic Neuropathies

Industrial chemicals and insecticides
Acrylamide
Carbon disulfide
Cyanide
n-Hexane
Organophosphates (cholinergic symptoms with delayed-onset neuropathy)
Trichloroethylene (facial numbness)
Tri-orthocresylphosphate
Metals
Lead (especially neuropathy of radial nerve, causing wristdrop)
Arsenic (Mees lines, sensory deficit)
Mercury
Thallium (ataxia, alopecia, seizures)
Pharmaceutical agents
Chloramphenicol
Cisplatin
Diphenylhydantoin
Disulfiram
Gold (may be acute)
Hydralazine
Isoniazid
Metronidazole
Vincristine

Some of the more common agents causing toxic neuropathies are listed in Table 228-4.

Lead poisoning in children typically produces symptoms of encephalopathy. On occasion, however, a peripheral neuropathy may precede the development of encephalopathic symptoms. Lead usually causes a motor neuropathy with only mild sensory impairment. The distribution of weakness is distal with patients having either footdrop or wristdrop. The diagnosis is suggested by a history of pica and may be confirmed by an elevated lead concentration in the blood. Treatment consists of removing the source of lead and administering a chelating agent. Long-term arsenic intoxication may cause paresthesias and symmetric distal weakness, primarily in the feet and legs. Sensation is decreased in a glove-and-stocking distribution, and the tendon reflexes are depressed. Transverse white striae (Mees lines) are seen in the fingernails 6 weeks after exposure. Cranial nerve involvement is unusual, and the CSF protein concentration is normal helping to differentiate arsenic poisoning from GBS.

CHAPTER 229
Rett Syndrome

Adapted from Alan K. Percy

SYNDROME CHARACTERISTICS

Clinical Features

Rett syndrome is a pervasive developmental disorder affecting young girls. After a period of apparently normal development, affected children reach a plateau and then experience a rapid decline in motor and cognitive function usually beginning at age 6 to 18 months. The principal clinical features are loss of purposeful hand use; development of stereotypic hand movements such as hand washing, hand wringing, and hand tapping (Fig. 229-1); and loss of communication and socialization skills. Generally, these children have developed the ability to speak a few words but, with onset of the disorder, meaningful verbal communication is lost. In addition, affected individuals maintain very poor eye contact, which has led to interpretation of their behavior as autistic. An acquired-type deceleration of head growth is noted as early as 3 months of life; other features include periodic breathing while wakeful including breath holding or hyperventilation or both. Seizures occur in many of these children and may consist of staring spells and complex partial and generalized tonic-clonic events. Pervasive growth failure including poor weight gain, short stature, and small hand and foot size is evident. In addition, the hands and feet tend to be markedly cooler and discolored (bluish) as compared to the remainder of the extremities. Often, diminished responses to pain are mentioned by parents.

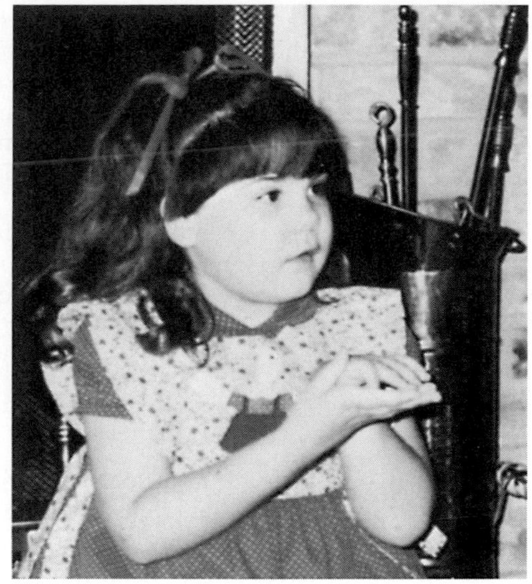

Figure 229-1. Photograph of a 5-year-old girl with Rett syndrome demonstrating the typical hand position associated with the disorder.

Although the behavioral mannerisms (hand stereotypies and periodic breathing) of children with Rett syndrome are confined to wakefulness, sleep is often interrupted, and periods of uncontrollable screaming are frequently reported by parents during affected children's first few years of life. A rather long, relatively stable phase during which the episodes of screaming and the behavioral mannerisms may become milder follows the early period of decline. Attentiveness and eye contact improve to the extent that communication may occur through gaze or eye pointing. In later childhood and early adolescence, scoliosis is common. Affected individuals may survive well into adulthood. Because this disorder has been recognized for only approximately 35 years and accurate clinical diagnosis has been possible only since the 1980s, the natural history of Rett syndrome has not been fully elucidated.

Pathophysiology

The pathophysiology of Rett syndrome is not understood well, although emerging evidence strongly supports a neurodevelopmental arrest in late gestation or early infancy. No biological marker is available to provide definitive diagnosis. Clinical assessment remains the sole basis for diagnosis. As a result, the spectrum of clinical expression has widened considerably with descriptions of several variant forms based on different patterns of expression. Clinical neurophysiologic studies have revealed progressive changes on electroencephalographic (EEG) tracings featuring slowing, loss of occipital dominant rhythm, and the appearance of multifocal spike and wave epileptiform activity. Previous reports of biogenic amine metabolite reduction in the cerebrospinal fluid (CSF) have not been substantiated. Elevated CSF beta–endorphin levels have been noted in most instances, but this finding is not specific to Rett syndrome. Abnormalities have also been described in glutamate and nerve growth factor levels in CSF and in acetylcholine, dopamine, and glutamate neurotransmitter systems in the brain.

Genetics

The occurrence of Rett syndrome almost exclusively in girls has led to the suggestion that it is an X-linked disorder that is lethal in boys, although the precise genetic mechanism is unknown. At present, the locus of interest is the distal long arm of the X chromosome Xq28. Few affected boys have been identified. The recurrence of Rett syndrome within individual families has been reported in less than 1% of cases. When recurrence has been described in more than one generation, the mode of transmission appears to be through the maternal side of the family. However, genealogic studies conducted in Sweden traced several families to specific homesteads through both maternal and paternal lines. The prevalence rate of between 1:10,000 and 1:15,000 exceeds that of phenylketonuria in female individuals.

Differential Diagnosis

The differential diagnosis of Rett syndrome includes infantile autism with which it has been most frequently confused. If the clinical criteria for autism and Rett syndrome are carefully applied, however, one should have no difficulty in making the distinction. In addition, all children with acquired deceleration of head growth and a diagnosis of progressive cerebral palsy should be carefully evaluated for the possibility of Rett syndrome. Angelman syndrome, often associated with a 15q deletion, may resemble Rett syndrome during early stages and should be excluded with appropriate cytogenetic testing. Finally, other neurodegenerative disorders such as infantile neuronal ceroid lipofuscinosis should be considered, and appropriate diagnostic tests should be conducted. Periodic breathing has been described in patients with Joubert syndrome. This condition can be differentiated from Rett syndrome by neuroimaging, however, as children with Joubert syndrome have structural abnormalities of the cerebellum. The only imaging abnormality noted in patients with Rett syndrome is mild to moderate cortical atrophy. Volumetric studies indicate specific reductions in frontal cortex and caudate nuclei.

Neuropathologic assessment has revealed intriguing abnormalities, in addition to reduced brain weight. The principal findings have been reduced pigmentation within neurons of the substantia nigra, reduced neuronal size, and reduced synaptic connections. These findings suggest a fundamental abnormality in brain development most likely occurring near the time of birth.

Treatment

No specific therapy is available for children with Rett syndrome. The majority of affected children achieve independent walking. Some will lose this capability in later stages and are susceptible to the complications of relative immobility including orthopedic deformities, particularly progressive scoliosis. Antiepileptic agents are indicated if seizures occur. Carbamazepine has been particularly effective; lamotrigine and valproate are suitable alternatives. Nutritional supplementation including gastrostomy feeding to promote adequate dietary intake may be required. Constipation is common and requires careful attention. Early childhood education and programs involving physical and occupational therapy should be tailored to individual children. Prolonged survival requires appropriate prospective care to minimize future medical and orthopedic complications.

11

Allergy and Immunology

CHAPTER 230

General Considerations of Allergies in Childhood

Adapted from Hugh A. Sampson
and Peyton A. Eggleston

CLASSIFICATION OF ALLERGY

Gell and Coombs classified allergic (hypersensitivity) reactions into four types in 1963. While this classification presumes that only one mechanism participates in the pathophysiology of immunologically mediated disease, it is now appreciated that this definition is too simplistic. Allergic diseases are more diverse immunologic responses. Nevertheless, the classification is helpful and is still used.

Type I (Anaphylactic Reactions)

IgE antibody can bind to the surface of mast cells, basophilic granulocytes, and certain antigen-presenting cells (e.g., macrophages, Langerhans cells). Exposure of these IgE-coated cells to antigen results in cell activation and release of potent cytokines and inflammatory mediators, which interact with blood vessels, bronchi, or mucus-secreting glands on an acute or chronic basis. Examples of this allergic reaction include anaphylactic reactions to insect stings and food-induced urticaria.

Type II (Cytotoxic Reactions)

IgG or IgM antibodies are formed by the patient to environmental or self (autoimmune) antigens. On subsequent exposure, antigen can bind to this antibody resulting in activation of complement. The cell can then be damaged or destroyed by the membrane attack complex (C5–C9). Examples of this allergic reaction include drug-induced leukopenia and hemolytic anemia.

Type III (Arthus or Immune Complex Reactions)

Circulating antigen can bind to IgG and IgM antibodies to form antigen-antibody complexes. Small complexes may remain harmlessly in the circulation, whereas large complexes are rapidly cleared by the reticuloendothelial system. Intermediate-size complexes, however, may be deposited in vessel walls and tissues. Vascular damage is then initiated by activation of complement, granulocytes, and platelets. The most common example of this reaction is serum sickness.

Type IV (Cell-Mediated Reactions)

Type IV reactions involve antigen-presenting cells (e.g., monocytes, macrophages, dendritic cells) and antigen-specific T lymphocytes. After primary exposure, T cells respond to subsequent exposure by proliferation and differentiation into cells capable of causing cytolysis (natural killer cells), or by recruiting other cytolytic cells (macrophages). Classic examples of these reactions are contact dermatitis from poison ivy or tuberculin skin tests.

PATHOGENESIS OF IGE-MEDIATED DISORDERS

Atopic disease is caused by type I, IgE-mediated reactions. IgE does not activate complement nor does it cross the placenta. Forty thousand to 90,000 IgE molecules can bind to the cell membrane of a mast or basophil. IgE is produced by plasma cells, primarily in the lymphoid tissue of the respiratory tract (tonsils and adenoids) and gut.

Studies have demonstrated two types of $CD4^+$ (T_H) cells based on the profile of cytokines they generate. T_H1 cells promote cell-mediated reactions by secreting interleukin-2 (IL-2), interferon-gamma, and granulocyte-macrophage colony-stimulating factor (GM-CSF); and T_H2 cells that promote immunoglobulin synthesis including IgE synthesis by secreting IL-4, IL-5, IL-6, IL-10, IL-13, and GM-CSF. B cells can differentiate into IgE-secreting plasma cells in the presence of allergen, antigen-presenting cells, and the appropriate antigen-presenting cell and T cell-derived cytokines. Exposure to any antigen causes IgE production in most individuals, but the response is normally turned off by suppressor T lymphocytes. Procedures that eliminate T-suppressor cells such as irradiation or cyclophosphamide promote the indefinite production of high-titer IgE antibodies in animal models.

Atopic diseases have a strong familial tendency. The approximate prevalence of atopic disease is 15% when no first-degree relatives have allergic disease, 33% when one first-degree relative is affected, and 68% when two or more first-degree relatives are atopic. No clear pattern of inheritance is found suggesting that the diseases are polygenic. Exposure to several environmental factors such as cigarette smoke, air pollutants, allergens (mites, foods, pollens, cockroaches, and molds) have been associated with an increased risk of atopic disease. In addition, specific IgE antibody responses are more frequently associated with specific HLA specificities such as HLA-Dw2 and HLA-B8.

Elevated serum IgE concentrations are not restricted to allergic disorders. With atopic disease, the IgE concentration is generally elevated in only 60% to 70% of patients and roughly correlates with disease severity. Individuals with no detectable serum or cell-bound IgE are apparently healthy, which suggests that IgE is not essential in maintaining good health.

After the mast cell or basophil responds to an allergen, release of numerous chemical mediators results in an immediate response (within 15–30 minutes), which includes vasodilation, increased vascular permeability, smooth-muscle constriction, and mucus secretion in the respiratory and gastrointestinal tracts. In addition, mast cell activation may result in a late-phase reaction (LPR), which lasts 12 to 48 hours. In the nose, for example, the LPR is responsible for persistent obstruction and hypersecretion of mucous. In the lung, LPR is associated with a persistent airflow obstruction that only partially responds to bronchodilator therapy. The exact mechanism of the LPR is unknown, but it is clearly important to the pathophysiology of chronic allergic disease.

CLINICAL PRESENTATION OF THE ATOPIC SYNDROME

The atopic disorders include atopic dermatitis, allergic rhinitis, and asthma. Each of these disorders has an underlying IgE-dependent mechanism, and, therefore, more than one can affect a patient. For instance, asthma occurs in 40% to 60% children with atopic dermatitis, and 80% to 90% of children with asthma have concomitant allergic rhinitis.

Disorders such as food allergy, drug allergy, insect hypersensitivity, urticaria, angioedema, and contact dermatitis are not included in the atopic syndrome. Epidemiologic studies have not confirmed the suggestion that insect hypersensitivity or drug allergy occur more frequently in atopic individuals.

Prevalence and Natural History

The cumulative prevalence of asthma among children is 8% to 12%. In Western societies, 50% of children with asthma have onset of their disease before age 3 years. Atopic dermatitis occurs in 10% to 12% of children with more than 85% of cases presenting before age 5 years. Studies have shown that the prevalence of allergic rhinitis is as high as 20 to 40% in children.

The natural history of atopic diseases is complex. Each disorder generally appears for the first time at a characteristic age, frequently becomes more severe over a period of months to years, then undergoes a period of prolonged remission. For example, asthma often begins by 4 years of age in the majority of children and may be outgrown by late adolescence only to recur in the mid-20s in approximately 25% of those affected.

Prediction and Prevention

The development of atopic disease depends on sufficient contact between a genetically predisposed host and an allergen. Sensitization may take weeks or years and depends on host genetic factors, allergen dose and time of exposure, and adjuvant factors such as infection, cigarette smoke, and environmental pollutants. Identification of subjects at risk and avoidance of allergen exposure early in life may reduce the incidence of atopic disease. For example, breast-feeding exclusively for the first 4 to 6 months of life may affect the natural history of atopic disease and postpone allergic symptoms until after the first or second year of life. Placing a lactating mother of a high-risk infant on a diet free of major allergens (eggs, milk, peanuts) may also be protective because food allergens can be transmitted in maternal breast milk. The addition of solid foods to an infant's diet in the first 4 months of life has been directly correlated with increased risk of developing food allergy and atopic disease.

Exposure to irritants or infection may also increase the risk of atopy. Studies show that infants exposed to tobacco smoke develop higher serum IgE levels and develop respiratory disease at an earlier age than infants in a nonsmoking environment. A few studies suggest that certain viral infections (e.g., respiratory syncytial virus, parainfluenza) may act as adjuvants for increased IgE responses to environmental allergens.

If patients remove themselves from pertinent allergens by controlling their environment or moving to an area of the country free of offending pollens or allergens, they often experience remission. Many develop sensitivities to new local allergens, so moving is not usually recommended.

DIAGNOSTIC EVALUATION

No single historical, physical, or laboratory finding is diagnostic of atopic disease. Developing a clear understanding of age of onset and progression of symptoms is important. Knowledge of local flora helps in making the diagnosis. For example, most tree pollens are released during early spring (February to March) and most grass pollens are released from late spring through midsummer. In the eastern and Midwestern United States, ragweed is a major source of pollen in late summer and early fall. High humidity provides favorable conditions for mold growth. House dust (dust mites, animal danders, molds, pollens) is nonseasonal. Domestic animals are common sources of potent allergens, but families often deny their pet causing symptoms. Foods such as cow's milk, eggs, and peanuts are frequent causes of allergic symptoms.

Many atopic diseases have abnormal findings on physical exam. These findings are covered in the subsequent chapters on specific allergic diseases.

Laboratory abnormalities such as peripheral blood eosinophilia (greater than 500 cells per microliter) often occurs in atopic patients with asthma and atopic dermatitis, but is not common in patients with allergic rhinitis. Eosinophilia in respiratory or gastrointestinal secretions highly suggests allergic disease. Secretions may be collected, dried on a microscope slide, and stained with Hansel stain, which stains eosinophils in a few minutes. While peripheral blood eosinophilia can be seen with other illnesses such as parasitic infections, secretory eosinophilia is seen in few other conditions.

Total serum IgE concentration is somewhat useful as a screening test for allergic disease, but this test suffers from low specificity. Normal values (0–100 IU/mL in childhood) are age-dependent with highest levels normally found in late adolescence. A concentration of greater than 100 IU/mL in the first year of life is correlated with the future development of atopic disease.

Specific sensitivity may be confirmed with immediate wheal-and-flare skin test results using such methods as prick, puncture, or scratch techniques. The resulting wheal size is determined in approximately 15 minutes and compared with sizes of positive and a negative controls. A positive skin test does not necessarily reflect clinical reactivity. Nevertheless, skin tests provide a rapid readout and are relatively inexpensive.

Serologic assays to measure allergen-specific IgE are available. Methods such as the RAST can measure circulating allergen-specific IgE antibodies. By incubating sera with allergens chemically coupled to a solid matrix and washing away nonspecific antibody, adherent (allergen-specific) antibody can then be detected by incubation with a radiolabeled (enzyme-linked or fluorescein-linked) antihuman IgE antibody. Studies indicate that high levels of allergen-specific IgE antibodies are more predictive of symptomatic sensitivity. Unlike skin testing, RAST (and similar type testing) carries no risk of anaphylaxis.

TREATMENT

Treatment of allergic diseases falls into three categories: allergen avoidance, symptomatic drug intervention, and allergen immunotherapy. Allergen avoidance is the treatment of choice, but compliance is difficult to obtain for indoor allergens and basically impossible for outdoor allergens. Drug therapy has become much more practical and sophisticated in the past decade. Immunotherapy may reverse specific hypersensitivities, but it is time-consuming, expensive, and has risks.

When total allergen avoidance is possible for long periods of time, IgE production may diminish and loss of reactivity ("outgrowing") may occur. Other forms of allergen avoidance include removal of the pets from the household, use of dust-mite barriers (encasings) for pillows and mattresses, removal of carpeting, and removal of nonwashable stuffed animals.

Drug intervention is the second arm of allergy therapy. Certain drugs prevent IgE-mediated activation of mast cells and basophils. Corticosteroids inhibit mast cell activation and interleukin production and also interfere with the LPR through direct effects on granulocyte chemotaxis. Antihistamines are antagonists that interfere with immediate reactions by blocking the effects of histamine released by mast cells and basophils.

Immunotherapy, or allergy-injection therapy, consists of repeated injections of allergenic material to increase the patient's tolerance of those allergens. Immunotherapy is indicated only for stinging insect hypersensitivity and for allergic rhinitis and asthma (where allergen-related symptoms are implicated by history and laboratory testing) The concentration of the allergen extract is gradually increased until high doses are tolerated. Immunotherapy carries a small (1%–5%) risk of systemic anaphylaxis.

CHAPTER 231
Asthma

Adapted from Peyton A. Eggleston

Asthma is a chronic inflammatory disorder of the airways that causes recurrent episodes of wheezing, breathlessness, chest tightness, and coughing. These episodes are associated with variable airflow obstruction that reverses spontaneously or with treatment.

Asthma is the most frequent cause for hospitalization and school absenteeism in children. Since the 1980s, the prevalence of asthma in the United States increased from 4.2% to approximately 7.5%. This may be related to more accurate diagnosis of asthma and increasing urbanization with exposure to air pollution. Death from asthma is, thankfully, uncommon in children but, in the 1990s, rates increased as much as 6% per year in the United States.

The median age of onset of asthma is 4 years, but more than 20% of children develop symptoms within the first year of life. One significant risk factor is childhood atopy or atopy in family members. Respiratory infections, especially with the respiratory syncytial virus (RSV), are a risk factor for future wheezing episodes; approximately 40% of children with RSV bronchiolitis can develop symptoms of chronic asthma.

In 60% of cases, asthma beginning in childhood resolves by young adult life. As many as 25% to 50% of those children who undergo remission in adolescence become symptomatic again as young adults. Heavy exposure to pollution, allergens, or cigarette smoke makes resolution less likely.

PATHOPHYSIOLOGY

Inflammation

Asthma is an inflammatory disease. The infiltrate in the airway and the surrounding parenchyma can be rich in eosinophils, neutrophils, basophils, and mononuclear cells. Bronchial smooth muscle is hypertrophied. Respiratory epithelium is desquamated, and together with inflammatory cells, it creates large mucus plugs that can block the airway lumen. The inflammatory process is due to mast cell activation by lymphokines or IgE-dependent mechanisms producing a variety of proinflammatory substances. These mediators result in an "immediate response" (within 15–30 minutes), which includes vasodilation, increased vascular permeability, smooth-muscle constriction, and mucus secretion in the respiratory tract. A late-phase reaction (LPR) within 2 to 4 hours after antigen exposure also occurs. Persistent airflow obstruction that responds poorly to beta agonist treatment is associated with this LPR.

Airway Hyperresponsiveness

The airway obstruction characteristic of asthma is called airway hyperresponsiveness. This hyperresponsiveness may be seen in response to "precipitants" of bronchospasm. These stimuli include irritants (cigarette smoke, odors, pollution), weather changes, and emotions. Viral infections (RSV, influenza, rhinovirus, parainfluenza) can also trigger severe attacks. Certain drugs (beta–blockers, aspirin) can cause airway obstruction. Exercise can cause obstruction due to hyperventilation and exposure to cold, dry air. Allergens cause attacks when specific IgE antibody is present.

PHARMACOTHERAPY FOR ASTHMA

Beta–Adrenergic Agonists

Beta–adrenergic agonists are the primary symptomatic therapy for asthma. Airway obstruction is rapidly reversed through their effects on the $beta_2$ receptor on bronchial smooth muscle. Some of the available drugs and their doses are listed in Table 231-1. The current drug of choice is albuterol.

In most cases, beta–adrenergic agonists should be inhaled. Effective bronchodilation can be achieved with doses ten to 20 times lower than with oral dosing. Toxicity can include tachycardia, palpitations, and central nervous system excitement and muscular tremor. Nebulized drugs can be given, but an inhaler (MDI, metered dose inhaler) is often easier to administer (even in very young children) when used with a reservoir device such as an Aerochamber (Monaghan, North Andover, MA). A reservoir device can be used with or without a mask.

Beta–adrenergic agonists inhibit immediate responses to allergens, exercise, and many inhaled irritants when given just before exposure. Short acting beta–adrenergic agonists cannot inhibit inflammation. They have little effect on the LPR. The role of these drugs is primarily "rescue" reversal of bronchoconstriction. Long-acting beta–adrenergic agonists are available and may have a role in the chronic therapy of persistent asthma (see below).

Anticholinergics

Anticholinergic drugs (muscarinic antagonists) are useful bronchodilators in acute asthma but are not effective when used chronically. Representative drugs include atropine, ipratropium, and glycopyrrolate. These drugs are potent bronchodilators with peak effects that are delayed for 30 to 60 minutes. Toxic effects (xerostomia, mydriasis, tachycardia, and abdominal pain) are less common with ipratropium than with atropine or glycopyrrolate.

Cromolyn

Cromolyn has no bronchodilator properties but can prevent allergen-induced asthma. It's function may be due to its ability to inhibit mast cell activation. Cromolyn can inhibit bronchospasm due to allergen, exercise, and sulfur dioxide. It can block both the early- and late-phase reactions. When used chronically, it causes slight improvement in airway reactivity and decreases disease activity. This effect requires approximately 2 to 4 weeks of therapy, and approximately 25% of patients do not benefit. Except for a rare allergic reaction, cromolyn is nontoxic. Nedocromil is a medication with very similar activity to cromolyn.

Theophylline

Theophylline (not shown in Table 231-1) is a weak bronchodilator associated with toxicity at high blood levels. Although it may still have an occasional role, studies have demonstrated that theophylline is inferior to beta agonists for therapy of acute asthma. A small number of patients may benefit from therapy with chronic theophylline.

Leukotriene Modifiers

Leukotrienes are inflammatory mediators released from mast cells, eosinophils, and basophils. Their effect is to cause smooth muscle contraction, increase vascular permeability, increase mucus secretion, and further activate inflammatory cells in the airway. The most effective medications (zafirlukast, monteleukast) competitively inhibit tissue effects of leukotrienes. These medications have been demonstrated to inhibit exercise-induced asthma and allergen-induced asthma. They are meant to be taken daily.

Corticosteroids

Corticosteroids are the most potent available drugs for asthma. The mechanism of their effectiveness in asthma may relate to inactivation of inflammatory cells. Acutely, their use can increase numbers of beta–adrenergic receptors on bronchial smooth muscle and lead to increased responsiveness to beta agonists. Inhaled and systemic steroids inhibit the allergen-induced LPR but have little effect on the immediate reaction.

Available preparations are listed in Table 231-1. Newer inhaled corticosteroids (fluticasone, budesonide) are approximately 100 times more potent than prednisone in antiinflammatory activity. These medications also have the benefit of being poorly absorbed from the respiratory tract and being rapidly cleared when absorbed from the gastrointestinal tract. This result is a wide therapeutic ratio and a recent increase in their application in chronic asthma.

Chronic systemic (oral) steroid therapy may be needed for some patients, but it is associated with potential growth suppression, adrenal suppression, decreased bone mass, and cataracts. These toxic effects are minimized by alternate-day therapy or by treatment with high-dose inhaled steroids. Chronic treatment with inhaled steroids at doses higher than 400 μg/day has been associated with growth retardation and decreased serum cortisol concentrations.

CHRONIC MANAGEMENT

The reader is referred to the National Asthma Education and Prevention Program Expert Panel Report 2: Guidelines for the Diagnosis and Management of Asthma (1997).

TABLE 231-1. Drugs Available for Asthma

Drug	Preparations available: Inhaled	Tablets	Liquid	Dose
Beta-adrenergic agonist				
Metaproterenol		10, 20 mg	10 mg/tsp	1–2 mg/kg/d divided into 3–4 daily doses
Albuterol		2, 4 mg	2 mg/tsp	0.4–0.6 mg/kg/d divided into 3 daily doses
Terbutaline		2.5, 5.0 mg	Not available	0.15 mg/kg/d divided into 3 daily doses
Metered-dose inhalers (MDI)				
Metaproterenol	650 μg/puff			1–2 puffs four times per day as needed
Albuterol	90 μg/puff			1–2 puffs four times per day as needed
Terbutaline	200 μg/puff			1–2 puffs four times per day as needed
Pirbuterol	200 μg/puff			1–2 puffs four times per day as needed
Bitolterol	370 μg/puff			1–2 puffs four times per day as needed
Salmetrol	21 μg/puff			1–2 puffs twice per day as needed
Nebulized solution				
Metaproterenol	50 mg/mL			0.1–0.3 mL in 2.5 ml normal saline four times per day as needed
Albuterol	5 mg/mL			1.25–2.5 mg per dose four times per day as needed
Terbutaline	1 mg/mL			0.5–1.5 mg in 2.5 mL normal saline four times per day as needed
Anticholinergic				
Nebulized solution				
Atropine	0.1–1.0 mg/mL			0.05 mg/kg per dose in 2.5 mL normal saline
Ipatropium	500 μm/2.5 mL			250 μg four times per day
Theophylline		100, 200, 300 mg (many formulations exist)	80 mg/15 mL (many formulations exist)	5–15 mg/kg/d to maintain peak serum concentration at 5–15 μg/mL
Aminophylline (approximately 80% theophylline)			25 mg/mL (IV)	3- to 6-mg/kg bolus, 1 mg/kg/hr infusion to maintain serum concentration at 10–20 μg/mL
Cromolyn	MDI: 800 μg/puff Nebulizer solution: 20 mg per ampule			2 puffs four times per day 1 nebulizer treatment four times per day
Nedocromil	MDI: 1.75 mg/puff			2 puffs four times per day
Leukotriene modifiers				
Zileuton		300, 600 mg		600 mg four times per day
Zafirlukast		20 mg		20 mg twice per day
Montelukast		10 mg, 5 mg chewable		5–10 mg/d
Corticosteroids				
Oral				
Prednisone		1–50 mg	5 mg/tsp	1–2 mg/kg/d for 5-day acute course
Prednisolone		5 mg	5, 15 mg/tsp	
Methylprednisolone		2–32 mg		
Dexamethasone		0.25–6.0 mg	Elixir: 0.5 mg/tsp Oral solution: 0.1–1.0 mg/mL	0.75 mg/kg/d for 5 days only
Inhaled				
Beclomethasone	42 μg/puff			2–4 puffs two to four times per day
Triamcinolone	100 μg/puff			1–2 puffs twice per day
Flunisolide	250 μg/puff			2 puffs twice per day
Fluticasone	44, 110, 220 μg/puff			2–4 puffs three times per day
Budesonide	200 μg/puff			1–2 puffs twice per day
Injection				
Prednisolone				1–2 mg/kg; then 1–2 mg/kg/d
Methylprednisolone				1–2 mg/kg; then 1–2 mg/kg/d

This monograph is available on the World Wide Web at http://www.nhlbi.nih.gov/guidelines/asthma/asthgdln.htm

In most cases, the diagnosis of asthma is a clinical one based on a history of episodic bronchospasm (coughing, wheezing) in response to certain stimuli with subsequent relief when the patient gets appropriate therapy. Patients may have a positive family history, eosinophilia, and an elevated serum total IgE. Allergy skin testing or RAST for common inhalant and food allergens may help to identify asthma triggers.

Allergic Aspects

Allergen avoidance is an essential first step in treating allergic asthma. The most common allergens associated with chronic asthma are dust mites, cats, dogs, molds, cockroaches, pollens, and foods.

To avoid dust mite allergen, airtight covers should be installed to cover mattresses and pillows completely. Bedding can be rendered mite-free by washing in hot water (55°C) or by dry cleaning; usually, mite reinfestation occurs within a few weeks. Wall-to-wall carpeting in children's bedrooms should be eliminated, as should excessive numbers of fuzzy toys near areas where children sleep.

Pets contribute potent allergens primarily from the animal's secretions. Pets should be eliminated from households with sensitized children. Washing pets every 1 to 2 weeks can reduce airborne allergens somewhat, but cat antigen does not disappear from settled dust for 6 months after the animal has been removed.

Mold antigens are ubiquitous in a home environment and more than 25% of asthmatic children have positive skin tests to mold extracts. The most effective way to remove mold and mildew is to remove contaminated material, to wash with 2% chlorine bleach solutions or benzalkonium, and to reduce home moisture content using air conditioning or dehumidifiers.

Cockroaches contribute important allergens, particularly in urban environments. Usually, elimination of the antigen requires pest control consultation and careful clean-up of the remaining insect parts and feces.

Stepped Management of Medications

Patients should have the severity of their asthma classified using the schema in Table 231-2. Symptoms of coughing and wheezing have the same significance in children. An asthma exacerbation is defined as a period of severe symptoms lasting hours to days and requiring additional medications to resolve. As asthma becomes more severe, intermittent episodes generally evolve to continuous symptoms.

Mild intermittent asthma exhibits no symptoms between episodes, and symptoms occur no more often than twice a week. If symptoms are present more than twice a week, affected children are said to have persistent asthma. Persistent asthma is then graded as mild, moderate, or severe, depending on the frequency of daytime and nighttime symptoms; interference with usual activity such as school, sports, or play; and detectable abnormalities in lung function tests. Nocturnal cough may be present but never more than two to three times a month in mild asthma. Notably, severe wheezing episodes may be seen in asthmatics regardless of their chronic severity.

Objective measurements of pulmonary functions are essential in managing asthma on a day-to-day basis. Home peak expiratory flow meters should be used to educate patients about symptoms, to establish a baseline for measuring exacerbations, and to adjust medications. Acutely, peak flow meters should be used to establish the severity of obstruction. The peak expiratory flow rate (PEFR) is inexpensive and convenient and correlates well with FEV_1 in a patient who is trained in the proper technique. Normal values are based on gender and standing height. These values can be found in reference books.

Classification of asthma according to the categories described can be used to plan therapy as shown in Table 231-3.

MILD INTERMITTENT ASTHMA

This is best treated with an inhaled beta-agonist as needed for symptoms. No daily medication is required. In nearly all children, inhaled (MDI) medication should be used with a spacer device. It may also be used as a prophylactic before exercise or exposure to allergen. If symptoms require more than two doses weekly (a new canister approximately every year), affected children should be considered to have persistent asthma, and additional medications in different therapeutic classes should be added.

MILD PERSISTENT ASTHMA

This should be treated with daily doses of a disease-controlling antiinflammatory medication, in addition to a short-acting beta-adrenergic agonist for use as needed. Low-dose inhaled steroids are preferred, but leukotriene modifiers and cromolyn or nedocromil are also appropriate medications.

MODERATE PERSISTENT ASTHMA

This should be treated with daily medications that induce long-term resolution. Moderate doses of inhaled steroids or lower-dose inhaled corticosteroids with a long-acting inhaled beta agonist is recommended. Leukotriene modifiers may be added. A short acting beta-agonist will be needed for relief of acute bronchospasm when it arises.

TABLE 231-2. Classification of Severity of Chronic Asthma[a]

Classification	Days with symptoms	Nights with symptoms	PEF (% best)[b] FEV_1 (% predicted)[c]	PEF variability[b]
Mild intermittent	≤2/wk	≤2/mo	≥80%	<20%
Mild persistent	>2/wk	3–4/mo	≥80%	20–30%
Moderate persistent	Daily Daily adrenergic inhaler Interferes with activity	≥1/wk	>60% but <80%	>30%
Severe persistent	Continual Limited activity Frequent exacerbations[c]	Frequent	≤60%	>30%

FEV_1, forced expiratory volume over 1 second; PEF, peak expiratory flow.
[a]The features of a given patient's severity are highly variable and may overlap severity grades. The presence of any one feature of a severity grade is sufficient to place a child in that severity category.
[b]For children older than 5 years who can use a spirometer or peak flowmeter.
[c]Patients at any severity level can experience mild, moderate, or severe exacerbations. An *exacerbation* is defined as an increase in symptoms lasting hours to days and requiring additional emergency medications.
Adapted from the National Heart, Lung and Blood Institute. National Asthma Education and Prevention Program. *Expert panel report 2: Guidelines for the diagnosis and management of asthma,* publication no. 97-4051, Bethesda, MD: National Institutes of Health, 1997.

TABLE 231-3. Recommended Chronic Medications for Different Severity Levels of Chronic Disease

Severity level	Symptomatic medication	Controller medication
Mild intermittent	Short-acting adrenergic agent	None
Mild persistent	Short-acting adrenergic agonist	Low-dose inhaled steroids *or* Cromolyn, nedocromil *or* Leukotriene modifiers
Moderate persistent	Short-acting adrenergic agonist	Moderate-dose inhaled steroids *or* Low-dose inhaled steroids *and* Long-acting adrenergic agonist *or* Low-dose inhaled steroids *And either* Leukotriene modifiers *or* Theophylline
Severe persistent	Short-acting adrenergic agonist	High-dose inhaled steroids *and* Long-acting adrenergic agonist

Severe Persistent Asthma

Severe asthma requires treatment with inhaled steroids in high doses (generally greater than 800 μg daily). In addition, a second drug for chronic use such as a long-acting beta–adrenergic agonist is usually required. If symptoms and pulmonary functions are not controlled with inhaled beta agonists, oral steroids (prednisone or equivalent) should be added every other day.

The goal of therapy is to normalize pulmonary function, to decrease peak flow variability, and to allow normal or near-normal activity with infrequent night symptoms and no absences from school.

TREATMENT OF ACUTE ASTHMA

The goal of treating acute asthma is to rapidly normalize pulmonary functions and to prevent progression of the attack. A scheme to assess severity in acute asthma is shown in Table 231-4. Generally, therapy for acute attacks should begin in the home or at school. Certain patients are at risk for life-threatening severe attacks. At times, these patients cannot be treated at home or school and should be brought to medical attention immediately. High-risk patients include those with prior intubation for asthma, two or more hospitalizations for asthma in the last year, three or more emergency department visits for asthma in the last year, hospitalization or emergency department use within the last month, a requirement for oral steroid therapy, a history of syncope or hypoxic seizures during an asthma attack, and a history of serious psychiatric or psychosocial problems.

Beginning at home (or school), in mild to moderate attacks, albuterol should be given by nebulization or metered-dose inhaler with a spacer. If a positive response is identified, albuterol should be given every 3 to 4 hours, and severity should be frequently reassessed. An incomplete response is indicated by persistent evidence of airway obstruction with wheezing and respiratory distress. The attending physician should then be contacted, oral prednisone (1–2 mg/kg per dose) should be given and beta-agonist treatment should continue. If severity subsides to mild over the next 4 hours, continued home treatment is appropriate. If moderate asthma continues, affected patients should be seen in the physician's office or in a hospital-based emergency department.

In the office or emergency department, oxygen should be administered together with nebulized albuterol every 20 minutes for 1 hour. If it has not been given already, prednisone (1–2 mg/kg) should be given. If the patient is unable to tolerate

TABLE 231-4. Estimation of Severity of Acute Exacerbations of Asthma

Manifestation	Mild	Moderate	Severe
Alertness	Normal	Agitated	May be drowsy
Dyspnea	Absent, speaks complete sentences	Speaks short phrases, soft short cry	Speaks short phrases, words
Pulsus paradoxus (mm Hg)	<10	10–25	25–40
Accessory muscle use	None	Retractions, sternocleidomastoid	Severe retractions, nasal flaring
Skin color	Good	Pale	Cyanotic
Auscultation	End-expiratory wheeze	Inspiratory, expiratory wheeze	Quiet breath sounds
O_2 saturation (%)	>95	91–95	<91
Pco_2 (mm Hg)	<42	<42	≥42
PEFR (% predicted or best)	>80	50–80	<50

PEFR, peak expiratory flow rate.
Adapted from the National Heart, Lung and Blood Institute. National Asthma Education and Prevention Program. *Expert panel report 2: Guidelines for the diagnosis and management of asthma,* publication no. 97-4051, Bethesda, MD: National Institutes of Health, 1997.

oral steroids, parenteral preparations can be used. Epinephrine, 0.01 mg/kg (maximum dose 0.3 mg; 1:1,000), should be given if such patients cannot generate a peak flow, have decreased consciousness, or cannot cooperate for treatment with nebulized drugs. If treatment is required for more than 4 hours or treatment response is poor, the patient should be hospitalized and therapy should be augmented with consideration of intravenous magnesium sulfate and continuous inhaled or intravenous beta-agonists in severely ill patients.

CHAPTER 232
Food Allergies

Adapted from Hugh A. Sampson

Adverse food reactions are often the result of food hypersensitivity (adverse immunologic responses) or food intolerance (adverse physiologic responses). Food intolerance makes up the majority of adverse food reactions and may be secondary to substances found in some foods, or a metabolic disorder of the host (e.g., lactose intolerance). Food hypersensitivity may be the result of IgE-mediated mechanisms or other less well-defined immunologic mechanisms.

PREVALENCE

The term *food allergy* should not be used to denote simply any adverse food reaction. When this occurs, the perceived prevalence of food allergy is far greater than actual prevalence. In Bock's survey of a general pediatric practice, 28% of the infants were reported to have experienced adverse food reactions by their third birthday. Symptoms, however, were only confirmed by oral food challenge in 8% of infants. Similarly, in four prospective studies from four different countries using appropriately performed milk challenges, 2.2% to 2.5% of infants were found to have cow's-milk allergy in the first 1 to 2 years of life.

Children with atopic disorders tend to have a higher prevalence of food allergy. In a study of children in a dermatology clinic with moderate to severe atopic dermatitis, approximately 40% were found to have skin symptoms provoked by food hypersensitivity. Studies of asthmatic children attending general pulmonary clinics suggest that 8% to 10% of such patients have food-induced wheezing.

PATHOGENESIS

The pathogenesis of food allergy involves three main factors: the food (or allergen), the gastrointestinal barrier and its handling of food, and affected individuals' genetic predisposition to developing an allergic response. In children, eggs, peanuts, milk, soy, wheat, and fish account for 85% to 90% of food allergy reactions.

In order to prevent intact foreign antigens from gaining access to the body, the gastrointestinal has both nonimmunologic and immunologic defense mechanisms. IgA in the gastrointestinal tract lumen binds foreign antigens such as food and impedes their absorption. Although more than 98% of ingested protein is blocked by the gastrointestinal barrier, minute amounts of intact antigens are absorbed and gain access to immune reactive cells. Most individuals, however, develop "tolerance" to ingested food antigens and allergy does not result. This tolerance is induced in T cells.

Antibody production (B cells) against food is a universal phenomenon and is not generally associated with hypersensitivity. Most antibodies to foods in clinically tolerant individuals are of the IgG class with high levels of IgE or IgA antibodies more likely to be an indicator of a pathologic process (e.g., cow's-milk allergy or celiac disease, respectively).

The increased susceptibility of young infants to food-allergic reactions appears to be the result of both immunologic and gastrointestinal tract immaturity. The relatively low concentration of secretory IgA in the intestine of young infants, together with large quantities of ingested proteins, contributes to the large amount of food antigens confronting gut-associated lymphoid tissue. In genetically predisposed infants, these antigens may stimulate excessive production of IgE antibodies or other abnormal immune responses.

Exclusive breast-feeding may prevent some food allergy and atopic dermatitis. Possible mechanisms are decreased exposure to foreign proteins, breast-milk sIgA that provides passive protection against foreign proteins and pathogens, and soluble factors in breast milk that may induce earlier maturation of the gastrointestinal tract barrier. Soluble factors in human milk may also stimulate lymphocytes to mature.

CLINICAL SYMPTOMS (Table 232-1)

Gastrointestinal Food Hypersensitivity

A number of gastrointestinal syndromes are associated with both IgE-mediated and nonIgE-mediated food allergies.

Oral Allergy Syndrome

Pruritus and edema of the lips, tongue, palate, and throat may be the first symptoms of a more generalized food-allergic reaction or may be the sole manifestations of ingesting a food allergen. Generally, this oral allergy syndrome occurs with the ingestion of fresh fruits and raw vegetables. These patients may have allergic

TABLE 232-1. Symptoms Substantiated by Controlled Food Challenges

Generalized anaphylaxis with cardiovascular collapse (sometimes exercise-associated)
Respiratory symptoms
Upper airway (rhinoconjunctivitis, laryngeal edema)
Lower airway (wheezing, asthma)
Cutaneous
Urticaria-angioedema
Atopic dermatitis
Exercise-associated urticaria
Dermatitis herpetiformis
Gastrointestinal symptoms
IgE-mediated (lip swelling, palatal itching, tongue swelling, nausea, abdominal pain, cramps, emesis, diarrhea)
Celiac disease and dermatitis herpetiformis
Protein-induced enterocolitis (vomiting, diarrhea, rarely shock)
Protein gastroenteropathy, especially to soy and milk (diarrhea, gross or occult blood loss, malabsorption, failure to thrive)
Protein-induced colitis (diarrhea, gross blood loss)
Heiner syndrome (pulmonary infiltrates, iron-deficiency anemia, emesis, diarrhea, and failure to thrive)
Colic (cow's milk–induced, allergen in breast milk)
Allergic eosinophilic gastroenteritis
Neurologic symptoms
Migraine

pollenosis. For example, oral symptoms after the ingestion of raw potatoes, carrots, celery, apples, and hazelnuts are associated with birch pollen allergy; and symptoms secondary to bananas and melons are associated with ragweed sensitivity. Many children can experience symptoms when ingesting raw, pitted fruit (e.g., cherries, peaches, plums) but have no reaction when such fruit has been cooked.

Gastrointestinal Anaphylaxis

Nausea, abdominal pain, cramps, vomiting, and (less frequently) diarrhea develop within minutes to 2 hours of ingesting a food allergen in IgE-mediated gastrointestinal allergy. Repeated ingestion, however, can result in partial desensitization of GI mast cells and subclinical symptoms such as poor appetite, periodic abdominal pain, and poor weight gain. Improved appetite and catch-up weight gain may follow elimination of the responsible food allergen.

Allergic Eosinophilic Gastroenteritis

Patients may present with postprandial vomiting, gastroesophageal reflux, abdominal pain, diarrhea, and weight loss. Approximately one-half of patients will have peripheral blood eosinophilia. NonIgE-mediated food hypersensitivity appears to be responsible for symptoms in most patients with allergic eosinophilic gastroenteritis but, in a subset, IgE-mediated food allergy is responsible for symptoms. Generally, patients with IgE-mediated food-induced symptoms have other atopic symptoms, elevated serum IgE levels, and skin-prick tests positive to a variety of foods and inhalants.

Approximately 40% of infants who are younger than 1 year and experience gastroesophageal reflux were found to have milk-induced allergic eosinophilic esophagitis and reflux. Elimination of cow's-milk formula led to resolution of symptoms.

Infantile Colic

Food hypersensitivity can be implicated in 15% of colicky infants. Most infants "outgrow" their sensitivity within 1 to 2 years.

Food-Induced Enterocolitis Syndrome

Young infants who are between ages 1 week and 3 months and have food hypersensitivity may present with protracted vomiting and diarrhea resulting in dehydration. Most often, cow's milk or soy proteins are responsible, but egg-, rice-, and peanut-induced enterocolitis has also been reported. Generally, stools of affected infants contain occult blood, eosinophils, and polymorphonuclear neutrophils. IgE food-specific antibodies are absent. Generally, elimination of the responsible food leads to resolution of symptoms within 72 hours. The diagnosis is confirmed by oral food challenge. Children with cow's-milk sensitivity should be placed on a hypoallergenic protein-hydrolysate formula until approximately 9 to 12 months of age because as many as 50% may develop a similar sensitivity to soy. The majority of these children appear to outgrow their hypersensitivity in 1 to 2 years.

Food-Induced Proctocolitis

These healthy appearing infants can present in the first few months of life with gross blood in the stool. This syndrome is generally due to cow's-milk or soy-protein hypersensitivity. In infants who are breast-fed, the reaction is to antigens passed in maternal breast milk. Mucosal lesions are confined to the distal large bowel. Generally, gross hematochezia resolves within 72 hours of appropriate food allergen elimination, but resolution of the mucosal lesions may take several weeks. Reintroduction of the responsible food leads to resumption of symptoms within hours to days. Food-induced proctocolitis resolves after 6 months to 2 years of allergen avoidance.

Food-Induced Enteropathy (Malabsorption) Syndromes

Excluding celiac disease (see Chapter 198), diarrhea (frequently fat and carbohydrate malabsorption), vomiting and poor weight gain in the first few months of life may be secondary to a variety of food proteins including those in cow's milk, soy, wheat and other cereal grains, and egg. Cow's-milk sensitivity appears to be the most frequent cause of this syndrome. Elimination from the diet brings about resolution of symptoms, but this process may require several days to weeks. Complete resolution of the intestinal lesions may require 6 to 18 months of food allergen avoidance.

Respiratory Reactions

Double-blind placebo-controlled oral food challenges (DBPCFC) can provoke both upper and lower respiratory symptoms. Food allergens may induce tearing and periorbital pruritus and erythema, nasal congestion, and rhinorrhea. Similarly, pulmonary function studies during DBPCFCs demonstrate significant drops in pulmonary function in those patients with a positive test.

Consumption of food allergens is rarely the main aggravating factor in chronic rhinoconjunctivitis and asthma. Asthmatic children with food-induced wheezing may be identified by an atopic dermatitis or a history of eczema.

Cutaneous Reactions

The skin is the most common target organ in IgE-mediated food hypersensitivity. Ingestion of food allergens may provoke rapid onset of cutaneous symptoms or aggravate more chronic conditions.

Urticaria-Angioedema

Acute urticaria and angioedema are among the most common symptoms of food-allergic reactions. The foods incriminated most commonly include eggs, milk, peanuts, and nuts in children, and fish, shellfish, nuts, and peanuts in adults. Food hypersensitivity is an uncommon (less than 10%) cause of chronic urticaria and angioedema (symptoms lasting longer than 6 weeks).

Atopic Dermatitis

IgE-mediated food allergy plays a role in approximately 25%–40% of children with moderate to severe atopic dermatitis. Repeated ingestion of food allergen leads to chronic inflammation and the typical eczematous lesions (see Chapter 233, Atopic Dermatitis).

Generalized Anaphylactic Reaction

Systemic anaphylaxis is an acute, potentially fatal, immunologically mediated reaction involving many organ systems. Systemic symptoms include tongue swelling and itching, palatal itching, throat itching and tightness, nausea, abdominal pain, emesis, diarrhea, dyspnea, wheezing, cyanosis, chest pain, urticaria, angioedema, hypotension, and shock. Peanuts, tree nuts, and seafood are most often responsible for severe life-threatening reactions. Food ingestion is also implicated as a co-factor in some cases of exercise-induced anaphylaxis.

DIAGNOSIS

The medical history should explore symptom type, severity, frequency, and timing after certain ingestions. Cofactors (e.g., exercise) relating to symptoms should also be sought. In general, symptoms occurring soon after ingestion are more likely to be due to food hypersensitivity than those that take hours or days to develop. There are no specific findings that are unique on the physical examination in individuals with food hypersensitivity, but the physical may exclude some disorders in the differential diagnosis.

Various diagnostic studies (e.g., radiographic studies) exclude many anatomic and metabolic abnormalities. Laboratory studies such as skin-prick tests and tests for IgE-specific food antibodies are of some value in determining the foods responsible for immediate, IgE-mediated hypersensitivity reactions.

Generally, to establish whether a patient has food hypersensitivity, a provocative oral food challenge is necessary. Food challenges may be openly performed, when both the patient and the physician know the contents of the challenge; may be single-blind, when only the physician is aware of the contents of the challenge; or may be double-blind, when neither the patient nor the physician knows the contents of the challenge. Placebo controls are necessary in the blinded challenges. Only the double-blind procedure is free of inherent bias on the part of the patient and the physician. Several studies comparing results of single-blind and double-blind challenges in the same patient population have demonstrated the necessity of removing observer bias. For research purposes, the DBPCFC should be the gold standard for diagnosing food allergy.

The DBPCFC is not practical for all settings. Table 232-2 outlines a more useful approach for the office setting.

TREATMENT

Strict avoidance of the offending food allergen is the only proven therapy for food sensitivity. Drugs may modify symptoms in some cases but are not curative.

TABLE 232-2. Evaluating Food Sensitivity

History and physical examination
History; Stress types of symptoms, timing, severity, and reproducibility.
Physical examination: Exclude many possibilities in the differential diagnosis.
Laboratory tests
Studies to be performed are suggested by the history and physical examination (e.g., radiography, breath hydrogen, sweat test).
Skin tests (prick technique with commercial extract or fresh food):
If negative (wheal <3 mm), immediate hypersensitivity is very unlikely, and further workup probably is unnecessary.
If positive (wheal >3 mm), proceed to the next step.
Strict allergen-avoidance diet for 2 weeks
Include foods suggested by the history for most sensitivities, as well as foods suggested by skin-prick tests for immediate hypersensitivity.
If improvement is unequivocal and only one major or one or two minor foods are involved, continue the restricted diet.
If improvement is equivocal or more than two foods are involved, refer patient to an allergist or gastroenterologist for evaluation.

Generally, infants sensitive to cow's milk can be managed adequately with hypoallergenic formulas such as Alimentum or Nutramigen. Most infants with IgE-mediated cow's-milk allergy can be given soy formulas, but infants with cow's-milk protein-induced enterocolitis syndrome develop sensitivity to soy in as many as 50% of cases. Most infants with food sensitivity can have their diets expanded appropriately (i.e., addition of fruits, vegetables, and meats) without difficulty. Adding only one new food every 3 to 5 days, however, is probably a useful practice.

Children older than 2 years rarely, if ever, require an elemental diet for treatment of food sensitivity, except for some children with allergic eosinophilic gastroenteritis. Generally, appropriate oral challenge studies reveal only one or two specific food sensitivities in more than 90% of cases. The most practical method for implementing strict allergen avoidance diets is to teach parents (and older patients) to carefully read food labels. A dietitian's assistance in suggesting alternative food preparation techniques and assuring a nutritionally sufficient diet is invaluable.

Caregivers of children with IgE-mediated food allergies need to be instructed in the care of allergic reactions in case of accidental ingestions. A formal emergency plan should be developed and injectable epinephrine (EpiPen or Ana Kit) should be available at all times. The Food Allergy Network [Fairfax, VA; tel. (800) 929-4040; www.foodallergy.org] has excellent educational material for patients, parents, schools, and physicians.

Strict allergen avoidance can lead to development of tolerance to offending foods. Virtually all young infants experiencing diarrhea in response to cow's milk or soy protein lose their sensitivity in 1 to 3 years. Infants who are younger than 2 years and experience mild reactions may be rechallenged every 4 to 6 months to ascertain whether symptoms persist. Older patients may be rechallenged every 1 to 2 years depending on the degree of difficulty in avoiding the food in question. Because loss of sensitivity varies with the antigen, rechallenging with some particularly offending foods (such as peanuts and shellfish) should be considered only in consultation with an allergist. In certain disorders such as celiac disease, restricted diets should be continued indefinitely.

CHAPTER 233
Atopic Dermatitis

Adapted from Hugh A. Sampson

EPIDEMIOLOGY

Studies suggest that atopic dermatitis affects between 12% and 15% of the pediatric population. Approximately 60% of affected patients develop symptoms within the first year of life, and approximately 90% develop symptoms within the first 5 years.

DEFINITION AND CLINICAL FEATURES

Atopic dermatitis is a chronic cutaneous inflammatory disorder. The skin symptoms generally present as an erythematous, papulovesicular eruption that progresses to a scaly, lichenified dermatitis over time. The distribution of the rash typically varies with age.

In infancy, the cheeks, wrists, and extensor surfaces of the arms and legs typically develop papulovesicular lesions. The scalp and postauricular area are frequently affected. Generally

TABLE 233-1. Diagnostic Features of Atopic Dermatitis

Major features*
Pruritus
Typical morphology and distribution
  Flexural lichenification or hyperlinearity in adults
  Facial and extensor involvement in infants and children
Chronic or chronically relapsing course
Personal or family history of atopy (asthma, allergic rhinitis, or atopic dermatitis)
Minor features*
Xerosis
Ichthyosis, palmar hyperlinearity, keratosis pilaris
Immediate (type I) skin test reactivity
Elevated serum IgE
Early age of onset
Tendency toward cutaneous infections (especially *Staphylococcus aureus* and herpes simplex), impaired cell-mediated immunity
Tendency toward nonspecific hand or foot dermatitis
Nipple eczema
Cheilitis
Recurrent conjunctivitis
Dennie-Morgan infraorbital fold
Keratoconus
Anterior subcapsular cataracts
Orbital darkening
Facial pallor, facial erythema
Pityriasis alba
Itch when sweating
Intolerance to wool and lipid solvents
Perifollicular accentuation
Food hypersensitivity
Course influenced by environmental/emotional factors
White dermographism, delayed blanch

*Must have three or more major and three or more minor criteria.

the diaper area is spared, even if the eczematous eruption involves the entire body.

In children (2–12 years), flexor surfaces, neck, wrists, and ankles are generally involved with dry maculopapular lesions being a more prominent feature. Pruritus and scratching lead to excoriations, hyperpigmentation, and lichenification.

In the teenaged patient and young adult, flexural surfaces, face (especially periorbital), hands, and feet are frequently involved. Extreme xerosis and lichenification are characteristic of this stage.

Unlike most dermatoses, atopic dermatitis has no primary skin lesion but is identified by a constellation of symptoms. The diagnostic features are presented in Table 233-1 with a modification for the young infant in Table 233-2.

TABLE 233-2. Diagnostic Features of Atopic Dermatitis for Infants

Major features*
Family history of atopic disease
Typical facial or extensor eczematous or lichenified dematitis
Evidence of pruritus
Minor features*
Xerosis, ichthyosis, hyperlinear palms
Perifollicular accentuation
Postauricular fissures
Chronic scalp scaling

*Must have three or more of both major and minor criteria.

No laboratory test exists that indicates atopic dermatitis. Peripheral blood eosinophilia is present in 5% to 20% and elevated total serum IgE concentrations are present in approximately 80% of patients. Test results for specific IgE antibodies to foods and inhalants are positive in at least 80% of pediatric patients.

PATHOPHYSIOLOGY

Itch is the dominant symptom in atopic dermatitis and the major cause of damaging excoriations and lichenification. The local release of inflammatory mediators is likely responsible for increased pruritus.

Increased transepidermal water loss is believed to be secondary to decreased sebum production and is also a universal feature. Sweating is thought to be abnormally increased in these patients.

IMMUNOLOGIC ABNORMALITIES

Abnormalities of both humoral and cellular immunity have been described in patients with atopic dermatitis. These include elevated serum IgE concentrations in approximately 80% of children; defective delayed-type skin responsiveness to various antigens; variably decreased lymphocyte responses to mitogens, recall antigens, and alloantigens *in vitro*; defective generation of cytotoxic T-lymphocyte response *in vitro*; and variably decreased phagocytic capacity and chemotaxis of neutrophils and monocytes. These defects generally fluctuate with disease activity and may revert to normal during long remissions.

The nearly constant presence of S. aureus (colonizing the skin in more than 90% of patients) suggests microbiocidal dysfunction. S. aureus can lead to flares of dermatitis, as well as skin infections. Flares may be related to hypersensitivity to Staphylococcus exotoxins.

Studies indicate depressed cell-mediated T_H1-type functions in patients with atopic dermatitis. There is increased susceptibility to certain viral infections: herpes simplex (eczema herpeticum), verruca vulgaris (common warts), molluscum contagiosum and, rarely, vaccinia. Dermatophyte infections are also more common in patients with atopic dermatitis. Eczematous lesions in atopic dermatitis show infiltration of $CD4^+$ T_H2-type lymphocytes. These cells antagonize T_H1-type responses, probably accounting for the depressed cell-mediated function seen in the skin.

ETIOLOGY

The etiology of atopic dermatitis is not entirely known. The interaction of allergens with allergen-specific IgE on the surface of mast cells and Langerhans cells leads to the release of a variety of inflammatory mediators. Mast cells release histamine, leukotriene C_4 (LTC_4), platelet-activating factor, tryptase, cytokines, and other factors that attract and activate inflammatory cells. IgE-bearing Langerhans cells have been shown to be highly efficient in activating T_H2-type lymphocytes. Repeated allergen exposure provokes chronic inflammation secondary to IgE-mediated mast cell and lymphocytic responses and contributes to the pathogenesis of atopic dermatitis.

Inhalant allergens (pollens, molds, and dust mites) may also play a role in IgE-induced pathology. Normal individuals passively sensitized to ragweed absorb sufficient pollen allergen via nasal challenge to produce a wheal-and-flare response at a distal skin site.

DIAGNOSIS

The diagnosis of atopic dermatitis is based on the presence of sufficient major and minor criteria (Tables 233-1–233-2). In the differential diagnosis of atopic dermatitis, seborrheic dermatitis and allergic contact dermatitis are confused most frequently. Seborrheic dermatitis often has a more frequent distribution in the axillae and diaper area, less prominent pruritus, and general absence of elevated serum total IgE and positive skin test results to foods and inhalants. Other less common disorders may be mistaken for atopic dermatitis: hyper-IgE syndrome, Wiskott–Aldrich syndrome, and Langerhans cell histiocytosis.

THERAPY

Many trigger factors are known to exacerbate flares of eczema. These include irritants (soaps, chemicals), heat and humidity, infection, allergens, stress, and sweating. Successful management relies on which triggers exist for each patient and instructing the patient and family on avoidance whenever possible.

Bathing in hot water and scrubbing vigorously with soap is a frequent source of irritation. Patients should be encouraged to bathe in tepid water (especially for hydration), avoid soap, and pat dry with soft absorbent towels. Clothing should be rinsed carefully after washing to remove all residual detergent.

Thermal change, exercise, or anxiety can induce sweating, generally leading to cutaneous pruritus, scratching, and subsequent skin changes. Measures taken to avoid sweating such as keeping the environment cool will prevent this.

Infection is typically suspected in the presence of acute weeping or crusted lesions and small superficial pustules, but it should also be suspected in recalcitrant cases of eczema. The most likely organism, Staphylococcus, may be resistant to multiple antibiotics and treatment is best guided by results of skin culture and sensitivity tests. When lesions fail to respond to oral antibiotics, herpes simplex infection should be considered. A Tzanck smear or viral culture can aid in diagnosis. Topical or systemic (oral or intravenous) acyclovir should be administered. Superimposed dermatophyte infections can lead to flares of dermatitis. These infections respond readily to either locally applied dacarbazine (Imidazole) creams or oral griseofulvin daily for 1 month.

Patients or their parents are generally aware that stress, anxiety, anger, and frustration provoke pruritus and flares of atopic dermatitis. Patients should be encouraged to verbalize their emotional conflicts and, occasionally, psychological counseling may be sought. In children, potential stressful situations in the home or school should be assessed and discussed.

Several general measures may be taken to reduce pruritus and consequent skin damage secondary to scratching. Fingernails should be trimmed short and cotton gloves may be worn at night. Skin hydration is of critical importance. Bathing for hydration in tepid water for 20 to 30 minutes followed by immediate application of an ointment or cream is the most effective form of therapy. Lubricant creams and ointments (Aquaphor, Cetaphil, Eucerin, Lubriderm, petrolatum, Vanicream, etc.) should be applied within 3 minutes of the child getting out of the tub to seal in moisture so that water absorbed into the stratum corneum does not evaporate.

Topical corticosteroids are the mainstay of therapy for atopic dermatitis. For general management, mid-strength corticosteroids such as 0.1% triamcinolone cream or ointment are optimal. Occasionally, more potent fluorinated corticosteroids are required to suppress an acute flare. Systemic corticosteroids should be avoided in this chronic dermatitis because many patients experience a rebound flare after a short course, which only leads to further requests for systemic therapy.

Several new immunomodulating agents are now FDA approved for use in children with moderate to severe atopic dermatitis. ELIDEL® (pimecrolimus) and PROTOPIC® (tacrolimus) are both highly effective and approved for use in children as young as 2 years old.

COURSE AND PROGNOSIS

The course of atopic dermatitis is marked by unexplained exacerbations and remissions. Recent studies indicate that the majority of patients "outgrow" their eczema but most retain some stigmata of the disorder throughout life. Less favorable prognostic signs include late onset and reverse pattern (involvement of extensor surfaces instead of flexors), severe widespread dermatitis in childhood, family history of atopic dermatitis, and associated allergic rhinitis or asthma. In general, the more severe the symptoms, the less likely is a permanent remission.

CHAPTER 234
Allergic Rhinitis

Adapted from F. Estelle R. Simons

Allergic rhinitis, or inflammation of the nasal mucosa, is the most common chronic disorder of the respiratory tract with physician-diagnosed allergic rhinitis occurring in up to 42% of 6-year-old children in the United States. Many patients with allergic rhinitis have concomitant asthma, allergic conjunctivitis, chronic sinusitis, or otitis media with effusion.

Seasonal allergic rhinitis is caused by nonflowering, wind-pollinated plants. In temperate climates, tree pollens cause symptoms in the early spring, grass pollens cause symptoms in the late spring and early summer, and ragweed and other weed pollens cause symptoms in the late summer and autumn. A priming effect on the nasal mucosa occurs after continued daily allergen exposure. Perennial allergic rhinitis is triggered by animal dander, house dust mites, and molds. In subtropical and tropical climates, pollens cause perennial, rather than seasonal, rhinitis. Food allergens seldom trigger allergic rhinitis symptoms.

PATHOPHYSIOLOGY

In allergic rhinitis, an immediate hypersensitivity response occurs in the nasal mucosa of a person who has become sensitized to inhaled allergens. Allergen-specific immunoglobulin E (IgE) binds to high-affinity receptors on mast cells and basophils. When the patient sensitized to an allergen is reexposed to it, an allergen-IgE antibody reaction occurs within minutes. The bridging of two or more mast cell or basophil-bound IgE molecules by allergen results in mast cell release of cytokines [including interleukin-4 (IL-4), IL-5, IL-13, and granulocyte-macrophage colony-stimulating factor] and chemical mediators of inflammation, both preformed (histamine, tryptase, kinins) and newly formed membrane-derived lipid mediators (prostaglandin D_2, leukotrienes C_4 and D_4), into the extracellular environment. This results in vascular dilitation with plasma exudation and leukocyte diapedesis and consequent mucosal edema. Parasympathetic reflexes are stimulated leading to glandular secretions and rhinorrhea. Stimulation of type C nociceptive nerve fibers results in nasal itching and reduction in the threshold for sneezing.

Two to 8 hours after initial exposure to allergen, and without further exposure, many patients have a late-phase response characterized by infiltration with eosinophils and neutrophils and by fibrin deposition. This response may be followed by infiltration of mononuclear cells such as lymphocytes, macrophages, and fibroblasts and even by tissue destruction.

CLINICAL DIAGNOSIS

The characteristic symptoms of allergic rhinitis are nasal congestion, paroxysmal sneezing, itching, and watery, profuse rhinorrhea. Other symptoms include noisy breathing, oronasal breathing, snoring, loss of olfaction or taste, itching of the palate or pharynx, and repeated throat clearing or cough secondary to drainage of nasal secretions into the pharynx. Ocular symptoms such as redness, itching, or tearing may also be present. Systemic symptoms include malaise and disturbed nocturnal sleep with subsequent daytime fatigue and decreased ability to concentrate and learn.

Children with allergic rhinitis may have allergic shiners, a term used to describe the dark discoloration of the infraorbital regions secondary to obstruction of venous drainage. If they are chronic oronasal breathers, they may have hypertrophied gingival mucosa and halitosis. In contrast to children who breathe through unobstructed nasal passages, they are more likely to have a gaping expression; a long, retrognathic facies with a high, narrow palate; and orthodontic anomalies such as posterior dental crossbite. Pharyngeal lymphoid tissue, adenoids, tonsils, and the lymphoid tissue of the anterior cervical region may be hypertrophied. If adenoidal hypertrophy is severe, obstructive sleep apnea and cor pulmonale may develop.

Examination of the nose of the child with allergic rhinitis sometimes reveals a transverse external wrinkle secondary to rubbing and dorsal manipulation of the nose, also known as the allergic salute. The nasal mucosa usually appears edematous and may be pale, violaceous, or red. Nasal polyps are rare in children; if they are observed, the diagnosis of cystic fibrosis must be ruled out. Examination using an otoscope is not always adequate, and flexible fiberoptic rhinoscopy may be required to differentiate allergic rhinitis from other disorders that cause chronic nasal symptoms (Table 234-1).

TABLE 234-1. Differential Diagnosis of Rhinitis

Allergic rhinitis: seasonal of perennial
Infection: viral or bacterial
Eosinophilic nonallergic rhinitis
Acute or chronic sinusitis
Adenoid hypertrophy
Foreign body
Congenital intranasal lesions (dermoid cysts, meningomyelocele, nasal glioma)
Choanal atresia
Ciliary dyskinesia
Vasomotor rhinitis
Rhinitis medicamentosa (topical decongestants, oral contraceptives, some antihypertensives, beta-adrenergic blockers)
Hormonal changes (pregnancy, hypothyroidism)
Anatomic variations, including nasal septal deviation
Trauma (septal hematoma, fracture of nasal bones, synechiae)
Cerebrospinal fluid rhinorrhea
Granulomatous disease (e.g., Wegener granulomatosis)
Nasal polyps
Neoplasms

DIAGNOSTIC TESTS

The diagnosis of allergic rhinitis can be confirmed by identifying eosinophils as the predominant cells in nasal secretions; these cells also predominate in eosinophilic nonallergic rhinitis.

Skin tests and measurements of allergen-specific IgE may be useful but should not be used to screen patients for allergic rhinitis, because the test results may be positive in patients who are sensitized but who do not have symptoms and do not require treatment.

MANAGEMENT

The management of allergic rhinitis consists of pharmacologic treatment to prevent or relieve symptoms, education of the child and family, avoidance of triggering factors for symptoms and, in some patients, down-regulation of the immune response to airborne allergens using immunotherapy (allergy shots).

In allergic rhinitis, the nasal mucosa is hyperresponsive to both specific (allergens) and nonspecific stimuli (cigarette smoke, paint fumes, perfumes, cold air, etc). Both types of triggers should be avoided. Air-conditioning units and high-efficiency particulate air filter units are helpful.

Major advances have occurred in the pharmacologic treatment of allergic rhinitis. H_1 receptor antagonists (antihistamines) relieve itching, sneezing, and rhinorrhea but are not particularly effective for relieving nasal congestion. Newer "non-sedating" antihistamines such as cetirizine, fexofenadine, or loratadine have a greatly improved side effect profile.

Intranasal sympathomimetics such as xylometazoline and oxymetazoline increase nasal patency and can be helpful acutely but may cause rebound congestion with long-term use (rhinitis medicamentosa). Orally administered sympathomimetics such as pseudoephedrine can cause adverse reactions (hypertension, agitation, hallucinations, and insomnia) and their use should be occasional, if at all, in children.

Disodium cromoglycate (cromolyn sodium) 2% solution (Nasalcrom®) is mildly effective with few side effects. It can prevent sneezing, rhinorrhea, and nasal itching when used four to six times per day.

Intranasal glucocorticoids such as beclomethasone dipropionate, flunisolide, triamcinolone, budesonide, fluticasone propionate, and mometasone furoate have a high ratio of topical to systemic activity and are very effective in the treatment of allergic rhinitis. They decrease sneezing, nasal discharge, itching, and nasal blockage. They act locally in the nasal mucosa by down-regulating cytokine gene expression and modulating the immune response. Effect is generally seen within a few days, but children with seasonal allergic rhinitis should begin using them before the pollen season starts.

Immunotherapy consisting of injections of increasing concentrations of a specific allergen may reduce morbidity and medication requirements in selected patients. The response to immunotherapy is allergen specific and dose related. Immunologic effects produced by immunotherapy include decreased early- and late-phase responses to nasal allergen challenge. The most common adverse effects are large local reactions at the injection sites. Generalized systemic reactions such as anaphylaxis or serum sickness rarely occur.

CHAPTER 235

Primary Immunodeficiency Diseases

Adapted from Howard M. Lederman and Jerry A. Winkelstein

NORMAL IMMUNE SYSTEM

Components of the immune system are found in all parts of the body but are concentrated in the thymus, bone marrow, lymph nodes, spleen, liver, and blood (Fig. 235-1). The integrated system of B lymphocytes, T lymphocytes, phagocytes, and the complement system form an important mechanism for the generation of a normal inflammatory response. This is vital for the host's defense against infection.

Lymphoid System

Lymphoid precursors differentiate along one of two mutually exclusive pathways to become B or T lymphocytes. B lymphocytes are the effector cells of humoral immunity. B lymphocyte differentiation begins with a series of immunoglobulin gene rearrangements to create large numbers of B-lymphocyte clones. Eventually, cytoplasmic immunoglobulin is expressed and the cells reach the preB-cell stage. Further rearrangement of immunoglobulin genes is associated with expression of surface IgM and IgD. At this stage, each B cell has unique antigenic specificity based on the cell membrane immunoglobulin receptor. When antigen binds to this surface immunoglobulin (antibody), B cells proliferate to form a clone of progeny with identical antibody specificity. Further differentiation into plasma cells leads to the secretion of IgM, IgG, IgA, or IgE. For most antigens, optimal B-cell differentiation into plasma cells requires the presence of T-lymphocyte helper cells (T-dependent antigens). Some antigens such as bacterial capsular polysaccharides can trigger B-cell differentiation in the absence of T lymphocytes (T-independent antigens). In all cases, CD4 helper T lymphocytes (T_H) are important modulators of B-cell function influencing the degree, duration, and quality (affinity and class distribution) of the antibody response.

The five major classes of immunoglobulins are IgM, IgG, IgA, IgE, and IgD. IgM is the first immunoglobulin produced in an immune response and is the most efficient activator of complement. IgG is the predominant serum immunoglobulin. It is transported across the placenta, possesses opsonic activity, and activates complement. IgA is secreted onto mucosal surfaces and prevents microbial adherence and penetration across these surfaces. IgE is a mediator of allergic disease but can play a role in host defense against parasitic infections.

T lymphocytes are the effectors for cell-mediated immunity. They serve to regulate both humoral and cell-mediated immunity. Differentiation of T lymphocytes occurs in the thymus. In the absence of antigen, T-lymphocyte clones with various antigenic specificities are generated by rearrangements of T-cell antigen receptor genes. After these gene rearrangements, the T-cell antigen receptor is expressed on the surface of the T lymphocyte.

T lymphocytes further mature along functionally distinct pathways. Initially, double-positive CD4/CD8 thymocytes differentiate into a CD4 subset that regulates immune responses (T_H) and a CD8 subset that functions as cytotoxic effectors in cell-mediated immunity [cytotoxic T lymphocytes (T_C)].

CD4 T lymphocytes carry out immunoregulatory functions by the release of soluble protein mediators [i.e., lymphokines, cytokines, or interleukins (ILs)]. When CD4 T_H lymphocytes proliferate, they differentiate into T_H1 or T_H2 cells, which have very different functions. T_H1 cells secrete cytokines that stimulate cell-mediated immune responses such as activation of macrophage bactericidal function, delayed-type hypersensitivity, and cytotoxicity. T_H2 cells secrete cytokines that drive B-cell proliferation resulting in antibody synthesis.

T_C cells are able to kill target cells such as virus-infected host cells, tumor cells, or the cells of a histoincompatible tissue graft. This is achieved by the cells reversibly binding and releasing cytotoxins into their target cell.

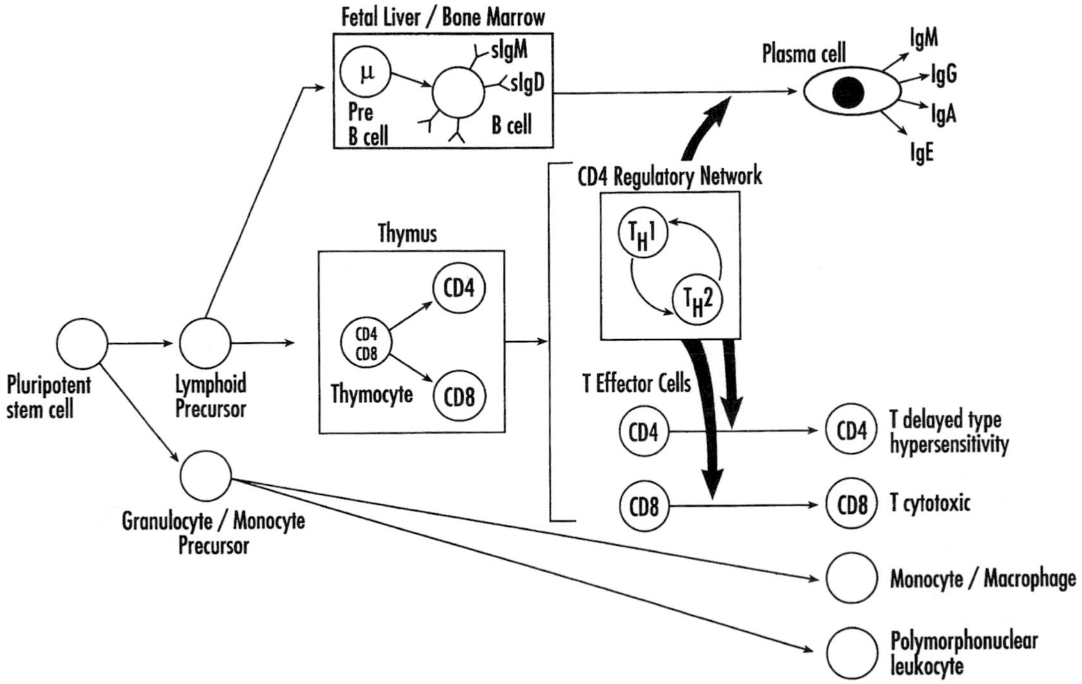

Figure 235-1. The cells of the immune system.

Phagocytic Cells

Phagocytic cells ingest foreign antigens and microorganisms. Some phagocytic cells are able to move to sites of microbial invasion or inflammation while others reside in fixed locations serving to clear microorganisms and other particulate matter from the circulation. Neutrophils and the cells of the monocyte-macrophage system are the most important phagocytes of the immune system. Monocytes and macrophages also present antigen to lymphoid cells and secrete a variety of proinflammatory substances including cytokines and complement components.

To function properly, phagocytic cells must attach to a substrate (adherence), move through tissues toward the site of microbial invasion (chemotaxis), attach to opsonized microbes and ingest them (phagocytosis), and finally kill the microbes (intracellular killing). Clinical disorders in which some of these necessary steps are defective are discussed in Chapter 238.

Complement System

The complement system refers to a number of serum proteins that mediate a variety of defensive and inflammatory responses. The majority of the biologically significant effects of the complement system are mediated by the third component (C3) and the terminal components (C5–C9). To subserve their biologic functions, C3 and C5 through C9 must first be activated via either the classical or alternative complement pathway.

Whether C3 is activated via the classical or alternative complement pathway, two fragments of unequal size are produced, C3a and C3b. C3a acts as an anaphylatoxin. Although most C3b is rapidly hydrolyzed, some binds to the surface of the activating cells and can act as an opsonin.

Further activation of C5 creates two additional cleavage products C5a and C5b. C5a can act as an anaphylatoxin. It also has potent chemotactic activity. C5b can combine with native C6. It can then initiate the formation of a membrane attack complex, a multimolecular assembly of C5b, C6, C7, C8, and C9. This complex is inserted into cell membranes and is responsible for the cytolytic and bactericidal actions of complement.

CLINICAL PRESENTATION OF PRIMARY IMMUNODEFICIENCY DISEASES

Collectively, the primary immunodeficiency diseases are not rare disorders. Manifestations can include increased susceptibility to infection, as well as autoimmune or chronic inflammatory disorders.

Increased Susceptibility to Infection

Children with primary immunodeficiency diseases most commonly present with an increased susceptibility to infection. Infections may not necessarily be more severe than in normal hosts but may be recurrent, chronic, or caused by an unusual organism (e.g., *Pneumocystis carinii*).

Infections with certain microorganisms are characteristically found in specific immunodeficiency diseases. For example, patients with abnormalities of cell-mediated immunity characteristically develop *P. carinii* pneumonia, disseminated fungal infections, mucocutaneous candidiasis, overwhelming viral infections, and severe mycobacterial disease. Patients with defects of antibody or complement more often have infections with pyogenic encapsulated bacteria. Patients with phagocytic defects develop bacterial and fungal infections of the skin and reticuloendothelial system. While helpful in directing the evaluation of suspected patients, these distinctions are not absolute. For example, a rare patient with an antibody deficiency can develop pneumocystis pneumonia or chronic enteroviral meningitis. Recurrent infections at a single anatomic site should always prompt consideration of other predisposing conditions such as ciliary dyskinesia, cystic fibrosis, bronchial obstruction, or a basilar skull fracture. Patterns of illness and screening tests for primary immunodeficiency disorders are outlined in Table 235-1.

Autoimmune and Inflammatory Disorders

Immunodeficiency may also lead to abnormal immunoregulatory mechanisms with the result being autoimmune or chronic inflammatory diseases. Patients with primary immunodeficiency diseases can present with disorders such as autoimmune hemolytic anemia or immune thrombocytopenia, autoimmune endocrinopathy, juvenile rheumatoid arthritis, a lupus-like illness, or inflammatory bowel disease. This type of presentation is most often seen in patients with common variable immunodeficiency, selective IgA deficiency, chronic mucocutaneous candidiasis, and deficiencies of the classical complement pathway.

Immunodeficiency Syndromes

Some immunodeficiencies can be seen as part of a syndrome complex (Table 235-2). For instance, children with the DiGeorge

TABLE 235-1. Patterns of Illness and Screening Tests for Primary Immunodeficiency

Disorder	Illnesses: *Infection*	Illnesses: *Other*	Diagnostic tests
Antibody	Sinopulmonary (pyogenic bacteria, viruses); gastrointestinal (enterovirus, giardia)	Autoimmune disease (autoantibodies, inflammatory bowel disease)	Quantitative immunoglobulin levels (IgG, IgA, IgM); antibody responses to immunization
Cell-mediated immunity	Pneumonia (pyogenic bacteria, *Pneumocystis carinii*, viruses); gastrointestinal (viruses); skin, mucous membranes (fungi)		Lymphocyte count; delayed-type hypersensitivity tests; T-lymphocyte subsets (CD4, CD8)
Complement	Sepsis and other blood-borne (streptococci, pneumococci, *Neisseria*)	Autoimmune disease (systemic lupus erythematosus, glomerulonephritis)	Total hemolytic complement (CH50)
Phagocytosis	Skin, reticuloendothelial system (staphylococci, enteric bacteria, fungi, mycobacteria)		White blood count and differential; nitroblue tetrazolium dye test

TABLE 235-2. Examples of Syndromes in which Immunodeficiency Occurs

Syndrome	Clinical presentation	Immunologic abnormality
Acrodermatitis enteropathica	Dermatitis, alopecia, diarrhea	Variable B- and T-lymphocyte deficiency
Ataxia-telangiectasia	Ataxia, telangiectasia	Variable B- and T-lymphocyte deficiency
Cartilage hair hypoplasia	Short-limbed dwarfism, sparse hair	Neutropenia, T-lymphocyte deficiency
Centromeric instability syndrome	Dysmorphic facies, ataxia, developmental delay	Variable B- and T-lymphocyte deficiency
Chédiak-Higashi syndrome	Oculocutaneous albinism	Abnormal neutrophil function
DiGeorge anomaly	Congenital heart disease, dysmorphic facies, hypoparathyroidism	T-lymphocyte deficiency
Hyperimmunoglobulin E syndrome	Coarse facies, eczematoid rash, elevated IgE	Neutrophil chemotactic defect
Ivemark syndrome	Heterotaxia Bilateral three-lobed lungs Midline liver Discordance of cardiac and abdominal situs Congenital heart disease	Asplenia
Polyendocrinopathy syndrome	Endocrine organ dysfunction	Mucocutaneous candidiasis
Wiskott-Aldrich syndrome	Thrombocytopenia, eczema	Variable B- and T-lymphocyte deficiency

anomaly are usually often initially identified because of the neonatal presentation of congenital heart disease or tetany. This leads to the recognition that they have a T-lymphocyte defect before any infections occur.

LABORATORY EVALUATION OF THE CHILD WITH SUSPECTED IMMUNODEFICIENCY

Indications for screening include any child with a history of severe, chronic or recurrent infections, infection caused by an unusual organism, autoimmune disorders, or recognition of an immunodeficiency syndrome. A diagnostic evaluation should also be considered for any child with infections that exceed the norm for the clinician's own experience considering such factors as day-care attendance, etc. As stated above, selection of which screening tests to perform should be based on the spectrum of problems in a given patient. Consideration must always be given to secondary immunodeficiencies (e.g., HIV infection or complications of medication therapy).

Examination of the Peripheral Blood Smear

Neutropenia may occur secondary to immunosuppressive drugs, infection, malnutrition, autoimmunity, or as a primary problem (congenital or cyclic neutropenia). A persistent neutrophilia with a predominance of immature forms is characteristic of leukocyte adhesion molecule deficiency, and abnormal cytoplasmic granules may be seen in the peripheral blood smear of patients with Chédiak–Higashi syndrome (see Chapter 238).

Lymphopenia may be a presenting feature of T-cell or combined immunodeficiency disorders such as severe combined immunodeficiency disease or DiGeorge syndrome.

Thrombocytopenia may occur as a secondary manifestation of immunodeficiency but is often a presenting manifestation of the Wiskott–Aldrich syndrome.

Examination of red blood cell morphology may reveal Howell–Jolly bodies suggestive of splenic dysfunction or asplenia. The absence of Howell–Jolly bodies, however, does not guarantee normal splenic function.

Evaluation of Humoral Immunity

The measurement of serum immunoglobulin levels is readily available, highly reliable, and relatively inexpensive. It is useful as a screening test because more than 80% of patients with primary disorders of immunity have abnormalities of serum immunoglobulins.

Quantitative measurements of serum IgG, IgA, and IgM can identify patients with panhypogammaglobulinemia, as well as those with deficiencies of an individual class of immunoglobulins such as selective IgA deficiency. Age-related normal values must always be used for comparison. In some instances, the total serum IgG may be normal or near-normal, but the patient may still have an IgG subclass deficiency. Thus, measurements of individual IgG subclasses should be performed when total serum IgG is normal in a child strongly suspected of humoral immunodeficiency.

Assessment of antibody function should always be included as part of the evaluation of humoral immunity. Antibody titers generated in response to childhood immunization with protein or polysaccharide antigens can be measured in selected reference laboratories.

If immunoglobulin levels and functional antibody titers are decreased, the evaluation should proceed with enumeration of B lymphocytes in the peripheral blood. Further specialized tests may be necessary to delineate the specific functional B-cell defect. These may include *in vitro* studies of mitogen or antigen-driven B-cell proliferation and immunoglobulin secretion.

Evaluation of Cell-Mediated Immunity

Findings such as lymphopenia or the lack of a thymus on a chest radiograph may be suggestive of a T-cell deficiency, if present. These findings, however, may be seen in normal children and may not necessarily be present in patients with T-lymphocyte defects.

Delayed-type hypersensitivity skin testing with a panel of antigens is an excellent screening method for older children (older than 12 months). It lacks predictive value in younger children. The presence of one or more positive delayed-type skin test results is generally indicative of intact cell-mediated immunity. Besides age of the patient, other significant limitations exist to this testing. For example, normal patients may have transient depression of delayed-type hypersensitivity with acute viral infections.

Enumeration of T-lymphocytes to provide quantitative information on total T ($CD2^+$ or $CD3^+$), T_H ($CD4^+$), and T_C ($CD8^+$) cells can be performed with monoclonal antibodies. Patients with severe combined immunodeficiency and DiGeorge anomaly generally have decreased numbers of both $CD4^+$ and $CD8^+$ T lymphocytes. Patients infected with the human immunodeficiency virus have decreased numbers of $CD4^+$ lymphocytes.

Other specialized tests of cell-mediated immunity include the measurement of lymphocyte proliferation *in vitro* after stimulation with mitogens, antigens, or allogeneic cells. Production of lymphokines and cytotoxic effector function can be measured as well.

Evaluation of Phagocytic Cells

Deficiencies may be characterized by abnormal phagocyte number or function. Disorders with abnormal cell numbers such as congenital agranulocytosis or cyclic neutropenia can be detected using the complete blood count and white cell differential.

Assessment of phagocytic cell function includes assays of phagocyte motility (chemotaxis), ingestion (phagocytosis), and intracellular killing (bactericidal activity). Selected tests are discussed in Chapter 238.

Evaluation of the Complement System

Most deficiencies of the classical activating pathway of C3, of C3 itself, and of the terminal components (C5, C6, C7, C8, and C9) can be detected using a total serum hemolytic complement (CH_{50}) assay. This assay depends on the functional integrity of C1 through C9. Therefore, a severe deficiency of any component leads to a marked reduction or absence of total hemolytic complement activity. Other assays exist to detect deficiencies of components of the alternative pathway. Highly specific assays have been developed for each of the individual components of the complement system. These assays have become widely available but care should be taken to have such tests performed by a reliable laboratory.

CHAPTER 236

Disorders of Humoral Immunity

Adapted from Howard M. Lederman

Antibodies may serve in host defense without the participation of other components of the immune system. These functions include neutralization of viruses and inhibition of microbial adherence. Antibody-mediated functions also exist such as activation of complement and opsonization for phagocytosis. When combined, these mechanisms are effective against extracellular pathogens such as encapsulated bacteria (e.g. *Streptococcus pneumoniae*). Humoral immunity is generally less important in the host's defense against intracellular bacteria, fungi, or protozoa.

X-LINKED AGAMMAGLOBULINEMIA

X-linked agammaglobulinemia (X-LA) is the prototypic disorder of humoral immunity. Male patients with this disease have severe panhypogammaglobulinemia with little or no humoral immune function but intact cell-mediated immunity. These patients have B-lymphocyte precursors (preB cells) but do not have mature B lymphocytes or plasma cells. T lymphocytes and all other components of the immune system are normal.

X-LA is caused by mutation of the gene on the X chromosome encoding a cytoplasmic tyrosine kinase (Bruton's tyrosine kinase). The absence of this tyrosine kinase results in a developmental arrest of B-lymphocyte maturation at the preB cell stage. In female carriers of X-LA, all mature B lymphocytes have inactivated the abnormal X chromosome because lack of expression of the normal gene blocks B-cell differentiation.

Boys with X-LA have normal numbers of T lymphocytes but have no detectable B lymphocytes. In contrast, infants with panhypogammaglobulinemia due to transient hypogammaglobulinemia or common variable immunodeficiency (see below) generally have normal numbers of B and T lymphocytes; children with severe combined immunodeficiency have decreased numbers of T lymphocytes with normal, decreased, or increased numbers of B cells; and children with HIV infection have decreased numbers of $CD4^+$ T lymphocytes.

Boys with X-LA are generally protected by transplacental IgG for the first 3 to 4 months of life. Thereafter, chronic and recurrent infections such as otitis media, pneumonia, diarrhea, and sinusitis begin to occur. *S. pneumoniae*, *H. influenzae*, and *Staphylococcus aureus* are the most frequently identified bacterial pathogens, but nontypable, unencapsulated *H. influenzae*, *Salmonellae*, *Pseudomonas*, and *Mycoplasma* infections occur with increased frequency. Deeper seeded infections such as bacterial meningitis, sepsis, and osteomyelitis occur in as many as 15% of untreated patients. Hypoplastic or absent tonsils, adenoids, or lymph nodes may be noted on physical examination, a marker of the absence of B lymphocytes.

Gamma globulin replacement therapy is highly effective in reducing the incidence of systemic bacterial infections. Enterovirus infections (coxsackie, echovirus, and polio) can cause chronic diarrhea, hepatitis, pneumonitis, and meningoencephalitis in patients with X-LA. These infections are often fatal in patients with X-LA, although therapy with extremely high doses of gamma globulin containing virus-specific antibodies has been helpful.

Early diagnosis of X-LA is critical to initiate gamma globulin therapy before the onset of chronic pulmonary disease or chronic enterovirus infections. Furthermore, families need to be provided with appropriate genetic counseling. Gamma globulin prophylaxis and an aggressive approach to febrile or inflammatory illnesses can result in a good prognosis in most patients.

IgG SUBCLASS DEFICIENCIES

Four subclasses of IgG exist. IgG1, IgG2, and IgG3 fix complement bind to monocytic Fc receptors and participate in antibody-dependent cellular cytotoxicity. The IgG response to protein antigens occurs within the IgG1 and IgG3 subclasses, IgG response to polysaccharide antigens is generally restricted to the IgG2 and IgG4 subclasses. Deficiencies of IgG2 and IgG4 may predispose the host to infections caused by encapsulated bacteria (*S. pneumoniae* and *H. influenzae*).

Deficiencies of IgG subclasses may occur in association with selective IgA deficiency, ataxia-telangiectasia, and Wiskott–Aldrich syndrome. Patients with IgG subclass deficiencies may have a borderline or low, normal total serum IgG level with recurrent sinopulmonary infections. Quantitation of IgG subclasses, in addition to measurement of antibody responses to protein (e.g., diphtheria and tetanus toxoids) and polysaccharide (e.g., pneumococcal) vaccines, should be the next steps in evaluating such a patient.

Some patients with selective deficiency of IgG2, IgG3, or IgG4, or deficiencies of IgG2 and IgG4, have recurrent pyogenic infections of the respiratory tract. They may benefit from antibiotic prophylaxis. Gamma globulin therapy can be used for patients who, in addition to subclass deficiency, also have documented deficiency of antibody production to protein and polysaccharide vaccines.

COMMON VARIABLE IMMUNODEFICIENCY

The term *common variable immunodeficiency* (CVID) refers to a heterogeneous group of disorders characterized by hypogammaglobulinemia. Unlike X-LA, B lymphocytes are frequently found in the peripheral blood and the hypogammaglobulinemia may be less profound. T-cell dysfunction and autoimmune diseases are expressed variably. Most patients have no recognizable pattern of inheritance, but other disorders of humoral immunity (e.g., IgA deficiency and transient hypogammaglobulinemia of infancy) occur at higher frequency among family members of patients with CVID than among the general population. Many patients with CVID have defects intrinsic to the B lymphocyte, but other patients have excessive T-lymphocyte suppressor function, inadequate T-lymphocyte helper function, or anti-B-lymphocyte antibodies.

Symptoms can be seen in early infancy, but most patients do not develop symptoms until after the first decade of life. Chronic or recurrent respiratory infections with encapsulated bacteria are the most common manifestations. As many as 30% to 60% of patients with CVID have chronic diarrhea due to infectious causes or idiopathic inflammatory bowel diseases. Giardia lamblia is a frequent gastrointestinal pathogen in patients with CVID. Patients with CVID have a variety of associated disorders, which are either infectious or due to disordered immunoregulation. Gastrointestinal and hematologic disorders predominate. An increased susceptibility to malignancy (particularly thymoma and lymphoma) in adults with CVID appears to exist, but the risk in children is not known.

Treatment of these patients is the same as for those with X-LA: replacement with gamma globulin and aggressive management of infections.

SELECTIVE IgA DEFICIENCY

Selective IgA deficiency is the most prevalent primary immunodeficiency disease occurring in approximately 1 of 600 individuals. Patients have a serum IgA level of less than 5 mg/dL, normal levels of other immunoglobulins, normal serum antibody responses, and normal cell-mediated immunity.

IgA is found in serum and is the predominant immunoglobulin on mucosal surfaces of the gastrointestinal and respiratory tracts. IgA inhibits microbial adherence, thus, preventing invasion into the systemic circulation. The majority of patients with IgA deficiency lack both serum and secretory IgA. IgA deficiency can be associated with infection, atopic disease, and rheumatic disorders.

Although some patients with selective IgA deficiency are more susceptible to infection, many asymptomatic individuals can be identified as IgA deficient by population-based screening. The most common infections in IgA-deficient patients are otitis media, sinusitis, bronchitis, pneumonia, and diarrhea; meningitis and bacterial sepsis are rare. A subset of patients with IgA-deficiency and deficiencies of IgG2 and IgG4 can experience severe and chronic sinopulmonary infections. Because IgG subclass deficiencies are treatable, IgG subclass measurement and IgG antibody responses should be included in the workup of all IgA-deficient patients. Chronic diarrhea, frequently from Giardia infection, can be seen in IgA deficiency.

Atopic diseases such as allergic rhinitis, asthma, urticaria, eczema, and food allergy have been reported to occur in as many as 50% of patients with selective IgA deficiency. A variety of rheumatic diseases (such as juvenile rheumatoid arthritis, systemic lupus erythematosus) have also been associated with selective IgA deficiency.

Children with low, but not absent, IgA (5–10 mg/dL) may share the same disease manifestations. Serum IgA levels have been shown to increase to within the normal range in more than 50% of these less severe cases. Symptoms subside in these patients.

Patients with IgA deficiency and associated IgG subclass deficiencies may benefit from immunoglobulin prophylaxis. However, use of commercial gamma globulin in patients with IgA deficiency requires caution. Some preparations may contain trace amounts of IgA, which can sensitize the patient, thereby inducing an IgG or IgE antiIgA antibody. This development is a relative, not an absolute, contraindication to gamma globulin therapy. For example, in such cases, an intravenous gamma globulin preparation that contains less than 0.01 g/L of IgA can be given with caution.

X-LINKED HYPER-IgM SYNDROME

Patients with X-linked hyper-IgM syndrome (XHIM) have normal or elevated serum IgM and IgD but are deficient in all other immunoglobulin classes. IgM levels are not consistently elevated in the first few months of life.

XHIM is caused by mutations of the gene for CD40 ligand, membrane protein expressed on the surface of activated T lymphocytes. Without CD40 ligand, T lymphocytes are unable to trigger B lymphocytes to switch their immunoglobulin production from IgM to IgG, IgA, or IgE. Patients have most of their peripheral blood B cells bearing IgM on their surface. Antibody responses to immunization may be present but are predominantly or exclusively IgM antibodies. *In vitro* cellular immune responses have been demonstrated to be abnormal in XHIM.

Recurrent infections of both pyogenic bacteria (e.g., *Streptococcus pneumoniae*), viruses, and opportunistic infections (such as *Pneumocystis carinii, Cryptosporidium,* and *Mycobacteria*) can occur. Patients with XHIM have a significant risk for developing neutropenia, sclerosing cholangitis, and lymphoid hyperplasia and malignancy.

TRANSIENT HYPOGAMMAGLOBULINEMIA OF INFANCY

Infants with transient hypogammaglobulinemia have delayed acquisition of normal serum immunoglobulin levels. This diagnosis can be established only in retrospect, after immunoglobulin levels become normal. Some patients will go on to have persistent abnormalities and may eventually be classified as having CVID, immunodeficiency with increased IgM, or selective IgA deficiency. A controversy exists as to whether transient hypogammaglobulinemia of infancy should be considered an immunodeficiency disease or a developmental variant.

Most symptomatic patients have chronic or recurrent infections of the respiratory and gastrointestinal tracts. Bacterial sepsis and meningitis are rare. Eczema and asthma have also been reported in some series.

Immunoglobulin levels may remain low for months to years, then eventually increase to within the normal range. Despite variable degree of panhypogammaglobulinemia, normal peripheral blood B lymphocytes are present in normal numbers.

Prophylactic antibiotics are sometimes needed for managing recurrent sinopulmonary infections, but most children do not need gamma globulin replacement.

CHAPTER 237
Complement Deficiencies

Adapted from Jerry A. Winkelstein

The complement system refers to a group of plasma proteins and cellular receptors that serve as important mediators of host defense and inflammation. A described deficiency exists for nearly all components of the complement system. Selected deficiencies are described in this chapter.

CLINICAL PRESENTATION

Patients with complement deficiencies can demonstrate differing clinical presentations. Most patients have increased susceptibility to infection, some have rheumatic disease, others have angioedema, and, rarely, some patients may be asymptomatic.

For those patients with increased susceptibility to infection, types of infections relate to the functions of the missing complement component(s). For example, patients with a deficiency of C3 (an opsonic ligand), are more susceptible to infections caused by encapsulated bacteria for which opsonization is the primary host defense (e.g., *Streptococcus pneumoniae, Streptococcus pyogenes*). Similarly, C5 through C9 form the membrane attack complex (MAC), important for serum bactericidal activity. Patients with deficiencies of C5, C6, C7, C8, or C9 are susceptible to gram-negative bacteria, notably Neisseria species. For this reason, it is reasonable to screen children with systemic meningococcal infections for the presence of a complement deficiency.

Rheumatic diseases in patients with complement deficiency include a lupus-like disorder, glomerulonephritis, dermatomyositis, anaphylactoid purpura, and vasculitis. The prevalence of these inflammatory disorders is highest in those patients with deficiencies of the classical activating pathway (C1, C4, and C2) and of C3.

Patients with a deficiency of one of the control proteins of the classical pathway, C1 esterase inhibitor, usually present with angioedema of the skin or mucous membranes.

Some patients with complement deficiencies are relatively asymptomatic and are typically ascertained by screening family members of complement-deficient patients.

SELECTED SPECIFIC DISORDERS

C1 Esterase Inhibitor Deficiency

Deficiency of C1 esterase inhibitor (C1-INH) is inherited in an autosomal dominant fashion and is responsible for hereditary angioedema (HAE). Eighty-five percent of patients have type I and are deficient in both C1-INH protein (5%–30% of normal) and C1-INH activity. In type II, a protein with reduced function is present in normal or elevated concentrations. In either type, serum levels of C4 are reduced both during and between attacks.

Submucosal or subcutaneous edema of the skin, respiratory tract, and gastrointestinal tract is the most common manifestation. In attacks involving the skin, the edema can vary from a few centimeters to involvement of a whole extremity. The face and genitalia may also be affected. The lesions are pale, are not usually warm, and are characteristically nonpruritic. Attacks usually progress for 1 to 2 days and resolve over an additional 2 to 3 days.

Attacks involving the respiratory tract can create life-threatening airway obstruction. The patients may experience a tightness in the throat with swelling of the tongue, buccal mucosa, oropharynx, and larynx. The gastrointestinal tract can be involved due to edema of the bowel wall. Symptoms can include vomiting and crampy abdominal pain. Trauma, anxiety, and stress are frequently cited as triggering events; more than one-half of patients are unable to identify a precipitator of the attack.

Management consists of both prophylaxis and treatment of attacks. Antifibrinolytic agents such as epsilon aminocaproic acid or its cyclic analogue, tranexamic acid, have been used with some success in the long-term prevention of attacks. More recently, androgen compounds such as danazol and stanozolol, which have attenuated androgenic potential, have been found to be effective for prophylaxis. These compounds seem to act by stimulating the synthesis of functionally intact C1-INH by the normal gene.

Epinephrine, antihistamines, and corticosteroids are of no proven benefit in interrupting attacks once they have begun. Infusion of partially purified C1-INH has been accompanied by resolution of edema and symptoms within a few hours.

C2 Deficiency

C2 deficiency is the most common of the inherited complement deficiencies. Homozygous deficiency of C2 occurs as frequently as 1 in 10,000 individuals. The clinical manifestations of C2 deficiency vary from individuals who are asymptomatic to individuals who have increased susceptibility to infection, rheumatic diseases, or both. The infections are mostly blood-borne and systemic (e.g., sepsis, meningitis, arthritis, and osteomyelitis) and caused by encapsulated bacteria. A variety of rheumatic diseases are associated with C2 deficiency. The most common disorders resemble SLE and discoid lupus.

C3 Deficiency

The clinical manifestations of C3 deficiency in humans include increased susceptibility to infection and rheumatic disorders. Patients with C3 deficiency have a variety of infections including pneumonia, bacteremia, meningitis, and osteomyelitis caused by encapsulated pyogenic bacteria. A number of patients have presented with arthralgias and vasculitic skin rashes and a clinical picture consistent with SLE. Renal disease has also been reported.

C4 Deficiency

Two loci (C4A and C4B) within the major histocompatibility complex encode for C4. Although the products of the two loci share some functional, structural, and antigenic characteristics that identify them as C4, other characteristics differ slightly. Total homozygous (deficient at both loci) C4 deficiency is rare. Clinical manifestations described include an SLE-like illness characterized by photosensitive skin rashes, renal disease, and, occasionally, arthritis and increased susceptibility to infection.

Approximately 1% of the population is homozygous deficient in C4A and 3% of the population is deficient in C4B. C4A and C4B differ in that C4A interacts more efficiently with proteins, and C4B interacts more efficiently with carbohydrates. Individuals who lack C4A seem to be more susceptible to immune complex diseases such as SLE. The prevalence of homozygous C4A deficiency in SLE is between 10% and 15%. Individuals who are deficient in C4B are perhaps more susceptible to blood-borne bacterial infections. The prevalence of C4B deficiency is increased in children with bacteremia and meningitis.

C5 Deficiency, C6 Deficiency, C7 Deficiency, C8 Deficiency, C9 Deficiency

Deficiencies of any of these terminal complement components causes a reduction in serum bactericidal activity. The most clinically important susceptibility is to systemic meningococcal or disseminated gonococcal infections.

Properdin Deficiency

Properdin is a control protein that stabilizes the alternative pathway enzymes that activate C3 and C5. Properdin deficiency is inherited as an X-linked recessive disorder. The only reported clinical manifestation of properdin deficiency is a marked increased susceptibility to systemic meningococcal infections.

CHAPTER 238
Functional Disorders of Granulocytes

Adapted from Donald C. Anderson and C. Wayne Smith

Two broad categories of functional granulocyte disorders have been delineated: those of impaired motility, recruitment, or localization of granulocytes to sites of infection, and those of defective ingestion or intracellular killing of microorganisms by granulocytes. In this latter group, granulocytes accumulate normally but are unable to eradicate invading microorganisms.

DISORDERS OF ADHERENCE AND MOTILITY

Granulocytes and other leukocytes preferentially adhere to vascular endothelium adjacent to an area of inflammation before migrating into surrounding tissues. This process is mediated by immunospecific adhesion molecules on leukocytes and endothelial cells. Several clinical entities characterized by diminished or enhanced cellular adherence properties have been identified.

Leukocyte Adhesion Deficiency

Leukocyte adhesion deficiency (LAD) is an autosomal recessive disorder characterized by recurrent bacterial infections, impaired pus formation, abnormal wound healing, and a spectrum of functional abnormalities in granulocytes, monocytes, and lymphoid cells.

Recurrent, necrotic, and indolent infections of skin, mucous membranes, and intestinal tract occur. Often small, erythematous, nonpustular skin lesions progress to large, well-demarcated, ulcerative craters, which heal slowly, possibly with eschars. Staphylococcal or gram-negative enteric bacterial organisms may be cultured from the lesions for several weeks despite antimicrobial therapy. In addition to infections such as perirectal abscesses and cellulitis, sepsis progressing from omphalitis associated with delayed umbilical cord detachment has been observed.

Other common respiratory infections include bacterial laryngotracheitis (Pseudomonas has been reported), recurrent pneumonitis, and sinusitis. Severe gingivitis or periodontitis is a major feature among all patients who survive infancy.

Inflammatory infiltrates are typically totally devoid of neutrophils. Most patients have peripheral blood leukocytosis of 5 to 20 times normal.

Inflammatory signs may be minimal before the development of septicemic episodes. Management, therefore, consists of aggressive local care and antibiotic therapy of any suspicious superficial inflammatory lesions. Prophylactic antibiotic regimens with trimethoprim-sulfamethoxazole (TMP-SMZ) may reduce the number of systemic infections. In clinical settings in which antibiotic or surgical interventions have been ineffective, leukocyte transfusions have been used successfully. Bone marrow transplantation with successful engraftment and apparent clinical recovery from disease has been achieved in several patients.

Chédiak–Higashi Syndrome

Chédiak–Higashi syndrome is an autosomal recessive disorder characterized by partial oculocutaneous albinism, the presence of giant lysosomal granules in all granular cell types, increased susceptibility to bacterial infection, variable occurrence of neutropenia and thrombocytopenia, and an accelerated lymphoma-like proliferative disorder generally occurring in the first decade of life. Infectious complications are attributable to both neutropenia and functional deficits of neutrophils, monocytes, and natural killer cells. Many individuals die within the first decade, primarily of infection. When a pathogen can be identified, *S. aureus* is the predominant one; group A streptococcus, gram-negative enterics (*Klebsiella, Pseudomonas*), *Aspergillus*, and *Candida* species are also reported.

Neutrophils, monocytes, and lymphocytes demonstrate large intracellular inclusions or granules, which are the pathologic hallmark of the disease. Analysis of bone marrow from patients suggest that these abnormal granules are formed during granulocyte maturation by the aggregation and fusion of azurophilic and specific granules. Such findings are consistent with a proposed membrane abnormality.

Defective neutrophil and monocyte chemotaxis is one of many functional abnormalities in Chédiak–Higashi syndrome. Despite a normal capacity to ingest organisms and a normal oxidative burst, neutrophils also have diminished intracellular killing of bacterial organisms. A selective impairment of the functions of natural killer cells may be responsible for the development of a lymphoproliferative syndrome in most patients.

Chédiak–Higashi syndrome is diagnosed by identifying the clinical features of the disorder, as well as large cytoplasmic inclusions in all granular cells including peripheral blood granulocytes. Neutropenia and thrombocytopenia are seen during the accelerated phase of disease. Splenomegaly and associated hypersplenism contribute to anemia and thrombocytopenia and may also contribute to neutropenia.

Successful bone marrow transplantation with reversal of the defect in natural killer activity has been reported in Chédiak–Higashi syndrome.

Shwachman–Diamond Syndrome

The Shwachman and Diamond syndrome includes exocrine pancreatic insufficiency, bone marrow hypoplasia with intermittent neutropenia, metaphyseal chondrodysplasia, growth retardation, and recurrent soft tissue infections. Diminished chemotaxis of neutrophils can be found in this syndrome.

DISORDERS OF INTRACELLULAR MICROBIAL KILLING

When a phagocyte engulfs a microorganism, there is an associated burst of oxidative activity, which leads to the evolution of superoxide, hydrogen peroxide, or other oxygen radicals. This respiratory burst requires a series of electron transfers using nicotinamide-adenine dinucleotide phosphate (NADPH) as the electron donor. It involves a flavin-adenine dinucleotide-containing flavoprotein and a unique cytochrome b. This system is associated with the plasma membrane of granulocytes or mononuclear phagocytes.

Chronic Granulomatosis Disease (CGD)

The CGDs are a genetically heterogeneous group of disorders of oxidative metabolism of phagocytes. CGD results in impairment of intracellular microbial killing. Its frequency is 1 in 1 million and CGD is identified most often in boys. Most patients develop recurrent soft tissue infections during the first year of life; a high proportion of these patients become clinically ill before age 3 months. Rarely, individuals may be clinically well until early adolescence or adulthood, possibly reflecting less deleterious genetic phenotypes.

The basis for abnormal oxygen-dependent microbicidal activity in CGD cells is directly related to impaired generation of superoxide anion and H_2O_2. Abnormal NADPH oxidase activity caused by one of several molecular defects represents the fundamental basis for diminished microbicidal function.

Historically, three genetic forms of CGD were described based on inheritance patterns and detection of the cytochrome b in phagocytes of affected patients: X-linked (approximately 70%), autosomal recessive (approximately 30%), and autosomal dominant (rare cases).

Patients with CGD have a predilection for infection caused by catalase-positive microorganisms such as *S. aureus*. Catalase-positive, gram-negative bacteria such as *E. coli, Klebsiella, Enterobacter* species, *Serratia marcescens, Salmonellae*, and *Pseudomonas* species may also account for infections. Fungal pathogens are involved in infections in approximately 20% of CGD patients with *Aspergillus* species (most common), *C. albicans* and *Torulopsis* species being represented. *Pneumocystis carinii* and *Mycobacterium* species may also cause infections.

The inability of circulating phagocytes to kill invading bacteria or fungi at sites of heavy colonization leads to the predictable features of CGD, which include surface infections, inflammatory lesions of skin or subcutaneous tissues, ulcerative stomatitis, pneumonitis, perianal abscesses, and conjunctivitis. Granulomas, the histopathologic hallmark of this disorder, commonly develop in lymph nodes, lungs, liver, spleen, gastrointestinal tract, and bone. Organisms can remain viable in tissue abscesses or granulomas accounting for delayed or refractory response to antimicrobial, surgical, or other therapeutic regimens. A history of sterile aspirates of superficial or deep-seated abscesses should alert the clinician to the possible diagnosis of CGD.

In general, CGD should be considered when a history of recurrent soft tissue or systemic infections beginning in infancy is elicited. Laboratory findings suggestive of CGD include leukocytosis, elevation of erythrocyte sedimentation rate, abnormal chest radiographs, and elevated serum levels of IgG, IgA, and IgM. Specific antibody synthesis and delayed hypersensitivity skin tests are generally normal. Evaluations of postmortem or biopsy tissues often reveal granulomas at sites of infection.

The definitive diagnostic test for CGD is the demonstration of impaired intracellular bactericidal activity by phagocytes. These tests require a specialized laboratory. Screening tests, however, such as the nitroblue tetrazolium (NBT) dye test are applicable for use in the general diagnostic laboratory. Oxidized NBT is colorless. When reduced by superoxide, it precipitates in the cytosol as blue formazan, which can be identified histochemically.

Management of CGD includes prevention of infection, as well as early identification and treatment of infection with antimicrobial and surgical therapies. Superficial lesions such as furuncles, paronychia, and areas of cellulitis should warrant concern, even with no fever or other systemic symptoms. Isolation of the etiologic agent from involved tissue should be a priority; this will direct the appropriate antimicrobial therapy. Incision and drainage of abscesses may be needed. Prolonged antibiotic courses (weeks to months) are necessary as microorganisms are sequestered but not killed within defective phagocytes. There is a high incidence of relapsing infections in CGD patients. Some centers recommend prolonged prophylactic antibiotic administration, but the overall benefit of this approach is unproven. Leukocyte transfusions may be used when there is rapidly progressive infection or failure of conventional medical and surgical therapy.

Recombinant interferon-gamma offers a potentially important advantage in the management of CGD. *In vitro* studies show that interferon-gamma enhances expression of cytochrome b 91-kd mRNA and superoxide production in phagocytic cells from normal and some X-linked CGD patients. *In vivo* studies have shown that patients receiving subcutaneous interferon-gamma have demonstrated a fourfold decreased risk for significant infection when compared to recipients receiving placebo.

Bone marrow transplantation has been attempted in a limited number of patients with CGD, yielding both unsuccessful and successful outcomes. Experimental advances in gene therapy for patients with CGD are ongoing.

CHAPTER 239
Combined Immunodeficiency Diseases

Adapted from Richard Hong

COMBINED DISEASE

The humoral (B cell) and cell-mediated (T cell) immune systems do not function independently. In the past, the term "combined immunodeficiency" was used to denote defects in both major arms of the immune system. With today's knowledge of the complex pathways of lymphocyte differentiation, antigen processing, cytokine secretion, and signal transduction, we know that, except for the "pure" B-cell diseases, which constitute some form of hypogammaglobulinemia, essentially all primary immunodeficiency is a combined disease.

Clinical Features

Infants with combined immunodeficiency disease (CID) often present with infections within the first months of life. Recurrent pneumonia, failure to thrive, chronic diarrhea, and persistent mucosal and cutaneous candidiasis are typical manifestations. These infants may have infections with all types of microorganisms, as well as opportunistic pathogens (Pneumocystis carinii). Many infants with CID will develop graft–versus–host disease (GVHD) after blood transfusions, which contain immunocompetent donor T lymphocytes. Maternal lymphocytes entering fetal circulation during gestation, labor, and delivery can also cause GVHD in infants with CID.

Immunologic Findings

Quantitative studies of lymphocytes (enumeration studies using monoclonal antibodies) and measurement of immunoglobulins levels should be performed when a combined immunodeficiency is suspected.

Qualitative studies often yield important information. For example, some individuals may have lymphocyte or immunoglobulin levels below the range of normal, yet these components can respond to antigenic challenge. Such patients are symptom free and are not unduly susceptible to infection.

When performed with care and proper training, a delayed hypersensitivity skin challenge can be an excellent measure of T-cell integrity. In the first few years of life, due to variability in the patient's sensitization to certain antigens, this test is not useful. *In vitro* tests, based on proliferative responses to mitogens, alloantigens, and antigens, are more sensitive and can be used at very young age. Of the three, reactivity to antigens is the most stringent and informative test of the T-cell system.

As further measures of T-cell function, cytolytic capability of T cells can be used to measure killer cell functions, as well as the release of cytokines after appropriate stimuli.

B-cell functionality is defined by total and functional antibody titers (to protein and polysaccharide antigens). Whenever there is a concern about the patient's immunity, neither the patient nor any member of the family should have a live virus vaccine.

Tests are available to aid in carrier diagnosis or to provide a diagnosis of a primary immunodeficiency *in utero*. Sampling chorionic villi in the first trimester of pregnancy provides DNA for molecular diagnoses. The genes for adenosine deaminase, purine nucleoside phosphorylase, X-linked SCID, Wiskott–Aldrich syndrome (WAS), and ataxia-telangiectasia (AT) (see below) have been identified and allow specific diagnosis. Probes for the deletions found in the DiGeorge anomaly can be used with sensitive techniques such as fluorescent in situ hybridization. Similar techniques are applied to blood samples from the parents or siblings to determine carrier status.

Amniotic fluid samples can be analyzed biochemically for purine salvage enzymes to detect adenosine deaminase or purine nucleoside phosphorylase deficiencies. After 18 weeks' gestation, blood samples can be taken directly from the fetus and examined by flow cytometry and *in vitro* proliferation and biochemical assays.

For X-linked diseases in which the gene has not been mapped, restriction fragment length polymorphism can be used to define carrier status.

Pathogenesis

Six basic steps describe the physiology of a competent immune response. These are: stem cell generation; T- and B-cell differentiation; surface receptor expression and transduction; cytokine response or secretion; cell traffic; and cell number homeostasis. A failure in any one of the steps results in immunodeficiency. In the past, many of the diseases, which are now defined to the level of enzyme deficiency or molecular defect, were considered SCID or combined immunodeficiency.

SELECTED SPECIFIC DISEASES

Combined Immunodeficiency Disease with Adenosine Deaminase Deficiency

ADA deficiency is an example of failure to maintain adequate numbers of lymphocytes (cell number homeostasis). In the pathway of normal purine metabolism, ADA catalyzes the conversion of adenosine to inosine and deoxyadenosine to deoxyinosine (Fig. 239-1). In ADA deficiency, deoxyadenosine accumulates in the serum and tissues. In individuals with ADA deficiency, all cells of the body lack the enzyme, but lymphocytes are particularly susceptible to damage. This is thought to be due to lymphocytes being efficient at phosphorylating deoxyadenosine to deoxyadenosine triphosphate, which is toxic to cells. Lymphocytes in this disorder basically poison themselves.

In some patients with ADA-negative CID, agammaglobulinemia and severe lymphopenia are present, but other patients may have less severe defects, likely related to different enzyme levels.

Bone marrow transplantation has been successful in ADA-negative patients with CID. As an alternative to transplantation,

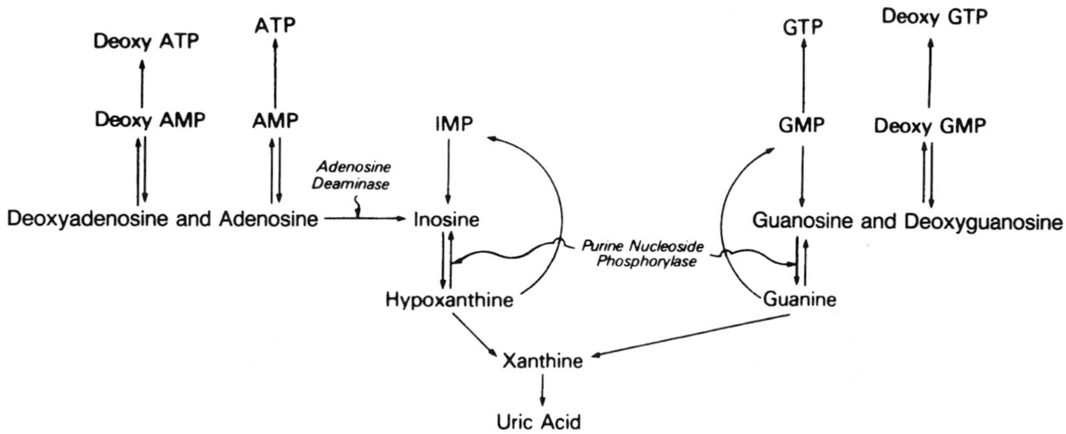

Figure 239-1. Purine catabolic pathway showing the positions at which the enzymes adenosine deaminase and purine nucleoside phosphorylase catalyze their respective reactions. The accumulation of the toxic triphosphates of deoxyadenosine and deoxyguanosine leads to the immunodeficiency in these disorders. AMP, adenosine monophosphate; ATP, adenosine triphosphate; GMP, guanosine monophosphate; GTP, guanosine triphosphate; IMP, inosine monophosphate.

however, enzyme replacement is possible in ADA-negative CID. Bovine ADA is conjugated with polyethylene glycol (PEG-ADA) and is given as weekly subcutaneous injections to ADA-negative patients with CID. The PEG conjugation renders the bovine enzyme less immunogenic and extends the serum half-life of the ADA. Treated patients have been shown to have an increase in lymphocyte numbers in the blood.

ADA deficiency is the first immunodeficiency disease to be treated by gene therapy. T-cell lines established from ADA-negative patients with CID have been "cured" *in vitro* after successful transfer of the human ADA gene using a recombinant retrovirus vector gene transfer system. A limited number of children have received monthly infusions of 1 billion transfected cells.

Combined Immunodeficiency Disease with Purine Nucleoside Phosphorylase Deficiency

Deficiency in the enzyme purine nucleoside phosphorylase (PNP) causes severely defective T-cell function. PNP is encoded by a gene on chromosome 14, and its deficiency is inherited as an autosomal recessive trait. The enzyme catalyzes the conversion of inosine to hypoxanthine and guanosine to guanine in the pathway of purine catabolism. This step in purine degradation immediately follows the step catalyzed by adenosine deaminase. The accumulation of deoxyguanosine triphosphate is the toxic compound that interferes with T-lymphocyte development and function.

PNP deficiency is usually associated with a defect in T-cell immunity with preservation of B-cell function and immunoglobulin production. These patients have profound T lymphopenia, skin-test anergy, and defective *in vitro* lymphocyte function test results. Thymic morphology is intact, as is the ability of the patients to produce isohemagglutinins and antibodies. The serum concentrations of IgM, IgG, and IgA may be normal. The immune deficiency in PNP deficiency may be progressive. Because PNP catalyzes the degradation of inosine and guanosine, the principal substrates for uric acid production, PNP deficiency, usually results in low levels of uric acid in the blood and urine, which provides a simple, convenient screening test for this disorder.

Bone marrow transplantation has successfully treated these patients. Repeated red blood cell transfusions that replace enzymes have provided limited benefit in some patients with PNP deficiency.

Ataxia-Telangiectasia

AT is an autosomal recessive disorder characterized by severe cerebellar ataxia, oculocutaneous telangiectasia, variable immunodeficiency, and a high incidence of malignancy. The disorder frequently results in profound disability, and the patient becomes almost totally dependent on others for care and feeding. Neurologic symptoms dominate the clinical picture with onset at approximately the time the child is learning to walk.

The cerebellar dysfunction is manifested early as ataxia and is followed by choreoathetosis, severe involuntary myoclonic jerking movements, and oculomotor abnormalities. The telangiectasia usually first appears on the bulbar conjunctiva when the child is between 2 and 5 years of age (Fig. 239-2). Then, they begin to appear on the skin of exposed areas and on areas of trauma such as the nasal bridge and flexor folds on the neck and extremities. Multiple endocrine abnormalities including hypogonadism can be seen. Cancer, predominantly, nonHodgkin's lymphoma, develops in as many as 15% of AT patients. Many patients have recurrent sinopulmonary infections.

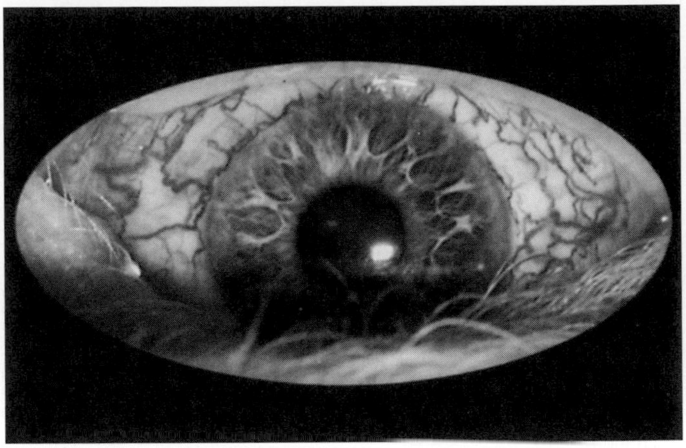

Figure 239-2. Striking telangiectasia on the bulbar conjunctiva of a 22-year-old patient with ataxia-telangiectasia. These dilated vessels typically appear between 2 and 5 years of age, first in the eye and later on cutaneous areas of chronic exposure or trauma.

The finding of the gene responsible for AT [AT mutated (ATM) located on the long arm of chromosome 11 (11q22–23)] has increased the accuracy of diagnosis, as well as serving to identify milder clinical variants of the disease. A very mild form of AT without many of the serious features previously described is found in 10% to 15% of families in the United Kingdom.

The ATM protein is involved in cell-cycle control, telomere length monitoring, and responses to DNA damage. The multifaceted role of the ATM protein in signal transduction, cell proliferation and growth, and activation of cell cycle checkpoints explains the multisystem nature of AT. Defects in both the T- and B-cell immune systems have been reported, but different patients may have varying degrees of immunodeficiency. The most consistent defects in humoral immunity are IgA deficiency in 75% and IgE deficiency in 85% of cases. IgG2 and IgG4 deficiency are also common. The T-cell system also has a variety of abnormalities including skin-test anergy in depressed lymphocyte proliferative responses. Depressed cytotoxic T-cell responses also occur.

No specific useful therapy corrects the multisystem manifestations of the disease. Immunoglobulin replacement therapy can cause a serious anaphylactic reaction in patients who are IgA deficient due to circulating antiIgA antibodies. Because patients are extremely radiosensitive, radiation therapy for their malignancies is contraindicated.

Wiskott–Aldrich Syndrome

WAS is an X-linked disorder consisting of the triad of recurrent infection with all classes of microorganisms, hemorrhage secondary to thrombocytopenia, and eczema of the skin. Bleeding episodes or symptoms caused by infection typically begin during the first 6 months of life. Patients with WAS may come to medical attention due to repeated episodes of otitis media or pneumonia caused by *Streptococcus pneumoniae* or *Haemophilus influenzae*. They are also prone to septicemia or meningitis with these organisms. *Candida albicans*, cytomegalovirus, and *Pneumocystis carinii* are also causes of significant infectious episodes in these children. Viral infections have been fatal in patients with WAS; disseminated herpes simplex, varicella and generalized vaccinia (after smallpox vaccination) have been reported.

Small platelets make the thrombocytopenia in WAS unique from other thrombocytopenic disorders. Bleeding accounts for approximately 30% of the mortality in WAS with intracranial hemorrhage being the greatest threat.

Eczema and other manifestations of autoimmunity make up another aspect of WAS. The autoimmune disorder may take on many forms including hemolytic anemia, a juvenile rheumatoid arthritis-like disorder and idiopathic thrombocytopenic, a purpura-like thrombocytopenia.

The incidence of malignancy is more than 100 times that of the normal population. Most cancers are non-Hodgkin's lymphomas with the brain involved in more than one-half of cases.

Patients with WAS have selective defects of each component of the immune system, rather than one more global defect that can occur in other diseases. Variable patterns of serum immunoglobulins are seen, with the most typical profile consisting of normal levels of IgG and IgA elevated to approximately twice normal levels, and IgM at approximately one-half the normal level. The serum half-life of IgM, IgG, IgA in patients with WAS is only one-third to one-half normal, so to keep serum levels normal, these proteins are synthesized at high rates. Antibody responses to some antigens (tetanus) are normal, whereas responses to others (polysaccharide antigens) are absent. Patients are, therefore, susceptible to infection with encapsulated organisms.

The cellular immune system also has selective defects in many functions. Despite normal or near-normal numbers of T lymphocytes in their blood and a normal ratio of $CD4^+$ to $CD8^+$ T cells, patients are anergic and T cell proliferation to antigens may be poor.

The monocytes from patients with WAS have defects in chemotaxis and cytotoxic function mediated by antibodies (antibody-dependent cell-mediated cytotoxicity).

A defective protein, named the WAS protein (WASp), is the cause of WAS. The now cloned gene maps to Xp11.22 and is responsible for causing cytoskeletal abnormalities, which impair T-cell response to antigen-presenting B cells.

HLA-matched bone marrow transplantation is the treatment of choice if a matched sibling donor is available. After transplantation, all of the manifestations of this disease are corrected. For patients lacking an HLA-identical sibling donor, T-cell-depleted, haploidentical bone marrow transplantation has been successful. The numbers of successful treatments with matched unrelated and cord blood donors are increasing.

Splenectomy cures the thrombocytopenia in more than 90% of patients, but prophylactic antibiotics or intravenous gamma globulin must be used regularly because these patients are more susceptible to overwhelming infection.

The autoaggressive syndrome may be difficult to treat. Nonsteroidal antiinflammatory drugs and corticosteroids are often used. As with all patients with severe T-cell immunodeficiency, all transfusions containing blood cells should be irradiated to prevent the development of GVHD.

DiGeorge Anomaly (CATCH-22)

DiGeorge anomaly (formerly DiGeorge syndrome) is a congenital immunodeficiency disease caused by the embryonic maldevelopment of structures derived from the first through sixth branchial pouches. Structures derived from the branchial pouches include portions of the ear and certain facial features, portions of the aortic arch and heart, the parathyroids and thyroid, and the thymus. Submicroscopic deletion of chromosome 22q11 is found in more than 90% of patients with DiGeorge anomaly. This characteristic is also seen in a familial congenital heart syndrome and velocardiofacial syndrome. DiGeorge anomaly is likely one phenotype of a spectrum of related chromosome 22 deletion disorders. The acronym CATCH-22 (cardiac defects, abnormal facies, thymic hypoplasia, cleft palate, and hypocalcemia resulting from chromosome 22q11 deletions) has been proposed for this group of defects.

Congenital heart lesions, particularly conotruncal defects are common presenting problems during the first 2 weeks of life. Abnormal calcium homeostasis caused by hypoparathyroidism occurs in nearly all patients, and hypocalcemic tetany is the most common initial problem. Facial abnormalities include microstomia, hypertelorism, upturned nose, posteriorly rotated and small low-set ears with notched pinnae, and downward slant of the eyes (Fig. 239-3). Approximately 25% have a significant immune deficit. These immunodeficiencies become clinically apparent later than the cardiac and metabolic complications, but, eventually, patients begin to experience an increased susceptibility to infections such as recurrent pneumonia, diarrhea, and candidiasis of the mouth, oropharynx, esophagus, and skin of the diaper area.

Immunologic defects are variable and, when they occur, they are the direct consequence of the failure of thymus development. Approximately 25% of DiGeorge anomaly patients have a

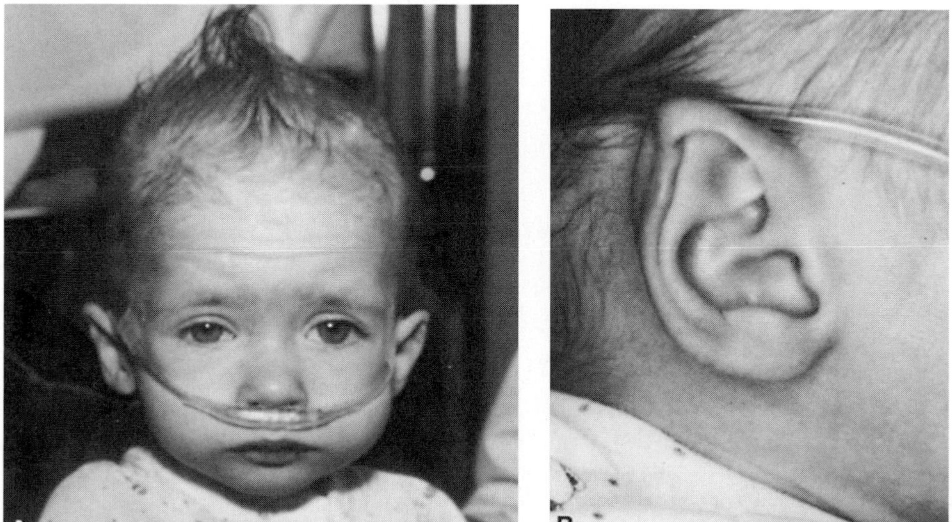

Figure 239-3. DiGeorge anomaly is a congenital disorder involving maldevelopment of the structures derived from the first through the sixth pharyngeal pouches during embryonic life. **A:** As a consequence, these children often have facial abnormalities as illustrated in this child with hypertelorism, defective low-set ears, hypoplastic mandible, and upward bowing of the upper lip. **B:** A close-up view of the ear shows notched pinna and deficient helix formation.

persistent immune defect such as low $CD4^+$ T cells (less than 400 per microliter) or decreased T cell response to phytohemagglutinin stimulation. The total lymphocyte count is usually normal, but it consists mostly of B cells and non-T cells. The morphology of the spleen and lymph nodes reflects the T lymphopenia with depletion seen in the usual thymic-dependent areas. Specific antibody responses are not present. Although the chromosomal deletion is known (22q11.2), thus far, the genetic mechanism has not been defined.

Despite the immune system compromise, patients with heart disease tolerate the surgical procedures very well. All blood products must be irradiated, however. When a deficiency state is confirmed, immunologic reconstitution can be attempted through thymus transplantation or bone marrow transplantation using a matched sibling.

12 Orthopedic Disorders

CHAPTER 240

Developmental Dysplasia of the Hip

Adapted from Paul D. Sponseller

CLINICAL FEATURES

The cause of developmental dysplasia of the hip (DDH) in an otherwise normal child is multifactorial. Mechanical factors within the uterine environment play a role. Therefore, the frequency is increased greatly in fetuses with breech presentation and in infants with oligohydramnios. These factors are associated with increased forces across the hip leading to malposition of the femoral head and acetabulum. Hormonal factors may play a role, as generalized ligamentous laxity occurs around the time of birth, caused by increased circulating estrogens and relaxin. Probably for this reason, the incidence of DDH is sixfold greater in girls than in boys. Interestingly, the left hip is involved more commonly than the right. Evidence for hereditary control of these and other factors lies in the fact that more than 20% of patients have a positive family history. A change in terminology from *congenital dislocation of the hip* to *DDH* has become widely accepted. The term *dysplasia* better describes the spectrum of severity of this disorder, which ranges from slight malformation to full dislocation of the hip. The term *developmental* acknowledges that some cases cannot be detected at birth and may occur later.

In order of their increasing severity, the three degrees of hip dysplasia are subluxatable, dislocatable, and dislocated. In the *subluxatable* hip, the femoral head rests in the acetabulum and can be partially dislocated during the examination. The *dislocatable* hip can be fully dislocated with manipulation but is normally located when a baby is at rest. In the *dislocated* hip, the femoral head rests in the dislocated position. The combined incidence of these three conditions is 1 in 60 births; the incidence of true dislocation is only 1 to 2 per 1,000 births.

DIAGNOSIS

Physical examination remains the key to the diagnosis of DDH. The signs in the newborn period usually include instability without significant fixed deformity; in later months, untreated dislocation becomes more fixed, and less instability and more limitation of certain motions occur. Specifically, Barlow and Ortolani signs should be sought in newborns (Fig. 240-1). These signs are defined as positive when the hip can be dislocated and relocated, respectively. Affected children should be relaxed when the tests are performed, and only one hip should be examined at a time. The pelvis should be stabilized with one hand, while the femur is controlled with the other hand, with fingers placed on the greater and lesser trochanters. With adduction and pressure directed posteriorly, the femur can be felt to slide out in the abnormal hip (Barlow sign; Fig. 240-1A) and then back in with abduction causing a dull clunk to be heard (Ortolani sign; Fig. 240-1B).

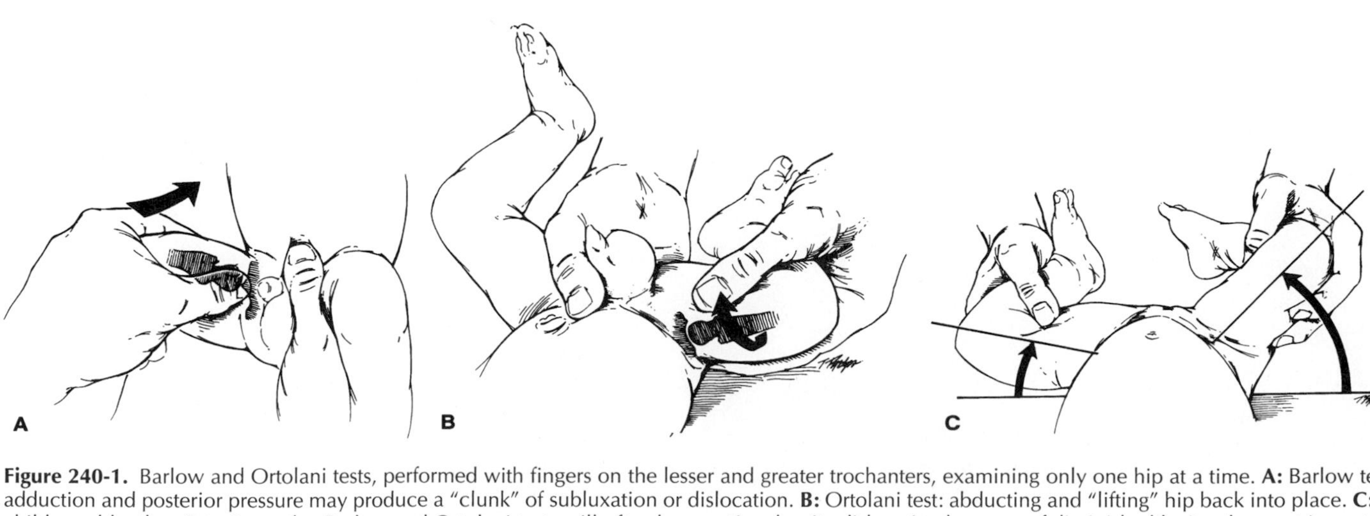

Figure 240-1. Barlow and Ortolani tests, performed with fingers on the lesser and greater trochanters, examining only one hip at a time. **A:** Barlow test: adduction and posterior pressure may produce a "clunk" of subluxation or dislocation. **B:** Ortolani test: abducting and "lifting" hip back into place. **C:** In children older than 3 to 6 months, Barlow and Ortolani tests will often be negative despite dislocation because of diminished laxity; the most important finding in this age group may be limitation of abduction.

ERRORS IN DIAGNOSIS

A common error made in DDH diagnosis is examining both hips at once, which impairs sensitivity. Another error is mistaking insignificant soft tissue "clicks" for the more important and palpable "clunk." These innocent clicks may result from movement of fascia over the greater trochanter or may originate from the meniscus or the patella. Approximately 60% of all unstable hips seen in newborns spontaneously normalize within the first 2 to 4 weeks after birth as perinatal laxity resolves. A severely dysplastic hip may have negative results on examination because of the lack of an acetabular shelf. Some cases of dysplasia are believed to develop after birth. For this reason, most large series have shown that not all abnormal hips can be detected by screening, even when it is performed by skilled examiners. The signs of a dysplastic hip change with time. If the hip remains dislocated, it cannot usually be relocated by the time an affected baby is 6 months old. Findings of asymmetry such as limitation of abduction (Fig. 240-1C) and apparent shortening of the thigh are more sensitive at this time. This last sign, known as *Allis sign* or the *Galeazzi sign*, is best noted by comparing the lengths of the two flexed thighs when they are held together. Asymmetry of skin folds by itself is an unreliable finding. When children begin to walk, a positive Trendelenburg sign is noted: When weight is borne on the unstable side, the pelvis inclines to the other side.

Before age 6 months, there is a lack of apparent bony changes and ultrasonography is the imaging modality of choice to detect DDH. Ultrasonography is indicated if the neonatal examination is abnormal or questionable and may be used later to guide treatment. After age 6 months, the increasing ossification of the femur renders ultrasonography less reliable, and plain films are preferred.

TREATMENT

Treatment involves different measures at different ages. The aim of all therapy is to restore contact between the femoral head and the acetabulum. Because of the high percentage of patients who experience spontaneous improvement of lax hip capsules in the early perinatal period, most orthopedists recommend observing a hip that is subject to subluxation and reexamining it at age 3 to 4 weeks. Dislocated hips should be treated at the time of diagnosis. Usually, the initial treatment is a brace that holds the hip in flexion and abduction such as the Pavlik harness, which allows some motion while it holds the hip reduced. The alignment should be checked by radiography in 1 to 2 weeks. The brace is worn until the results of clinical and radiologic examinations are normal, an interval equal to approximately one to two times an affected child's age at diagnosis. If treatment is begun after affected children have reached age 6 months, they are usually too large and strong to tolerate the brace. At that point, reduction is performed under general anesthesia. Closed reduction is attempted first and is usually checked with an arthrogram. If it is successful, the reduction is held in a spica cast for a number of months. If closed reduction is unsuccessful, open reduction should be performed.

COMPLICATIONS

Possible complications of DDH include persistent dysplasia from failure of normal development, recurrent dislocation, and avascular necrosis of the femoral head. The latter condition, which is the most serious complication of DDH, is caused by obstruction of the epiphyseal vessels by excess pressure or capsular stretch. Avascular necrosis is more likely to occur when a hip is reduced in a patient who is older than 6 months and requires excessive traction or abduction to reduce the hip. The earlier treatment is carried out, the better is the resultant hip development, and the safer is each of the steps in treatment. Thus, careful, methodical early screening at well child visits can decrease the need for complex orthopedic procedures later.

CHAPTER 241
Transient (Toxic) Synovitis of the Hip

Adapted from Paul D. Sponseller

Transient (toxic) synovitis of the hip is a self-limited condition that represents the most common cause of an irritable hip in children. It is a clinical diagnosis of exclusion that presents as a painful limp or hip pain of acute or insidious onset, usually occurring unilaterally. The most common age range for the condition is 2 to 6 years, but it has been described in patients ranging from ages 1 to 15. Spasm occurs on testing of hip range of motion, particularly with internal rotation. The temperature, white blood cell (WBC) count, and erythrocyte sedimentation rate may be normal or slightly elevated. The cause of the condition is unknown; although an immune mechanism or viral infection is postulated. The differential diagnosis should include septic arthritis, osteomyelitis, and Legg-Calvé-Perthes disease. Juvenile monoarthritic rheumatoid arthritis and slipped capital femoral epiphysis (SCFE) should also be considered. Admission to the hospital, observation, and possible early aspiration should be undertaken if septic arthritis cannot be ruled out. Treatment consists of bed rest with analgesic agents provided, as needed, for 2 to 7 days. Sometimes, if the diagnosis is clear, therapy can be accomplished on an outpatient basis with frequent follow-up. Persistence of the symptoms beyond 1 week should prompt reevaluation, although bed rest for as long as 1 month has occasionally been required.

CHAPTER 242
Legg–Calvé–Perthes Disease (Coxa Plana)

Adapted from Paul D. Sponseller

Legg–Calvé–Perthes disease is characterized by ischemic (avascular) necrosis of the proximal femoral epiphysis with later resorption. The amount of the femur that is rendered ischemic varies and affects the outcome. Ischemia is followed by reossification with or without collapse of the femoral head. Recent evidence indicates that some cases may be caused by a subclinical hypercoagulable state such as a deficiency of antithrombotic factors S or C or a decrease in fibrinolysis. Legg–Calvé–Perthes disease usually, but not exclusively, affects children between ages 4 and 8. Boys are affected four times as often as girls and 15% of all cases are bilateral. As a group, affected patients have slightly shorter stature and delayed bone age as compared to their peers.

CLINICAL PRESENTATIONS

Usually, the clinical presentation of this disorder is a limp with minimal pain of either short or long duration. The pain is not as acute or severe as that of transient synovitis or septic arthritis. Motions that are especially limited include internal rotation and abduction. These movements may be resisted by mild spasm or guarding. In the earliest stage, radiographic results may be normal or reveal that the affected femoral epiphysis is slightly smaller as compared to the contralateral side as a result of its failure to grow after becoming avascular. Later, a narrow crescentic lucency, seen best on the lateral view, may be observed; it is the result of a tiny fracture of the subchondral bone. This view reveals the extent of bone involved (Fig. 242-1A–C).

DIFFERENTIAL DIAGNOSIS

The differential diagnosis should include transient synovitis, septic arthritis, hematogenous osteomyelitis, various types of hemoglobinopathy, Gaucher disease, hypothyroidism, and the epiphyseal dysplasias. Often, the latter two conditions are

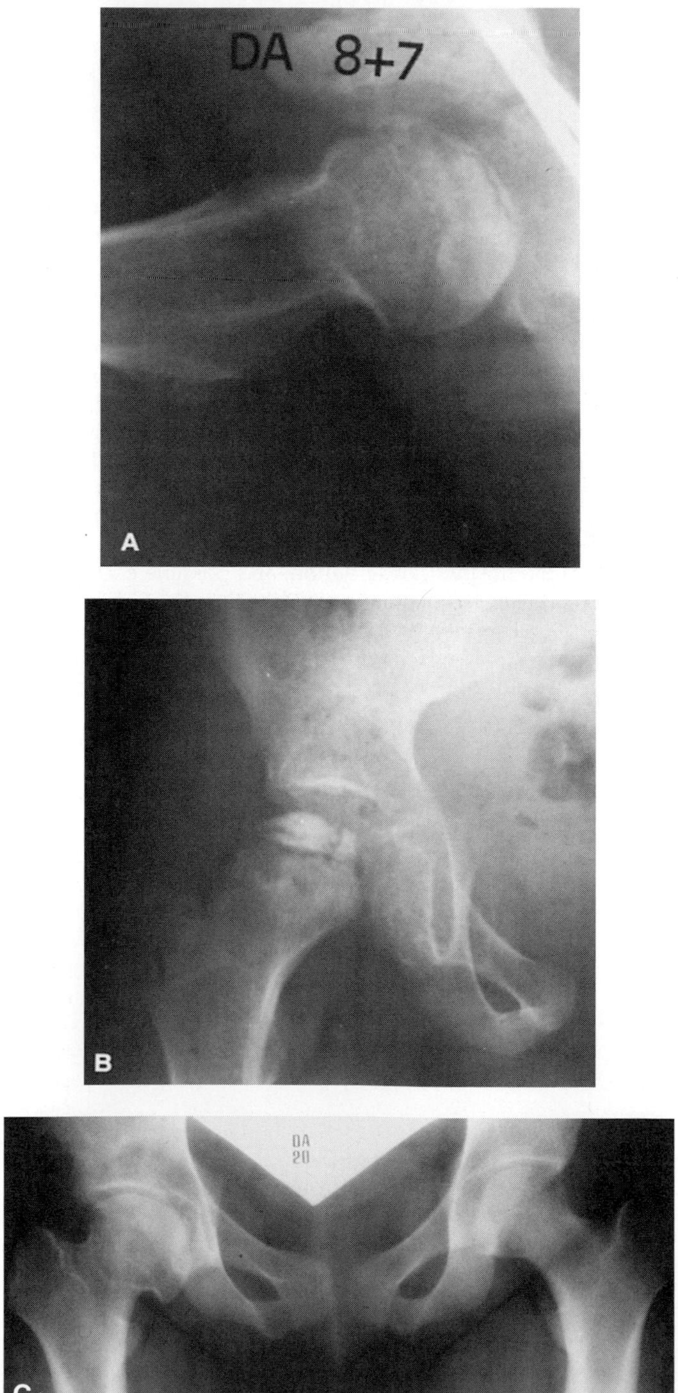

Figure 242-1. A: Early Legg–Calvé–Perthes disease showing subchondral "crescent." **B:** Later, resorption and apparent collapse of the femoral head are evident. **C:** Finally, restoration of the spherically ossified femoral head is seen here at age 20, although the femoral neck is slightly short.

temporally symmetric bilaterally, whereas Legg–Calvé–Perthes disease is not.

TREATMENT

Treatment follows two principles: containment of the femoral head within the acetabulum and maintenance of range of motion. Children younger than 6 years or those who have involvement of less than one-half the femoral head may be observed without active treatment if a full range of motion is preserved because this range signals containment, and patients in this age group have a good prognosis. Aggressive treatment is indicated for patients who have involvement of more than one-half the femoral head and are older than 6 years.

CONTAINMENT

Containment may be achieved by the use of an orthosis or by surgery. Orthoses produce abduction with or without internal rotation. The orthosis used most commonly is the Scottish Rite brace, which does not extend below the knees (Fig. 242-2). Affected children are allowed to perform any activity that is possible in the brace. The orthosis should be worn until early reossification is seen. Generally, surgical treatment is more effective in achieving containment than the brace. Surgery does not speed the healing of the femoral head but causes it to reossify in a more spherical fashion. Typically, children with Legg–Calvé–Perthes disease have intermittent mild aching in the hip for 1 to 2 years until reossification is complete, but then they are virtually asymptomatic throughout childhood. Symptoms may develop later in adulthood depending on the degree of femoral head deformation.

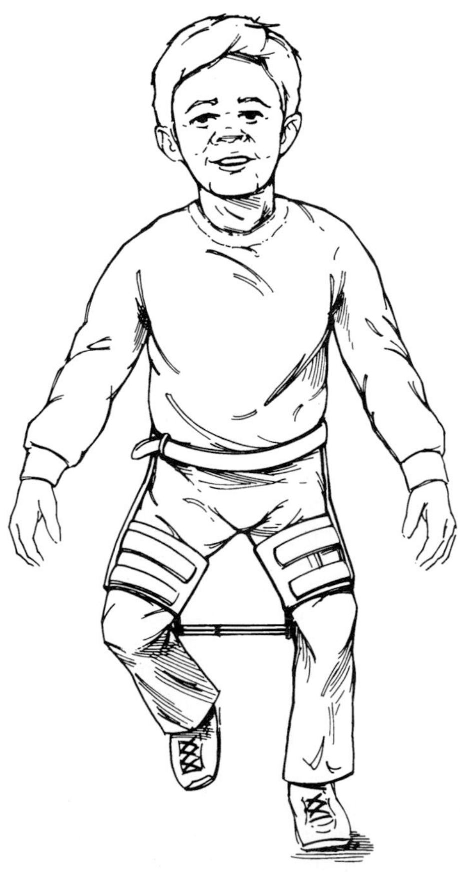

Figure 242-2. Scottish Rite brace for Legg–Calvé–Perthes disease produces containment by abduction and allows free knee motion.

CHAPTER 243

Slipped Capital Femoral Epiphysis

Adapted from Paul D. Sponseller

Slipped capital femoral epiphysis (SCFE) is a growth-plate disorder that occurs near the age of skeletal maturity and involves a three-dimensional displacement of the epiphysis (posteriorly, medially, and inferiorly). In other words, the femur is rotated externally from under the epiphysis. The periosteum at this age is thin and less able to resist the shearing forces. The cause appears to involve both mechanical and biological factors. Usually, SCFE occurs without severe sudden force or trauma. Mechanically, in most affected children, increased stress occurs as a result of obesity and abnormal posterior rotation of the femoral head and neck. Possible biological causes include hormonal factors and delayed growth-plate maturation, which may account for the associated obesity. Increased growth hormone levels have been associated with decreased physeal shear strength, and hypothyroidism has been found in some cases. Usually, SCFE occurs during the growth spurt and before menarche in girls. The condition is rare with a frequency of 1 in 100,000 to 8 in 100,000. It is more common in men and in blacks. Approximately one-fourth to one-third of all affected children experience bilateral involvement but usually not simultaneously.

CLINICAL PRESENTATIONS

The clinical presentation varies with the acuity of the process. Most affected children exhibit a limp and endure varying degrees of aching or pain. The discomfort may be in the groin, but it is often referred to the thigh or knee. Many patients are dismissed for an apparent knee complaint with no obvious cause, only to have the true hip pathology discovered later with worsening of the slip. This paradoxic distribution of pain is attributed to referral within the femoral nerve distribution, which involves both the hip and knee joints. Some patients have acute, severe pain and inability to walk or move the hip. Abduction, internal rotation, and flexion are the motions that are most limited. A characteristic finding is external rotation of the hip with flexion, which is caused by the preexisting posterior rotation and the slip itself. Apparent limb shortening as a result of the proximal displacement of the metaphysis may be present.

LABORATORY FINDINGS

The earliest radiographic findings are widening and irregularity of the growth plate and osteopenia of the femur. Later, displacement of the epiphysis occurs and is best seen on the frog-leg lateral view of the pelvis. On the AP view, a line drawn

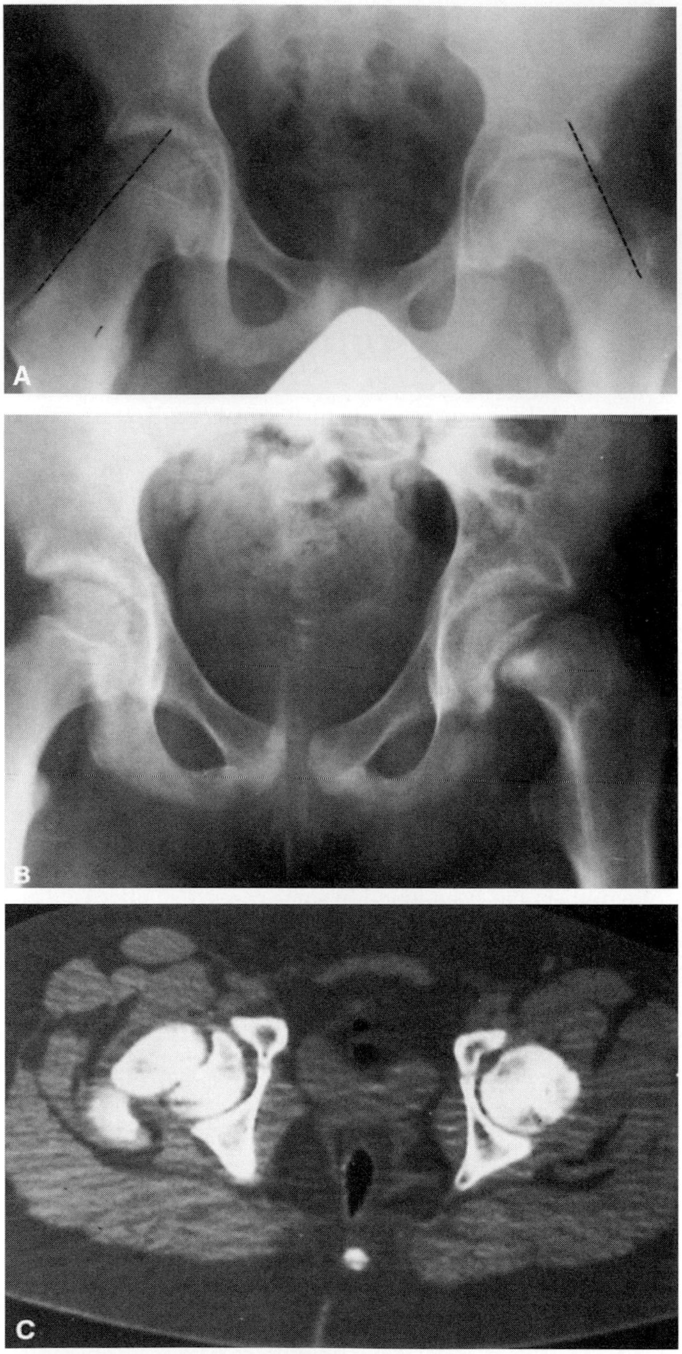

Figure 243-1. Radiographic findings in slipped capital femoral epiphysis. **A:** A line drawn along the superior-lateral femoral neck intersects less than the normal 20% of the epiphysis on the left (affected) side. **B:** A more severe slip showing that the femoral neck subluxates laterally and superiorly with respect to the epiphysis. **C:** Computed tomographic (CT) scan most clearly shows the direction of the slip. This figure shows *in situ* fixation with a single screw, the preferred method for slips of mild to moderate degree and even many cases of severe degree.

through the upper margin of the narrowest portion of the neck should intersect at least 20% of the epiphysis (Fig. 243-1). This point is important because, with remodeling during chronic slipping, a step-off at the junction of the epiphysis and metaphysis may be absent. The severity of the slip is graded as mild (less than 33%), moderate (33%–50%), or severe (greater than 50%). Later changes may include avascular necrosis of the epiphysis or chondrolysis (i.e., joint-space narrowing).

TREATMENT

Treatment centers on preventing further slippage, usually by placing affected patients immediately at bed rest and obtaining a prompt orthopedic consultation. Surgery (pinning) is intended to stabilize the upper femur and to cause the growth plate to close. Realignment of the slip is not safe in chronic cases because the forces necessary to accomplish realignment may produce avascular necrosis by disrupting the blood supply to the epiphysis. The contralateral side should be monitored by affected patients' parents for symptoms of SCFE and should be pinned early if such symptoms occur. Long-term follow-up reveals no early degenerative change unless chondrolysis or avascular necrosis occurs; each has an incidence of 1% to 5% and produces disability during adolescence. However, even in the absence of these complications, degenerative joint disease may occur in middle age.

CHAPTER 244
Femoral Anteversion

Adapted from Paul D. Sponseller

Increased femoral anteversion is one of a spectrum of torsional deformities that affect the alignment of the knee and foot with the body and may lead to toeing-in. The differential diagnosis of toeing-in includes this disorder and internal tibial torsion and foot deformities such as metatarsus adductus (Table 244-1). Increased anteversion of the femur is defined as an increase in the angle between the plane of the femoral neck and the plane of the knee (Fig. 244-1). Normally, this angle is approximately 30 degrees at birth and declines to 15 degrees by age 10. Femoral anteversion persists in some neuromuscular conditions, presumably as a result of lack of remodeling forces. The type discussed here is isolated idiopathic femoral anteversion.

On physical examination, affected patients appear to toe-in unless compensatory external tibial torsion is present. The patellae also face medially ("squint"). Radiographically, the femoral head and neck appear to be relatively straight on an AP film with the patella forward. Computed tomography (CT) is the best device for measuring femoral anteversion directly.

The natural history of femoral anteversion is benign. In a few patients, it may contribute to patellar malalignment, however, it does not impair function. Anteversion later in life has not been linked to arthritis of the hip or knee. Treatment of increased anteversion typically consists of observation. Children older than age 8 can develop restriction from prolonged W-sitting (with the knees touching and the legs folded under), which may impair remodeling. Affected children should be instructed to sit in the tailor position (with the feet tucked under and the knees out to the side). Orthotics and braces such as cables and bars are not effective in derotating the femur. Femoral osteotomy, proximally or distally, is the only truly effective therapy. It should be performed only in children who are older than age 8 and have a functional disability as a result of patellar malalignment or, rarely, in older children with a persistent concern regarding their appearance.

TABLE 244-1. Differential Diagnosis of Common Pediatric Symptoms

Limp
- Pain
  - Septic arthritis-osteomyelitis
  - Transient synovitis
  - Juvenile rheumatoid arthritis
  - Migratory polyarthritis (immunologic)
  - Legg–Calvé–Perthes disease
  - Slipped capital femoral epiphysis
  - Meniscus tear
  - Idiopathic chondrolysis of the hip
  - Osgood–Schlatter disease
  - Impacted fracture
  - Spinal disorder
- Weakness
  - Congenital dislocation of the hip
  - Myopathy
  - Polio
  - Cerebral palsy–myelomeningocele
  - Spinal cord compression
- Limitation of motion
  - Legg–Perthes disease–slipped capital femoral epiphysis (old)
  - Posttraumatic muscle contracture
  - Posttraumatic joint contracture
- Leg-length inequality
  - Idiopathic hemihypertrophy
  - Posttraumatic malunion or growth-plate closure
  - Neuromuscular
    - Cerebral palsy
    - Polio
  - Neurofibromatosis
  - Congenital limb deficiency
  - Ollier disease
  - Arteriovenous malformation

Knee pain
- Musculotendinous
  - Patellofemoral stress syndrome
  - Osgood–Schlatter disease
  - Patellar-quadriceps tendinitis
  - Iliotibial band syndrome
- Bony-cartilaginous
  - Meniscus tear
  - Discoid meniscus
  - Osteochondritis dissecans
  - Tibial spine fracture–physeal injury
- Miscellaneous
  - Infection
  - Tumor
  - Connective tissue disorder
  - Hip disorder

Childhood back pain
- Developmental-acquired
  - Scheuermann kyphosis
  - Spondylolysis-spondylolisthesis
  - Herniated nucleus pulposus
  - Fracture of vertebral body
  - Muscle strain
- Infectious
  - Vertebral body osteomyelitis
  - Discitis
  - Tuberculosis
- Neoplastic
  - Osteoid osteoma
  - Osteoblastoma-osteosarcoma
  - Leukemia-lymphoma
  - Eosinophilic granuloma
  - Ewing sarcoma–neuroblastoma
  - Spinal cord tumor

Internal rotation of the lower extremity: toeing-in
- Femoral
  - Anteversion
  - Muscular-capsular
- Tibial torsion
- Metatarsus adductus
- Clubfoot, partially treated
- Neuromuscular disorder

Flatfoot
- Flexible-idiopathic
- Tarsal coalition
- Juvenile rheumatoid arthritis
- Congenital vertical talus
- Marfan syndrome
- Neuromuscular disorders

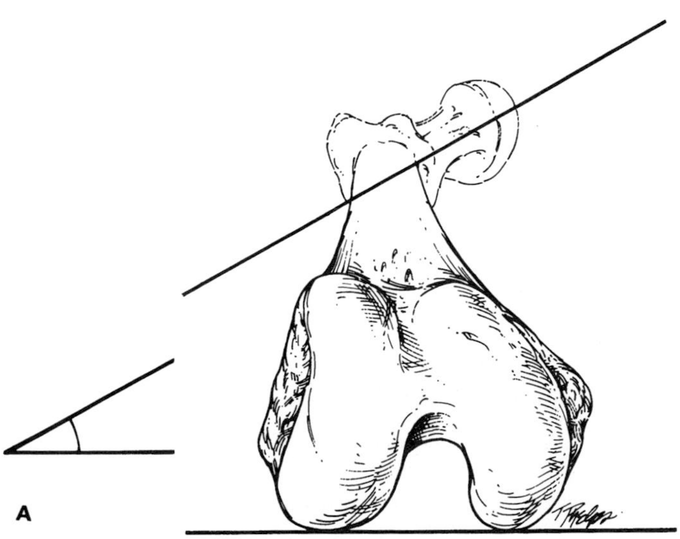

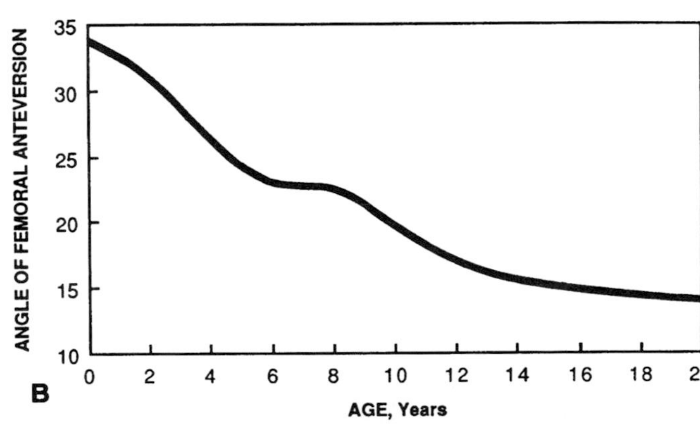

Figure 244-1. A: Femoral anteversion is defined as the rotation of the femoral neck forward (in comparison with the distal condyles), as seen in this view down the axis of the femur. **B:** The curve shows the normal decrease in femoral anteversion with age.

CHAPTER 245
Patellofemoral Problems

Adapted from Paul D. Sponseller

The patellofemoral joint is subject to repeated high loads of laterally and posteriorly directed forces. Chondromalacia refers specifically to the appearance of softening and degeneration of the patellar cartilage. Patellar subluxation refers to partial lateral displacement of the patella. The terms *patellofemoral stress syndrome*, *patellar malalignment*, and *excessive lateral pressure syndrome* refer to the abnormal mechanics causing stress concentration and pain.

The patellofemoral force may be as great as 2.5 times body weight and is greatest in flexion. The average tibiofemoral angle is angled approximately 6 degrees outward, which the patella must follow. The quadriceps-patella mechanism itself is angled away from the midline of the body, as measured by the Q (quadriceps) angle from the anterosuperior spine to the patella to the tibial tubercle (Fig. 245-1A). These high forces and asymmetric loads cause minor variations to become significant, especially when repeated over high numbers of cycles as a part of daily living. Laxity of the medial side of the patellar restraints contributes to subluxation or dislocation. Possible factors contributing to patellar pathology are shown in Fig. 245-1B. Usually, these factors cause greater stress on the lateral side of the patella and, sometimes, decreased medial patellofemoral contact. Cartilage degeneration occurs as a result of the decreased contact beginning in the deep layers centrally and medially and becoming visible later.

CLINICAL PRESENTATIONS

Clinically, problems with the patella cause aching that is greatest in the anteromedial knee region, on the medial side or center of the patella. Usually, this pain is worse with stair climbing or prolonged sitting. Crepitus may be felt, but it may be painless in some patients and is not pathologic in itself. "Catching" or "locking" may be noted and might represent pain-induced inhibition or mechanical phenomena. A feeling of "giving way" may be described by the patient, especially with subluxation of the patella.

PHYSICAL EXAMINATION

On physical examination, the most reliable way to test patellar tenderness is by direct compression of each facet against the femur. Contraction of the quadriceps and patella against resistance is nonspecific because it may be painful even in normal persons. Effusion is present only if patellar degenerative changes or extreme overuse has occurred. Reproducing patellar subluxation with laterally directed pressure may cause apprehension. The Q angle, femoral anteversion, and tibial torsion should be checked. Usually, radiographic results are nonspecific, but lateral displacement or tilt of the patella may be occasionally seen on the sunrise view.

Patellofemoral stress disorders are common in patients between the ages of 10 and 20, but they often become less symptomatic later. Usually, they do not progress to osteoarthritis. Other diagnoses to consider are shown in Table 245-1.

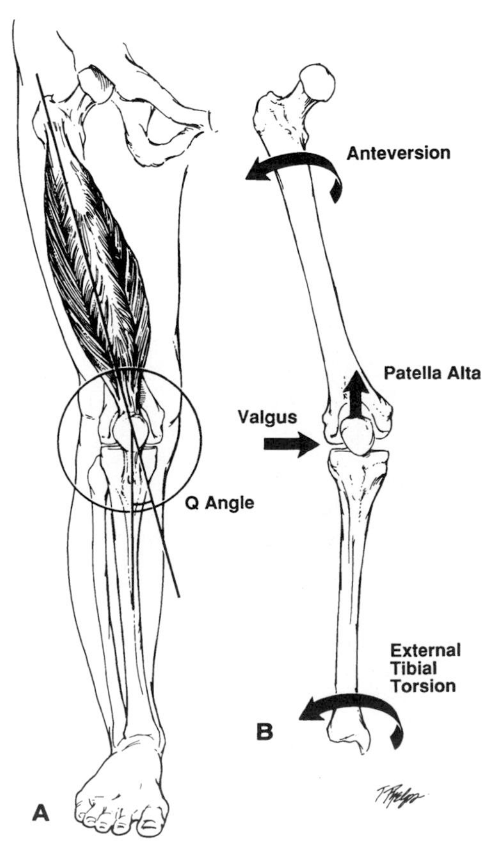

Figure 245-1. A: The Q angle, measured from anterior superior iliac spine to center of patella to tibial tubercle. **B:** Factors that may contribute to excess patellofemoral stress.

TABLE 245-1. Differential Diagnosis of Patellofemoral Stress Disorders
Synovial fold or "plica"
Medial meniscus tear
Tendinitis of the quadriceps or patellar tendon
Osteochondritis dissecans of the patella or distal femur

TREATMENT

Treatment consists of altering the abnormal stresses that are occurring. Modification may include decreasing activities performed with the knees flexed, especially those that cause pain (i.e., stair climbing, prolonged sitting, and bicycling). Temporary rest from sports and the use of nonsteroidal antiinflammatory agents may be necessary. Exercises to strengthen the medial (stabilizing) part of the quadriceps may be beneficial. Hamstrings and rectus femoris muscles, if they are tight, should be stretched to decrease preload on the extensors. Arch supports may help if severe flexible flatfoot is contributing to tibial torsion. Surgical measures include release of a tight lateral patellar retinaculum, medial soft tissue tightening, tibial tubercle transfer, or correction of genu valgum, knee anteversion, or patella alta if it is severe. These measures produce satisfactory pain relief in 75% to 90% of patients.

Patellar dislocations may be acute, recurrent or, rarely, habitual. Almost always, they occur in the lateral direction. Acute dislocations are associated with significant swelling and medial knee pain and with a history of significant outward or rotating force. They should be treated for extension with a lateral knee immobilizer until symptom-free, except in skeletally mature patients with bony avulsion. Recurrent subluxation is common, causes less pain and swelling, and often occurs with minimal force. A realignment operation (as described) is the only effective way to stop frequent and bothersome episodes.

CHAPTER 246
Osgood–Schlatter Disease

Adapted from Paul D. Sponseller

Osgood–Schlatter disease is a traction-induced inflammation of the tibial tubercle. It is a reaction of the bone and cartilage of this region to high stress. The tibial tubercle is a downward extension of the proximal tibial epiphysis. It develops an ossification center in patients between ages 9 and 13, but it does not ossify completely until they are 15 to 17 years old. Within this age range, repetitive stresses can gradually deform the outer surface of the tubercle plastically causing it to enlarge and become locally inflamed (Fig. 246-1). Tenderness and swelling are localized to this region. Symptoms are worse with running, jumping, or kneeling. Treatment involves decreasing activity to a tolerable level and occasionally using a knee immobilizer, crutches, and ice after activity in severe cases. The patient may be vulnerable to recurrence of symptoms for up to 2 years until the tubercle matures. If affected children and their families are informed of this likelihood, individual regulation of activities can be effective.

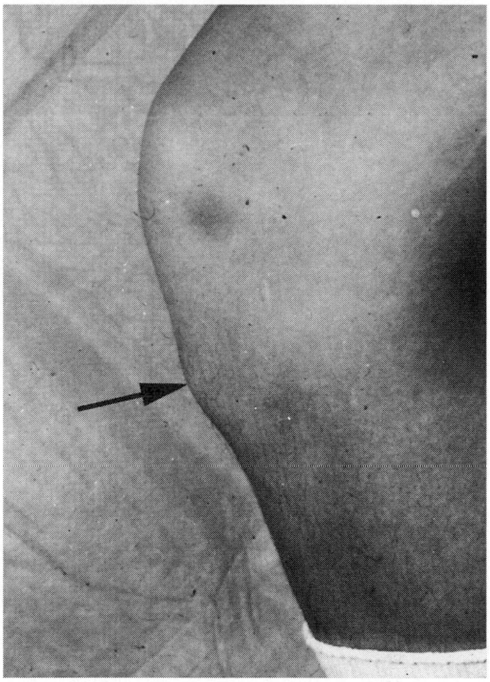

Figure 246-1. Osgood–Schlatter "disease" often produces an enlargement of the tibial tubercle (*arrow*).

Usually, activities of daily living and even some sports are tolerated using daily stretching of tight quadriceps and hamstrings and occasional antiinflammatory agents. Complete avulsion of the tubercle is extremely rare and seems to be related more to sudden stress than to apophysitis.

CHAPTER 247
Genu Varum

Adapted from Paul D. Sponseller

Genu varum, or "bowed leg" of up to 20 degrees, is normal in children until age 18 months. Normally, it does not significantly increase after walking begins. After the child reaches the age of 24 months, genu valgum normally develops (see below). The differential diagnosis of genu varum (physiologic bowing) includes Blount disease, rickets, posttraumatic growth-plate disturbance, enchondromatosis, achondroplasia, and other skeletal dysplasias.

Indications for radiographs in children with genu varum are shown in Table 247-1. Radiographic findings of benign genu varus include symmetric bowing of the tibia and femur, a normal-appearing growth plate without narrowing or step-off, and a generalized, rather than focal, outward bowing (Fig. 247-1).

TABLE 247-1. Indications for Radiographs in Children with Genu Varum
Bowing present after age 2 or progressive after age 1
Severe or asymmetric bowing
High risk groups (obese children, early walkers)

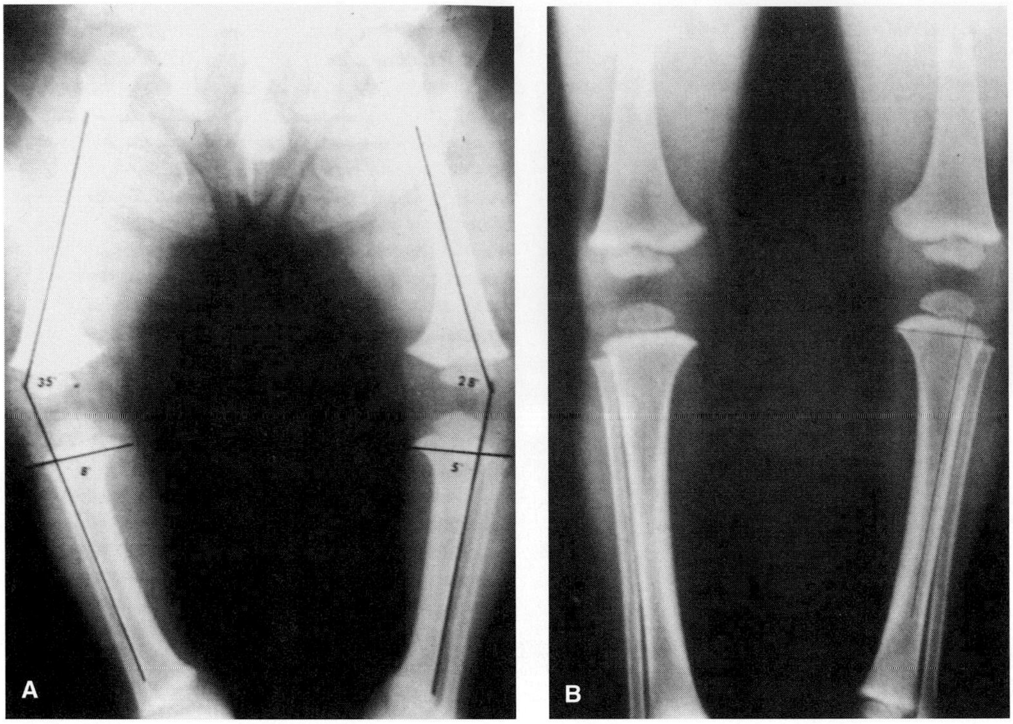

Figure 247-1. Note improvement in physiologic bowing between age 18 months (**A**) and 24 months (**B**) without treatment.

Treatment involves observation to verify resolution. Measurement of the angle on physical examination should be performed with the child standing and may also be accomplished by measuring the distance between the femoral condyles or of the AP tibiofemoral angle. These methods are not as accurate as are radiographs, but they are a practical way of observing change in patients when the presumptive diagnosis is physiologic genu varum.

CHAPTER 248

Blount's Disease

Adapted from Paul D. Sponseller

Tibia vara, also known as *Blount disease*, is an idiopathic, probably mechanical deficiency in the medial tibial growth plate that may be unilateral or bilateral. The ratio of genu varum (physiologic bowing) to Blount disease is more than 1,000:1. Initially, it may present in two different age groups: infants and adolescents.

Untreated infantile tibia vara is almost always progressive with evidence of outward angulation, flexion, internal rotation, and abnormal lateral knee laxity. Radiography demonstrates progressive depression of the medial metaphysis, the growth plate, and the epiphysis. Fusion of the medial metaphysis to the epiphysis may occur in severe cases. A helpful early distinction in tibia vara is the focal nature of the change with sharp angulation of the proximal tibial metaphysis resulting in a metaphyseal-diaphyseal angle of 11 to 16 degrees or more, measured as shown in Fig. 248-1. It is a specific sign because such localized angulation occurs in less than 5% of children with physiologic bowing but is seen in essentially all those with Blount disease.

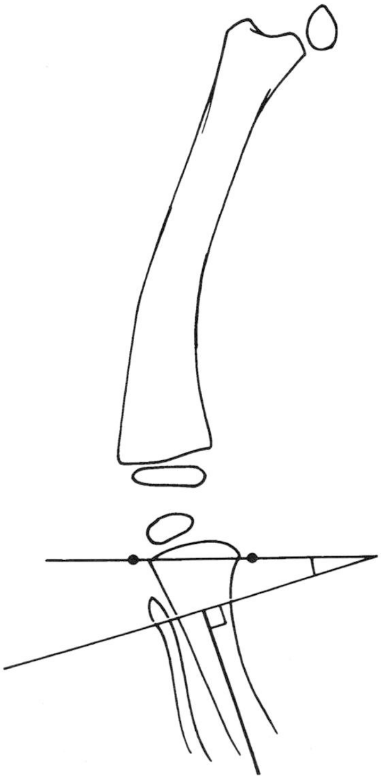

Figure 248-1. Metaphyseal-diaphyseal angle. The angle is formed by the line of the tibial shaft and the line between the medial and lateral beaks of the proximal tibial metaphysis. (Redrawn with permission from Levine AM. Physiologic bowing and tibia varum. *J Bone Joint Surg* 1982;64A:1159.)

Night-brace treatment, though not formally proven to be effective, is usually used for mild but definite cases of Blount disease. Valgus rotational osteotomy of the tibia is indicated if the angulation persists beyond 3 years. Recurrence is common if treatment begins after age 4, if the epiphysis is fragmented, or if an affected child is obese. Persistent tibia vara leads to early degenerative change.

Adolescent tibia vara has its onset in children older than age 9. It is most common in obese boys. Probably, it is caused by decreased growth of the medial tibial physis resulting from excessive medial stresses. Radiography shows medial femoral and tibial bowing. Bracing is not practical in these obese adolescents. Treatment involves osteotomy to realign the limb or lateral growth-plate closure to allow growth to "catch up" medially.

CHAPTER 249

Genu Valgum

Adapted from Paul D. Sponseller

Genu valgum of the knee is normal in children older than age 2, reaches a mean of 12 degrees at age 3, and remains approximately constant at a mean of approximately 7 degrees in boys and 9 degrees in girls after age 8. Night bracing may be helpful in children with angulation exceeding 20 degrees. If the angle remains greater than 15 degrees when the child reaches age 10, early growth-plate stapling or later osteotomy of the affected region may be indicated. Valgus of the proximal tibia often follows medial metaphyseal fractures, but it frequently corrects spontaneously.

CHAPTER 250

Internal Tibial Torsion

Adapted from Paul D. Sponseller

Internal tibial torsion is the most common cause of toeing-in among children ages 1 to 3. Tibial torsion is determined by measuring the angle between the foot and the thigh with the ankle and knee positioned at 90 degrees. Normally, the foot rotates externally with age (Fig. 250-1). The differential diagnosis includes metatarsus adductus, femoral anteversion, and neuromuscular disorders. For making these distinctions, the foot, as well as the hip, should be examined (Fig. 250-1A–C). Tibial torsion improves naturally with growth, but this improvement often takes years. Because of our improved knowledge of the benign natural history of this condition, bracing is only rarely used. Studies have shown that braces cannot apply significant rotational force to the tibia because the corrective force is taken up in the foot, knee, and hip joints. The improvement that was previously attributed to the brace is primarily the result of normal growth patterns. Correction is a slow process and often frustrates parents. Primary care physicians should be confident in allaying parental anxiety about toeing-in caused by tibial torsion. Children may have varying degrees of toeing-in and some may catch a foot when they run. Fortunately, this improves as the bone grows longer and straighter. Most children outgrow this problem over time, and minor persistent internal torsion has not shown to be detrimental.

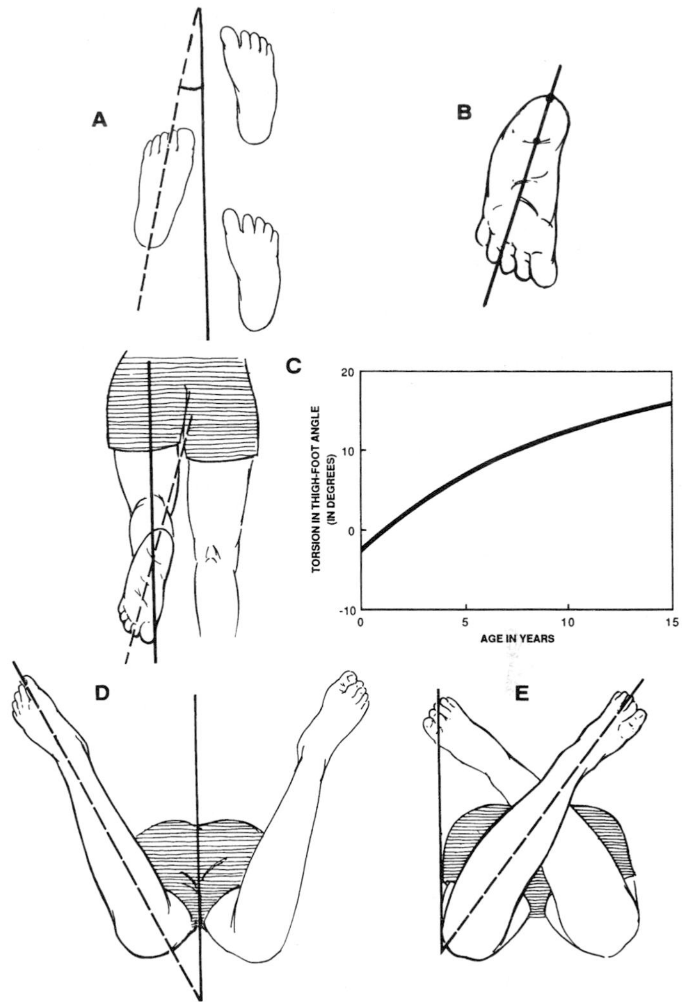

Figure 250-1. Assessment of torsional deformities. **A:** Angle of progression (the angle between the foot and the line of gait)—summation of femoral, knee, tibial, and foot relationships. **B:** Assessment of metatarsus adductus. Normally, the heel bisector falls between the second and third toe space. **C:** Thigh-foot angle and its variation with age. This is a reflection of tibial torsion. Measurement of internal (**D**) and external (**E**) rotation of the hip. If external rotation is less than 20 degrees, "in-toeing" may come from femoral anteversion or hip capsular contractures. (Redrawn with permission from Staheli LT, et al. Lower-extremity rotational problems in children. *J Bone Joint Surg* 1985;67A:41.)

CHAPTER 251

Limb-Length Inequality

Adapted from Paul D. Sponseller

Limb-length differences are best screened by palpating the heights of the iliac crests with the hips and knees straight. Any discrepancy may be confirmed with a tape measure held between the anterior superior iliac spine and the inferior edge of the medial malleolus. Most commonly, apparent differences in the lengths of the lower limbs in children are due to measurement error, as affected patients have difficulty in lying still and in holding hips and knees straight. In the normal population, differences of 1 cm between the two sides are not uncommon findings.

Discrepancies of up to 2 cm in adults (or a proportionately smaller amount in children) have been shown to have no ill effects on gait or joints and do not need treatment. Larger discrepancies should be confirmed with a radiographic film (scanogram) or with a computed tomographic (CT) scan. Causes of true, significant discrepancy greater than 2 cm may include hemihypertrophy, hemiatrophy, coxa vara, hip dysplasia, or growth-plate damage, to name a few. Because hemihypertrophy has been associated with Wilms tumor in some cases, these patients should be examined with abdominal ultrasonography two to three times per year. Treatment of significant limb-length inequalities may include a lift, an epiphyseodesis of the long side if growth remains, or a surgical shortening or lengthening procedure.

CHAPTER 252
Metatarsus Adductus

Adapted from Paul D. Sponseller

Metatarsus adductus, or isolated idiopathic adduction of the metatarsals, is also known as *metatarsus varus* or *C-foot*. In contrast to conditions seen in clubfoot, in metatarsus adductus, the hindfoot is normal or angled outward slightly. The ankle joint itself has normal dorsiflexion and plantar flexion (Fig. 252-1). The probable cause of this condition is medially directed intrauterine pressure. Children with metatarsus adductus may also have an increased incidence of other molding deformities such as congenital dislocation of the hip or torticollis. Metatarsus adductus deformity should be differentiated from skewfoot, which involves severe outward deviation of the hindfoot, treatment of which is much more difficult.

The natural history of untreated metatarsus adductus is spontaneous correction in 85% of children with the persistence of mild adduction in 10% and more pronounced adduction in 5%. In one longitudinal study of 2,000 feet in newborns followed until maturity, no patients had symptomatic adduction in adulthood. Those cases that will resolve spontaneously cannot be predicted, even on the basis of severity or rigidity.

Usually, manipulative correction is successful anytime during the first 8 months of life. Some orthopedists prefer observation with stretching for the first 6 to 8 months, followed by corrective casts or splints if the condition persists beyond this time. The casts are changed every 1 to 2 weeks until the defect is clinically corrected; then a "holding cast" is applied for 2 weeks. Osteotomy for very late-presenting adduction in children older than age 3 is rarely necessary.

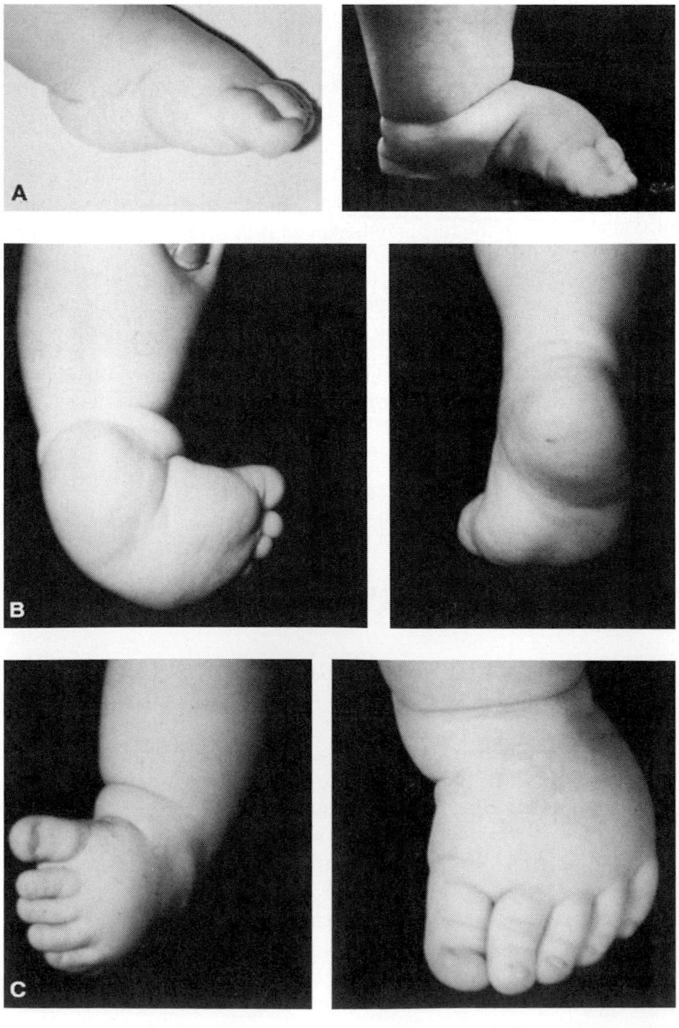

Figure 252-1. Comparison of clubfoot (*left*) and metatarsus adductus (*right*). **A:** Lateral view showing the equinus present only in clubfoot. **B:** Posterior view showing the hindfoot varus in clubfoot but not in metatarsus adductus. **C:** Anterior view showing adduction in both feet with the varus also present in clubfoot.

CHAPTER 253
Clubfoot

Adapted from Paul D. Sponseller

Talipes equinovarus congenita, or clubfoot, is a more complex disorder involving not only metatarsal adduction but also abnormalities of the hind part of the foot including malrotation of the calcaneus under the talus and equinus (plantar flexion) of the ankle. The incidence is 1 in 1,000, and it is more common in men than in women. Clubfoot may be unilateral or bilateral. Its cause is unknown but appears to be related to a primary defect of local connective tissue or a very early insult to the leg muscles or tarsal bones.

Physical examination reveals a small foot, and the combination of deformities often results in a 90-degree rotation of the forefoot in all planes so that the leg and foot truly resemble the shape of a club. A deep crease is present on the medial border of the foot. The deformity may initially be correctable to the neutral position only in the neonatal period, and the range of motion in all planes is limited. Although not necessary in the typical case, radiography shows an abnormal parallelism of the talus and calcaneus.

Clubfoot ranges from a mild, "postural," and easily correctable condition to one that is severe and resistant to treatment. A trial of cast correction is indicated in all cases. This treatment is most successful when started in the perinatal period when ligamentous laxity is greatest with the casts being changed every few days. Overall, casting is effective in approximately one-third to one-half of all patients. Surgery is indicated in the others and involves complete release of all bony malalignments and tendon contractures; it is performed most commonly between the ages of 6 and 12 months.

CHAPTER 254
Flatfoot (Pes Planovalgus)

Adapted from Paul D. Sponseller

The condition called *flatfoot* can be divided into flexible and rigid types. The flexible type is very common in children and usually causes no symptoms. Development of the arch of the foot spontaneously occurs during the first 8 years of life in most children. The arch of the foot is restored when weight bearing is relieved. Inward-outward motion is normal. In contrast, rigid flatfoot may be caused by tarsal coalition, a vertical talus, neuromuscular imbalance (which, occasionally, may also be flexible), or arthritis of the foot.

The cause of the usual type of flexible flatfoot is ligamentous laxity with mild secondary bony changes. No primary muscle abnormality exists. Treatment is not indicated in asymptomatic cases of flexible flatfoot; prospective studies have shown that no orthotic or special shoe can produce a lasting change in pediatric flatfoot. Such devices may be indicated for rigid or neuromuscular flatfoot but not in asymptomatic children who have flexible flatfoot. The heel cord should be stretched if it is tight. Soft tissue reconstruction or osteotomy is rarely indicated. It should be emphasized to parents that shoes are primarily for protection; "corrective shoes" have no effect on flatfoot; and shoes should be flat, flexible, porous, and high-topped to prevent them from slipping off the foot.

CHAPTER 255
Childhood Back Pain

Adapted from Paul D. Sponseller

Although popular wisdom formerly held that back pain in children almost always had a serious underlying cause, more recent studies have shown that nonspecific back pain is common in children with only one-fifth eventually given a diagnosis of a specific cause. Nevertheless, potential problems should be ruled out. Careful neurologic examination is necessary in evaluating children for back pain, as is an assessment of spinal flexibility and deformity. The differential diagnoses listed in Table 244-1 are the conditions most commonly encountered.

MUSCULOLIGAMENTOUS PAIN

All the components of a child's spine (i.e., discs, ligaments, muscles, and joint capsules) are flexible and easily conform to the extreme spinal positions that are encountered daily in the schoolyard or on the playing field. After the child reaches approximately 12 years, generally the spine loses some of its flexibility and, during the teenage years, further "stiffening" may take place. Muscular or ligamentous back pain is almost never observed in children who are younger than 10 years. This diagnosis should be reserved for an older child (often involved in a new physical activity) who has lumbar area pain for which no other specific cause can be elucidated. To warrant this diagnosis, affected children should have pain localized to the lumbar area, a normal neurologic examination, normal results on radiography of the lumbar spine and, in some instances, normal bone scan results.

Once the diagnosis has been made, the treatment of musculoligamentous pain involves rest from any activity that causes the pain. The use of ice in the first 24 hours after onset is helpful; thereafter, heat is usually more efficacious. Once the pain has resolved, exercises should be used to strengthen the abdominal musculature and the lumbar muscles before sports activity is resumed. A lumbosacral corset is often helpful in the acute stage and, for a few months thereafter, when affected children are participating in sports to protect the low back and its muscles from the extremes of spinal movement. Once low-back pain has resolved, physicians should stress the importance of warming up before participating in sports activities. The persistence of pain requires further investigation for unusual causes of back pain.

SPONDYLOLYSIS AND SPONDYLOLISTHESIS

Spondylolysis is a common anatomic cause of back pain in children typically resulting from a stress fracture of the pars interarticularis segment of the vertebra. This thin segment of bone between the facet joints is subjected to high forces, especially with marked lordosis of the lumbar spine or with heavy lifting. The overall incidence in the general population is approximately 6%. Most of these stress fractures likely occur in the early school years, though symptoms most frequently occur when children are in their early teenage years. A much higher frequency of spondylolysis occurs in children who participate in gymnastics, wrestling, and weight-lifting activities at times approaching 20% for participants in these sports.

Most commonly, symptoms include pain in the lumbar area after or during a sports activity and a concomitant limitation of lumbar spine motion. If affected children have a chronic spondylolysis, the pain is often intermittent; if the spondylolysis is acute, the pain is more severe the first time it is noted. Occasionally, radiation of pain along the sciatic nerve distribution into the lateral calf or dorsum of the foot may be present.

The physical examination may be unremarkable. Usually, limitation of lateral spine flexion toward the side of the spondylolysis occurs and may be associated with limited forward flexion from back pain. Back pain may be produced by straight-leg raising, but radiation of pain into the legs with this maneuver is rare. The results of the neurologic examination are normal.

Often, the diagnosis can be made by lumbar spine radiographs (Fig. 255-1). The most common locations of spondylolysis are L4 and L5. Often, spondylolysis can be visualized by AP and lateral radiographic views, but oblique views are usually more definitive. It may be prudent to refer children suspected of having spondylolysis to an orthopedic surgeon for further evaluation and radiographic studies. Treatment initially involves rest from activity. Often, a lumbosacral corset is helpful for a few weeks until pain resolves. Some teenagers with spondylolysis prefer to wear the corset during sports activities as added protection, even after acute back pain resolves. Children should be followed with serial radiography during the growing years to rule out development of a progressive slip. Generally, fusion for spondylolysis is not needed. With the exception of occasional episodes of low-back pain, teenagers are able to participate in any sport that does not repetitively lead to back pain after playing.

Spondylolisthesis occurs in some children who have spondylolysis. This condition results from forward slipping of a superior vertebra on the inferior vertebra, most commonly, slipping of L5 on the sacrum (Fig. 255-2). Worsening of this slip coincides with growth of the spine and generally subsides once growth is completed. Because the slip of the vertebra progresses forward, the posterior elements (i.e., the spinous process and inferior facets) remain behind, attached to the adjacent vertebrae by ligaments. The combination of excessive motion of the posterior elements and forward vertebral slipping may lead to irritation of L5 or S1 nerve roots. Because this slipping is usually slow, the nerve root irritation may present only as progressive tightening of the hamstrings. Affected children may note difficulty in touching their toes or reaching objects on the floor. If one side of the spine is affected more than the other, scoliosis may also be present.

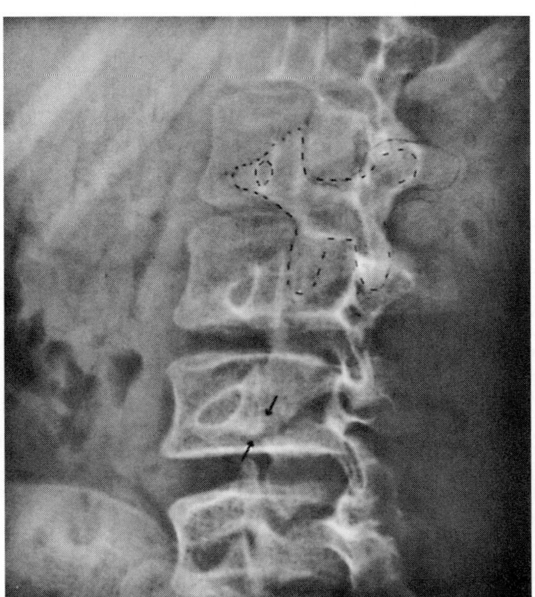

Figure 255-1. Spondylolysis. Oblique film of lumbar spine shows defect in pars interarticularis of L4 (*arrows*). Note that the posterior elements of a vertebra resemble a Scottie dog in this view, as outlined. The nose, eyes, ears, neck, and body are the transverse process, pedicle, pedicle superior articular process, pars interarticularis, and lamina, respectively. Spondylolysis appears as a break in the "neck" region.

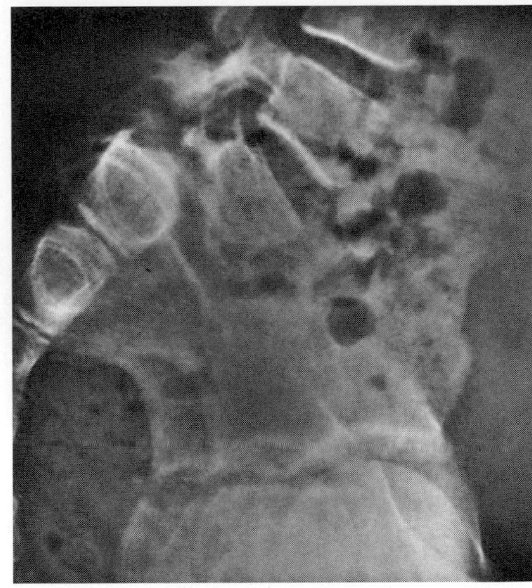

Figure 255-2. Severe vertebral slips, as shown here, lead to hamstring spasm and leg pain, as well as to back pain. Surgery is needed.

On physical examination, the most striking finding is limitation in straight-leg raising because of the hamstring spasm. Radiation of pain into the calf or foot with straight-leg raising may indicate more advanced nerve root irritation. A definite diagnosis can be made on the basis of plain radiography, most easily in the lateral view. If the vertebral slip is greater than 50%, posterior lumbosacral fusion is indicated. If the slip is less than 50%, initial management is directed toward relief of back pain and hamstring spasm using rest and corset therapy, as with spondylolysis. If the pain does not respond to conservative treatment, fusion may be needed. If the pain improves with conservative treatment, a corset may be used for sports activities, and follow-up lateral lumbosacral radiography at 6- to 9-month intervals is recommended until growth is complete or a worsening slip can be identified. If progression of the slip occurs, fusion is indicated.

INTERVERTEBRAL DISC HERNIATION

Herniation of the intervertebral disc is a common cause of back and leg pain in middle-aged adults. In this age group, disc protrusion occurs posteriorly with the protruded disc compressing the nerve roots or the cauda equina. If similar forces are applied to the spine of skeletally immature children, the disc will not always rupture posteriorly, but a fracture of the ring apophysis of the vertebral body may occur causing the extrusion of disc material anteriorly (Fig. 255-3). Most affected children have back pain without radiation into the leg or calf. If nerve-root pain also occurs, a small avulsion fracture of the ring apophysis posterolaterally might be present in a position that causes nerve-root compression. The diagnosis of an old disc injury in children can

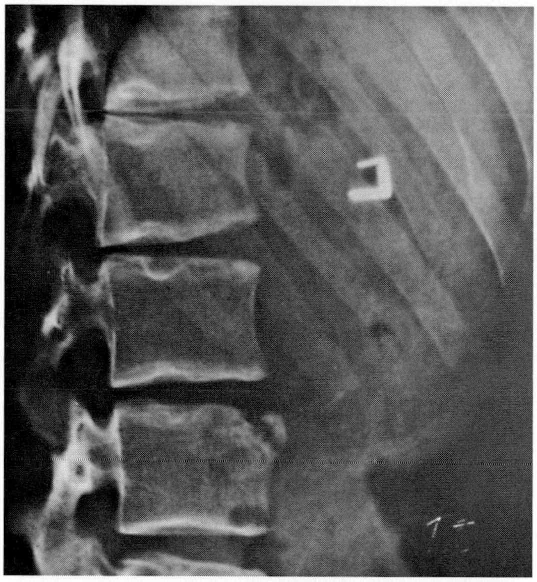

Figure 255-3. A disc rupture in skeletally immature children will lead to disruption of the apophysis or vertebral growth area, as shown here.

be confirmed by radiographic findings of a narrowed lumbar disc adjacent to a vertebral end plate that has some irregular pattern of ossification.

If no neurologic defect is present, treatment consists of symptomatic care, usually rest, until the pain resolves. If the condition is the result of a vehicular accident, evaluation for the development of an ileus should be performed. If both leg pain and back pain are present, magnetic resonance imaging (MRI) or computed tomographic (CT)-myelography should be performed to localize any neural compression, which could be relieved by surgical treatment.

DISCITIS

Discitis may present in a wide variety of ways. Severe back pain with limitation of back movements is common in older children, whereas younger children may simply refuse to walk or may limp. Usually, the cause of this disc inflammation is bacterial infection. The vascular anatomy of the growing disc varies from that of the adult, and the common bacteremias of childhood can infect the disc more readily than the vertebral body itself. Approximately 50% of affected children have positive blood culture results at the time of their acute pain with *Staphylococcus aureus* as the organism most commonly identified. Despite this finding, milder forms of discitis often appear to resolve without the need for antibiotics.

The most striking finding on physical examination in discitis patients is marked stiffness of the spine that is notable with attempts at flexion. Often, fever is present. The results of the neurologic examination are normal. In the early stages, radiographs of the spine appear normal. Usually, a few weeks after the onset of pain, narrowing of a single disc may be seen on radiography. Often, the sedimentation rate and white blood cell (WBC) count are elevated. A technetium Tc 99m bone scan typically reveals increased uptake at the involved level and should be performed whenever discitis is suspected. If the bone scan results are positive and the age and clinical presentation are typical, needle aspiration or open biopsy of the involved disc is not generally necessary.

Treatment decisions in cases of discitis revolve around choosing between antibiotics or a body jacket brace or cast. If a positive blood culture result has been obtained, antibiotics should be used for 3 to 6 weeks. Some prefer to use antibiotics in children who have significant pain or a positive bone scan result, even if no bacteremia has been demonstrated. Bed rest should be instituted at the time of presentation if significant spasm is present. If the spasm persists for more than a few days, a body jacket brace or cast will allow for immobilization and ambulation on a limited basis. Discitis rarely develops into vertebral osteomyelitis with local bone destruction. Usually, the involved vertebral bodies eventually fuse together after the infection resolves.

CHAPTER 256
Scoliosis

Adapted from Paul D. Sponseller

Scoliosis is a lateral curvature of the spine. The two forms of scoliosis are postural and structural. Postural scoliosis results from spinal factors outside the spine such as leg-length discrepancy or hip disorders. In these cases, if the leg lengths are equalized or if the child sits, the spine becomes straight indicating that no structural change has occurred. Structural scoliosis is of greater concern, because it involves not only a lateral spinal curvature, but also a rotation of the vertebrae involved in the lateral curve. The most common causes of scoliosis are shown in Table 256-1.

Congenital scoliosis is present at birth, though the diagnosis is not often made at that time. It may be associated with other birth defects or may present as an isolated condition. Because the genitourinary system arises embryologically from the same region as that of the spine, approximately 30% of children with a congenital spinal deformity have an associated genitourinary abnormality. The most common anomaly is unilateral renal agenesis; therefore, sonography or intravenous pyelography should be performed on all patients who have congenital scoliosis or kyphosis. Although active treatment of a unilateral kidney may not be necessary, an important adjunct is appropriate cautioning against the child's participation in contact sports that may lead to kidney injury. The treatment of congenital scoliosis consists of serial radiographic follow-up to determine whether the deformity is worsening. If no curve progression occurs, further treatment is not generally needed. If worsening of 5 to 10 degrees or more is documented, surgical fusion is necessary, regardless of an affected child's age. Brace treatment may be useful to prevent worsening of curves above or below the congenital scoliosis, but it is not indicated for the congenital scoliosis itself.

Neuromuscular scoliosis is spinal deformity associated with a wide variety of neurologic or muscular diseases such as cerebral palsy, muscular dystrophy, myelomeningocele, and poliomyelitis. Spinal curvature, secondary to muscular imbalance, is

TABLE 256-1. Causes of Scoliosis

Idiopathic	80%
Neuromuscular	10%
Congenital	5%
Miscellaneous (connective tissue disorders, genetic diseases)	5%

classically C-shaped and extends to include the pelvis, which is not usually the case in idiopathic scoliosis. Scoliosis is present more often and tends to worsen more quickly in patients who do not walk because of their neuromuscular disease. With continued progression, sitting balance becomes further impaired, and the child may need to use one arm or hand to assist in sitting. Treatment centers on preservation of sitting ability and pulmonary function. Although wearing a brace is often useful, surgical fusion is frequently indicated to preserve function.

Idiopathic scoliosis is generally found in healthy children. Scoliosis requiring treatment is approximately eight times more frequent in girls than in boys, however, the incidence of mild curves is approximately equal. A family history of curvature of the spine is found in as many as 70% of all children with scoliosis, though the exact mode of inheritance has not been determined. Although the cause of idiopathic scoliosis remains elusive, a combination of growth asymmetry and postural imbalance is believed to be important. Minor abnormalities in the postural control center in the brainstem have been demonstrated in children with mild scoliosis. Once the curve begins to develop in response to this impaired postural feedback, growth asymmetry likely occurs. Growth is slower when increased pressure is exerted on the growth areas. Because more pressure is exerted on the concave growing areas than on the convex side, the convexity grows more quickly leading to increasing curve size. This theory accounts for the observation that curves worsen most during the rapid adolescent growth spurt, which is the time when most of these curves are diagnosed.

The key to early detection of scoliosis is careful assessment of the entire trunk for asymmetry. Affected children should be examined with their back clearly exposed. Table 256-2 lists the recommendations for spinal deformity evaluation. Figures 256-1–2 demonstrate the standing and forward bending examination for scoliosis. In approximately 50% of children with uneven shoulder height, no spinal deformity is present on radiography. The view from the caudal aspect allows ready detection of prominence of the thoracic ribs, whereas forward bending or viewing from the head down is better for suspected lumbar curves. Both thoracic and lumbar regions should be checked. In the office, the amount of rib hump can be measured by means of an inclinometer placed at the apex of the curve with an affected child bending forward. If the inclinometer measurement is 5 degrees or less, the scoliosis is rarely significant and radiographs are not usually needed. If the inclinometer reading exceeds 6 to 7 degrees, standing posteroanterior and lateral radiography is indicated for better assessment.

TABLE 256-2. Spinal Deformity Evaluation

Examine in swimming suit or similar clothing to expose back.
Observe asymmetry on trunk examination: shoulder height, scapular height, waistline equality, levelness of pelvis, leg-length difference, forward bending (both side and front-back).
Measure rib prominence with inclinometer (optional).
Assess skeletal maturity (e.g., age of menses onset).
Obtain standing posteroanterior radiograph of the spine if asymmetry is seen.
Measure using Cobb method.
Recommend follow-up or treatment (none if the curve is less than 25 degrees and growth is complete).
If growth is not complete and the curve is less than 25 degrees, obtain repeat radiographs in 4 to 15 months (see text).
If scoliosis of more than 25 degrees is seen and growth is not complete, consider a brace.
If scoliosis of more than 40 degrees is seen, consider surgery.

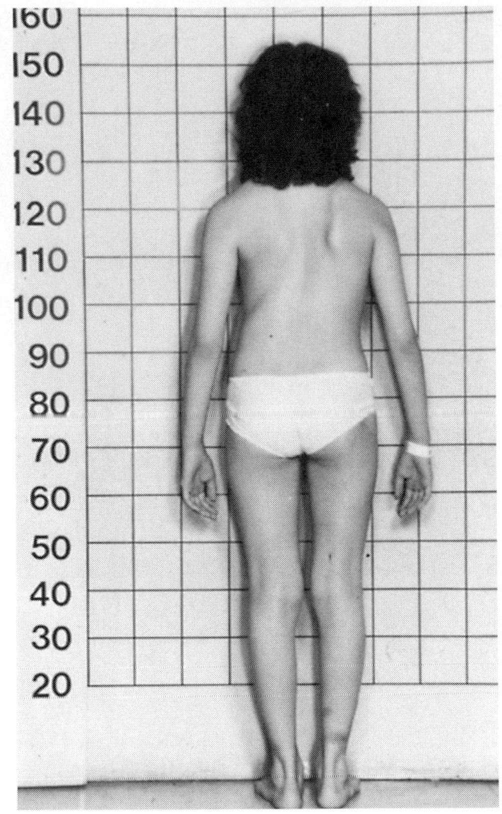

Figure 256-1. In examining for scoliosis, asymmetry of the trunk (shoulders, scapular height, waist area, pelvic height) should be carefully noted.

The magnitude of the scoliosis is measured radiographically by the Cobb method (Fig. 256-3A). This measurement should always be performed on an erect posteroanterior spine radiograph. The error of measurement for this method is approximately 5 degrees. Because no active treatment is needed until the curve reaches 25 degrees, the time estimate for a follow-up radiograph, once the diagnosis has been made, is 25 minus the

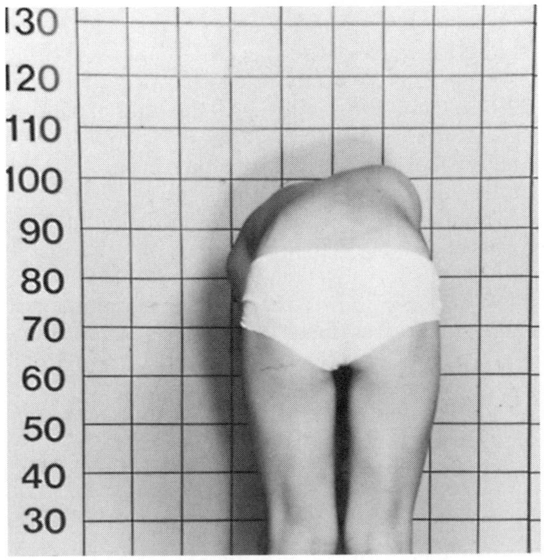

Figure 256-2. The forward-bending examination will detect even very small curvatures. The prominence is produced by chest-wall asymmetry, the result of vertebral-body rotation in the curved segment of the spine.

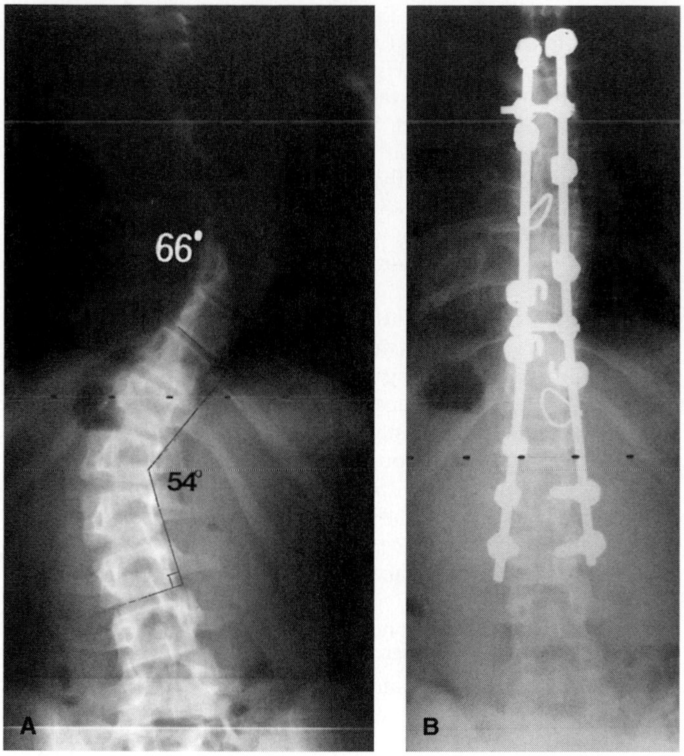

Figure 256-3. A standing posteroanterior radiograph of the spine is the correct film to use in quantitating the magnitude of scoliosis. **A:** The Cobb method of measurement is routinely used and is obtained as shown on this radiograph. **B:** The postoperative result after spinal correction and fusion in the same patient.

present curve magnitude. This result provides an estimate of the number of months that may pass until another radiograph is indicated. This time estimate is based on the premise that during the adolescent growth spurt, annual curve progression is 5 to 10 degrees or approximately 1 degree per month. Completion of growth or skeletal maturity can be most accurately assessed with bone age radiography of the hand and wrist. From the clinical standpoint, girls who have been menstruating for 2 years essentially have completed their spinal growth.

The treatment of scoliosis is based on three fundamental principles (Table 256-3). If affected children are skeletally mature and have a curvature of less than 25 degrees, no further evaluation or treatment of scoliosis is needed. If the scoliosis is 25 degrees or more and such children are still growing, brace treatment is generally recommended and is successful in approximately 80% of the patients who actually wear the brace as prescribed. Spinal exercises alone will not be successful in stopping curve progression. Once the brace treatment begins, it is continued until growth is complete. Usually, the brace is worn 18 to 23 hours daily. Physical activity is not limited by scoliosis, and affected children can often participate in sports activities while wearing their brace. Wearing a brace is considered successful if it prevents further progression, rather than providing correction of the curve, as long-term follow-up studies have shown that the final size of the curve is virtually the same as before brace treatment begins. Despite some earlier controversy about the efficacy of bracing, prospective randomized studies published within the last few years have shown bracing to be an effective treatment method.

TABLE 256-3. Principles of Scoliosis that Guide Treatment

Curves of more than 25 degrees are likely to increase if an affected child is still growing.
Curves of 40 to 50 degrees are likely to increase even after growth is complete.
Some degree of clinical pulmonary restriction may begin to be noticeable in thoracic curves of more than approximately 75 degrees.

Although children and parents are often dismayed by our inability to straighten the spine nonoperatively, if curves can be kept at less than 35 to 40 degrees by the time growth is completed, most cases of scoliosis will not worsen in adult life. If the thoracic curve is greater than 50 degrees or the lumbar curve is greater than 40 degrees at the time growth is completed, progression will usually continue at a rate of approximately 1 degree annually, and surgery will often be recommended.

Surgical treatment is recommended for curves that are greater than 40 degrees, particularly in children who are not fully grown. Usually, the surgical treatment used consists of instrumentation of the curved area of the spine combined with posterior spinal fusion of the instrumented area (Fig. 256-3B). Generally, correction of the scoliosis is at least 50%. Failure of fusion occurs in only approximately 1% of affected teenagers. Fusion is complete by 6 months after surgery, at which time such teenagers can return to almost all physical activities, except tackle football, wrestling, and gymnastics. Teenagers should be encouraged to return to activity, including physical education class in school, to deemphasize the psychological potential for disability after this surgery.

If the thoracic scoliosis exceeds 50 degrees, patients commonly have diminished vital capacity and residual lung volumes on pulmonary function testing. Even with surgical correction of the scoliosis, pulmonary function will postoperatively change little because of the persistence of chest wall or rib deformities that have occurred as a result of the scoliosis. Therefore, scoliosis should be prevented from progressing to this point if possible.

Pain is rare in adolescents who have idiopathic scoliosis. Although it may result from degenerative changes that are present by the time such patients are middle-aged, pain that occurs during adolescence is an indication for further evaluation. Such patients should be questioned in detail about the nature of the pain. If it is severe, limits activities, or requires frequent analgesics, a workup is indicated. If the neurologic examination is normal, a technetium Tc 99m bone scan should be performed to screen for discitis, stress fracture, osteoid osteoma, or other bone tumors. If spinal flexion is limited and a neurologic deficit is discovered, magnetic resonance imaging (MRI) or computed tomographic (CT)-myelography is necessary to rule out intraspinal pathology. Although all these conditions may cause scoliosis, the curvature will straighten as soon as its underlying cause is treated. Therefore, physicians should evaluate patients thoroughly for treatable causes of scoliosis before making a diagnosis of idiopathic scoliosis and instituting brace treatment or recommending spinal fusion.

CHAPTER 257
Kyphosis

Adapted from Paul D. Sponseller

Normal spinal sagittal contours consist of lordosis in the cervical and lumbar spinal segments to balance the kyphosis that is present in the thoracic area. Sometimes, the term *kyphosis* is used to describe those abnormal conditions in which increased rounding of the back is present in the thoracic or thoracolumbar area. Usually, parents complain about a child's posture. Assessment of apparent excessive kyphosis should include a forward-bending examination, viewed from the side, to determine whether the back is flexible or rigid in the rounded segment (Fig. 257-1). The kyphosis may be discovered to be a rib prominence associated with a scoliosis. Similarly, mild to moderate scoliosis is commonly seen with moderate and marked kyphosis, so careful examination for both conditions is necessary.

The least serious type of kyphosis is postural round back. This is most commonly seen in the preadolescent years. It occurs more often in children who are taller than their peers and in girls whose breasts have developed earlier than their friends. This condition is a flexible, increased kyphosis that can be voluntarily straightened by the child and can be corrected with hyperextension positioning. This group of spinal deformities can be treated with exercises alone. Active hyperextension of the trunk and sit-ups to decrease lumbar lordosis are useful in improving trunk control. As long as no fixed deformity is established, as an affected teenager's body image improves, so will the rounding of the upper back.

Usually, a more fixed and less flexible thoracic or thoracolumbar kyphosis is called *Scheuermann disease*. This condition most commonly occurs in teenage boys. Attempts to correct this kyphosis passively are unsuccessful, and a large lumbar lordosis is often associated with it. Lateral radiography of the spine will demonstrate irregularity of numerous disc spaces and anterior vertebral body wedging (Fig. 257-2). To establish the diagnosis of Scheuermann kyphosis radiographically, at least 5 degrees of wedging in three adjacent vertebrae should be demonstrated. The Cobb method is also used to measure the amount of kyphosis present. Normally, the amount of kyphosis from T3 to T12 is between 20 and 45 degrees. If the kyphosis is present in the thoracolumbar area, which normally appears straight on lateral radiography, measurements greater than 10 degrees are abnormal.

If wedging is present, little correction can be achieved with thoracic spine hyperextension; if the lateral thoracic kyphosis is 55 to 60 degrees, bracing is indicated while the child is still growing. A Milwaukee brace, which uses a neck ring, in addition to trunk pads, is the gold standard, but for kyphoses low in the thoracic spine, a more unobtrusive underarm brace may be used. Unlike scoliosis, in which little correction results from bracing, in kyphosis, approximately 50% improvement can be anticipated after 1 year of full-time brace wear. Once this degree of correction is obtained, nighttime brace wear is generally sufficient until growth is complete.

Increased thoracic kyphosis does not cause abnormalities in pulmonary function. The principal problem seen later in Scheuermann disease is pain in the low thoracic spine after an affected patient has been standing for some time. If the kyphosis exceeds 70 degrees by the time such a patient has stopped growing, spinal instrumentation and fusion, as with scoliosis, can provide excellent correction with a significant improvement in appearance.

Congenital kyphosis is less common than congenital scoliosis but almost always requires early spinal fusion surgery. If the congenital kyphosis progresses unchecked, spinal cord compression at the apex of the kyphosis is common. As with congenital scoliosis, evaluation for associated genitourinary abnormalities should be performed.

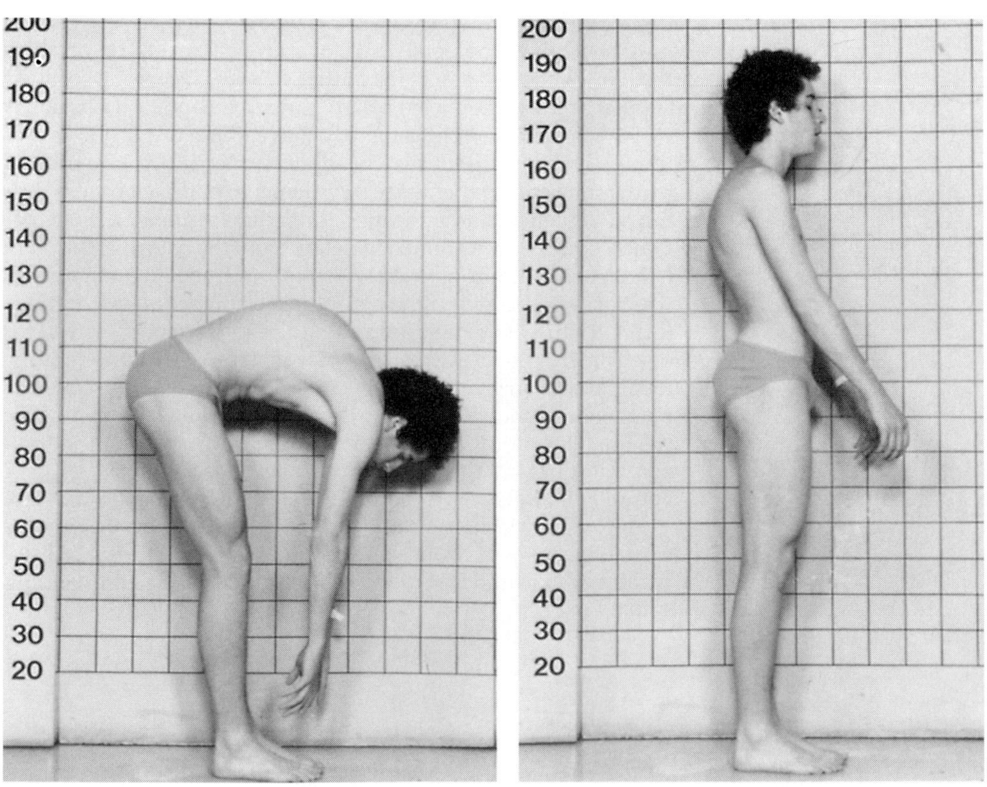

Figure 257-1. The examination for kyphosis should also include a forward-bending test to help determine the rigidity and severity of the kyphosis, which may be hidden more easily in the upright position.

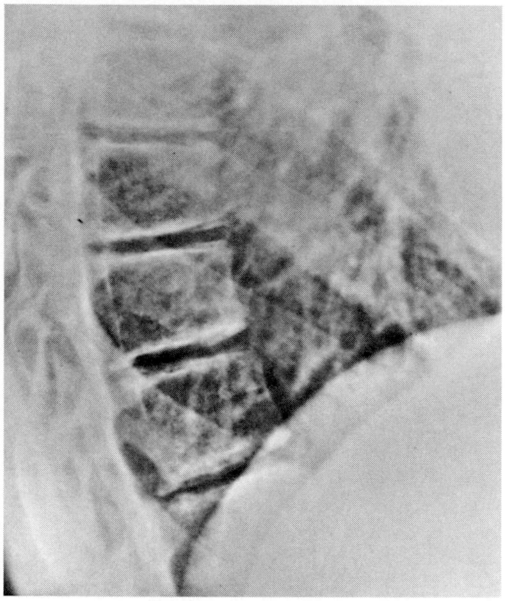

Figure 257-2. Lateral spine radiograph demonstrating the disc irregularities and anterior vertebral body wedging seen in Scheuermann disease.

CHAPTER 258

Cervical Spine Problems

Adapted from Paul D. Sponseller

Evaluation of the cervical spine, because of its many normal variations on radiography, is often confusing. As seen on lateral cervical spine radiography, the anterior and superior corner of each vertebral body is normally the last part to ossify, sometimes giving the appearance of a small compression fracture. Full ossification and development of the odontoid process are not complete in young children and may give the appearance of being maldeveloped. The spine of children younger than age 10 is much more flexible than that of teenagers or older adults. As much as 3 mm of anterior movement of C2 on C3 with flexion is normal in this group, whereas no such movement should be present in adults. In fact, under experimental conditions, the newborn spine can stretch about 5 cm (2 in.) before it fails, whereas the adult spinal cord can stretch only 1.25 cm (0.5 in.) before it ruptures. Because of this difference in elasticity, infants who are involved in automobile accidents may sustain spinal cord injury without apparent spinal fracture. The proper use of car-seating supports for these very young children decreases the risk of these devastating injuries (see Chapter 45, Injury Prevention and Control).

Children with Down syndrome comprise a special group that commonly has instability of the atlantoaxial region. If this instability persists unrecognized, spinal cord compression with myelopathy may result leading to leg weakness and lessened walking ability. Lateral cervical flexion-extension radiography should be performed at age 5 years in all children who have Down syndrome and are involved in activities involving forceful flexion of the neck or impact to the head. Although approximately 15% of such children will have some evidence of atlantoaxial instability, the majority do not need fusion surgery but can have periodic follow-up by neurologic examination. If the first radiograph reveals increased laxity (greater than 5 mm distance between the odontoid and the atlas), films should be repeated every 2 years. If no laxity is seen, repeat radiography is not recommended as long as no signs of spasticity or symptoms of neck pain occur. Atlantoaxial posterior fusion is recommended if a neurologic deficit or excessive instability (greater than 8 mm) is present.

CHAPTER 259

Torticollis

Adapted from Paul D. Sponseller

Most commonly, torticollis is present at or near the time of birth and results from a contracture of one of the sternocleidomastoid muscles. An affected child's head will be tilted toward the side of the contracture with the chin rotated away from the contracted side, because the origin of the contracted muscle is on the mastoid process. The cause of torticollis is not well defined, but the incidence is higher in children with breech presentation and forceps delivery. Commonly, a fusiform, firm mass is palpable in the body of the contracted muscle. Often, affected children have plagiocephaly, or asymmetry of face and skull development. If the neck range of motion can be returned to normal by age 1 year, this facial asymmetry will disappear. If the torticollis is untreated until later in childhood, the eyes and ears will never become level.

Cervical spine radiography should be evaluated to ensure that the position of the head is not the result of congenital spine abnormalities such as hemivertebrae. If the bony cervical spine is normal, stretching exercises should be instituted shortly after birth. These exercises are designed to stretch the contracted sternocleidomastoid muscle and should be taught to parents of affected children by a knowledgeable physical therapist. Although one of the parents should be asked to do these stretching exercises at home, initial weekly checkups by the therapist or the physician can help to ensure compliance. If a significant contracture persists by the time such patients reach age 1, despite stretching exercises, surgical treatment to lengthen the sternocleidomastoid muscle is appropriate. Even after surgical release, some stretching and (at times) bracing will continue to be needed as the child grows.

CHAPTER 260

Klippel–Feil Syndrome/Sprengel Deformity

Adapted from Paul D. Sponseller

Failure of normal vertebral segmentation in the cervical spine is known as *Klippel–Feil syndrome*, defined as congenital fusion of at least two cervical vertebrae (Fig. 260-1). In the milder forms, when only one or two levels are involved, diagnosis may be delayed until the teenage years and, even then, may be made only when the neck is examined radiographically for other reasons. In more severely involved children, however, the neck is very

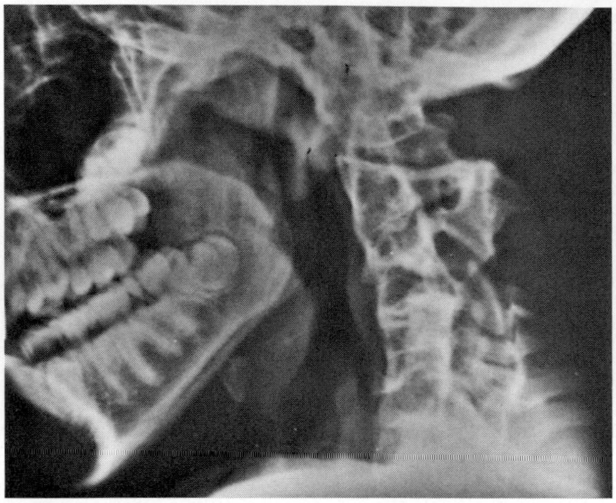

Figure 260-1. Klippel-Feil syndrome results from incomplete segmentation of the cervical vertebrae. Often, Sprengel deformity of the scapulae is associated with this syndrome.

short, and webbing appears to be present. Often, Klippel–Feil syndrome is associated with Sprengel deformity, which is a congenital elevation of the scapula. In this deformity, the pectoralis major muscle may be underdeveloped and scapular winging may occur as a result of serratus anterior muscle palsy.

Associated genitourinary abnormalities may be present, and sonography or intravenous pyelography is indicated when the diagnosis of Klippel–Feil syndrome is made. Little specific treatment is available for this syndrome. Because of the congenital fusion of several segments of the cervical spine, instability may occur at the levels that move. If this instability is excessive or if neurologic deficits are present, fusing the unstable segment is necessary. Surgical fusion may also be needed in adult life for degenerative changes at the moveable segments. In more involved cases, contact sports should be avoided, because any neck injury in a child with Klippel–Feil syndrome is more likely to be serious as a result of the limited flexibility of the cervical area.

CHAPTER 261
Nursemaid's Elbow

Adapted from Paul D. Sponseller

Annular ligament entrapment, known as *nursemaid's elbow*, consists of elbow pain after longitudinal traction on a pronated, extended elbow in children between the ages of 2 and 7. A snap may or may not be heard. It has been suggested that the annular ligament of the radial head slips partially over the radial head, the narrowest portion being prominent when pronated (Fig. 261-1). Usually, radiography shows no bony abnormality or displacement. An elbow fracture or septic arthritis should be ruled out, especially if the mechanism of injury is a fall rather than traction. Usually, treatment is reduction by stabilizing the elbow with one hand, with a finger placed over the radial head for palpation, followed by gentle firm flexion until a click is felt. Affected children should begin using the elbow within minutes. Usually, immobilization is not carried out and is not necessary in first-time cases.

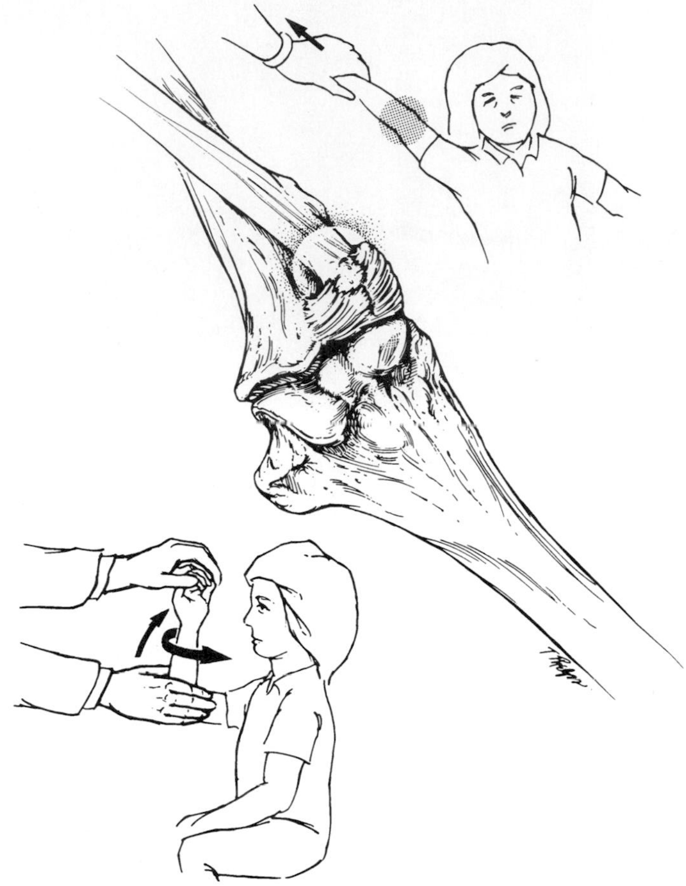

Figure 261-1. "Pulled elbow" represents subluxation of the radial head through a partially torn annular ligament. Method of injury (*above*) and method of reduction (*below*).

CHAPTER 262
Osteogenesis Imperfecta

Adapted from Paul D. Sponseller

Osteogenesis imperfecta encompasses a spectrum of diseases that are the end result of defects in collagen or proteoglycan synthesis. These diseases result in bones that have thin cortices and multiple fractures. Short stature, blue sclerae, middle-ear deafness, abnormal dentition, and thin skin may coexist. Usually, inheritance is dominant, occasionally is recessive, but is frequently the result of spontaneous mutation. Tiny fractures occur to cause bowing of long bones and scoliosis. Child abuse should be considered in the differential diagnosis, and the absence of pelvic deformities or wormian cranial bones in children who are subjected to abuse may be helpful. Aids to mobility and preventive bracing can be very helpful in preventing fractures. Occasionally, intramedullary rods that elongate with growth are needed. Fortunately, the frequency of fractures diminishes with age.

CHAPTER 263

Benign Bone Tumors

Adapted from Paul D. Sponseller

Benign or malignant musculoskeletal tumors can be classified according to their tissue of origin (Table 263-1). The history and physical examination are rarely definitive. Many tumors become evident after trauma when a new prominence is noted or when pathologic fracture occurs through weakened bone. Some idea of the benign or malignant nature of a tumor can be gained from the following radiographic features (Table 263-2). Leukemia presents with musculoskeletal complaints 20% of the time, and radiographic findings include osteopenia, sclerotic or lytic lesions, lucent metaphyseal bands, or periosteal new bone.

Radiographic studies must be tailored to the differential diagnosis. Computed tomographic (CT) may show internal consistency, soft tissue spread, and extent of the lesion. Technetium Tc 99m bone scans reveal lesions in the remainder of the skeleton, bony involvement with soft tissue lesions, and bone turnover or activity of questionable lesions. Angiograms may be helpful to determine whether the tumor involves a vascular bundle. Magnetic Resonance Imaging (MRI) is helpful in assessing soft tissue involvement.

The location of a lesion is meaningful, and a diagram of the location of common bone lesions is presented in Fig. 263-1. Generally, laboratory studies are not specific; the sedimentation rate and complete blood count are abnormal in several of the aforementioned tumors, and often the alkaline phosphatase level is elevated in patients with osteogenic sarcoma. The treatment of musculoskeletal tumors defies simplification. The most important generalization is that any patient requiring surgery should be under the care of a surgeon who has had experience in this area.

UNICAMERAL BONE CYST

A unicameral bone cyst is a benign, smooth, well-marginated lucency that is fairly centrally located in the metaphysis of children between ages 2 and 15 (Fig. 263-2). Usually, it is not recognized until a fracture occurs through the cyst. The fracture should be allowed to heal, and the lesion can be observed if it is small and is located in a bone that does not bear weight; otherwise, it can be injected with steroids or bone-inducing substance. The latter two treatments produce results equal to or better than open bone grafting. The natural history of these defects is spontaneous regression during late adolescence.

TABLE 263-1. Musculoskeletal Neoplasms

Origin	Benign	Malignant
Cartilage	Chondroblastoma Enchondroma Chondromyxoid fibroma Osteochondroma	Chondrosarcoma*
Bone	Osteoid osteoma Osteoblastoma	Osteosarcoma
Marrow elements	Lipoma	Ewing sarcoma Reticulum cell sarcoma Liposarcoma* Plasma cell Myeloma
Fibrous connective tissue	Desmoplastic fibroma Fibrous cortical defect	Fibrosarcoma
Skeletal muscle		Rhabdomyosarcoma
Neurogenous tissue	Neurilemma Neurofibroma	Neuroblastoma
Unclear	Giant cell tumor*	Adamantinoma

*Rarely occurs in children.

TABLE 263-2. Radiographic Features of Malignant Tumors

Rapid spread
Lack of local containment
Vague zone of transition between lesion and normal bone
Soft tissue mass in the presence of a bone tumor
Calcification of the cartilage matrix
Fluffy opacification (Osteosarcoma)
Lesions crossing epiphyseal plates*

*May also represent infection.

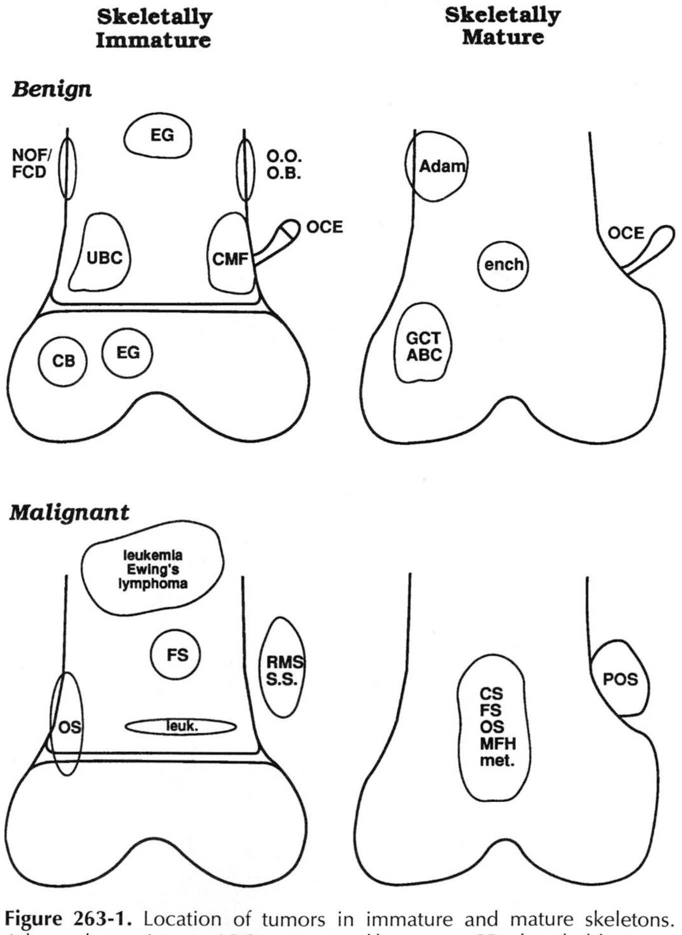

Figure 263-1. Location of tumors in immature and mature skeletons. Adam, adamantinoma; ABC, aneurysmal bone cyst; CB, chondroblastoma; CMF, chondromyxoid fibroma; CS, chondrosarcoma; EG, eosinophilic granuloma; ench, enchondroma; FCD, fibrous cortical defect; FS, fibrosarcoma; GCT, giant cell tumor; leuk., leukemia; met., metastasis; MFH, malignant fibrous histiocytoma; NOF, nonossifying fibroma; O.B., osteoblastoma; OCE, osteocartilaginous exostosis; O.O., osteoid osteoma; OS, osteogenic sarcoma; P, parosteal; RMS, rhabdomyosarcoma; S.S., synovial sarcoma; UBC, unicameral bone cyst.

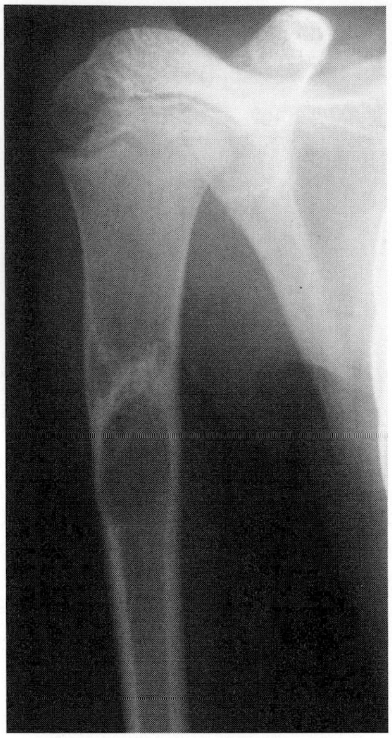

Figure 263-2. Unicameral bone cyst in the proximal humerus of a 9-year-old. Often, it is located closer to the growth plate.

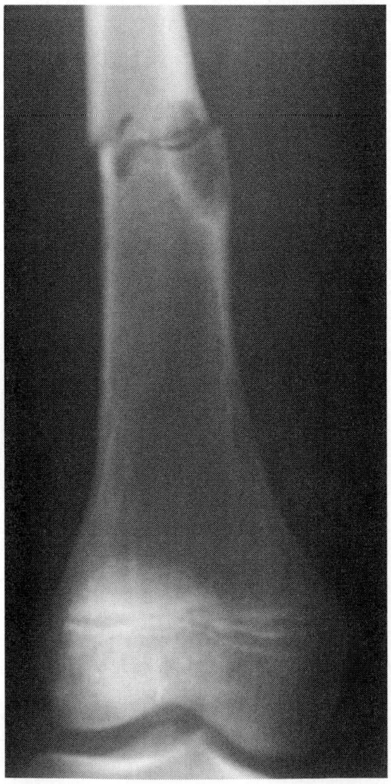

Figure 263-3. Fibrous cortical defects with pathologic fracture. Note two lesions on the medial side within one wall of the cortex and expanding it.

FIBROUS CORTICAL DEFECTS

Fibrous cortical defects are benign, well-marginated lucencies located in (and, occasionally, slightly expanding) the cortex. Usually, one radiographic view can show that these lesions are not central in bone (Fig. 263-3). They are present in as many as one-third of all young children at some time and disappear with age. In a weight-bearing bone, the risk of fracture is appreciable if the lesion is greater than approximately 3 cm in length and more than one-half the width of the bone. Lesions this large should be protected by limiting activities, if possible, or by performing bone grafting.

CHAPTER 264
Osteomyelitis and Septic Arthritis

Adapted from Paul D. Sponseller

HEMATOGENOUS OSTEOMYELITIS

Acute hematogenous osteomyelitis includes processes that have been operating for a week or less at the time of diagnosis. After infancy, this condition occurs more frequently in boys than in girls, presumably because trauma plays a role in increasing susceptibility. The peak ages of occurrence are infancy (younger than 1 year) and preadolescence (9 to 11 years). The incidence declines in adulthood because of the change in vascular supply of bone. The sites most commonly affected are the femur and tibia, each of which accounts for one-third of all cases, followed by the humerus, calcaneus, and pelvis. The metaphysis is the region involved most often, and spread may occur from this point to involve any other portion.

Pathophysiology

The metaphyseal vascular channels form loops near the growth plate. Blood flow is slowed, and the capillary basement membrane and reticuloendothelial system are deficient in these regions. Experimental bacteremias have been shown to produce foci of infection only in these areas. Trauma likely plays more than a circumstantial role, as experimentally traumatized areas are more susceptible to the development of osteomyelitis. Only approximately one-fourth of all cases have a demonstrable source such as cutaneous, aural, or respiratory seeding.

After a focus of infection is initiated, local inflammation is followed by spread up and down the medullary canal. The growth plate in children has no bridging vessels and acts as a barrier to spread in most cases. The germinal cells are on the epiphyseal side and, therefore, are spared. In the first year of life, however, the transphyseal vessels that exist allow spread to proceed up to the epiphysis and into the joint. These facts have two implications. First, growth-plate damage is more likely during the first year of life. Second, in children of this age, septic arthritis may follow osteomyelitis in any metaphyseal location, whereas in older children without transphyseal vessels, it occurs only in locations where the joint capsule extends over the growth plate (i.e., the shoulder, elbow, and hip). At skeletal maturity with growth-plate closure, this barrier is again eliminated, although hematogenous osteomyelitis is rare after this point. As intramedullary pressure increases, pus dissects through the haversian system elevating the periosteum and producing a subperiosteal, then soft tissue, abscess. The elevated periosteum may be radiographically apparent within 1 to 2 weeks.

Clinical Characteristics

Clinical diagnosis remains key despite the availability of new imaging techniques. Affected children may appear well or may have systemic involvement ranging from malaise to shock. Often, refusal to bear weight is an early symptom. The very earliest sign is fever and local bone tenderness, followed later by a fluctuant mass if a subperiosteal or soft tissue abscess has developed. Spread to adjacent joints should be ruled out by palpation and range of motion evaluation. Usually, passive motion of the extremity is not significantly resisted unless a soft tissue abscess or joint involvement is present. Increased suspicion should be aroused with neonates, who are more often afebrile and may first be noted to have a swollen or motionless limb. Vertebral or pelvic osteomyelitis may present as abdominal pain and can resemble the more common septic arthritis of the hip.

Unlike septic arthritis, the organisms involved in hematogenous osteomyelitis vary slightly with the age of affected patients. In all age groups, the predominant organism is *S. aureus*, although *Streptococcus pneumoniae* and *Haemophilus* species must be considered. *S. aureus* infection is associated with a higher recurrence rate than other organisms. *Salmonella* should be considered in patients with sickle cell anemia, although *S. aureus* infection is still more common in these patients. Blood culture results during the acute phase are positive approximately 40% to 50% of the time, and direct cultures of pus or bone are positive only 60% to 80% of the time, which may be the result of prior antibiotic use, errors in sampling or processing, or autoeradication of the organism.

Diagnosis

The differential diagnosis primarily includes neoplasm, contusion, nondisplaced fracture, and sickle cell crisis. Elevated white blood cell (WBC) counts and sedimentation rates are helpful but not diagnostic. Serum antibody titers may be helpful, but their sensitivity is a problem. Radiography at the earliest stage may show soft tissue swelling. Osteopenia or lysis may appear after 7 to 10 days, followed by new bone formation at the borders of the process. Bone scanning has been widely used in the last two decades, but the subtleties of its use have been recognized only recently. The tracer that is most widely used is technetium Tc 99m methylene diphosphonate because of its speed, cost, and sensitivity. Immediate scans for flow and blood pool should be obtained, as should later skeletal images. Results of the scan may be normal in the very early stages, but the procedure should be repeated after 48 hours if clinically indicated.

Cold or photopenic areas are important because they may indicate avascular sites, especially when adjacent areas of increased uptake accompany them. Cellulitis may cause confusion but does not usually show bony localization on delayed images. The overall accuracy of nuclear imaging is approximately 60% to 90%. It may be much lower in neonates, however, according to some reports. These studies have their greatest value when localization for aspiration is difficult. The role of magnetic resonance imaging (MRI) has yet to be defined.

Aspiration is indicated in all cases to identify the pathogen and, in some cases, to decompress localized purulence. It should be performed with a large-diameter needle. The anesthetic may be local, intravenous, or general, as indicated. In sequence, the extraosseous soft tissues, periosteum, and (if necessary) intramedullary canal should be assessed for purulent localization. Fluoroscopy may be useful in deep lesions if radiographic changes are evident. Experiments in animals have shown that aspiration of bone alone does not cause a bone scan result to become positive.

Treatment

Treatment involves the delivery of an appropriate antibiotic to all infected tissue. Therefore, avascular abscesses may require surgical decompression if aspiration cannot accomplish drainage. Antibiotic therapy can be divided into initial and definitive periods. In the initial phase, broad-spectrum antibiotics including antistaphylococcal agents such as nafcillin or oxacillin (150–200 mg/kg/day) are indicated. Vancomycin should be used if resistance is suspected. In neonates, an aminoglycoside should be added. In children who are younger than 3 years and have osteomyelitis associated with septic arthritis, cefuroxime may be used to cover *Haemophilus influenzae*. In the definitive period, the most effective, least toxic antibiotic effective against the isolated organism should be given for 4 to 6 weeks. It may be administered by the oral route if affected patients are clinically improved and compliant, and if adequate blood levels can be documented.

Surgery is reserved for cases in which affected children are systemically ill or worsening under medical treatment or in which an abscess has been demonstrated. An abscess or avascular tissue should be removed to allow antibiotic penetration, and usually the wound is closed over a drain. Complications include recurrence (10% overall; 6% at 6 months), minor growth acceleration, growth-plate damage, and fracture through weakened bone.

SEPTIC ARTHRITIS

Slightly more common than hematogenous osteomyelitis, septic arthritis may have more disastrous long-term consequences if effective treatment is delayed. Most cases occur in infants and younger children with nearly one-half of all affected patients younger than age 3. A high index of suspicion for septic arthritis should be maintained in sick neonatal patients, for they show few signs. The hip is the joint most commonly involved in infants, as compared to the knee in older children. The spread may be from the bloodstream or from an adjacent osteomyelitis, especially in the hip and shoulder where the capsular insertion extends over the growth plate onto the metaphysis. Many theories, including alteration of joint fluid by toxins from both the neutrophils and the bacteria, have been advanced to explain the pathogenesis of joint destruction.

The spectrum of causative organisms in septic arthritis is somewhat broader than that of hematogenous osteomyelitis, which may be related to the greater frequency of this condition. Overall, *S. aureus* remains the most common causative organism. In patients between ages 1 month and 5 years, however, *H. influenzae* is also common. The use of the vaccine against this organism appears to have reduced, although not eliminated, this organism as a cause of septic arthritis in the toddler. The streptococci *Escherichia coli*, *Proteus*, and other organisms should also be considered. The yield of organisms from aspiration is approximately 60% to 80%. Gonococcal arthritis also occurs in children. Usually, it becomes evident after the systemic and febrile phase of the illness and should be distinguished from the more common gonococcal migratory multiple arthralgia or tenosynovitis. An average of two to three joints, most commonly the wrists and knees, are affected.

Clinical Characteristics

Clinical findings vary with the age of affected patients. In infants, fever, failure to feed, and tachycardia may be present. Subtle changes in position, unilateral swelling of an extremity or a joint, asymmetry of soft tissue folds, and pain with range of motion may serve as clues. In older children, the signs are more localized.

Diagnosis

Aspiration with a large needle should be performed if any reasonable suspicion of septic arthritis exists, both for diagnosis and, in some cases, for treatment. In such deep joints as the hip, injection of radiopaque dye should be used to confirm the position of the needle, especially if the aspirated fluid is normal. This ensures that joint fluid was actually obtained, and it also helps to distinguish joint infection from septic involvement of the bursa underneath the nearby psoas muscle. Usually, the WBC count in fluid obtained from patients with septic arthritis ranges from 50,000 to 250,000 with 95% polymorphonuclear leukocytes. Elevated lactate levels may be helpful in cases in which WBC counts are borderline. The differential diagnosis includes toxic synovitis of the hip in which pain, fever, leukocytosis, and spasm are more moderate and do not escalate on serial observations. However, at times the two conditions are indistinguishable, and aspiration should be performed. Lyme arthritis, rheumatoid arthritis, cellulitis, traumatic synovitis, and the migratory multiple arthralgias of rheumatic fever should be considered. A sympathetic effusion may also occur from adjacent osteomyelitis.

The role of arthrotomy versus aspiration in confirmed cases of septic arthritis is controversial. The key feature is removal of deleterious enzymes and restoration of effective synovial perfusion. Because the decision not to operate requires the ability to monitor and aspirate repeatedly as needed, the use of arthrotomy is probably preferable in deep joints that are difficult to assess such as the hip and shoulder; in young patients in whom examination is difficult; and when the fluid obtained is viscous or has a very high WBC count. The surgical procedure should include irrigation, drainage, and closure, which may be performed arthroscopically in the knee, shoulder, and ankle. Direct instillation of antibiotics has no benefit.

Treatment

Early effective treatment is very important. The chance of achieving good results dramatically declines if treatment is initiated after the symptoms have been present for 4 days. Antibiotics should be continued for 4 to 6 weeks. Treatment of gonococcal arthritis consists of aspiration and closed irrigation followed by 3 days of intravenous penicillin and 4 days of ampicillin or amoxicillin. Oral treatment alone with one of these drugs for 7 days is acceptable in compliant patients after a loading dose has been given. Whether the joint should be immobilized or treated with continuous passive motion is controversial; however, the latter modality is practiced less commonly. Contractures should be prevented, and abduction of the hip decreases the likelihood of dislocation. Complications include permanent destruction of cartilage and, in the hip, avascular necrosis with resorption or overgrowth of the femoral head. Complications are more frequent in young infants.

CHAPTER 265

Puncture Wounds

Adapted from Paul D. Sponseller

Puncture wounds to the foot are significant in that they may involve *Pseudomonas* infection, which occurs with colonization of a sock or a sneaker by this organism. The wound should be inspected, and foreign material should be removed. If the bone or joint is contaminated, debridement and antibiotic therapy should be begun. Otherwise, affected patients should be seen in 3 to 5 days or at least should be instructed to return if symptoms of infection occur.

CHAPTER 266

Injuries

Adapted from Paul D. Sponseller

Children's bones differ from those of adults both biomechanically and physiologically. Mechanically, immature bone is more porous, and the pores serve to limit crack propagation. Instead of complete fractures, children often have involvement of only part of the cortex such as in a buckle fracture from compression or a greenstick fracture from tension. Another biomechanical feature of children's skeletons is that the ligaments are stronger than either the bone or the growth plate. Injuries that would produce dislocations or sprains in adults (e.g., elbow dislocation or medial collateral ligament tear of the knee, respectively)

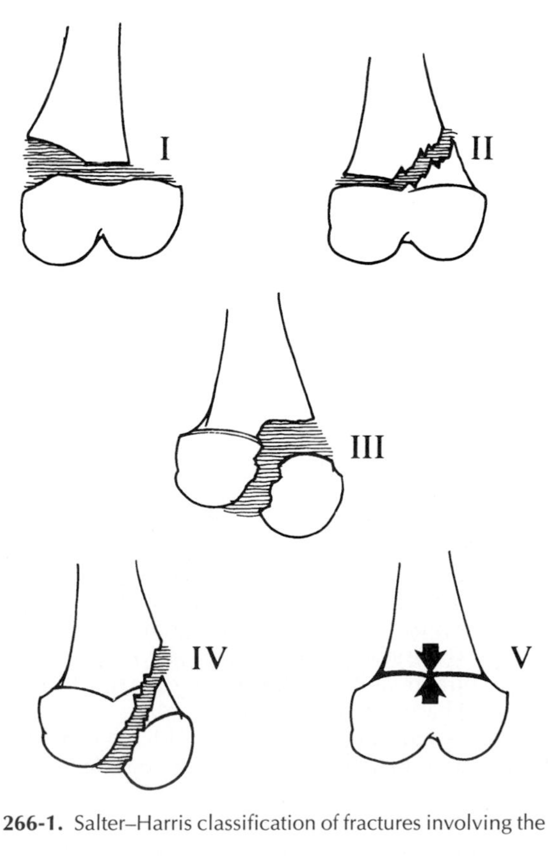

Figure 266-1. Salter–Harris classification of fractures involving the growth plate.

produce different patterns in children (i.e., supracondylar humeral fractures or femoral physeal separations, respectively).

Physiologic differences include union rates, remodeling, overgrowth, and growth-plate injuries. Nonunion is nearly nonexistent in children occurring only in open fractures with extensive soft tissue loss and periosteal stripping. Bone union times range from 3 weeks in infants to 3 months in adolescents. Remodeling of angulation and displacement is an impressive tendency until the early teenage years. It is most effective in the metaphysis, where angulation does not create as much deformity as in the midshaft.

Another physiologic feature of children's fractures is growth stimulation, which occurs because of hyperemia and continues for approximately 18 months after the fracture occurs. In contrast, growth arrest may occur if the growth plate is crushed or crossed by the fracture. The Salter–Harris classification (Fig. 266-1) was developed to predict the risk for growth arrest. Because types I and II do not cross the germinal layers, the risk of growth-plate damage with these injuries is minimal. In types III and IV, the fracture crosses the plate, but anatomic reduction may diminish the risk of plate closure. In type V, the crushing cannot be reversed.

Basic evaluation of specific injuries should include three features: (a) assessment of the entire limb to rule out other fractures or dislocation above or below the joint; (b) assessment of neurovascular status including sensation, motor function and pulses, capillary refill, and temperature; (c) assessment of the site of injury.

HAND INJURIES

Injuries to the hand are common in children. Fractures of the phalangeal and metacarpal shafts can be splinted if they are minimally angled and stable, but rotational alignment should be checked by observing the fingernails with the fingers flexed and extended. They should be aligned similarly if no malrotation is present. "Buddy taping" helps to minimize malrotation. Growth-plate or epiphyseal fractures may be splinted if they are nondisplaced but should be referred if they are displaced. Dorsally dislocated interphalangeal joints may be reduced and viewed radiographically to rule out fracture. If they are stable enough to allow active range of motion, they should be splinted for 3 weeks with an aluminum splint. Immobilization of the metacarpophalangeal joints should be in 50 to 90 degrees of flexion to minimize stiffness, and the interphalangeal joints should be in mild flexion of approximately 20 degrees. Laceration of the palm and digits may sever a flexor tendon, and active range of motion of each joint should be checked to ensure that this has not occurred.

SCAPHOID FRACTURES

The scaphoid bone ossifies when a child is 6 years old. Scaphoid fractures in children may develop nonunion if they are not recognized. However, they occur less often in children than in adults. "Snuff box" tenderness may be indicative of a scaphoid injury and warrants further radiographic evaluation. Placing a thumb spica splint is an excellent way to stabilize the joint until formal orthopedic evaluation can take place.

FOREARM FRACTURES

Forearm fractures are very common in children. Nondisplaced buckle fractures of one or both bones should be treated with a short arm cast for 3 or 4 weeks. Greenstick fractures represent tension or rotational failures with less intrinsic stability, and they should be held in a long arm cast for 6 weeks. Completion of the greenstick fracture is not necessary as long as angulation can be controlled. With any forearm fracture, the wrist and elbow joints should be checked because dislocation may occur at one of these locations to compensate for fracture malalignment (Fig. 266-2A). The ossification patterns of the elbow and wrist are complex. If a radiographic text is not available, comparison films of the contralateral side may clarify abnormalities (Fig. 266-2E).

CLAVICLE FRACTURES

Usually, the clavicle fractures at the junction of the middle and distal thirds. Neurovascular damage to the underlying brachial plexus and subclavian vessels is rare but should be considered. Usually, the periosteal sleeve is intact, and remodeling is excellent. Treatment consists of preventing movement with a sling for 4 weeks in children and 6 weeks in teenagers.

KNEE LIGAMENT INJURIES

Knee ligament injuries are rare in children. Usually, femoral growth-plate separation occurs instead of collateral ligament damage. The tibial growth plate is protected because the collateral ligaments insert distal to it. Any trauma resulting in a swollen knee in a growing child (i.e., ages 7–13 years) should be examined to rule out avulsion of the tibial intercondylar eminence because this eminence represents the insertion of the anterior cruciate ligament and is a serious injury (Fig. 266-2B).

Partial fractures of the medial proximal tibial metaphysis are notorious for later developing outward angulation as a result of medial tibial growth-plate overactivity. Care should be taken to obtain good initial fracture alignment, and parents will accept this outward angulation better if they are forewarned that it may occur despite adequate care. Some of the angulation may decrease with time, but osteotomy may be performed near maturity if significant deformity persists (Fig. 266-2C–D).

ANKLE INJURIES

Several types of ankle injuries are common with injuries of the distal fibula predominating. If a bone fragment is nondisplaced, diagnosis is made by palpating for tenderness at the growth plate, not by obtaining stress films. Three weeks in a short leg cast is the usual treatment; the intent is more to increase patient mobility than to decrease instability. On the tibial side, the anterolateral quadrant of the distal tibial physis is the last to close, and this area may be avulsed with rotation. It should be reduced if it is displaced.

SOFT TISSUE INJURIES

Soft tissue trauma of the extremities may be encountered in the emergency department, and foreign penetration should be considered. Occasionally, palpation and radiography at soft tissue settings may help. Glass is seen only if it has a high lead content. Exploration for deeper foreign bodies may be very frustrating unless it is done surgically under adequate regional or general anesthesia. Contusions to areas with thick subcutaneous fat may produce permanent depression of the area secondary to fat necrosis.

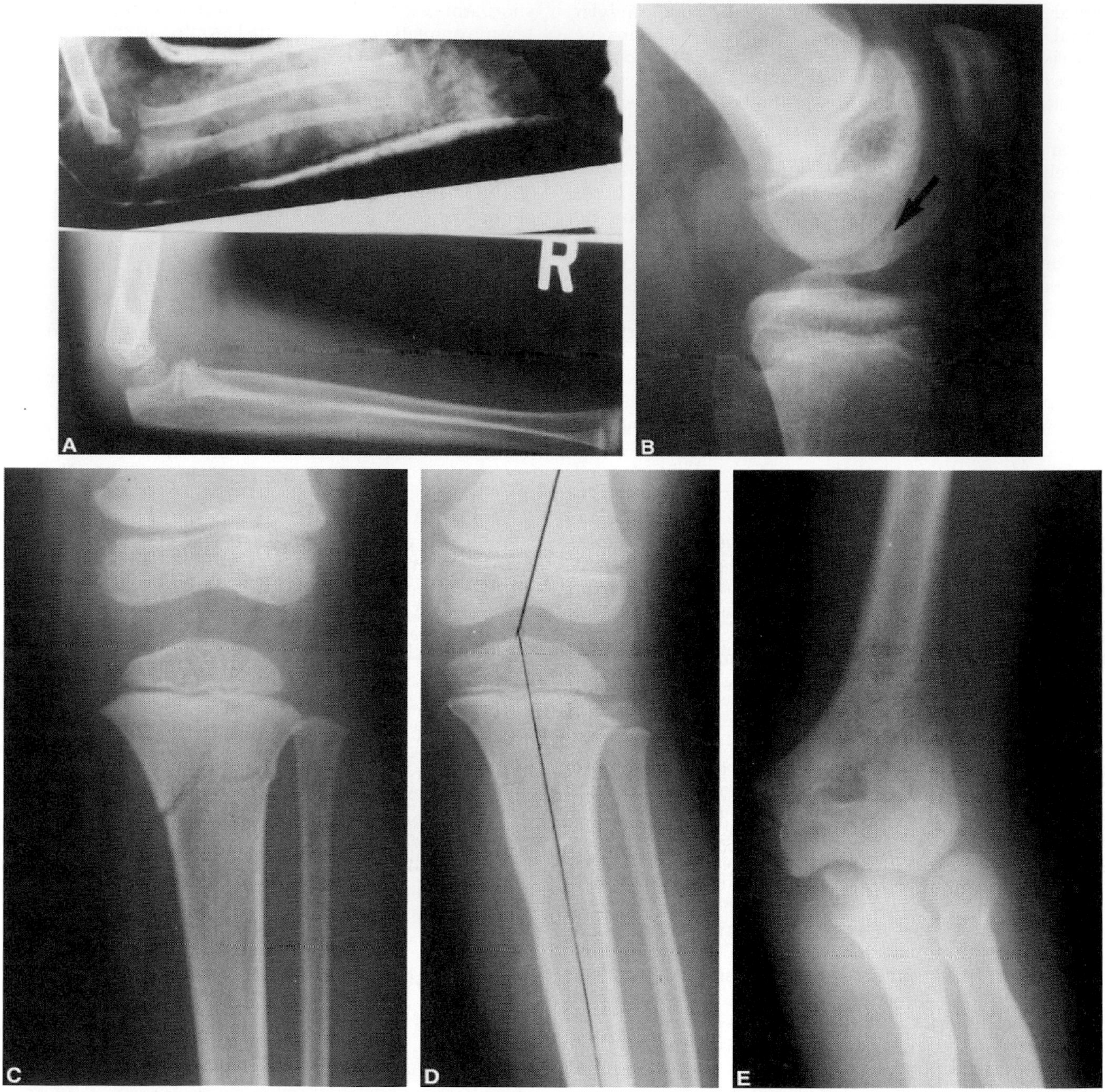

Figure 266-2. Avoiding four common pitfalls in evaluating musculoskeletal trauma. **A:** Always check the joint above and below a fracture. This Monteggia fracture of the ulna is reduced, but the radial head fracture was missed. The radial head should line up with the capitellum, as it does in the elbow on the right. **B:** In a child's swollen knee, check the lateral film for a tibial spine avulsion fracture. It may be obscured partially by the overlying femoral condyles. **C,D:** A proximal tibial fracture may result in valgus deformity even when initially reduced well. **E:** Obtain comparison views when uncertain. This round ossicle in the medial joint space appears to belong there and was missed by an orthopedist, but it actually represents the medial epicondyle trapped inside the joint.

OPEN FRACTURES, DISLOCATIONS, AND COMPARTMENT SYNDROMES

Open fractures, dislocations, and compartment syndromes (the last in particular) should be treated as quickly as possible for best results. Open fractures allow bacteria to come in contact with damaged tissue, which is an ideal culture medium. They should be irrigated down to bone within 6 hours to decrease the rate of infection and, if extensive, should be left open for several days for drainage and further débridement, unless they are small and clean.

Dislocations of almost all major joints constitute emergencies because nerves and vessels are stretched, and further swelling can add to the problem. The ulnar, median, and radial nerves and the brachial artery are involved at the elbow, the sciatic nerve is involved at the hip, and the popliteal artery is involved at the knee. Fractures that occur near these areas have similar implications.

Compartment syndromes have been increasingly recognized in the last two decades and occur most commonly in the forearm, leg, and buttock. Such syndromes develop when injury increases the tissue pressure within a closed fascial compartment above the capillary perfusion pressure (usually 30–45 mm Hg) resulting in ischemia and swelling. The earliest sign is excessive pain on passive stretch of the involved muscles within the compartment, followed by sensory loss and paresthesias of the involved nerves, and weakness of the muscle. Loss of pulses is a very late sign, and it indicates that pressure has risen above large arteriolar systolic pressure. Confirmation is obtained by measurement of the pressures using a hydrostatic or electronic apparatus. Treatment involves release of the tight fascia with later skin closure when swelling resolves (if possible) or skin grafting (if not possible).

FRACTURES WITH MALPOSITION

Fractures with malposition may have to be stabilized so that an affected child can be transported to a consultant. Materials used for this purpose may be improvised, or plaster splints over soft wadding may be used. In general, fractures should be splinted in the position in which they present, with the exception of femur fractures, which can be placed in longitudinal traction with a splint.

MUSCLE CONTUSIONS

Muscle contusions occur most frequently in the quadriceps, upper arm, or shoulder muscles. They may be intensely painful. Compartment syndromes are rare in these regions. Treatment consists of limitation of hemorrhage by rest, ice packing, and elastic bandage wrapping. Active range of motion should be instituted in 1 to 3 days, but passive range of motion (i.e., stretching) should be avoided because it may cause further damage. Strength rehabilitation is instituted after motion is regained. Myositis ossificans (i.e., intramuscular calcification and ossification) may follow this injury but usually does not limit function.

13
Rheumatologic Disorders

CHAPTER 267
Juvenile Rheumatoid Arthritis

Adapted from James T. Cassidy

JRA is the most common pediatric connective tissue disease having arthritis as the principal manifestation (Table 267-1). It is one of the most frequent chronic childhood illnesses and a leading cause of disability and blindness. The etiology of JRA is unknown. Likely, it does not represent a single disorder but rather a spectrum of diseases of diverse pathogenesis. Antibodies and cellular immune reactivity to type II collagen have been demonstrated in children with JRA. Children with JRA may form antibodies to surface membrane antigens on T cells of the suppressor-inducer type.

CLINICAL CHARACTERISTICS AND TYPES OF DISEASE

Although onset of JRA before age 6 months is unusual, the mean age at onset is characteristically young (1–3 years) with a substantial number of cases beginning throughout childhood and young adolescence. Girls are affected at least twice as frequently as boys.

Fatigue, low-grade fever, anorexia, weight loss, and failure to grow are common at onset of the disease in moderate to severely affected children. Often, morning stiffness, musculoskeletal gelling after inactivity, and night pain are encountered in uncontrolled disease. Affected children may not always communicate these symptoms to their parents. They may present, instead, with increased irritability, a posture of guarding the joints, a limp, or refusal to walk.

TABLE 267-1. Frequency of the Pediatric Rheumatic Diseases in 12,939 Children, 1992–1995

Disease	Number of cases (%)
Juvenile rheumatoid arthritis	2,071 (16)
Connective tissue diseases	1,409 (11)
Spondyloarthropathy and reactive arthritis	1,080 (8)
Infectious arthritis and osteomyelitis	471 (4)
Chronic pain syndromes	1,577 (12)
Hypermobility and overuse syndromes	607 (5)
Other diseases	5,724 (44)

Courtesy of Suzanne Bowyer, M.D., Pediatric Rheumatology Database Research Group.

TABLE 267-2. Classification of Types of Onsets of Juvenile Rheumatoid Arthritis

Sign/symptom of onset	Polyarthritis	Oligoarthritis (pauciarticular disease)	Systemic disease
Frequency of cases	30–40%	50–60%	10–15%
Number of joints involved	≥5	≤4	Variable
Gender ratio (F:M)	3:1	5:1	1:1
Systemic involvement	Moderate involvement	Not present	Prominent
Occurrence of chronic uveitis	5%	20%	Rare
Frequency of seropositivity			
Rheumatoid factors	10% (increases with age)	Rare	Rare
Antinuclear antibodies	40–50%	75–85%*	10%
Course	Systemic disease generally mild; possible unremitting articular involvement	Systemic disease absent; major cause of morbidity is uveitis	Systemic disease often self-limited; arthritis is chronic and destructive in 50%
Prognosis	Guarded to moderately good	Excellent except for eyesight	Moderate to poor

*In girls with uveitis.

Tenosynovitis and myositis are also accompaniments of active disease. Rheumatoid nodules may occur on the tendons or subcutaneously over pressure points. They are found particularly in children who have widespread polyarthritis, are older at onset, and have prominent small-joint disease. These patients typically have an unrelenting course with early development of bony erosions and RF seropositivity.

The classification of JRA is based on recognition of at least three distinct types of onsets of the disease (Table 267-2). Of note, a few children have onset of JRA with severe constitutional and systemic disease. The systemic signs and symptoms may precede the appearance of overt arthritis by weeks, months, or even years. A hallmark of this type of disease is a high-spiking fever, often combined with a rheumatoid rash. Temperature elevations occur once or twice daily, often in late afternoon or evening, to a level of 39°C or higher with a quick return to baseline temperature or lower. This quotidian pattern is highly suggestive of a diagnosis of JRA.

The rash of JRA develops with this fever and consists of 2- to 5-mm erythematous morbilliform macules (Fig. 267-1). It is most commonly seen in the trunk and proximal extremities and over pressure areas, but it may occur on the face, palms, or soles. Generally, the rash is not pruritic; its most characteristic feature is its transient nature. This rash may also be seen in some children with polyarthritis at onset, but it is never seen in children with oligoarthritis. Sometimes, the rash can be elicited by rubbing or scratching the skin (Koebner phenomenon).

Usually, children with systemic onset have hepatosplenomegaly and lymphadenopathy. Pericarditis, hepatitis, and other visceral disease may occur. Pulmonary involvement consists of a wide spectrum of abnormalities such as pleuritis and effusion, interstitial fibrosis, and hemosiderosis. The central nervous system (CNS) may be affected, but distinguishing encephalopathy from drug toxicity, viral infection, or other complications of the systemic illness and fever may be difficult.

Laboratory Examination

Children with active disease develop a normocytic, hypochromic anemia characteristic of the chronic anemia of inflammation. Often, it is moderately severe with the hemoglobin in the range of 7 to 10 g/dL. Leukocytosis and thrombocytosis are common with active disease. These findings are either not seen or are much less pronounced in children with oligoarthritis.

Often, the acute-phase reactants are elevated in concentration at onset of the disease and are moderately useful in following the course of the disease. The Westergren erythrocyte sedimentation rate (ESR), C-reactive protein level, and immunoglobulin concentrations reflect inflammatory activity. Usually, serum complement components are elevated at onset and with exacerbations.

Tests for rheumatoid factors (RFs) are positive in children with JRA less frequently than in adults with rheumatoid arthritis. RFs are IgM macroglobulins with antigenic specificity directed against components of IgG. Approximately 10% of children with JRA eventually become seropositive, even though few children

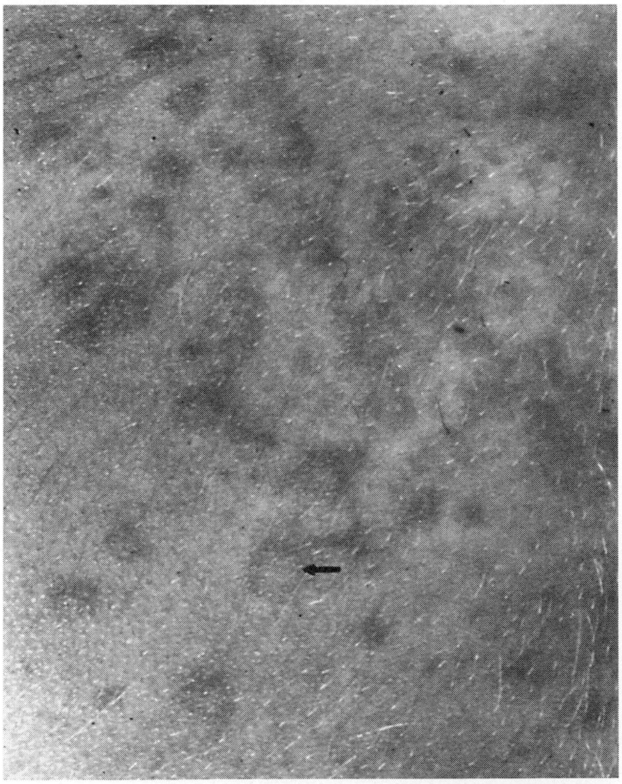

Figure 267-1. Rash of systemic-onset juvenile rheumatoid arthritis. This 4-year-old girl presented with high-spiking fever that occurred once a day accompanied by a transient nonpruritic rash. An area of active maculopapular rash on her back was salmon pink in color. The arrow points to central clearing in a lesion. (Reprinted with permission from Cassidy JT. Juvenile rheumatoid arthritis. In: Kelley WN, Harris ED Jr, Ruddy S, Sledge CB, eds. Textbook of rheumatology. Philadelphia: Saunders, 1997: 1211.)

at onset of JRA are seropositive. RFs tend to be present in children who are older at onset or in older children and in those who have prominent symmetric polyarthritis with involvement of the small joints, subcutaneous rheumatoid nodules, articular erosions, and a poor functional outcome.

Antinuclear antibody (ANA) seropositivity is present in at least 45% of children with JRA. Usually, the pattern of fluorescent staining is homogeneous or speckled; generally, the titer is low to moderate. The presence of these antibodies is significantly correlated with development of chronic uveitis. They are found less commonly in older boys and in children with systemic disease. A positive ANA determination is a valuable diagnostic measure in children suspected of having JRA because ANAs are not frequently found in other childhood illnesses except for the rheumatic diseases and transient acute viral disease.

Usually, the synovial fluid white cell count is moderately elevated in the range of 10,000 to 20,000 cells per microliter. Synovial glucose concentration is low. Complement levels may be depressed indicating intrasynovial complement activation.

Generally, urinalysis is normal in children with JRA except for those few who have a mild glomerulitis at onset. Proteinuria may occur with fever. However, persistent proteinuria may be the first evidence of drug toxicity or amyloidosis. Some children develop renal papillary necrosis related to therapy and dehydration during the course of the disease.

Radiologic Examination

Children with JRA exhibit a wide range of distinctive radiologic findings. Early changes consist of soft tissue swelling, juxtaarticular osteoporosis, and periosteal new-bone apposition. Development of the ossification centers may be accelerated or premature epiphyseal closure leading to stunting of bone growth may occur.

Cervical spine disease is characteristic of JRA. The upper cervical segments are principally affected with apophyseal joint fusion and atlantoaxial subluxation (Fig. 267-2). The lower vertebrae may also be involved with failure to grow normally. Fractures, particularly of the long bones and vertebrae, occur in children who develop generalized osteopenia.

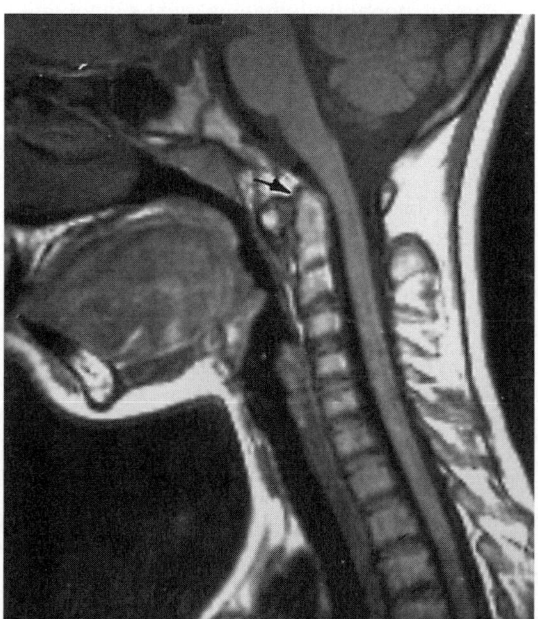

Figure 267-2. Magnetic resonance image (MRI) of the cervical spine of a child with 7 mm of atlantoaxial subluxation. The odontoid is beginning to impinge on the upper cervical cord (*arrow*).

TABLE 267-3. Comparison of ACR and EULAR Criteria for Idiopathic Arthritis in Children

Entity	ACR (JRA)	EULAR (JCA)
Age at onset	≤16 yr	≤16 yr
Definition of arthritis	Yes	No
Duration of disease	≥6 wk	≥3 mo
Onset type	3	3
Course subtype	9	No
Inclusion of JAS, psoriatic arthritis, and IBD	No	Yes
Exclusion of other forms of juvenile arthritis	Yes	Yes

ACR, American College of Rheumatology; EULAR, European League Against Rheumatism; IBD, inflammatory bowel disease; JAS, juvenile ankylosing spondylitis; JCA, juvenile chronic arthritis; JRA, juvenile rheumatoid arthritis.

Generally, routine radiographic studies are sufficient to delineate this progression of changes in evaluating affected children's response to a management program. However, magnetic resonance imaging (MRI) is more precise than routine radiographic examination in delineating soft tissue abnormalities in response to abnormal bone growth or fusion and in detecting early cartilage or bone destruction.

Diagnosis

JRA classification criteria of the American College of Rheumatology and juvenile chronic arthritis criteria of the European League Against Rheumatism are compared in Table 267-3. JRA is defined as onset of idiopathic peripheral arthritis in children younger than 16 years. Arthritis is clinically defined by swelling or effusion or the presence of two or more of the following signs: limitation of range of motion, tenderness or pain on motion, and increased heat in one or more joints. Often, JRA is a diagnosis of exclusion and, therefore, similar diseases must be considered (Table 267-4). Generally, the differential diagnosis includes other rheumatic and connective tissue diseases, especially rheumatic fever, SLE, and ankylosing spondylitis.

Treatment

Conservative management of JRA attempts to control clinical manifestations of the disease and to prevent or minimize deformity. Ideally, this approach involves a multidisciplinary team that follows affected children throughout the course of their illness. Management should be family centered, community based, and coordinated. Prognosis is good to excellent for most children with JRA, so the philosophy of management should initially stress the simplest, safest, and most conservative measures. If this treatment proves inadequate, other therapeutic modalities should be chosen (Table 267-5).

Nonsteroidal antiinflammatory drugs (NSAIDs) are effective in suppressing inflammation and fever. Because of the risk of Reye syndrome, pediatric rheumatologists often prefer nonsteroidal drugs such as ibuprofen, naproxen, and tolmetin to aspirin. The first two can also be prescribed as a suspension, which is particularly useful for younger children. All children with JRA should receive yearly influenza vaccines and should be immune to varicella.

TABLE 267-4. Diagnostic Classification of Juvenile Arthritis

Connective tissue diseases
Juvenile rheumatoid arthritis
Systemic lupus erythematosus
Dermatomyositis
Vasculitis
Scleroderma
Psoriatic arthritis
Seronegative spondyloarthropathies
Juvenile ankylosing spondylitis
Reiter disease
Inflammatory bowel disease
Infectious arthritis
Bacterial arthritis (including staphylococcal, gonorrhea, tuberculosis)
Viral arthritis
Fungal arthritis
Lyme disease
Reactive arthritis
Rheumatic fever
Post-*Yersinia* arthritis
Rheumatic diseases associated with immunodeficiency
Congenital anomalies and genetically determined abnormalities of the musculoskeletal system
Constitutional diseases of bone
Lysosomal storage diseases
Heritable disorders of collagen and fibrous connective tissue
Amyloidosis
Nonrheumatic conditions of bones and joints
Traumatic arthritis
Reflex neurovascular dystrophy
Legg–Calvé–Perthes disease
Slipped capital femoral epiphysis
Toxic synovitis of the hip
Osteochondritis dissecans
Patellofemoral pain syndromes
Plant-thorn synovitis
Hematologic diseases
Sickle cell anemia
Hemophilia
Thalassemia
Leukemia and lymphoma
Neoplastic diseases
Neuroblastoma
Malignant and benign tumors of cartilage, bone, and synovium
Histiocytosis
Arthromyalgia
Growing pains
Idiopathic pain syndromes

TABLE 267-5. Management of Children with Juvenile Rheumatoid Arthritis

Medication program: suppression of inflammation
Nonsteroidal antiinflammatory drugs
Hydroxychloroquine
Methotrexate
Glucocorticoid drugs
Immunosuppressive drugs
Preservation of function and prevention of deformities
Local and general rest
Physical therapy
Occupational therapy
Orthopedic surgery: preventive and reconstructive
Psychosocial development
Peer group relationships and schooling
Counseling of patients and families
Involvement of community agencies
Maintenance of adequate nutrition
Coordinated care

Methotrexate has become the most successful and safe approach to advanced drug treatment of severe or resistant polyarthritis. In a large, multinational, double-blind, randomized trial, a weekly dose of 10 mg/m^2 markedly reduced the articular severity index as compared to placebo. This drug is attractive for pediatric use because it is given only once a week orally as a pill or liquid and it has no proven oncogenic potential or untoward risk of sterility. Toxicity is monitored by periodic complete blood cell counts and liver enzyme determinations.

Glucocorticoid drugs should be reserved for treatment of severely involved children who are recalcitrant to more conservative therapeutic regimens. Many toxicities (e.g., Cushing syndrome) and severely retarded growth are associated with steroid use. Steroids are indicated for resistant or life-threatening disease and its complications such as pericarditis. Ophthalmic administration is indicated for treatment of chronic uveitis. Often, intraarticular steroid is used to achieve specific goals of a physical therapy program or for persistent monoarticular or oligoarticular involvement.

Physical and Occupational Therapy

Maintenance of function and prevention of deformity cannot be overemphasized in the total management of children with JRA. Appropriate prescriptions for physical and occupational therapy, a balanced program of rest and activity, and selective splinting are used. Normal play should be encouraged. Only unacceptable levels of stress on inflamed weight-bearing joints should be limited. Children with cervical spine disease should wear a padded plastic collar when traveling in an automobile or studying.

COMPLICATIONS

Chronic Uveitis

One of the most serious complications of JRA is the development of a chronic nongranulomatous uveitis involving the iris, ciliary body and, occasionally, the posterior choroid. Usually, this disease is bilateral and, in 20% of involved children, leads to blindness in the affected eye. Characteristically, chronic uveitis has an insidious, asymptomatic onset and is diagnosed only by routine ophthalmologic and slit-lamp examinations at onset of the disease. These examinations should be repeated at frequent intervals during the first years after onset. Chronic uveitis is confined to children with polyarthritis or oligoarthritis. It tends to occur particularly in young girls who experience early age of onset and limited joint disease and are ANA-seropositive.

Growth Retardation

Disturbances of growth and normal development are complications of any chronic disease such as JRA. Linear growth is retarded during periods of active disease and with the use of glucocorticoid drugs. Localized growth retardation may also occur in specific areas such as the jaw (micrognathia). Unequal leg or arm lengths develop with monoarticular disease involving a single limb. Often, delayed development of secondary sexual characteristics occurs. Psychosocial retardation may be a frequent and potentially severe complication. Psychological regression to a more infantile pattern is present in most children who experience moderate to severe disease.

Course and Prognosis

In general, 85% of children who develop JRA experience a satisfactory recovery from their disease and enter adult life without serious functional disability, although as many as 45% may have continuing low-grade activity. A small percentage of patients whose disease has gone into remission have a recurrence of arthritis during the adult years. As many as 15% of children, however, enter adulthood with moderate to significant functional disability. Children most at risk are those who have had late-onset polyarthritis, symmetric involvement of the small joints of the hands or feet, unremitting activity of the joint disease, early appearance of erosions, or prominent systemic manifestations and development of RF seropositivity and subcutaneous nodules. Progressive hip disease is also a major cause of long-term disability.

CHAPTER 268

Systemic Lupus Erythematosus

Adapted from James T. Cassidy

Systemic Lupus Erythematosus (SLE) is a multisystem disease in which widespread inflammatory involvement of the connective tissues and immune-complex vasculitis occur. It is a prototypic example of autoimmunity in humans and results from abnormal immunologic hyperreactivity and an immunogenetic predisposition to the disease.

CLINICAL CHARACTERISTICS

Although SLE can develop at any age, onset in children usually occurs after age 5 and becomes increasingly common during the adolescent years. The female–to–male ratio is approximately 8:1 except in the youngest children, when relatively more boys are affected.

The manifestations of SLE vary (Table 268-1) and present with any degree of severity from an acute, rapidly fatal illness to insidious, chronic disability with multisystem exacerbations. In more than three-fourths of affected children, SLE is diagnosed within the first 6 months after onset because of the acute nature of the illness, but diagnosis is often delayed by 4 to 5 years in some patients.

Fever, malaise, and weight loss are common. Each exacerbation of the disease tends to mimic previous episodes. If serious renal disease develops, it usually does so within 2 years after onset. The major exception to the predictability of SLE is seen in the occurrence of CNS illness, which may intervene at any time in approximately one-third of affected children.

A malar erythematous rash in a butterfly distribution across the bridge of the nose and over each cheek is characteristic of an acute onset or exacerbation (Fig. 268-1). Other forms of cutaneous and mucocutaneous involvement are common and vary in character and distribution. Raynaud phenomenon is frequent in SLE. It may result in digital ulceration and gangrene in a few affected children. The risk of developing osteonecrosis, particularly of the femoral heads, is common and is worsened by glucocorticoid therapy.

Arthritis affects the majority of children with SLE and commonly involves the small joints of the hands, wrists, elbows,

TABLE 268-1. Clinical Presentation and Course of Systemic Lupus Erythematosus in Children

Presentation	At onset (%)	During course (%)
Nephritis	84	86
Hypertension	10	28
Arthritis	72	76
Dermatitis	69	76
Malar erythema	51	56
Photosensitivity	16	16
Alopecia	16	20
Oral or nasopharyngeal ulcerations	12	16
Pericarditis	40	47
Pleuritis	31	36
Central nervous system disease	9	31
Raynaud phenomenon	16	24
Hepatomegaly	43	47
Splenomegaly	20	20
Anemia	43	47
Leukopenia	60	71
Thrombocytopenia	22	24

Modified from Cassidy JT, Sullivan DB, Petty RE, et al. Lupus nephritis and encephalopathy: prognosis in 58 children. *Arthritis Rheum* 1977;20:316.

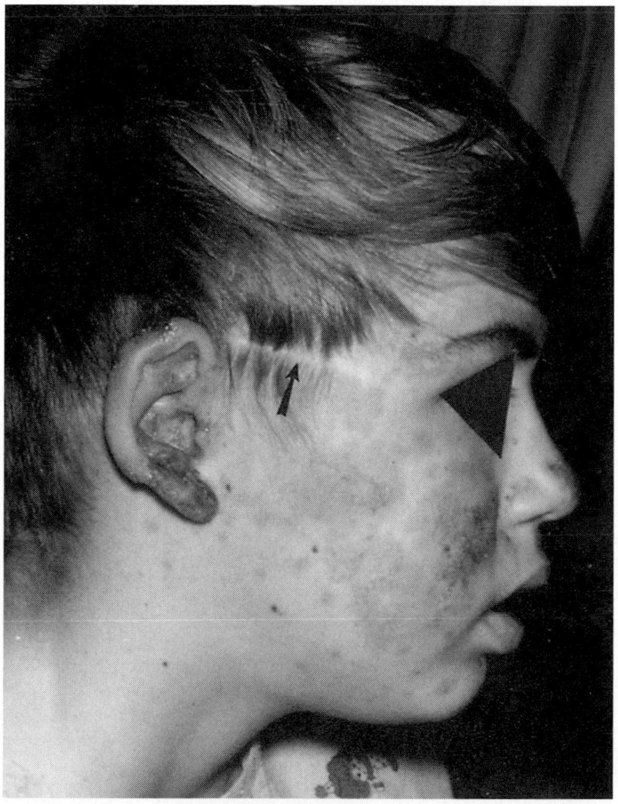

Figure 268-1. Excoriating erythematous facial rash of acute systemic lupus erythematosus in a 14-year-old boy. The crusting lesions are seen over the nose, malar areas, cheeks, and earlobes. Clear area corresponds to eyeglass frames (*arrow*) confirming the role of photosensitivity in the genesis of this lesion.

shoulders, knees, and ankles. Characteristically, this arthritis is transient and may be migratory. Often, pain is more severe than is supported by objective changes. The arthritis of SLE is almost never erosive, and it does not often result in permanent deformity.

Pericarditis is the most common manifestation of cardiac involvement. Affected children may also experience congestive heart failure, arrhythmias, or myocardial infarction. Valvular insufficiency develops in a few cases, and a sterile verrucous endocarditis (Libman–Sacks) is particularly characteristic of SLE. Echocardiography is a sensitive method of confirming its presence. Pleuritis is also common and may involve the diaphragmatic pleurae, along with a basilar pneumonitis. Pulmonary hemorrhage is rare but can be fatal.

Often, abdominal pain presents a diagnostic dilemma in children with SLE, especially in those who are under treatment with glucocorticoids and in whom peptic ulcer disease is a consideration. Mesenteric thrombosis and acute pancreatitis are life-threatening events. Hepatomegaly and splenomegaly are common, and splenic infarction may occur. Chronic active hepatitis is associated with SLE in an overlap syndrome.

Disease of the central nervous system (CNS) and peripheral nervous system is a common cause of morbidity. Pseudotumor cerebri may be a complication of SLE or the glucocorticoid therapy. Variously, recurrent headaches, seizures, chorea, or frank psychoses are encountered. Intracranial hemorrhage may result from hypertension, thrombocytopenia, or thrombosis associated with antiphospholipid antibodies. Systemic polyneuropathy, the Guillain–Barré syndrome, transverse myelopathy, or involvement of specific cranial nerves has been reported.

Some involvement of the kidneys is present in virtually all children with SLE. Even moderately severe nephritis may not be detected early by the presence of an abnormal urinary sediment, proteinuria, or changes in the creatinine clearance. Evidence of active immune-complex disease such as increased levels of antinative DNA antibodies or hypocomplementemia correlates with active nephritis in most patients.

In the diagnosis of lupus nephritis, microscopical interpretation of a renal biopsy is categorized by the World Health Organization as type I, normal; type II, mesangial; type III, focal proliferative; type IV, diffuse proliferative; type V, membranous; and type VI, sclerosing disease. The relation of specific types of involvement to prognosis and eventual renal failure is shown in Table 268-2. Thus, renal biopsy to delineate the type of nephritis is warranted in the majority of children with SLE unless no clinical evidence of significant involvement of the kidney is present, as usually the safest approach to long-term therapy is based on careful evaluation of the renal status. Serious renal lesions are believed to be more common in children with SLE than in adults, and prognosis for renal disease is more guarded.

LABORATORY EXAMINATION

Generally, the acute-phase indices are increased in active systemic disease. Otherwise unexplained leukopenia is particularly characteristic of SLE. The majority of affected children are leukopenic at onset with neutrophils predominating in the peripheral count. During the course of the illness, the white blood cell (WBC) count does not often become elevated to an appropriate degree, even with serious infection or bacteremia. Thrombocytopenia and acute hemolytic anemia may also be present. Often, Coombs tests are sensitive in such children. Besides systemic disease, other causes of anemia include menorrhagia, septicemia, and gastrointestinal bleeding. SLE may present as thrombocytopenic purpura.

ANAs are present in most children with SLE and are generally found in high titer in a homogeneous pattern. A peripheral nuclear pattern is virtually synonymous with the presence of antinative DNA antibodies. AntiRo antibodies are characteristic of subacute cutaneous lupus and the neonatal lupus syndromes and are associated with the development of pulmonary disease and nephritis. AntiSm antibodies are also diagnostic of SLE or of an associated syndrome and correlate with isolated CNS disease.

Rheumatoid factors (RFs) and other antitissue antibodies such as antithyroglobulin are often positive in children with SLE. Cold agglutinins or cryoglobulins may result in peripheral anoxia such as Raynaud phenomenon. Affected children are predisposed to repeated episodes of thrombosis by antiphospholipid antibodies or circulating lupus anticoagulants that cross-react with a phospholipid antigen of the VDRL test for syphilis. Young people with a biological false-positive test for syphilis are at risk for developing SLE.

Components of both the classic and alternative complement pathways are consumed in the presence of active immune-complex vasculitis. The hemolytic complement determination or CH_{50} reflects the status of the total complement cascade; C3 concentration appears to be depressed less frequently, but a falling concentration of C4 is usually a reliable indicator of active disease.

DIAGNOSIS

Diagnostic suspicion of SLE in children depends on recognizing an episodic, multisystem constellation of clinical disease strongly associated with persistent antinuclear antibody (ANA) seropositivity. Eleven criteria have been chosen by the American College of Rheumatology for the classification of SLE. They are listed in Table 268-3.

The differential diagnosis of SLE should consider juvenile rheumatoid arthritis (JRA), other forms of acute glomerulonephritis, hemolytic anemia, leukemia, allergic or contact dermatitis, an idiopathic seizure disorder, mononucleosis, acute

TABLE 268-2. Classification of Lupus Nephritis

Type of renal disease	Remission	Nephrotic syndrome	Renal failure	Uremic deaths
Glomerular lesions				
Mesangial	+	–	–	–
Focal proliferative	++	+	+	+
Diffuse proliferative	+	++	++	+++
Membranous	+	+++	++	+
Extraglomerular lesions	+	+	++	++

–, absent; +, minimal; ++, moderate; +++, severe.

TABLE 268-3. Criteria for Classification of Systemic Lupus Erythematosus*

Malar (butterfly) rash
Discoid-lupus rash
Photosensitivity
Oral or nasal mucocutaneous ulcerations
Nonerosive arthritis
Nephritis
Proteinuria >0.5 g/d
Cellular casts
Encephalopathy
Seizures
Psychosis
Pleuritis or pericarditis
Cytopenia
Positive immunoserology
Antibodies to nDNA
Antibodies to Sm nuclear antigen
Biological false-positive test for syphilis
Positive antinuclear antibody test

*Four of 11 criteria provide a sensitivity of 96% and a specificity of 96% for systemic lupus erythematosus.

rheumatic fever with carditis, and septicemia. SLE remains the great masquerader.

TREATMENT

Long-term supportive care of children with SLE includes adequate nutrition, fluid and electrolyte balance, early recognition and treatment of infections, and control of hypertension. Fevers and potential infection should be promptly evaluated. Pneumonitis, septicemia, and pyelonephritis are of particular concern.

Because SLE is a serious disease, children with SLE benefit from contact with the same medical team over the course of the illness. This team should emphasize the rationale supporting the treatment program and should encourage prophylactic measures of avoiding excessive sunlight, unnecessary drug exposure, and transfusion. Appropriate photoprotective clothing and sunscreens are prescribed. Affected children's general activities and interactions with peer groups should not be restrained unnecessarily.

Nonsteroidal antiinflammatory drugs (NSAIDs) (e.g., naproxen) are useful in treating minor manifestations of SLE such as arthralgia and myalgia. Hydroxychloroquine is an adjunctive medication that helps to control photosensitive dermatitis or moderates glucocorticoid dosage. Glucocorticoid drugs are the mainstay of the basic regimen, and prednisone is the preferred analogue. A negative purified protein derivative test for tuberculosis should be verified before affected children are started on prednisone. The minimum prednisone dose to achieve the goals of the treatment program is initiated at onset and maintained during the course of the disease. Low-dose therapy, defined as 0.5 mg/kg/day in divided doses, is used to treat noninfectious fever, dermatitis, arthritis, or serositis. Usually, these manifestations are promptly suppressed. Often, weeks are required for improvement in anemia or the serologic tests reflecting active immune-complex disease. Low-dose glucocorticoid programs often control clinical disease in children with mesangial or focal glomerulonephritis.

High-dose prednisone therapy, defined as 1 to 2 mg/kg/day in divided doses, is used for lupus crisis, CNS disease, acute hemolytic anemia, or the more severe forms of nephritis. Hypertension, azotemia, and preexisting psychosis are relative contraindications to prolonged high-dosage regimens. Results of treatment are monitored by the clinical course of affected children and by periodic assessment of antinative DNA antibodies and serum complement levels. Exacerbation of the disease during a steroid taper is signaled by a deterioration of the serologic indices.

Intravenous methylprednisolone pulse therapy may be indicated in an acute exacerbation of the disease to avoid increasing the daily steroid intake. Immunosuppressive agents are necessary in some affected children. Although azathioprine has been used extensively, data suggest that intravenous pulse cyclophosphamide is preferable, especially in children with severe nephritis. Dialysis and kidney transplantation have been successfully used in end-stage renal disease.

COURSE AND PROGNOSIS

Prognosis in children with SLE has improved substantially since the 1960s; therefore, a guardedly optimistic attitude toward this disease is warranted. An estimated 85% to 90% of children with SLE will survive over a 10-year period, but survivorship in children with diffuse proliferative glomerulonephritis is less favorable at 70% for 10 years. Infection has replaced severe nephritis and CNS disease as the leading cause of death in children with SLE. Malignant hypertension, gastrointestinal bleeding or perforation, acute pancreatitis, and pulmonary hemorrhage are also serious complications of the disease or of its treatment.

SLE is characterized by repeated exacerbations and remissions; often, active disease is prolonged over many years. Generalizations concerning prognosis for specific children are especially unwise during the first 1 to 2 years after diagnosis. Later, a more reliable estimate can be offered to families of affected children on the basis of the degree of systemic activity and its response to therapy and on the severity of nephritis, systemic vasculitis, and parenchymal organ involvement. Prognosis for life or function is poorest in diffuse proliferative nephritis or the organic brain syndrome, and it is best in minimal systemic disease and mesangial nephritis and with a prompt sustained response to glucocorticoid therapy.

DRUG-INDUCED SYSTEMIC LUPUS ERYTHEMATOSUS

In some affected children, acute SLE is precipitated or preceded by a drug reaction. Agents most frequently implicated in this outcome are hydralazine, isoniazid, penicillin, sulfonamides, and anticonvulsant medications. The most frequent clinical manifestations in drug-induced SLE are cutaneous and pleuropericardial. CNS disease and nephritis are uncommon. In most instances, drug-induced SLE is a self-limited illness that abates on withdrawal of the offending agent. Antibodies to native DNA are not present, but antiDNA-histone reactivity is present in 95% of affected patients. The serum complement concentration remains normal. Although the precise immunologic mechanisms have not been elucidated, some of these medications (e.g., hydralazine) may sensitize cutaneous DNA to degradation by UV light. A drug reaction may also precipitate clinical manifestations indistinguishable from idiopathic SLE.

CHAPTER 269

Sjögren Syndrome

Adapted from James T. Cassidy

The diagnosis of Sjögren syndrome (SS) is based on a triad of findings: (a) the sicca syndrome (dry eyes and dry mouth), (b) a connective tissue disease [usually Systemic Lupus Erythematosus (SLE) or scleroderma], and (c) high titers of autoantibodies [usually rheumatoid factors (RFs) or antinuclear antibodies (ANAs)]. SS can be divided into two forms: a primary disease, in which a defined connective tissue disease is not present, and a secondary disease, in which a connective tissue disease is prominent. The secondary form of the disorder is far less common in children with rheumatic diseases than in adults. The primary disorder is very rare and may present as recurrent bilateral parotid swelling. It has been reported in children as young as 5 and is much more common in girls than boys.

Pathophysiologically, SS appears to be an extreme example of uncontrolled B-cell hyperactivity to a variety of antigens in conjunction with decreased T-cell responsiveness and suppression. Skin tests for delayed hypersensitivity are impaired, and *in vitro* measures of lymphocyte transformation are decreased. HLA-B8 and -DR3 are strongly associated with development of this syndrome.

CLINICAL CHARACTERISTICS

SS is a multisystem disorder that often involves many organ systems (Table 269-1). It is insidious in onset in many patients and is slowly progressive. The sicca component is the dominant symptomatic feature of SS and is directly related to lymphocytic infiltration of the lacrimal and salivary glands, although more widespread involvement of the entire upper respiratory tract, larynx, stomach, and genitourinary systems may be present. Patients with SS may also have achlorhydria or may develop pancreatitis, hepatobiliary disease, chronic active hepatitis, or evidence of active vasculitis. Renal tubular abnormalities related to hypergammaglobulinemia or lymphocytic infiltration may be present and can result in renal tubular acidosis. Hyposthenuria unresponsive to vasopressin occurs with decreased permeability of the distal convoluted tubules and collecting ducts to water. Other patients develop a chronic interstitial nephritis.

TABLE 269-1. Associated Features of Sjögren Syndrome

Sicca complex
Bilateral parotid enlargement
Hashimoto thyroiditis
Lymphoid myositis
Achlorhydria
Hyposthenuria and renal tubular acidosis
Hepatomegaly
Pancreatitis
Celiac syndrome
Connective tissue disease
Systemic lupus erythematosus
Vasculitis
Raynaud phenomenon
Nonthrombocytopenic purpura
Chronic active hepatitis
Autoantibodies
Rheumatoid factors
Antinuclear antibodies
Antibodies to SS-A, SS-B, and rheumatoid arthritis preciptin
Antisalivary duct antibodies
Antitissue antibodies
Malignancy
Pseudolymphoma
Lymphoma
Macroglobulinemia

LABORATORY EXAMINATION

Anemia, thrombocytopenia, and persistent leukopenia may be present in approximately one-third of affected patients. Almost always, a striking polyclonal hypergammaglobulinemia is found. All patients have high titers of RFs or other autoantibodies such as ANA in which a speckled or nucleolar pattern is frequently found.

Most individuals with SS have circulating antibodies directed against small nuclear or cytoplasmic ribonucleoprotein antigens that are termed SS-A (Ro) and SS-B (La). Often, rheumatoid arthritis precipitin is present. Other antitissue antibodies including antiparietal cell and antithyroid antibodies are found in 40% of patients.

DIAGNOSIS

Diagnosis is made by demonstrating the cardinal features of the sicca complex. The mucous membranes are dry. Inadequate tearing is documented by Schirmer test, which demonstrates decreased wetting of a filter paper strip placed in the conjunctival sac. Sialography with contrast media or scintigraphy of the salivary glands with ^{99m}Tc are positive. Diagnosis may be confirmed by biopsy of the labial mucosa to demonstrate the characteristic round cell infiltration in the minor salivary glands.

TREATMENT

Treatment of the sicca complex is primarily symptomatic. Affected children may benefit from the use of artificial tears, saline nasal douches, or the use of sour-lemon drops to provide relief from the xerostomia. Glucocorticoid and immunosuppressive agents can be considered if life-threatening complications occur. When SS is secondary to an established connective tissue disease, treatment is directed toward that disorder.

CHAPTER 270

Dermatomyositis

Adapted from James T. Cassidy

Dermatomyositis occurs in approximately 5% of affected children newly referred to a pediatric rheumatology clinic. The disease is slightly more common in girls than boys, at a ratio of approximately 1.6:1.0. The disease can present at any age, but onset is especially common from the fourth to the tenth years.

Current investigations suggest that dermatomyositis is autoimmune in pathogenesis with both humoral and cell-mediated abnormalities. Immune-complex vasculitis may be an initiating or perpetuating event. Immunoglobulins and complement are deposited in the walls of small blood vessels and in skeletal muscles. An immunogenetic predisposition to the development of dermatomyositis may be present. Dermatomyositis has also occurred in patients with selective IgA deficiency and C2 complement component deficiency. It has developed after vaccination and as a hypersensitivity reaction to drugs, sunburn, or infections (e.g., coxsackie B virus or toxoplasmosis). An acute transient inflammatory myositis occurs in otherwise normal children after certain viral infections, especially influenza. A similar myositis has been described in a few children with agammaglobulinemia in association with echovirus infection.

CLINICAL CHARACTERISTICS

Table 270-1 lists characteristic clinical features of dermatomyositis in children. Most patients have prominent constitutional symptoms of fatigue, malaise, weight loss, anorexia, and low-grade unexplained fever. The proximal limb-girdle muscles of the lower extremities are initially affected, the shoulder girdle and proximal arm muscles are the entities next most frequently involved. Affected children may be unable to hold the head upright or to maintain a sitting posture because of weakness of the anterior neck flexors and back muscles. The distal muscles of the extremities may be involved later in the disease or in children in whom the disease has an acute onset. Affected children may stop walking or be unable to dress or climb stairs or may complain of either vague or specific muscle pain. Such children show a pronounced inability to get up from the floor (a positive Gower sign) or to rise from their bed unaided.

Involvement of the pharyngeal, hypopharyngeal, and palatal muscles develops in 10% of children with dermatomyositis. Dysphonia and difficulty in swallowing may be related to this involvement and also to esophageal hypomotility. Palatal speech or regurgitation of liquids through the nose are early signs of impending respiratory difficulty and aspiration. Profound involvement of the thoracic and respiratory muscles occurs in a few children and leads to increasing dyspnea at rest, aspiration, or death.

The classic dermatomyositis rash is seen in the majority of affected children and may be the first sign of the disease; in the remainder, it is less characteristic but usually suggests the diagnosis (Fig. 270-1). The severity of cutaneous involvement

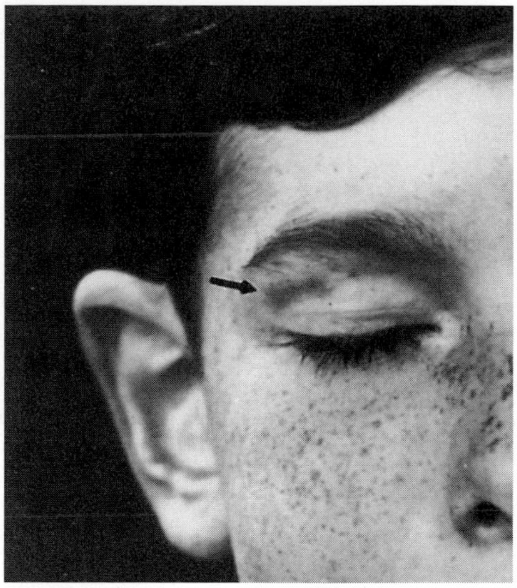

Figure 270-1. Violaceous suffusion of the upper eyelid (*arrow*) in a boy with active juvenile dermatomyositis.

is variable. The rash is most distinctive over the upper eyelids, the malar areas, and the dorsal surfaces of the knuckles, elbows, and knees. Often, at onset of the disease, indurative edema of the skin and subcutaneous tissues is present. Later manifestations include thinning and atrophy of the accessory epidermal structures with loss of hair and development of telangiectases.

TABLE 270-1. Clinical Features Associated with Dermatomyositis in Childhood

Muscle weakness
Proximal pelvic girdle (95%)
Proximal shoulder girdle (75%)
Neck flexors (60%)
Pharyngeal muscles (30%)
Distal muscles of the extremities (30%)
Facial and extraocular muscles (5%)
Muscle contractures and atrophy (60%)
Muscle pain and tenderness (50%)
Skin lesions (85%)
Hellotrope rash of eyelids
Malar rash
Subcutaneous and periorbital edema
Periungual and articular rash (Gottron papules)
Raynaud phenomenon (20%)
Arthritis and arthralgia (25%)
Dysphagia, other gastrointestinal symptoms (10%)
Calcinosis (40%)
Pulmonary fibrosis (5%)

LABORATORY EXAMINATION

The acute-phase reactants such as the erythrocyte sedimentation rate (ESR) and C-reactive protein determination tend to correlate with the degree of clinical inflammation. Anemia is uncommon at onset, except in children with gastrointestinal bleeding. Generally, urinalysis results are normal, but a few affected children have microscopic hematuria. Antinuclear antibodies (ANAs) are variably present in these children. One-half of the affected children have circulating immune complexes at onset.

The three most important diagnostic laboratory abnormalities are shown in Table 270-2. The levels of the serum muscle enzymes are important for diagnosis and in monitoring effective therapy. Generally, a panel of the creatine kinase (CK), aspartate transaminase, alanine transaminase, and aldolase is initially followed. The level of increase in serum concentrations ranges from 20 to 40 times normal for the CK or aspartate transaminase. Usually, the appearance of MB bands on the isozyme pattern of CK in children with dermatomyositis is interpreted as evidence of regenerative striated muscle and not of cardiac damage.

Electromyography aids in confirming the diagnosis of dermatomyositis in selected children and helps to determine the best

TABLE 270-2. Common Laboratory Abnormalities Dermatomyositis

Elevated serum muscle enzyme levels	98%
Abnormal electromyographic changes	96%
Characteristic abnormalities on muscle biopsy	70%

TABLE 270-3. Diagnostic Criteria for Dermatomyositis

Progressive symmetric weakness of proximal limb-girdle and anterior neck flexor muscles
Classic dermatitis of eyelids, metacarpophalangeal and proximal interphalangeal joints, elbows, knees, and medial mallcoli
Elevation of serum muscle enzymes
Electromyographic demonstration of myopathy and denervation
Muscle biopsy showing inflammatory myositis

site for a muscle biopsy. Electromyography changes are those of myopathy and denervation. Magnetic resonance imaging (MRI) results are also abnormal and distinguish between unaffected and affected muscles.

Although seldom necessary for diagnosis, a muscle biopsy is generally indicated in the initial assessment of affected children to support long-term glucocorticoid therapy (or eventually immunosuppressive drugs) and to provide an assessment of prognosis.

DIFFERENTIAL DIAGNOSIS

Dermatomyositis is diagnosed on the basis of an acute onset of proximal limb-girdle muscle weakness accompanied by a characteristic dermatitis (Table 270-3). The differential diagnosis of dermatomyositis ensures little clinical confusion with the acute systemic onset of JRA or with SLE. However, mild forms of dermatomyositis with a prominent degree of arthritis may be confused with either of these two diseases. Scleroderma presents unique diagnostic problems because approximately one-fifth of affected children present with a primary myositis not unlike that seen in dermatomyositis. An occasional child develops an overlap syndrome with varying features of the other connective tissue diseases. Eosinophilic fasciitis and mixed connective tissue disease (MCTD) are distinctive syndromes within this category.

The muscular dystrophies are diagnostic considerations in early disease. In these disorders, an insidious onset, progressive or remitting disease, a positive family history, and a selective, predictable pattern of muscle involvement should be present. Dermatitis is absent. The serum CK is increased in first-degree relatives of children with muscular dystrophy and especially in the mothers of children with X-linked disorders. Other congenital myopathies, myotonias, and hypotonic syndromes; the metabolic and endocrine myopathies; paroxysmal myoglobulinuria, thyrotoxic myopathy, and myasthenia gravis must also be considered.

Poliomyelitis and the Guillain–Barré syndrome, in addition to influenza, coxsackievirus, and echovirus disease, are other diagnostic possibilities in children with the acute onset of severe pain and muscle weakness. Trichinosis and toxoplasmosis cause myositis of varying severity, and severe pustular acne may be associated with inflammation of muscle. Rhabdomyolysis may follow an acute infection, trauma, or extreme muscular excretion with an acute onset characterized by profound weakness, myoglobinuria and, occasionally, oliguria and renal failure.

TREATMENT

General supportive care and a coordinated team approach are necessary to manage this serious disease. Treatment should include a program of graduated rest and positioning, along with physical therapy to minimize contractures. Generally, prednisone is necessary and is given in a dosage of approximately 2 mg/kg/day in divided doses for at least the first month after diagnosis. If clinical response is acceptable and the serum muscle enzyme concentrations decrease, a lower dosage of approximately 1 mg/kg/day is instituted. Thereafter, the prednisone dose is slowly tapered by frequent monitoring of improvement in the clinical status of affected children, the degree of muscle weakness documented by objective testing, and the serum muscle enzyme concentrations. Myositis is not satisfactorily controlled until serum muscle enzymes return to normal (or near normal) levels and remain there while the steroid is tapered during an increase in such children's prescribed level of physical activity. Because long-term steroid administration is accompanied by significant toxicity in growing children, the glucocorticoid dose should be lowered as quickly as possible concomitant with continued improvement in indices of the disease. The initial or early use of intravenous methylprednisolone pulse therapy may minimize steroid toxicity and eventual muscle atrophy and calcinosis. During the course of the disease, progressive healing of the myositis and the extent of the rash may not correlate.

Acute gastrointestinal complications occur in a minority of affected children and may not be controlled well by glucocorticoid therapy. These complications have been an important cause of death. Often, respiratory insufficiency with or without aspiration is a preterminal event. Cutaneous ulcerations are seen in children and, likewise, are poor prognostic signs. These acute complications, along with disease that is steroid-unresponsive, are indications for the use of immunosuppressive agents. Methotrexate has been successful therapy in resistant children. Intravenous cyclophosphamide, cyclosporin A, and repeated steroid-pulse therapy have also been used.

COURSE AND PROGNOSIS

The course of dermatomyositis can be divided into four characteristic clinical phases (Table 270-4). Approximately three-fourths of affected children follow a uniphasic course that lasts from 8 months to 2 years. The remainder continue to have acute exacerbations and remissions; some of these patients eventually develop a clinical disease more typical of systemic vasculitis. A small number of affected children, late in the course, assume more of the characteristics of scleroderma with profound sclerodactyly and cutaneous atrophy. Lipoatrophy, acanthosis nigricans, or a recurrence of arthritis may develop. Even years after onset, other affected children have persistent (if only moderate) elevations of serum muscle enzymes and demonstrate characteristic histopathologic features of the disease on muscle biopsies.

Long-term survival in dermatomyositis approaches 90%. If death occurs, it is often within the first years after onset.

TABLE 270-4. Clinical Phases of Childhood Dermatomyositis

Prodromal period with nonspecific symptoms (weeks to months)
Progressive muscle weakness and rash (days to weeks)
Persistent weakness, rash, and active myositis (up to 2 years)
Recovery with residual muscle atrophy and contractures with or without calcinosis

Adapted from Hanson V. Dermatomyositis, scleroderma, and polyarteritis nodosa. *Clin Rheum Dis* 1976;2:445.

TABLE 270-5. Prognosis for Dermatomyositis

Recovery with no disability	65%
Minimal atrophy or contractures	25%
Calcinosis*	20%
Wheelchair dependence	5%
Death	7%

*Children with calcinosis also are included in the other categories.

Average affected children are expected to progressively improve to an acceptable functional recovery (Table 270-5). During this period, physical therapy is intensified to normalize function and to minimize development of contractures secondary to muscle weakness or atrophy. Muscle-strengthening exercises should be added to the program only when acute inflammation subsides. Functional outcome appears best in children who have been seen early and vigorously treated. Most survivors function independently as adults, although some have residual atrophy of skin or muscle groups.

Late in the disease, during the healing phase, approximately one-half of affected children develop calcinosis of the skin and subcutaneous tissues about the joints and within the interfascial planes of the muscles. The calcium salts have been identified as hydroxyapatite or fluorapatite. Many therapeutic approaches to calcinosis have been tried, none have been uniformly successful. Surgical excision of calcium tumors in areas of ulceration or pressure can be performed if necessary.

CHAPTER 271
Scleroderma

Adapted from James T. Cassidy

A classification of the sclerodermas is presented in Table 271-1. In all these disorders, girls are affected more often than boys, and the conditions demonstrate no peak age of onset during childhood.

TABLE 271-1. Classification of Scleroderma

Systemic disease
Scleroderma
Diffuse
Localized
Overlap syndromes
Sclerodermatomyositis or other connective tissue diseases
Mixed connective tissue disease
Localized disease
Morphea
Linear scleroderma
Eosinophilic fascitis

SYSTEMIC SCLERODERMA

An idiopathic angiitis appears to be the basic lesion of scleroderma and involves the lungs, heart, and kidneys, in addition to the skin and gastrointestinal tract. Systemic scleroderma exhibits thinning of the epidermis and atrophy of the dermal appendages, an increased density and thickness of collagen deposition, and a predominance of embryonal fibers. Telangiectases about the face, upper trunk, and on the palms appear during the early phases of the disease as further evidence of vascular involvement.

Clinical Characteristics

Often, diagnosis in children with scleroderma is delayed for years because of the subtle and insidious nature of the onset. The presentation is characterized by the appearance of Raynaud phenomenon, thinning and atrophy of the skin of the hands or face, or the development of cutaneous telangiectases (Table 271-2). Tightening and thickening of the skin is virtually universal at onset and becomes more generalized. Raynaud phenomenon with a two- or three-color change occurs in most children and may antedate the onset of cutaneous abnormalities. It is characterized by obstructive digital arterial disease and sympathetic hyperactivity that are often regressive. Many children have arthralgia, and a few present with objective arthritis or contractures about the joints. Muscle pain and tenderness are present in approximately 20% of patients. However, elevation of the serum muscle enzyme level tends to be only mild to moderate. Cardiac involvement with arrhythmias may develop during the course of the disease, and often congestive heart failure is a terminal event. Dyspnea on exertion may be related to skin tightness, intercostal muscle weakness, or intrinsic pulmonary disease.

Laboratory Examination

Often, routine laboratory studies of scleroderma are normal. Antinuclear antibodies (ANAs) are found in most affected children and are characterized by high-titered speckled patterns. Distinct antigenic specificity may be present: anticentromere in localized systemic scleroderma [the CREST (calcinosis, Raynaud phenomenon, esophageal abnormalities, sclerodactyly,

TABLE 271-2. Clinical Manifestations in Children with Systemic Scleroderma

Organ system	Frequency of involvement (%)
Skin	
Ulceration	30
Subcutaneous calcification	60
Telangiectases	30
Pigmentation	20
Digital arteries (Raynaud phenomenon)	75
Musculoskeletal	
Contractures	75
Resorption of digital tufts	60
Muscle weakness	40
Muscle atrophy	40
Gastrointestinal tract	
Abnormal esophageal motility	75
Colonic sacculations	20
Duodenal dilatation	5
Pulmonary tract	
Abnormal diffusion	75
Abnormal vital capacity	70
Heart	
Electrocardiographic abnormalities	30
Cardiomegaly	15
Congestive failure	15

and telangiectases) syndrome], antiScl 70 (topoisomerase 1) in diffuse systemic scleroderma, or nucleolar antibodies.

Plethysmography is abnormal in affected digits in children with Raynaud phenomenon and documents both the obstructive vascular disease and involvement of the sympathetic nervous system.

Pulmonary diffusion and spirometry are sensitive measures of involvement of the respiratory tract. These studies are abnormal in many children at onset and are progressive. Usually, upper gastrointestinal films document disordered motility of the distal esophagus. Balloon esophageal motility and pH probe studies are more sensitive indicators of the degree of abnormality in these children.

Differential Diagnosis

Diagnosis of systemic scleroderma is based on demonstration of the classic cutaneous findings of skin tightening of the face, hands, and feet; telangiectases; Raynaud phenomenon; and the presence of visceral disease, usually gastrointestinal or pulmonary. The differential diagnosis includes dermatomyositis, Systemic Lupus Erythematosus (SLE), overlap syndromes, and, less frequently, Juvenile Rheumatoid Arthritis (JRA). Children with localized systemic scleroderma (CREST syndrome) have prominent calcinosis, Raynaud phenomenon, esophageal abnormalities, sclerodactyly, and telangiectases. Such patients were once thought to have a more favorable prognosis; however, evidence for this judgment is not confirmed in more recent studies.

Numerous other entities mimic or duplicate abnormalities found in scleroderma. Scleroderma-like disease has developed as a toxic reaction to vinyl chloride, bleomycin, and pentazocine. It has also occurred in epidemic proportions and with many deaths in Spain secondary to contaminated cooking oil (rapeseed oil). Occasionally, it is encountered as a component of graft–versus–host disease in bone marrow transplantation patients. Scleroderma-like changes may be seen in children with phenylketonuria and progeria.

Treatment

Of the connective tissue diseases, scleroderma presents the most difficulty in treatment. NSAIDs are helpful for relieving musculoskeletal pain and stiffness. Colchicine may be useful. Children who present with gastrointestinal problems demand special therapeutic considerations for esophageal stricture or obstruction, reflux esophagitis, or malabsorption.

Raynaud phenomenon is managed with alpha-blocking agents such as phenoxybenzamine or with calcium-channel blockers such as nifedipine or verapamil. Children with prominent Raynaud phenomenon need to dress seasonally and avoid cold liquids and objects that exacerbate not only the peripheral arteriolar constriction but also vascular spasm within viscera. If prescribed early, D-penicillamine may be useful in managing cutaneous manifestations of the disease. Vigorous physical therapy to prevent contractures is important.

Glucocorticoid drugs are probably contraindicated in most of such children. The agents may exacerbate small-blood-vessel disease and renal involvement with hypertension. Renal failure and acute hypertensive encephalopathy may supervene as potentially fatal complications in a few children. These events seem most likely to occur early in the course of the disease. Angiotensin-converting enzyme inhibitors are crucial in managing hypertensive crisis. Some investigators also recommend early treatment of the angiitis of scleroderma by these drugs.

Course and Prognosis

Often, the outcome of scleroderma is poor, but survival has not been precisely determined because of the rarity of the disease in children. The prognosis is not judged to be any more favorable than that in adults, in whom it is only 35% after 7 years. However, children may live decades after onset; therefore, an optimistic, but realistic, attitude should be taken in discussions with parents.

LOCALIZED SCLERODERMA

Localized scleroderma is much more common than systemic disease. Fibrosis of connective tissues in morphea is limited to the dermis, subdermis, and superficial striated muscles. This variant is subcategorized into plaque, generalized, bullous, or deep morphea. Morphea is characterized by one or more circumscribed cutaneous lesions marked by hypopigmentation and induration surrounded by hyperpigmentation. Erythema and acute inflammatory edema are present, especially at the margins. These lesions are located anywhere on the trunk or extremities. Affected children may complain of paresthesia or pain over the involved areas. Each lesion may enlarge centrifugally or can coalesce and involve larger areas of skin.

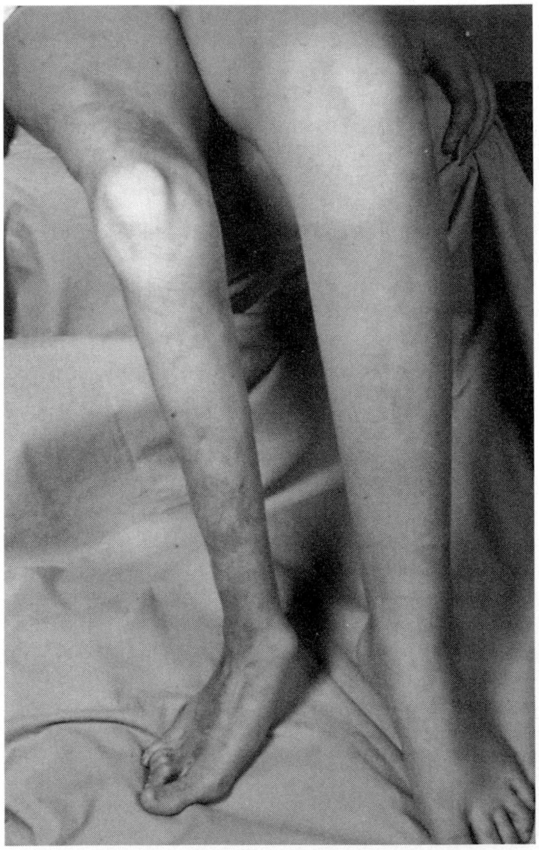

Figure 271-1. Severe linear scleroderma affecting the right leg of an adolescent girl. This lesion involves not just the skin but the deeper subcutaneous tissues, fascia, muscle, and bone. It resulted in the deformity shown and a 7.5-cm shortening of that limb. (Reprinted with permission from Cassidy JT. SLE, juvenile dermatomyositis, scleroderma, and vasculitis. In: Kelley WN, Harris ED Jr, Ruddy S, Sledge CB, eds. *Textbook of rheumatology.* Philadelphia: Saunders, 1997:1253.)

Hide-binding from fibrosis of the involved skin and subcutaneous tissues may become extensive and can result in marked contractures of an extremity. Active disease may undergo exacerbations and remissions for many months to years, although lesions tend to regress slowly with age. Local emollients and glucocorticoid ointments may result in some improvement. D-Penicillamine may be effective if used early in the more generalized form of morphea. Systemic antibiotics are reportedly effective in a few studies.

Linear scleroderma (or linear morphea) primarily develops in the first two decades of life. The disorder is characterized by the presence of one or more areas of linear involvement of the skin of the head, trunk, or extremities. Because lesions of the face or scalp may look like scars from dueling, the term en coup-de-sabre has been used to describe them. Often, underlying muscle and bone are involved in the pattern of fibrosis and inflammation in this form of the disease with localized growth abnormalities, deformity, or contractures of joints. Often, linear scleroderma affects only one side of the body, producing hemiatrophy of the involved parts (Fig. 271-1). This lack of normal growth and development produces the most severe disabilities (e.g., hemifacial atrophy, failure of an extremity to grow in proportion to its opposite member, and severe joint contractures).

Laboratory abnormalities in localized scleroderma are few. ANAs are positive in approximately 50% of affected children. Antibodies to centromere or Scl-70 are not generally present in the localized forms of the disease.

Linear scleroderma may regress without treatment or with time. Although linear lesions may improve with age, significant abnormalities of local growth persist, particularly if deep tissues and bone are involved. Occasionally, visceral disease or seizures develop late in the course of the disease. In a few affected children, the disease evolves into a syndrome overlapping with another connective tissue disease such as SLE.

CHAPTER 272
Idiopathic Vasculitis

Adapted from James T. Cassidy

Although vasculitis is a prominent and almost universal component of the connective tissue diseases, distinct types of idiopathic vasculitis are encountered in children (Table 272-1). All forms of vasculitis, except for Henoch–Schönlein syndrome and Kawasaki disease, are rare in children. These clinical entities are discussed separately. A few of the other idiopathic vasculitic conditions will be discussed below.

TABLE 272-1. Classification of Idiopathic Vasculitis

Necrotizing vasculitis or medium and small arteries
Polyarteritis nodosa
Kawasaki disease
Necrotizing arteritis of small vessels
Hypersensitivity angiitis
Henoch-Schönlein purpura
Granulomatous vasculitis
Allergic necrotizing granulomatrosis
Wegener granulomatosis
Giant cell arteritis
Systemic giant cell arteritis
Takayasu arteritis
Cranial arteritis

POLYARTERITIS NODOSA (PAN)

Clinical Characteristics

No single pattern of clinical presentation is characteristic and, frequently, the onset is insidious. Constitutional symptoms of fever and weight loss may be the presenting complaints (Table 272-2). Often, renal, gastrointestinal, nervous system, and cardiac disease initially occur. Dermatitis, although characteristic, includes a spectrum of lesions of purpura, gangrene of the distal parts of the extremities, and erythematous, painful nodules. The initial clinical diagnosis of PAN may be renovascular hypertension or an acute abdomen. Frequently, severe, symmetric sensorimotor peripheral neuropathy (mononeuritis multiplex) is observed.

Laboratory Examination

Often, the level of anemia, leukocytosis, elevation of the erythrocyte sedimentation rate (ESR), concentration of the serum immunoglobulins, and urinary sediment changes reflect the extent of multisystem involvement. Usually, a firm diagnosis is based on characteristic histologic changes in a biopsy specimen or an angiogram showing multiple aneurysms.

Treatment

Glucocorticoid administration is the primary approach to the management of PAN. Usually, prednisone is first prescribed in suppressive amounts in the range of 1 to 2 mg/kg/day in divided doses. The degree of cardiac or renal involvement or the presence of hypertension modulates therapeutic aggressiveness. Extensive systemic involvement, particularly of the intraabdominal vessels with aneurysms or thrombosis, is generally an indication for the addition of cyclophosphamide.

Course and Prognosis

The course of PAN is highly variable, and death is most commonly secondary to renal failure, myocardial infarction, or hypertensive encephalopathy. Children with more restricted organ involvement have better prognoses. Cogan syndrome is very rare and is characterized by ocular and inner-ear vasculitis. Affected patients present with interstitial keratitis, vertigo, tinnitus, and deafness. Serous otitis media may also be seen in children in association with PAN.

TABLE 272-2. Clinical Manifestations of Polyarteritis

Manifestation	Percentage of patients
Constitutional signs and symptoms	75
Musculoskeletal involvement	75
Leukocytosis, eosinophilia	75
Dermatitis	60
Peripheral neuropathy	40
Mesenteric involvement	40
Central nervous system disease	30
Pulmonary disease	25
Nephritis and hypertension	25
Myocardial infarction	20

WEGENER GRANULOMATOSIS

Clinical Characteristics

Wegener granulomatosis is a very rare syndrome in children, although it has been described in children as young as 3 months. It is characterized by a necrotizing granulomatous angiitis involving both the respiratory tract (sinuses, nasal passages, and lungs) and the kidneys. Characteristic granulomatosis may also be found in skin, heart, CNS, gastrointestinal tract, and synovia. Constitutional symptoms are almost always prominent.

Unexplained sinopulmonary pain, rhinorrhea, mucosal ulceration, or bleeding from the upper respiratory tract may be the presenting sign. Hemoptysis and pleuritic pain are frequent. Chest films demonstrate multiform pulmonary infiltrates and nodules. Computed tomographic (CT) scans may reveal erosion of nasal cartilage and bone. Most affected patients have moderate to severe renal disease that is progressive if untreated. Hypertension may be less common than in other types of nephritis.

Differential Diagnosis

The differential diagnosis includes the other forms of vasculitis, sarcoidosis, berylliosis, Loeffler syndrome, tuberculosis, disseminated fungal disease, syphilis, or lymphoma. Clinically, Goodpasture syndrome and other rare forms of granulomatous arteritis are easily confused with Wegener granulomatosis. Diagnosis is established by microscopical examination of a biopsy of an affected organ (usually the nasal mucosa) or of an open lung biopsy. Granulomas and a necrotizing vasculitis with leukocytic, lymphocytic, and giant cell infiltration are seen.

Treatment and Prognosis

Glucocorticoid treatment had some effect early in the disease, but more recent trials support therapy with cyclophosphamide for managing affected patients. A dramatic response to cyclophosphamide use has altered the outcome of this otherwise fatal disease to one of remission, if not cure, in the adult series reported from the National Institutes of Health. More recent consideration is being given to use of other immunosuppressive agents with less toxicity such as methotrexate and trimethoprim-sulfamethoxazole. Historically, death from renal or pulmonary disease occurred with only rare long-term survival.

TAKAYASU ARTERITIS

Clinical Characteristics

Takayasu arteritis is a giant cell arteritis predominantly seen in teenage girls. Stenosis, occlusion, dilation, and aneurysm formation are confined to the aorta, its major branches, and the pulmonary arteries. This disease has been called pulseless disease because of the obliteration of the radial pulses or reverse coarctation. Hypertension is frequent. Usually, the acute-phase reactants and the white blood cell (WBC) count are elevated. Takayasu arteritis appears to be more common in Asians, Latinos, blacks, and Sephardic Jews. The female–to–male ratio is 8:1. Unidentified environmental or genetic factors may play a role in its pathogenesis. Occasionally, it is seen in families of children with other connective tissue diseases, and it has been reported in monozygotic twin sisters.

Treatment

Nonsteroidal antiinflammatory drugs (NSAIDs) are useful in managing the symptoms of affected patients during the acute early phases of the illness. Generally, glucocorticoid drugs are indicated for early disease, along with consideration of weekly methotrexate pulse therapy. Aggressive control of hypertension is essential. Anticoagulants or antiplatelet agents may be indicated for widespread chronic occlusion of vessels. Vessel grafts have been successful late in the course of the disease.

Course

The course of Takayasu arteritis may be limited lasting 3 to 6 months or can be prolonged over many years. Often, early diagnosis is difficult because of its insidious onset, and an erroneous diagnosis [e.g., systemic onset Juvenile Rheumatoid Arthritis (JRA), acute rheumatic fever] may be made. Eventually, signs of vascular insufficiency suggest the correct diagnosis, which can then be confirmed by angiography or magnetic resonance imaging (MRI). Calcification may be seen in the affected vessels on plain-film radiography.

CHAPTER 273
Behçet Syndrome

Adapted from James T. Cassidy

This syndrome consists of a triad of recurrent uveitis, mucocutaneous ulcerations, and genital ulcerations. However, arriving at absolute certainty of this diagnosis in affected children is difficult unless involvement of the central nervous syndrome (CNS) is present. Additional features include arthritis, gastrointestinal disease, and cardiovascular involvement. No etiology has been identified. An infectious cause has been advanced because of the geographic foci of the disease.

CLINICAL CHARACTERISTICS

This disorder affects men more frequently than women. The most common age at onset is 18 to 40 years. Occurrence of the disease in children as young as 2 years has been reported. Commonly, a nondestructive polyarthritis occurs in approximately 75% of affected children. The peripheral joint disease may be either symmetric or asymmetric. Large joints such as the knees are most frequently affected, but small joints may be involved. Multiple recurrences of synovitis, particularly in the knees and ankles, develop during a period of several years, but bony erosions and functional disability are uncommon. Frequently, fever and erythema nodosum accompany the arthritis.

Aphthous stomatitis is common, as are ulcerative lesions of the mucous membranes of the upper and lower gastrointestinal tracts. The oral ulcerations are fairly painful and interfere with swallowing and speech. Similar ulcerations occur in the genitourinary tract and are accompanied by a sterile pyuria. These lesions may resemble herpes simplex or the Stevens–Johnson syndrome. An incorrect diagnosis of regional enteritis or ulcerative colitis may have been made. Behçet syndrome can be clinically confused with Reiter syndrome.

Involvement of the eye includes photophobia, pain, conjunctivitis, and blurred vision. Uveitis is common. Scleritis, retinal vasculitis, and optic neuritis develop and lead to blindness.

CNS disease ranges from trivial neurologic signs to confusion to papilledema and pseudotumor cerebri. These disorders occur in approximately one-fourth of the patients and are divided into five syndromes: pseudotumor cerebri, meningoencephalitis, brainstem involvement, dementia, and changes in personality and behavior.

LABORATORY EXAMINATION

Cerebrospinal fluid abnormalities include pleocytosis and increased concentrations of protein. Hypergammaglobulinemia is characteristic. Autoantibodies reacting with mucosal cells have been demonstrated in some patients. HLA associations include B5 in North American studies and an increased prevalence of B27 in others, although the frequency of spondylitis does not appear to be increased.

TREATMENT

Treatment is difficult and puzzling because the course is punctuated by frequent remissions. Reports suggest that immunosuppressive or alkylating agents (chlorambucil) may be indicated, along with glucocorticoid drugs.

COURSE AND PROGNOSIS

The course of Behçet syndrome is highly variable. Active disease may span a period of a few weeks or can extend to several years, and the pattern of involvement is characterized by frequent remissions and exacerbations. Often, prognosis is directly related to the extent of CNS disease.

CHAPTER 274
Henoch–Schönlein Syndrome

Adapted from W. Allan Walker and Leslie M. Higuchi

Henoch–Schönlein syndrome is thought to be an immune-mediated vasculitic disorder. Abnormalities in patients include deposition of immunoglobulin A (IgA) in affected organs and elevated serum IgA concentrations. One unifying hypothesis speculates that IgA, IgG, and other plasma proteins form aggregates that activate the alternative pathway of the complement system; subsequently, complement activation and the deposition of IgA in target organs may initiate the release of a cascade of inflammatory mediators including vasoactive prostaglandins leading to tissue injury. Leukocytoclastic vasculitis with small vessel perivascular infiltration of neutrophils and mononuclear cells is noted on biopsy of skin lesions.

Some authors have postulated that factor XIII may play a role in the pathogenesis of Henoch–Schönlein syndrome. One proposed hypothesis suggests that proteases released during the local tissue inflammatory response may degrade factor XIII, resulting in tissue fibrin deposition and contributing to the development of vasculitis.

Although the etiology remains unknown, several predisposing factors have been suggested. Upper respiratory infections precede the onset of illness in at least 50% of children with the syndrome. Infectious agents reported include streptococci, parvovirus, adenovirus, Mycoplasma pneumoniae, Yersinia, Legionella, Epstein–Barr virus, and varicella. Vaccination against measles, cholera, yellow fever, typhoid, and paratyphoid A and B preceded Henoch–Schönlein syndrome in other cases. Additional implicated factors reported include insect bites and exposure to cold.

Reports of familial occurrence of Henoch–Schönlein syndrome may imply a genetic connection, but because families may also have similar environmental exposures, such evidence is only circumstantial. In children transplanted for end-stage renal failure associated with Henoch–Schönlein syndrome, the increased recurrence of disease in living related donor allografts also suggests a genetic predisposition.

CLINICAL CHARACTERISTICS

The typical clinical presentation is that of a previously well child who develops the distinctive rash accompanied by other organ involvement (Table 274-1). The manifestations may occur simultaneously or sequentially over a period of several days or weeks. Early in the illness, patients commonly experience malaise and low-grade fever. One-half of the patients initially present with the skin rash, which is essential to the clinical diagnosis and

TABLE 274-1. Organ Involvement in Henoch-Schönlein Syndrome

Skin
Purpura typically on the buttocks and lower extremities
Erythema multiforme
Vesicular eruptions and bullae
Nonpitting edema (35% to 70%)
Common in children younger than 3 years
Affected areas are tender and distorted
Predilection for the scalp, ears, periorbital region, and the dorsum of the hands and feet
Gastrointestinal system
Colicky abdominal pain (70%)
Ileus (40%)
Vomiting (25%)
Hepatomegaly (10%)
Intussusception (3%)
Common in older children and ileoileal in 65% of cases
Gastrointestinal bleeding
Melena or guaiac-positive stools (56%)
Hematemesis (10%)
Massive gastrointestinal hemorrhage (5%)
Bowel infarction or perforation
Pancreatitis
Hydrops of the gallbladder
Protein-losing enteropathy
Ileal stricture formation (late finding)
Renal system (20% to 60%)
Microscopic hematuria (60%)
Gross hematuria (40%)
Nephrotic syndrome (30%)
Mild proteinuria (25%)
Acute nephritis with hypertension (15%)
Neurologic system
Headaches and behavioral changes (31%)
Seizures, focal neurologic deficits, and peripheral neuropathies (2% to 8%)

occurs in all pediatric patients with the syndrome. The classic rash begins as localized or generalized urticarial wheals that are replaced by erythematous macules or maculopapules. Subsequently, petechiae and larger purpuric areas form. Often, the purpuric lesions are palpable and described as raised papules or plaques that, similar to stages of ecchymoses, evolve from red-purple to yellow and then to purple-brown before fading over several days. The lesions usually arise in crops, and new crops may arise at different times, resulting in a polymorphic appearance with varying stages of eruption simultaneously present. Typically, the rash is nonpruritic and favors pressure-dependent areas with a characteristic distribution of the lower extremities and the buttocks, but it can also involve the upper extremities, face, and trunk. The rash can be transient or persist for weeks and may recur.

Arthralgia or arthritis develops in 65% to 85% of patients and is the presenting symptom or sign of the illness preceding the rash in 17% to 25% of patients. The nonmigratory joint involvement is usually periarticular; erythema and warmth of the joint are uncommon. Joint involvement more commonly affects the knees and ankles than the smaller joints of the fingers and wrists and is usually self-limited without residual sequelae.

Reporting of acute scrotal findings ranges from 2% to 38% of male subjects with Henoch–Schönlein syndrome and is rarely the initial presenting symptom or sign. Clinical findings include pain, tenderness, and swelling of the involved testicle or scrotum. Surgical exploration has demonstrated localized vasculitis and bleeding into the affected testes. The presentation can mimic symptoms and signs of testicular torsion, and surgical evaluation may be indicated.

Gastrointestinal manifestations appear in as many as three-fourths of patients. They may precede the rash in 15% of cases creating difficulty in establishing the diagnosis of Henoch–Schönlein syndrome. Other findings include renal involvement and neurological symptoms (Table 274-1). Rare organ complications such as pulmonary or intramuscular hemorrhage, ureteral vasculitis with stenosis, and carditis have been attributed to Henoch–Schönlein syndrome.

LABORATORY DATA

No pathognomonic laboratory tests are available to confirm the diagnosis of Henoch–Schönlein syndrome. Laboratory evaluation can assist with the exclusion of other diagnoses and the assessment of organ involvement.

A leukocytosis of 10,000 to 20,000 cells per microliter is noted in two-thirds of patients with an accompanying left shift seen in one-half of patients. Anemia can occur, possibly resulting from intestinal blood loss. The erythrocyte sedimentation rate and platelet count may be normal or elevated. The prothrombin time and partial thromboplastin time are normal, but factor XIII (fibrin-stabilizing factor) is usually decreased and normalizes with the resolution of the disease. Serum IgA is elevated during the acute illness in approximately 50% of patients, and serum IgG and IgM may be normal or elevated. Assay results for antinuclear antibodies and rheumatoid factor (RF) are negative. Approximately one-third of patients develop a low total hemolytic complement level (CH_{50}), associated with normal C3 and C4 levels and low properdin levels.

Urinalysis should be performed on all patients with Henoch–Schönlein syndrome and may demonstrate red or white blood cells, cellular casts, or protein. Serum creatinine and blood urea nitrogen levels may be elevated suggesting renal insufficiency associated with glomerulonephritis. Indications for a renal biopsy include the presence of nephrotic syndrome; a rapidly progressive deterioration in renal function; and persistent nephritic syndrome with macroscopic hematuria, hypertension, or renal insufficiency. Electrolyte abnormalities and hypoalbuminemia may be present secondary to either renal disease or protein-losing enteropathy. Stool examination may reveal evidence of blood loss.

When gastrointestinal symptoms are present, contrast radiologic studies of the gastrointestinal tract usually demonstrate small bowel involvement with thickened folds, pseudotumors, hypomotility, and "thumbprinting," which is characteristic of submucosal hemorrhages. Abnormalities of the terminal ileum resembling Crohn's ileal involvement may be seen, but colonic findings are unusual. Ultrasound evaluation for intussusception may be helpful given its noninvasive nature and its ability to identify intussusceptions proximal to the ileocolic location, often missed by air or liquid contrast enemas. The ultrasound appearance of intussusception is that of a rounded mass with echocentric structures resembling a target. Furthermore, ultrasound can demonstrate intestinal wall thickening and abnormal peristalsis, which are highly suggestive of Henoch–Schönlein syndrome.

DIFFERENTIAL DIAGNOSIS

In the presence of the characteristic constellation of clinical findings of Henoch–Schönlein syndrome, the diagnosis is easily made. However, diagnostic dilemmas arise when only one symptom or sign is evident and, depending on the presentation, other causes for similar skin lesions, abdominal pain, nephritis, and arthritis must be considered.

Petechiae or purpuric rashes may be associated with septicemia, idiopathic thrombocytopenic purpura, hemolytic uremic syndrome, bacterial endocarditis, acute poststreptococcal glomerulonephritis, leukemia, and coagulopathies. Laboratory evaluation with positive blood culture results, abnormal platelet and coagulation study results, or low C3 levels may differentiate these disorders from Henoch–Schönlein syndrome.

Entities including systemic lupus erythematosus, polyarteritis nodosa, and Wegener granulomatosis are associated with vasculitic rashes. In addition to the clinical course, assays for serum complement, antinuclear and antideoxyribonuclease antibodies, and antineutrophil cytoplasmic antibodies may be helpful. Rheumatoid arthritis and rheumatic fever may present with joint pain accompanied by skin rashes, but can often be differentiated from Henoch–Schönlein syndrome by clinical and laboratory evaluation.

Patients with IgA nephropathy, or Berger disease, present with a glomerulonephritis with immunologic and histopathologic findings similar to those seen in Henoch–Schönlein syndrome. Whether these two illnesses are actually the same underlying condition is controversial. Observations of both disorders occurring in the same patient, within the same family, or in identical twins in which one developed Henoch–Schönlein syndrome and the other IgA nephropathy support the hypothesis that these two entities are variants of the same disease. However, the age distribution and typical clinical presentations differ between IgA nephropathy and Henoch–Schönlein syndrome. As a result, some authorities consider these two entities to be the same illness, whereas others suggest that the disorders are different entities but may share a common pathogenesis.

TREATMENT

Treatment is largely supportive. Most children with Henoch–Schönlein syndrome may be followed as outpatients. Admission to the hospital may be indicated if children develop conditions of greater concern such as colicky abdominal pain suggestive of intussusception, gastrointestinal hemorrhage, significant renal disease, or changes in mental status. In the acute care of the ill patient, management includes adequate hydration and monitoring for potential complications. Some authors suggest nonsteroidal antiinflammatory drugs for relief of joint and soft tissue discomfort, but caution should be exercised in the setting of prominent abdominal symptoms or renal insufficiency.

The use of corticosteroid therapy in the management of the manifestations and complications of Henoch–Schönlein syndrome is controversial. Favorable anecdotal evidence suggests a role for a short course of prednisone in a dose of 1 to 2 mg/kg/day to hasten improvement of abdominal pain. However, other retrospective studies have shown that the abdominal pain in children with Henoch–Schönlein syndrome tends to resolve within 3 to 7 days with or without corticosteroid administration, and the duration of illness is not altered by corticosteroids. Some authors advocate that corticosteroids may reduce the incidence of intussusception. Improvement of gastrointestinal manifestations after intravenous immunoglobulin administration has been reported in individual cases, but no formal studies examining its effectiveness have yet been performed. Clinical manifestations of Henoch–Schönlein syndrome, especially abdominal symptoms, significantly improved after 3 days of factor XIII concentrate administration in one study. Further investigation is needed to determine the potential usefulness of factor XIII therapy.

If nephropathy is present, monitoring should focus on fluid and electrolyte balance, salt intake, and blood pressure measurements. At present, no proven therapy exists for the prevention or treatment of nephropathy associated with Henoch–Schönlein syndrome. Several studies have examined whether early corticosteroid administration prevents nephropathy. Results of these studies often conflict and are difficult to interpret, precluding making any formal recommendations. Suggested therapies for patients with severe renal involvement include intravenous immunoglobulin, plasmapheresis, and corticosteroids, alone or in combination with immunosuppressive agents such as azathioprine, cyclophosphamide, or cyclosporine or with antiplatelet agents such as dipyridamole.

CLINICAL COURSE AND PROGNOSIS

In the absence of significant renal, gastrointestinal, or neurologic complications, the clinical course is usually self-limited with an excellent prognosis. Symptoms may persist for an average of 4 weeks with a duration ranging from 3 days to 2 years. Recurrences occur in 40% of patients, usually within 6 weeks of onset, but they have been reported up to years later. Children younger than 2 years follow a milder, shorter clinical course with fewer recurrences and renal and gastrointestinal manifestations than their older peers.

The reported long-term morbidity is primarily secondary to renal complications. Microscopic hematuria alone or in combination with mild proteinuria is usually associated with a good renal outcome. On the other hand, in patients with nephritic, nephrotic, or both syndromes, 44% develop long-term impairment of renal function. Furthermore, patients with crescent formation in more than 50% of glomeruli on renal biopsy tend to have a poorer outcome. End-stage renal failure is reported to develop in as many as 2% to 5% of patients. Given that the progression of renal disease may not develop for years, long-term follow-up is necessary in patients with renal involvement. Mortality in Henoch–Schönlein syndrome is less than 1% and is caused by severe gastrointestinal, renal, pulmonary, or neurologic involvement.

PART

IV

Pediatrician's Companion: Things You Forget to Remember

CHAPTER 275

Dysmorphology: Selected Syndromes and Associations

Adapted from Amy Feldman Lewanda and Ethylin Wang Jabs

A *syndrome* is a constellation of features that occur together and have a common cause. An *association* describes the sporadic occurrence of two or more features more often than their individual frequencies would suggest. The underlying cause of such associations is unknown. A *sequence* defines a condition that results from a single initiating defect leading to a series of subsequent abnormalities. The majority of the conditions reviewed in this chapter have a genetic basis and are caused by chromosomal abnormalities or single gene defects. Several other conditions are caused by environmental effects *in utero.* As more becomes known about their molecular etiology, the distinctions between traditional groupings will change.

This chapter provides information and photographs for selected conditions. More extensive compendiums and descriptions are available in Jones's *Smith's Recognizable Patterns of Human Malformation* (Saunders), Gorlin et al.'s *Syndromes of the Head and Neck* (Oxford University Press), and Online Mendelian Inheritance in Man (http://www.ncbi.nlm.nih.gov/omim/).

AMNIOTIC BAND SEQUENCE, OR DISRUPTION COMPLEX

Key Features

Facial clefting
Annular constriction of limbs or digits
Limb or digital amputations
Pseudosyndactyly
Strands of amnion on infant or placenta

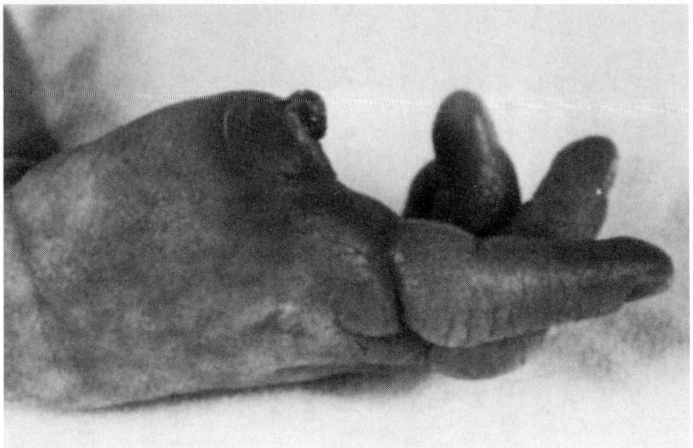

Other Findings

Features of fetal akinesia caused by constriction

COMMENTS

Amniotic band sequence occurs in 1 in 5,000 to 15,000 newborns. Elevated amnionic alpha-fetoprotein levels are often found. Due to the variable nature of this disruption sequence, findings may be quite disparate between patients. Findings depend on the degree of entanglement, the body part(s) involved, and the timing of insult.

PERFORMANCE

Affected individuals usually have normal intelligence. However, cases with cranial constriction and central nervous system defects would be expected to have some intellectual impairment.

ETIOLOGY

Occurrence of amniotic band sequence or disruption complex is usually sporadic with a low risk of recurrence. Rare cases have been associated with maternal trauma during pregnancy.

DIABETIC EMBRYOPATHY (INFANT OF A DIABETIC MOTHER)

Key Features

Macrosomia
Cardiac septal hypertrophy
Other congenital heart disease [ventricular septal defect (VSD)]
Caudal regression (hypoplasia of sacrum and lower extremities)
Hypoglycemia, hypocalcemia in the newborn period

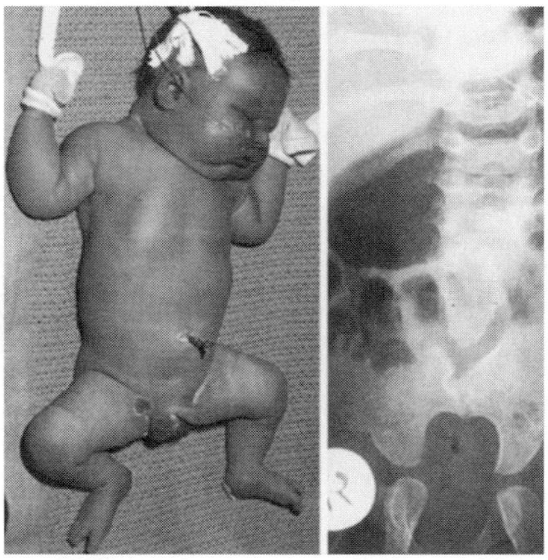

Other Findings

Malformation of external ear
Cleft lip, palate, or both
Rib and vertebral defects
Single umbilical artery
Central nervous system abnormalities

COMMENTS

The rate of fetal complications appears to be higher in constitutional diabetics than in women who become diabetic only during pregnancy (gestational diabetics). Because of the macrosomia, these infants are at higher risk for birth trauma and birth asphyxia, which occurs in 25%.

PERFORMANCE

Mental retardation is not significantly increased; however, an increased risk exists for cerebral palsy and epilepsy. Such impairments are believed to be on the basis of birth trauma, asphyxia, pregnancy complications, or central nervous system defects.

ETIOLOGY

Maternal hyperglycemia during pregnancy is the cause.

FETAL ALCOHOL SYNDROME

Key Features

Growth retardation
Microcephaly
Small palpebral fissures
Short nose
Smooth philtrum
Thin upper lip
Cardiac defects [VSD, atrial septal defect (ASD)]
Hypoplastic fifth fingernails

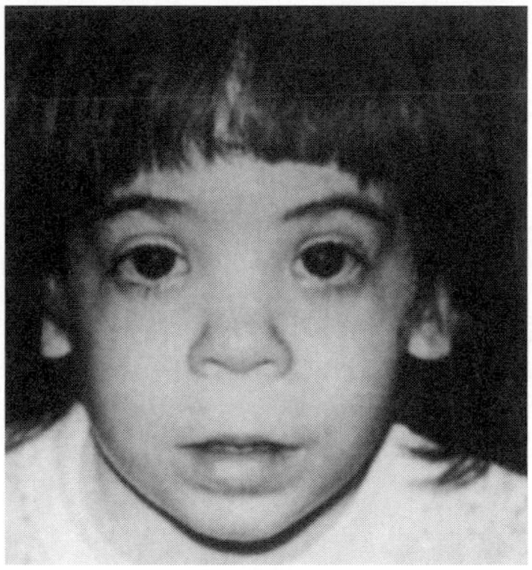

Other Findings

Ptosis
Microphthalmia
Optic nerve hypoplasia
Cleft lip or cleft palate
Cervical spine defects
Joint abnormalities
Short fourth and fifth metacarpals
Central nervous system (CNS) abnormalities

COMMENTS

Fetal alcohol syndrome is estimated to occur in 1 in 500 to 1,000 live births. Features of this condition range from mild (referred to as fetal alcohol effects) to severe (fetal alcohol syndrome). The degree of involvement depends, in part, on the amount of alcohol consumed during pregnancy, as well as the timing of exposure. Thirty percent to 50% of children of chronic alcoholic women (consumers of 6–8 drinks or more per day) are estimated to have mental retardation. Infants may present with tremulousness and irritability, and children may have fine motor dysfunction and hyperactivity.

PERFORMANCE

Mental retardation, behavioral abnormalities, and language delays are common, and range in severity depending on degree of prenatal exposure. The average IQ of an individual with fetal alcohol syndrome is 67.

ETIOLOGY

Maternal ingestion of alcohol during the pregnancy is the cause.

TRISOMY 13 SYNDROME (PATAU SYNDROME)

Key Features

Microcephaly with sloping forehead
Cutis aplasia of scalp (localized scalp defects)
Microphthalmia
Cleft lip, palate, or both
Postaxial polydactyly
Fingers flexed and overlapping
Nails hyperconvex
Cardiac malformations (VSD, PDA, ASD, dextrocardia)

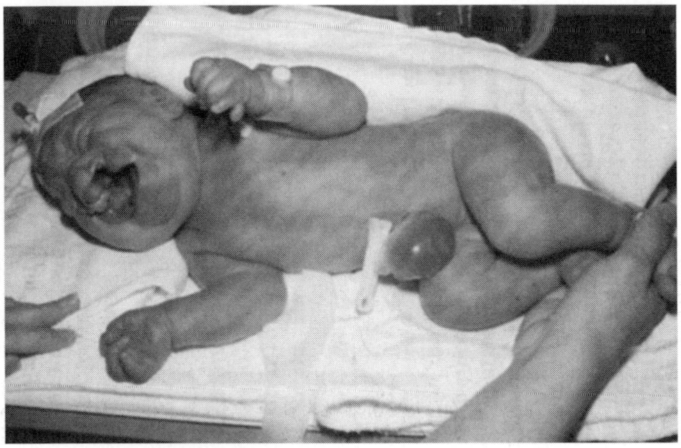

Other Findings

Low birth weight
Holoprosencephaly
Iris coloboma
Dysplastic ears
Omphalocele
Genital abnormalities (cryptorchidism, bicornuate uterus)
Polycystic kidney or other renal defects
Seizures, agenesis of corpus callosum

COMMENTS

Trisomy 13 syndrome occurs in approximately 1 in 5,000 to 12,000 live births.

PERFORMANCE

Prognosis is extremely poor with more than 50% mortality within the first month. Survivors have severe mental retardation, failure to thrive, and often have seizures.

ETIOLOGY

Trisomy for all or most of chromosome 13 is present. More than three-fourths of cases result from chromosomal nondisjunction and are associated with advanced maternal age. Trisomy 13 due to a translocation is another cause and imparts a higher recurrence risk for the parents (approximately 10% for a carrier). Five percent of all cases are mosaic (in which another normal cell line is present, in addition to the trisomic cell line). Trisomy 13 constitutes approximately 1% of all recognized spontaneous abortions.

TRISOMY 18 SYNDROME (EDWARDS SYNDROME)

Key Features

Low birth weight
Lack of subcutaneous fat
Prominent occiput
Narrow bifrontal diameter of forehead
Small palpebral fissures
Low-set, malformed ears
Micrognathia
Short sternum
Clenched hands with overlapping digits
Limited hip abduction
Short dorsiflexed halluces
Cardiac defects (VSD, ASD, PDA)

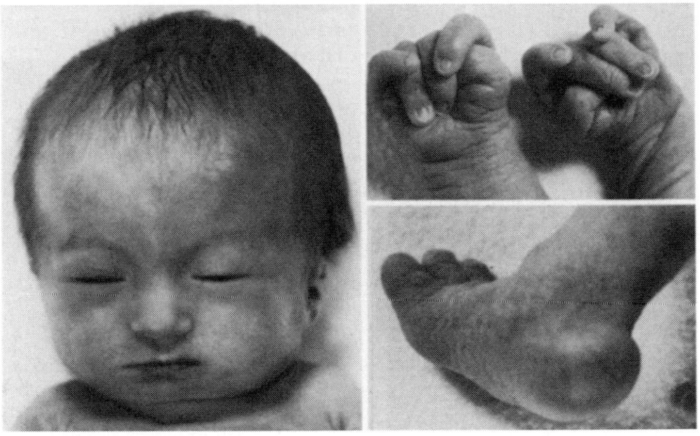

Other Findings

Microcephaly
Clefting of lip, palate, or both
Rocker-bottom feet
Cardiac valvular abnormalities, coarctation of the aorta
Abdominal, inguinal, or diaphragmatic hernia
Renal abnormalities
Genital abnormalities

COMMENTS

Trisomy 18 syndrome occurs in approximately 1 in 3,000 to 7,000 live births. In the newborn period, babies have a poor suck and hypotonia, which is followed by failure to thrive and hypertonia.

PERFORMANCE

Mortality is 50% in the first weeks of life with less than 10% surviving the first year. Survivors have severe mental retardation.

ETIOLOGY

Trisomy for all or most of chromosome 18 is present. Eighty percent of cases are caused by chromosomal nondisjunction and are associated with advanced maternal age. If the trisomy is found to be caused by a translocation, parental karyotypes should be obtained to rule out an inherited defect. Trisomy may be partial (involving only a portion of the chromosome) or mosaic. Both would be expected to show a variable and generally less severe phenotype.

TRISOMY 21 SYNDROME (DOWN SYNDROME)

Key Features

Brachycephaly
Upslanting palpebral fissures*
Epicanthal folds
Flattened facial profile*
Small, rounded ears*
Excess nuchal skin*
Congenital cardiac anomalies in 40% to 50% (endocardial cushion defect, VSD, PDA)
Dysplasia of pelvis*
Hyperflexibility of joints*
Brachydactyly
Clinodactyly of fifth fingers (dysplasia of midphalanx)*
Single transverse palmar crease (simian crease)*
Hypotonia,* poor Moro reflex*

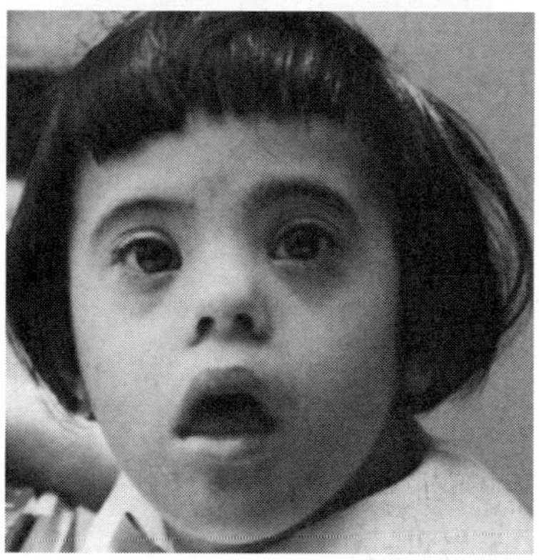

Other Findings

Short stature
Brushfield spots (speckling of the iris)
Wide gap between first and second toes

COMMENTS

Trisomy 21 is the most common autosomal chromosome abnormality in liveborn infants and occurs in approximately 1 in 700 to 800 newborns with frequencies increasing with advanced maternal age. In 90% of neonates with Down syndrome, ten key features (indicated by asterisks) are found. These features designate the Hall criteria for diagnosis. Also, an increased risk exists for duodenal atresia, Hirschprung disease, leukemia, hypothyroidism, atlantoaxial instability, and premature aging.

PERFORMANCE

All individuals are mentally retarded, although a considerable range of severity occurs (average IQ of 30–50). Early intervention programs have been beneficial in helping these children to achieve to their maximum potential.

ETIOLOGY

Trisomy for all or part of chromosome 21 is present. The majority of cases (almost 95%) are caused by full trisomy, usually caused by maternal meiosis I nondisjunction with the remainder made up of translocation cases (2%) and mosaic Down syndrome (3%). Each parent of a child with translocation Down syndrome should have karyotype analysis to rule out the small possibility of being a translocation carrier, which could carry as high as 100% risk of recurrence for a translocation involving both chromosomes 21.

TURNER SYNDROME (XO)

Key Features

Short stature
Prominent or low-set ears
Excess nuchal skin (broad-based neck), low posterior hairline
Broad chest with widely spaced nipples
Cubitus valgus (increased carrying angle of arms)
Dorsal lymphedema of hands and feet (most evident in the newborn period)
Congenital heart disease (bicuspid aortic valve, coarctation of aorta)
Ovarian dysgenesis (primary or secondary amenorrhea)
Renal abnormalities (horseshoe kidney)
Hypertension

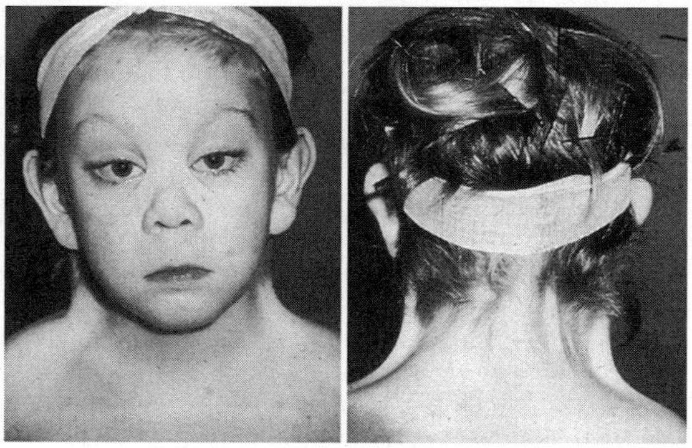

Other Findings

Ptosis, epicanthal folds
Narrow palate
Poor breast development
Hypoplastic, hyperconvex nails
Short fourth metacarpal/metatarsal
Pigmented nevi
Hearing impairment
Hypothyroidism

COMMENTS

The attrition rate of Turner syndrome fetuses is extremely high with only approximately 5% to 10% surviving to birth. The occurrence of Turner syndrome is 1 in 2,000 to 6,000 live births. The adult height, when untreated, is usually less than 144 cm. Ultimate height achievement has been greatly improved by combination therapy with growth hormone and oxandrolone. Additional hormonal treatment with estrogen may allow for menstrual cycling, although fertility remains greatly reduced.

PERFORMANCE

Turner syndrome individuals are usually of normal intelligence with a mean IQ of 90. They may have specific deficits in the areas of visual–spatial organization, psychomotor coordination, and social interaction.

ETIOLOGY

Loss of one X chromosome leading to a 45,X chromosome complement with the paternal sex chromosome most commonly lost occurs in 50% of cases. Mosaicism may lead to more complex karyotypes including 46,XX/45,X or 46,XY/45,X. A ring chromosome X with loss of some associated genes, as well as isochromosome Xp with loss of genetic material from the long arm can lead to similar phenotypes depending on the amount of the deleted material. The finding of any Y chromosome material is significant because of the increased risk of gonadoblastoma.

KLINEFELTER SYNDROME (XXY)

Key Features

Eunuchoid habitus
Gynecomastia
Hypogonadism
Long limbs

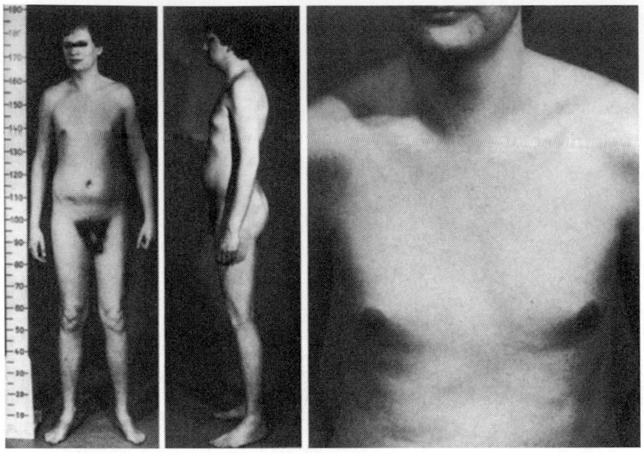

Other Findings

Scoliosis
Infertility

COMMENTS

Klinefelter syndrome affects approximately 1 in 500 male infants. Individuals with the syndrome have a mean height of 177.4 cm and a reduced upper to lower segment ratio. Most boys have inadequate or partial puberty, and they should be considered for testosterone replacement therapy beginning in the early teen years to promote more normal adult development. This replacement therapy has traditionally been given intramuscularly, although newer, transdermal delivery systems are now available. The frequency of breast carcinoma in men with Klinefelter syndrome is 66 times that of normal men and approaches the risk in women.

PERFORMANCE

IQ usually ranges from 85 to 90. Behavior problems, particularly immaturity and insecurity, are common, as are difficulties with expressive language, auditory processing, and auditory memory.

ETIOLOGY

The presence of an extra X chromosome is noted in boys and men. This may be caused by nondisjunction in the mother (the risk of which increases with maternal age) or in the father (whose risk does not increase with advancing paternal age). Chromosomal mosaicism may also be seen in which the XXY cell line is found in conjunction with a normal XY cell line leading to an improved prognosis for testicular function.

FRAGILE X SYNDROME

Key Features

Macrocephaly
Long face
Large ears
High arched palate
Macroorchidism (after puberty)

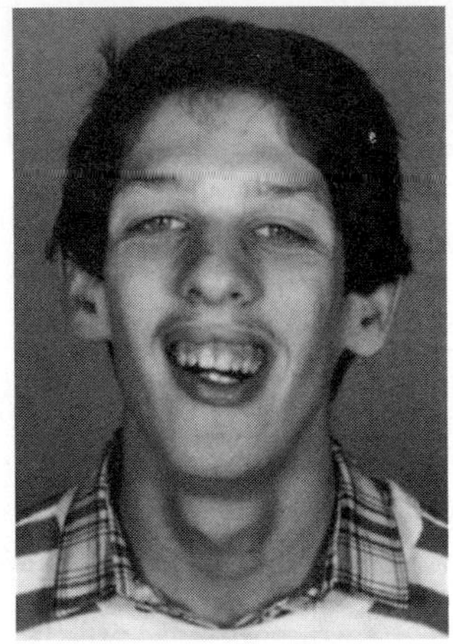

Other Findings

Prominent nasal bridge extending to the nasal tip
Prominent jaw
Joint laxity

COMMENTS

Fragile X syndrome is believed to be the most common form of heritable mental retardation. It occurs in approximately 1 in 1,000 to 1,500 boys and 1 in 2,000 to 2,500 girls. Female heterozygotes have an increased risk for developmental delay and behavioral abnormalities, but are usually less affected than males. It should be considered in the differential diagnosis of early overgrowth syndromes.

PERFORMANCE

All males affected with the fragile X syndrome have developmental delays, speech delays, or both. IQs of affected boys usually range from 30 to 55. Hyperactivity and autistic behaviors are frequent, as are poor motor coordination and temper tantrums.

ETIOLOGY

Fragile X was first detected as a gap or constriction in the X chromosome when cells from patients were grown in folate-deficient media and karyotyped. This chromosomal abnormality is caused by an expansion of the *FMR1* (familial mental retardation 1) gene at chromosome Xp27.3. The gene normally contains fewer than 50 trinucleotide CGG repeats. Individuals who carry 50 to 200 repeats are said to have the premutation and are at an increased risk for having affected children. Clinical symptoms of the fragile X syndrome become apparent when the repeat length has expanded to 200 or more repeats or when these repeats are methylated. Increased methylation of a gene can cause the gene to be inactivated.

CRI DU CHAT SYNDROME (5P-, DELETION 5P)

Key Features

Low birth weight and growth retardation
Microcephaly
Rounded face
Epicanthal folds
Hypertelorism
High-pitched, catlike cry
Single transverse palmar crease
Hypotonia

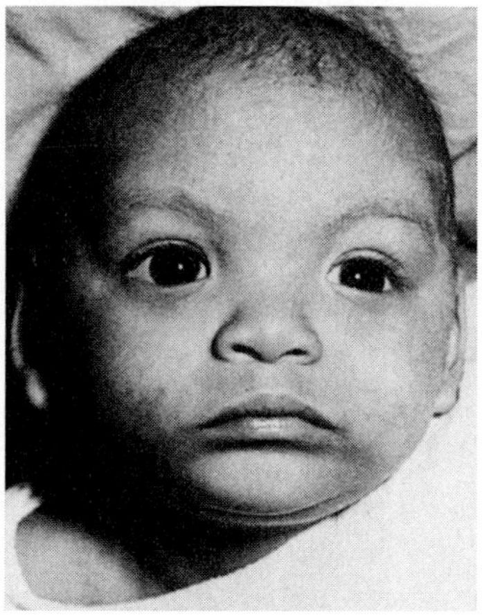

Other Findings

Dysplastic ears
Malocclusion
Congenital heart disease
Scoliosis

COMMENTS

Cri du chat syndrome occurs in 1 in 20,000 to 50,000 live births. The cat-like cry characteristic of this disorder is believed to be caused by abnormal laryngeal development and tends to disappear with age.

PERFORMANCE

Patients with cri du chat syndrome are mentally retarded. They have significant behavioral abnormalities including self-injurious tendencies, hypersensitivity to sound, and repetitive movements. In general, they can, with appropriate intervention, learn to communicate their needs, interact with others, and become independently mobile.

ETIOLOGY

Deletion of the short arm of chromosome 5 is present. The critical region for the high-pitched cry appears to be at 5p15.3 with the remaining features caused by deletion of 5p15.2. In *de novo* deletions (which account for 85% of cases), the vast majority are paternal in origin. The remaining 15% of cases are caused by inherited unbalanced translocation from a carrier parent.

ACHONDROPLASIA

Key Features

Short stature (mean adult height for men is 131 cm and for women is 124 cm)
Macrocephaly, frontal bossing
Narrowed foramen magnum
Depressed nasal bridge
Progressive narrowing of lumbar interpedicular distance
Lumbar lordosis
Rhizomelic limb shortening
Trident hand (fingers cannot appose one another)

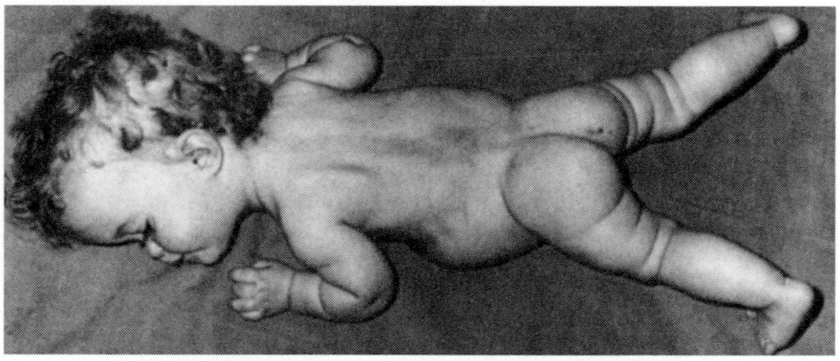

Other Findings

Hydrocephalus
Cuboid-shaped vertebral bodies
Small iliac wings and narrow sciatic notches
Bowed legs

COMMENTS

Achondroplasia is the most common skeletal dysplasia in humans occurring in 1 in 15,000 live births. Early motor progress may be delayed. Because of the small foramen magnum and narrowed lower spinal canal, patients are predisposed to neurosurgical complications.

PERFORMANCE

Intelligence is usually normal.

ETIOLOGY

Achondroplasia is an autosomal dominant condition. Mutations of the fibroblast growth factor receptor 3 (*FGFR3*) gene at chromosome 4p16.3 are responsible for achondroplasia, as well as related conditions hypochondroplasia (mild) and thanatophoric dysplasia (severe and lethal). A single mutation accounts for almost all cases of achondroplasia. Eighty percent to 90% of cases represent new mutations, all occurring in the father's sperm, and are associated with advanced paternal age.

ALAGILLE SYNDROME (ARTERIOHEPATIC DYSPLASIA)

Key Features

Broad forehead
Deep-set eyes
Ocular abnormality (posterior embryotoxin)
Long straight nose with flattened tip
Prominent chin
Peripheral pulmonic stenosis
Intrahepatic biliary atresia
Butterfly vertebrae

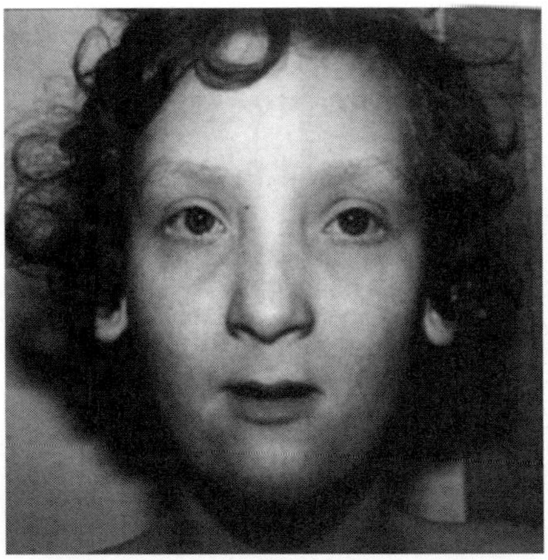

Other Findings

Growth retardation
Retinal degeneration
Cardiac defects
Renal abnormalities

COMMENTS

Patients usually present with direct hyperbilirubinemia in the neonatal period, and a number have undergone liver transplantation.

PERFORMANCE

A few individuals have mild mental retardation.

ETIOLOGY

Alagille syndrome is an autosomal dominant condition. Mutations have been found in the *JAGGED1* gene, which is located at chromosome 20p12.

ANGELMAN SYNDROME

Key Features

Microbrachycephaly
Hypopigmentation, blond hair, pale blue eyes
Large mouth with tongue protrusion
Prognathism
Awkward gait with arms upheld and flexed at the wrists and elbows
Seizures
Absence of speech

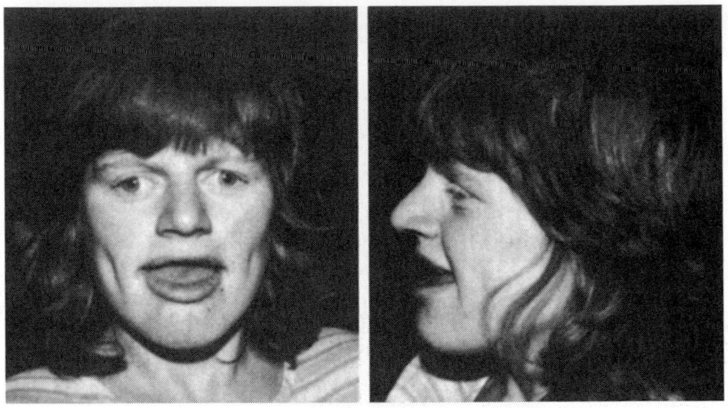

Other Findings

Strabismus
Scoliosis
Unprovoked bursts of laughter
Electroencephalographic abnormalities

COMMENTS

Angelman syndrome has also been called the *happy puppet syndrome* because of the unusual gait and unprovoked laughter. Affected individuals are usually unable to communicate verbally, but some may communicate by sign language.

PERFORMANCE

Patients have severe mental retardation.

ETIOLOGY

An interstitial deletion of chromosome 15q11–q13 accounts for 60% to 80% of cases. This region is known to show genomic imprinting, meaning that the parental origin of the deleted material affects the phenotypic expression. In Angelman syndrome, the deleted material is always maternal in origin, as opposed to the Prader–Willi syndrome, in which the same deleted segment is paternal. Deletions may be large enough to detect cytogenetically, or may require molecular methods [FISH (fluorescent *in situ* hybridization)] to detect.

A much less frequent cause of Angelman syndrome is lack of the maternal genetic material via paternal uniparental isodisomy. In this case, the individual inherits both chromosomes 15 from the father with no genetic contribution from the mother. Even though two copies of the genetic information are present, a lack of maternal genetic input still exists.

Mutations of the E6-AP ubiquitin-protein ligase gene are one cause of Angelman syndrome.

APERT SYNDROME

Key Features

Craniosynostosis
Brachycephaly with flat occiput
Wide, late-closing anterior fontanelle
Frontal bossing
Downslanting palpebral fissures
Shallow orbits with proptosis
Midface hypoplasia
High-arched, narrow palate
"Mitten-type" syndactyly of hands and feet

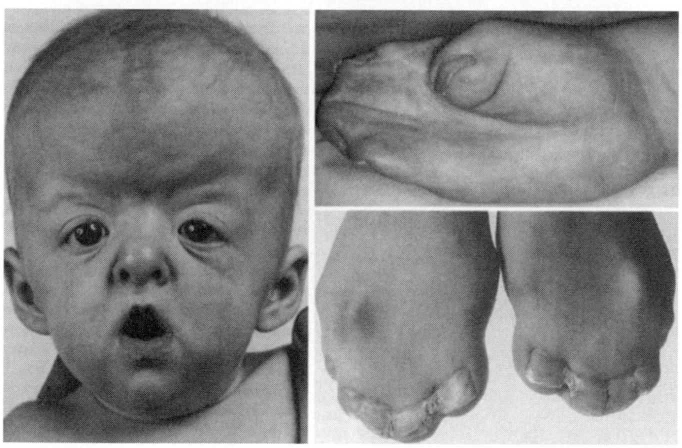

Other Findings

Cervical fusions
Progressive ankyloses of elbows, shoulders, hips
Cardiac defects
Genitourinary defects
Gastrointestinal or respiratory abnormalities
Hearing loss secondary to chronic otitis media
Central nervous system abnormalities
Moderate to severe acne (trunk and arms at adolescence)

COMMENTS

Birth prevalence is estimated to be 1 in 160,000. Affected individuals are typically born with fused coronal sutures and a large patent midline skull defect where the sagittal and metopic sutures would normally form. Because this gap takes 2 to 3 years to fill in with bone, the incidence of increased intracranial pressure is low in the first years of life. Some patients have complete osseous and cutaneous fusion of digits. Most patients undergo multiple cranial and hand and feet reconstruction procedures.

PERFORMANCE

A significant percentage of patients have mental retardation, which is not believed to be solely caused by increased intracranial pressure and may reflect, in part, the increased incidence of CNS malformations.

ETIOLOGY

Apert syndrome is an autosomal dominant condition caused by mutations in the fibroblast growth factor receptor 2 (*FGFR2*) gene on chromosome 10q25–q26. The majority of cases result from new mutations, although at least 1 three-generation family has been reported. Sporadic cases are associated with *de novo* mutations in the father's sperm and with increased paternal age.

BARDET–BIEDL SYNDROME

Key Features

Obesity
Short stature
Retinal dystrophy
Other ocular defects (myopia, astigmatism, nystagmus, cataracts, glaucoma, retinitis pigmentosa)
Postaxial polydactyly
Renal abnormalities (abnormal calyces, communicating cysts, fetal lobulations)
Hypogonadism

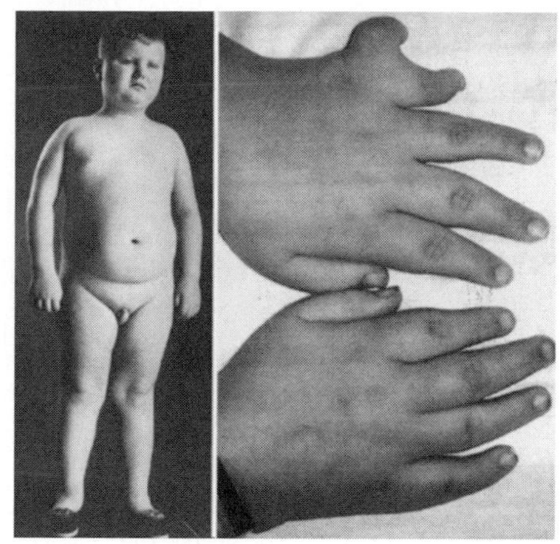

Other Findings

Brachydactyly
Short, broad feet
Hearing deficit
Asthma
Psychological and neurologic disorders

COMMENTS

The highest incidence of Bardet–Biedl syndrome has been reported in the Middle East (1 in 13,500) with much less frequent occurrence in Switzerland (1 in 160,000). Retinal dystrophy is present in 100% of patients with visual disturbances beginning in childhood. More than 70% are blind by age 20. Early visual changes can be detected by electroretinography. Renal failure develops in a small but significant number. The Lawrence Moon syndrome is another autosomal recessive condition with pigmentary retinopathy, hypogonadism, spastic paraplegia, and mental retardation, but no polydactyly.

PERFORMANCE

Mental deficiency occurs in more than three-fourths of patients. Delay of gross and fine motor skills is common, as are both dyspraxia and clumsiness. Speech delay is also seen in the majority of patients and appears amenable to speech therapy. Inappropriate mannerisms and affect are common.

ETIOLOGY

Bardet–Biedl syndrome is inherited as an autosomal recessive condition with heterogeneity. Four loci have been identified to date. *BBS1* is located on chromosome 11q13, *BBS2* at 16q21, *BBS3* at 3p13–p12, and *BBS4* at 15q22–q23. A number of families do not show linkage to any of these sites indicating that other causative loci still exist. Significant interfamial and intrafamilial variation in phenotype exists with only subtle differences attributable to the various loci.

BECKWITH–WIEDEMANN SYNDROME

Key Features

Macrosomia
Nevus flammeus of forehead and eyelids
Linear ear creases
Indentations on posterior pinnae
Macroglossia
Abdominal wall defects (diastasis recti, umbilical hernia, or omphalocele)
Organomegaly
Hypoglycemia in the newborn period

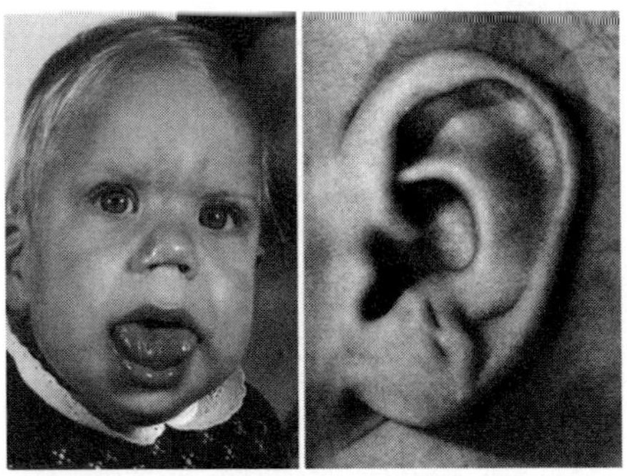

Other Findings

Hemihypertrophy
Large fontanelles
Diaphragmatic hernia
Advanced bone age
Polycythemia in the newborn period

COMMENTS

Beckwith–Wiedemann syndrome occurs in approximately 1 in 15,000 live births. An increased rate of both polyhydramnios and prematurity exists. Babies are usually large at birth (average weight, 4 kg; average length, 52.6 cm), but tend to level off closer to upper normal ranges as they get older. Advanced bone age is similarly more pronounced in the first few years of life. These children are at increased risk of malignancy, specifically Wilms tumor, hepatoblastoma, and gonadoblastoma, and should be followed with abdominal ultrasounds and serum alpha-fetoprotein levels every 6 months until age 6. The risk of malignancy is more significantly increased in those patients who also have hemihypertrophy.

PERFORMANCE

Intellect is normal in most cases, but a minority of patients has intellectual impairment ranging from mild to severe. It is thought that some of these cases are explainable by prematurity, hypoglycemic insult, or chromosome abnormalities documented in a few patients.

ETIOLOGY

Most cases are sporadic, but a significant percentage is inherited in an autosomal dominant manner. The gene has been localized to chromosome 11p15. The maternal copy of the gene is normally imprinted, or inactive, so the single paternal gene provides normal function. Beckwith–Wiedemann syndrome results if the paternal copy is duplicated or a translocation causes activation of the normally quiescent maternal gene. Evidence exists for the insulin-like growth factor–2 gene and a tumor-suppressor gene in this chromosomal region.

BLOOM SYNDROME

Key Features

Prenatal-onset growth deficiency
Small, narrow facies
Facial erythema and telangiectasia (exacerbated by sunlight)
Protruding ears
High-pitched voice
Predisposition to malignancy

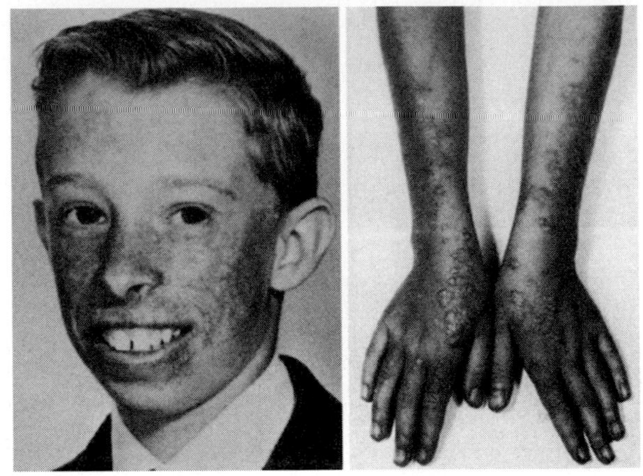

Other Findings

Absence of upper lateral incisors
Café au lait spots
Immunoglobulin deficiency

COMMENTS

Bloom syndrome is most common in Ashkenazi Jewish individuals with a carrier frequency believed to be at least 1 in 100 in that population. Skin lesions present on the nose, lips, malar areas, forearms, dorsa of hands, and back of neck and ears. Malignancy occurs in approximately 25% of those with Bloom syndrome and is the major cause of death. Leukemias are frequent, and a variety of solid tumor types have been described. Men are usually infertile because of insufficient spermatogenesis.

PERFORMANCE

Patients may show mild mental retardation or learning disabilities, although the majority is of normal intelligence.

ETIOLOGY

Bloom syndrome is an autosomal recessive condition with its gene, a member of the RecQ helicase family, located at chromosome 15q26.1. Chromosome analysis shows increased sister chromatid exchange considered diagnostic of this condition.

CORNELIA DE LANGE SYNDROME (BRACHMANN–DE LANGE SYNDROME)

Key Features

Microbrachycephaly
Bushy eyebrows with synophrys
Long, curly eyelashes
Depressed nasal bridge, anteverted nares
Thin upper lip, long philtrum
Downturned corners of mouth
Hirsutism, low posterior hairline
Limb defects including syndactyly, oligodactyly, micromelia, phocomelia
Cryptorchidism

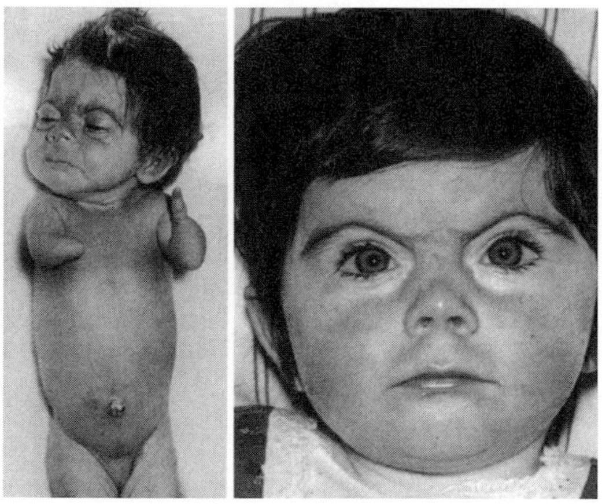

Other Findings

Ocular abnormalities (myopia, nystagmus)
High-arched palate
Hearing loss
Mandibular spur, 13 ribs
Cardiac defect (VSD)
Gastrointestinal abnormalities (reflux, malrotation, pyloric stenosis)
Delayed osseus maturation
Low-pitched, growling cry
Hypertonicity
Seizures

COMMENTS

Cornelia de Lange syndrome occurs in approximately 1 in 10,000 to 20,000 live births. In addition to prenatal onset growth deficiency, feeding difficulties are frequent, and affected individuals often fail to thrive because of persistent vomiting and other gastrointestinal disturbances. Those followed beyond 13 years of age had normal onset of puberty.

PERFORMANCE

Average IQ is 53 with the range being 30 to 86. Some individuals have autistic or self-destructive behaviors.

ETIOLOGY

Usually, Cornelia de Lange syndrome occurs sporadically. Cases of autosomal dominant inheritance have been reported. Patients with abnormalities of the chromosome 3q26.3 region show features similar to the syndrome indicating a possible causative gene in this area.

CROUZON SYNDROME

Key Features

Craniosynostosis, usually coronal synostosis
Brachycephaly
Proptosis due to shallow orbits
Hypertelorism
Strabismus
Beaked nose
Midface hypoplasia
High, narrow palate
Prognathism

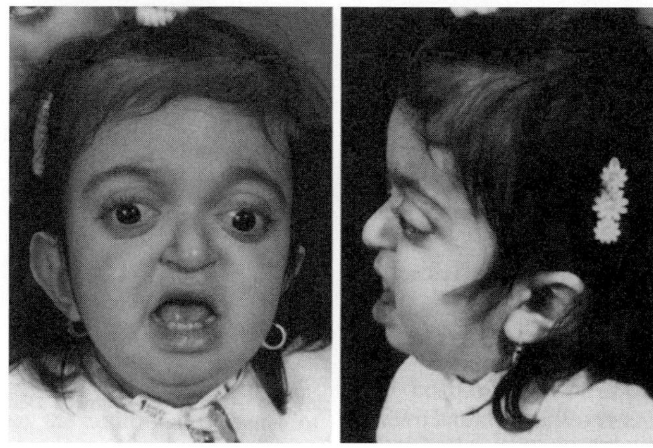

Other Findings

Conductive hearing loss
Dental malocclusion
Acanthosis nigricans

COMMENTS

Birth prevalence has been estimated at 1 in 25,000 live births. The phenotype is highly variable, and some patients are only diagnosed after the birth of a more severely affected child.

PERFORMANCE

Mental retardation has been reported in a small percentage of patients. Surgical correction of increased intracranial pressure caused by craniosynostosis is indicated to avoid intellectual compromise.

ETIOLOGY

Crouzon syndrome is inherited as an autosomal dominant condition. Crouzon syndrome is caused by mutations of the fibroblast growth factor receptor gene family. Most mutations have been reported in the *FGFR2* gene; however, some patients with Crouzon syndrome with the additional finding of acanthosis nigricans have a mutation in *FGFR3*. Pfeiffer syndrome (craniosynostosis and broad thumbs and toes) is a similar autosomal dominant condition that can be caused by mutations in the *FGFR1*, *FGFR2*, or *FGFR3* gene. Some patients with Pfeiffer syndrome carry an identical *FGFR2* mutation similar to that seen in Crouzon patients. Different *FGFR2* mutations cause Apert syndrome.

EHLERS–DANLOS SYNDROME

Key Features

Skin hyperextensibility and easy bruising
Joint hypermobility leading to sprains and joint dislocations
Increased tissue fragility (leading to formation of widened, atrophic scars)
Velvety feel to skin
Thin, translucent skin and hollow organ (aorta, intestine, uterus) fragility and rupture (type 4 Ehlers–Danlos syndrome)

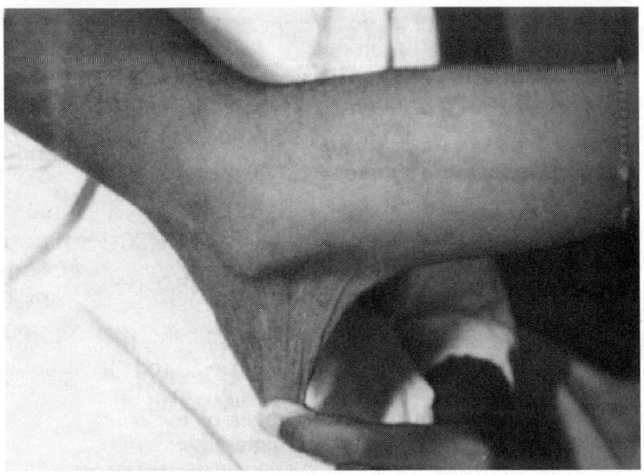

Other Findings

Small, mobile subcutaneous nodules (may represent adipose or mucinous material)
Mitral valve prolapse
Chronic joint and limb pain
Postsurgical complications (incisional hernias)
Preterm birth caused by premature rupture of membranes

COMMENTS

The Ehlers–Danlos syndromes are a group of inherited connective tissue disorders. Previously, ten forms were named, but revised nosology now recognizes six separate conditions: type 1 (classic), type 2 (hypermobility), type 3 (vascular), type 4 (kyphoscoliosis), type 5 (arthrochalasia), and type 6 (dermatosparaxis). The latter three types are considerably less common. The vascular form carries the highest risk of early death from rupture of the aorta and may have significant morbidity from rupture of intestines or midsized arteries.

PERFORMANCE

Intelligence is usually normal, although some mental deficiency has been reported. Psychosocial functioning is affected with increased incidence of anxiety and depression.

ETIOLOGY

Ehlers–Danlos syndrome types are thought to be distinct from one another, and some forms have shown further genetic heterogeneity. The classic form is caused by a defect in type V collagen and is autosomal dominant. The vascular form is also dominant and is caused by defects of type III collagen.

MARFAN SYNDROME

Key Features

Skeletal*: Tall stature, long slender limbs, arachnodactyly, scoliosis, joint hypermobility, pectus excavatum or carinatum, pes planus, reduced upper to lower segment ratio, Walker–Murdoch wrist sign (the ability of the fifth finger and thumb to overlap when encircling the opposite wrist), and Steinburg thumb sign (the ability of the nail of the thumb to project beyond the ulnar aspect of the palm when the hand is clenched without assistance).
Ocular*: Lens subluxation (typically upward), myopia, retinal detachment
Cardiac*: Aortic dilatation, dissection, or both, aortic regurgitation, mitral valve prolapse
Skin and integument*: Striae, hernias (inguinal, umbilical, ventral, incisional)

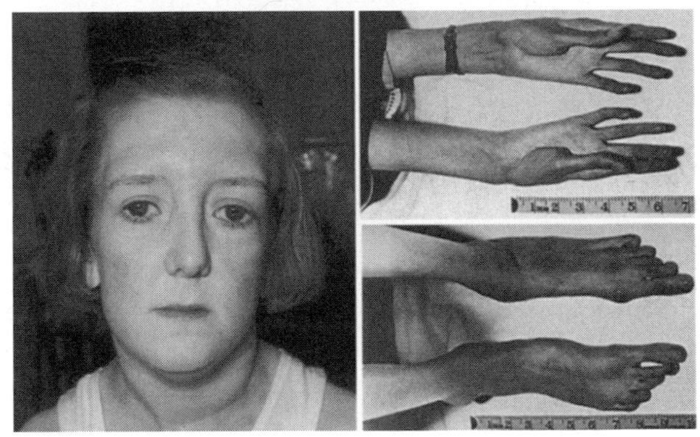

Other Findings

Dolichocephaly
Dural ectasia*
Narrow, high-arched palate
Spontaneous pneumothorax

COMMENTS

Marfan syndrome occurs in approximately 1 in 10,000 individuals in the United States. Expression is highly variable. The most severely affected individuals present with cardiac abnormalities in early infancy (infantile Marfan syndrome). Individuals with Marfan syndrome are at risk for early death caused by aortic dissection and may be treated with beta-blockers to prevent further aortic dilatation or with surgical replacement of the aortic root if dilatation is severe. Diagnosis requires positive findings in three of the five categories marked by asterisks (two with major criteria and involvement of a third, or mutation present in the *fibrillin* gene and one major criterion and involvement of a second).

PERFORMANCE

Intelligence is normal, although some neuropsychological deficits (including learning disabilities and attention deficit disorder) occur with increased frequency.

ETIOLOGY

Marfan syndrome is inherited as an autosomal dominant condition with wide variation of expression. The disorder is caused by mutations in the *fibrillin* gene located at chromosome 15q21.1. Approximately 25% to 30% of new cases are sporadic. A paternal age effect has been demonstrated.

MILLER–DIEKER LISSENCEPHALY SYNDROME

Key Features

Lissencephaly ("smooth brain")
Heterotopias
Absent/hypoplastic corpus callosum
Microcephaly with bitemporal narrowing
Vertical furrowing of forehead with crying
Small, anteverted nose
Long philtrum
Thin prominent upper lip

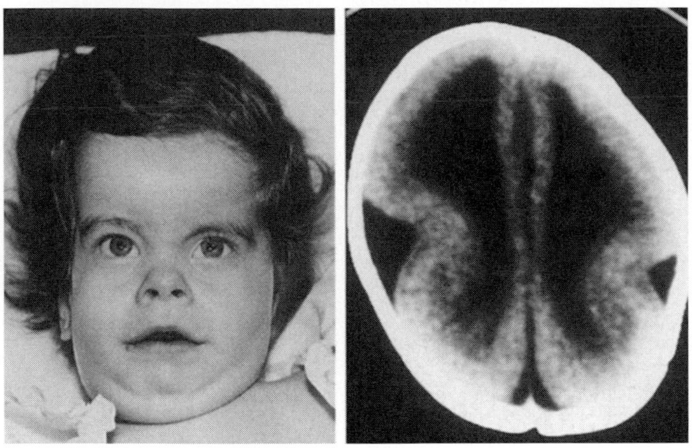

Other Findings

Cardiac defects
Cryptorchidism

COMMENTS
Lissencephaly is pachygyria/agyria resulting from deficiency of neuronal migration. Patients have significant seizures, failure to thrive, and feeding problems. Survival is greatly reduced and death usually occurs before 2 years of age.

PERFORMANCE
Patients have severe mental retardation.

ETIOLOGY
Miller–Dieker lissencephaly syndrome is caused by a deletion of chromosome 17p13.3 in 90% of patients and can be detected by FISH. The gene shows significant homology to beta subunits of heterotrimeric G proteins suggesting that it may be involved in a signal transduction pathway crucial for cerebral development.

NEUROFIBROMATOSIS SYNDROME

Key Features

Café au lait spots (six measuring at least 5 mm before puberty or 15 mm after puberty*)
Lisch nodules (hamartomas of the iris)*
Neurofibromas (two cutaneous or one plexiform type*)
Optic glioma*
Inguinal or axillary freckling*
Bony lesions (pseudoarthrosis, sphenoid wing dysplasia)*

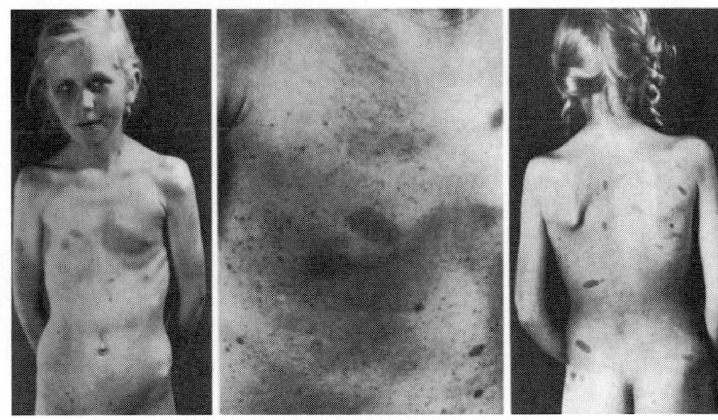

Other Findings

Macrocephaly
Scoliosis
Pheochromocytoma
Tumors of the central nervous system

COMMENTS
Neurofibromatosis type 1 (NF1), also called *von Recklinghausen disease*, occurs in approximately 1 in 3,000 live births. The diagnosis of NF1 is considered to be established in anyone having two key features (positive family history and those marked by an asterisk). Skin findings may or may not be present at birth and tend to progress during childhood. Neurofibromas may become more numerous and prominent during puberty and pregnancy. Each neurofibroma has a 5% lifetime risk for malignant degeneration, so vigilance is advised for any pain, bleeding, or changes in color or size of an existing growth. Neurofibromatosis type 2 (NF2) is a distinct disorder marked by multiple intracranial tumors and less prominent skin findings.

PERFORMANCE
A small percentage (5%–8%) of patients are mentally retarded; a greater number (25%–50%) have more subtle difficulties such as learning disabilities, hyperactivity, or speech problems.

ETIOLOGY
Neurofibromatosis syndrome is inherited as an autosomal dominant condition caused by mutations of the neurofibromatosis gene, *NF1*, at chromosome 17q11.2. Approximately one-half of individuals with NF1 represent a new mutation, and a paternal age effect has been noted in these cases. The risk for an affected individual to have an affected child is 50%; however, expression is quite variable, and offspring may be affected to a greater or lesser extent than the parent. NF2 is caused by mutations of the *merlin* gene on chromosome 22.

NOONAN SYNDROME

Key Features

Short stature
Downslanting palpebral fissures
Ptosis
Low-set, malformed ears
Short or broad-based (webbed) neck
Shield chest
Cardiac abnormalities (pulmonic stenosis)
Cryptorchidism

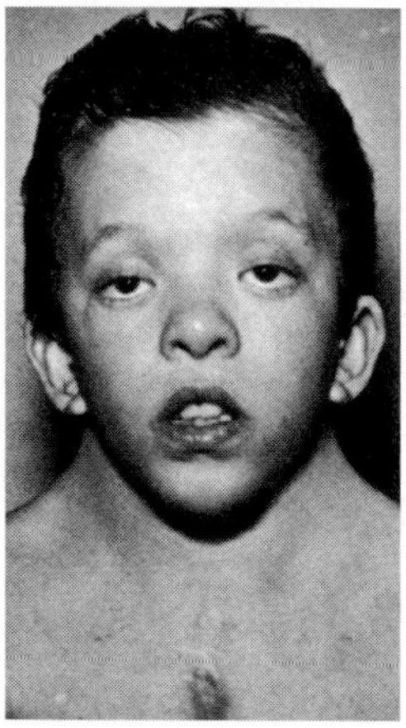

Other Findings

Pectus excavatum or carinatum
Cubitus valgus
Edema of dorsal aspects of hands and feet
Hearing loss
Malignant hyperthermia (sometimes called *King syndrome* when present)
Bleeding diathesis (von Willebrand disease, platelet dysfunction, or defects of intrinsic pathway)

COMMENTS

Noonan syndrome has been referred to as *male Turner syndrome* because many features are similar in these two conditions. However, Noonan syndrome can occur in both sexes and is a separate entity from Turner syndrome. It is thought to be fairly common with a frequency of approximately 1 in 1,000 to 2,500.

PERFORMANCE

Mental retardation is present in at least one-fourth of patients. However, learning disabilities, language delay, and articulation problems are frequent.

ETIOLOGY

Noonan syndrome is usually sporadic; however, autosomal dominant transmission has been described. A gene for this condition has been mapped to chromosome 12q22-qter. Genetic heterogeneity is suggested by the fact that not all familial cases map to this region.

OSTEOGENESIS IMPERFECTA SYNDROME

Key Features

Increased bone fragility with multiple fractures
Short stature
Blue sclerae
Hearing loss
Dentinogenesis imperfecta (translucent/opalescent teeth with increased susceptibility to caries)
Bowing of limbs
Joint hyperextensibility

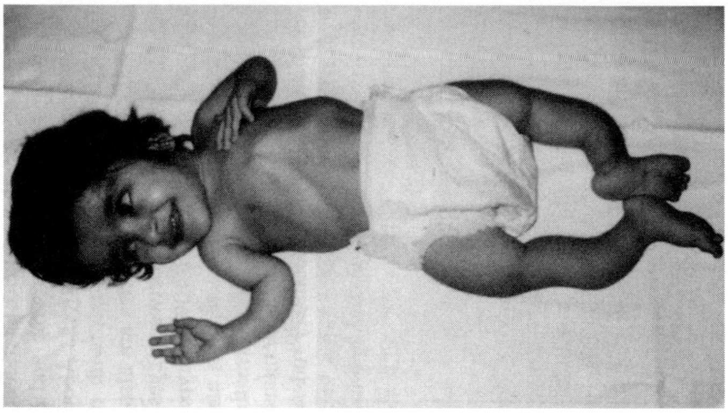

Other Findings

Wormian bones of skull
Scoliosis
Easy bruisability

COMMENTS

Osteogenesis imperfecta syndrome represents a group of disorders with increased bone fragility. These disorders are divided into four types, and each is divided into subtypes indicating the presence or absence of features such as blue sclerae and dental abnormalities. Type I is generally mild to moderate in severity, type II is the severe perinatal lethal form, type III is described as progressively deforming, and type IV involves bone fragility without characteristic features of type I.

PERFORMANCE

Infants with type II disease are usually stillborn or die in the early perinatal period. For other forms, intelligence is generally normal.

ETIOLOGY

Mutations in the genes contributing to the formation of type I collagen have been found in all forms. Mutations in both *COL1A1* and *COL1A2* have been identified in all types. These conditions are usually dominant, and many represent new mutations with a paternal age effect. However, recessive inheritance has been described for some of the rarer type II and III subtypes.

PRADER–WILLI SYNDROME

Key Features

Obesity
Almond-shaped palpebral fissures
Hypogonadism
Small hands and feet
Hypotonia in infancy

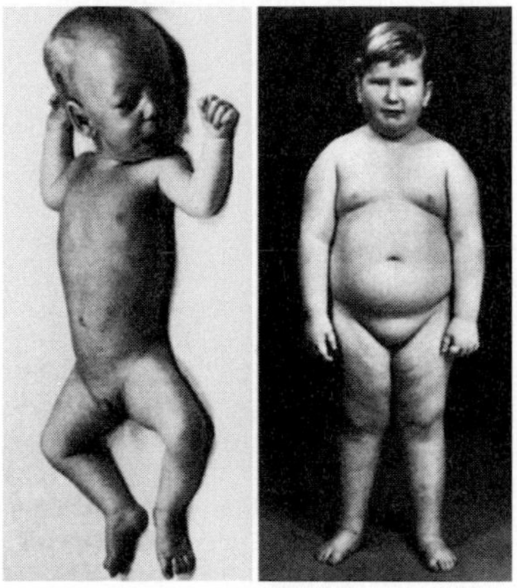

Other Findings

Narrow bifrontal diameter
Strabismus
Frequent skin picking leading to scabs and scars

COMMENTS

The incidence of Prader–Willi syndrome is approximately 1 in 16,000 live births. These patients are hypotonic at birth. They often have failure to thrive in infancy and may require tube feedings. However, by 6 months to 6 years of age, appetite increases, and they rapidly begin to put on weight leading to obesity.

PERFORMANCE

Mild to moderate mental retardation is present. Behavior problems are frequent and include excessive eating, rage behaviors (especially when denied food), and eating unusual foodstuffs. Psychiatric problems may develop in adolescents.

ETIOLOGY

Deletion of chromosome 15q11–q13 is detectable by high-resolution chromosome analysis or FISH in 70%. The deleted segment is always paternal, in contrast to the Angelman syndrome in which the maternal copy of the same chromosome segment is deleted. In a small percentage of cases, the patient has inherited both copies of chromosome 15 from the mother (uniparental disomy) leading to a functional deletion of paternal information. This contiguous gene syndrome results from inactivity of the paternal copies of the imprinted small ribonucleoprotein N gene (*SNRPN*), the *necdin* gene, and possibly other genes on 15q11.

SMITH–LEMLI–OPITZ SYNDROME

Key Features

Microcephaly
Ptosis
Anteverted nares and broad nasal tip
Syndactyly of second and third toes
Genital abnormalities (hypospadias, cryptorchidism, bifid or hypoplastic scrotum)
Renal abnormalities

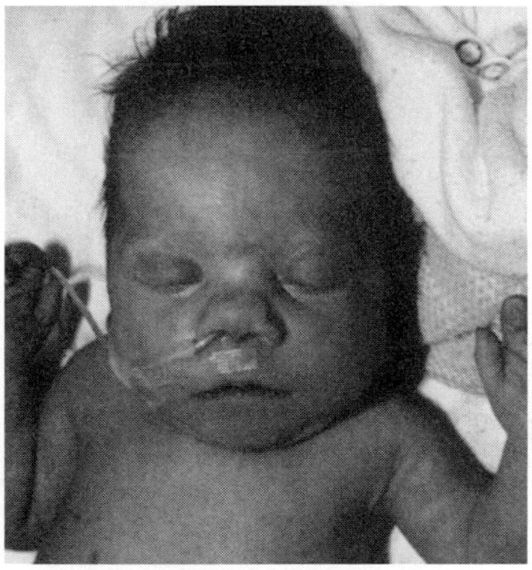

Other Findings

Cardiac defects
Seizures
Polydactyly

COMMENTS

Babies with Smith–Lemli–Opitz syndrome have severe failure to thrive, irritability, and abnormalities of muscle tone (initially hypotonic with hypertonicity developing with time). Approximately 20% die within the first year of life, and 50% die by age 18 months.

PERFORMANCE

Moderate to severe mental retardation is present.

ETIOLOGY

Smith–Lemli–Opitz syndrome is inherited in an autosomal recessive manner. The disorder is caused by a defect in cholesterol biosynthesis leading to a low blood cholesterol levels and dramatic elevations of the cholesterol precursor 7-dehydrocholesterol (which is the basis for diagnostic blood testing). Cholesterol supplementation is being used with amelioration of some of the symptoms (such as irritability). Prenatal cholesterol supplementation of women carrying affected fetuses has been attempted, although no formal results are available as to its effectiveness.

STICKLER SYNDROME (HEREDITARY ARTHROOPHTHALMOPATHY)

Key Features

Flat facies, maxillary hypoplasia
Severe, progressive myopia (may lead to retinal detachment)
Deafness (conductive or sensorineural)
Robin sequence (micrognathia and rounded palatal cleft)
Rhizomelic limb shortening
Enlargement of wrist, knee, and ankle joints at birth

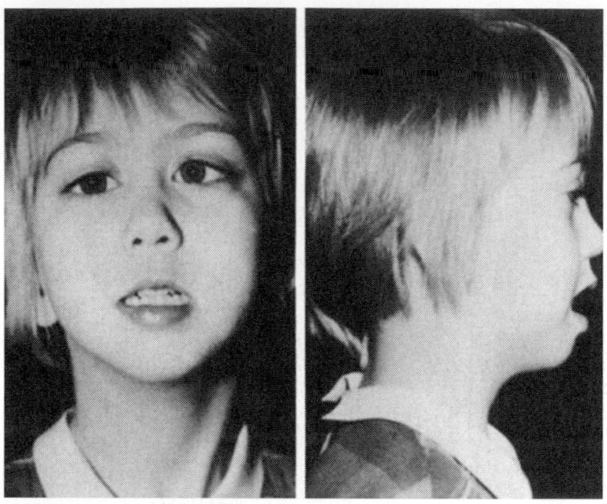

Other Findings

Mitral valve prolapse
Scoliosis
Arthritis
Hyperextensible joints
Mild spondyloepiphyseal dysplasia

COMMENTS

Any newborn with the Robin sequence should be evaluated to rule out the Stickler syndrome. Ocular involvement is progressive and severe. Arthritis becomes a problem in young adulthood.

PERFORMANCE

Mental retardation has been reported in some patients but is not considered a frequent finding.

ETIOLOGY

Stickler syndrome is an autosomal dominant condition. Stickler syndrome can be caused by mutations in the gene for type II collagen (*COL2A1*) located at chromosome 12q13.11–q13.2.

TUBEROUS SCLEROSIS SYNDROME

Key Features

Glioma-angioma lesions in the cortex and white matter*
Fibrous plaque on forehead*
Hamartomas of the retina*
Fibrous-angiomatous lesions of the cheeks*
White macules (ash leaf spots)
Shagreen patch
Café au lait spots
Pit-shaped enamel defects of labial premolar surface
Ungual fibromas*
Cyst-like areas of phalanges
Seizures

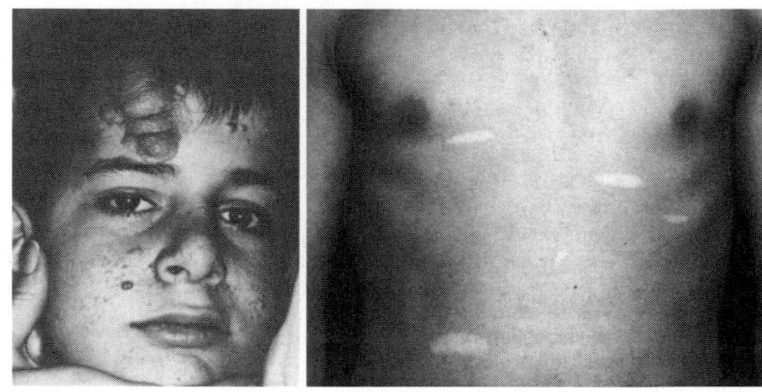

Other Findings

Infantile spasms
Intracranial mineralization in basal ganglia and periventricular region
Cardiac rhabdomyoma
Renal angiomyolipomas or cysts

COMMENTS

The occurrence of tuberous sclerosis syndrome is 1 in 10,000 live births. Only one of the features with an asterisk, or two or more other features are required for diagnosis. Facial nodular lesions are present in 50% of children by 5 years, whereas white macules are present at birth or in early infancy. Malignant transformation may occur, and approximately 6% of patients develop a brain tumor. Patients have behavioral problems and autism.

PERFORMANCE

Mental impairment is present in 69% of patients. Mental retardation and seizures are related to the extent of hamartomatous involvement of the brain.

ETIOLOGY

Tuberous sclerosis syndrome is an autosomal dominant condition with 50% to 60% of cases representing *de novo* mutations. Two genes causing tuberous sclerosis syndrome have been identified: *TCS1* on chromosome 9q34 and *TCS2* on chromosome 16p13.3. Contiguous to the *TCS2* gene on chromosome 16q13 is the autosomal dominant polycystic kidney disease gene. In angiomyolipomas and lymphangiomyomatosis, a loss of heterozygosity (mutation in one gene is already present, followed by the loss of the second gene of the pair) of *TCS1* occurs.

VELO–CARDIO–FACIAL SYNDROME (SHPRINTZEN SYNDROME)

Key Features

Cleft of the secondary palate
Velopharyngeal incompetence
Prominent nose
Narrow palpebral fissures
Retruded mandible
Slender and hyperextensible hands and fingers
Cardiac defects (VSD, TOF, right aortic arch)

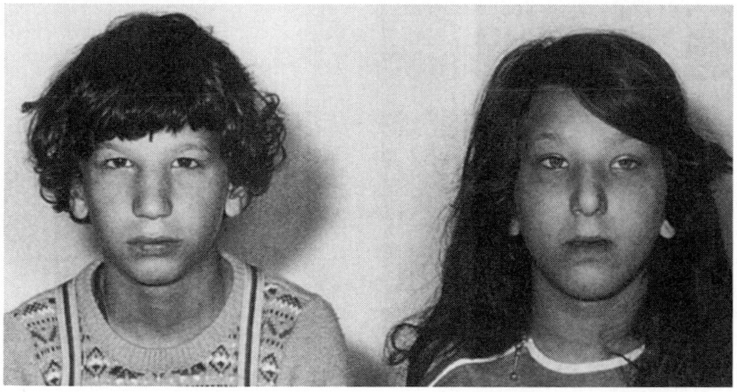

Other Findings

Minor auricular anomalies
Hypoplastic and elongated malar area
Medial displacement of the internal carotid arteries
Scoliosis
Hypernasal speech
Psychiatric disorders

COMMENTS

Hypotonia in infancy is frequent with transient hypocalcemia.

PERFORMANCE

Learning disabilities and mild intellectual impairment (IQ of 70–90) is present. Speech development is often delayed, and language is impaired. Socialization skills may surpass intellectual skills.

ETIOLOGY

Velo–cardio–facial syndrome is inherited as an autosomal dominant condition. Affected individuals have an interstitial deletion of chromosome 22q11.21–q11.23 and are monosomic for this region. The deletion is detected by FISH. The same region is deleted in some cases of DiGeorge syndrome, a condition that variably includes lateral displacement of inner canthi with short palpebral fissures, short philtrum, micrognathia, ear anomalies, and defects of development of the thymus, parathyroids, and great vessels.

WILLIAMS SYNDROME (WILLIAM–BEUREN SYNDROME)

Key Features

Periorbital soft tissue fullness
Blue irides with stellate pattern
Medial eyebrow flare
Anteverted nares
Long philtrum
Prominent, thick lips with mouth held open
Cardiac abnormalities (supravalvular aortic stenosis, peripheral pulmonic stenosis, pulmonary valve stenosis, ASD, VSD)

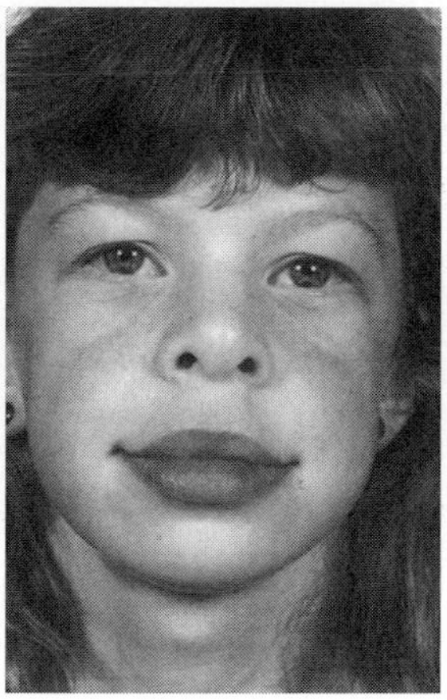

Other Findings

Mild short stature
Hoarse, husky voice
Renal anomalies, artery stenosis
Hypoplastic nails
Friendly, "cocktail party" personality
Hypercalcemia in infancy

COMMENTS

Feeding difficulties are frequent in infants with the Williams syndrome. Adults are at risk for additional medical problems including hypertension, gastrointestinal difficulties (gastrointestinal bleeding, constipation, diverticulosis), urinary tract infections, and joint contractures.

PERFORMANCE

Mental retardation occurs with an IQ usually in the 50s. Language skills are less affected than cognitive skills and may hide the extent of the patient's mental impairment.

ETIOLOGY

Cases of Williams syndrome are usually sporadic, although dominant inheritance has been reported. This condition is a contiguous gene syndrome that is located at chromosome 7q11.23. Deletions and mutations occur in the *elastin* gene. Another gene involved in its pathogenesis is *LIM-kinase-1*. It has been proposed that loss of this gene is the basis for impaired visuospatial constructive cognition and that loss of the *elastin* gene leads to vascular abnormalities. The replication factor C2 gene has also been found to be deleted.

ZELLWEGER SYNDROME (CEREBRO–HEPATO–RENAL SYNDROME)

Key Features

Large fontanelles
High forehead
Flat occiput
Flat facies
Gross defects of early brain development
Anteverted nares
Hepatomegaly with dysgenesis
Albuminuria with small cysts

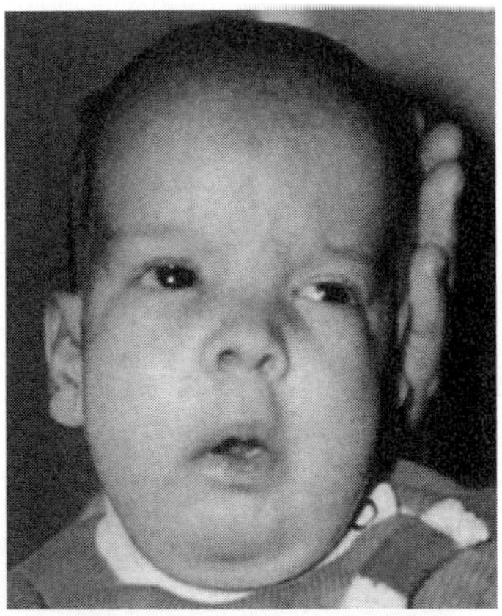

Other Findings

Congenital cataracts
Retinal pigmentary changes
Decreased weight
Cardiac defects (PDA, septal changes)
Variable contractures
Stippling of patellae

COMMENTS

Most infants with Zellweger syndrome are born with breech presentation and present with failure to thrive. They are found to have variable elevated serum iron levels and evidence of iron storage, pipecolic acidemia, abnormal bile acids, and absent liver peroxisomes. Diagnosis is based on biochemical studies including decreased dihydroxyacetone phosphate acyltransferase activity in fibroblasts and blood cells, a lowered plasmalogen biosynthesis, accumulation of unmetabolized very long-chain fatty acids, and an absence of catalase-containing subcellular particles in fibroblasts.

PERFORMANCE

The vast majority of infants die within the first year of life. Survivors have severe mental retardation and seizures.

ETIOLOGY

Zellweger syndrome is inherited as an autosomal recessive condition. The condition is heterogeneous and is caused by mutations in any of several different genes involved in peroxisome biogenesis. Peroxin genes can be mutated and have been mapped to chromosomes 12, 8, and 6. Mutations have been found in the peroxisomal membrane protein PMP70 at chromosome 1p22–p21. Another locus is suspected at chromosome 7q11.23 where chromosomal aberrations have been detected.

CHARGE

Key Features

*C*oloboma of retina, lens, choroid, or optic nerve
*H*eart defect (TOF, PDA, VSD, ASD)
*A*tresia choanae
*R*etardation of growth, development, or both
*G*enital abnormalities in male infants (cryptorchidism, microphallus)
*E*ar abnormalities or deafness

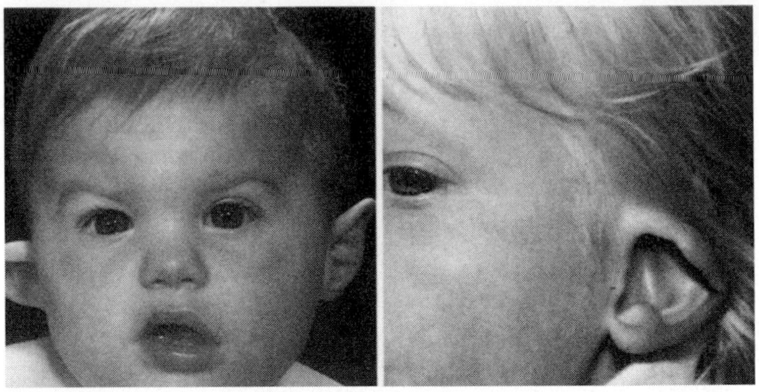

Other Findings

Cleft lip or cleft palate
Micrognathia
Multiple cranial nerve abnormalities
Facial palsy
Tracheoesophageal fistula
Hypocalcemia

COMMENTS

In infants with CHARGE, feeding problems are frequent, and some patients die in infancy.

PERFORMANCE

Almost all patients have some degree of mental retardation ranging from mild to profound. Concomitant central nervous system malformations may be found including holoprosencephaly.

ETIOLOGY

The cause of CHARGE is unknown but is thought to be caused by an insult during the second month of gestation, possibly affecting the neural crest cells. This condition is usually a sporadic occurrence within a family, although familial cases have been reported.

VATER/VACTERL

Key Features

*V*ertebral defects
*A*nal atresia (imperforate anus)
*C*ardiac defects
*T*racheo*e*sophageal fistula
*R*enal, radial, or both kinds of dysplasia
*L*imb abnormality

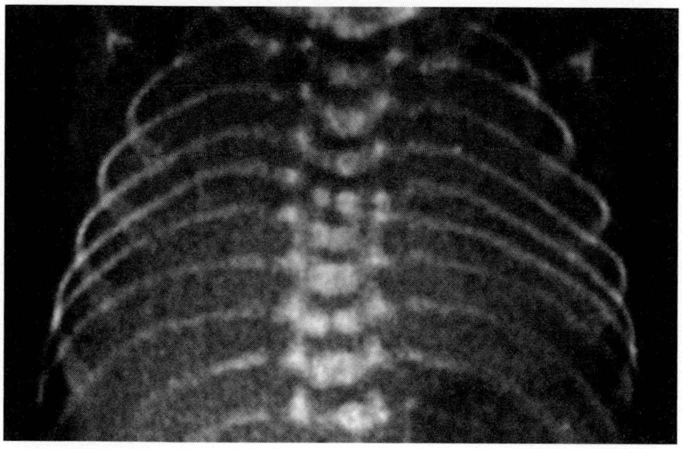

Other Findings

Single umbilical artery
Genital abnormalities
Growth retardation
Ear abnormalities

COMMENTS
The nonrandom association of vertebral defects, anal defects, tracheoesophageal fistula, and renal and radial abnormalities was initially designated as *VATER association* but has been expanded to *VACTERL* to recognize the increased incidence of cardiac and limb defects. These patients do not usually show facial dysmorphism. The presence of at least three of the features is considered necessary for diagnosis.

PERFORMANCE
Intelligence is usually normal.

ETIOLOGY
The association is usually sporadic with increased occurrence in infants of diabetic mothers.

CHAPTER 276

Laboratory Values

Adapted from Michael A. Barone

The following reference values for laboratory tests represent guidelines. Reference ranges typically vary from one institution to the next depending on the laboratory method used. Where applicable, conventional units and International System (IS) units are listed with conversion factors.

ABBREVIATIONS

CI	confidence interval
F	female
Hb	hemoglobin
M	male
MCHC	mean corpuscular hemoglobin concentration
MCV	mean corpuscular volume
RBC	red blood cell
SD	standard deviation
WBC	white blood cell

TABLE 276-1. Blood

Test	Conventional units reference range	Conversion factor	SI units reference range
Alanine aminotransferase (ALT)	0–5 yr: 7–46 U/L >5 yr: 6–39		0–5 yr: 7–46 U/L >5 yr: 6–39
Albumin	Premature, 24 hr: 1.5–3.0 g/dL Term, 6 d: 2.5–3.4 1–3 yr: 3.4–4.2 4–6 yr: 3.5–5.2 7–19 yr: 3.7–5.6	g/dL × 10 = g/L	Premature, 24 hr: 15–30 g/L Term, 6 d: 25–34 1–3 yr: 34–42 4–6 yr: 35–52 7–19 yr: 37–56
Alkaline phosphatase	Infant: 150–420 U/L 2–10 yr: 100–320 11–18 yr (M): 100–390 11–18 yr (F): 100–320 Adult: 30–120		Infant: 150–420 U/L 2–10 yr: 100–320 11–18 yr (M): 100–390 11–18 yr (F): 100–320 Adult: 30–120
Ammonia nitrogen	Newborn: 90–150 μg/dL 0–2 wk: 79–129 >1 mo: 29–70 Thereafter: 0–50	μg/dL × 0.714 = μmol/L	Newborn: 64–107 μmol/L 0–2 wk: 56–92 >1 mo: 21–50 Thereafter: 0–35.7
Amylase	Newborn: 5–65 U/L Thereafter: 0–130		Newborn: 5–65 U/L Thereafter: 0–130
Anion gap	7–14 mEq/L		7–14 nmol/L
Aspartate aminotransferase (AST)	0–2 yr: 23–65 U/L 2–8 yr: 23–58 8–14 yr: 16–46 >14 yr: 16–38		0–2 yr: 23–65 U/L 2–8 yr: 23–58 8–14 yr: 16–46 >14 yr: 16–38
Bicarbonate	Premature: 18–26 mEq/L <2 yr: 20–25 >2 yr: 22–26		Premature: 18–26 mmol/L <2 yr: 20–25 >2 yr: 22–26
Bilirubin (total)	*Preterm* / *Term* Cord: <2 / <2 mg/dL 0–1 d: <8 / <6 1–2 d: <12 / <8 3–5 d: <16 / <12 Thereafter: <2 / <1	mg/dL × 17.1 μmol/L	*Preterm* / *Term* Cord: <34 / <34 μmol/L 0–1 d: <137 / <103 1–2 d: <205 / <137 3–5 d: <274 / <205 Thereafter: <34 / <17
Bilirubin (conjugated)	0–0.2 mg/dL	mg/dL × 17.1 = μmol/L	0–3.4 μmol/L
Calcium (ionized)	<7 d: 4.52–6.32 mg/dL Adult: 4.68–5.28	mg/dL × 0.25 = nmol/L	<7 d: 1.13–1.58 nmol/L Adult: 1.17–1.32
Calcium (total)	Preterm <1 wk: 6–10 mg/dL Term <1 wk: 7–12 Child: 8.0–10.5 Adult: 8.5–10.5	mg/dL × 0.25 = mmol/L	Preterm <1 wk: 1.5–2.5 mmol/L Term <1 wk: 1.75–3.0 Child: 2.0–2.6 Adult: 2.1–2.6
Carbon dioxide (CO_2 content)	Cord blood: 14–22 mEq/L Infant/child: 20–24 Adult: 24–30		Cord blood: 14–22 mmol/L Infant/child: 20–24 Adult: 24–30
Chloride	Pediatric: 99–111 mEq/L Adult: 96–109		Pediatric: 99–111 mmol/L Adult: 96–109
Cholesterol	<1 yr: 93–260 mg/dL 1–5 yr: 97–213 6–19 yr: 97–263 >20 yr: 116–360	mg/dL × 0.0259 = mmol/L	<1 yr: 2.4–6.7 mmol/L 1–5 yr: 2.5–5.5 6–19 yr: 2.5–6.8 >20 yr: 3.0–9.3
Complement, total hemolytic (CH_{50})	75–160 U/mL		75–160 U/mL
Creatine kinase	Newborn: 76–600 U/L Adult (M): 38–174 Adult (F): 96–140		Newborn: 76–600 U/L Adult (M): 38–174 Adult (F): 96–140
Creatinine	Cord blood: 0.6–1.2 mg/dL Newborn: 0.3–1.0 Infant: 0.2–0.4 Child: 0.3–0.7 Adolescent: 0.5–1.0 Adult (M): 0.6–1.3 Adult (F): 0.5–1.2	mg/dL × 88.4 = μmol/L	Cord blood: 53–106 μmol/L Newborn: 27–88 Infant: 18–35 Child: 27–62 Adolescent: 44–88 Adult (M): 53–115 Adult (F): 44–106
Erythrocyte sedimentation rate	Newborn (0–48 hr): 0–4 mm/hr Child: 4–20 mm/hr Adult (M): 0–10 mm/hr Adult (F): 0–20 mm/hr		
Fibrinogen	200–400 mg/dL		

(*continued*)

TABLE 276-1. *(Continued)*

Test	Conventional units reference range	Conversion factor	SI units reference range
Gamma glutamyl transferase	Cord blood: 19–270 U/L 0–3 wk: 0–130 3 wk to 3 mo: 4–120 3 mo to 1 yr (M): 5–65 3 mo to 1 yr (F): 5–35 1–15 yr: 0–23 Adult (M): 11–50 Adult (F): 7–32		Cord blood: 19–270 U/L 0–3 wk: 0–130 3 wk to 3 mo: 4–120 3 mo to 1 yr (M): 5–65 3 mo to 1 yr (F): 5–35 1–15 yr: 0–23 Adult (M): 11–50 Adult (F): 7–32
Glucose	Premature: 45–100 mg/dL Full term: 45–120 1 wk to 16 yr: 60–105 >16 yr: 70–115	mg/dL × 0.0555 = mmol/L	Premature: 2.49–5.55 mmol/L Full term: 2.49–6.66 1 wk to 16 yr: 3.33–5.83 >16 yr: 3.89–6.38
Growth hormone (somatotropin)	1 d: 5–53 ng/mL 1 wk: 5–27 1–12 mo: 2–10 Fasting Child/adult: <0.7–6.0		1 d: 5–53 μg/L 1 wk: 5–27 1–12 mo: 2–10 Fasting Child/adult: <0.7–6.0
Hemoglobin A1C	3.0–7.7% of total Hb		0.030–0.077 fraction of total Hb
Immunoglobulin G, M, A (95% CI)	*IgG*	*IgM*	*IgA*
Cord blood	636–1,606 mg/dL	6.3–25 mg/dL	1.4–3.6 mg/dL
1 mo	251–906	20–87	1.3–53
2 mo	206–601	17–105	2.8–47
3 mo	176–581	24–89	4.6–46.0
4 mo	196–558	27–101	4.4–73.0
5 mo	172–814	33–108	8.1–84.0
6 mo	215–704	35–102	8.1–68.0
7–9 mo	217–904	34–126	11–90
10–12 mo	294–1,069	41–149	16–84
1 yr	345–1,213	43–173	14–106
2 yr	424–1,051	48–168	14–123
3 yr	441–1,135	47–200	22–159
4–5 yr	463–1,236	43–196	25–154
6–8 yr	633–1,280	48–207	33–202
9–10 yr	608–1,572	52–242	45–236
Adult	639–1,349	56–352	70–312

Immunoglobulin G subclasses (mg/dL) 95% CI *Age*	*IgG1*	*IgG2*	*IgG3*	*IgG4*
0–1 yr	190–620	30–140	9–62	6–63
1–2 yr	230–710	30–170	11–98	4–43
2–3 yr	280–830	40–240	6–130	3–120
3–4 yr	350–790	50–260	9–98	5–180
4–6 yr	360–810	60–310	9–160	9–160
6–8 yr	280–1,120	30–630	40–250	11–620
8–10 yr	280–1,740	80–550	22–320	10–170
10–13 yr	270–1,290	110–550	13–250	7–530
13 yr to adult	280–1,020	60–790	14–240	11–330

Test	Conventional units reference range	Conversion factor	SI units reference range
Immunoglobulin E (IU/mL) (95% CI)			
0 d	0.04–1.28		
6 wk	0.08–6.12		
3 mo	0.18–3.76		
6 mo	0.44–16.3		
9 mo	0.76–7.31		
1 yr	0.80–15.2		
2 yr	0.31–29.5		
3 yr	0.19–16.9		
4 yr	1.07–68.9		
7 yr	1.03–161.3		
10 yr	0.98–570.6		
14 yr	2.06–195.2		
17–85 yr	1.53–114.0		
Insulin (fasting)	1.8–24.6 μU/mL		1.8–24.6 mU/L
Iron	Newborn: 100–250 μg/dL Infant: 40–100 Child: 50–120 Adult (M): 65–170 Adult (F): 50–170	μg/dL × 0.179 = μmol/L	Newborn: 18–45 μmol/L Infant: 7–18 Child: 9–22 Adult (M): 12–30 Adult (F): 9–30

(continued)

TABLE 276-1. *(Continued)*

Test	Conventional units reference range	Conversion factor	SI units reference range
Lactate	Venous: 5–20 mg/dL	mg/dL × 0.111 = mmol/L	Venous: 0.55–2.2 mmol/L
	Arterial: 5–14		Arterial: 0.55–1.6
Lactate dehydrogenase	Newborn: 160–1,500 U/L		Newborn: 160–1,500 U/L
	Infant: 150–360		Infant: 150–360
	Child: 150–300		Child: 150–300
	Adult: 0–250		Adult: 0–250
Lead	<10 μg/dL	μg/dL × 0.0483 = μmol/L	<0.48 μmol/L
Lipase	1–5 yr: 18–98 U/L		1–5 yr: 18–98 U/L
	6–12 yr: 21–120		6–12 yr: 21–120
	13–18 yr: 26–144		13–18 yr: 26–144
	Adult: 30–160		Adult: 30–160
Magnesium	1.3–2.0 mEq/L	mEq/L × 0.411 = mmol/L	0.53–0.82 mmol/L
Methemogloblin	<0.3 g/dL	g/dL × 154 = μmol/L	<46 μmol/L
Osmolality	285–295 mOsm/kg		285–295 mmol/kg
Partial thromboplastin time (activated) (APTT)	Preterm: 80–168 sec		
	Term: 31.3–54.3		
	Child/adult: 26.6–40.3		
Phosphorus (inorganic)	0–5 d: 4.8–8.2 mg/dL	mg/dL × 0.323 = mmol/L	0–5 d: 1.55–2.65 mmol/L
	1–3 yr: 3.8–6.5		1–3 yr: 1.25–2.1
	4–11 yr: 3.7–5.6		4–11 yr: 1.2–1.8
	12–15 yr: 2.9–5.4		12–15 yr: 0.95–1.75
	16–19 yr: 2.7–4.7		16–19 yr: 0.90–1.50
Potassium	<10 d: 4–6 mEq/L		<10 d: 4–6 mmol/L
	≥10 d: 3.5–5.0		≥10 d: 3.5–5.0
Prealbumin	Newborn to 6 wk: 4–36 mg/dL		
	6 wk to 16 yr: 13–27		
	Adult: 18–45		
Protein, total	Preterm: 4.3–7.6 g/dL	g/dL × 10 = g/L	Preterm: 43–76 g/L
	Term: 4.6–7.4		Term: 46–74 g/L
	1–3 mo: 4.7–7.4		1–3 mo: 47–74
	3–12 mo: 5.0–7.5		3–12 mo: 50–75
	1–15 yr: 6.5–8.6		1–15 yr: 65–86
Prothrombin time (PT)	Preterm: 11–17 sec		
	Term: 10–16 sec		
	Adult: 10 sec		
Pyruvate	0.3–0.9 mg/dL	mg/dL × 0.11 mmol/L	0.03–0.10 mmol/L
Sodium	Premature: 135–146 mEq/L		Premature: 135–146 mmol/L
	Older: 135–148		Older: 135–148
Thyroid-stimulating hormone (TSH)	Cord blood: <2.5–17.4 mIU/mL		Cord blood: <2.5–17.4 μU/L
	1–3 d: <2.5–13.3		1–3 d: <2.5–13.3
	1–4 wk: 0.6–10.0		1–4 wk: 0.6–10.0
	1–12 mo: 0.6–6.3		1–12 mo: 0.6–6.3
	1–15 yr: 0.6–6.3		1–15 yr: 0.6–6.3
	16–50 yr: 0.2–7.6		16–50 yr: 0.2–7.6
Thyroxine (T_4), total	Cord: 7.4–13.0 μg/dL	μg/dL × 12.9 = nmol/L	Cord: 95–168 nmol/L
	<1 mo: 7.0–22.6		<1 mo: 90–292
	1 mo to 1 yr: 7.2–16.5		1 mo to 1 yr: 93–213
	1–5 yr: 7.3–15.0		1–5 yr: 94–194
	5–10 yr: 6.4–13.3		5–10 yr: 83–172
	10–15 yr: 5.6–11.7		10–15 yr: 72–151
	Adult: 4.3–12.5		Adult: 55–161
Thyroxine (T_4), free	1–10 d: 0.6–2.0 ng/dL	ng/dL × 12.9 = pmol/L	1–10 d: 7.74–25.8 pmol/L
	>10 d: 0.7–1.7		>10 d: 9.03–21.9
Urea nitrogen	5–21 mg/dL	mg/dL × 0.36 = mmol/L	2.0–7.6 mmol/L
Uric acid	0–2 yr: 2.4–6.4 mg/dL	mg/dL × 0.058 = mmol/L	0–2 yr: 0.14–0.38 mmol/L
	2–12 yr: 2.4–5.9		2–12 yr: 0.14–0.35
	12–14 yr: 2.4–6.4		12–14 yr: 0.14–0.38
	Adult (M): 3.5–7.2		Adult (M): 0.20–0.43
	Adult (F): 2.4–6.4		Adult (F): 0.14–0.38
Vitamin D (1,25 dihydroxy)	25–45 pg/mL	pg/mL × 2.4 = pmol/L	60–108 pmol/L

TABLE 276-2. Age-Specific Indices for Hematology

Age	Hgb (g/dL)		Hematocrit (%)		MCV (fl)		MCHC (g/dL RBC)		Reticulocyte (%)	Platelets (1,000 per mm^3) mean (±SD) [range]
	Mean	*−2 SD*[a]	*Mean*	*−2 SD*[a]	*Mean*	*−2 SD*[a]	*Mean*	*−2 SD*[a]		
18–21 wk gestation[b]	11.69	9.2	37.3	28.7	131.1	109.2				234 (±57)
22–25 wk gestation[b]	12.2	9	38.59	30.7	125.1	109.4				247 (±59)
26–29 wk gestation[b]	12.91	10.2	40.88	32	118.5	102.6				242 (±69)
>30 wk gestation[b]	13.64	9.2	43.55	29.2	114.4	95.7				232 (±87)
Term (cord blood)	16.5	13.5	51	42	108	98	33	30	3–7	290
1–3 days	18.5	14.5	56	45	108	95	33	29	1.8–4.6	192
1 wk	17.5	13.5	54	42	107	88	33	28	0–1	248
2 wk	16.5	12.5	51	39	105	86	33	28	0–1	252
1 mo	14	10	43	31	104	85	33	29	0–1	
2 mo	11.5	9	35	28	96	77	33	29	0–2	280
3–6 mo	11.5	9.5	35	29	91	74	33	30	0.7–2.3	
6–24 mo	12	10.5	36	33	78	70	33	30		[150–300]
2–6 yr	12.5	11.5	37	34	81	75	34	31	0.5–1.0	[150–300]
6–12 yr	13.5	11.5	40	35	86	77	34	31	0.5–1.0	[150–300]
12–18 yr (male)	14.5	13	43	37	88	78	34	31	0.5–1.0	[150–300]
12–18 yr (female)	14	12	41	36	90	78	34	31	0.5-1.0	[150–300]

[a] At −2 SD from mean, approximately 95% of the population is encompassed.
[b] Forestier F, Daffos F, Catherine N, Renard M, Andreaux JP. Developmental hematopoiesis in normal human fetal blood. *Blood* 1991;77:2360.
Data compiled from normal reference values in Nathan DG, Orkin SH. *Nathan and Oski's hematology of infancy and childhood,* 5th ed. Philadelphia: Saunders, 1998.

TABLE 276-3. Cerebrospinal Fluid

Cell count range

Preterm: 0–25 WBC × 10^6 cells per liter (57% polymorphonuclears)
Term: 0–22 WBC × 10^6 cells per liter (61% polymorphonuclears)
Child: 0–7 WBC × 10^6 cells per liter (5% polymorphonuclears)

Cell count percentiles

Age	Total WBC			Polymorphonuclears			Monocytes		
	25%	*50%*	*75%*	*25%*	*50%*	*75%*	*25%*	*50%*	*75%*
<6 wk	0.50	2.57	5.16	0	0	2.42	0	0.83	2.71
6 wk to 3 mo	0.34	1.86	3.75	0	0	0.66	0	0.96	2.78
3–6 mo	0	1.11	2.31	0	0	0.40	0	0.43	1.64
6–12 mo	0.41	1.47	3.25	0	0	0.52	0.03	0.93	2.32
>12 mo	0	0.68	1.82	0	0	0	0	0.25	1.45

Test	SI reference range	Conventional units reference range
Glucose	Preterm: 1.3–3.5 mmol/L Term: 1.9–6.6 Child: 2.2–4.4	Preterm: 24–63 mg/dL Term: 34–119 Child: 40–80
Protein	Preterm: 0.65–1.50 g/L Term: 0.20–1.70 Child: 0.05–0.40	Preterm: 65–150 mg/dL Term: 20–170 Child: 5–40
Pressure	<200 mm H_2O	<200 mm H_2O

Subject Index

B

D

N

U

V

W

X

Y

Z